W9-BEO-179

Features

Over 40 animations will help you to master the hardest topics in nutrition. Topics covered include digestion, protein synthesis, emulsification of fat, effects of insulin within the cell, cancer, and more.

Applied **Nutri-Cases** will allow you to view multiple dimensions to the health and nutrition dilemmas presented in each character.

Quizzing & Testing gives you the opportunity to track your progress with hundreds of practice quiz and test questions.

A healthy approach to diet analysis

MyDiet Analysis

If your instructor has ordered MyNutritionLab with MyDietAnalysis, you will have access to this application; otherwise, you may purchase it online. MyDietAnalysis offers an accurate and easy-to-use program for your diet analysis needs. It has been tailored for use by students in college and university nutrition courses.

MyDietAnalysis features a database of nearly 20,000 foods, including ethnic foods, name-brand fast foods, and convenience foods. The program allows you to create multiple profiles allowing you to analyze various diets and energy expenditures. The program provides for a variety of reports based on personal food intake and activity level for up to seven days to make this analysis easier for you to complete.

Nutrition: A Functional Approach

Second Canadian Edition

Nutrition: A Functional Approach

Second Canadian Edition

Janice Thompson, PhD, FACSM
University of New Mexico

Melinda Manore, PhD, RD, FACSM
Oregon State University

Judy Sheeshka, PhD, RD
University of Guelph

Pearson Canada
Toronto

Library and Archives Canada Cataloguing in Publication

Thompson, Janice, 1962–
    Nutrition: a functional approach / Janice Thompson, Melinda Manore, Judy Sheeshka. — 2nd Canadian ed.

Includes index.
ISBN 978-0-321-52433-1

    1. Nutrition—Textbooks. I. Manore, Melinda, 1951– II. Sheeshka, Judy Diane, 1952– III. Title.
QP141.T46 2010   613.2   C2008-904270-0

Copyright © 2010, 2007 Pearson Education Canada, a division of Pearson Canada Inc., Toronto, Ontario.

Pearson Benjamin Cummings. All rights reserved. This publication is protected by copyright and permission should be obtained from the publisher prior to any prohibited reproduction, storage in a retrieval system, or transmission in any form or by any means, electronic, mechanical, photocopying, recording, or likewise. For information regarding permission, write to the Permissions Department.

Original edition, entitled *Nutrition: An Applied Approach,* published by Pearson Education, Inc., publishing as Pearson Benjamin Cummings. Copyright © 2005 Pearson Education, Inc. This edition is authorized for sale only in Canada.

ISBN-13: 978-0-321-52433-1
ISBN-10: 0-321-52433-0

Vice President, Editorial Director: Gary Bennett
Acquisitions Editors: Carolin Sweig, Michelle Sartor
Marketing Manager: Colleen Gauthier
Developmental Editor: Paul Donnelly
Production Editor: Patricia Jones
Copy Editor: Cat Haggert
Proofreader: Dawn Hunter
Production Coordinators: Patricia Ciardullo, Lynn O'Rourke
Permissions and Photo Researcher: Terri Rothman, M.L.S.
Art Director: Julia Hall
Cover and Interior Designer: Anthony Leung
Cover Image: Getty Images

Statistics Canada information is used with the permission of Statistics Canada. Users are forbidden to copy the data and redisseminate them, in an original or modified form, for commercial purposes, without permission from Statistics Canada. Information on the availability of the wide range of data from Statistics Canada can be obtained from Statistics Canada's Regional Offices, its World Wide Web site at www.statcan.ca, and its toll-free access number 1-800-263-1136.

1 2 3 4 5   12 11 10 09

Printed and bound in the United States of America.

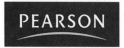

Brief Contents

Contents

Chapter 4   Carbohydrates: Bountiful Sources of Energy and Nutrients 111

Chapter 6   Proteins: Crucial Components of All Body Tissues 193

Chapter 8 Nutrients That May Function As Antioxidants 265

Chapter 9 Nutrients Involved in Bone Health 309

Welcome to *Nutrition: A Functional Approach,* Second Canadian Edition!

Why We Wrote the Book

Nutrition gets a lot of press. Pick up a newspaper and you'll read the latest findings from studies published in *The Lancet* or the *New England Journal of Medicine.* Turn on the TV and you'll hear a Canadian medical expert talk about the rising rates of childhood obesity. Pick up a magazine and read the latest debate over the use of antioxidant supplements. How do you navigate through the endless recommendations and come up with a way of eating that's right for you—one that supports your physical activity, allows you to maintain a healthful weight, and helps you avoid chronic disease? How do these recommendations apply to us in Canada, with our regulatory systems and marketplace?

What Is Unique About *Nutrition: A Functional Approach*?

For many years, Canadian instructors have been using U.S. textbooks and struggling to adapt the content for Canadian audiences. This second edition of *Nutrition: A Functional Approach* is an updated Canadian adaptation of the U.S. textbook *Nutrition: An Applied Approach,* written by Janice Thompson and Melinda Manore. It provides health facts and figures, nutrition research, and food and nutrition issues in a uniquely Canadian context.

Nutrition: A Functional Approach, **Second Canadian Edition,** is based on the conviction that both students and instructors would benefit from an accurate and clear textbook that links nutrients to their functional benefit. As authors and instructors, we know that students have a natural interest in their bodies, their health, their weight, and their success in sports and other activities. By demonstrating how nutrition is related to these interests, *Nutrition: A Functional Approach,* **Second Canadian Edition,** empowers students to reach their personal, health, and fitness goals. We used several strategies to capture students' interest, including the use of Canadian statistics and issues, a functional organization, and a variety of pedagogical features and activities. In addition, throughout the chapters, material is presented in a lively narrative that continually links the facts to students' situations, lifestyles, and goals. Information on current events and research keeps the inquisitive spark alive, illustrating that nutrition is not a "dead" science, but rather the source of considerable debate.

The content of *Nutrition: A Functional Approach,* **Second Canadian Edition,** is appropriate for those students who may be taking an introductory nutrition course out of their own personal interest as well as those embarking on a career in the nutritional sciences. For example, there is more in-depth information to challenge students who have a more advanced understanding of biochemistry and math. We present the "science side" in an easy-to-read, friendly narrative with engaging features that reduce students' fear and encourage them to apply the material to their lives.

New to the Second Canadian Edition

Nutrition: A Functional Approach, **Second Canadian Edition,** provides food and nutrition issues and nutrition research in a Canadian context. The scientific content of the text has been revised to better suit Canadian nutrition courses.

Canadian Issues

The Canadian regulatory system and policies are substantially different from those in the United States, and the Canadian culture contributes to a difference in perspective. This text has been revised to reflect these differences. For example:

- Chapter 1 provides information on the roles of dietitians and the various designations used across Canada (e.g., PDt., R.D.).

- Chapter 2 looks at Canadian food labels and explains the guidelines for nutrient content claims and health claims. The history of food guides in Canada and Canada's 2007 *Eating Well with Canada's Food Guide* are outlined, along with supporting programs such as the Heart and Stroke Foundation of Canada's *Health Check™*.

- Chapter 3 contains recent research on CCK, celiac disease, and irritable bowel syndrome. The Nutrition Debate on probiotics has been updated to include prebiotics.

- Chapter 4 contains updated sections on the glycemic index, glycemic load, and added sugars. Data from the Canadian Community Health Survey 2004 on carbohydrate and dietary fibre intakes are now provided. There is a new section on "prediabetes".

- In Chapter 5, the more technically-correct term *lipids* now replaces the term *fats* in portions of the text where the "chemistry" of these compounds is discussed. The term *fats* is retained in discussions of foods and solid fats. New figures have been added, along with more detail on the digestion, absorption, and transportation of lipids in the body, including more information on phospholipids, secretin, bile acids, micelles, and lipoproteins. A new table on the energy and fat intakes of Canadians compares the Nutrition Canada survey data (1972) to the data from the Canadian Community Health Survey version 2 (2004). There is new information on possible health benefits from omega-3 fatty acids (EPA and DHA), including possible slower rates of cognitive decline and possible protection against macular degeneration. A new table providing the omega-3 fatty acid content of fish, and new guidance from Health Canada on eating fish twice a week and choosing fish high in omega-3 FA and low in mercury are also included in this edition. New guidelines for food manufacturers and the restaurant industry from the Trans Fat Task Force, and trans fat enforcement/monitoring by Health Canada, are discussed. A new Highlight featuring one food scientist's attempts to create an acceptable alternative to trans fats is included.

- Chapter 6 contains updated information on Protein Energy Malnutrition and the protein intakes of Canadians (from the Canadian Community Health Survey, v.2).

- Chapter 7 includes the latest figures on sodium consumption among Canadians, as well as the updated guidelines for preventing hypertension (high blood pressure).

- Chapter 8 includes new information about antioxidants in tea and coffee, factors that may reduce cancer risk and factors that may increase cancer risk, and updated statistics on cancer and cardiovascular disease.

- Chapter 9 contains new data on the calcium intakes of Canadians, from the Canadian Community Health Survey (2004). More details on the conversion of various forms of vitamin D from inactive to active forms in several body tissues (e.g., brain, breast, prostate, etc.), and on the possible role of vitamin D in preventing certain cancers, heart disease, and some autoimmune diseases (such as multiple sclerosis, type 1 diabetes) are provided. There is a discussion of the controversy over the DRIs for vitamin D, and updated data on the cost of treating osteoporosis in Canada and medications available (a new once-yearly intravenous infusion). Lastly, new sections on cancer-induced bone loss and recommendations for ways to prevent osteoporosis among cancer patients have been added to this edition.

- Chapter 10 features new photos of conditions associated with nutrient deficiencies, to better illustrate these terms (e.g., pellagra, beriberi, etc.), and more description of the consequences of these nutrient deficiencies. Updated research on choline is provided.
- Chapter 11 has new information on the usefulness of measuring waist circumferences, updated information on prescription drugs to treat obesity, and a new topic, sarcopenic obesity.
- Chapter 12 has updated information on creatine, chromium, and carnitine, plus new data on the physical activity level of Canadians.
- In Chapter 13, "eating disorders—not otherwise specified (ED-NOS)" has been added as one of the three main categories of eating disorders. More recent research on the influence of media images on the way that women feel about their bodies, as well as new evidence of a role for biology in anorexia nervosa, has been added. Information on the Female Athlete Triad has also been updated.
- Throughout Chapter 14, there has been a clarification of food safety and food quality, and food-borne illness and food spoilage. Under "Government Regulations," the role of public health inspectors in monitoring food safety in eating and drinking establishments has been added, along with a sample of the notices that restaurants in some municipalities post so consumers will know whether an establishment passed its safety inspection or not. A new section on FATTOM—an acronym for the six conditions for bacteria to growth—has been added, and the section on "durable life" information has been updated.
- Chapter 15 provides updated recommendations for weight gain during pregnancy. Folate recommendations have been updated and more information on neural tube defects, including a description and picture of spina bifida, are provided. Updated guidelines for caffeine during pregnancy, and a new Highlight on the Safety of Herbal Teas during Pregnancy has been added. The section on Fetal Alcohol Syndrome, now called Fetal Alcohol Spectrum Disorder (FASD), has been updated, and a new section on food-borne illnesses with serious consequences during pregnancy, plus a list of foods for pregnant women to avoid, has been added. Lastly, new recommendations for introducing solid foods into infants' diets have been provided.

Canadian Research

The latest Canadian research findings are incorporated throughout the text to examine emerging issues. The specific contributions of Canadian researchers to our understanding of the role of nutrition in disease are highlighted. For example:

- Chapter 1 presents findings from the 2004 Canadian Community Health Survey on overweight and obesity rates among children and adults.
- Chapter 4 provides recent insights into the glycemic index and glycemic load, developed by Dr. David Jenkins and Dr. Tom Wolever at the University of Toronto. A new Highlight on Dr. Timothy Kieffer at University of British Columbia and his research on leptin and type 2 diabetes has been added.
- Canada led the world in requiring the disclosure of the trans fat content of food on food labels, and in Chapter 5 we feature an interview on this subject with the internationally renowned Canadian researcher Dr. Bruce Holub. Dr. Alejandro Marangoni's ground-breaking research on a substitute for trans fats in baked products is also featured.
- Chapter 9 includes the latest Canadian research on bone health from the Canadian Multicentre Osteoporosis Study and a feature interview with Dr. Susan Whiting, a leading expert from the University of Saskatchewan. The international impact of Canadian research is also highlighted through an interview with Dr. Stanley Zlotkin. He has developed a micronutrient supplement called *Sprinkles*™ that is having tremendous success in preventing

iron-deficiency anemia, rickets, and other debilitating conditions in developing countries.

- Chapter 11 includes a new Highlight on Dr. Linda McCargar at the University of Alberta and her research on body composition, specifically, sarcopenic obesity.

- Chapter 15 features the research of Dr. Debbie O'Connor from the University of Toronto, and the controversy about folate supplementation possibly masking vitamin B12 deficiencies.

Content Is Applied to Life

Because students are most interested in how nutrition applies to their own lives, we have developed several learning tools throughout the book to illustrate real-life implications of nutrition. For instance, to teach students the effect of vitamins and minerals in the body, we organized the micronutrients chapters according to their function. We also developed nutrition debates, math activities, and nutrition label activities that encourage students to put the information they've just learned into practice.

Functional Organization

Students have traditionally learned about micronutrients by memorizing each one along with their deficiency symptoms and toxicity syndromes. We have found with this traditional approach that they quickly forget the information they have learned, and they never really understand why micronutrients are important. To respond to this problem, we decided to illustrate the immediate health issues and physiological functions of vitamins and minerals by discussing them within the context of fluid and electrolyte balance, antioxidant function, bone health, and energy metabolism and blood formation. We've found, through our own experience teaching and through extensive class testing, that this functional approach helps students to think about these micronutrients on a conceptual level, enabling them to answer the questions "Why are vitamins and minerals important?" and "What do they do?" This approach also promotes better retention of the material and application to real life.

You Do the Math

You Do the Math boxes show students how to perform nutritional calculations, such as determining their own body mass index (BMI), step by step. Knowledge of these calculations helps students determine their own nutritional needs.

Nutrition Label Activities

Nutrition Label Activities teach students how to read and evaluate labels from real food products so they can make educated choices about the foods they eat. Students can use the skills they learn when they do their food shopping.

▶ YOU DO THE MATH

Using the % Daily Values (%DV) to Calculate Specific Amounts of Calcium and Iron

The %DV can be used to calculate specific amounts of any nutrient listed on the label. Let's say you are a 23-year-old male. You are interested in meeting the DRI standards for both calcium and iron, and you are curious about how much of the food shown in Figure 2.3 contributes to your daily intake of these two nutrients. We will use Table 2.3 and Figure 2.3 to assist us in these calculations.

a. *Calcium:* The %DV for calcium listed on the label is 2%. As you can see in Table 2.3, the RDI for calcium is 1100 mg. By multiplying the %DV by 1100 mg, you will get the total amount of calcium (in milligrams) in 1 serving of this food:

$$2\% = 0.02$$
$$0.02 \times 1100 \text{ mg} = 22 \text{ mg}$$

How do we know how much this food contributes to your calcium requirement as described by the DRI standards? By looking at the tables in Appendix H, you can see that the Adequate Intake (AI) for calcium for a man 23 years of age is 1000 mg. By dividing the amount of calcium in milligrams in 1 serving of this food by the AI for calcium (1000 mg) and multiplying by 100, you will get the percentage of your AI for calcium from this food:

$$22 \text{ mg}/1000 \text{ mg} \times 100 = 2.2\%$$
of your AI for calcium

b. *Iron:* The %DV for iron listed on the label is 35%. As you can see in Table 2.3, the RDI for iron is 14 mg. By multiplying the %DV by 14 mg, you

of iron in milligrams in 1 serving of this food by the RDA for iron (8 mg) and multiplying by 100, you will get the percentage of your RDA for iron from this food:

$$4.9 \text{ mg}/8 \text{ mg} \times 100 = 61\% \text{ of your RDA}$$
for iron

These calculations are very helpful when you need to determine how a food meets your individual nutrient needs based on your gender and age. The % daily values are a helpful guide in determining whether a food is high or low in a given nutrient, and the calculations just shown can further assist you when you do not eat a 2000-Calorie (8400 kJ) diet or you want to determine how well your diet is meeting the DRI standards.

By comparing labels from different foods, you can start planning a more nutritious diet today. Try looking at the two labels in Figure 2.4 to decide which food is a better choice. First, decide which nutrients are most important to you. Let's assume you are trying to eat foods with more dietary fibre and iron. The label on the left shows that Cereal A contains 1 gram of dietary fibre and 30% of the DV for iron per serving. The label on the right shows that Cereal B contains 6 grams of dietary fibre and 60% of the DV for iron per serving. For these two nutrients, Cereal B, on the right, would clearly be the more nutritious choice.

Notice that Cereal B is a denser cereal, though. One serving of Cereal B is 25 biscuits, or approximately 1 cup; this weighs 55 grams and contains 270 Calories when served with 125 mL (1/2 cup) of 2% milk.

▶ NUTRITION LABEL ACTIVITY

Recognizing Carbohydrates on the Label

Figure 4.11 shows labels for two breakfast cereals. Cereal A, on the left, is processed and sweetened, and Cereal B, on the right, is a whole-grain product with little added sugar.

- Check each label to locate the amount of total carbohydrate. For Cereal A, the total carbohydrate is 30 grams, and for Cereal B it is 22 grams for the same serving size.

- Look at the information listed as subgroups under Carbohydrate. The label for Cereal A shows that the cereal contains 1 gram of dietary fibre, 8 grams of sugars, and 21 grams of starch per serving.
- The label for Cereal B lists only the fibre (3 grams) and sugars (1 gram) per serving. In this case, the amount of

Nutrition Facts (A) Serving 1 cup (30 g)		
Amount	Cereal Only	With 1/2 cup 2% milk
Calories	120	180
		% Daily Value
Fat 0 g*	0%	4%
Saturated 0 g	0%	8%
+ Trans 0 g		
Cholesterol 0 g	0%	3%
Sodium 160 mg	7%	10%
Carbohydrate 30 g	10%	12%
Fibre 1 g	4%	4%
Sugars 8 g		
Starch 21 g		
Protein 3 g		
Vitamin A	0%	8%
Vitamin C	0%	0%
Calcium	10%	20%
Iron	30%	30%
Vitamin D	0%	25%
Thiamin	45%	50%
Riboflavin	35%	50%

Nutrition Facts (B) Serving 1 cup (30 g)		
Amount	Cereal Only	With 1/2 cup 2% milk
Calories	120	180
		% Daily Value
Fat 2 g*	3%	7%
Saturated 0.4 g	2%	10%
+ Trans 0 g		
Cholesterol 0 g	0%	2%
Sodium 280 mg	12%	14%
Carbohydrate 22 g	7%	9%
Fibre 3 g	12%	12%
Sugars 1 g		
Starch		
Protein 4 g		
Vitamin A	0%	7%
Vitamin C	0%	0%
Calcium	9%	22%
Iron	30%	30%
Vitamin D	0%	25%
Thiamin	40%	44%
Riboflavin	2%	15%

Teaching How to Evaluate Nutrition Information

One of our goals with *Nutrition: A Functional Approach,* **Second Canadian Edition,** is to teach students how to evaluate the nutrition information they encounter every day. Each chapter discusses how to find and evaluate reliable sources for nutrition facts, and provides references students can trust for answers to common nutrition questions. In addition, the following features help to debunk some commonly held myths about nutrition.

Test Yourself Questions

A brief **Test Yourself** quiz at the beginning of each chapter piques students' interest in the topics to be covered by raising and dispelling common myths about nutrition. The answers to these questions can be found at the end of each chapter.

Nutrition Myth or Fact

Nutrition Myth or Fact boxes provide the facts behind the hype on many current nutrition and dietary issues. They dispel common misconceptions and teach students how to critically evaluate information on the internet, in the mass media, and from their peers.

Nutrition Debates

Nutrition Debates contain in-depth coverage of current events and hot topics, such as vitamin and mineral supplementation. By presenting both sides of the argument, these debates encourage students to think critically about controversial issues and become more informed and discriminating consumers of nutrition and health information.

Captivating Student Interest

In order to capture students' interest and motivate them to read on, we have created chapter-opening scenarios and Highlight boxes that stimulate students' curiosity, and we have included appealing and informative illustrations and photos that draw students into the text and create an engaging learning environment.

Chapter-Opening Scenarios

Each chapter opens with a real-life story that teaches students about the sometimes life-altering effects of diet and exercise. These scenarios grab students' attention and motivate them to delve deeper into the chapter material.

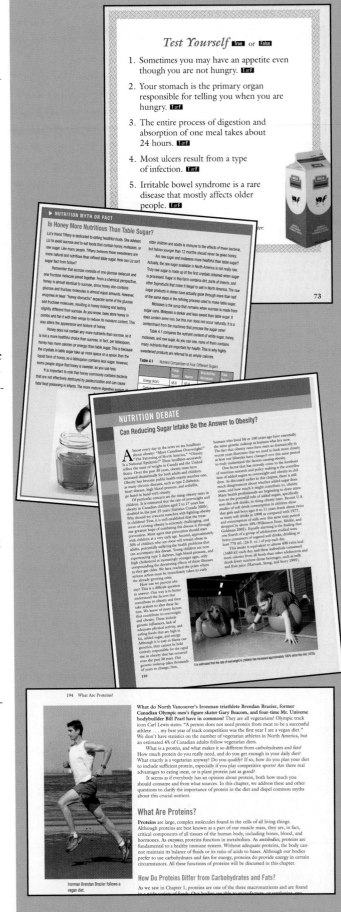

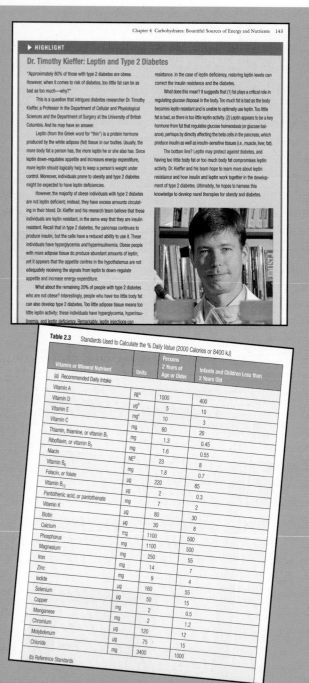

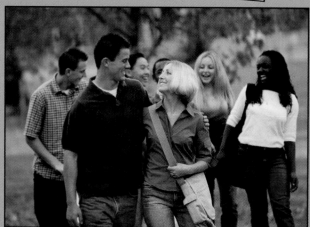

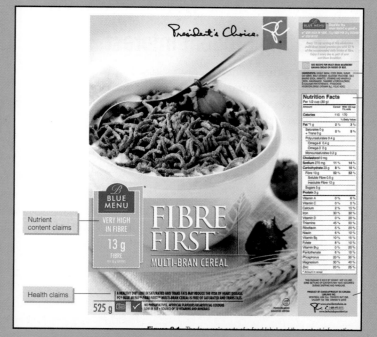

Highlight Boxes

Highlight boxes provide further insight into topics that students will recognize from the mass media and popular culture, such as mad cow disease or sports beverages. These boxes discuss the nutritional facts and theories behind these often complex issues.

Art, Photos, and Tables

The art program was specially designed to walk students through the body's processing of nutrients. Insets on digestion diagrams illustrate context, so students understand where in the body a given process is located. The photos were chosen to provide illustration for conditions created by nutrient deficiencies, as well as to show students foods that they may not immediately think of as good sources for specific nutrients. Tables integrate nutrition information, and special figures act as "shopper's guides," indicating foods that are good sources of Dietary Reference Intakes of specific vitamins and minerals.

Support for the Student

In writing *Nutrition: A Functional Approach*, **Second Canadian Edition**, we worked to develop pedagogical features that would benefit students by helping them learn and remember all the information in the chapter. These features help students review the material they just learned, find more information, check their understanding of the material, and stay focused on the most important points.

Chapter Objectives

Chapter objectives help students stay focused by listing the most important concepts in the chapter. After reading the chapter, students can go back and review the objectives to make sure that they understand each point.

Recaps

We have placed **Recap** paragraphs throughout each chapter of the text. The Recaps rephrase what students just learned in the preceding sections, providing a quick summary and using new wording to help students remember the concept (not just the words) before moving on to the next topic.

Test Yourself Answers

Answers to each chapter's **Test Yourself** questions are located after the review questions at the end of the chapter. Using the Test Yourself answers, students can evaluate their responses to these basic, but sometimes deceiving, questions about nutrition.

Chapter Summaries

Our chapter summaries provide quick reviews of the major points and topics covered in each chapter. By going through the chapter summaries, students can determine whether they have understood information about the chapter's main concepts.

Review Questions

Review questions at the end of each chapter allow students to assess their retention and understanding of the material they have covered in the chapter. Answers to multiple choice review questions appear at the end of the book; answers to the short answer questions are found in MyNutritionLab.

Web Links and References

Web Links at the end of each chapter provide students with connections for further information and study. The comprehensive references for each chapter appear at the end of the book.

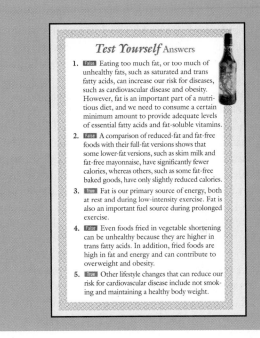

Recap: The six classes of nutrients found in foods are carbohydrates, lipids or fats, proteins, vitamins, minerals, and water. Carbohydrates, lipids, and proteins are referred to as the energy-yielding nutrients, as they provide our bodies with the energy necessary to thrive. Carbohydrates are the primary energy source for our bodies; fats are a source of fat-soluble vitamins and essential fatty acids and act as energy storage molecules; and proteins support tissue growth, repair, and maintenance.

Test Yourself Answers

1. False Eating too much fat, or too much of unhealthy fats, such as saturated and trans fatty acids, can increase our risk for diseases, such as cardiovascular disease and obesity. However, fat is an important part of a nutritious diet, and we need to consume a certain minimum amount to provide adequate levels of essential fatty acids and fat-soluble vitamins.

2. False A comparison of reduced-fat and fat-free foods with their full-fat versions shows that some lower-fat versions, such as skim milk and fat-free mayonnaise, have significantly fewer calories, whereas others, such as some fat-free baked goods, have only slightly reduced calories.

3. True Fat is our primary source of energy, both at rest and during low-intensity exercise. Fat is also an important fuel source during prolonged exercise.

4. False Even foods fried in vegetable shortening can be unhealthy because they are higher in trans fatty acids. In addition, fried foods are high in fat and energy and can contribute to overweight and obesity.

5. True Other lifestyle changes that can reduce our risk for cardiovascular disease include not smoking and maintaining a healthy body weight.

Supplements Help Students and Instructors

Instructors and students have access to a wide variety of supplementary material to facilitate teaching, help learning and retention, and contribute to the classroom experience.

Instructor's Resource CD-ROM

The Instructor's Resource CD-ROM includes all of the following instructor supplements in one convenient package:

- *Instructor's Manual:* The Instructor's Manual contains chapter summaries, objectives, lecture outlines, and activity ideas, including a Nutrition Debate activity for each chapter.
- *Pearson TestGen:* Over 1200 test questions, including multiple choice, true/false, short answer, and essay questions, are provided in TestGen format. TestGen is a testing software that enables instructors to view and edit existing questions, add questions, generate tests, and distribute the tests in a variety of formats. Powerful search and sort functions make it easy to locate questions and arrange them in any order desired. TestGen also enables instructors to administer tests on a local area network, have the tests graded electronically, and have the results prepared in electronic or printed reports. TestGen is compatible with Windows and Macintosh operating systems, and can be downloaded from the TestGen website located at www.pearsoned.com/testgen. Contact your local sales representative for details and access.
- *PowerPoints:* PowerPoint presentations offer an outline of the key points for each chapter.
- *Image Library:* The Image Library consists of JPEG files of most of the figures and tables from the text.
- *CBC/Pearson Education Canada Video Library:* This collection of videos and video cases includes segments from CBC programs that deal with current issues in nutrition. Students are able to access the videos, the cases, and the discussion questions to accompany the segments on our password-protected Video Central website. The cases and answers to the discussion questions are also provided in the Instructor's Manual.

These instructor supplements are also available for download from a password-protected section of Pearson Education Canada's online catalogue (vig.pearsoned.ca). Navigate to your book's catalogue page to view a list of the supplements that are available. See your local sales representative for details and access.

CourseSmart

CourseSmart is a new way for instructors and students to access textbooks online anytime from anywhere. With thousands of titles across hundreds of courses, CourseSmart helps instructors choose the best textbook for their class and give their students a new option for buying the assigned textbook as a lower cost eTextbook. For more information, visit www.coursesmart.com.

MyNutritionLab

This online standard course management system is loaded with teaching and learning resources that make giving assignments and tracking student progress easy. MyNutritionLab features a wealth of pre-loaded content for instructors including PowerPoint slides, Test Bank, questions, Instructor's Manual material, and more. Features for students include interactive label activities, animations, and drag-and-drop activities. Research Navigator, which provides three databases of credible and reliable source materials, is also included.

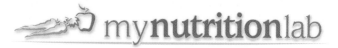

MyDietAnalysis

MyDietAnalysis offers an accurate, reliable, and easy-to-use program for students' diet analysis needs. Available on CD-ROM or online, the program allows students to track their diet and activity and to generate and submit reports electronically. Developed by the nutrition database experts at ESHA Research, Inc. and tailored for use in university nutrition courses, **MyDietAnalysis** features a database of nearly 20 000 foods and multiple reports.

Pearson Advantage

For qualified adopters, Pearson Education is proud to introduce the **Pearson Advantage.** The Pearson Advantage is the first integrated Canadian service program committed to meeting the customization, training, and support needs for your course. Our commitments are made in writing and in consultation with faculty. Your local Pearson Education sales representative can provide you with more details on this service program.

Technology Specialists

Pearson's Technology Specialists work with faculty and campus course designers to ensure that Pearson technology products, assessment tools, and online course materials are tailored to meet your specific needs. This highly qualified team is dedicated to helping schools take full advantage of a wide range of educational resources, by assisting in the integration of a variety of instructional materials and media formats. Your local Pearson Education sales representative can provide you with more details on this service program.

Acknowledgments

This book would not have been possible without the written contributions and information retrieval skills of my research assistants, Maxine Fung, Kelly Matheson, Jessica Wegener, Alison Campbell, and June Matthews. Their creativity and writing skills are much appreciated. I am also very grateful for the assistance of food safety experts Mary Alton Mackey and Dr. Bonnie Lacroix in rewriting sections of Chapter 14.

I am very grateful to the outstanding researchers who agreed to be interviewed and featured in this book: Dr. Tim Kieffer at UBC, Dr. Linda McCargar at the University of Alberta, Dr. Susan Whiting at the University of Saskatchewan, Dr. Bruce Holub and Dr. Alejandro Marangoni at the University of Guelph, Dr. Stanley Zlotkin and Dr. Deborah O'Connor at the University of Toronto and the Hospital for Sick Children, and Dr. Valerie Tarasuk at the University of Toronto.

The talented staff at Pearson Education Canada need to be acknowledged for their dedication to this project, their writing and editorial skills, and their patience. Developmental Editor Paul Donnelly was invaluable in providing guidance about the content and in eliciting great feedback from the peer reviewers. Copy Editor Cat Haggert provided her exceptional editing skills. Trish Jones, Trish Ciardullo, and Lynn O'Rourke efficiently guided the manuscript through the production process, and Colleen Gauthier managed the marketing and sales teams through the final stages of the process. Charlotte Morrison-Reed worked tirelessly on MyNutritionLab. I am indebted to Carolin Sweig, Acquisitions Editor, for her support and dedication to the preparation of the second edition.

I am grateful to the following people for their valued input and assistance in reviewing this book and for their contributions to the text supplements.

Rhonda Bell, *University of Alberta*
Jesse Colbeck *University of Alberta*
Eithne Dunbar, *St. Lawrence College*
Matthew Durant, *Acadia University*
Natalie Hamilton, *Seneca College*
Gail Hammond, *University of British Columbia*
Christine Johnson, *St. Francis Xavier University*
Vineet Johnson, *Capilano College*
Paul LeBlanc, *Brock University*
Jane Mackie, *Trent University*
Karen McLaren, *Canadore College*
Susan Whiting, *University of Saskatchewan*

—*Judy Sheeshka, October 2008*

About the Authors

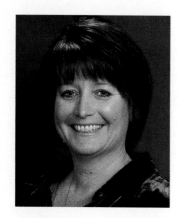

Janice Thompson earned a PhD at Arizona State University in exercise science with an emphasis in exercise physiology and nutrition. She is currently a research assistant professor at the University of New Mexico Health Sciences Center in the Department of Internal Medicine. As the Director of the Office of Native American Diabetes Programs, she conducts research on how nutrition and physical activity interventions reduce diabetes risk in Native American populations. She also mentors junior faculty in research and teaches nutrition courses.

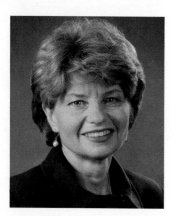

Melinda Manore earned a doctorate in human nutrition with a minor in exercise physiology at Oregon State University, and a master's degree in health education from the University of Oregon. She is a professor in the Department of Nutrition and Exercise Sciences at Oregon State University, where she teaches and conducts research in the area of nutrition and exercise. Prior to her tenure at Oregon State, she taught at Arizona State University for seventeen years. Melinda's areas of specialization include nutritional requirements and issues for active women, nutrition assessment, and the role that nutrition and exercise play in health, energy balance, obesity, and disordered eating.

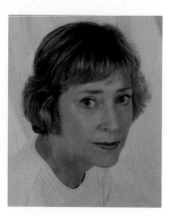

Judy Sheeshka earned a PhD in Applied Human Nutrition at the University of Guelph, where she currently is an Associate Professor. Her research interests include nutrition policy, behaviour change theory, and risk perception. She has been actively involved in the Canadian Foundation for Dietetic Research and is an Editor-in-Chief for the *American Journal of Health Promotion*.

Nutrition: A Functional Approach

Second Canadian Edition

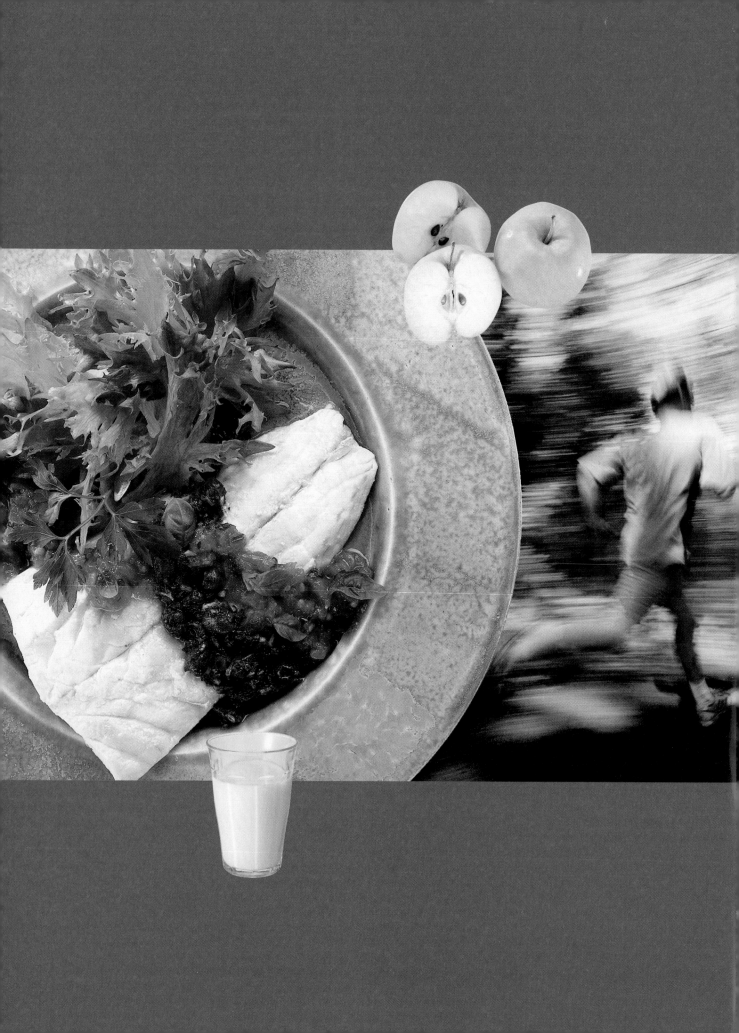

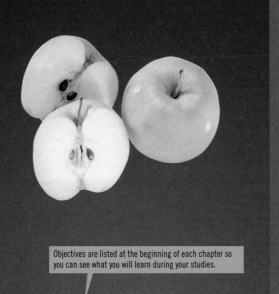

Objectives are listed at the beginning of each chapter so you can see what you will learn during your studies.

CHAPTER 1

The Role of Nutrition in Our Health

CHAPTER OBJECTIVES

After reading this chapter you will be able to:

1. Discuss why nutrition is important to health, pp. 4–8.

2. Identify the six classes of nutrients, p. 9.

3. Discuss the three classes of nutrients that provide energy for the body to work, pp. 9–13.

4. Describe how vitamins and minerals differ from each other, pp. 13–17.

5. Explain the purpose of the Dietary Reference Intakes, pp. 17–21.

6. Describe four sources of reliable nutrition information, pp. 21–25.

Test Yourself questions are a "roadmap" showing what will be covered in each chapter

Test Yourself True or False

1. The term *malnutrition* refers to both nutrient deficiencies and overnutrition. T or F

2. Proteins are a major energy source for our bodies. T or F

3. Fat-soluble vitamins must be consumed daily to support optimal health. T or F

4. Tolerable Upper Intake Levels are set because some nutrients can be toxic if consumed in excess. T or F

5. In Canada, a nutritionist has the same qualifications as a registered dietitian. T or F

Test Yourself answers can be found at the end of the chapter.

Like most people, you've probably been offered nutrition-related advice from well-meaning friends and self-professed "experts." Perhaps you found the advice helpful, or maybe it turned out to be all wrong. Where can you go for reliable advice about nutrition? What exactly is nutrition anyway, and why does what we eat have such an influence on our health? In this chapter, we'll begin to answer these questions, and you'll gain a deeper understanding as you work through the rest of this book. Our goal, by the time you finish this course, is for you to be better qualified to determine your own nutritional needs.

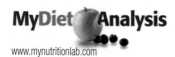

www.mynutritionlab.com

nutrition The science that studies food and how food nourishes our bodies and influences our health.

Key terms are highlighted in the margins and defined where they first appear.

What Is Nutrition?

If you think that the word *nutrition* means pretty much the same thing as *food*, you're right—partially. But the word has a broader meaning that will gradually become clear as you make your way in this course. Specifically, **nutrition** is the science that studies food and how food nourishes our bodies and influences our health. It encompasses how we consume, digest, metabolize, and store nutrients and how these nutrients affect our bodies. Nutrition also involves studying the factors that influence our eating patterns, making recommendations about the amount of each type of food we should eat, attempting to maintain food safety, and addressing issues related to the global food supply. You can think of nutrition, then, as the discipline that encompasses everything about food.

Nutrition is a relatively new scientific discipline. Although food has played a major role in the lives of humans since the beginning of time, the importance of nutrition to our health has been formally recognized and studied only for the past one hundred years or so. Early research in nutrition focused on making the link between nutrient deficiencies and illness. For instance, the cause of scurvy, which is a vitamin C deficiency, was discovered in the mid-1700s. At that time, however, vitamin C had not been identified—what was known was that some ingredient found in citrus fruits could prevent scurvy. Another example of early discoveries in nutrition is presented in the Highlight box on "Solving the Mystery of Pellagra." As was the case with scurvy and vitamin C, this early research was able to pinpoint a nutrient-deficiency disease and foods that could prevent it; it would only be later in the twentieth century that the exact nutrient responsible for the deficiency symptoms would be discovered. Thus, unlike such sciences as physics and mathematics, the majority of discoveries in the field of nutrition are relatively recent, and we still have much to learn.

Why Is Nutrition Important?

Thousands of years ago, people in some cultures believed that the proper diet could cure criminal behaviour, cast out devils, and bring us into alignment with the divine. Although modern science has failed to find evidence to support these claims, we do know that proper nutrition can help us improve our health, prevent certain diseases, achieve and maintain a desirable weight, and maintain our energy and vitality. As you'll learn in Chapter 3, there is some truth in the adage "you are what you eat." Most of the substances you take into your body are broken down and reassembled into your brain cells, bones, muscles—all of your tissues and organs. Think about it: if you eat three meals a day, then by this time next year, you'll have had more than a thousand chances to influence your body's makeup! Let's take a closer look at how nutrition supports health.

Nutrition Is One of Several Factors Contributing to Health

Health can be defined in many ways. Traditionally, health simply referred to the absence of disease. However, as we have learned more about our health and what it means to live a healthy lifestyle, our definition of health has expanded. The World Health Organization defines it as "A state of complete physical, mental and social

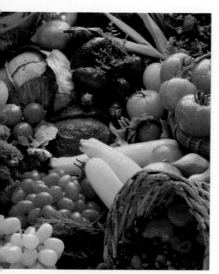

The study of nutrition encompasses everything about food.

The text contains several boxes to help you apply what you've learned.

▶ **HIGHLIGHT**

Solving the Mystery of Pellagra

In the first few years of the twentieth century, Dr. Joseph Goldberger successfully controlled outbreaks of several fatal infectious diseases, from yellow fever in Louisiana to typhus in Mexico. So it wasn't surprising that, in 1914, the Surgeon General of the United States chose him to tackle another disease thought to be infectious that was raging throughout the South. Called pellagra, the disease was characterized by a skin rash, diarrhea, and mental impairment. At the time, it afflicted more than 50 000 people each year, and in about 10% of cases, it resulted in death.

Goldberger began studying the disease by carefully observing its occurrence in groups of people. He asked, if the disease is infectious, then why would it occur in prison inmates yet leave their guards unaffected? Why, in fact, did it overwhelmingly affect impoverished U.S. Southerners while leaving their affluent (and well-fed) neighbours healthy? Could a dietary deficiency cause pellagra?

Finally he found an inexpensive and widely available substance—brewer's yeast—that cured the disease.

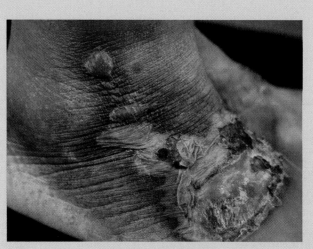

Pellagra is often characterized by a scaly skin rash.

In 1937, eight years after Goldberger's death, scientists identified the precise nutrient that was deficient in the diet of pellagra patients: niacin, one of the B vitamins, which is plentiful in brewer's yeast.

Source: Based on Howard Markel, "The New Yorker Who Changed the Diet of the South," *New York Times,* 12 August 2003, p. D5.

well-being and not merely the absence of disease or infirmity." **Health** is now considered a multidimensional process that includes physical activity and occupational, social, emotional, intellectual, and spiritual health (Figure 1.1). Health is not an endpoint in our lives but an active process we can work on every day.

In this book, we focus on two critical aspects of health: nutrition and physical activity. The two are so closely related that you can think of them as two sides of the same coin: our overall state of nutrition is influenced by how much energy we expend doing daily activities, and our level of physical activity has a major impact on how we use the nutrients in our food. We can perform more strenuous activities for longer periods when we eat a nutritious diet, whereas an inadequate or excessive food intake can make us lethargic. A poor diet, inadequate or excessive physical activity, or a combination of these also can lead to serious health problems. Finally, several studies have suggested that nutrition and regular physical activity can increase feelings of well-being and reduce feelings of anxiety and depression. In other words, wholesome food and physical activity feel good!

health A multidimensional process that includes physical activity and occupational, social, emotional, intellectual, and spiritual health.

A Nutritious Diet Can Prevent Some Diseases and Reduce Your Risk for Others

Early work in the area of nutrition focused on nutrient deficiencies and how we can prevent them. As you read in the Highlight box on pellagra, nutrient deficiencies can cause serious, even life-threatening, illnesses; such diseases as scurvy, goiter, and rickets are other examples. The discoveries of the causes of nutrient deficiencies have aided nutrition experts in developing guidelines for diets that can prevent deficiency diseases. An ample food supply and the fortification of foods with nutrients have ensured that the majority of nutrient-deficiency diseases are no longer of concern in

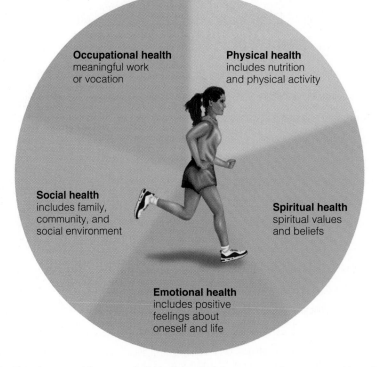

Figure 1.1   Many factors contribute to an individual's health. Primary among these are a nutritious diet and regular physical activity.

developed countries. However, these diseases are still major problems in many developing nations. Some of the nutritional issues affecting developing nations will be discussed throughout this book in Highlight boxes on Global Nutrition.

In addition to preventing diseases related to nutrient deficiencies, a nutritious diet can reduce your risk for certain chronic diseases. In Canada, the United States, New Zealand, and the United Kingdom, the prevalence of obesity, type 2 diabetes mellitus, and some cancers have dramatically increased over the past 20 years (Raine 2004). Figure 1.2 shows that within each age category, the percentage of Canadian adults who

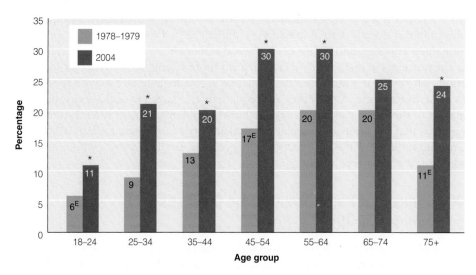

Figure 1.2   Obesity rates among Canadian adults, by age group, 1978–79 versus 2004.

* Significantly higher than estimate for 1978–79 ($p < 0.05$)

E Coefficient of variation 16.6% to 33.3% (interpret with caution)

(Adapted from Statistics Canada publication "Measured obesity, Adult obesity in Canada: Measured height and weight", 2004, no. 1, Catalogue 82-620, July 6, 2005, page 19, available at www.statcan.ca/english/research/82-620-MIE/2005001/articles/adults/aobesity.htm. Accessed January 2006.)

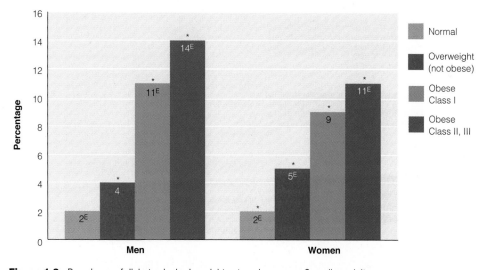

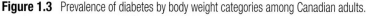

Figure 1.3 Prevalence of diabetes by body weight categories among Canadian adults.

* Significantly higher than estimate for normal ($p < 0.05$)

E Coefficient of variation 16.6% to 33.3% (interpret with caution)

(Adapted from Statistics Canada publication "Measured obesity, Adult obesity in Canada: Measured height and weight", 2004, no. 1, Catalogue 82-620, July 6, 2005, page 19, available at www.statcan.ca/english/research/82-620-MIE/2005001/articles/adults/aobesity.htm. Accessed January 2006.)

were obese was higher in 2004 than in 1978–79. Overall, 23.1% of adults (an estimated 5.5 million) were obese when heights and weights were measured in the 2004 Canadian Community Health Survey, compared with 13.8% in the 1978–79 Canada Health Survey. Another 36.1% (an estimated 8.6 million adults) were categorized as being overweight, meaning that more than half (59.2%) of Canadians aged 18 and older were either overweight or obese. Figure 1.3 shows that diabetes is more prevalent in people who are overweight and obese, compared with people who have normal body weights. (Obesity Class I, II, and III refer to increasing levels of body fat.) Chapter 11 examines overweight and obesity, and the health risks of these conditions, in more detail.

Similarly, the proportion of children and adolescents who are overweight or obese has increased in the past 25 years. Figure 1.4 shows that 8% were obese and

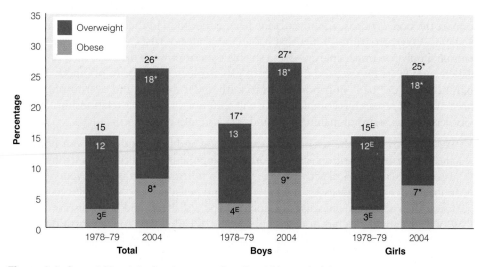

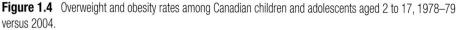

Figure 1.4 Overweight and obesity rates among Canadian children and adolescents aged 2 to 17, 1978–79 versus 2004.

* Significantly higher than estimate for 1978–79 ($p < 0.05$)

E Coefficient of variation 16.6% to 33.3% (interpret with caution)

(Adapted from Statistics Canada publication "Measured obesity, Overweight Canadian children and adolescents", 2004, no. 1, Catalogue 82-620, July 6, 2005, page 19, available at www.statcan.ca/english/research/82-620-MIE/2005001/articles/child/cobesity.htm. Accessed January 2006.)

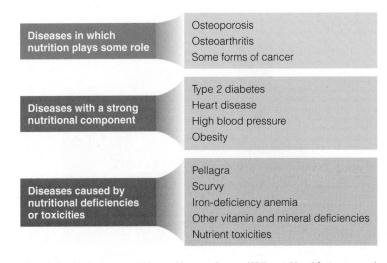

Figure 1.5 The relationship between nutrition and human disease. While nutritional factors are only marginally implicated in the diseases on the top, they are strongly linked to the development of the diseases in the middle row and truly causative of those on the bottom.

18% were overweight in 2004, compared with only 3% who were obese and 12% who were overweight in 1978–79. The implications of this trend for the health of children and adolescents are discussed in more detail in Chapter 16.

We know that obesity and its accompanying diseases are significantly affected by nutrition and activity: regularly consuming foods that are high in total energy (kilocalories or kilojoules), total fat, and saturated fat and low in fibre, fruits, vegetables, and whole grains is associated with an increased risk for obesity, heart disease, type 2 diabetes, and some forms of cancer. The imbalance of consuming too much food and exercising too little also greatly increases our risk for these diseases. Throughout this text, we will discuss in more detail how nutrition and physical activity affect the development of obesity and other chronic diseases.

Nutrition appears to play a role in many diseases. Its role can vary from a mild influence, to a strong association, to directly causing a disease (Figure 1.5). For instance, **undernutrition**—meaning a diet that lacks energy or specific essential nutrients—is known to cause deficiency diseases, such as anemia and scurvy. **Essential nutrients** are ones that can't be manufactured by the human body at all, or not in amounts sufficient to meet the body's needs, and must come from either food in the diet or nutrient supplements. **Overnutrition**—a diet that has an imbalance of fats, carbohydrates, and proteins or simply too much energy—has a strong association with diseases, such as type 2 diabetes and heart disease, and it appears to play a role in some forms of cancer. Thus, **malnutrition**, or "bad" nutrition, refers to both undernutrition and overnutrition. As more nutrition research is completed, we will continue to uncover relationships between various forms of malnutrition and various types of diseases.

undernutrition A diet that lacks energy or specific essential nutrients.

essential nutrients Nutrients that must come from food or nutrient supplements because they are not manufactured by the body at all or not in amounts sufficient to meet the body's needs.

overnutrition A diet that has an imbalance of fats, carbohydrates, and proteins or simply too much energy.

malnutrition Any condition associated with undernutrition or overnutrition.

> **Recap:** Nutrition is the science that studies food and how food affects our body and our health. Nutrition is an important component of health and is strongly associated with physical activity. One goal of a nutritious diet is to prevent nutrient-deficiency diseases, such as scurvy and pellagra; a second goal is to lower the risk for chronic diseases, such as type 2 diabetes and heart disease. Both nutrient-deficiency diseases and chronic disease linked to overnutrition are types of malnutrition found in developed and developing nations.

What Are Nutrients?

A glass of milk or a spoonful of peanut butter may seem as if it is all one substance, but in reality most foods are made up of many different chemicals. Some of these chemicals are probably not useful to the body, whereas others are critical to human

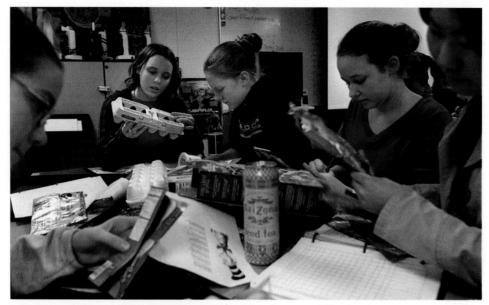

In this text you will learn how to read labels to assist you in meeting your nutritional goals.

growth and function. These latter chemicals are referred to as **nutrients**. Six classes of nutrients are found in the foods we eat (Figure 1.6):

nutrients Chemicals found in foods that are critical to human growth and function.

- carbohydrates
- lipids (fats)
- proteins
- vitamins
- minerals
- water

The four classes of **organic** nutrients contain an element called carbon that is an essential component of all living organisms. Minerals and water are **inorganic** because they do not contain carbon. Both organic and inorganic nutrients are equally important for sustaining life but differ in their structures, functions, and basic chemistry.

organic A substance or nutrient that contains the element carbon.
inorganic A substance or nutrient that does not contain the element carbon.

Carbohydrates, Fats, and Proteins Are Nutrients That Provide Energy

Carbohydrates, fats, and proteins are the only classes of nutrients in foods that provide energy. By this we mean that these nutrients break down and reassemble into a fuel that our body uses to support physical activity and basic functioning. Although taking a multivitamin and a glass of water might be beneficial in other ways, it will not provide you with the energy you need to do your 20 minutes on the stairclimber! The three energy-yielding nutrients are also referred to as **macronutrients**. *Macro* means "large," and our bodies need relatively large amounts of these nutrients to support normal function and health.

macronutrients Nutrients that our bodies need in relatively large amounts to support normal function and health. Carbohydrates, fats, and proteins are macronutrients.

We express energy in units of kilocalories (kcal) or kilojoules (kJ). Refer to the Highlight box "What Is a Calorie?" for an explanation of energy and these units of measurement. Both carbohydrates and proteins provide 4 kilocalories (17 kJ) per gram, while fats provide 9 kilocalories (37 kJ) per gram. Thus, for every gram of fat we consume, we obtain more than twice the energy as compared with a gram of carbohydrate or protein. Refer to the You Do the Math box to learn how to calculate the energy contribution of carbohydrate, fat, and protein in a given food.

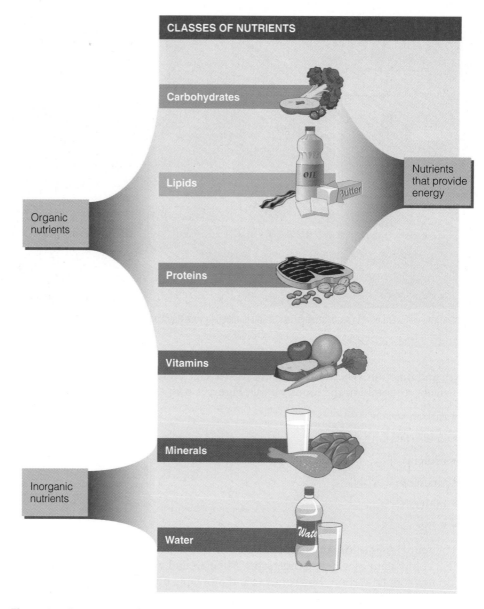

Figure 1.6 The six classes of nutrients found in the foods we consume.

carbohydrates The primary fuel source for our bodies, particularly for our brain and for physical exercise.

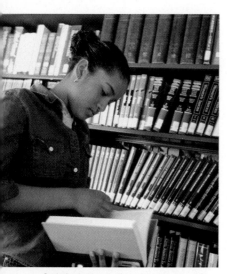

Carbohydrates are the primary source of fuel for our bodies, particularly for our brain.

Carbohydrates Are a Primary Fuel Source

Carbohydrates are the primary source of fuel for our bodies, particularly for our brain and during physical exercise (Figure 1.7). A close look at the word *carbohydrate* reveals the chemical structure of this nutrient. *Carbo-* refers to carbon, and *-hydrate* refers to water. You may remember that water is made up of hydrogen and oxygen. Thus, carbohydrates are composed of chains of carbon, hydrogen, and oxygen.

Carbohydrates are abundant in a wide variety of foods; rice, wheat, and other grains, as well as vegetables, contain carbohydrates. Fruits contain natural sugars that are carbohydrates. Carbohydrates are also found in legumes (including lentils, dry beans, and peas), milk and other dairy products, seeds, and nuts. Dietary fibre is a type of carbohydrate that does not provide energy but has a functional role in the intestine. Carbohydrates and their role in health are the subject of Chapter 4.

> ▶ **HIGHLIGHT**

What Is a Calorie?

Confused by the terms *energy*, *kilocalorie*, and *Calorie*? Should these terms be used interchangeably? What do they really mean? The brief review provided in this highlight should broaden your understanding. First, some precise definitions:

- *Energy* is defined as the capacity to do work. We derive energy from the energy-containing nutrients in the foods we eat; namely, carbohydrates, fats, and proteins.
- A *kilocalorie* (kcal), or *Calorie* (Cal), is the amount of heat required to raise the temperature of 1 kilogram of water by 1 degree Celsius. It is a unit of measurement we use to quantify the amount of energy in food that can be supplied to the body. For instance, we say that energy found in 1 gram of carbohydrate is equal to 4 kcal or 4 Cal.

- In Canada, we also use the *International System of Units (SI)*. The exact conversion is 1 kcal (or 1 Cal) = 4.184 *kilojoules (kJ)*. For approximate calculations, you can use 1 kcal = 4.2 kJ. In general, energy measured in kJ should be rounded to the nearest 10 kJ.

It is most appropriate to use the term *energy* when you are referring to the general concept of energy intake or energy expenditure. If you are discussing the specific units related to energy, use either *kilocalories* or *kilojoules*. The new food labels in Canada use Calorie (upper-case C); we have chosen to use kcal as the unit of measurement throughout this book.

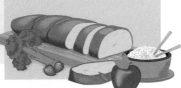

Carbohydrates
- Primary source of energy for body
- Composed of carbon, hydrogen, and oxygen

lipids An important energy source for our bodies at rest and during low-intensity exercise.

Figure 1.7 Carbohydrates are a primary source of energy for our bodies and are found in a wide variety of foods.

Lipids Provide Energy and Other Essential Nutrients

Lipids are another important source of energy for our bodies (Figure 1.8). Lipids are a diverse group of organic substances that are insoluble in water. Lipids include triglycerides (more commonly called fats), phospholipids, and sterols. Like carbohydrates, lipids are composed of carbon, hydrogen, and oxygen; however, they contain proportionally much less oxygen and water than carbohydrates do. This quality allows them to pack together tightly, which explains why they yield more energy per gram than either carbohydrates or proteins.

Lipids are an important energy source for our bodies at rest and during low-intensity exercise. Our body is capable of storing large amounts of fat as triglycerides in adipose tissue. These fat stores can be broken down for energy during periods of fasting, such as while we are asleep. Foods that contain fats are also important in providing fat-soluble vitamins and essential fatty acids.

Dietary fats come in a variety of forms. Solid fats include butter, lard, vegetable shortening, and margarine. Liquid fats are referred to as oils and include corn, safflower, canola, and olive oils. Cholesterol is a form of lipid that is synthesized in our

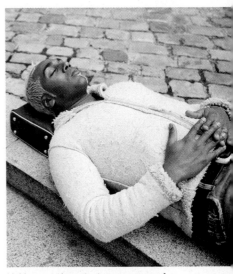

Lipids are an important energy source for our bodies at rest and can be broken down for energy during periods of fasting, such as while we are asleep.

▶ **YOU DO THE MATH**

Calculating the Energy Contributions of Carbohydrate, Fat, and Protein

Have you ever wondered how you can determine the percentage of the total energy you eat that comes from carbohydrate, fat, or protein? You can use a simple equation to calculate these values. To begin, you need to know how much energy you consume and how many grams of carbohydrate, fat, and protein you eat. You also need to know the kilocalorie (energy) value of each of these nutrients. Remember that the energy value for carbohydrate and protein is 4 kilocalories (17 kJ) per gram, and the energy value for fat is 9 kilocalories (37 kJ) per gram. Working along with the following example will help you perform the calculations for yourself:

1. Let's say you have completed a personal diet analysis, and you consume 2500 kcal (10 500 kJ) per day. From your diet analysis, you also find that you consume 300 grams of carbohydrates, 90 grams of fat, and 123 grams of protein.

2. To calculate your percentage of total energy that comes from carbohydrate, you must do two things:

   a. Take your total grams of carbohydrate and multiply by the energy value for carbohydrate to give you how many kilocalories of carbohydrate you have consumed.

   300 grams of carbohydrate × 4 kcal
   (17 kJ) per gram

   = 1200 kilocalories (5040 kJ)
   of carbohydrate

   b. Take the kilocalories of carbohydrate that you have consumed, divide this number by the total number of kilocalories consumed, and multiply by 100. This will give you the percentage of the total energy you consume that comes from carbohydrate.

   (1200 kcal ÷ 2500 kcal) or

   (5040 kJ ÷ 10 500 kJ) × 100 = 48%
   of your total energy comes from
   carbohydrate

3. To calculate the percentage of your total energy that comes from fat, you follow the same steps but use the energy value for fat:

   a. Take your total grams of fat and multiply by the energy value for fat to find the Calories of fat consumed.

   90 grams of fat × 9 kcal (37 kJ)
   per gram

   = 810 kcal (3400 kJ) of fat

   b. Take the Calories of fat you have consumed, divide this number by the total number of Calories you consumed, and multiply by 100 to get the percentage of total energy you consume that comes from fat.

   (810 kcal ÷ 2500 kcal) or

   (3400 kJ ÷ 10 500 kJ) × 100 = approx.
   32% of your total energy comes from fat

Now try these steps to calculate the percentage of the total energy you consume that comes from protein. The sum of your percentages for carbohydrate, fat, and protein should add up to 100%. These calculations will be very useful throughout this course as you learn more about how to plan a nutritious diet and how to read labels to assist you in meeting your nutrition goals. Later in this book, in Chapter 11, you will learn how to estimate your unique energy needs and determine the ideal amount of energy you need from carbohydrate, fat, and protein.

bodies, and it can also be consumed in the diet. Chapter 5 provides an introduction to lipids.

Proteins Support Tissue Growth, Repair, and Maintenance

proteins The only macronutrient that contains nitrogen; the basic building blocks of proteins are amino acids.

Proteins also contain carbon, hydrogen, and oxygen, but they are different from carbohydrates and fats in that they contain the element *nitrogen* (Figure 1.9). These four elements assemble into small building blocks known as amino acids. We break down dietary proteins into amino acids and reassemble them to build our own body proteins—for instance, the proteins in our muscles and blood.

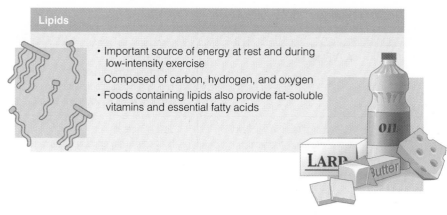

Lipids

- Important source of energy at rest and during low-intensity exercise
- Composed of carbon, hydrogen, and oxygen
- Foods containing lipids also provide fat-soluble vitamins and essential fatty acids

Figure 1.8 Lipids are an important energy source during rest and low-intensity exercise. Foods containing fat also provide other important nutrients.

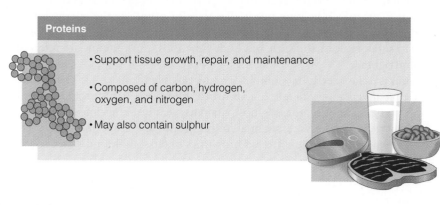

Proteins

- Support tissue growth, repair, and maintenance
- Composed of carbon, hydrogen, oxygen, and nitrogen
- May also contain sulphur

Figure 1.9 Proteins contain nitrogen in addition to carbon, hydrogen, and oxygen. Proteins support the growth, repair, and maintenance of body tissues.

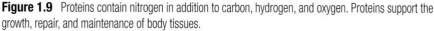

Meats are an excellent source of proteins.

Although proteins can provide energy, they are not a primary source of energy for our bodies. Proteins play a major role in building new cells and tissues, maintaining the structure and strength of bone, repairing damaged structures, and assisting in regulating metabolism and fluid balance. Some proteins are digestive enzymes and hormones (e.g., insulin).

Proteins are found in many foods. Meats and dairy products are important sources of protein, but we also obtain small amounts of protein from vegetables and whole grains. Seeds, nuts, and legumes are good sources of protein. Proteins are reviewed in Chapter 6.

Recap: The six classes of nutrients found in foods are carbohydrates, lipids or fats, proteins, vitamins, minerals, and water. Carbohydrates, lipids, and proteins are referred to as the energy-yielding nutrients, as they provide our bodies with the energy necessary to thrive. Carbohydrates are the primary energy source for our bodies; fats are a source of fat-soluble vitamins and essential fatty acids and act as energy storage molecules; and proteins support tissue growth, repair, and maintenance.

Vitamins Assist in the Regulation of Biological Processes

Vitamins are organic compounds that assist us in regulating our bodies' processes. Vitamins are critical in building and maintaining healthy bone and muscle tissue, supporting our immune system so we can fight illness and disease, and ensuring

vitamins Organic compounds that assist us in regulating our bodies' processes.

Table 1.1   Overview of Vitamins

Type	Names	Distinguishing Features
Fat-soluble	A, D, E, and K	Soluble in fat Stored in the human body Toxicity can occur from consuming excess amounts, which accumulate in the body
Water-soluble	C, B vitamins (thiamin, riboflavin, niacin, vitamin B_6, vitamin B_{12}, pantothenic acid, biotin, and folate)	Soluble in water Not stored to any extent in the human body Excess excreted in urine Toxicity generally occurs only as a result of vitamin supplementation

healthy vision. They also assist in maintaining the health of our blood. Contrary to popular belief, vitamins do not contain energy (or kilocalories); however, vitamins do play an important role in helping our bodies to release and use the energy found in carbohydrates, fats, and proteins. Because we need relatively small amounts of these nutrients to support normal health and body functions, the vitamins are referred to as **micronutrients**.

Vitamins are classified as fat-soluble or water-soluble (Table 1.1). Their solubility in water or fat affects how vitamins are absorbed, transported, and stored in our bodies. As our bodies cannot synthesize most vitamins, we must consume them in our diets. Both types of vitamins are essential for our health and are found in a variety of foods. Let's now review the different properties of fat-soluble and water-soluble vitamins.

micronutrients Nutrients needed in relatively small amounts to support normal health and body functions. Vitamins and some minerals are micronutrients.

Fat-Soluble Vitamins Are Stored in the Body

Vitamins A, D, E, and K are **fat-soluble vitamins**. As you will learn in more detail in Chapter 3, fat-soluble vitamins are absorbed in our intestines along with dietary fat. They are then transported to the liver or other organs, where they are either used or stored for later use.

Our ability to store fat-soluble vitamins sets them apart from the water-soluble vitamins. Because we are capable of storing fat-soluble vitamins, we do not have to consume the recommended intakes of these nutrients on a daily or weekly basis. As long as our diet contains the average amounts recommended over a given time, our intake of these vitamins will be sufficient to support healthy body functions.

fat-soluble vitamins Vitamins that are not soluble in water but are soluble in fat. These are vitamins A, D, E, and K.

Storing fat-soluble vitamins in our bodies can have its disadvantages. Consuming large amounts of these vitamins, particularly from supplements, can cause an excessive buildup and lead to dangerously toxic levels. Toxicity can occur relatively quickly for some of these vitamins. Toxicity symptoms include damage to our hair, skin, bone, eyes, and nervous system.

Even though we can store fat-soluble vitamins, deficiencies can and do occur, although they are relatively uncommon. Eating too little fat in our diet or excreting these vitamins from our digestive tract along with undigested fat can lead to deficiencies. Using mineral oil as a laxative can result in a significant loss of fat-soluble vitamins in our feces. Diets that are extremely low in fat, as well as diseases that prevent the normal absorption of fat, can also result in fat-soluble-vitamin deficiencies. Deficiencies of fat-soluble vitamins can lead to serious health problems, such as night blindness and osteoporosis and even death in the most severe cases.

Fat-soluble vitamins are found in a variety of fat-containing foods. Meats, dairy products, vegetable oils, avocados, nuts, and seeds are all potentially good sources. You will learn more about the specific functions, toxicity and deficiency symptoms, and food sources of these vitamins in Chapters 7 through 10.

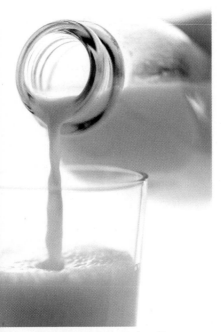

Fat-soluble vitamins are found in a variety of fat-containing foods, including dairy products.

Water-Soluble Vitamins Should Be Consumed Daily or Weekly

In contrast to the fat-soluble vitamins, **water-soluble vitamins** dissolve in water. Vitamin C and the B vitamins (thiamin, riboflavin, niacin, vitamin B_6, vitamin B_{12}, pantothenic acid, biotin, and folate) are absorbed through the intestinal wall directly into the bloodstream. These vitamins then travel to the cells of the body where they are needed.

water-soluble vitamins Vitamins that are soluble in water. These include vitamin C and the B vitamins. Some are destroyed by heat or light.

Precisely because these vitamins dissolve in water, our bodies cannot store large amounts of them. Our kidneys filter out any excess water-soluble vitamins we consume, and we then excrete this excess in our urine. Because we cannot store large amounts of these vitamins, toxicity rarely occurs when we consume excess amounts in our diet. We *can* consume toxic levels of these nutrients through supplementation, however, if we consume higher amounts than our bodies can eliminate.

Another consequence of our inability to store large amounts of water-soluble vitamins is that we need to consume adequate amounts of these nutrients on a daily or weekly basis. If we do not regularly consume these nutrients in our diets, deficiency symptoms and even disease can result fairly quickly. However, this does not mean that we must take vitamin supplements to obtain adequate amounts of these nutrients. The water-soluble vitamins are abundant in many foods, including whole grains, fruits, vegetables, meat, and dairy products. They can be destroyed by cooking and poor food storage practices, such as exposure to light, however. The toxicity symptoms, deficiency diseases, and food sources of these vitamins are described in detail in Chapters 7 through 10 in relation to their specific functions.

> **Recap:** Vitamins are organic compounds that assist with regulating many body processes. Fat-soluble vitamins are soluble in fat and include vitamins A, D, E, and K. We can store fat-soluble vitamins in our liver and in adipose and other fatty tissues. Water-soluble vitamins are soluble in water and include vitamin C and the B vitamins (thiamin, riboflavin, niacin, vitamin B_6, vitamin B_{12}, pantothenic acid, biotin, and folate). We excrete excess amounts of water-soluble vitamins in our urine.

Minerals Assist in the Regulation of Many Body Functions

Minerals are inorganic substances, meaning that they do not contain carbon. Some important dietary minerals include sodium, potassium, calcium, magnesium, and iron. Minerals are different from the macronutrients and vitamins in that they are

minerals Inorganic substances that are not broken down during digestion and absorption and are not destroyed by heat or light. Minerals assist in the regulation of many body processes and are classified as major minerals or trace minerals.

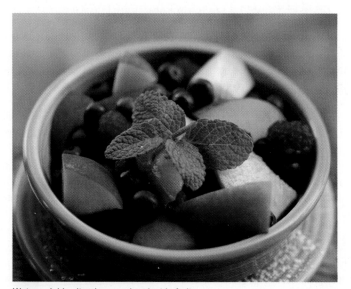

Water-soluble vitamins are abundant in fruits.

Table 1.2   Overview of Minerals

Type	Names	Distinguishing Features
Major minerals	Calcium, phosphorus, magnesium, sodium, potassium, chloride, sulphur	Needed in amounts greater than 100 mg/day in our diets Amount present in the human body is greater than 5 g (or 5000 mg)
Trace minerals	Iron, zinc, copper, manganese, selenium, iodine, fluoride, chromium, molybdenum	Needed in amounts less than 100 mg/day in our diets Amount present in the human body is less than 5 g (or 5000 mg)

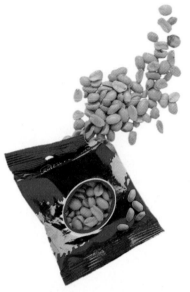

Peanuts are a good source of magnesium and phosphorus, which play an important role in the formation and maintenance of the skeleton.

major minerals Minerals we need to consume in amounts of at least 100 mg per day and of which the total amount in our bodies is at least 5 grams.

trace minerals Minerals we need to consume in amounts less than 100 mg per day and of which the total amount in our bodies is less than 5 grams.

not broken down during digestion or when our bodies use them to promote normal function; they are also not destroyed by heat or light. Thus, all minerals maintain their structure no matter what environment they are in. This means that the calcium in our bones is the same as the calcium in the milk we drink, and the sodium in our cells is the same as the sodium in our table salt. Like vitamins, minerals are also known as micronutrients.

Minerals have many important functions in our bodies. They assist in regulating fluids and producing energy, are essential to the health of our bones and blood, and help rid our body of harmful byproducts of metabolism. Chapters 7 through 10 discuss the various minerals and the roles they play in maintaining human health and function.

Minerals are classified according to the amounts we need in our diet and how much of the mineral is found in our bodies. The two categories of minerals in our diets and bodies are the major minerals and the trace minerals (Table 1.2).

Major Minerals Are Required in Amounts Greater than 100 Milligrams per Day

Major minerals earned their name from the fact that we need to consume at least 100 milligrams (mg) per day of these minerals in our diets and because the total amount found in our bodies is at least 5 grams (or 5000 mg). The major minerals calcium, phosphorus, and magnesium play an important role in the formation and maintenance of our skeletons. Sodium, potassium, and chloride play critical roles in fluid balance, while sulphur is primarily recognized as a component of specific vitamins and amino acids. Food sources of major minerals are varied and include meats, dairy products, fresh fruits and vegetables, and nuts.

Trace Minerals Are Required in Amounts Less than 100 Milligrams per Day

Trace minerals are those we need to consume in amounts less than 100 mg per day, and the total amount of these minerals in our bodies is less than 5 grams (or 5000 mg). The trace minerals discussed in this textbook are iron, zinc, copper, manganese, selenium, iodine, fluoride, and chromium. Iron is important in maintaining the health of our blood and supporting oxygen transport to all parts of our bodies. Zinc has numerous functions, including ensuring reproductive health and appropriate cell growth and development. Copper, manganese, and selenium play roles in the antioxidant function, while iodine is critical for the adequate production of hormones that control body temperature regulation, metabolic rate, and growth. Fluoride helps reduce tooth decay and strengthens our bones and teeth. Chromium is necessary for the proper metabolism of carbohydrates and fats. Food sources of the trace minerals are the same as those for major minerals.

Water Supports All Body Functions

Water is an inorganic nutrient that is vital for our survival. We consume water in its pure form; in juices, soups, and other liquids; and in solid foods, such as fruits and vegetables. Adequate water intake ensures the proper balance of fluid both inside and outside our cells, and it also assists in the regulation of nerve impulses, muscle contractions, nutrient transport, and excretion of waste products. Because of the key role that water plays in our health, Chapter 7 focuses on water and its function in our bodies.

> **Recap:** Minerals are inorganic elements that maintain their structure throughout the processes of digestion, absorption, and metabolism. Major minerals are needed in amounts greater than 100 mg per day, and the total amount found in our bodies is at least 5 grams (or 5000 mg). Trace minerals are needed in amounts less than 100 mg per day, and the total amount found in our bodies is less than 5 grams (or 5000 mg). Minerals play critical roles in virtually all aspects of human health and function. Water is critical for our survival and is important for regulating nervous impulses, muscle contractions, nutrient transport, and excretion of waste products.

How Can I Figure Out My Nutrient Needs?

Now that you know the six classes of nutrients, you are probably wondering how much of each you need each day. But before you can learn more about specific nutrients and how to plan your own healthful diet, you need to become familiar with current dietary standards and how these standards shape nutrition recommendations.

Use the Dietary Reference Intakes to Check Your Nutrient Intake

In the past, the dietary standards in Canada were called the Recommended Nutrient Intakes (RNIs), and the standards in the United States were referred to as the Recommended Dietary Allowances (RDAs). These standards were used to define recommended intake values for various nutrients and could be used to plan diets for both individuals and groups. They were developed from the perspective of preventing nutrient-deficiency diseases; however, in most developed countries, these diseases are now extremely rare. Thus, much of our current work in nutrition is focused on the associations between nutrition and health. We want to learn more about the role of nutrition in preventing and reducing the risks for chronic diseases, such as diabetes, heart disease, and cancer, and to design diets that promote optimal health. In response to these changes in focus, a new set of reference values has been developed to replace the RNI and RDA values. These new reference values in both Canada and the United States are termed the **Dietary Reference Intakes (DRIs)** (Figure 1.10).

Dietary Reference Intakes (DRIs) A set of nutritional reference values for Canada and the United States that apply to healthy people.

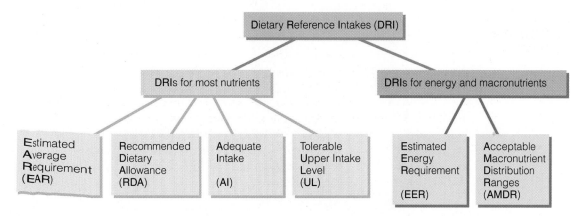

Figure 1.10 The Dietary Reference Intakes (DRIs) for all nutrients. Note that the Estimated Energy Requirement (EER) applies only to energy, and the Acceptable Macronutrient Distribution Ranges (AMDR) apply only to the macronutrients and alcohol.

These standards were developed to include and expand on the former values and to set new recommendation standards for nutrients that did not have reference values.

The DRIs are dietary standards for healthy people only; they do not apply to people with diseases or to those who are suffering from nutrient deficiencies. Like the RNIs and RDAs, they identify the amount of a nutrient needed to prevent deficiency diseases in healthy individuals, but they also consider how much of this nutrient may reduce the risk for chronic diseases in healthy people. The DRIs establish an upper level of safety for nutrients and an international standard for both Canada and the United States.

The DRIs for most nutrients consist of four values:

- Estimated Average Requirement (EAR)
- Recommended Dietary Allowances (RDA)
- Adequate Intake (AI)
- Tolerable Upper Intake Level (UL)

In the case of energy and the macronutrients, different standards are used. The standards for energy and the macronutrients include the Estimated Energy Requirement (EER) and the Acceptable Macronutrient Distribution Ranges (AMDR). Let's now define each of these DRI values.

The Estimated Average Requirement Guides the Recommended Dietary Allowance

Estimated Average Requirement (EAR)
The average daily nutrient intake level estimated to meet the requirement of half of the healthy individuals in a particular life stage and gender group.

The **Estimated Average Requirement (EAR)** represents the average daily nutrient intake level estimated to meet the requirement of half the healthy individuals in a particular life stage and gender group (Institute of Medicine 2003). Figure 1.11 provides a graph representing this value. As an example, the EAR for phosphorus for women between the ages of 19 and 30 years represents the average daily intake of phosphorus that meets the requirement of half the women in this age group. The EAR is used by scientists to statistically define the Recommended Dietary Allowance (RDA) for a given nutrient. Obviously, if the EAR meets the needs of only half the people in a group, then the recommended intake will be higher.

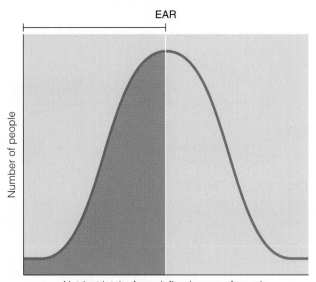

Figure 1.11 The Estimated Average Requirement (EAR) represents the average daily nutrient intake level that meets the requirements of half the healthy individuals in a given group.

The Recommended Dietary Allowance Meets the Needs of Nearly All Healthy People

As previously introduced, the Recommended Nutrient Intake (RNI) was the term previously used to refer to all nutrient recommendations in Canada, and the **Recommended Dietary Allowance (RDA)** was the term used in the United States. The RDA is now considered one of many reference standards within the larger umbrella of the DRIs. The RDA represents the average daily nutrient intake level that meets the nutrient requirements of 97% to 98% of healthy individuals in a particular life stage and gender group (Figure 1.12) (Institute of Medicine 2003). For example, the RDA for phosphorus is 700 mg per day for women between the ages of 19 and 30 years. This amount of phosphorus will meet the nutrient requirements of almost all women in this age category.

Again, scientists use the EAR to statistically establish the RDA. In fact, if an EAR cannot be determined for a nutrient, then this nutrient cannot have an RDA. When this occurs, an Adequate Intake value is determined for a nutrient.

Recommended Dietary Allowance (RDA) The average daily nutrient intake level that meets the nutrient requirements of 97% to 98% of healthy individuals in a particular life stage and gender group.

The Adequate Intake Is Based on Estimates of Nutrient Intakes

The **Adequate Intake (AI)** value is a recommended average daily nutrient intake level based on observed or experimentally determined estimates of nutrient intake by a group of healthy people (Institute of Medicine 2003). These estimates are assumed to be adequate and are used when an RDA cannot be determined. There are numerous nutrients that have an AI value, including calcium, vitamin D, vitamin K, and fluoride. More research needs to be done on human requirements for the nutrients assigned an AI value so that an EAR, and subsequently an RDA, can be established.

In addition to establishing RDA and AI values for nutrients, an upper level of safety for nutrients, or Tolerable Upper Intake Level, has also been defined.

Adequate Intake (AI) A recommended average daily nutrient intake level based on observed or experimentally determined estimates of nutrient intake by a group of healthy people.

The Tolerable Upper Intake Level Is the Highest Level That Poses No Health Risk

The **Tolerable Upper Intake Level (UL)** is the highest average daily nutrient intake level likely to pose no risk of adverse health effects to almost all individuals in a particular life stage and gender group (Institute of Medicine 2003). This does not mean that we should consume this intake level or that we will receive more benefits from a

Tolerable Upper Intake Level (UL) The highest average daily nutrient intake level likely to pose no risk of adverse health effects to almost all individuals in a particular life stage and gender group.

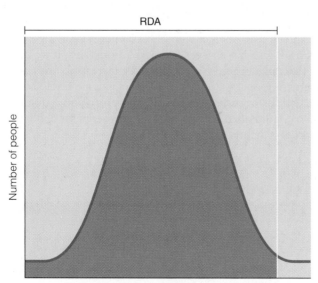

Figure 1.12 The Recommended Dietary Allowance (RDA). The RDA represents the average daily nutrient intake level that meets the requirements of almost all (97% to 98%) healthy individuals in a given life stage and gender group.

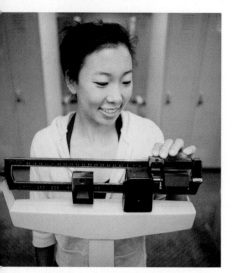

Knowing your daily Estimated Energy Requirement (EER) is a helpful way to maintain a healthy body weight. Your EER is defined by your age, gender, weight, height, and physical activity level.

Estimated Energy Requirement (EER) The average dietary energy intake that is predicted to maintain energy balance in healthy reference adults.

Acceptable Macronutrient Distribution Ranges (AMDR) Ranges of intakes for energy sources associated with reduced risk of chronic disease while providing adequate intakes of essential nutrients.

nutrient by meeting or exceeding the UL. In fact, as our intake of a nutrient increases in amounts above the UL, the potential for toxic effects and health risks increases. The UL value is a helpful guide to assist you in determining the highest average intake level that is deemed safe for a given nutrient.

> **Recap:** The Dietary Reference Intakes (DRIs) are dietary standards for nutrients established for healthy people in a particular life stage and gender group. The Estimated Average Requirement (EAR) represents the nutrient intake level that meets the requirement of half the healthy individuals in a group. The Recommended Dietary Allowances (RDA) represent the nutrient intake level that meets the requirements of 97% to 98% of healthy individuals in a group. The Adequate Intake (AI) is a recommended nutrient intake level based on estimates of nutrient intake by a group of healthy people when not enough information is available to set an RDA. The Tolerable Upper Intake Level (UL) is the highest daily nutrient intake level that likely poses no risk of adverse health effects to almost all individuals in a group.

The Estimated Energy Requirement Is the Intake Predicted to Maintain a Healthy Weight

The **Estimated Energy Requirement (EER)** is defined as the average dietary energy intake that is predicted to maintain energy balance in healthy reference adults. Reference adults are men 19 to 30 years old, 1.75 metres (5′9″) in height and 70 kg (154 lb.) in weight, and women of the same age who are 1.63 metres (5′4″) tall and weigh 57 kg (126 lb.). This dietary intake is defined by a person's age, gender, weight, height, and level of physical activity that is consistent with good health (Institute of Medicine 2002). It is recommended that an individual maintain an active lifestyle to maintain health and decrease risk for chronic diseases; thus, the EER for an active person is higher than the EER for an inactive person even if all other factors (age, gender, etc.) are the same.

The Acceptable Macronutrient Distribution Ranges Are Associated with Reduced Risk for Chronic Diseases

The **Acceptable Macronutrient Distribution Ranges (AMDR)** are ranges of intakes for energy sources that are associated with reduced risk of chronic disease while providing adequate intakes of essential nutrients (Institute of Medicine 2002). The AMDR is expressed as a percentage of total energy or as a percentage of total Calories. The AMDR also has a lower and upper boundary; if we consume nutrients above or below this range, there is a potential for increasing our risk for chronic diseases and for increasing our risk of consuming inadequate levels of nutrients essential for health. The AMDR for carbohydrate, fat, and protein for adults are listed in Table 1.3. (The recommended intakes of macronutrients for children and adolescents are discussed in Chapter 16.)

Table 1.3 Acceptable Macronutrient Distribution Ranges (AMDR) for Adults

Nutrient	AMDR*
Carbohydrate	45%–65%
Fat	20%–35%
Protein	10%–35%

Source: Institute of Medicine, Food and Nutrition Board, *Dietary Reference Intakes for Energy, Carbohydrates, Fiber, Fat, Protein and Amino Acids (Macronutrients),* Washington, DC: National Academies Press, 2002.

* AMDR values expressed as percentage of total energy or as percentage of total kcal.

Calculating Your Unique Nutrient Needs

The primary goal of dietary planning is to develop a diet or eating plan that is nutritionally adequate, meaning that the chances of consuming too little or too much of any nutrient are very low. By eating foods that give you nutrient intakes that meet the RDA or AI values, you help your body to maintain a healthy weight, support your daily physical activity, and prevent nutrient deficiencies and toxicities.

The DRI values are listed in Appendix H; they are also reviewed with each nutrient as it is introduced throughout this text. Find your life stage group and gender in the left-hand column of the Appendix, and then simply look across to see each nutrient's value for you. Using the DRI values in conjunction with diet planning tools, such as *Eating Well with Canada's Food Guide,* will ensure a healthful and adequate diet. Chapter 2 provides details on how you can use these tools to develop a healthful diet.

> **Recap:** The Estimated Energy Requirement (EER) is the average daily energy intake that is predicted to maintain energy balance in a healthy adult. The EER is defined by a person's age, gender, weight, height, and physical activity level. The Acceptable Macronutrient Distribution Ranges (AMDR) are ranges of intakes for particular energy sources that are associated with reduced risk of chronic disease while also providing adequate intakes of essential nutrients. The DRI values can be used to plan diets that are nutritionally adequate and healthful.

Nutrition Advice: Whom Can You Trust?

After reading this chapter, you can see that one of the major nutritional concerns in North America is our high risk for many chronic diseases. One result of this concern has been the publication of an almost overwhelming quantity of nutritional information on television shows and websites; in newspapers, magazines, newsletters, and journals; and in many other forums. In addition to this information overload, we continually discover that the nutritional messages from these supposedly expert sources are confusing, dissimilar, or even contradictory. Because early studies need to be followed by experiments to verify findings, studies can be contradictory! If you are wondering how to sort nutritional fact from fiction, the following discussion should help.

Trustworthy Experts Are Educated and Credentialed

A considerable number of health professionals can assist us with reliable and accurate nutrition information. It is not possible to list in this chapter all individuals who can provide information. The following is a list of a few groups that provide reputable nutrition information:

- Registered dietitian—A registered dietitian (RD) is a health professional with a baccalaureate (bachelor's) degree in foods and nutrition from a university program accredited by the Dietitians of Canada (DC). After finishing this undergraduate degree, the individual needs to complete a dietetic internship or equivalent practicum experience. (At some universities, the dietetic internship is integrated into the undergraduate degree program.) The final steps are to successfully complete the Canadian Dietetic Registration Examination and to become registered with a provincial regulatory body. As is the case for other health professionals, provincially mandated colleges or registration boards ensure public safety. These colleges monitor the competence of members, protect the public from unsafe or unethical dietetic practice, respond to complaints from the public, and discipline members when necessary. The title *dietitian* is legally protected in each province so that only qualified practitioners with the appropriate education can use it. Look for the professional designation RD,

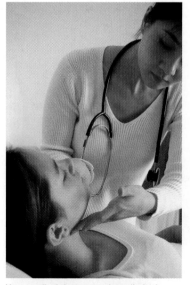

Your medical doctor may have limited experience and training in the area of nutrition, but he or she can refer you to a registered dietitian (RD) to assist you in meeting your dietary needs.

PDt, or RDt (or the French equivalent Dt.P). To find registered dietitians in your community, check the Dietitians of Canada website, www.dietitians.ca. See the Highlight box on "What Does a Registered Dietitian Do?" for more information on RDs.

- Nutritionist—The title *nutritionist* (e.g., a public health nutritionist) is protected for dietitians in some provinces but not in most, so people with different levels of training and knowledge can call themselves nutritionists. Unqualified people sometimes use the terms *registered* or *certified* with a variation of *nutrition* as a title. To make sure a person is a qualified nutrition professional, contact the Dietitians of Canada or the provincial regulatory body in your area.

- Professional with an advanced degree (a master's degree [MSc, MAN, MHSc, MScAHN] or doctoral degree [PhD]) in nutrition—Many individuals are educated and experienced in nutrition and hold an advanced degree. Some of these individuals teach at community colleges and universities or work in fitness and health settings. Not all of these individuals are registered dietitians. Such individuals who do not have a registered dietitian designation (RD, PDt, RDt, or Dt.P) are very knowledgeable about nutrition and health, but they are not qualified to provide clinical dietary counselling or treatment for individuals with diseases or illnesses.

- Medical doctor—A medical doctor, also called a physician or MD, is educated, trained, and licensed to practise medicine in Canada. This individual typically has limited experience and training in the area of nutrition. However, if you become ill, the medical doctor is usually one of the first health professionals you'll see for an accurate medical diagnosis. If you require a dietary plan to treat an illness or disease, most medical doctors will refer you to an RD to assist you in meeting your dietary needs.

Government Sources of Information Are Trustworthy

Federal, provincial or territorial, and municipal government health agencies have been restructured quite a bit in the past 20 years to better address the health problems related to malnutrition in Canada. These agencies are funded with taxpayer dollars, and some also provide financial support for research in the areas of nutrition and health. The following are just a few of the main government agencies affiliated with Health Canada:

Office of Nutrition Policy and Promotion, Health Products and Food Branch, Health Canada This office conducts reviews of nutrition policy and recommendations. For example, guidelines for determining healthy weights, infant feeding recommendations, nutrition labelling guidelines, and *Eating Well with Canada's Food Guide* are all available at this website. Visit www.hc-sc.gc.ca/fn-an/nutrition/index-eng.php to learn more about food and nutrition policy in Canada.

Natural Health Products Directorate, Health Products and Food Branch, Health Canada The mission of this directorate is "to ensure that all Canadians have ready access to natural health products that are safe, effective and of high quality, while respecting freedom of choice and philosophical and cultural diversity." To learn more about the regulation of natural health products in Canada, visit www.hc-sc.gc.ca/dhp-mps/prodnatur/index-eng.php.

Canadian Food Inspection Agency, Bureau of Food Safety and Consumer Protection The Canadian food supply is inspected by this agency, which reports to Health Canada. Food recalls, mad cow disease, biotechnology, and food package labelling requirements for manufacturers are some of the topics that you can find at www.inspection.gc.ca.

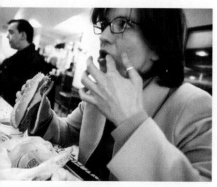

Lifestyle behaviours, such as eating an unhealthy diet, can increase your risk for chronic disease.

▶ **HIGHLIGHT**

What Does a Dietitian Do?

Dietitians play a major role in health care, industry, government, and education. Dietitians influence policy development; direct nutrition programs; manage quality food services; and provide information and counsel that allow clients, including the consumer, to make informed decisions about their nutrition and food choices. Dietitians are essential members of the health care team and practise in a wide range of diverse workplaces. Dietitians work

- In health care facilities, including hospitals and nursing homes, community health centres, and home care
- In the community
- In foodservice management
- In private practice
- In industry
- In government, education and research

Clinical Dietitians identify nutrition problems and assess the nutritional status of patients; develop care plans and monitor the effectiveness of nutrition interventions; and counsel patients on special diet modifications.

Public Health Nutritionists/Dietitians; Dietitians working in Community Health Centres or Aboriginal Health assess the nutritional needs of populations; identify community nutrition problems; and develop health promotion strategies, nutrition education programs, and healthy eating resources. They work with individuals and groups to improve their nutritional well-being; prevent nutrition-related disease; increase access to food; and enhance personal control of health.

Administrative Dietitians manage food production, distribution, and service of high quality meals/snacks, ensuring adherence to sanitation and safety standards and a cost effective operation. They manage food service departments in hospitals and other health care facilities, schools, universities, and businesses and may be employed by contract food companies.

Consulting Dietitians provide expertise in nutrition to promote health and prevent disease, counselling services for nutrition-related diseases and disorders, and management advice to food service operations. They operate their own private consulting practices or businesses and work with individuals, groups, workplaces, and media.

. . .

Source: Excerpts from Dietitians of Canada. www.dietitians.ca/public/content/career_in_nutrition/where_do_dietitians_work.asp accessed September 2008. Reprinted with permission from Dietitians of Canada. All rights reserved.

Public Health Agency of Canada The federal government created this national agency, with a Chief Public Health Officer for Canada, in the wake of the Walkerton, Ontario, experience with a deadly microorganism (E. coli O157:H7) in its water supply, the Severe Acute Respiratory Syndrome (SARS) crisis, and the avian flu outbreak in British Columbia. Its mandate is to prevent disease and injury and to promote health by monitoring trends in chronic infectious and non-infectious diseases and by conducting research. Learn more about this agency at www.phac-aspc.gc.ca.

U.S. Sources The United States government and large national not-for-profit health agencies have the resources to organize and disseminate the most recent and reliable information on nutrition and health. Among the most recognized and respected of these agencies are the National Institutes of Health and the Centers for Disease Control and Prevention.

The **National Institutes of Health (NIH)** is the world's leading medical research centre and the focal point for medical research in the United States. The mission of the NIH is to uncover new knowledge that leads to better health for

National Institutes of Health (NIH) The world's leading medical centre and the focal point for medical research in the United States.

everyone. The NIH has many institutes and centres, including the following, that investigate a broad array of nutrition-related health issues:

- National Cancer Institute (NCI)
- National Eye Institute (NEI)
- National Heart, Lung, and Blood Institute (NHLBI)
- National Institute of Diabetes and Digestive and Kidney Diseases (NIDDK)
- National Center for Complementary and Alternative Medicine (NCCAM)
- NIH headquarters are located in Bethesda, Maryland. To find out more about the NIH, go to www.nih.gov.

The **Centers for Disease Control and Prevention (CDC)** is the leading federal agency to protect the health and safety of people. The CDC is located in Atlanta, Georgia, and works in the areas of health promotion, disease prevention and control, and environmental health. Among its many activities, the CDC supports two large national surveys that monitor the health, lifestyle behaviours, and food and nutrient intakes of Americans—The Behavioral Risk Factor Surveillance System (BRFSS) and The National Health and Nutrition Examination Survey (NHANES). Unfortunately, we have no similar nutrition and food-monitoring systems in Canada to track changes in what people are eating and trends in nutrition issues over time. To learn more about the CDC, go to www.cdc.gov.

> **Centers for Disease Control and Prevention (CDC)** The leading federal agency in the United States that protects the health and safety of people. Its mission is to promote health and quality of life by preventing and controlling disease, injury, and disability.

Professional Organizations Provide Reliable Nutrition Information

A number of professional organizations have members who are qualified nutrition professionals, scientists, and educators. These organizations publish cutting-edge nutrition research studies and educational information in journals that are accessible in most university and medical libraries. Some of these organizations include the following:

- Dietitians of Canada (DC)—This is the national professional organization for dietitians in Canada, and membership is voluntary. DC promotes dietitians as credible sources of nutrition advice, organizes an annual national Nutrition Month campaign, and represents the profession when policy issues related to health and nutrition are being discussed in the public domain. It publishes the *Canadian Journal of Dietetic Practice and Research*. Visit its website at www.dietitians.ca.

- Canadian Society for Nutritional Sciences (CSNS)—The Society represents nutritional scientists in academia, government, industry, hospitals, and research institutes. The purpose of the CSNS is to acquire, share, and encourage the use of knowledge in the science of nutrition. Visit the CSNS website at www.nutritionalsciences.ca.

- Canadian Society of Nutrition Management (CSNM)—This is the professional association for nutrition managers, who complete two-year accredited programs in food and nutrition management. To learn more about the role of nutrition managers in promoting sound nutrition, visit the CSNM website at www.csnm.ca.

- International Society for Behavioral Nutrition and Physical Activity (ISBNPA)—This professional organization was formed in 2000 to bring together researchers interested in nutrition and physical activity. Its goals include increasing our understanding of the determinants of healthy eating and physical activity behaviours and developing successful intervention programs. You can learn more about this organization at www.isbnpa.org.

- American Dietetic Association (ADA)—This is the largest organization of food and nutrition professionals in the United States. The mission of this organization is to promote nutrition, health, and well-being. The ADA publishes a professional journal called the *Journal of the American Dietetic Association;* information about ADA can be found at www.eatright.org.

- American Society for Nutrition (ASN)—The goal of the ASN is to improve the quality of life through the science of nutrition. The ASN publishes a professional journal called the *American Journal of Clinical Nutrition,* which focuses on basic and clinical studies in the area of human nutrition. More information about the ASN can be found at www.nutrition.org.

- Society for Nutrition Education (SNE)—SNE is dedicated to promoting healthy, sustainable food choices in communities through nutrition research and education. The primary goals of SNE are to educate individuals, communities, and professionals about nutrition education and to influence policy makers about nutrition, food, and health. The professional journal of SNE is the *Journal of Nutrition Education and Behavior.* Information about SNE can be found at www.sne.org.

- American College of Sports Medicine (ACSM)—The ACSM is the leading sports medicine and exercise science organization in the world. The mission of the ACSM is to advance and integrate scientific research to provide educational and practical applications of exercise science and sports medicine. Many members are nutrition professionals who combine their nutrition and exercise expertise to promote health and athletic performance. *Medicine and Science in Sports and Exercise* is the professional journal of the ACSM. You can learn more about the ACSM at www.acsm.org.

If you aren't sure whether or not the source of your information is reliable, or you can't tell whether the results of a particular study apply to you, how do you find out? What if two studies seem sound, but their findings contradict each other? The Nutrition Debate at the end of this chapter (page 29) explains how you can become a more informed and critical consumer of nutrition-related research.

Recap: Registered dietitians are professionals who have completed an accredited undergraduate program and dietetic internship or comparable practical experience. Look for the professional designation RD, PDt, or RDt (or the French equivalent Dt.P) to ensure an individual is qualified to provide nutrition advice. Dietitians of Canada, and other professional associations, such as the American Dietetic Association and the Society for Nutrition Education, are excellent sources of reliable nutrition information. Health Canada is the lead federal agency responsible for protecting people's health. Its affiliated agencies include the Canadian Food Inspection Agency and the Public Health Agency of Canada.

CHAPTER SUMMARY

- Nutrition is the science of food and how food nourishes the body and affects health.

- Nutrition is an important component of health, and nutrition plays a critical role in eliminating nutrient-deficiency diseases and can help reduce our risks for various chronic diseases.

- Nutrients are chemicals found in food that are critical to human growth and function.

- The six classes of nutrients found in the foods we eat are carbohydrates, fats, proteins, vitamins, minerals, and water.

- The nutrients that provide energy for our bodies are the macronutrients: carbohydrates, fats, and proteins.

- Carbohydrates are composed of carbon, hydrogen, and oxygen. Carbohydrates are the primary energy source for our bodies, particularly our brains.

CHAPTER SUMMARY

- Fats provide us with fat-soluble vitamins and essential fatty acids in addition to storing large quantities of energy.

- Proteins can provide energy if needed, but they are not a primary fuel source. Proteins support tissue growth, repair, and maintenance.

- Vitamins assist with the regulation of body processes.

- Fat-soluble vitamins can be stored in our tissues; these include vitamins A, D, E, and K.

- Water-soluble vitamins are soluble in water, and we excrete excess amounts in our urine. These include vitamin C and the B vitamins (thiamin, riboflavin, niacin, vitamin B_6, vitamin B_{12}, pantothenic acid, biotin, and folate).

- Minerals are inorganic substances that are not changed by digestion or other metabolic processes.

- Major minerals are found in our bodies in amounts greater than 5 grams (or 5000 mg), and we need to consume at least 100 mg of these minerals each day.

- Trace minerals are found in our bodies in amounts less than 5 grams (or 5000 mg), and we need to consume less than 100 mg of these minerals each day.

- Water is critical to support numerous body functions, including fluid balance, conduction of nervous impulses, and muscle contraction.

- The Dietary Reference Intakes (DRIs) are reference standards for nutrient intakes for healthy people in Canada and the United States.

- The DRIs can be used for dietary planning for individuals and groups.

- The DRIs include the Estimated Average Requirement, the Recommended Dietary Allowance, the Adequate Intake, and the Tolerable Upper Intake Level.

- Potentially good sources of reliable nutrition information include individuals who are registered dietitians or those who hold an advanced degree in nutrition.

- Registered dietitians are professionals who have completed an accredited undergraduate program and dietetic internship or comparable practical experience. They are trustworthy sources of nutrition information.

- Health Canada is the lead federal agency that protects the health and safety of Canadians.

- When looking for information on the internet, be wary of website addresses ending in .com. Look for .org (organization), .edu (educational institution), or .gov (government) for dependable sources of information.

*my*nutritionlab Go to MyNutritionLab at www.pearsoned.ca/mynutritionlab and enrich your understanding of nutrition! You'll find key animations, interactive exercises, access to My DietAnalysis, and much more.

REVIEW QUESTIONS

Quizzes

1. Vitamins A and C, thiamin, calcium, and magnesium are considered
   a. water-soluble vitamins.
   b. fat-soluble vitamins.
   c. energy nutrients.
   d. micronutrients.

2. The term *malnutrition* refers to
   a. undernutrition caused by not consuming enough energy from food.
   b. overnutrition caused by eating too much food.
   c. undernutrition resulting from inadequate nutrient intakes.
   d. all of the above.

3. Ten grams of fat
   a. contain 40 kcal (170 kJ) of energy.

   b. constitute the Dietary Reference Intake for an average adult male.
   c. contain 90 kcal (370 kJ) of energy.
   d. constitute the Tolerable Upper Intake Level for an average adult male.

4. Which of the following statements about hypotheses is true?
   a. Hypotheses can be tested by clinical trials
   b. "Many inactive people have high blood pressure" is an example of a hypothesis
   c. If the results of multiple experiments consistently support a hypothesis, it is confirmed as fact
   d. "A high-protein diet increases the risk for porous bones" is an example of a hypothesis

5. Choose the incorrect statement about vitamins:
   a. Vitamins A, D, E, and K are fat-soluble vitamins
   b. Water-soluble vitamins can never be toxic
   c. Fat-soluble vitamins are stored in the human body
   d. Vitamins are organic compounds

6. Carbohydrates, fats, and proteins have all of the following in common EXCEPT
   a. they contain carbon, hydrogen, and oxygen.
   b. they break down and reassemble into a fuel that is used by the body.
   c. they are all primary sources of energy.
   d. they are referred to as macronutrients.

7. Which DRI value is based on the average daily nutrient intake level that meets the nutrient requirements of most healthy individuals in a given life stage and gender group?
   a. Adequate Intake
   b. Estimated Average Requirement
   c. Tolerable Upper Intake Level
   d. Recommended Dietary Allowance

8. Which of the following is *not* a function of minerals in the body?
   a. Assist in fluid regulation
   b. Help rid the body of harmful metabolism byproducts
   c. Produce energy
   d. Help maintain bone and blood health

9. Choose the correct statement:
   a. Minerals are organic substances
   b. All vitamins are fat-soluble
   c. Proteins contain only hydrogen, oxygen, and carbon
   d. Fats are insoluble in water

10. Explain the difference between a trace mineral and a major mineral.

11. Compare the Estimated Average Requirement with the Recommended Dietary Allowance.

12. Your uncle has learned that you are taking a nutrition course and asks, "How can I find reliable nutrition information?" How would you answer?

13. Your mother, who is a self-described "chocolate addict," phones you. She has read in the newspaper a summary of a research study suggesting that the consumption of a moderate amount of bittersweet chocolate reduces the risk of heart disease in older women. You ask her who funded the research. She says she doesn't know and asks you why it would matter. Explain why such information is important.

14. Intrigued by the idea of a research study on chocolate, you obtain a copy of the full report. In it, you learn that
    • twelve women participated in the study;
    • the women's ages ranged from 65 to 78;
    • the women had all been diagnosed with high blood pressure;
    • they all described themselves as sedentary; and
    • six of the twelve smoked at least half a pack of cigarettes a day, but the others did not smoke.

    Your mother is 51 years old, walks daily, and takes a weekly swim class. Her blood pressure is on the upper end of the normal range. She does not smoke. Identify at least three aspects of the study that would cause you to doubt its relevance to your mother.

CASE STUDY

Now that you have had the chance to learn the basics about the importance and role of nutrition in our health, let's meet Cory, a 19-year-old male. Cory is living away from home for the first time and he is finding it difficult to balance his energy intake with his energy expenditure. Cory finds that he is eating slightly more than in the past and that he is less physically active. After recording his intake for three days, Cory discovers he is consuming, on average, 2900 kilocalories per day. Carbohydrates, fat, and protein are present in the amounts of 486 grams, 77 grams, and 65 grams, respectively.

a. Calculate the percentage of total energy that comes from carbohydrate, fat, and protein. (Hint: the sum of the percentages should total 100%.)

b. Refer to the Acceptable Macronutrient Distribution Ranges (AMDR). Do Cory's nutrient intakes fall within the ranges?

c. Based on the above information, including your energy intake calculations, is Cory's diet classified as undernutrition or overnutrition? What risks are associated with this diet?

d. The importance of micronutrients, both vitamins and minerals, is often overlooked. To demonstrate to Cory the importance of consuming adequate levels of vitamins and minerals, list two beneficial roles of each. What foods are generally good sources of both micronutrients?

e. List three people or places you would advise Cory to go to for nutrition advice. Give reasons for your choices.

WEB LINKS

www.hc-sc.gc.ca/fn-an/nutrition/index-eng.php
Health Canada
Search this site for food and nutrition guidelines and policies and for reports and statistics on the health of Canadians.

www.dietitians.ca
Dietitians of Canada (DC)
You can ask nutrition and diet questions or get the names of qualified dietitians in your community from this national professional organization.

www.nih.gov
National Institutes of Health (NIH)
Find out more about the National Institutes of Health, an agency under the U.S. Department of Health and Human Services.

www.eatright.org
American Dietetic Association (ADA)
This is the largest organization of food and nutrition professionals in the United States, and it has an excellent selection of consumer publications.

www.nutrition.gov
U.S. Department of Agriculture (USDA)
This website is designed for consumers who want more information about nutrition, food, and health from sources that they know will be credible and trustworthy. Visit this site for access to databases, recipes, interactive tools, and specialized information for people of all ages.

www.cdc.gov
Centers for Disease Control and Prevention (CDC)
Visit this site for additional information about the leading federal agency in the United States that protects the health and safety of people.

www.nutrition.org
The American Society for Nutrition (ASN)
Learn more about the American Society for Nutrition and its goal to improve the quality of life through the science of nutrition.

Test Yourself Answers

1. `True` The term *malnutrition* means "bad nutrition" and includes both undernutrition and overnutrition.

2. `False` Carbohydrates and fats are the major energy sources for our bodies.

3. `False` Fat-soluble vitamins can be stored in the fatty tissues of the body and thus don't need to be consumed every day.

4. `True` The Tolerable Upper Intake Levels exist because some vitamins and minerals can be toxic when large amounts are taken as dietary supplements.

5. `False` The term *nutritionist* is not protected in Canada and can be used by people with little formal training in nutrition. The term *registered dietitian* is a protected term and can only be used by people who have completed an accredited undergraduate program and dietetic internship or comparable practical experience.

www.sne.org
Society for Nutrition Education (SNE)
Go to this site for further information about the Society for Nutritional Education and its goals to educate individuals, communities, and professionals about nutrition education and influence policy makers about nutrition, food, and health.

www.acsm.org
American College of Sports Medicine (ACSM)
Obtain information about the leading sports medicine and exercise science organization in the world.

Research Study Results: Whom Can We Believe?

"Reduce your fat intake! Make sure at least 60% of your diet comes from carbohydrates!" "Eat more protein and fat! Carbohydrates cause obesity!"

Do you ever feel overwhelmed by the abundant and often conflicting advice in media reports related to nutrition? If so, you are not alone. In addition to hearing about the "high-carb, low-carb" controversy, we've been told that calcium supplements are essential to prevent bone loss and that calcium supplements have no effect on bone loss; that high fluid intake prevents constipation and that high fluid intake has no effect on constipation. For years, we were told that coffee and tea could be bad for our health; now, it appears that coffee is not unhealthy and tea may actually contain nutrients that are beneficial! When even nutrition researchers cannot agree, whom can we believe?

Recall that we acknowledged at the beginning of this chapter that nutrition is a relatively young science. New experiments are being designed every day to determine how nutrition affects our health, and new discoveries are being made. So just as Dr. Goldberger's experiments toppled the theory that pellagra was caused by germs, the results of current experiments will topple the theories we hold today. Viewing conflicting evidence as essential to the advancement of our understanding may help you to feel more comfortable with the contradictions. In fact, controversy is what stimulates researchers to explore unknown areas and attempt to solve the mysteries of nutrition and health.

It is important to recognize that media reports rarely include a thorough review of the research findings on a given topic. Typically, they focus only on the most recent study. Thus, one article in a newspaper or magazine should never be taken as absolute fact on any topic.

To become a more educated consumer and informed critic of nutrition reports in the media, you need to understand the research process and how the results of different types of studies should be interpreted. Let's now learn more about research.

Research Involves Applying the Scientific Method

The *scientific method* is a multistep process that involves observation, experimentation, and development of a theory. This method was developed as a way to apply standardized procedures to minimize the influence of personal prejudices and biases on our understanding of natural phenomena. Thus, this method is used to perform quality research studies in any discipline, including nutrition.

Observation of a Phenomenon Initiates the Research Process

The first step in the scientific method is the observation and description of a phenomenon. As an example, let's say you are working in a health care office that caters to mostly elderly clients. You have observed that many of the elderly have high blood pressure. After talking with a large number of clients, you notice a pattern developing in that those who report being more physically active are also those having lower blood pressure readings. This observation leads you to question the relationship that might exist between physical activity and blood pressure. Your next step is to develop a *hypothesis,* or possible explanation for your observation.

A Hypothesis is a Possible Explanation for an Observation

A hypothesis is also sometimes referred to as a research question. In this example, your hypothesis would be something like, "Regular physical activity lowers blood pressure in elderly people." You must generate a hypothesis before you can conduct experiments to determine what factors may explain your observation.

Experiments Are Conducted to Test Research Hypotheses

An *experiment* is a scientific study that is conducted to test a research question or hypothesis. In the case of your hypothesis, we could design a variety of research studies to determine the impact of regular physical activity on blood pressure in elderly people. Later in this debate, we will review the different types of research that can be done to assist us in answering your question.

A well-designed experiment attempts to control for factors that may coincidentally influence the results. In the case of your research study, it is well known that weight loss can reduce blood pressure in people with high blood pressure. Thus, in performing your experiment on the effects of exercise on blood pressure, you would want to control for weight loss. You could do this by making sure people eat enough food so that they do not lose weight during your study.

It is important to emphasize that one research study does not prove or disprove a hypothesis. Ideally, multiple experiments are conducted over many years to thoroughly examine a hypothesis. Science exists to allow us to continue to challenge existing hypotheses and expand what we currently know by providing new facts.

A Theory May Be Developed Following Extensive Research

If multiple experiments do not support a hypothesis, then the hypothesis is rejected or modified. On the other hand, if the results of multiple experiments consistently support a hypothesis, then it is possible to develop a theory. A *theory* represents a hypothesis or group of related hypotheses that have been confirmed through repeated scientific experiments. Theories are strongly accepted principles, but they can be challenged and changed as a result of applying the scientific method. Remember that centuries ago, it was theorized that the Earth was flat. People were so convinced of this that they refused to sail beyond known boundaries because they believed they would fall off the edge. Only after multiple explorers challenged this theory was it discovered that the Earth is round. We continue to apply the scientific method today to test hypotheses and challenge theories.

Various Types of Research Studies Tell Us Different Stories

You have just learned that the scientific method is applied to test a hypothesis. Establishing nutrition guidelines and understanding the role of nutrition in health involves constant experimentation. Depending upon how the research study is designed, we can gather information that tells us different stories. Let's now learn more about the different types of research conducted and what they tell us.

Epidemiological Studies Inform Us of Existing Relationships

Epidemiological studies are also referred to as observational studies. These types of studies involve assessing nutritional habits, disease trends, or other health phenomena of large populations and determining the factors that may influence these phenomena. The Canadian Community Health Survey (CCHS) introduced earlier in this chapter is an example of an epidemiological study. Epidemiological studies are very important in helping us study populations and health trends in large groups. However, these studies can only indicate relationships between factors, and the results do not indicate a cause-and-effect relationship.

Using a hypothesis that "regular physical activity lowers blood pressure in elderly people" as an example, we can gain a better understanding of what epidemiological studies can tell us. Let's say you are working with a researcher who has access to the CCHS database. Based on the original hypothesis, you conduct an experiment that includes gathering blood pressure and physical activity information from all of the elderly study participants in the CCHS database. After studying the data,

you find that the blood pressure values of physically active elderly people are lower than those of inactive elderly people. These results do not indicate that regular physical activity reduces blood pressure or that inactivity causes high blood pressure. All these results can tell us is that there is a relationship between higher physical activity and lower blood pressure in elderly people.

Laboratory Studies

Laboratory studies generally involve experiments with animals. In many cases, animal studies provide preliminary information that can assist us in designing and implementing human studies. Animal studies also are used to conduct research that cannot be done with humans. For instance, it is possible to study nutritional deficiencies in animals by causing a deficiency and studying its adverse health effects over the lifespan of the animal; this type of experiment is not acceptable to do in humans. One drawback of animal studies is that the results may not apply directly to humans. However, these studies can guide us in determining how we need to proceed to design experiments with humans.

Human Studies

The two primary types of studies conducted with humans are case control studies and clinical trials. *Case control studies* are epidemiological studies done on a smaller scale. Case control studies involve comparing a group of individuals who have a particular condition (for instance, elderly people with high blood pressure) with a similar group who don't have this condition (for instance, elderly people with low blood pressure). This comparison allows the researcher to identify factors other than the defined condition that differ between the two groups. By identifying these factors, researchers can gain a better understanding of things that may cause and help prevent disease. In the case of your experiment, you may find that elderly people with low blood pressure are not only more physically active, but they also eat more fruits and vegetables and less sodium. These findings indicate that other factors in addition to physical activity may play a role in affecting the blood pressure levels of elderly people.

Clinical trials are tightly controlled experiments in which an intervention is given to determine its effect on a given disease or health condition. Interventions can include medications, nutritional supplements, controlled diets, or exercise programs. Clinical trials have an experimental group, who are given the intervention, and a control group, who are not given the intervention. The responses of the intervention group are compared with those of the control group. In the case of your experiment, you could assign one group of elderly people with high blood pressure to an exercise program and assign a second group of elderly people with high blood pressure to a program where no exercise is done. After the exercise program is completed, you can measure the blood pressure of the elderly people who exercised to those who did not exercise. If the blood pressure of the intervention group decreased and was statistically lower than the blood pressure of the control group, you can feel confident that the exercise program caused a decrease in blood pressure.

There are other important things to consider when conducting a quality clinical trial. Ideally, it is best to randomly assign research participants to intervention and control groups. Randomizing participants is like flipping a coin or drawing names from a hat; doing this reduces prejudice or bias within each group. If possible, it is also important to "blind" both researchers and participants to the treatment being given. A *double-blind experiment* is one in which neither researchers nor participants know which group is really getting the treatment. Blinding helps prevent the researcher from seeing only the results he or she wants to see, even if these results do not actually occur. In the case of testing medications or nutrient supplements, the blinding process can be assisted by giving the control group a placebo. A *placebo* is an imitation treatment that has no effect on participants; for instance, a sugar pill may be given in place of a vitamin supplement.

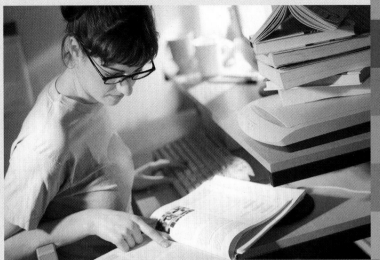

To become a more educated consumer and informed critic of nutrition reports in the media, you need to understand the research process and how the results of different types of studies should be interpreted.

Use Your Knowledge of Research to Help You Evaluate Media Reports

How can all this research information assist you in becoming a better consumer and critic of media reports? By having a better understanding of the research process and types of research conducted, you are more capable of discerning the truth or fallacy within media reports. Keep the following points in mind when examining any media report:

- Who is reporting the information? Is it an article in a newspaper or magazine, or on the internet? If the report is made by a person or group who may financially benefit from your buying their products, you should be skeptical of the reported results. Also, many people who write for popular magazines and newspapers are not trained in science and are capable of misinterpreting research results.

- Is the report based on reputable research studies? Did the research follow the scientific method, and were the results reported in a reputable scientific journal? Ideally, the journal is peer-reviewed; that is, the articles are critiqued by other specialists working in the same scientific field. A reputable

report should include the reference, or source of the information, and identify researchers by name. This allows the reader to investigate the original study and determine its merit. Reputable journals include the *Canadian Journal of Dietetic Practice and Research, American Journal of Clinical Nutrition, Journal of Nutrition, Journal of the American Dietetic Association, Canadian Medical Association Journal, New England Journal of Medicine, The Lancet, British Medical Journal,* and *Journal of the American Medical Association*.

- Is the report based on testimonials about personal experiences? Are sweeping conclusions made from only one study? Be aware of personal testimonials, as they are fraught with bias. In addition, one study cannot answer all of our questions or prove any hypothesis, and the findings from individual studies should be placed in their proper perspective.

- Are the claims in the report too good to be true? Are claims made about curing disease or treating a multitude of conditions? If something sounds too good to be true, it probably is. Claims about curing diseases or treating many conditions with one product should be a signal to question the validity of the report.

Throughout this text we provide you with information to assist you in becoming a more educated consumer regarding nutrition. You will learn about labelling guidelines, the proper use of supplements, and whether various nutrition topics are myths or facts. Armed with this knowledge, you will become more confident when trying to determine whom you can believe when it comes to nutrition claims in the media.

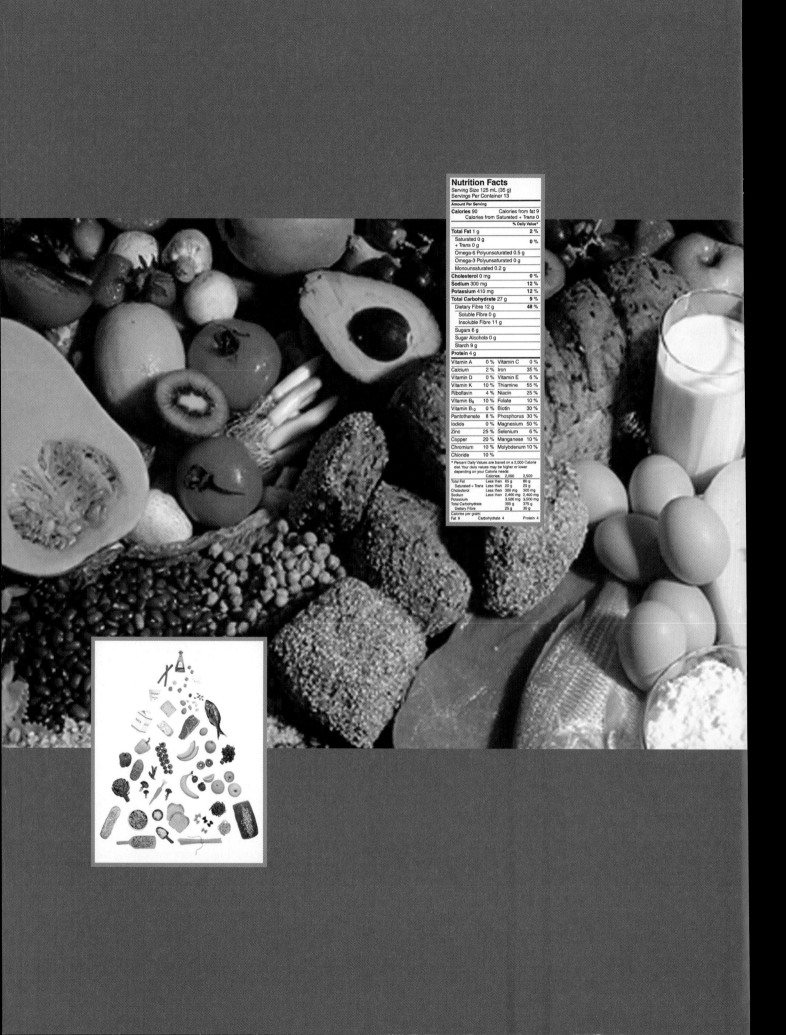

Nutrition Facts

Serving Size 125 mL (35 g)
Servings Per Container 13

Amount Per Serving		
Calories 90	Calories from fat 9	
	Calories from Saturated + Trans 0	
		% Daily Value*
Total Fat 1 g		**2 %**
Saturated 0 g		**0 %**
+ Trans 0 g		
Omega-6 Polyunsaturated 0.5 g		
Omega-3 Polyunsaturated 0 g		
Monounsaturated 0.2 g		
Cholesterol 0 mg		**0 %**
Sodium 300 mg		**12 %**
Potassium 410 mg		**12 %**
Total Carbohydrate 27 g		**9 %**
Dietary Fibre 12 g		**48 %**
Soluble Fibre 0 g		
Insoluble Fibre 11 g		
Sugars 6 g		
Sugar Alcohols 0 g		
Starch 9 g		
Protein 4 g		

Vitamin A	0 %	Vitamin C	0 %
Calcium	2 %	Iron	35 %
Vitamin D	0 %	Vitamin E	6 %
Vitamin K	10 %	Thiamine	55 %
Riboflavin	4 %	Niacin	25 %
Vitamin B$_6$	10 %	Folate	10 %
Vitamin B$_{12}$	0 %	Biotin	30 %
Pantothenate	8 %	Phosphorus	30 %
Iodide	0 %	Magnesium	50 %
Zinc	25 %	Selenium	6 %
Copper	20 %	Manganese	10 %
Chromium	10 %	Molybdenum	10 %
Chloride	10 %		

* Percent Daily Values are based on a 2,000 Calorie diet. Your daily values may be higher or lower depending on your Calorie needs:

		Calories:	2,000	2,500
Total Fat		Less than	65 g	80 g
Saturated + Trans		Less than	20 g	25 g
Cholesterol		Less than	300 mg	300 mg
Sodium		Less than	2,400 mg	2,400 mg
Potassium			3,500 mg	3,500 mg
Total Carbohydrate			300 g	375 g
Dietary Fibre			25 g	30 g

Calories per gram:
Fat 9   Carbohydrate 4   Protein 4

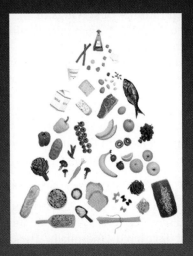

CHAPTER 2

Planning a Nutritious Diet

CHAPTER OBJECTIVES

After reading this chapter you will be able to:

1. Describe the four characteristics of a nutritious diet, pp. 34–36.

2. Interpret the Nutrition Facts table on a food label, pp. 37–46.

3. Use the food groups and recommended number of servings of each in *Eating Well with Canada's Food Guide* to plan a nutritious diet, pp. 47–54.

4. Describe the key features of the new *Eating Well with Canada's Food Guide: First Nations, Inuit and Métis*, pp. 54–56.

5. Name at least four ways to apply guidelines for healthy eating when eating out, pp. 65–66.

Test Yourself True or False

1. A nutritious diet can include most foods. **T or F**

2. Food labels are the most commonly used tool for choosing healthy foods. **T or F**

3. The portion sizes used in *Eating Well with Canada's Food Guide* are based on the average portion sizes eaten by Canadians. **T or F**

4. Manufacturers must list the ingredients in packaged food in descending order by weight. **T or F**

5. Manufacturers can claim that eating their food products helps prevent diseases, like cancer. **T or F**

Test Yourself answers can be found at the end of the chapter.

Guess how many Canadians eat the recommended number of servings of vegetables and fruits, on average, each day? In the Canadian Community Health Survey cycle 2.2, conducted in 2004, only 29% of children aged 4 to 8 years met the recommended minimum of 5 servings of vegetables and fruit each day (Health Canada 2007). Only about one half of the adults surveyed reported eating an average of 5 or more servings daily.

Why are vegetables and fruit important? Do you eat at least 5 servings every day? What factors do you think contribute to poor diets? If a friend asked your advice about trying to lose weight, and you noticed her skipping lunch in the cafeteria in favour of a diet pop from the vending machine, what might you say to her?

Many factors contribute to the confusion surrounding healthful eating. First, nutrition is a relatively young science. In contrast to physics, chemistry, and astronomy, which have been studied for thousands of years, the science of nutrition emerged around 1900, with the first vitamin being discovered in 1897. New findings on the benefits of foods and components of food are discovered almost daily. These new findings contribute to regular changes in how we define a nutritious diet. Second, as stated in Chapter 1, the popular media typically report the results of only selected studies, usually the most recent. This practice does not give a complete picture of all the research conducted in any given area. Indeed, the results of a single study are often misleading. Third, there is no one right way for everyone to eat what is healthy and acceptable. We are individuals with unique needs, food preferences, and cultural influences. For example, a person with diabetes may benefit from eating lower amounts of added sugars and higher amounts of protein or monounsaturated fats than a person without diabetes. People following certain religious practices may limit or avoid foods like specific meats and dairy products. Thus there are many different ways to design a nutritious diet to fit individual needs.

Given all this potential confusion, it's a good thing there are tools to guide us in designing a healthful diet. In this chapter, we introduce these tools, including the Nutrition Facts table, *Eating Well with Canada's Food Guide*, and others. Before we explore the question of how to design a nutritious diet, however, we should first make sure we understand what a nutritious diet *is*.

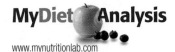

www.mynutritionlab.com

nutritious diet A diet that provides the proper combination of energy and nutrients and is adequate, moderate, balanced, and varied.

adequate diet A diet that provides enough of the energy, nutrients, and fibre to maintain a person's health.

What Is a Nutritious Diet?

A **nutritious diet** provides the proper combination of energy and nutrients. It has four characteristics: it is adequate, moderate, balanced, and varied. Whether you are young or old, overweight or underweight, healthy or ill, if you keep in mind these characteristics of a nutritious diet, you will be able to consciously select foods that provide you with the optimal combination of nutrients and energy each day.

A Nutritious Diet Is Adequate

An **adequate diet** provides enough of the energy, nutrients, and fibre to maintain a person's health. A diet may be inadequate in only one area. For example, many people in Canada do not eat enough vegetables although their intake of breads, meats, fruits, and dairy products may be sufficient. By failing to eat enough vegetables, these people are not consuming enough of many of the important nutrients found in vegetables, such as fibre, vitamin C, beta carotene, and potassium. However, their intake of protein, fat, carbohydrate, and calcium may be adequate. In fact, many people who eat too few vegetables are overweight or obese, which means they are eating a diet that exceeds their energy needs but may not be adequate in the nutrients found predominantly in vegetables.

Conversely, a generalized state of undernutrition can occur if a person's diet contains an inadequate level of several nutrients for a long period. This situation occurs when a person severely limits his or her food intake to avoid gaining weight. For example, many teenage girls and young women follow a very restrictive eating

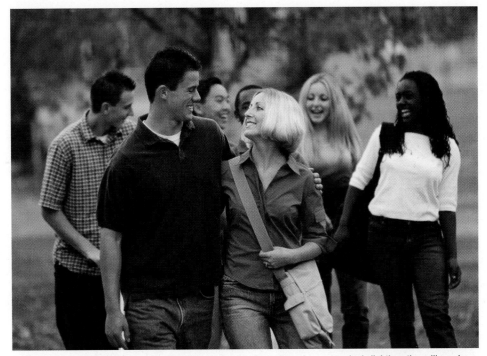

A diet that is adequate for one person may not be adequate for another. A woman who is lightly active will require less energy per day than a highly active male.

pattern to maintain a thin figure. They may skip multiple meals each day, avoid foods that contain any fat, and limit their meals to only a few foods, such as a bagel, a banana, a diet pop, or a small green salad. This type of restrictive eating pattern practised over a prolonged period can cause low energy levels and loss of bone and hair, impair memory and cognitive function, and cause menstrual dysfunction.

Many people have small appetites, especially seniors and young children, and it is important that they get as many nutrients as possible before they feel full. For these people, a nutritious diet is one that is nutrient dense or nutrient rich. **Nutrient density** refers to the relative amount of nutrients per amount of energy (or number of kilocalories). Thus, a nutrient-dense or nutrient-rich diet includes foods that are rich in nutrients and limits foods that provide plentiful energy but few nutrients.

nutrient density The relative amount of nutrients per amount of energy (or number of kilocalories).

A Nutritious Diet Is Moderate

Moderation is the key to a nutritious diet. **Moderation** refers to eating the right amounts of foods to maintain a healthy weight and to optimize the body's metabolic processes. For example, some people drink a lot of sugared soft drinks, as they enjoy the sweet taste and carbonation. It is not uncommon for people to drink 1 litre (about 35 fl. oz.) of pop on some days. Drinking this much contributes an extra 435 kcal (1820 kJ) of energy to a person's diet but provides no nutrients (i.e., it is not a nutrient-dense choice). To maintain weight, a person would need to either reduce his or her food intake, exercise more, or both to make up for these extra kilocalories. This could lead to a person cutting nutritious food choices from his or her diet. By consuming a more moderate amount of pop, or switching to diet soft drinks or water, people can consume more nutritious foods and maintain a healthy body weight.

moderation Eating the right amounts of foods to maintain a healthy weight and to optimize the body's metabolic processes.

A Nutritious Diet Is Balanced

A **balanced diet** is one that contains the combinations of foods that provide the proper balance of nutrients. As you will learn in this course, our bodies need many

balanced diet A diet that contains the combinations of foods that provide the proper balance of nutrients.

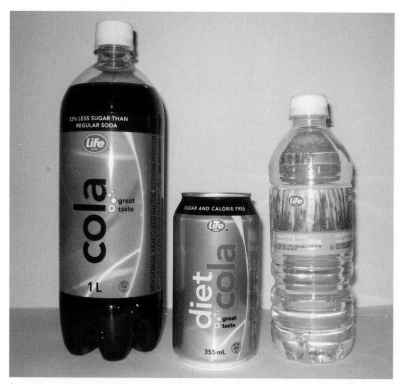

Choosing a smaller-size drink of pop, or switching to diet pop, helps to maintain a healthy body weight. Better yet—drink water to quench your thirst!

types of foods in varying amounts to maintain health. For example, vegetables are excellent sources of fibre, vitamin C, beta carotene, potassium, and magnesium.

In contrast, meats are not good sources of these nutrients. However, meats are excellent sources of protein, iron, zinc, and copper. By eating the proper balance of nutritious foods, including fruits, vegetables, and meats (or meat substitutes), we can be confident that we are consuming the proper balance of the nutrients we need to maintain health.

When we balance our food intake with our energy needs, we can maintain a stable body weight. For example, a small woman who is lightly active may require approximately 1700 to 2000 kilocalories (7100 to 8400 kJ) of energy each day to support her body's functions. In contrast, a highly active male athlete may require more than 4000 kilocalories (16 700 kJ) of energy each day to support his body's demands. These two individuals differ greatly in their activity levels and in their quantity of body fat and muscle mass, which means they require very different levels of fat, carbohydrate, protein, and other nutrients to support their daily needs.

A Nutritious Diet Is Varied

variety Eating many different foods each day.

Variety refers to eating many different foods each day. There are literally thousands of foods we can choose from each day. Trying new foods on a regular basis can assist us in eating a more varied diet. For example, try a new green vegetable each week. Or try putting spinach on your turkey sandwich in place of iceberg lettuce. By selecting a variety of foods, we optimize our chances of consuming the multitude of nutrients our bodies need. As an added benefit, eating a varied diet prevents boredom and avoids our getting into a "food rut." Later in this chapter we provide suggestions for eating a varied diet.

> **Recap:** A nutritious diet provides adequate nutrients and energy, and it includes only moderate amounts of foods that are less nutritious. It also includes an appropriate balance of foods and a wide variety of foods to ensure that many different nutrients are provided.

What Tools Can Help Me Plan a Nutritious Diet?

Many people feel it is impossible to eat a nutritious diet. They may believe that the foods they would need to eat are too expensive or not available to them, or they may feel too busy to do the necessary planning, shopping, and cooking. Some people rely on dietary supplements to get enough nutrients instead of focusing on eating a variety of foods. But is it really that difficult to eat a nutritious diet?

Although planning and maintaining a nutritious diet is not as simple as eating whatever you want, most of us can do it with a little practice and a little help. Let's look now at some tools for planning a nutritious diet.

Canada's Food Labels Have Changed!

For many years, Canada's food labels looked quite different from the labels on American food products. Canadian labels were required to have ingredient lists but didn't have to include Nutrition Information panels. Some products, such as breakfast cereals, voluntarily carried Nutrition Information panels—but the nutrient amounts were given for serving sizes that differed from product to product, making comparisons between similar products difficult. Consumers were a bit mystified about the numbers as well. What did 480 mg of sodium really mean? Was 9 g of fat per serving anything to worry about? What did it mean in terms of the overall amount of fat a person should have in one day? Consumers frequently commented that the U.S. food labels, which expressed nutrient contents as percentages of amounts needed each day, were easier to understand than Canadian labels.

At the same time, Canadian food manufacturers were frustrated that they couldn't claim that there may be health benefits associated with eating their products but manufacturers could in the United States. They also complained that they had to have two separate packaging formats for their products, one for products sold in the United States and one with bilingual labels (English and French) for products sold in Canada. This added extra costs to their manufacturing processes.

In late 2002, the Canadian government announced a new set of labelling regulations that became mandatory for all prepackaged foods on December 12, 2007. These new regulations specify which foods need a food label, provide detailed descriptions of the information that must be included on the food label, and outline the food products that are exempt from carrying nutrition information on their food labels. The latter are shown in Table 2.1.

Table 2.1   Examples of Foods Exempt from Carrying Nutrition Information

The following are examples of foods that are exempt from carrying a Nutrition Information panel:

- Such foods as spices and coffee, where the amounts of nutrients required on the label would be 0
- Alcoholic drinks (with an alcohol content of more than 0.5%)
- Fresh vegetables or fruits, with no added ingredients
- Fresh meats
- Foods sold at roadside stands, craft shows, flea markets, fairs, or farmers' markets by the person who prepared and processed them
- Individual servings of food sold for immediate consumption, such as salads and sandwiches, that have not been treated or packaged to extend their durable life
- One-bite candies or desserts
- Prepackaged individual portions of food intended to be served with meals or snacks by a restaurant or other commercial enterprise
- Some cow and goat milk products sold in refillable glass containers

(*Source: Canada Gazette,* Vol. 137, No. 1, January 1, 2003, Food and Drug Act: Regulations Amending the Food and Drug Regulations, B.01.401, http://canadagazette.gc.ca/partII/2003/20030101/html/sor11-e.html. Reproduced with the permission of the Minister of Public Works and Government Services Canada, 2008.)

Food labels allow food manufacturers to communicate directly with purchasers, and allow consumers to compare similar products. The food label has three main purposes (Health Canada 2003):

- To give basic product information, including a list of ingredients, product weight or net quantity, best-before or expiry dates, grade or quality, country of origin, and the name and address of the manufacturer, dealer, or importer. Some manufacturers include 1–800 phone numbers or website addresses for consumers to contact them directly with product-related questions.

- To provide health, safety, and nutrition information. This includes nutrition information, such as the amount and type of fats, proteins, carbohydrates, vitamins, and minerals present in a specified serving size (in the Nutrition Facts table). The label may also give instructions for safe storage and handling of the product.

- To provide a means for marketing or promoting the product by such claims as "low fat," "cholesterol free," "high source of fibre," "product of Canada," "no preservatives added," and so on.

Food Labels Can Have Four Main Components

The new labels on packaged foods can have four main parts, as shown in Figure 2.1. The figure also shows the contact information.

1. *Ingredient list:* The ingredients must be listed in descending order by weight. This means that the first product listed in the ingredient list is the predominant ingredient, by weight (not volume amount), in that food. This information is

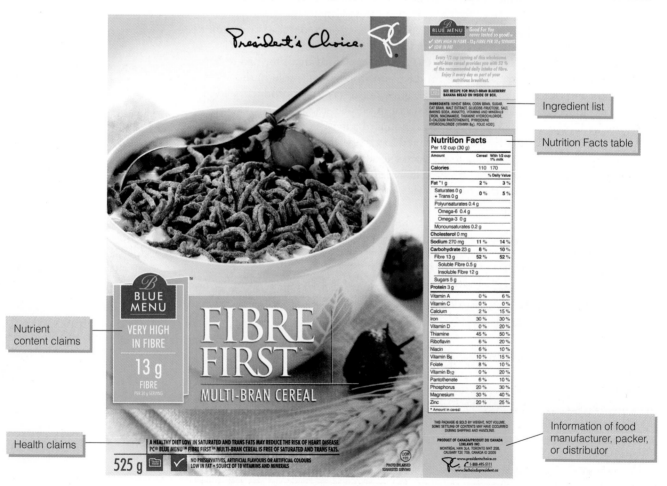

Figure 2.1 The four main parts of a food label and the contact information.
(Courtesy of President's Choice®, www.presidentschoice.ca.)

How to use Canada's Food Guide

The Food Guide shows how many servings to choose from each food group every day and how much food makes a serving.

	Recommended Number of Food Guide Servings per day			
	Children 2-3 years old	Children 4-13 years old	Teens and Adults (Females)	(Males)
Vegetables and Fruit Fresh, frozen and canned.	4	5-6	7-8	7-10
Grain Products	3	4-6	6-7	7-8
Milk and Alternatives	2	2-4	Teens **3-4** Adults (19-50 years) **2** Adults (51+ years) **3**	Teens **3-4** Adults (19-50 years) **2** Adults (51+ years) **3**
Meat and Alternatives	1	1-2	2	3

Figure 2.6 *Eating Well with Canada's Food Guide* recommended number of *Food Guide* servings per day from each of the four food groups. (*Eating Well with Canada's Food Guide* (2007), Health Canada. Reproduced with the permission of the Minister of Public Works and Government Services Canada, 2008.)

age categories for adults, ages 19–50 years and 51+ years, and both list the recommended number of servings from each food group for men and women separately.

This is the first time that *Canada's Food Guide* has tailored Food Guide Servings per day to nine different age and sex groups, to help ensure that consumers who follow the guide are eating the recommended amounts of various nutrients each day while preventing obesity.

What Is One *Food Guide* Serving in *Eating Well with Canada's Food Guide?*

What is considered 1 *Food Guide* Serving in *Eating Well with Canada's Food Guide?* The middle panel in *Canada's Food Guide* (Figure 2.7) shows examples of serving sizes for foods in each group.

A serving of vegetables is 250 mL (1 cup) of raw leafy vegetables, such as uncooked spinach or 125 mL (1/2 cup) of chopped fresh, frozen, or canned vegetables, such as broccoli or squash. A serving from the Grain Products group is defined as 1 slice of bread, 1/2 of a regular pita or hamburger bun, or 30 g (1 oz.) of cold cereal. Fortified soy beverages (250 mL or 1 cup) and kefir (175 g or 3/4 cup) are now included in the Milk and Alternatives group. A serving of cooked lean meat, fish, shellfish, or poultry is 75 g (2.5 oz.), which is approximately the size of a deck of cards. A serving of meat alternatives could be 2 eggs, 30 mL (2 Tbsp) peanut butter, 150 grams or 175 mL (3/4 cup) tofu, 175 mL (3/4 cup) cooked legumes, or 60 mL (1/4 cup) nuts and seeds. Although it may seem unnatural or inconvenient to measure our food servings, understanding the size of a serving is critical to planning a nutritious diet.

It is important to understand that there is no standardized definition of a serving size for any food. A serving size as defined in *Canada's Food Guide* may not be equal

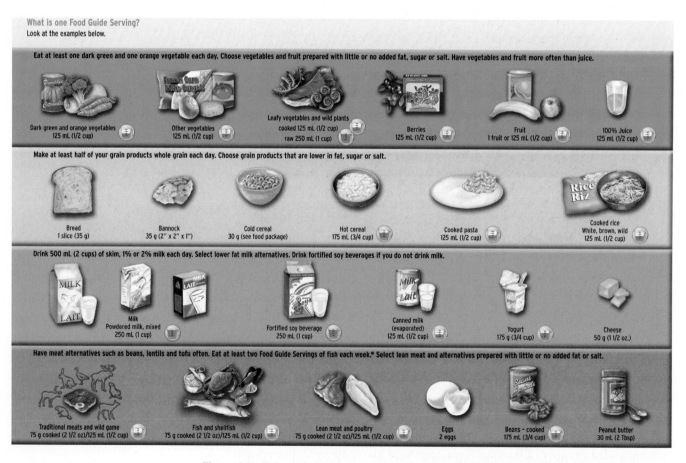

Figure 2.7 *Eating Well with Canada's Food Guide* suggested serving sizes. The amount shown for each food represents 1 *Food Guide* serving. (*Eating Well with Canada's Food Guide* (2007), Health Canada. Reproduced with the permission of the Minister of Public Works and Government Services Canada, 2008.)

to a serving size listed on a food label. In addition, a "medium-sized" vegetable or fruit may be much smaller than the vegetables and fruit that we buy. Try the Nutrition Label Activity to see how well you know the recommended portion sizes in *Eating Well with Canada's Food Guide*.

Make Each *Food Guide* Serving Count . . . Wherever You Are—At Home, at School, at Work or When Eating Out!

Accompanying each of the four food groups are recommendations for the best quality, most nutrient-rich food choices to help reduce the risk of chronic disease and obesity.

Vegetables and Fruit

- Choose one dark green and one orange vegetable each day.
  - Go for dark green vegetables, such as broccoli, romaine lettuce, and spinach.
  - Go for orange vegetables, such as carrots, sweet potatoes, and winter squash.
- Choose vegetables and fruit prepared with little or no added fat, sugar, or salt.
  - Enjoy vegetables steamed, baked, or stir-fried instead of deep-fried.
- Have vegetables and fruit more often than juice.

Vegetables and Fruit are grouped together because they are good sources of carbohydrate, dietary fibre, vitamins A and C, folate, potassium, and magnesium. Dark green and orange vegetables and fruit are especially rich in vitamins A and C. These foods also contain differing amounts and types of naturally occurring chemicals called phytochemicals that enhance our health. A detailed explanation of phytochemicals is presented in Chapter 8.

Grain Products

- Make at least half your grain products whole grain each day.
  - Eat a variety of whole grains, such as barley, brown rice, oats, quinoa, and wild rice.
  - Enjoy whole grain breads, oatmeal, or whole wheat pasta.
- Choose grain products that are lower in fat, sugar, or salt.
  - Compare the Nutrition Facts table on labels to make wise choices.
  - Enjoy the true taste of grain products. When adding sauces or spreads, use small amounts.

Bread, cereal, rice, and pasta are clustered together in the Grain Products food group because they provide complex carbohydrates and dietary fibre, and they are good sources of the nutrients riboflavin, thiamin, niacin, iron, folate, zinc, protein, and magnesium. Whole-grain products are especially good sources of dietary fibre and the nutrients listed, while enriched products have some of the nutrients lost in processing added back into the final product.

Milk and Alternatives

- Drink skim, 1%, or 2% milk each day.
  - Have 500 mL (16 fl. oz. or 2 cups) of milk every day for adequate vitamin D.
  - Drink fortified soy beverages if you do not drink milk.
- Select lower-fat milk alternatives.
  - Compare the Nutrition Facts table on yogurts or cheeses to make wise choices.

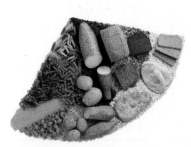

Eating a diet rich in whole-grain foods, like whole wheat bread and brown rice, can enhance your overall health.

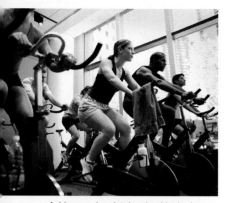

Achieve and maintain a healthy body weight by enjoying regular physical activity and healthy eating.

The Milk and Alternatives food group contains foods that are good sources of calcium, phosphorus, riboflavin, protein, and vitamin B$_{12}$. In addition, many of these foods are also fortified with vitamins D and A. Lower-fat products have the same levels of these nutrients as their full-fat counterparts, with only the fat removed. If you don't consume milk products, you will need to replace them with other foods that provide calcium, such as calcium-fortified orange juice and soy milk, turnip greens, broccoli, kale, black-eyed peas, or sardines. A diet that lacks adequate amounts of calcium may put you at risk for excessive bone loss and its related health consequences (see Chapter 9).

Meat and Alternatives

- Have meat alternatives, such as beans, lentils, and tofu, often.
- Eat at least 2 *Food Guide* Servings of fish each week.
  - Choose such fish as char, herring, mackerel, salmon, sardines, and trout.
- Select lean meat and alternatives prepared with little or no added fat or salt.
  - Trim the visible fat from meats. Remove the skin on poultry.
  - Use cooking methods, such as roasting, baking, or poaching, that require little or no added fat.
  - If you eat luncheon meats, sausages, or prepackaged meats, choose those lower in salt (sodium) and fat.

The Meat and Alternatives food group consists of foods that are good sources of protein, phosphorus, vitamin B$_6$, vitamin B$_{12}$, zinc, magnesium, iron, niacin, riboflavin, and thiamin. Dried peas, beans, and lentils are called legumes and are promoted because they are high in dietary fibre and low in fat. Meats, particularly processed meat products, and poultry can be high in saturated fats; leaner cuts of meat, low-fat processed meat products, skinless poultry, and fish are recommended.

In the previous version of *Canada's Food Guide* (1992), there was a paragraph about "Other Foods"—foods and beverages that were not part of any food group. They included foods that were high in fat, sugar, or salt; beverages, such as tea, coffee, and soft drinks; and seasonings and condiments. The new *Eating Well with Canada's Food Guide* encourages consumers to eat well by

Limiting foods and beverages high in calories, fat, sugar or salt (sodium) such as cakes and pastries, chocolate and candies, cookies and granola bars, doughnuts and muffins, ice cream and frozen desserts, french fries, potato chips, nachos and other salty snacks, alcohol, fruit flavoured drinks, soft drinks, sports and energy drinks, and sweetened hot or cold drinks.

Guidance on choosing appropriate amounts of healthier oils and fats is also provided in *Canada's Food Guide*:

- Include a small amount—30 to 45 mL (2 to 3 Tbsp)—of unsaturated fat each day. This includes salad dressings, margarine, mayonnaise, and oil used for cooking.
- Use vegetable oils, such as canola, olive, and soybean.
- Choose soft margarines that are low in saturated and trans fats.
- Limit butter, hard margarine, lard, and shortening.

Advice for Different Ages and Stages

On the back of the *Food Guide* is a panel that provides specific advice for children, women of childbearing age, and men and women over 50. Parents are advised not to limit the fat intake of young children who need energy to support their growth and development. All women who could become pregnant are advised to take a multivitamin supplement containing folic acid every day. Pregnant women need to ensure that they also have iron in their multivitamin supplement. Finally, men and women over the age of 50 are advised to consume the recommended servings of food groups and take a daily vitamin D supplement of 10 μg (400 IU). This is the first time that *Canada's Food Guide* has recommended that certain groups supplement their food intakes with specific vitamins and minerals.

Eat Well and Be Active Today and Every Day!

The last panel of the *Food Guide* (Figure 2.8) encourages people to think about their activity levels in addition to their food intakes. Table 2.4 lists some ways that you can incorporate *Canada's Food Guide* into your daily life.

Advice for different ages and stages...

Children	Women of childbearing age	Men and women over 50
Following *Canada's Food Guide* helps children grow and thrive. Young children have small appetites and need calories for growth and development. • Serve small nutritious meals and snacks each day. • Do not restrict nutritious foods because of their fat content. Offer a variety of foods from the four food groups. • Most of all... be a good role model.	All women who could become pregnant and those who are pregnant or breastfeeding need a multivitamin containing **folic acid** every day. Pregnant women need to ensure that their multivitamin also contains **iron**. A health care professional can help you find the multivitamin that's right for you. Pregnant and breastfeeding women need more calories. Include an extra 2 to 3 Food Guide Servings each day. **Here are two examples:** • Have fruit and yogurt for a snack, or • Have an extra slice of toast at breakfast and an extra glass of milk at supper.	The need for **vitamin D** increases after the age of 50. In addition to following *Canada's Food Guide*, everyone over the age of 50 should take a daily vitamin D supplement of 10 μg (400 IU).

How do I count Food Guide Servings in a meal?

Here is an example:

Vegetable and beef stir-fry with rice, a glass of milk and an apple for dessert		
250 mL (1 cup) mixed broccoli, carrot and sweet red pepper	=	2 **Vegetables and Fruit** Food Guide Servings
75 g (2 ½ oz.) lean beef	=	1 **Meat and Alternatives** Food Guide Serving
250 mL (1 cup) brown rice	=	2 **Grain Products** Food Guide Servings
5 mL (1 tsp) canola oil	=	part of your **Oils and Fats** intake for the day
250 mL (1 cup) 1% milk	=	1 **Milk and Alternatives** Food Guide Serving
1 apple	=	1 **Vegetables and Fruit** Food Guide Serving

Figure 2.8 *Eating Well with Canada's Food Guide* activity recommendations for better health and a healthy body weight. (*Eating Well with Canada's Food Guide* (2007), Health Canada. Reproduced with the permission of the Minister of Public Works and Government Services Canada, 2008.)

Table 2.4   Ways to Incorporate *Eating Well with Canada's Food Guide* into Your Daily Life

If You Normally Do This:	Try Doing This Instead:
Watch television when you get home at night	Do 30 minutes of stretching or lifting of hand weights in front of the television
Drive to and from the store down the block	Walk to and from the store
Go out to lunch with friends	Take a 15- or 30-minute walk with your friends at lunchtime three days each week
Make your sandwich with white bread	Use whole wheat bread or some other bread made from whole grains
Eat white rice or fried rice with your meal	Eat brown rice or try wild rice
Choose cookies or a candy bar for a snack	Choose a fresh nectarine, peach, apple, orange, or banana for a snack
Order french fries with your hamburger	Order a green salad with low-fat salad dressing on the side instead of french fries
Spread butter or margarine on your white toast each morning	Spread fresh fruit compote on whole-grain toast
Order a bacon double cheeseburger at your favourite restaurant	Order a turkey burger or grilled chicken sandwich, without the cheese and bacon, and add lettuce and tomato
Drink non-diet soft drinks to quench your thirst	Drink diet soft drinks, iced tea, or iced water with a slice of lemon
Eat salted potato chips and pickles with your favourite sandwich	Eat carrot slices and crowns of fresh broccoli and cauliflower dipped in low-fat or non-fat ranch dressing

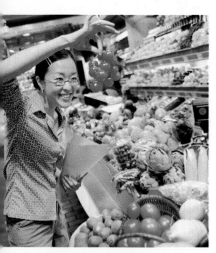

When grocery shopping, try to select foods that are moderate in fat.

Get Personalized *Food Guide* Information!

For the first time, consumers can visit *Canada's Food Guide* online at www.hc-sc .gc.ca/fn-an/food-guide-aliment/index-eng.php and tour the *Guide* or use interactive tools. Fill in your age, sex, food preferences, and favourite ways to be active in *My Food Guide* to get a customized version of *Canada's Food Guide*.

Recap: *Eating Well with Canada's Food Guide* can be used to plan a nutritious diet—one that provides adequate nutrients and energy and includes only moderate amounts of foods that are less nutritious. Following the advice in *Canada's Food Guide* will ensure your diet has a wide variety of foods and an appropriate balance of foods from the four food groups. The recommended number of servings from the four food groups—Vegetables and Fruit; Grain Products; Milk and Alternatives; and Meat and Alternatives—depends on your age and sex. The serving sizes of foods listed in *Canada's Food Guide* may be smaller than the amounts we normally eat or are served. Use the interactive tool provided on Health Canada's website to create your own customized *My Food Guide*.

Eating Well with Canada's Food Guide: First Nations, Inuit and Métis

For the first time, Health Canada has produced a food guide specifically for Aboriginal peoples: *Eating Well with Canada's Food Guide: First Nations, Inuit and Métis* (Figure 2.9).

▶ **NUTRITION MYTH OR FACT**

Binge Drinking Can Be Harmful

The effects of excessive alcohol consumption are well known. Alcohol is an addictive, toxic substance that can cause liver cirrhosis and brain damage, increase our risk for certain cancers and heart disease, and lead to numerous birth defects (called Fetal Alcohol Spectrum Disorder, or FASD) if consumed during pregnancy. (See Chapter 15 for more on FASD.) Although alcohol provides energy—7 kilocalories or 29 kJ per gram—and is therefore considered a food, it is not considered a nutrient, as it is not essential to our bodies and performs no necessary functions.

Because alcohol contributes energy without nutrients and increases our risk for some diseases, *Canada's Food Guide* recommends that you limit your alcohol intake. This generally means no more than one drink per day for women and two drinks for men. A drink is defined as

- 355 mL (12 fl. oz.) of regular beer (about 150 kcal or 630 kJ);
- 150 mL (5 fl. oz.) of wine (about 100 kcal or 420 kJ);
- 45 mL (1.5 fl. oz.) of 80-proof distilled spirits (hard liquor, such as vodka or whisky; about 100 kcal or 420 kJ).

By the way, drinking seven or eight drinks in one night and abstaining for six nights does not average out to moderate drinking! This type of behaviour, called binge drinking, is defined as the consumption of at least four drinks in a row for women and at least five for men.

Binge drinking is common among college and university students and occurs more frequently in people with a past drinking history, with a family history of alcohol abuse, and in members of athletic teams, fraternities, and sororities (Weschsler et al. 1995; Weschsler et al. 2000)

Binge drinking causes a rapid accumulation of alcohol in the blood, and this can lead to dehydration, loss of consciousness, and damage to the brain and heart. In addition to these negative effects on health, the behavioural consequences of binge drinking can include damaged property, academic problems, unprotected sex, injuries, and drinking and driving.

Some studies show that regular, moderate consumption of red wine with food reduces the risk for heart disease (Wollin and Jones 2001). Less expensive brands of wine may be more effective, as the grapes have been fermented with their skins on longer and therefore more beneficial compounds are extracted. Moderate consumption of beer also has documented health benefits.

Although drinking red wine and beer may have some health benefits, you can decrease your risk for heart disease much more effectively by eating a nutritious diet and exercising regularly. If you don't drink, don't start. If you do drink, do so in moderation.

Notice that this version of *Canada's Food Guide* uses a circle rather than a rainbow format, and the centre of the circle illustrates various traditional ways in which Aboriginal peoples are physically active. Foods enjoyed by these cultural groups, such as bannock, fiddleheads, seaweed, and traditional game meats, are included within the four food groups.

The USDA *MyPyramid*

The U.S. Department of Agriculture's *MyPyramid: Steps to a Healthier You* (USDA and USDHHS 2005) is the American counterpart to *Eating Well with Canada's Food Guide*. As you can see in Figure 2.10, the pyramid has six sections that represent five food groups plus oils and includes a stylized figure climbing stairs to represent the importance of daily physical activity. *MyPyramid*, which replaces the USDA Food Guide Pyramid, was designed with seven concepts in mind:

1. *One size doesn't fit all.* Unlike previous food guides intended to be general guides suitable for all healthy people, the new guide is very simple and has no numbers. The simple form is meant as a reminder to people that healthy eating and physical activity are important every day. Consumers can explore the

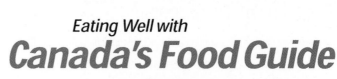

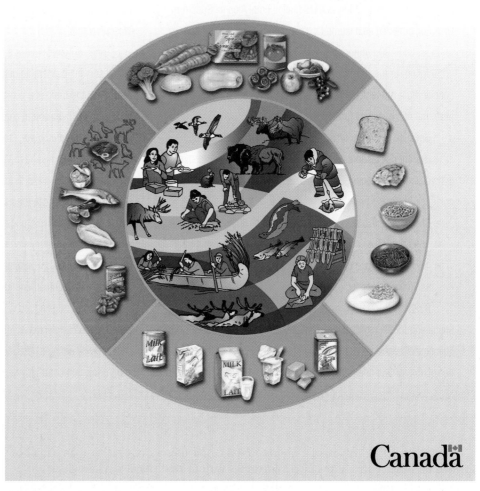

Figure 2.9 *Eating Well with Canada's Food Guide: First Nations, Inuit and Métis. (Eating Well with Canada's Food Guide: First Nations, Métis, Inuit 2007. Health Canada. © Reproduced with the permission of the Minister of Public Works and Government Services Canada, 2008. HC Pub.:3426, Cat.:H34-159/2007E-PDF, ISBN:0-662-44562-7.)*

pyramid on an interactive website and get specific information on their diets and advice on physical activity.

2. *Activity.* The steps on the side of *MyPyramid*, and the stylized figure climbing them, symbolize the importance of regular physical activity.

3. *Moderation.* The wider bases of each section contain foods with little or no solid fats or added sugars. Foods with solid fats and added sugars are placed in the narrower tops of each section, showing that "the more active you are, the more of these foods can fit into your diet" (USDA and USDHHS 2005).

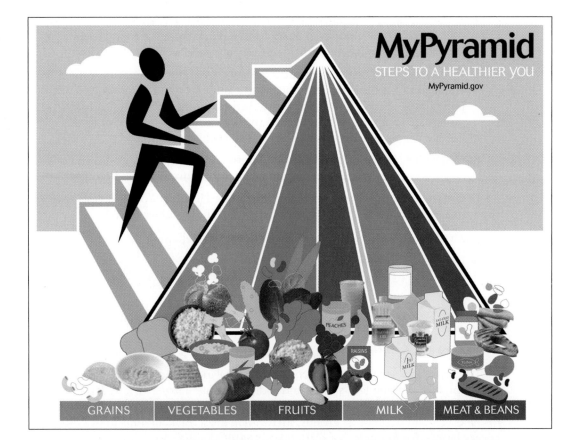

Figure 2.10 The USDA's *MyPyramid*. (USDA, US Department of Agriculture, Center for Nutrition Policy and Promotion, April 2005, CNPP-15, www.mypyramid.gov/downloads/MiniPoster.pdf, accessed January 2006.)

4. *Personalization.* Consumers can visit the interactive website to receive personalized advice on the amount of energy and servings from the food groups that are right for them based on their age, sex, and level of physical activity.

5. *Proportionality.* The relative widths of the bases of the food group sections are intended as a general guide to the relative amounts of different foods to eat. For example, the section for Grains is the largest, the Vegetables and Milk groups are approximately equal, and the Oils section is tiny. A visit to the website will provide more specific, personalized information.

6. *Variety.* The different-coloured sections for each of the food groups and oils are meant to convey that a healthy diet includes foods from all food groups.

7. *Gradual improvement.* The slogan "Steps to a Healthier You" suggests that small steps every day can lead to a better diet and healthier lifestyle.

Each of the five food groups has catchy slogans as well:

- *Grains*—"Make half your grains whole"
- *Vegetables*—"Vary your veggies"
- *Fruits*—"Focus on fruits"
- *Milk*—"Get your calcium-rich foods"
- *Meat and Beans*—"Go lean with protein"

There are also specific recommendations for balancing food intake with physical activity and for limiting fats, sugars, and sodium. Unlike *Eating Well with Canada's Food Guide,* which gives recommended numbers of daily servings for each food group for nine age- and sex-specific groups, *MyPyramid* gives total amounts for 12 different energy levels—for example, for a 2000 kcal (8400 kJ) diet, the recommendation is to eat 6 ounces of Grains every day; for a 2800 kcal (11 720 kJ) diet, it is 7 ounces a day. Amounts for the Meat and Beans food group are given in 1-ounce (30 g) equivalents—for example, 1 ounce of lean meat, poultry, or fish is equivalent to 1 egg, 15 mL (1 Tbsp) peanut butter, 65 mL (1/4 cup) cooked dry beans, or 15 g (1/2 oz.) of nuts or seeds. In a 2000 kcal (8400 kJ) diet, 5 1/2-ounce equivalents a day are suggested. It is interesting to note that in *MyPyramid,* legumes (dried peas, beans, and lentils) are included in both the Vegetables and Meat and Beans food groups whereas in *Canada's Food Guide* legumes are part of the Meat and Alternatives group.

The *Dietary Guidelines for Americans* (USDA and USDHHS 2005) has a total of 41 recommendations, including some written specifically for certain subgroups of the population, such as pregnant women. The key recommendations for the general public are found in Appendix I of this book.

Other Food Guides

Other countries have developed their own tools to teach their consumers how to follow their dietary guidelines. For example, Figures 2.11(a), 2.11(b), and 2.11(c) on page 61 show the food guides of Sweden, Australia, and China, respectively.

The Mediterranean Diet, which is itself a variation on the old U.S. model, has enjoyed considerable popularity. Does it deserve its reputation as a healthy diet? Check out the Highlight box to learn more about the Mediterranean Diet.

Diet Plans

As you already have learned, there is no single diet that is right for all individuals. By using *Canada's Food Guide,* each of us can plan a nutritious diet that fits our personal preferences and lifestyle. That said, a few diets do seem to improve health for a majority of people. The 5 to 10 a Day for Better Health program and the DASH

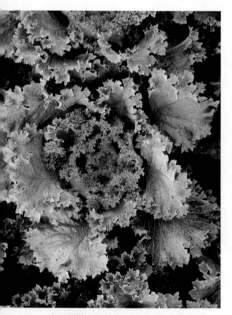
In addition to dairy products, kale is a good source of calcium.

▶ **HIGHLIGHT**

The Mediterranean Diet and Pyramid

The traditional Mediterranean-style pattern of eating has received significant attention in recent years, as the rates of cardiovascular disease in many Mediterranean countries are substantially lower than rates in Canada and the United States. There is actually not a single Mediterranean Diet, as this region of the world includes Portugal, Spain, Italy, France, Greece, Turkey, and Israel. Each of these countries has different dietary patterns; however, there are similarities that have led nutrition researchers to speculate that this type of diet is more healthful than the typical North American diet:

- Meats, eggs, and sweets are eaten only a few times each week, making the diet low in saturated fats and refined sugars.
- The predominant fat used for cooking and flavour is olive oil, making the diet high in monounsaturated fats.
- Foods eaten daily include grains, such as bread, pasta, couscous, and bulgur; fruits; beans and other legumes; nuts; vegetables; and cheese and yogurt. These choices make this diet high in fibre and rich in vitamins and minerals.

As you can see in Figure 2.12 on page 61, the base of the Mediterranean Diet Pyramid includes breads, cereals, and other grains. In this respect, as well as in the daily intake of fruits and vegetables, it is similar to the old U.S. Food Guide Pyramid. But the Mediterranean model differs in several important aspects. It includes beans, other legumes, and nuts daily; fish, poultry, and eggs are eaten a few times each week (not daily); and red meat is eaten only a few times each month. The Mediterranean Diet Pyramid highlights cheese and yogurt as the primary dairy sources, recommends daily consumption of olive oil, and includes wine with meals. It also emphasizes physical activity.

Interestingly, the Mediterranean Diet is not lower in fat; in fact, about 40% of the total energy in this diet is derived from fat, which is slightly higher than the 20%–35% of total energy recommended in Canada and the United States. This fact has led some nutritionists to

criticize the Mediterranean Diet. Supporters point out that the majority of fats in the Mediterranean Diet are healthier fats than the animal fats found in North American diets, which makes the Mediterranean Diet more protective against cardiovascular disease. The potential benefits of the Mediterranean Diet in reducing our cholesterol levels and reducing our risk for heart disease are discussed in Chapter 5.

Can following a traditional Mediterranean-style diet really improve your health? There is general agreement among researchers that eating a Mediterranean-style diet that includes more fruits and vegetables, less meat, and fewer high-fat dairy products does reduce the risks for heart disease and some cancers. PREDIMED, a recent randomized controlled trial with 372 people at high risk for cardiovascular disease, compared the effects of a traditional Mediterranean Diet and a low-fat diet on the primary prevention of coronary heart disease (Fito et al. 2007). The study found that blood levels of oxidized low-density lipoprotein, which is commonly used as a marker of coronary heart disease, were lower in the group that was following that Mediterranean Diet than in the group following the low-fat diet. (See Chapter 5 for a discussion of blood lipid components.)

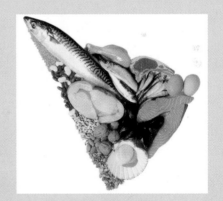

Seafood, meat, poultry, dry beans, eggs, and nuts are examples of foods that are high in protein.

diet are two such diet plans, and we review them here. Try one out for a while, and see if the design works for you!

The 5 to 10 a Day for Better Health Campaign

Canada's **5 to 10 a Day for Better Health program** is a media campaign designed to make children, teens, and adults, both male and female, aware of the health benefits of eating vegetables and fruit, and to promote greater consumption of

5 to 10 a Day for Better Health program A Canadian media campaign designed to make people aware of the health benefits of eating vegetables and fruits and to encourage people to eat more produce.

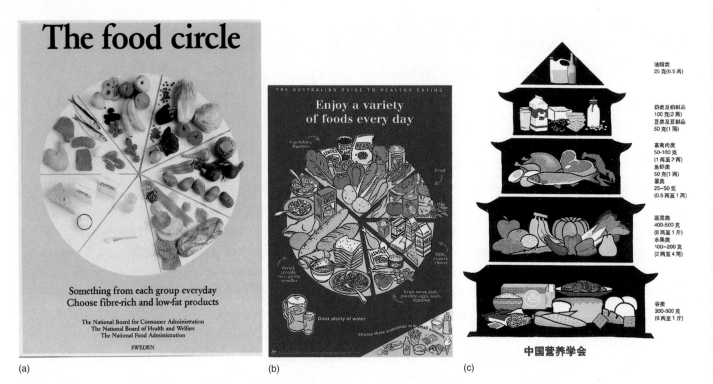

(a)   (b)   (c)

Figure 2.11 Food circles from (a) Sweden and (b) Australia, (c) and a food pagoda from China. (Reprinted from the *Journal of the Dietetic Association,* v.102(4), J. Painter, J-H Rah, Y-K Lee, "Comparison of International Food Guide Pictorial Representations," 483–489. © 2002, with permission from the American Dietetic Association.)

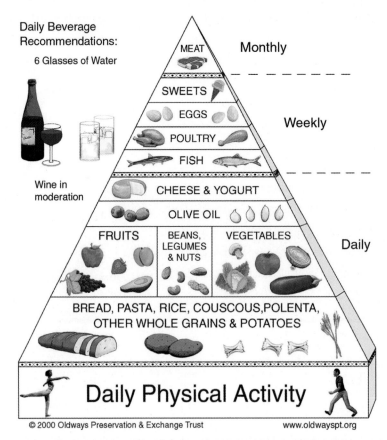

Figure 2.12 The Mediterranean Diet Pyramid. (© 2000 Oldways Preservation and Exchange Trust, The Food Issues Think Tank, Healthy Eating Pyramids & Other Tools, www.oldwayspt.org, accessed September 2002.)

vegetables and fruit. The Heart and Stroke Foundation of Canada, the Canadian Cancer Society, and the Canadian Produce Marketing Association are involved in the campaign, which uses public service announcements on radio and television, posters, and other strategies to get its messages out to consumers.

The DASH Diet Plan

The **DASH diet** resulted from a large research study funded by the National Institutes of Health (NIH) in the United States. DASH stands for Dietary Approaches to Stop Hypertension. Thus, this study was designed to assess the effects of the DASH diet on high blood pressure. Table 2.5 shows the DASH eating plan for a 2000 kcal (8400 kJ) diet. This plan is similar to the goals of *Eating Well with Canada's Food Guide* and the U.S. *MyPyramid* in that it is low in fat and high in fibre. The sodium content of the DASH diet is about 3 grams (or 3000 mg) of sodium, which is slightly less than the average sodium intake in the United States but about the same as average intakes in Canada.

The results of this study convincingly illustrated that eating the DASH diet has a very positive impact on blood pressure (Appel et al. 1997). Normal blood pressure is equal to, or lower than, 120/80 millimetres of mercury (mm Hg). For the study participants overall, systolic blood pressure (the top number) decreased by an average of 5.5 mm Hg and diastolic blood pressure (the bottom number) decreased by an average of 3.0 mm Hg. For the study participants who had high blood pressure, systolic blood pressure dropped an average of 11.4 mm Hg and diastolic blood pressure dropped by an average of 5.5 mm Hg. These decreases occurred within the first two weeks of eating the DASH diet and were maintained throughout the duration of the study. Researchers estimated that if all Americans followed the DASH diet plan and experienced reductions in blood pressure similar to this study, then heart disease would be reduced by 15% and the number of strokes would be 27% lower.

DASH diet The diet developed in response to research into hypertension funded by the U.S. National Institutes of Health (NIH); stands for Dietary Approaches to Stop Hypertension.

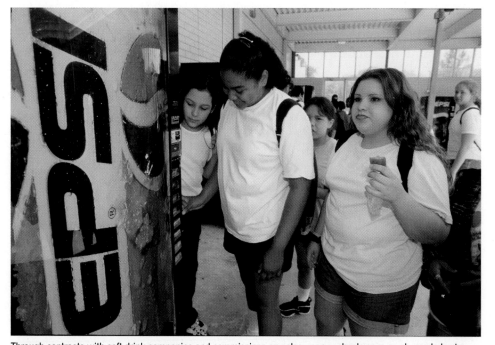

Through contracts with soft drink companies and commissions on sales, many schools earn much-needed extra revenue. However, recent studies have linked childhood obesity to soft drink consumption. In response to these findings Ontario has banned soft drinks in school vending machines in elementary schools.

Table 2.5   The DASH Eating Plan

Food Group	Daily Servings	Serving Size
Grains and grain products	7–8	1 slice bread 250 mL (1 cup) ready-to-eat cereal* 125 mL (1/2 cup) cooked rice, pasta, or cereal
Vegetables	4–5	250 mL (1 cup) raw leafy vegetables 125 mL (1/2 cup) cooked vegetable 180 mL (6 fl. oz.) vegetable juice
Fruits	4–5	1 medium fruit 65 mL (1/4 cup) dried fruit 125 mL (1/2 cup) fresh, frozen, or canned fruit 180 mL (6 fl. oz.) fruit juice
Low-fat or fat-free dairy foods	2–3	250 mL (8 fl. oz.) milk 250 mL (1 cup) yogurt 45 g (1 1/2 oz.) cheese Lean meats, poultry, and fish 2 or less 90 g (3 oz.) cooked lean meats, skinless poultry, or fish
Nuts, seeds, and dry beans	4–5 per week	75 mL (1/3 cup) or 45 g (1 1/2 oz.) nuts 15 mL (1 Tbsp) or 15 g (1/2 oz.) seeds 125 mL (1/2 cup) cooked dry beans
Fats and oils**	2–3	5 mL (1 tsp) soft margarine 15 mL (1 Tbsp) low-fat mayonnaise 30 mL (2 Tbsp) light salad dressing 5 mL (1 tsp) vegetable oil
Sweets	5 per week	15 mL (1 Tbsp) sugar 15 mL (1 Tbsp) jelly or jam 15 g (1/2 oz.) jelly beans 250 mL (8 fl. oz.) lemonade

Source: US Department of Health and Human Services, National Institutes of Health National Heart, Lung, and Blood Institute, NIH Publication No. 03-4082, revised May 2003.

Note: The plan is based on 2000 kcal (8400 kJ) per day. The number of servings in a food group may differ from the number listed, depending upon your own energy needs.

*Servings sizes vary between 125 and 315 mL (1/2 and 1 1/4 cups). Check the product's nutrition label.

**Fat content changes serving counts for fats and oils. For example, 15 mL (1 Tbsp) of regular salad dressing equals 1 serving; 15 mL of a low-fat dressing equals 1/2 serving; 15 mL of fat-free dressing equals 0 servings.

Further study of the DASH diet has found that blood pressure decreases even more if sodium intake is reduced below 3000 mg per day. A second study was conducted in which participants ate a DASH diet that provided either 3300 mg (average U.S. intake), 2400 mg (upper recommended intake), or 1500 mg of sodium each day (Sacks et al. 2001). After one month on this diet, all people eating the DASH diet saw a significant decrease in their blood pressure; however, those who ate the lowest-sodium version of the DASH diet experienced the largest decrease. These results indicate that eating a diet low in sodium and high in fruits and vegetables reduces blood pressure and decreases your risk for heart disease and stroke.

Recap: The 5 to 10 a Day for Better Health program and the DASH diet are two examples of healthy food plans. High fruit and vegetable consumption has been linked to cancer prevention and reduced risk of heart disease. The DASH diet was designed to reduce blood pressure in people with hypertension. It is similar to *Canada's Food Guide* with an emphasis on vegetables and fruit; it also is designed to keep sodium intakes to 3000 mg or less each day. The DASH diet has been shown to significantly decrease blood pressure.

Other Diet Plans

Other diet plans are available to consumers, and many of these may or may not have been researched to determine their health benefits. Some of these plans, such as Weight Watchers, have been marketed specifically for weight loss; many weight loss plans can be adapted to achieve healthy weight maintenance. It is inappropriate to endorse one specific diet plan for all people, as our nutritional needs and preferences are diverse and cannot be met by a single plan. Each person must make his or her own decisions about nutritious diet choices based on personal preferences, ethnic considerations, activity level, cost, and convenience.

When planning a nutritious diet for yourself, you need to look closely at any diet plan to determine if it meets the guidelines reviewed in this book. You can use *Eating Well with Canada's Food Guide* as a standard for comparison, and you also need to look at any diet plan to determine whether it emphasizes the principles of adequacy, moderation, balance, variety, and nutrient density.

Choose Foods High in Nutrient Density   As a general guideline, you should choose foods rich in nutrients—foods that have a high nutrient density. This means eating foods that give you the highest amount of nutrients for the least amount of energy (or kcal). As an example, three Oreo cookies provide the same number of Calories as the combination of a medium banana and 125 mL (1/2 cup) of fresh blackberries. Yet as you might guess, the density of nutrients in the fruit is far superior, giving you more true nourishment per kcal (Figure 2.13).

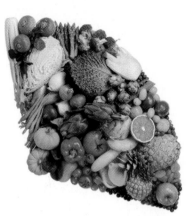

It is important to eat the recommended number of servings of vegetables and fruit every day.

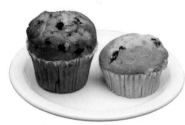

Although the serving size of a "medium" muffin in the *Food Guide* is 42 g (1 1/2 oz.), many muffins sold today range in size from 56 to 224 g (2 to 8 oz.).

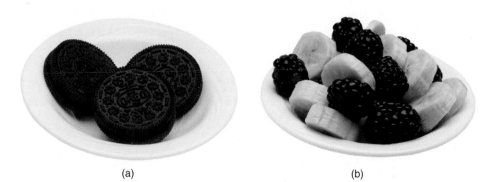

(a)   (b)

Figure 2.13 Examples of foods that are low and high in nutrient density. (a) Three Oreo cookies. (b) The combination of one medium banana and 125 mL (1/2 cup) fresh blackberries. Each bowl of food provides approximately 145 kcal (600 kJ). The cookies provide 56 kcal (230 kJ) from fat (6.2 grams), 1 gram of fibre, and very few vitamins and minerals. The fruit combination provides almost 7 grams of fibre, 8 kcal (32 kJ) from fat (0.85 grams), and a significant amount of other nutrients, such as potassium (608 mg), vitamin A (21 RE), and vitamin C (26 mg). For our limited daily energy budget, the fruit is richer in nutrients (more nutrient dense) and a more healthful choice. (Calculated by using USDA Nutrient Database for Standard Reference, Release 15, September 2002.)

Table 2.6   A Comparison of One Day's Meals that Contain Foods High in Nutrient Density to Meals that Contain Foods Low in Nutrient Density

Meals with Foods High in Nutrient Density	Meals with Foods Low in Nutrient Density
Breakfast:	**Breakfast:**
250 mL (1 cup) cooked oatmeal with 125 mL (4 fl. oz.) skim milk	250 mL (1 cup) puffed rice cereal with 125 mL (4 fl. oz.) whole milk
1 slice whole wheat toast with 5 mL (1 tsp) butter	1 slice white toast with 5 mL (1 tsp) butter
175 mL (6 fl. oz.) grapefruit juice	175 mL (6 fl. oz.) grape drink
Snack:	**Snack:**
1 peeled orange	355 mL (12 fl. oz.) can orange pop
250 mL (1 cup) non-fat yogurt	45 g (1 1/2 oz.) cheddar cheese
Lunch:	**Lunch:**
Turkey sandwich:	Hamburger:
90 g (3 oz.) turkey breast	90 g (3 oz.) cooked regular ground beef
2 slices whole-grain bread	1 white hamburger bun
10 mL (2 tsp) Dijon mustard	10 mL (2 tsp) Dijon mustard
3 slices fresh tomato	15 mL (1 Tbsp) tomato ketchup
2 leaves red leaf lettuce	2 leaves iceberg lettuce
250 mL (1 cup) baby carrots with broccoli crowns	1 snack-sized bag potato chips
	500 mL (16 fl. oz.) cola soft drink
Snack:	**Snack:**
1/2 whole wheat bagel	3 chocolate sandwich cookies
15 mL (1 Tbsp) peanut butter	355 mL (12 fl. oz.) can diet pop
1 medium apple	10 Gummi Bears candy
Dinner:	**Dinner:**
Spinach salad:	Green salad:
250 mL (1 cup) spinach leaves	250 mL (1 cup) iceberg lettuce
60 mL (1/4 cup) diced tomatoes	60 mL (1/4 cup) diced tomatoes
60 mL (1/4 cup) green pepper	5 mL (1 tsp) green onions
125 mL (1/2 cup) kidney beans	60 mL (1/4 cup) bacon bits
15 mL (1 Tbsp) fat-free Italian dressing	15 mL (1 Tbsp) regular ranch dressing
90 g (3 oz.) broiled chicken breast	90 g (3 oz.) beef round steak, breaded and fried
125 mL (1/2 cup) cooked brown rice	125 mL (1/2 cup) cooked white rice
125 mL (1/2 cup) steamed broccoli	125 mL (1/2 cup) kernel corn
250 mL (8 fl. oz.) skim milk	250 mL (8 fl. oz.) iced tea

Note: The conversions between Imperial and metric measures used here are not exact but are common conversions used in recipes and on food products in Canada. The exact conversions are slightly different in the United States (e.g., 1 fl. oz. = 29.57 mL; 8 fl. oz. = 1 cup = 237 mL) and in Canada (1 fl. oz. = 28.41 mL; 8 fl. oz. = 1 cup = 227 mL). As a result, U.S. volume measures are slightly larger (approximately 4%) than Canadian measures.

A helpful analogy for selecting nutrient-dense foods is shopping for clothes on a tight budget. If you had only $40 in your clothing budget, you would most likely buy two pairs of pants on sale for $20 each instead of one pair of pants for $40. Because you can only afford a certain number of Calories each day to maintain a healthy weight, it makes sense to maximize the nutrients you can get for each Calorie you consume. Table 2.6 provides a comparison of one day of meals that are high in nutrient density with meals that are low in nutrient density. This example can assist you in selecting the most nutrient-rich foods when planning your meals.

Can Eating Out Be Part of a Nutritious Diet?

How much of your food budget do you spend each week on restaurant meals? According to Statistics Canada, Canadian households spent an average of $124 weekly for food in 2001; 30% of their food dollars were on restaurant meals and 70% was spent on food purchased from stores (Statistics Canada 2003).

The Hidden Costs of Eating Out

Table 2.7 shows the nutrient content of some selected meals and snacks from Tim Hortons and Wendy's restaurants in Canada. As you can see, a Wendy's Grilled Chicken Go Wrap has only 250 kcal (1050 kJ), while the Mandarin Chicken Salad has 540 kcal (2270 kJ). A Tim Horton's meal of the B.L.T. sandwich, small iced cappucino (made with cream), and a chocolate glazed donut provides 960 kcal

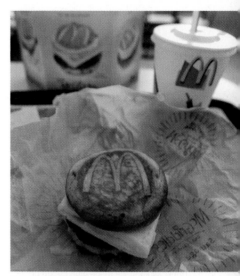

Foods served at fast food chains are often high in Calories, total fat, and sodium.

Table 2.7   Nutritional Value of Selected Fast Foods in Canada

Menu Item	Total Calories	Fat (% of Calories)	Total Fat (grams)	Saturated Fat (grams)	Trans Fat (grams)	Sodium (mg)
Tim Hortons						
Chocolate glazed donut	260	35	10	4.5	0.1	300
Old fashion plain	260	66	19	9	0.1	230
Raisin bran muffin	360	25	10	1.5	0	790
12-grain bagel	330	24.5	9	1	0	580
Raisin tea biscuit	290	31	10	2	0	590
Vanilla yogurt and berries	160	11	2	1.5	0	45
Ham & Swiss Cheese sandwich	440	24.5	12	5	0.2	1690
B.L.T.	450	36	18	5	0.1	850
Chicken Salad	380	21	9	1.5	0.2	980
Iced Capuccino – cream (small)	250	40	11	6	0.4	50
Iced Capuccino – milk (small)	150	9	1.5	1	0	35
Wendy's						
1/4 lb Hamburger	430	42	20	7	1	850
Ultimate Chicken Grill	320	20	7	1.5	0.1	950
Homestyle Chicken Breast Sandwich	430	33.5	16	2.5	0.1	1110
Grilled Chicken Go Wrap	250	36	10	3.5	0.3	700
Small Fries	270	43	13	2.0	0.1	240
Large Fries	480	41	22	3.5	0.2	410
Mandarin Chicken Salad	540	42	25	3.0	0.5	1260

Sources: Wendy's Nutritional Information is taken from the website www.wendys.ca and is based on standard U.S. product formulations. Variations may occur due to differences in suppliers, ingredient substitutions, recipe revisions, product assembly at the restaurant level and/or season of the year. Text products are not included. This information is effective as of October 1, 2007; Tim Hortons nutritional information used with permission of The TDL Group Corporation, www.timhortons.com

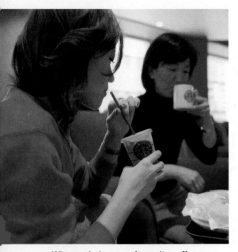

When ordering your favourite coffee drink, avoid those made with cream or whipping cream and request reduced-fat or skim milk instead.

(4030 kJ) and 39 grams of fat—about one-half of the energy to support an entire day's need for a small, lightly active woman! Similar meals at other fast food chains can also be high in energy, not to mention fat, saturated fat, and sodium.

It is not only the fast-food restaurants that serve large portions. Most sit-down restaurants serve meals that include bread with butter, a salad with dressing, and large portions of the main course. If an appetizer or a dessert is also eaten, along with alcoholic beverages, it can be easy to consume 2000 kcal (8400 kJ) at one meal.

Does this mean that eating out cannot be part of a nutritious diet? No. By becoming an educated consumer and making wise meal choices, you can enjoy both a nutritious meal and the social benefits of eating out with friends.

The Sensible Way to Eat Out

Most restaurants, even fast-food restaurants, offer lower-fat menu items that you can choose. For instance, an order of Wendy's Grilled Chicken Go Wrap, a small side of fries, and a diet beverage or water provides 520 kcal (2180 kJ) and only 23 grams of fat (or 32% of energy from fat). To provide some vegetables for the day, you could add a side salad with low-fat or non-fat salad dressing. Other fast-food restaurants also offer smaller portions, sandwiches made with whole-grain bread, grilled chicken or other lean meats, and side salads. Many sit-down restaurants offer "light" or "lite" menu items, such as grilled chicken and a variety of vegetables, which are usually a much better choice than eating from the regular menu.

Here are some other suggestions on how to eat out in moderation. Practise some of these suggestions every time you eat out:

- Avoid whole-milk lattés and other coffee drinks with cream or whipping cream; select reduced-fat or skim milk to add to your favourite coffee drink.

- Avoid eating appetizers that are breaded, fried, or filled with cheese or meat; you may want to skip the appetizer completely. Alternatively, you may want to order a healthful appetizer as an entrée instead of a larger meal.

- Share an entrée with a friend! Many restaurants serve entrées large enough for two people.

- Order broth-based soups instead of cream-based soups.

- Order any meat dish grilled or broiled, and avoid fried or breaded meat dishes.

- If you order a meat dish, select lean cuts of meat, such as chicken or turkey breast, extra-lean ground beef, pork loin chop, or filet mignon.

- Order a meatless dish filled with vegetables and whole grains. Avoid dishes with cream sauces and a lot of cheese.

- Order a salad with low-fat or non-fat dressing served on the side. Many restaurants smother their salads in dressing, and you will eat less by controlling how much you put on the salad.

- Order steamed vegetables on the side instead of potatoes or rice. If you order potatoes, make sure you get a baked potato (with very little butter or sour cream on the side).

- Order beverages with few or no calories, such as water, tea, herbal tea, or diet drinks.

- Eat no more than half of what you are served, and take the rest home for another meal.

- Skip dessert or share one dessert with several friends! Another healthful alternative is to order fresh fruit for dessert.

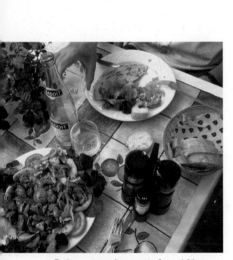

Eating out can be a part of a nutritious diet if you are careful to choose wisely.

Recap: Healthful ways to eat out include choosing menu items that are smaller in size, ordering meats that are grilled or broiled, avoiding fried foods, choosing items with steamed vegetables, avoiding energy-rich appetizers and desserts, and eating less than half of the food you are served.

CHAPTER SUMMARY

- A nutritious diet provides adequate energy, nutrients, and fibre to maintain health.

- A nutritious diet is moderate in the amounts of foods eaten. Foods that contain a lot of fat and sugar should be eaten only in moderation to maintain a healthy weight.

- A nutritious diet contains the proper balance of food groups and nutrients to maintain health.

- A nutritious diet provides a variety of foods every day.

- The Nutrition Facts table on a food label contains important nutrition information about serving size, servings per package, total Calories per serving, a list of various macronutrients, vitamins, and minerals, and the % daily values (%DV) for the nutrients listed.

- *Eating Well with Canada's Food Guide* is the major tool for consumers to use to plan nutritious diets. It was developed by Health Canada to be consistent with the DRIs. It is available in 10 languages in addition to English and French.

- *Eating Well with Canada's Food Guide* has four food groups: Vegetables and Fruit, Grain Products, Milk and Alternatives, and Meat and Alternatives.

- *Eating Well with Canada's Food Guide* contains the recommended number of servings for each food group for nine age and sex categories.

- Specific serving sizes are given for foods in each food group of *Canada's Food Guide*. There is no standard definition for a serving size, and the serving sizes listed in *Canada's Food Guide* are generally smaller than those listed on food labels and what most of us eat.

- The U.S. Department of Agriculture's *MyPyramid: Steps to a Healthier You* (USDA 2005) has six sections that represent five food groups plus oils and includes a stylized figure climbing stairs to represent the importance of daily physical activity

- Some researchers recommend that people follow a traditional Mediterranean Diet, which contains less red meat and dairy products and more legumes, healthy fats, and wine than the traditional North American diet. This diet, and daily physical activity, may help protect against heart attacks and some cancers.

- The 5 to 10 a Day for Better Health program is a major public health initiative promoting the intake of a combination of 5 to 10 servings of fruits and vegetables every day to reduce the risk for cancer and other chronic diseases.

- The DASH (Dietary Approaches to Stop Hypertension) diet is high in fibre, low in fat, and moderate in sodium, and includes 8 to 10 servings of fruits and vegetables each day. Eating the DASH diet can significantly decrease blood pressure, a benefit to people with high blood pressure.

- Eating out is challenging because of the high fat content and large serving sizes of many fast-food and sit-down restaurant menu items.

- Behaviours that can improve the quality of your diet when eating out include choosing lower-fat meats that are grilled or broiled, eating vegetables and salads as side or main dishes, asking for low-fat salad dressing on the side, skipping high-fat desserts and appetizers, and drinking low- or non-caloric beverages.

mynutritionlab Go to MyNutritionLab at www.pearsoned.ca/mynutritionlab and enrich your understanding of nutrition! You'll find key animations, interactive exercises, access to My DietAnalysis, and much more.

REVIEW QUESTIONS

Quizzes

1. The Nutrition Facts table identifies which of the following?
   a. All of the nutrients and Calories in the package of food.
   b. The Recommended Dietary Allowance for each nutrient found in the package of food.
   c. A footnote identifying the Tolerable Upper Intake Level for each nutrient found in the package of food.
   d. The % daily values of select nutrients in a serving of the packaged food.

2. An adequate diet
   a. provides enough energy to meet minimum daily requirements.
   b. provides enough of the energy, nutrients, and fibre to maintain a person's health.

   c. provides a sufficient variety of nutrients to maintain a healthy weight and to optimize our body's metabolic processes.
   d. contains combinations of foods that provide healthful proportions of nutrients.

3. Which of the following are required on labels for foods intended for infants and children less than two years of age?
   a. Saturated and trans fats
   b. Starch and fibre
   c. Cholesterol and trans fats
   d. Protein and iron

4. The Health Check symbol on a package tells you that the food
   a. meets a set of criteria by the Canadian Heart and Stroke Foundation for a "heart-healthy" choice.

b. has been approved by the Canadian Diabetes Association for diets for people with diabetes.

c. meets Health Canada's criteria for a nutritious food choice.

d. is part of the DASH eating plan for people with high blood pressure.

5. What does it mean to choose foods for their nutrient density?

a. Dense foods, such as peanut butter or chicken, are more nutritious choices than transparent foods, such as mineral water or gelatin

b. Foods with a lot of nutrients relative to their energy content, such as fish, are more nutritious choices than foods with less nutrients, such as candy

c. Energy-dense foods, such as cheesecake, should be avoided

d. Fat makes foods dense, and thus foods high in fat should be avoided

6. Choose the correct statement.

a. Percent daily values indicate the amount a nutrient should contribute to your overall energy intake per day

b. Ingredients must be listed in ascending order by weight

c. If omega-3 polyunsaturated fats are listed, omega-6 polyunsaturated fats must be listed as well

d. Health claims relate to the amount of nutrient in a food

7. List ways to make eating out healthy. Hint: Think of what you order when you're out to dinner and describe ways you could tweak the meal to make it healthy and lower the number of calories consumed.

8. How can percent daily values aid in making healthy food choices?

9. Defend the statement that no single diet can be appropriate for every person.

10. Describe the main characteristics of a traditional Mediterranean Diet.

11. Your little sister, Laura, comes home in tears because her elementary school has removed the vending machine with all of her favourite recess snacks. Laura is a healthy, active Grade 4 student who always brings a packed lunch with nutrient-dense foods, like sandwiches, vegetables, and fruit. She whines that removing vending machines isn't fair. Do you agree?

12. Vending machines are a source of extra income for many schools as the schools receive a percentage of the profits from sales (Heuter 2002). Is this situation a conflict of interest for schools? Although schools cannot control what students choose to eat, should they be held accountable for making these nutrient-void snacks so readily available? If you were on the committee deciding the fate of elementary school vending machines, what side would you be on, and what would your arguments be?

CASE STUDY

Now that you've had the opportunity to learn about nutritious diet planning, let's discuss Katie, a 20-year-old university student who lives in an apartment with one roommate. Since moving away from home, Katie has found it difficult to eat regular, nutritious meals. She often finds herself in the grocery store lost at the thought of having to make decisions about which product to purchase. The choices are seemingly endless!

a. What tools are available directly on the product package to aid Katie in making healthy food choices?

b. Katie decides to purchase a large meat lasagna to last her several meals. The whole meat lasagna is 1.2 kg (1200g). One portion (300g) contains 390 Calories and 13 grams of fat.

i. If Katie eats one half of the meat lasagna at dinner, how many grams of fat did she consume?

ii. If Katie's recommended intake of fat is 65 grams, what is her percent daily value of fat from the meat lasagna?

c. According to *Canada's Food Guide*, how many servings from each food group should she aim to consume each day? List several healthy food choices found at the grocery store for each group (remember to think about why they are healthy choices).

d. List several foods that you would advise Katie to purchase sparingly.

WEB LINKS

www.dietitians.ca
Dietitians of Canada
Click on Nutrition Challenges and take the Healthy Way Challenge and test your knowledge to see whether you are "portion-wise."

www.hc-sc.gc.ca/fn-an/label-etiquet/nutrition/cons/interactive_e.html
Health Canada's Interactive Nutrition Label
This interactive site can help you learn about the new food label. When you think you know the parts of the label, take the interactive quiz!

www.5to10aday.com
5 to 10 a Day for Better Health
Visit this site to learn more about Canada's 5 to 10 a Day program to promote vegetable and fruit consumption.

www.healthcheck.org
Heart and Stroke Foundation of Canada
Developed by the Heart and Stroke Foundation, Health Check is a non-profit food information program to promote healthy food choices. More than 1500 food products in Canada carry the Health Check logo and a message explaining how the food fits into a healthy diet.

www.wendys.ca
Wendy's
Select different beverages and foods to see their nutrient contents.

www.timhortons.com
Tim Hortons
Trying selecting various food and beverage items to see the amounts of energy and nutrients they contain.

www.inspection.gc.ca
Canadian Food Inspection Agency
If you are interested in more information about the new food labels in Canada, health claims, and so on, this is the place to find it.

www.health.gov/dietaryguidelines/
The Dietary Guidelines for Americans 2005
The latest dietary guidelines for American consumers are listed here.

www.mypyramid.gov
United States Department of Agriculture (USDA)
This interactive website outlines the 2005 USDA *MyPyramid: Steps to a Healthier You*. Try MyPyramid Tracker at www.mypyramidtracker.gov for an in-depth look at your diet quality and physical activity.

www.healthcanada.gc.ca/foodguide
Health Canada, Office of Nutrition Policy and Promotion
Learn more about *Eating Well with Canada's Food Guide* and other Canadian health policies.

www.oldwayspt.org
Oldways Preservation and Exchange Trust
Find different variations of ethnic and cultural food pyramids.

www.fruitsandveggiesmatter.gov
Fruits and Veggies—More Matters Program
The National Cancer Institute, Centers for Disease Control and Prevention, Department of Health and Human Services, the U.S. government, and other partners have collaborated on a new program to replace the old U.S. 5-A-Day Program.

www.nih.gov
The National Institutes of Health (NIH, part of the U.S. Department of Health and Human Services)

Test Yourself Answers

1. **True** A nutritious diet can include less nutritious foods in moderation, if the overall diet follows *Canada's Food Guide* and is well-balanced, varied, adequate, and includes foods in moderation.

2. **True** Most people say they read food labels to help them choose which foods to buy. However, research suggests that many people don't understand the information on food labels very well.

3. **False** *Canada's Food Guide* uses serving sizes that were developed many years ago. In the past decade, portions of foods we typically eat at home and in restaurants have become larger. The result is that most of us now are used to eating larger servings or portions than those recommended in *Canada's Food Guide*.

4. **True** The ingredients are listed in descending order by weight, not volume. This means that heavier ingredients, such as sugars, often appear before lighter ingredients, such as flour, in the ingredient list.

5. **False** The new legislation for health claims allows manufacturers to state that their products contain certain nutrients that are associated with reduced risks of some diseases. But they are not permitted to suggest that eating their product can prevent or treat a disease.

Search this site to learn more about the DASH diet (Dietary Approaches to Stop Hypertension).

http://hin.nhlbi.nih.gov/portion
The National Institutes of Health (NIH) Portion Distortion Quiz
Take this short quiz to see if you know how today's food portions compare with those of 20 years ago.

www.eatright.org
The American Dietetic Association
Visit the food and nutrition information section of this website for additional resources to help you achieve a healthy lifestyle.

www.hsph.harvard.edu
The Harvard School of Public Health
Search this site to learn more about the Healthy Eating Pyramid, an alternative to the USDA Food Guide Pyramid.

Should the Canadian Government Regulate the Food Industry to Combat the Obesity Epidemic?

As you learned in the first chapter, obesity is now considered an epidemic in North America and around the world. The dramatic rise in obesity not only is contributing to bulging waistlines but also is responsible for overwhelming burdens related to health care costs, emotional distress, and societal prejudice. What can we do to fight obesity and its extensive societal and medical consequences? Who is responsible for contributing to the obesity epidemic, and who should be held accountable to combat it?

For many years, all accountability for obesity has been placed on the obese person. These individuals have been portrayed as lazy, gluttonous, and having no will power. Losing weight has been portrayed as being as simple as eating less energy than you expend. Thus, weight loss has been viewed as the responsibility of the obese individuals; they should just eat less and exercise more, and they would not be obese.

Research has now shown that weight loss is not quite this simple. Friedman (2003) points out that obesity has a strong genetic component. For centuries, people who were regularly exposed to famine adapted so that they could readily store fat and survive when food was scarce. When a person with a strong genetic tendency toward obesity lives in an environment with ample food and inadequate physical activity, weight gain is virtually inevitable. In addition, the drive to eat is complex and is stimulated by weight loss. Thus, it is simply not enough just to eat less, exercise more, and lose weight. Many believe we are now living in a "toxic" environment, one that makes living a healthful life incredibly challenging for most people and almost impossible for some.

Because of these challenges, there is a growing trend to hold someone or something accountable for this toxic environment. Recent lawsuits in the United States have targeted fast-food chains and food manufacturers. Obese citizens have attempted to sue fast-food restaurants for serving foods that are high in fat, energy, and sugar. Food manufacturers are being sued because of the junk foods they produce and market to children. Recent history has shown us that litigation can be a powerful tool to bring attention to a major public health problem, as has occurred with smoking and the tobacco industry.

Suing food producers and restaurants may be even more challenging than suing the tobacco industry, however, as food is something we need to survive. In addition, proponents of the food and restaurant industry argue that people know that fast food and junk food is not nutritious and that it is up to individuals to moderate their intake of these foods.

Another approach to combating obesity is the proposed application of taxes on non-nutritious foods. The so-called sin tax has been applied to cigarettes and alcohol. The basic premise is to apply a small tax on soft drinks and snack foods, and then use the revenues from this tax to fund nutrition and physical activity programs across the country (Jacobson and Brownell 2000). This tax would be small enough that it would

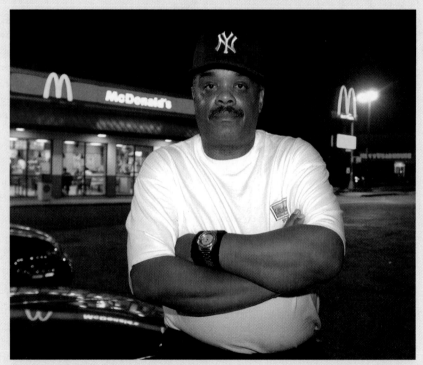

In 2002, Caesar Barber was the initial plaintiff in a class action suit in the United States against four food franchises, including McDonald's. He claimed that they contributed to his weight as well as other health problems by serving fatty foods. A U.S. federal court later threw out the lawsuit.

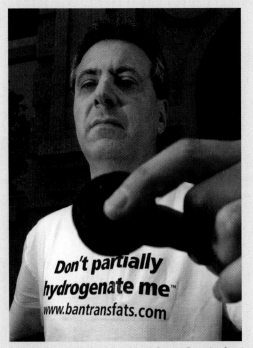

Attorney Stephen Joseph filed suit in a Marin County Superior Court seeking a ban on Oreo sales in California. He claimed that the cookies were unhealthy because they contained trans fat. He later dropped his suit when he learned that Kraft was working on ways to reduce the trans fat in the cookie.

not negatively affect food sales, but it could potentially generate millions, even billions, of dollars in revenue that could be used to fund a variety of health-promotion programs. To date, there has been no widespread support of this proposed approach.

A growing number of people believe that the Canadian and U.S. governments should step forward and lead the way in combating obesity. Federal governments are capable of applying taxes to foods, regulating the types of foods sold in stores and restaurants, and controlling the information listed on food labels. With obesity such a prominent health problem in North America, many wonder why governments don't support more health-promotion initiatives to take an active role in preventing and combating this disease.

The issues surrounding the role of government in regulating our food intake are complex and controversial. Many people stand strongly against any governmental control over what we eat. People pride themselves on individuality and personal freedoms, and they are averse to governmental control on personal behaviours. Thus, many feel that the government should play no role in what or how we eat. In addition, food companies hold a great deal of political clout, and these companies support our political candidates and contribute money to government officials, health care professionals, and media outlets. In fact, the politics of food make it very difficult for the federal government to place controls or demands on the food industry. The message of "eat less" does not bode well for food manufacturers and restaurant owners.

These politics are discussed in detail by Marion Nestle (2002), who describes how the food industry influences nutrition and health in the United States and makes suggestions as to how we can modify public policies to promote healthier lives. Some of these suggestions include the following:

- Mount a national campaign to "eat less, move more."
- End the sale of pop, chocolate bars, and other foods with minimal nutrition value in schools.
- Require fast-food restaurants to provide nutrition information labels on food wrappers and packages.
- Restrict television advertising of foods with minimal nutritional value.
- Apply taxes to soft drinks and other junk foods, and reduce the cost of fruits and vegetables.

How do you feel about this debate? To what level (if any) do you feel the government should be involved in regulating the food industry? What are you willing to give up or demand to fight the obesity epidemic? Are you willing to pay taxes on foods with minimal nutritional value? Should the food industry be held accountable for selling foods that are not nutritious and contribute to the obesity epidemic? These are questions that each of us may need to answer in the coming years. The obesity epidemic will not be quelled without a fight. It is up to all of us to determine whether we should fight this epidemic, and if so, just how we can fight it.

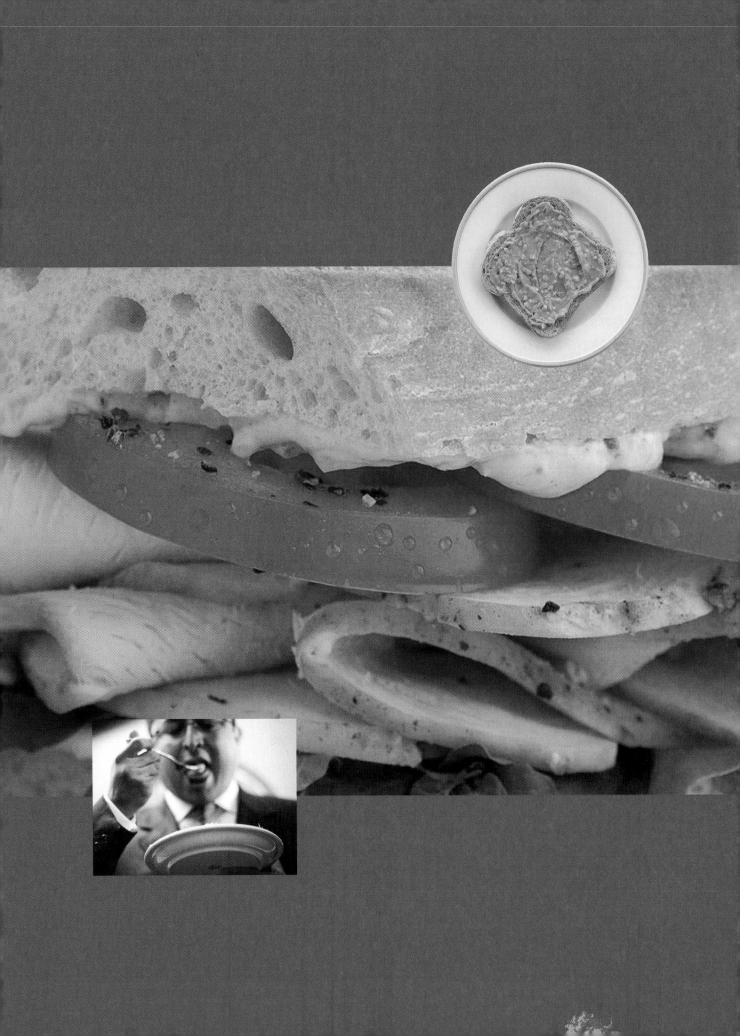

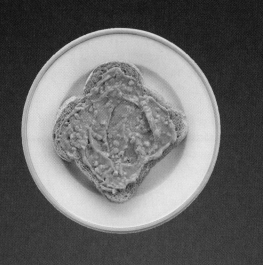

CHAPTER 3

What Happens to the Food We Eat?

CHAPTER OBJECTIVES

After reading this chapter you will be able to:

1. Distinguish between appetite and hunger, describing the mechanisms that stimulate each, pp. 75–78.

2. Draw a picture of the gastrointestinal tract, including all major and accessory organs, pp. 78–81.

3. Describe the contribution of each organ of the gastrointestinal system to the digestion, absorption, and elimination of food, pp. 81–83.

4. Identify some of the enzymes involved in digesting foods and list the source of these enzymes, pp. 83–93.

5. Describe the causes, symptoms, and treatments of gastroesophageal reflux disease and ulcers, pp. 95–98.

6. Describe three warning signs of dehydration resulting from diarrhea, pp. 102–104.

Test Yourself True or False

1. Sometimes you may have an appetite even though you are not hungry. **T or F**

2. Your stomach is the primary organ responsible for telling you when you are hungry. **T or F**

3. The entire process of digestion and absorption of one meal takes about 24 hours. **T or F**

4. Most ulcers result from a type of infection. **T or F**

5. Irritable bowel syndrome is a rare disease that mostly affects older people. **T or F**

Test Yourself answers can be found at the end of the chapter.

Do you know people who say they can't eat certain foods without experiencing upset stomach and diarrhea? Do you think these symptoms are "all in their head"? After all, how could common foods that most people eat every day make someone else sick? How do we actually digest and absorb foods? If you had a food-related illness, what do you think would change in your life? How would you feel about shopping for food, dining out, or accepting an invitation to dinner with friends?

Our ability to properly digest and absorb foods is critical to health and optimal function. It is important to understand not only what happens to the foods we eat, but also why we eat and how disorders related to digestion, absorption, and elimination of food affect our health. We begin this chapter with a look at why we want to eat. We then introduce the gastrointestinal system and explore what happens to the food we eat. Finally, we look at some disorders that are related to the digestion, absorption, and elimination of food.

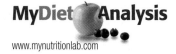

www.mynutritionlab.com

Why Do We Eat?

Food provides us with energy, and the heat our body generates from this energy helps keep our bodies at the temperature required to maintain the proper chemical functions needed for life. Food gives us the molecular building blocks we need to manufacture new tissues for growth and repair, thereby keeping us healthy. Considering the importance of food, it makes sense that our bodies would employ a variety of mechanisms to make us want to eat.

Food Stimulates Our Senses

You've just finished eating at your favourite Thai restaurant. As you walk back to the block where you parked your car, you pass a bakery window displaying several cakes and pies, each of which looks more enticing than the last. Through the door wafts a complex aroma of coffee, cinnamon, and chocolate. You stop. Are you hungry? You must be, because you go inside and buy a slice of chocolate torte and an espresso. Later that night, when the caffeine from the chocolate and espresso keeps you awake, you wonder why you succumbed.

The answer is that food stimulates our senses. Foods that are artfully prepared, arranged, or ornamented, with several different shapes and colours, appeal to our sense of sight. Advertisers know this and spend millions of dollars annually in Canada to promote and package foods in an appealing way. The aromas of foods like freshly brewed coffee and baked goods can also be powerful stimulants. Much of our ability to *taste* foods actually comes from our sense of smell. This is why foods are not as appealing when we are sick with a cold, because our ability to smell is blunted. Interestingly, our sense of smell is so acute that newborn babies can distinguish the scent of their own mother's breast milk from that of other mothers. Of all our senses, taste is the most important in determining what foods we choose to eat. Certain tastes, such as for sweet foods, are almost universally appealing, while others, such as the astringent taste of foods like spinach and kale, are quite individual. Texture is also important in food choices, as it stimulates nerve endings sensitive to touch in our mouth and on our tongue: do you prefer mashed potatoes, thick french fries, or rippled potato chips? Even your sense of hearing can be stimulated by foods, from the fizz of pop to the crunch of peanuts to the "snap, crackle, and pop" of Rice Krispies cereal.

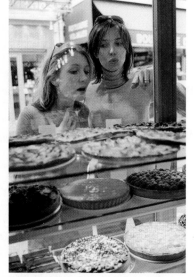

Food stimulates our senses. Foods that are artfully prepared, arranged, or decorated, like the cakes and pies in this bakery display case, appeal to our sense of sight.

Recap: A number of factors stimulate us to eat. Our senses of sight, smell, and taste are stimulated by foods. The texture of foods can also stimulate us to eat or may cause some foods to be unappealing. These four factors interact to motivate us to eat.

Psychosocial Factors Arouse Appetite

If it wasn't hunger that lured you into that bakery, it was probably appetite. **Appetite** is a psychological desire to consume specific foods. It is aroused by environmental cues—such as the sight of chocolate cake or the smell of coffee—and is usually not related to hunger. Appetite is generally related to pleasant sensations associated with food and is often linked to strong cravings for particular foods in the absence of hunger. **Hunger** is considered a basic physiologic sensation, a drive that prompts us to find food and eat. Although we try to define appetite and hunger as two separate entities, many times they overlap, and characteristics of appetite and hunger are different for many people. Hunger is discussed in more detail in the following section.

In addition to environmental cues, our brains associate certain foods with certain events, like birthday parties, or holidays, such as Thanksgiving; this can stimulate our appetite. At these times, society gives us permission to eat more than usual and to eat "forbidden" foods. For some people, being in a certain location, such as at a baseball game or in a movie theatre, can trigger appetite. Others may be triggered by the time of day or by an activity, such as watching television or studying. Many people feel an increase in their appetite when they are under stress. Even when we feel full after a large meal, our appetite can motivate us to eat a delicious dessert.

If you are trying to lose weight or to maintain your present weight, it is important to stay aware, as you go through a day, of whether you are truly hungry or whether you simply have an appetite. If you decide it is your appetite, try to get away from the trigger. For instance, in the previous scenario, you could have simply walked away from the bakery. By the time you'd reached your car, you would probably have forgotten the sights and smells of the bakery and would be aware of how full you felt from your Thai meal. Remember that, because appetite is presumed to be a psychological mechanism, you can train yourself to stop or ignore its cues when you want to avoid its consequences. Some studies suggest that appetite may have a genetic component and may be involved in food selection.

appetite A psychological desire to consume specific foods.

hunger A physiologic sensation that prompts us to eat.

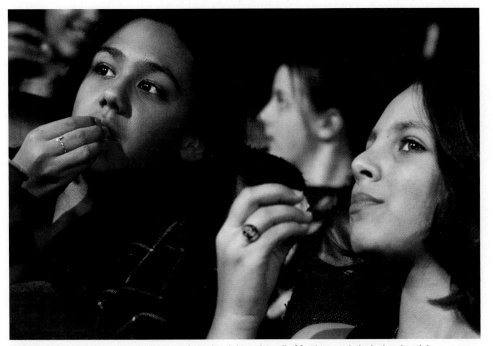

Appetite is aroused by environmental cues, from the sight and smell of food to psychological and social associations.

Recap: Appetite is thought to be a psychological desire to consume certain foods and is generally related to pleasant sensations associated with food. Appetite typically involves cravings for foods in the absence of hunger. Environments and moods contribute to appetite. For people trying to lose weight, it is important to ignore the cues of appetite to avoid overeating.

Various Factors Affect Hunger and Satiation

A number of factors influence whether we experience feelings of hunger or fullness (satiation). Signals from our brain, certain chemicals produced by our bodies, and even the amount and type of food we eat interact to cause us to feel hungry or full. Let's review these factors now.

Signals from the Brain Cause Hunger and Satiation

• Hormonal Control
  of Digestion

Because *hunger* is a physiologic sensation that prompts us to find food and eat, it is more often felt as a negative or an unpleasant sensation in which the physical drive to eat is very strong. The signal arises from within us, rather than in response to environmental stimuli, and is not typically associated with a specific food. A broad variety of foods appeal to us when we are really hungry.

One of the major organs affecting our sensation of hunger is the brain. That's right—it's not our stomachs but our brains that tell us when we're hungry. The region of brain tissue that is responsible for prompting us to seek food is called the **hypothalamus** (Figure 3.1). It triggers hunger by integrating signals from nerve cells throughout our bodies. One important signal comes from specialized cells lining the stomach and small intestine that perceive whether these organs are empty or distended by the presence of food. These cells sense changes in pressure and fullness in the stomach and small intestine and send signals to the hypothalamus. For instance, if you have not eaten for many hours and your stomach and small intestine do not contain food, signals are sent to the hypothalamus indicating it is "time to eat," which causes you to experience the sensation of hunger.

hypothalamus A region of the forebrain below the thalamus where visceral sensations, such as hunger and thirst, are regulated.

Our blood glucose levels, which reflect our bodies' most readily available fuel supply, are another primary signal affecting hunger. Falling blood glucose levels are accompanied by a change in insulin and glucagon levels. Insulin and glucagon are hormones produced in the pancreas and are responsible for maintaining blood glucose levels. These signals are relayed to the hypothalamus in the brain, where they trigger the sense that we need to eat to supply our bodies with more energy. Some people get irritable or feel a little faint when their blood glucose drops to a certain level. The level of blood glucose is related to when we last ate a meal, how active we are, and our individual metabolisms.

hormone Chemical messenger that is secreted into the bloodstream by one of the many glands of the body and acts as a regulator of the physiologic processes at a site remote from the gland that secreted it.

After we eat, the hypothalamus picks up the sensation of a distended stomach, other signals from the gut, and a rise in blood glucose levels. When it integrates these signals, you have the experience of feeling full, or *satiated*. However, as we saw in our previous scenario, even though our brain sends us clear signals about hunger, most of us become adept at ignoring them . . . and eat when we are not truly hungry.

Chemicals Called Hormones Affect Hunger and Satiation

A variety of hormones and hormone-like substances signal the hypothalamus to cause us to feel hungry or satiated. **Hormones** are chemical messengers that are secreted into the bloodstream in response to a stimulus or signal by one of the many *glands* of the body. Hormones travel in the

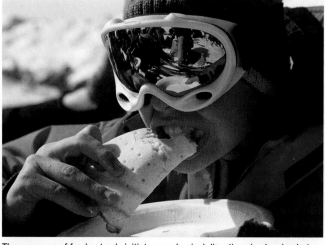

The presence of food not only initiates mechanical digestion via chewing but also initiates chemical digestion through the secretion of various substances throughout the gastrointestinal tract.

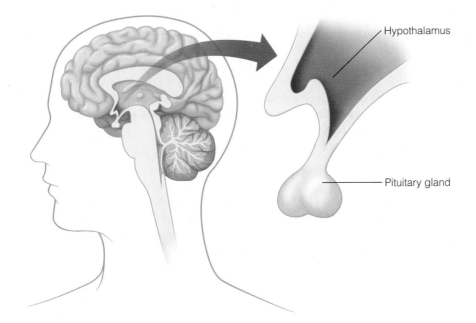

Hypothalamus

Pituitary gland

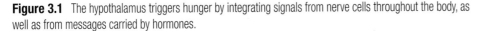

Figure 3.1 The hypothalamus triggers hunger by integrating signals from nerve cells throughout the body, as well as from messages carried by hormones.

bloodstream and exert a regulatory effect on another organ. Examples of signals include falling or rising fuels within the blood, such as blood glucose, and chemical and nervous signals from the gut and the liver. The levels of hormones in the blood then signal the hypothalamus to stimulate hunger or satiation. Examples of hormones and hormone-like substances that stimulate food intake include neuropeptide Y and galanin; those that create feelings of satiety include leptin, cholecystokinin (CCK), and serotonin (Bell and Rolls 2001).

A Canadian researcher, Dr. Larry Grovum, has tested the gut hormone CCK in pigs, which have digestive tracts that are similar to those of humans. When he injected this hormone into pigs at low dosages, it stimulated the receptors in the brain that trigger satiety; the pigs ate less at meals and had reduced appetites between. Grovum predicts that CCK supplements for humans may be safe and effective appetite suppressants in the future (University of Guelph 2007). The effects of CCK on satiety are known to be short-lived, whereas the appetite-suppressing effects of the intestine's release of the hormone PYY_{3-36} may continue for 24 hours (Batterham et al. 2002). In addition to hormones, gastric and gut peptides—chains of amino acids that are intermediate products of protein digestion—are also known to work with hormones and hormone-like substances in regulating appetite. The gastric peptide ghrelin stimulates the secretion of neuropeptide Y, which in turn causes people to feel hungry and to eat. Ghrelin appears to be activated two hours after eating and to be associated with insulin concentrations, but the mechanisms are not yet known (Blom et al. 2005). This is an area of intensive research, and the findings may one day enable us to use therapeutic measures to treat overeating and obesity.

The Amount and Type of Food We Eat Can Affect Hunger and Satiation

Foods containing protein have the highest satiety value (Bell and Rolls 2001). This means that a ham sandwich will cause us to feel satiated for a longer time than will a tossed salad and toast, even if both meals have exactly the same number of Calories. Recent research suggests that high-fat diets have a higher satiety value than previously thought. One of the reasons people may lose weight on high-protein diets is that these diets are often high in fat as well; the combined effects of both macronutrients helps people to feel full sooner than they would with a high-carbohydrate meal. High-carbohydrate diets have the lowest satiety, and people can consume quite a few calories before feeling full!

Another factor affecting hunger is how bulky the meal is—that is, how much fibre and water is within the food. Bulky meals tend to stretch the stomach and small intestine, which sends signals back to the hypothalamus telling us that we are full, so we stop eating. Beverages tend to be less satisfying than semisolid foods, and semisolid foods have a lower satiety value than solid foods. For example, if you were to eat a bunch of grapes, you would feel a greater sense of fullness than if you drank a glass of grape juice (Zorrilla 1998).

> **Recap:** In contrast to appetite, hunger is a physiologic sensation triggered by the hypothalamus in response to cues about stomach and intestinal distension, levels of energy substrates in the blood, and the release of certain hormones and hormone-like substances. High-protein and high-fat foods make us feel satiated for longer periods, and bulky meals fill us up quickly, causing the distension that signals us to stop eating.

Are We Really What We Eat?

You've no doubt heard the saying that "you are what you eat." Is this scientifically true? To answer that question, and to better understand how we digest and process foods, we'll need to look at how our body is organized (Figure 3.2).

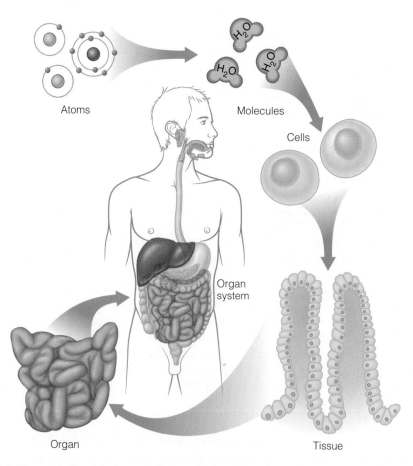

Figure 3.2 The organization of the human body. Atoms bind together to form molecules, and the body's cells are composed of molecules of the foods we eat. Cells join to form tissues, one or more types of which form organs. Body systems, such as the gastrointestinal system, are made up of several organs that perform discrete functions. For example, the small intestine is the primary site of chemical breakdown of food into molecules.

Atoms Bond to Form Molecules

Like all substances on Earth, our bodies are made up of *atoms*. Atoms are small units of matter that cannot be broken down by natural means. Atoms almost constantly bind to each other in nature. When they do, they form groups called *molecules*. For example, a molecule of water is composed of two atoms of hydrogen and an atom of oxygen, which is abbreviated H_2O.

Food Is Composed of Molecules

Molecules are critical to human life, as every particle of food we eat is composed of molecules. During digestion, we chew our food, mix it with saliva, churn it around in our stomachs, and mix it with the digestive enzymes in our small intestines. These actions result in breaking our food down into small molecules. Thus, the ultimate goal of digestion is to break the food we eat into small enough molecules that they can be easily transported through the gastrointestinal wall into the body and then travel more freely through our bloodstreams to help build the structures of our bodies and provide the energy we need to live.

> **Recap:** Our bodies are made up of atoms, which are small units of matter. Atoms group together to form molecules. The food we eat is composed of molecules. The ultimate goal of digestion is to break food into molecules small enough to be passed through the gastrointestinal tract walls and easily transported to the cells as needed.

Molecules Join to Form Cells

Whereas atoms are the smallest units of matter and make up both living and nonliving things, **cells** are the smallest units of life. That is, cells can grow, reproduce themselves, and perform certain basic functions, such as taking in nutrients, transmitting impulses, producing chemicals, and excreting wastes. The human body is composed of billions of cells that are constantly replacing themselves, destroying worn or damaged cells and manufacturing new ones. To support this constant demand for new cells, we need a ready supply of nutrient molecules, such as simple sugars, amino acids, and fatty acids, to serve as building blocks. These building blocks are the molecules that come from the breakdown of foods. All cells, whether of the skin, bones, or brain, are made of the same basic molecules of amino acids, sugars, and fatty acids that are also the main components of the foods we eat.

cell The smallest unit of matter that exhibits the properties of living things, such as growth, reproduction, and metabolism.

Cells Are Encased in a Functional Membrane

Cells are encased by a membrane called the **cell membrane**, or *plasma membrane* (Figure 3.3). This membrane is the outer covering of the cell and defines the cell's boundaries. It encloses the cell's contents and acts as a gatekeeper, either allowing or denying the entry and exit of molecules, such as nutrients and wastes.

Cell membranes comprise two layers. Each layer is made of molecules called *phospholipids*. Phospholipids consist of a long lipid "tail" bound to a round phospholipid "head." The phosphate head is **hydrophilic** (water loving and water soluble) and interacts with water, whereas the lipid tail is **hydrophobic** (dislikes water and is not water soluble) and repels water. In the cell membrane, the lipid tails of each layer face each other, forming the membrane interior, whereas the phosphate heads face either the extracellular environment or the cell's interior. Located throughout the membrane are molecules of another lipid, cholesterol, which help keep the membrane flexible. The membrane also contains various proteins that assist in transport of nutrients and other substances across the cell membrane and in the manufacture of certain chemicals.

Recall that the cell membrane is the gatekeeper that, along with its proteins, determines what goes into and out of the cell. This means cell membranes are *selectively permeable*, allowing only some compounds to enter and leave the cell.

cell membrane The boundary of an animal cell, composed of a phospholipid bilayer that separates its internal cytoplasm and organelles from the external environment.

hydrophilic Attracted to or soluble in water.
hydrophobic Not attracted to or soluble in water.

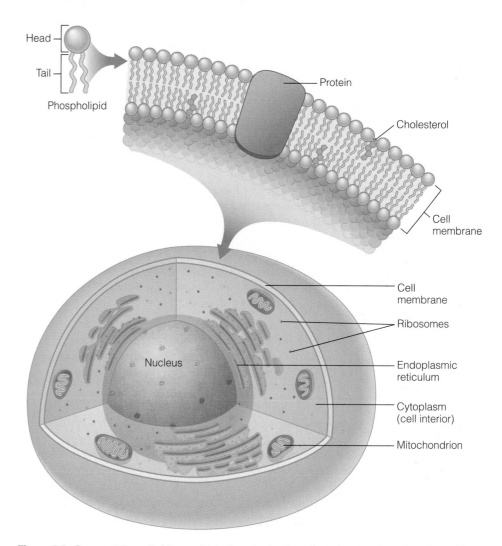

Figure 3.3 Representative cell of the small intestine, showing the cell membrane and a variety of organelles. The cell membrane is made up of phospholipid molecules, each composed of two fatty acid tails and a phosphate head. The two layers of the membrane align such that the fatty acid tails form the interior and the phosphate heads interact with the exterior aqueous environment. Inside the cell are the liquid cytoplasm and a variety of organelles.

Cells Contain Organelles That Support Life

cytoplasm The liquid within an animal cell.
organelle A tiny "organ" within a cell that performs a discrete function necessary to the cell.

Enclosed by the cell membrane is a liquid called **cytoplasm** and a variety of **organelles** (see Figure 3.3). These tiny structures accomplish some surprisingly sophisticated functions. A full description of the roles of these organelles is beyond the scope of this book, but a brief review of some of them and their functions related to nutrition is as follows:

- *Nucleus.* Our genetic information, in the form of deoxyribonucleic acid (DNA), is located in the nucleus. The cell nucleus is dark coloured because DNA is a huge molecule that is tightly packed within it. A cell's DNA contains the instructions that the cell uses to make certain proteins.

- *Ribosomes.* Ribosomes are structures the cell uses to make needed proteins.

- *Endoplasmic reticulum (ER).* The endoplasmic reticulum is important in the synthesis of proteins and lipids and the storage of the mineral calcium. The ER looks like a maze of interconnected channels.

- *Mitochondria.* Often called the cell's powerhouse, mitochondria produce the energy molecule ATP (adenosine triphosphate) from basic food components. ATP can be thought of as a stored form of energy, drawn upon as we need it. Cells that have high energy needs contain more mitochondria than cells with lower energy needs.

Recap: Cells are the smallest units of life. They perform all critical body functions, such as reproducing new cells, utilizing nutrients, transmitting nervous impulses, and excreting waste products. Cells are encased in a cell membrane that acts as a gatekeeper for the cell. Cells contain organelles, which are tiny structures that perform many functions, such as making proteins, storing nutrients, and producing energy.

Cells Join to Form Tissues and Organs

Cells of a single type, such as muscle cells, join together to form functional groupings of cells called **tissues**. We'll introduce some of the unique tissues of our gastrointestinal tract later in this chapter. In general, several types of tissues join together to form **organs**, which are sophisticated structures that perform a unique body function. The stomach and small intestine are examples of organs.

Organs Make Up Functional Body Systems

Organs are further grouped into **systems** that perform integrated functions. The stomach, for example, is an organ that is part of the gastrointestinal system. It holds and partially digests a meal, but it can't perform all system functions—digestion, absorption, and elimination—by itself. These functions require several organs working together in an integrated system. In the next section, we describe how the organs of the gastrointestinal system actually work together to accomplish digestion and absorption of foods and elimination of waste products.

Recap: Different cell types give rise to different tissue types and ultimately to different kinds of organs. Body systems, such as the gastrointestinal system, depend on many different organs to carry out all the varied functions they perform.

Digestion, Absorption, and Elimination Occur in the GI Tract

When we eat, the food we consume is digested, then the useful nutrients are absorbed, and, finally, the waste products are eliminated. But what does each of these processes really entail? In the simplest terms, **digestion** is the process by which foods are broken down into their component molecules, either mechanically or chemically. **Absorption** is the process of taking these products of digestion through the wall of the intestine for entry into the bloodstream or lymph system (described on p. 89). **Elimination** is the process by which the undigested and unabsorbed portions of food and waste products are removed from the body.

The processes of digestion, absorption, and elimination occur in the **gastrointestinal (GI) tract**, the organs of which work together to process foods. The GI tract is a long, muscular tube; if held out straight, an adult GI tract would be approximately 4.5 metres (about 15 feet) in length. Food within this tube is digested; in other words, food is broken down into molecules small enough to be absorbed by the cells lining the GI tract and thereby passed into the bloodstream to be transported through the body.

The GI tract begins at the mouth and ends at the anus (Figure 3.4). It is composed of several distinct organs, including the mouth, esophagus, stomach, small

tissue A grouping of similar cells that performs a particular set of functions; for example, muscle tissue.
organ A body structure composed of two or more tissues and performing a specific function; for example, the esophagus.

system A group of organs that work together to perform a unique function; for example, the gastrointestinal system.

Animations

- Human Digestive System
- Digestive System
- Gastrointestinal Tract Activities

digestion The process by which foods are broken down into their component molecules, either mechanically or chemically.
absorption The physiologic process by which molecules of food are taken from the gastrointestinal tract into the bloodstream to be carried to different parts of the body.
elimination The process by which the undigested and unabsorbed portions of food and waste products are removed from the body.
gastrointestinal (GI) tract A long, muscular tube consisting of several organs: the mouth, esophagus, stomach, small intestine, and large intestine.

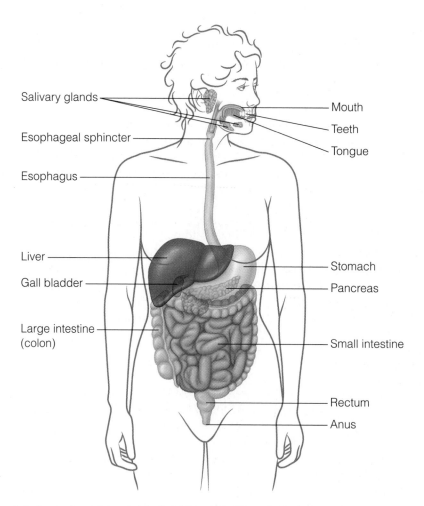

Salivary glands

Esophageal sphincter

Esophagus

Liver

Gall bladder

Large intestine
(colon)

Mouth

Teeth

Tongue

Stomach

Pancreas

Small intestine

Rectum

Anus

Figure 3.4 An overview of the gastrointestinal (GI) tract. The GI tract begins in the mouth and ends at the anus and is composed of numerous organs.

sphincter A tight ring of muscle separating some of the organs of the GI tract and opening in response to nerve signals indicating that food is ready to pass into the next section.

intestine, and large intestine (also called the colon or large bowel). These organs are kept somewhat separated by muscular **sphincters**, which are tight rings of muscle that open when a nerve signal indicates that food is ready to pass into the next section. Sphincters control the rate at which food flows from one organ to the next and prevent backflow. Surrounding the GI tract are several accessory organs, including the salivary glands, liver, pancreas, and gallbladder, each of which has a specific role in digestion and absorption of nutrients.

Now let's take a look at the role of each of these organs in processing the food we eat. Imagine that you ate a turkey sandwich for lunch today. It contained two slices of bread spread with mayonnaise, some turkey, two lettuce leaves, and a slice of tomato. Let's travel along with the sandwich and see what happens as it enters your GI tract and is digested into your body.

Recap: Digestion is the process by which foods are broken down into molecules. Absorption is the process of taking the products of digestion across the GI tract walls and into the body. Elimination is the process by which undigested food, unabsorbed nutrients, and waste products are excreted from the body. These processes take place in the gastrointestinal (GI) tract. The organs of the GI tract include the mouth, esophagus, stomach, small intestine, and large intestine (also called the colon or large bowel). Accessory organs, such as the pancreas, gallbladder, and liver, assist with digestion and absorption of nutrients.

Digestion Begins in the Mouth

Believe it or not, the first step in the digestive process is not your first bite of that sandwich. It is your first thought about what you wanted for lunch and your first whiff of turkey and freshly baked bread as you stood in line at the deli. In this **cephalic phase** of digestion, hunger and appetite work together to prepare the GI tract to digest food. The nervous system stimulates the release of digestive juices in preparation for food entering the GI tract, and sometimes we experience some involuntary movement commonly called hunger pangs.

Now, let's stop smelling that sandwich and take a bite and chew! Chewing is very important because it moistens the food with saliva and mechanically breaks it down into pieces small enough to swallow (Figure 3.5). Thus, chewing initiates the mechanical digestion of food. The tough coatings or skins surrounding the lettuce fibres and tomato seeds are also broken open, facilitating digestion. This is especially important when eating foods that are high in fibre, such as whole grains, fruits, vegetables, and legumes.

When we chew, everything in the sandwich mixes together: the protein in the turkey; the carbohydrates in the bread, lettuce, and tomato; the fat in the mayonnaise; and the vitamins and minerals in all the foods. The presence of food not only initiates mechanical digestion via chewing but also initiates chemical digestion through the secretion of various substances throughout the gastrointestinal tract. As our teeth cut and grind the different foods in the sandwich, more surface area is exposed to the digestive juices in our mouth. Foremost among these is **saliva**, which you secrete from your **salivary glands**. Saliva not only moistens your food but also begins the process of chemical breakdown. One component of saliva is salivary *amylase*, an enzyme that starts the process of carbohydrate digestion in the mouth. Saliva also contains other components, such as antibodies that protect the body from foreign bacteria entering the mouth and keep the oral cavity free from infection.

Salivary amylase is the first of many **enzymes** that assist our body in digesting and absorbing food. Since we will encounter many enzymes on our journey through the GI tract, let's discuss them briefly here. Enzymes are complex proteins that induce chemical changes in other substances to speed up bodily processes. Enzymes can be reused since they essentially are unchanged by the chemical reactions they catalyze. Imagine them as facilitators: a chemical reaction that might take an hour to occur independently might happen in a few seconds with the help of one or more enzymes. The action of enzymes can result in the production of new substances or assist in

cephalic phase Earliest phase of digestion in which the brain thinks about and prepares the digestive organs for the consumption of food.

saliva A mixture of water, mucus, enzymes, and other chemicals that moistens the mouth and food, binds food particles together, and begins the digestion of carbohydrates.

salivary glands A group of glands found under and behind the tongue and beneath the jaw that release saliva continually, as well as in response to the thought, sight, smell, or presence of food.

enzymes Small proteins that act on other chemicals to speed up body processes but are not apparently changed during those processes.

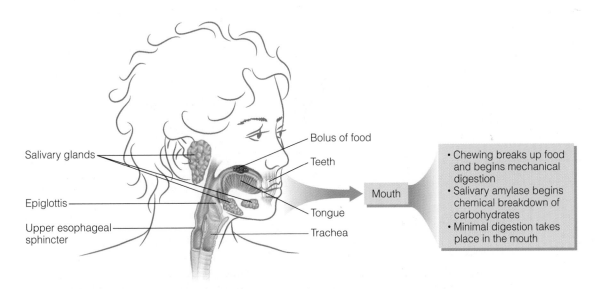

Figure 3.5 Where your food is now: the mouth. Chewing moistens food and mechanically breaks it down into pieces small enough to swallow, while salivary amylase begins the chemical digestion of carbohydrates.

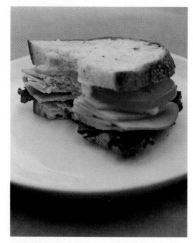

Digestion of a sandwich starts before you even take a bite.

breaking substances apart. We make hundreds of enzymes in our bodies, and the process of digestion—as well as many other biochemical processes that go on in our bodies—could not happen without them. Enzyme names often end in *-ase* (as in amylase), so they will be easy to recognize as we go through the digestive process.

In reality, very little digestion occurs in the mouth. This is because we do not hold food in our mouths for very long and because not all the enzymes needed to break down our food are present in our saliva. Salivary amylase starts the digestion of carbohydrates in the mouth, and this digestion continues in the esophagus and the stomach. Once the salivary amylase mixes with the stomach acids, it is destroyed.

Recap: The cephalic phase of digestion involves hunger and appetite working together to prepare the GI tract for digestion and absorption before you take your first bite of food. Chewing initiates mechanical digestion of food by breaking it into smaller components and mixing all nutrients together. Chewing also stimulates chemical digestion through the secretion of digestive juices, such as saliva. Saliva moistens food and starts the process of carbohydrate digestion through the action of the enzyme salivary amylase. This action continues during the transport of food through the esophagus and stops when food mixes with stomach acids.

The Esophagus Propels Food into the Stomach

Now that our sandwich is soft and moist in our mouths, it is time to swallow (Figure 3.6). Most of us take swallowing for granted. However, it is a very complex process involving voluntary and involuntary motion. A tiny flap of tissue called the *epiglottis* acts like a trapdoor covering the entrance to the trachea (or windpipe). The epiglottis is normally open, allowing us to breathe freely even while chewing (Figure 3.6a). As our bite of sandwich moves to the very back of the mouth it is now called a **bolus** of food. Our brain is sent a signal to temporarily raise the soft palate and close the openings to our nasal passages, preventing the aspiration of food or liquid into our sinuses (Figure 3.6b). The brain also signals the epiglottis to close during swallowing so food and liquid cannot enter our trachea. Sometimes this

bolus A mouthful of chewed and moistened food that has been swallowed.

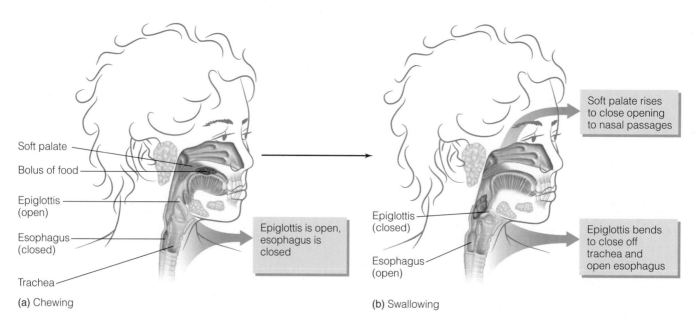

Soft palate
Bolus of food
Epiglottis (open)
Esophagus (closed)
Trachea

(a) Chewing

Epiglottis is open, esophagus is closed

Soft palate rises to close opening to nasal passages

Epiglottis (closed)
Esophagus (open)

Epiglottis bends to close off trachea and open esophagus

(b) Swallowing

Figure 3.6 Chewing and swallowing are complex processes. (a) During the process of chewing, the epiglottis is open and the esophagus is closed so that we can continue to breathe as we chew. (b) During swallowing, the epiglottis closes so that food does not enter the trachea and obstruct our breathing. The soft palate also rises to seal off our nasal passages to prevent aspiration of food or liquid into the sinuses.

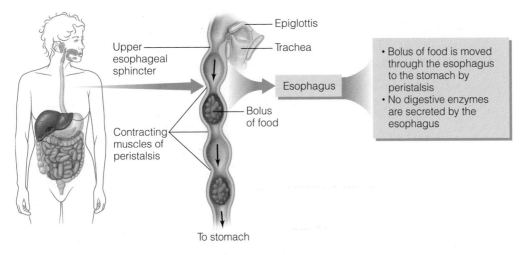

Figure 3.7 Where your food is now: the esophagus. Peristalsis, the rhythmic contraction and relaxation of both circular and longitudinal muscles in the esophagus, propels food toward the stomach. Peristalsis occurs throughout the GI tract.

protective mechanism goes awry, for instance when we try to eat and talk at the same time—sometimes referred to as "food going down the wrong way." When this happens, we experience the sensation of choking and typically cough involuntarily and repeatedly until the offending food or liquid is expelled from the trachea.

As the trachea closes, the **esophagus** opens. This muscular tube connects and transports food from the mouth to the stomach (Figure 3.7). It does this by contracting two sets of muscles: inner sheets of circular muscle squeeze the food, while outer sheets of longitudinal muscle push food along the length of the tube. Together, these rhythmic waves of squeezing and pushing are called **peristalsis**. We will see shortly that peristalsis occurs throughout the GI tract.

Gravity has a small effect in helping to transport food down the esophagus, which is one reason that it is wise to avoid reclining immediately after eating a meal. Together, peristalsis and gravity can transport a bite of food from our mouth to the opening of the stomach in five to eight seconds. At the end of the esophagus is a sphincter muscle, the *lower esophageal sphincter*, or cardiac sphincter (Figure 3.8) which is normally tightly closed. When food reaches the end of the esophagus, this sphincter relaxes to allow the passage of very small amounts of food into the stomach. In some people, this sphincter is continually somewhat relaxed. Later in the chapter, we'll discuss this disorder and the unpleasant symptoms caused when this sphincter does not function properly.

Recap: Swallowing causes our nasal passages to close and the epiglottis to cover our trachea to prevent food from entering our sinuses and lungs. The esophagus opens as the trachea closes. The esophagus is a muscular tube that transports food from the mouth to the stomach. The rhythmic waves of muscles surrounding the esophagus, called peristalsis, push food toward the stomach. Gravity helps move food toward the stomach to a lesser extent. Once food reaches the stomach, the lower esophageal sphincter (or cardiac sphincter) opens to allow food into the stomach.

The Stomach Mixes, Digests, and Holds Food

The **stomach** is a J-shaped organ. The size of the stomach is fairly individual; in general, its volume is about 180 mL (6 fl. oz.) when it is empty. When the stomach is full, it can expand to hold about 1 litre (about 32 fl. oz.) (Kim et al. 2001). Before any food reaches the stomach, the brain sends signals telling it to be ready for the

esophagus Muscular tube of the GI tract connecting the back of the mouth to the stomach.

peristalsis Waves of squeezing and pushing contractions that move food in one direction through the length of the GI tract.

stomach A J-shaped organ where food is partially digested, churned, and held until its release into the small intestine.

gastric juice Acidic liquid secreted within the stomach; it contains hydrochloric acid, pepsin, water, and other compounds.

denature A term used to describe the action of unfolding proteins. Proteins must be denatured before they can be digested.

chyme Semifluid mass consisting of partially digested food, water, and gastric juices.

food to arrive. The hormone gastrin is secreted after you eat a meal; this hormone acts on gastric cells and stimulates them to secrete digestive juices. The stomach also prepares for your sandwich by secreting **gastric juice**, which contains several important compounds:

- *Hydrochloric acid (HCl)* keeps the stomach interior very acidic—the pH of gastric juice is about 2.0, the same as lemon juice. This acid is extremely important for digestion because it starts to **denature** proteins, which means it destroys the bonds that maintain the three-dimensional structure of proteins. HCl also converts *pepsinogen*, an inactive substance, into the active enzyme *pepsin*, which assists in protein digestion. HCl performs another important function: it kills many bacteria and germs that may have entered your body with your sandwich.

- *Pepsin* begins to digest proteins into smaller components. Recall that salivary amylase begins to digest carbohydrates in the mouth. In contrast, proteins and fats enter the stomach largely unchanged. Pepsin begins the digestion of protein and activates many other GI enzymes needed to digest your meal.

- *Gastric lipase* is one enzyme responsible for fat digestion. Thus, it begins to break apart the fat in the turkey and the mayonnaise in your sandwich. Only minimal digestion of fat occurs in the stomach because not much gastric lipase is produced in adults. (This enzyme is more important in babies.)

- Cells in the stomach wall also secrete *mucus,* a thick white fluid that protects its lining from being digested by the HCl and pepsin.

With these gastric juices already present, the chemical digestion of proteins and fats begins as soon as food enters your stomach (Figure 3.8). The stomach has several other jobs, too. One is to mix and churn the food until it becomes a liquid called **chyme**. The stomach has three bands of muscles—longitudinal, circular, and diagonal—which give it the strongest muscles of any organ in the GI tract. This physical mixing and churning of food is another example of mechanical digestion that takes place in the gastrointestinal tract. Enzymes can access the liquid chyme more easily than more solid forms of food. This access allows chemical digestion to take place more easily.

Although most absorption occurs in the small intestine, the stomach lining does begin absorbing a few substances. These include water, some medium-chain fatty acids (Davidson 2003), and some drugs, including Aspirin and alcohol.

Another of your stomach's jobs is to store your sandwich (or what's left of it!) while the next part of the digestive tract, the small intestine, gets ready for the next wave of food. Remember that the stomach can hold about 1 litre (32 fl. oz.) of food. If this amount suddenly moved into the small intestine all at once, it would overwhelm it.

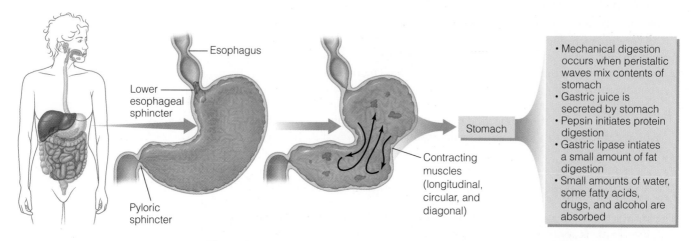

Figure 3.8 Where your food is now: the stomach. In the stomach, the protein and fat in your sandwich begin to be digested. Your meal is churned into chyme and held until release into the small intestine.

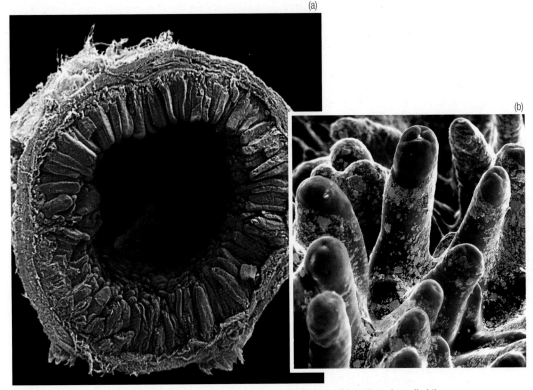

(a)

(b)

The small intestine. (a) The interior of the small intestine. (b) The wall of the small intestine, also called the mucosal membrane, has thousands of folds and fingerlike projections called villi that increase its surface area more than 500 times, significantly increasing the small intestine's absorptive capacity.

The pyloric sphincter regulates the release of food (chyme) from the stomach into the first part of the small intestine, called the duodenum. It opens and quickly closes about three times a minute to let tiny amounts of chyme (about 5 mL or 1 tsp) enter the duodenum. The remaining chyme is held in the stomach until it all passes through the pyloric sphincter—within about two hours (see Figure 3.8).

> **Recap:** The stomach prepares itself for digestion by secreting gastric juice. Gastric juice contains substances that assist in digestion, including hydrochloric acid and the enzymes pepsin and gastric lipase. The stomach wall also secretes mucus to protect the stomach's lining from digestion by HCl and enzymes. Digestion of proteins and minimal digestion of fats begins in the stomach. The stomach mixes food into a liquidy substance called chyme, which is more easily digested than solid food. The stomach holds the acidic chyme and releases it periodically into the small intestine through the pyloric sphincter in very small amounts (about 5 mL or 1 tsp).

Most of Digestion and Absorption Occurs in the Small Intestine

The **small intestine** is the longest portion of the GI tract, accounting for about two thirds (about 3 metres or 10 feet) of its length. However, at only 2.5 cm (1 in.) in diameter, it is comparatively narrow.

   The small intestine is composed of three sections (Figure 3.9). The *duodenum* is the section of the small intestine that is connected via the pyloric sphincter to the stomach. The *jejunum* is the middle portion, and the last portion is the *ileum*. It connects to the large intestine at another sphincter, called the *ileocecal valve*.

   Most of digestion and absorption take place in the small intestine. Here, food is broken down into its smallest components, molecules that the body can then absorb into its internal environment. In this next section we review a variety of accessory

small intestine The longest portion of the GI tract, where most digestion and absorption takes place.

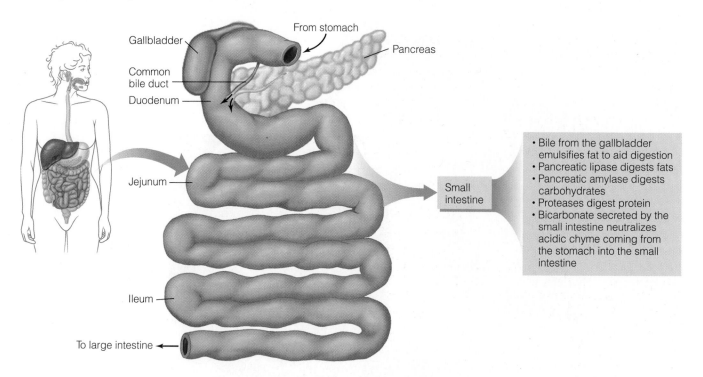

Labels on figure: Gallbladder, Common bile duct, Duodenum, Jejunum, Ileum, To large intestine, From stomach, Pancreas, Small intestine

Text box:
- Bile from the gallbladder emulsifies fat to aid digestion
- Pancreatic lipase digests fats
- Pancreatic amylase digests carbohydrates
- Proteases digest protein
- Bicarbonate secreted by the small intestine neutralizes acidic chyme coming from the stomach into the small intestine

Figure 3.9 Where your food is now: the small intestine. Here, most of the digestion and absorption of the nutrients in your sandwich take place.

organs, enzymes, and unique anatomical features of the small intestine that permit maximal absorption of most nutrients.

The Gallbladder and Pancreas Aid in Digestion

Now let's get back to your sandwich. As the fat from the turkey and mayonnaise enters the small intestine, a hormone called cholecystokinin (or CCK) is released in response to the presence of protein and fat. This substance signals an accessory organ, the **gallbladder**, to contract. The gallbladder is located beneath the liver (see Figure 3.4), and it concentrates and stores a greenish fluid, **bile**, produced by the liver. Contraction of the gallbladder sends bile through the *common bile duct* into the duodenum. Bile then *emulsifies* the fat; that is, it reduces the fat into smaller globules and disperses them so they are more accessible to digestive enzymes.

The **pancreas**, another accessory organ, manufactures, holds, and secretes digestive enzymes. It is located behind the stomach (see Figure 3.4). Enzymes secreted by the pancreas include *pancreatic amylase*, which continues the digestion of carbohydrates, and *pancreatic lipase*, which continues the digestion of fats. *Proteases,* such as trypsin, are secreted in pancreatic juice to digest proteins. The pancreas is also responsible for manufacturing hormones that are important in metabolism. Insulin and glucagon, two hormones necessary to regulate the amount of glucose in the blood, are produced by the pancreas.

Another essential role of the pancreas is to secrete bicarbonate into the duodenum. Bicarbonate is a base and, like all bases, is capable of neutralizing acids. Recall that chyme leaving the stomach is very acidic. The pancreatic bicarbonate neutralizes this acidic chyme so that the pancreatic enzymes will work effectively and to ensure that the lining of the duodenum is not eroded. Thus, the pH in the small intestine is approximately neutral (7 pH).

Now the protein, carbohydrate, and fat in your sandwich have been processed into a liquid that contains molecules of nutrients small enough for absorption. This molecular "soup" continues to move along the small intestine via peristalsis, encountering the absorptive cells of the intestinal lining along the way.

gallbladder A tissue sac beneath the liver that concentrates and stores bile and secretes it into the small intestine.

bile Fluid produced by the liver and stored in the gallbladder; it emulsifies fats in the small intestine.

pancreas An accessory organ located behind the stomach; it secretes digestive enzymes that break down proteins, carbohydrates, and fats.

A Specialized Lining Enables the Small Intestine to Absorb Food

The wall of the small intestine is especially well suited for absorption. If you looked at the inside of the lining, which is also referred to as the mucosal membrane, you would notice that it is heavily folded (Figure 3.10). This feature increases the surface area of the small intestine and allows it to absorb more nutrients than if it were smooth. Within these larger folds, you would notice even smaller fingerlike projections called *villi*, whose constant movement helps them to encounter and trap nutrient molecules. Inside each villus are *capillaries*, or tiny blood vessels, and a **lacteal**, which is a small lymph vessel. (The role of the lymphatic system is presented on page 91.) These vessels take up the final products of digestion. Water-soluble nutrients are absorbed directly into the bloodstream, while most fat-soluble nutrients are absorbed into lymph. Covering these villi are specialized cells covered with hairlike structures called *microvilli*. The microvilli look like tiny brushes and are sometimes referred to as the **brush border**. These intricate folds increase the surface area of the small intestine by more than 500 times, which tremendously increases the absorptive capacity of the small intestine.

The deep crypt glands found between villi secrete intestinal juices into the small intestine. These intestinal juices contain enzymes that break down carbohydrate, fat, and protein into smaller components. The goblet cells found on the surface of the villi secrete mucus to protect the cells lining the small intestine from being harmed by digestive juices.

lacteal A small lymph vessel located inside of the villi of the small intestine.

brush border Term that describes the microvilli of the small intestine's lining. These microvilli tremendously increase the small intestine's absorptive capacity.

- Passive Transport
- Selective Permeability

Intestinal Cells Readily Absorb Vitamins, Minerals, and Water

The turkey sandwich you ate contained several vitamins and minerals in addition to protein, carbohydrate, and fat. For instance, the bread contained B vitamins and

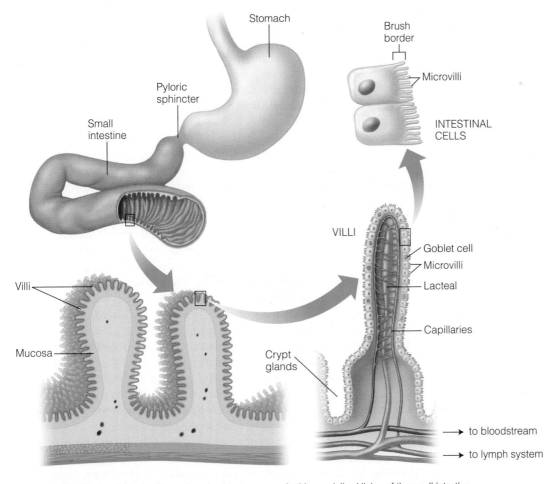

Figure 3.10 The brush border. Absorption of nutrients occurs via this specialized lining of the small intestine.

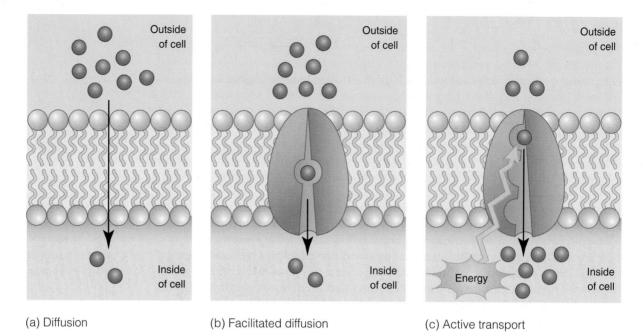

(a) Diffusion

(b) Facilitated diffusion

(c) Active transport

Figure 3.11 Nutrient absorption by (a) simple diffusion, (b) facilitated diffusion, and (c) active transport.

iron, and the tomato contained vitamin C. If you had a glass of milk with your sandwich, you also consumed the mineral calcium as well as vitamins A and D. The turkey contained some of the mineral zinc. Most of the sandwich also contained small amounts of sodium, potassium, and chloride.

Approximately three to four hours after you ate your turkey sandwich, the protein, fat, and carbohydrates it contained have been digested and the end products, as well as the vitamins and minerals, are ready to be removed from the lumen (interior) of the small intestine. They must pass through the cells of the intestinal wall to reach the bloodstream or lymphatic vessels that carry them through the body. This process of absorbing nutrients across the intestinal wall is typically one of simple diffusion or active transport (see Figure 3.11).

Vitamins and minerals do not have to be broken down or digested in the same way as macronutrients because they are already small enough to be readily absorbed by *simple diffusion*—sometimes called *passive diffusion*—across the intestinal wall. Some water-soluble vitamins, such as the B vitamins and vitamin C, are absorbed by *facilitated diffusion,* which requires specific carriers to take them from one side of the cell wall to the other. This helps to ensure that the vitamins get absorbed from the small intestine. Such nutrients as glucose and amino acids need *active transport*, a process requiring energy, to be moved across the cell wall.

Minerals are absorbed all along the small intestine, and in some cases in the large intestine as well, by a wide variety of mechanisms. For example, the absorption of sodium, potassium, and chloride is regulated by nerves and hormones working together to maintain water and salt balance (see Chapter 7). These minerals are absorbed in both the small and large intestines. Iron absorption increases or decreases according to the body's needs. One way the body regulates the amount of iron absorbed is by holding the iron in the mucosal cell until needed. The cells turn over every 24 to 72 hours, so any excess iron can be lost as the cell is sloughed off. There is also a specialized protein in the membrane of intestinal cells that can transport needed iron into the body (see Chapter 10). Zinc, copper, and manganese can each be absorbed with the help of a carrier protein, but they can also pass through the intestinal cells unassisted.

Finally, a large component of food is water, and of course you also drink lots of water throughout the day. Water is readily absorbed along the entire length of the GI tract because it is a small molecule that can easily pass through the cell membrane. However, as we will see shortly, a significant percentage of water is absorbed in the large intestine.

Blood and Lymph Transport Nutrients and Fluids

Our bodies have two main fluids that transport nutrients, water, and waste products throughout the body. These fluids are blood and lymph. Blood travels through the cardiovascular system, and lymph travels through the lymphatic system (Figure 3.12). The oxygen we inhale into our lungs is carried by our red blood cells. This oxygen-rich blood then travels to the heart, where it is pumped out to our body. Blood travels to all our tissues to deliver nutrients and other materials and pick up waste products. As blood travels through the GI tract, it picks up most nutrients and fluids that are absorbed through the wall of the small intestine. The lymphatic vessels pick up most fats and fat-soluble vitamins and fluids that have escaped from the cardiovascular system and transport them in the lymph. The contents of the lymph eventually enter the bloodstream in an area near the heart where the lymphatic and blood vessels join together.

As blood leaves the GI system, it is transported to the liver. The role of the liver in digestion is described in the following section. The waste products picked up by the blood as it circulates around the body are filtered and excreted by the kidneys. In addition, much of the carbon dioxide remaining in the blood once it reaches the lungs is exhaled into the outside air, making room for oxygen to attach to the red blood cells and repeat this cycle of circulation again.

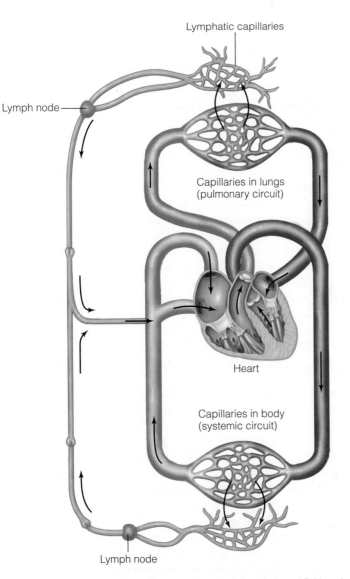

Figure 3.12 Blood travels through the cardiovascular system to transport nutrients and fluids and pick up waste products. Lymph travels through the lymphatic system and transports most fats and fat-soluble vitamins.

The Liver Regulates Blood Nutrients

liver The largest accessory organ of the GI tract and one of the most important organs of the body. Its functions include producing bile, processing nutrient-rich blood from the small intestine, and detoxifying harmful substances.

Once nutrients are absorbed from the small intestine, most enter the *portal vein*, which carries them to the **liver**. The liver is a triangular, wedge-shaped organ of about 1.4 kg (3 lb.) of tissue that rests almost entirely within the protection of the rib cage on the right side of the body (see Figure 3.4). The liver is the largest accessory organ of the digestive tract; it is also one of the most important organs in the body, performing more than 500 discrete functions. One function of the liver is to receive the products of digestion, and then release into the bloodstream those nutrients needed throughout the body. The liver also processes and stores monosaccharides, triglycerides (fats), and amino acids, and plays a major role in regulating these energy nutrients. For instance, after we eat a meal, the liver picks up excess glucose from the blood and stores it as glycogen, releasing it into the bloodstream when we need energy later in the day. It also stores certain vitamins and manufactures blood proteins. The liver can even make glucose from various food nutrients when necessary to make sure that our blood glucose levels stay constant. Thus, the liver plays a major role in regulating the level and type of fuel or energy nutrients circulating in our blood.

Have you ever wondered why people who abuse alcohol are at risk for damaging their liver? That's because another of its functions is to filter the blood, removing wastes and toxins like alcohol, medications, and other drugs. When you drink, your liver works hard to replace the cells poisoned with alcohol, but, over time, scar tissue forms. The scar tissue blocks the free flow of blood through the liver, so that any further toxins accumulate in the blood, causing confusion, coma, and, ultimately, death.

Another important job of the liver is to synthesize many of the chemicals used by the body in carrying out metabolic processes. For example, the liver synthesizes bile, which is then concentrated and stored in the gallbladder until needed to emulsify fats so they can be digested.

> **Recap:** Most digestion and absorption occurs in the small intestine. The small intestine comprises three sections: the duodenum, the jejunum, and the ileum. The gallbladder concentrates and stores bile, which is produced by the liver. Bile emulsifies fat into pieces that are more easily digested. The pancreas synthesizes and secretes digestive enzymes that break down carbohydrates, fats, and proteins into their basic building blocks: sugars, fatty acids, and amino acids. The lining of the small intestine is heavily folded, with the surface area expanded by villi and microvilli. Nutrients are absorbed across the mucosal membrane by various processes and enter either the lymph or the bloodstream. The liver processes all nutrients absorbed from the small intestine and stores and regulates monosaccharides (p. 112), fatty acids (p. 154), and amino acids (p. 194).

The Large Intestine Holds Food Waste Until It Is Excreted

large intestine The final organ of the GI tract, consisting of the cecum, colon, rectum, and anal canal, and in which most water is absorbed and feces are formed.

The **large intestine** is a thick, tubelike structure that frames the small intestine on three-and-a-half sides (Figure 3.13). It begins with a tissue sac called the *cecum*, which explains the name of the sphincter—the *ileocecal valve*—which connects it to the ileum of the small intestine. From the cecum, the large intestine continues up along the left side of the small intestine as the *ascending colon*. The *transverse colon* runs across the top of the small intestine, and then the *descending colon* comes down on the right. The *sigmoid colon* is the last segment of the colon, and extends from the bottom right corner to the *rectum*. The last segment of the large intestine is the *anal canal*, which is about 4 cm (1.5 in.) long.

What has happened to our turkey sandwich? The undigested and unabsorbed food components finally reach the large intestine. By this time, the digestive mass entering the large intestine does not resemble the chyme that left the stomach several hours before. This is because a majority of the nutrients have been absorbed, leaving mostly indigestible food material, such as fibre, bacteria, and water. The intestinal

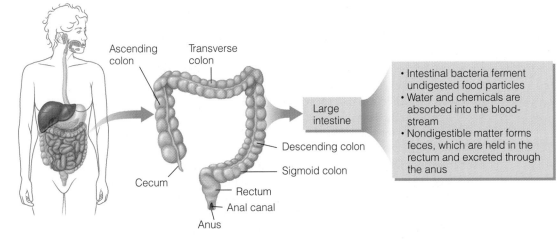

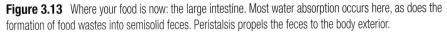

Figure 3.13 Where your food is now: the large intestine. Most water absorption occurs here, as does the formation of food wastes into semisolid feces. Peristalsis propels the feces to the body exterior.

bacteria are normal and helpful residents, since they ferment some of the nutrients from your sandwich. The byproducts of this fermentation, such as short-chain fatty acids, are reabsorbed into the body where they return to the liver and are either stored or used as needed. The bacteria living in our large intestine are so helpful that, as discussed in the Nutrition Debate at the end of this chapter, many people consume them deliberately! The main functions of the large intestine are to hold the digestive mass for 12 to 24 hours, and during that time to absorb nutrients and water from it, leaving a semisolid mass called *feces*. Peristalsis occurs weakly to move the feces through the colon, except for one or more stronger waves of peristalsis each day that force the feces more powerfully toward the rectum for elimination through the anus. This elimination of feces is called a bowel movement.

> **Recap:** The large intestine comprises seven sections: the cecum, ascending colon, transverse colon, descending colon, sigmoid colon, rectum, and the anal canal. Small amounts of undigested food, indigestible food material, bacteria, and water enter the large intestine from the small intestine. The bacteria assist with final fermentation of any remaining digestible food products; this fermentation causes some gas production. The main functions of the large intestine are to hold the digestive mass and absorb any remaining nutrients and water over a 12- to 24-hour period. The remaining substance, a semisolid mass called feces, is then eliminated from the body through the anus.

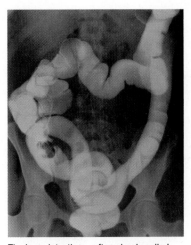

The large intestine—often simply called the colon or bowel—is a thick, tubelike structure that stores the undigested mass leaving the small intestine and absorbs any remaining nutrients and water.

How Does the Body Coordinate and Regulate Digestion?

To complete your picture of the gastrointestinal system, it might help to think of your body as a manufacturing plant with the GI tract as its assembly line. Here, all the raw, unprocessed materials (foods) needed by the manufacturing plant to synthesize new products arrive. As the raw materials are processed, they are broken down into usable parts. These parts are then sent to other departments to be reassembled into new products. Wastes and unwanted parts are excreted at the end of the assembly line. Now that you can identify the organs involved in this process and the jobs they each perform, you might be wondering—who's the boss? In other words, what organ or system directs and coordinates all of these interrelated processes? The answer is the neuromuscular system. Each of its two components, the nervous and muscular systems, is an essential partner in coordinating and regulating the digestion, absorption, and elimination of food.

The Muscles of the Gastrointestinal Tract Mix and Move Food

The purpose of the muscles of the GI tract is to mix food and move it in one direction; that is, from the mouth toward the anus. When food is present, nerves respond to the stretching of the tract walls and send signals to its muscles, stimulating peristalsis. As with the assembly line, the entire GI tract functions together so that materials are moved in one direction in a coordinated manner and wastes are removed as needed.

To process the large amount of food we consume daily, we use both voluntary and involuntary muscles. Muscles in the mouth are primarily voluntary; that is, they are under our conscious control. Once we swallow, involuntary muscles largely take over to propel food through the rest of the GI tract until we use voluntary muscles to expel feces from our bodies. The involuntary muscles enable us to continue digesting and absorbing our food while we're working, exercising, and even sleeping. Let's now reveal the master controller behind these involuntary muscular actions.

The Enteric Nerves Coordinate and Regulate Digestive Activities

The nervous system in your body is like the wiring and communications system in the manufacturing plant. It enables communication between the assembly line and all other departments, allowing the transfer of messages about when to start and stop various functions, how to operate, and what is needed in other parts of the manufacturing plant. Within this communications system, the central nervous system (CNS) is like the main control desk, and each body system or region has its own branch nerves. The CNS is composed of the brain and spinal cord. As discussed earlier in this chapter, the hypothalamus of the brain plays an important role in control of hunger and satiation.

There is also an intricate system of nerves and other structures outside of the CNS; this system is called the peripheral nervous system. The nerves of the GI tract are found within the peripheral nervous system and are collectively known as the **enteric nervous system**.

enteric nervous system The nerves of the GI tract.

Enteric nerves work both independently of and in collaboration with the CNS. For example, they can respond independently to signals produced within the GI tract without first relaying them to the CNS for interpretation or assistance. On the other hand, many jobs require the involvement of the CNS. For instance, as we discussed earlier, special nerves in the GI tract pick up mechanical signals indicating how far the tract wall is stretched, that is, how full it is. These receptors signal the brain that your digestive tract is full, and then your brain sends out messages that prompt you to stop eating. Another type of enteric nerve picks up chemical signals about how acidic the digestive environment is or if protein or fat is present. The CNS receives and responds to these signals, sending out a message to the pancreas to secrete enzymes for fat and protein digestion, for example.

All along the GI tract are a series of glands that secrete digestive juices, mucus, and water. These secretions are also under nervous system control. When food digestion products reach various locations within the GI tract, these glands are stimulated to release digestive enzymes, mucus, or water and electrolytes. For example, as chyme moves from the stomach into the small intestine, neural signals are sent to stimulate the pancreas, gallbladder, and mucosal cells lining the intestinal tract. These signals cause these glands and cells to secrete digestive enzymes, bile, bicarbonate, and water, secretions necessary to continue digestion in the small intestine.

> **Recap:** The coordination and regulation of digestion is directed by the neuromuscular system. The muscles of the GI tract mix food and move it from the mouth to the anus. Voluntary muscles, which are under our conscious control, assist us with chewing and swallowing and with expelling waste from our bodies. Once food is swallowed, the involuntary muscles along the entire length of the GI tract function together so that materials are moved in one direction in a coordinated manner. The enteric nerves of the GI tract work with the central nervous system to achieve digestion, absorption, and elimination of wastes.

What Disorders Are Related to Digestion, Absorption, and Elimination?

Considering the complexity of digestion, absorption, and elimination, it's no wonder that sometimes things go wrong. Disorders of the neuromuscular system, hormonal imbalances, infections, allergies, and a host of other disorders can disturb gastrointestinal functioning, as can merely consuming the wrong types or amounts of food for our unique needs. Whenever there is a problem with the GI tract, the digestion and absorption of nutrients can be affected. If absorption of a nutrient is less than optimal for a long time, malnutrition can result. Let's look more closely at some GI tract disorders and what you might be able to do if they affect you.

Heartburn and Gastroesophageal Reflux Disease (GERD)

When you eat food, your stomach secretes hydrochloric acid to start the gastric phase of the digestive process. In many people, the amount of HCl secreted is occasionally excessive or the gastroesophageal sphincter opens too soon. In either case, the result is that HCl seeps back up into the esophagus (Figure 3.14). Although the stomach is protected from HCl by a thick coat of mucus, the esophagus does not have this mucus coating. Thus, the HCl burns it. When this happens, a person experiences a painful sensation in the region of his or her chest above the sternum (breastbone). This condition is commonly called **heartburn**. People often take over-the-counter antacids to neutralize the HCl, thereby relieving the heartburn. A non-drug approach is to repeatedly swallow: this action causes any acid within the esophagus to be swept down into the stomach, eventually relieving the symptoms.

Gastroesophageal reflux disease (GERD) is a more painful type of heartburn that occurs more than twice per week. GERD affects about 13% of Canadians and, like heartburn, occurs when HCl flows back from the stomach into the esophagus. Although people who experience occasional heartburn usually have no structural abnormalities, many people with GERD have an overly relaxed or damaged lower esophageal sphincter or damage to the esophagus itself. Symptoms of GERD include persistent heartburn and acid regurgitation. Some people have GERD without heartburn and instead experience chest pain, trouble swallowing, burning in the mouth, the feeling that food is stuck in the throat, or hoarseness in the morning (NDDIC May 2007).

The exact causes of GERD are unknown. However, a number of factors may contribute, including the following (NDDIC May 2007):

- A *hiatal hernia*, which occurs when the upper part of the stomach lies above the diaphragm muscle. Normally, the diaphragm muscle separates the stomach from the chest and helps keep acid from coming into the esophagus. Stomach acid can more easily enter the esophagus in people with a hiatal hernia.

- Cigarette smoking.

- Alcohol use.

- Overweight.

- Pregnancy.

- Foods, such as citrus fruits, chocolate, caffeinated drinks, fried foods, garlic and onions, spicy foods, and tomato-based foods, such as chili, pizza, and spaghetti sauce.

- Large, high-fat meals. These meals stay in the stomach longer and increase stomach pressure, making it more likely that acid will be pushed up into the esophagus.

- Lying down soon after a meal. This is almost certain to bring on symptoms, since it positions the body so that it is easier for the stomach acid to back up into the esophagus.

heartburn The painful sensation that occurs over the sternum when hydrochloric acid backs up from the stomach into the lower esophagus.

gastroesophageal reflux disease (GERD) A painful type of heartburn that occurs more than twice per week.

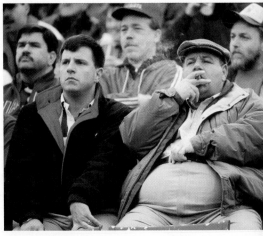

Although the exact causes of gastroesophageal reflux disease (GERD) are unknown, smoking and being overweight may be contributing factors.

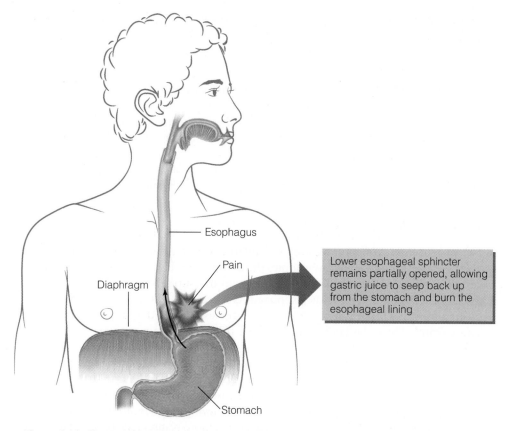

Figure 3.14 The mechanism of heartburn and gastroesophageal reflux disease is the same: acidic gastric juices seep backward through an open or a relaxed sphincter into the lower portion of the esophagus, burning its lining. The pain is felt above the sternum, over the heart.

There are ways to reduce the symptoms of GERD. One way is to identify the types of foods or situations that trigger episodes, and then avoid them. Eating smaller meals also helps. After a meal, waiting at least three hours before lying down is recommended. Some people relieve their nighttime symptoms by elevating the head of the bed 10 to 15 cm (4 to 6 in.), for instance, by placing a wedge between the mattress and the box spring. This keeps the chest area elevated and minimizes the amount of acid that can back up into the esophagus. It is also suggested that if people smoke, they should stop, and that if they are overweight, they should lose that weight. Taking an antacid before a meal can help prevent symptoms if a person accidentally eats an offending food, and there are also many other medications now prescribed to treat GERD. Many of these medications are reviewed in the Highlight box on page 98.

Another class of medications available both over the counter and by prescription are the H$_2$ blockers. Brand names include Tagamet, Pepcid AC, Axid, and Zantac 75. Prescription names include cimetidine, famotidine, and ranitidine. These medications work by stopping acid production before it starts. They do this by blocking the binding of histamine, a chemical produced during digestion, to H$_2$ receptor sites in the stomach. Most of these products can be taken 30 minutes to an hour before you expect to eat foods that may cause heartburn and can be taken to relieve heartburn once it has started. They do not relieve symptoms for at least 45 minutes after they are taken, as they cannot neutralize acid that is already in the stomach. Thus, antacids provide faster relief than H$_2$ blockers. However, if people are taking both antacids and H$_2$ blockers, they should stagger these and take the H$_2$ blockers at least one hour before consuming antacids. These products should also not be taken for more than two weeks continuously and are not recommended for children younger than 12 years of age. Potential side effects include diarrhea, constipation, headache, fatigue, mental confusion, drowsiness, and muscle aches (Marsh 1997).

The most effective medications currently available in Canada to treat GERD are proton pump inhibitors. These are available by prescription only and are marketed under the brand names of Losec, Prevacid, Pantoloc, Pariet, and Nexium. These drugs block the proton pump that is responsible for the secretion of gastric acid. These drugs are effective in reducing stomach acid production and in healing the damage caused as a result of GERD. Side effects are minimal and include mild dizziness, headache, nausea, rash, and diarrhea.

It is important to treat GERD, as it can cause serious health problems. GERD can lead to bleeding and ulcers in the esophagus. Scar tissue can develop in the esophagus, making swallowing very difficult. Some people can also develop a condition called Barrett's esophagus, which is characterized by severe damage to the cells lining the lower part of the esophagus and can lead to cancer. Asthma can also be aggravated or even caused by GERD.

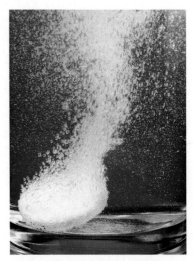

Antacids neutralize hydrochloric acid, thereby relieving heartburn.

> **Recap:** Heartburn is caused by the seepage of gastric juices into the esophagus. Gastroesophageal reflux disease (or GERD) is a painful type of heartburn that occurs more than twice per week. Factors contributing to GERD include a hiatal hernia; cigarette smoking; overweight; alcohol use; pregnancy; spicy, acidic, and fatty foods; large meals; and lying down after a meal. GERD can be treated by changing these factors and with medications. GERD can cause serious health consequences, such as esophageal bleeding, ulcers, and cancer.

Ulcers

A **peptic ulcer** is an area of the GI tract that has been eroded away by a combination of hydrochloric acid and the enzyme pepsin. In almost all cases, it is located in the stomach area (*gastric ulcer*) or the part of the duodenum closest to the stomach (*duodenal ulcer*). It causes a burning pain in the abdominal area, typically one to three hours after eating a meal. In serious cases, eroded blood vessels bleed into the GI tract, causing vomiting of blood or blood in the stools, as well as anemia. If the ulcer entirely perforates the tract wall, stomach contents can leak into the abdominal cavity, causing a life-threatening infection.

peptic ulcer An area of the GI tract that has been eroded away by the acidic gastric juices of the stomach. The two main causes of peptic ulcers are an *H. pylori* infection or use of non-steroidal anti-inflammatory drugs.

The bacterium *Helicobacter pylori* (*H. pylori*) plays a key role in development of most peptic ulcers, which include both gastric and duodenal ulcers (Chan and Leung 2002). Almost all people have this bacterium in their gastrointestinal tracts. It appears that *H. pylori* infects about 20% of people younger than 40 years of age and about 50% of people older than 60 years of age (NDDIC October 2004). Most people with *H. pylori* infection do not develop ulcers, and the reason for this is not known.

Because of the role of *H. pylori* in ulcer development, treatment usually involves antibiotics and other types of medications to reduce gastric secretions. Antacids are used to weaken the gastric acid, and the same medications used to treat GERD can be used to treat peptic ulcers. Special diets are not recommended as often as they once were because they do not reduce acid secretion. In fact, we now know that ulcers are not caused by stress or eating spicy foods.

Although most peptic ulcers are caused by *H. pylori* infection, some are caused by prolonged use of non-steroidal anti-inflammatory drugs (NSAIDs); these drugs include pain relievers, such as Aspirin, ibuprofen, and naproxen sodium. Acetaminophen use does not cause ulcers. The NSAIDs appear to cause ulcers by preventing the stomach from protecting itself from acidic gastric juices. Ulcers caused by NSAID use generally heal once a person stops taking the medication (NDDIC October 2004).

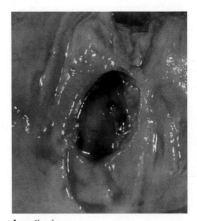

A peptic ulcer.

> **Recap:** Peptic ulcers are located in the stomach or duodenum and are caused by erosion of the GI tract by hydrochloric acid and pepsin. Peptic ulcers are painful and can lead to serious health consequences, such as internal bleeding, anemia, and potentially fatal infections. The two major causes of peptic ulcers are *Helicobacter pylori* infection and the use of non-steroidal anti-inflammatory drugs. Peptic ulcers are treated with medications.

> ▶ **HIGHLIGHT**

Medications Used to Treat Heartburn and GERD

A multitude of medications are currently available to treat GERD. Some of these are available over the counter, while others can be obtained with a prescription from your doctor. These medications work in different ways, and for many people a combination of medications is needed to treat their symptoms.

Antacids have been commonly used to treat heartburn and mild symptoms of GERD. Antacids include such products as Rolaids, Tums, Alka-Seltzer, Maalox, Pepto-Bismol, and Mylanta. These products work by neutralizing stomach acid and inhibiting the production of pepsin. They typically contain a combination of three salts—magnesium, aluminum, and calcium—combined with hydroxide or bicarbonate ions. One advantage of antacids is that they work relatively quickly to relieve symptoms; relief is virtually immediate upon consumption. Their action does not last very long, however, as they only work for about 20 to 60 minutes when taken on an empty stomach, or possibly up to three hours following a meal (Maton and Burton 1999). Because of their short-term action, antacids are often taken in combination with longer-acting medications that will be discussed shortly. Antacids also do not repair damage done to the esophagus.

Antacids are relatively safe for most people, but they do have potential side effects. These side effects are more common in people who take larger doses of antacids on a regular basis but are less common with occasional antacids use. Diarrhea is one of the most common side effects of antacid that contain magnesium. Constipation and aluminum retention can occur with antacids containing aluminum. In fact, people with kidney disease and renal failure cannot clear the aluminum, which may build up in the brain and body tissues, causing brain damage. Long-term use of high doses of aluminum-containing antacids is associated with bone loss and osteoporosis. Constipation, belching, intestinal gas, and high blood calcium levels can result from taking antacids containing calcium. These side effects occur more often in people with renal failure. People who consume a lot of dairy products and take vitamin D supplements should not consume large amounts of calcium-containing antacids, as these actions can lead to milk-alkali syndrome. This syndrome causes irritability, headache, distaste for milk, nausea, vomiting, and weakness and can lead to death (Maton and Burton 1999).

Food Allergies and Intolerances

Food allergies and intolerances have recently received a lot of attention in the media. You may have heard of allergies to foods like peanuts, eggs, dairy, or shellfish. You have also probably heard of food intolerances, such as lactose intolerance. What is the difference between a food allergy and a food intolerance? According to the U.S. National Institute of Allergy and Infectious Diseases, a **food allergy** is an actual allergic reaction to food or a hypersensitivity to a food caused by an activation of the immune system (NIAID 2003). A **food intolerance** is GI discomfort (for example, gas, pain, diarrhea, or constipation) caused by foods. A food intolerance can lead to symptoms that mimic a food allergy, but food intolerances are not caused by an immune system reaction. An example is lactose intolerance, which is discussed in Chapter 4. Food allergies are relatively rare, affecting about 8% of children and 1% to 2% of adults. Food intolerances are much more common.

food allergy An allergic reaction to food, caused by an activation of the immune system.

food intolerance Gastrointestinal discomfort caused by certain foods that is not a result of an immune system reaction.

Celiac Disease

Celiac disease, also known as *celiac sprue*, is a genetic disorder characterized by a total intolerance for gluten, a protein found in wheat, rye, triticale, and barley. It is considered to be a Caucasian disease caused by an uncontrolled immune response and is associated with the HLA-DQ2 gene. An estimated 25% of Caucasians have this gene, but, interestingly, only about 1% will develop celiac disease (American Physiological Society 2006). When a person with this disorder eats one of these grains, immune cells in the small intestine respond to the gluten as if it were a poison and cause an inflammatory response. The response destroys the gluten but in the

celiac disease A genetic disorder characterized by a total intolerance for gluten that causes an immune reaction that damages the lining of the small intestine.

process erodes the lining of the small intestine. If the person is unaware of the disorder and continues to eat gluten, repeated immune reactions cause even more damage. The villi of the small intestine become greatly decreased so there is less absorptive surface area and the enzymes located at the brush border of the small intestine become reduced. When this happens, the person becomes unable to absorb protein, fats, carbohydrate, and certain vitamins and minerals properly—a condition known as *malabsorption*. Over time, malabsorption can lead to malnutrition (poor nutrient status). Deficiencies of vitamins A, D, E, and K, iron, folic acid, and calcium are common in those suffering from celiac disease (Murray 1999).

Symptoms of this disease often mimic those of other intestinal disturbances, like irritable bowel syndrome (discussed shortly), and so the condition is often misdiagnosed. Some of the symptoms of celiac disease include fatty stools (due to poor fat absorption); frequent stools, either watery or hard, with an odd odour; cramping, anemia, pallor, weight loss, fatigue, and irritability.

Currently there is no cure for celiac disease. Treatment is with a special diet that excludes wheat, rye, triticale, and barley. Oats are allowed, but they are often contaminated with wheat flour from processing and even that small amount of wheat can cause the immune response and damage to intestinal villi. Corn, rice, tapioca, potato, arrowroot, cassava, and gluten-free breads may be used in the diet to supply the person with needed carbohydrate. Promising new research may be on the horizon, though. A team of Dutch researchers has found that an enzyme, prolyl endoprotease, produced commercially from a common fungus and used in the food industry, may "detoxify" gluten by breaking it down in the stomach before it reaches the small intestine (Stepniak et al. 2006). This enzyme works well in the acidic environment of the stomach and works 60 times faster than other enzymes that have been studied.

Besides the obvious sources of gluten—cereals, pasta, and breads—people with celiac disease must also be aware of hidden sources in packaged and processed foods. Gluten is often used as a filler or thickener and can be found in such foods as sausages, soups, ice creams, and soy sauce. People with celiac disease need to read labels carefully and contact manufacturers when they are in doubt about a product's ingredients. Eating out requires learning to ask questions about how dishes are prepared and educating family, friends, and restaurant chefs to ensure that they will avoid gluten-containing foods in preparing meals.

For most people, sticking to a gluten-free diet will stop the symptoms and allow the intestinal surface to heal. Within a few days of avoiding gluten, people begin to feel better, but it can take anywhere from three months to up to two years for the villi to fully regenerate.

It is estimated that about 1 in 200 Canadians have celiac disease, but some researchers believe the prevalence is considerably higher (Canadian Society of Intestinal Research 2008). That's because some people have few symptoms and aren't diagnosed. Celiac disease is most often diagnosed in children, and diagnosing it early helps avoid growth delays caused by malabsorption.

There appears to be a genetic link, as people with relatives with celiac disease are more at risk for acquiring this condition themselves. Research shows that more than 90% of people diagnosed with celiac disease have a particular gene, HLA-DQ2, that is believed to trigger the immune response to gluten. Although it is more common in Caucasians, it can develop in almost anyone at any point in his or her life. People sometimes develop celiac disease after an illness or pregnancy (Murray 1999).

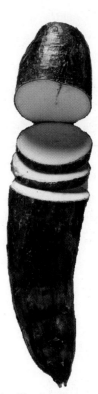

For people with celiac disease, cassava is a good gluten-free source of carbohydrates.

Food Allergies

Although much less common than food intolerances, a number of people suffer from food allergies. You may have heard stories of people being allergic to something as common as peanuts. This is the case for Liz. She was out to dinner with her parents, celebrating her birthday, when the dessert cart came around. The caramel custard looked heavenly and was probably a safe choice, but she asked the waiter just to be sure that it contained no peanuts. He checked with the chef, then returned and assured her

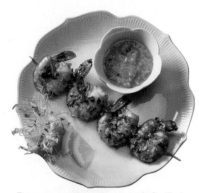

For some people, eating a meal of grilled shrimp with peanut sauce would cause a severe allergic reaction.

that, no, the custard was peanut-free—but within minutes of consuming it, Liz's skin became flushed, and she struggled to breathe. As her parents were dialling 911, she lost consciousness. Fortunately, the paramedics arrived within minutes and were able to resuscitate her. It was subsequently determined that, unknown to the chef, the spoon that his prep cook had used to scoop the baked custard into serving bowls had been resting on a cutting board where he had chopped peanuts for a different dessert. Just this small exposure to peanuts was enough to cause a severe allergic reaction in Liz.

How can a food that most people consume regularly, such as peanuts, shellfish, eggs, or milk, cause some people to suffer an allergic reaction? The answer lies with the immune system. In Liz's case, a trace amount of peanut stimulated immune cells throughout her body to release their inflammatory chemicals. In celiac disease, the inflammation is localized in the small intestine, so the damage is limited. This is true of many food allergies, as well. For instance, some people's lips swell when they eat melon, whereas others develop a rash whenever they eat eggs. What made Liz's experience so terrifyingly different was that the inflammation was so widespread, affecting essentially all of her body systems and sending her into a state called *anaphylactic shock*. Left untreated, anaphylactic shock is nearly always fatal, so many people with known food allergies always carry with them a kit containing an injection of a powerful stimulant called epinephrine. This drug can reduce symptoms long enough to allow the victim to get emergency medical care.

Health Canada, the Canadian Food Inspection Agency (CFIA), and medical experts have agreed upon nine foods or substances that are the most common causes of food allergies (Health Canada 2005). These "priority food allergens" are peanuts, tree nuts (e.g., Brazil nut, hazelnut), sesame seeds, soy, milk, eggs, fish (including crustaceans and shellfish), wheat and other cereal grains that contain gluten, and sulphites. For these nine allergens, Health Canada and the CFIA have jointly produced an excellent series of pamphlets for consumers. They can be downloaded at no cost from www.inspection.gc.ca/english/fssa/labeti/allerg/allerge.shtml.

As we learned in Chapter 2, food labels on packaged products must include a list of ingredients in a product, in descending order by weight. The CFIA looks for "undeclared allergens"—that is, food allergens that are in a product but have not been listed on its labels—to protect consumers from life-threatening allergic reactions. When they discover undeclared allergens, they issue a recall of the food product and a warning to the public is posted on the CFIA website.

Health Canada has a Food Allergen Program that conducts research into new laboratory methods for detecting undeclared allergens in food products. To help affected consumers avoid products that pose a risk, the department has also proposed changes to the Food and Drug Regulations that would require manufacturers to use on food labels the common names of foods and food components that can cause life-threatening allergic reactions.

Recap: Food allergies are a hypersensitivity to food caused by an immune reaction. Food allergies occur in about 8% of children and 1% to 2% of adults in Canada. Celiac disease is a genetic disorder that causes an intolerance to gluten, a protein found in wheat, rye, triticale, and barley. People with celiac disease cannot eat gluten, as it causes an immune reaction that damages the lining of the small intestine and leads to malabsorption of nutrients and malnutrition. Other foods that may cause allergies include peanuts, milk, eggs, and shellfish. Food allergies can cause mild symptoms, such as hives and swelling, or have serious consequences, such as anaphylactic shock. Food allergies and celiac disease can be treated only by avoiding foods that cause the immune reactions.

inflammatory bowel disease A term that includes two different diseases with unknown causes that trigger inflammation and swelling of the intestine: Crohn's disease and ulcerative colitis.

Inflammatory Bowel Disease

Inflammatory bowel disease (IBD) describes two quite different diseases with no known causes that trigger inflammation (swelling and redness) in the intestines: Crohn's disease and ulcerative colitis. It's estimated that 200 000 men, women, and children in Canada suffer from IBD (Crohn's and Colitis Foundation of Canada 2008).

In Crohn's disease, the last part of the small intestine, the end part of the ileum, is usually affected, but it can occur in patches in any part of the gastrointestinal tract. In 30% to 50% of cases, the colon or large bowel is also affected. The inflammation occurs in several layers of tissue through to the muscle, causing dilated blood vessels and extensive tissue damage. Sometimes the intestine becomes narrow and blocked, causing muscle spasms and requiring immediate medical attention. Because Crohn's disease affects the small intestine, the damage to the absorptive surface may interfere with nutrient absorption and lead to weight loss and diarrhea with unabsorbed fat (steatorrhea).

Ulcerative colitis usually involves only the colon and always begins at the anus or rectum and then continues up the colon for varying distances. The inflammation is generally limited to the inner mucosa of the colon, interfering with normal water reabsorption and frequently causing bloody diarrhea.

The inflammation in both conditions can lead to muscle spasms, cramping, abdominal pain, and fever. When small amounts of blood are lost because of tears in the lining of the intestine and chronic bloody diarrhea, people can develop anemia over time. Inflammatory bowel disease may also be accompanied by other conditions, such as joint pain and arthritis, skin and mouth sores, liver disease, kidney stones, and eye inflammations. Surgery to remove badly damaged sections of the intestine or blockages is sometimes needed for people with inflammatory bowel disease.

Irritable Bowel Syndrome

Irritable bowel syndrome (IBS) is a disorder that interferes with normal functions of the colon (sometimes called the bowel). Symptoms include abdominal cramps, bloating, and (1) constipation, or (2) diarrhea, or (3) both constipation and diarrhea (Spiller 2007). It is one of the most common disorders diagnosed by doctors, with approximately 6% of Canadians being diagnosed with IBS (Hauschildt 2001). More women than men appear to develop IBS, which typically first appears around 20 years of age (Spiller 2007).

However, it can occur in children. It may unexpectedly clear up for a long time and then reoccur. Recent research suggests that both men and women with asthma are more likely to suffer from IBS across all age groups, suggesting that there may be some common feature between the two diseases.

There is no known cause of IBS. For some people, it appears their colon is more sensitive to certain foods or stress. The immune system may also trigger symptoms of IBS. Whatever the cause, the normal movement of the colon appears to be disrupted. In some people with IBS, food moves too quickly through the colon and fluid cannot be absorbed fast enough, which causes diarrhea. In others, the movement of the colon is too slow and too much fluid is absorbed, leading to constipation. Some people alternate between both conditions.

It is important not to confuse IBS and IBD. There is no inflammation in IBS. Factors that are linked with IBS include the following:

- caffeinated drinks, such as tea, coffee, and colas
- foods, such as chocolate, alcohol, dairy products, and wheat
- large meals
- certain medications
- stress

Some women with IBS find that their symptoms worsen during their menstrual period, indicating a possible link between reproductive hormones and IBS.

If you think you have IBS, it is important to have a complete physical examination to rule out any other health problems. Treatment options include certain medications to treat diarrhea or constipation, stress management, regular physical activity,

irritable bowel syndrome A disorder that interferes with normal functions of the colon. Symptoms include abdominal cramps, bloating, and constipation or diarrhea.

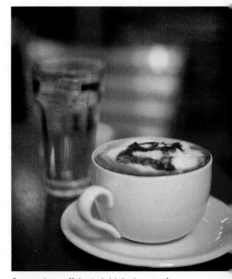

Consuming caffeinated drinks is one of several factors that have been linked with irritable bowel syndrome (IBS), a disorder that interferes with normal functions of the colon.

smaller meals, a higher-fibre diet, at least six to eight glasses of water each day, and avoidance of foods that exacerbate symptoms (NDDIC September 2007). Although IBS is uncomfortable, it does not appear to endanger long-term health. However, severe IBS can be disabling and prevent people from leading normal lives; thus, accurate diagnosis and effective treatment is critical to treat this disorder.

> **Recap:** Irritable bowel syndrome (IBS) causes abdominal cramps, bloating, and constipation or diarrhea. The causes of IBS are unknown. Factors linked to IBS include stress; consumption of caffeinated drinks and such foods as chocolate, dairy, alcohol, and wheat; large meals; and certain medications. IBS can be treated with medications, stress management, regular exercise, a high-fibre diet, at least six to eight glasses of water per day, and avoidance of irritating foods.

Diarrhea and Constipation

diarrhea A condition characterized by the frequent passage of loose, watery stools.

Diarrhea is the frequent passage (more than three times in one day) of loose, watery stools. Other symptoms may include cramping, abdominal pain, bloating, nausea, fever, and blood in the stools. Diarrhea is usually caused by an infection of the gastrointestinal tract, a chronic disease, stress, food intolerances, reactions to medications, or as a result of a bowel disorder (NDDIC March 2007).

Acute diarrhea lasts less than three weeks and is usually caused by an infection from bacteria, a virus, or a parasite. Chronic diarrhea, which lasts more than three weeks, is usually caused by intolerances or allergies to cow's milk, irritable bowel syndrome, or diseases, such as celiac disease.

Whatever the cause, diarrhea can be harmful if it persists for a long period because the person can lose large quantities of water and electrolytes and become severely dehydrated. Table 3.1 reviews the symptoms of dehydration in both adults and children. Diarrhea is particularly dangerous in infants and young children. In fact, a child can die from dehydration in just a few days. Adults, particularly older adults, can also become dangerously ill if severely dehydrated. Table 3.2 lists warning signs that occur with diarrhea; if you experience or observe any of these signs, see a doctor immediately.

A condition referred to as *traveller's diarrhea* has become a common health concern due to the expansion in global travel. Traveller's diarrhea is discussed in the Highlight box on page 104.

constipation A condition characterized by the absence of bowel movements for a time that is significantly longer than normal for the individual. When a bowel movement does occur, stools are usually small, hard, and difficult to pass.

In contrast, **constipation** is typically defined as a condition in which no stools are passed for two or more days; however, it is important to recognize that many people normally experience bowel movements only every second or third day. Thus, the definition of constipation varies from one person to another. In addition to being infrequent, the stools are usually hard, small, and somewhat difficult to pass.

Table 3.1   Symptoms of Dehydration in Adults and Children

Symptoms in Adults	Symptoms in Children
Thirst	Dry mouth and tongue
Light-headedness	No tears when crying
Less frequent urination	No wet diapers for 3 hours or more
Dark-coloured urine	High fever
Fatigue	Sunken abdomen, eyes, or cheeks
Dry skin	Irritable or listless
	Skin that does not flatten when pinched and released

Source: National Digestive Diseases Information Clearinghouse (NDDIC), Diarrhea, NIH Publication No. 01–2749, 2001, January, http://digestive.niddk.nih.gov/ddiseases/pubs/diarrhea/index.htm (accessed August 2003).

Table 3.2 Signs Occurring with Diarrhea That Indicate the Need for a Doctor

Danger Signs for Adults	Danger Signs for Children
Diarrhea lasts more than three days.	Diarrhea lasts more than 24 hours.
Severe pain is felt in abdomen or rectum.	Fever is present at a temperature of 38.6°C (101.4°F) or higher.
Fever is present at a temperature of 39°C (102°F) or higher.	There is blood or pus in the stools, or stools are black.
There is blood in the stools, or stools look black and tarry.	There are symptoms of dehydration.
There are symptoms of dehydration.	

Source: National Digestive Diseases Information Clearinghouse (NDDIC), Diarrhea, NIH Publication No. 01–2749, 2001, January, http://digestive.niddk.nih.gov/ddiseases/pubs/diarrhea/index.htm (accessed August 2003).

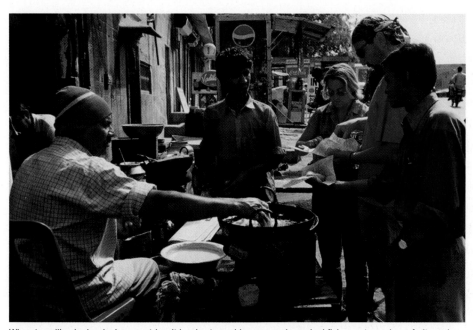

When travelling in developing countries, it is wise to avoid raw or undercooked fish, meats, and raw fruits and vegetables. Tap water, ice made from tap water, and unpasteurized milk and dairy products should also be avoided.

Constipation is frequent in people who have disorders affecting the nervous system, and in which the muscles of the large bowel do not receive the appropriate nerve signals needed for involuntary muscle movement to occur. For these individuals, drug therapy is often needed to keep the large bowel functioning.

Many people experience temporary constipation at some point in their lives in response to a variety of causes. Often people have trouble with it when they travel, when their schedule is disrupted, if they change their diet, or if they are on certain medications. Increasing fibre and fluid in the diet is one of the mainstays of preventing constipation. Five to 10 servings of fruits and vegetables each day and 5 or more servings of whole grains are helpful to most people. If you eat breakfast cereal, make sure you buy a cereal containing at least 2 to 3 grams of fibre per serving. The dietary recommendation for fibre and the role it plays in maintaining healthy elimination is discussed in detail in Chapter 4. Staying well hydrated by drinking lots of water and exercising will also help reduce the risk of constipation.

Recap: Diarrhea is the frequent passage of loose or watery stools, whereas constipation is failure to have a bowel movement for two or more days or within a time that is normal for the individual. Diarrhea should be treated quickly to avoid dehydration or even death. Constipation can be treated with medications or by exercising and increasing your intake of fibre and water.

▶ **HIGHLIGHT**

Global Nutrition: Traveller's Diarrhea—What Is It and How Can I Prevent It?

Diarrhea is the rapid movement of fecal matter through the large intestine, often accompanied by large volumes of water. Traveller's diarrhea is experienced by some people travelling to countries outside of their own and is usually caused by viral or bacterial infections. Diarrhea represents the body's way of ridding itself of the invasive agent. The large intestine and even some of the small intestine become irritated by the microbes and the body's defence against them. This irritation leads to increased secretion of fluid and increased motility of the large intestine, causing watery stools and a higher than normal frequency of bowel movements.

People generally get traveller's diarrhea from consuming water or food that is contaminated with fecal matter. High-risk destinations include developing countries in Africa, Asia, Latin America, and the Middle East. Low-risk destinations include the United States, most European countries, Canada, Japan, Australia, and New Zealand. Very risky foods include any raw or undercooked fish, meats, and raw fruits and vegetables. Tap water, ice made from tap water, and unpasteurized milk and dairy products are also common sources of infection.

Traveller's diarrhea may start about 5 to 15 days after you arrive at your destination. Symptoms include fatigue, lack of appetite, abdominal cramps, and watery diarrhea. In some cases, you may also experience nausea, vomiting, and low-grade fever. Usually, this diarrhea passes within four to six days, and people recover completely. However, infants and toddlers, older adults, and people with AIDS (acquired immunodeficiency syndrome), cancer, or other disorders that weaken their immune system are at greater risk for serious illness and may not recover as well. This is also true for people with digestive disorders, such as celiac disease and ulcers (Stanley 1999).

What can you do to prevent traveller's diarrhea? Because the primary cause is contaminated water and food, avoiding the risky foods described above can help reduce your risk of contracting this illness. In general, it is smart to assume that all local water and foods and beverages exposed to or cleaned with local water are contaminated and should be avoided. Brand-name bottled waters, wine, beer, and beverages made with boiling water are typically safe, but beware of using ice made from local water. It is important to remember to wipe all bottles clean and dry them before drinking bottled beverages. All food should be well cooked, fruit from which the peel is removed is generally safe, and raw vegetables and those with high water content (such as lettuce) should not be eaten.

Antibiotics can also be taken before your trip to avoid traveller's diarrhea. This prevention option should be discussed with your physician before travel. Many bacteria are now resistant to antibiotic treatment, and this option is not always safe or effective for everyone.

CHAPTER SUMMARY

- Food stimulates our senses of smell, taste, and sight; this motivates us to eat.
- Appetite is a psychological desire to consume specific foods; this desire is motivated by the environment and pleasant thoughts about food.
- Hunger is a physiologic drive that prompts us to eat.
- The hypothalamus in the brain interacts with signals from the gastrointestinal tract and levels of blood nutrients to signal when we are hungry or satiated.

- Hormones are chemical messengers secreted by glands in the body that signal the hypothalamus to stimulate hunger or satiation.
- Foods that contain fibre, water, and large amounts of protein have the highest satiety value.
- Atoms are small units of matter, and they bond together to form molecules.
- The primary goal of digestion is to break food into molecules small enough to be absorbed and transported throughout the body.

- Cells are the smallest units of life, and the human body comprises billions of cells. We build cells from the nutrients we absorb as a result of digesting food.
- Cells are encased in a cell membrane, which acts as a gatekeeper to determine which substances go into and out of the cell.
- Cells contain organelles, which are tiny structures that perform highly sophisticated functions. The nucleus, ribosomes, and mitochondria are examples of organelles.
- Cells of a single type join together to form tissues. Several types of tissues join together to form organs, such as the liver.
- Organs group together to form systems that perform integrated functions. The gastrointestinal system and the central nervous system are examples.
- Digestion is the process of breaking down foods into molecules; absorption is the process of taking molecules of food into the body; and elimination is the process of removing undigested and unabsorbed food and waste products from the body.
- In the mouth, chewing starts mechanical digestion of food. Saliva contains salivary amylase, which is an enzyme that initiates the chemical digestion of carbohydrates.
- Food moves down to the stomach through the esophagus via a process called peristalsis. Peristalsis involves the rhythmic waves of squeezing and pushing food through the gastrointestinal tract.
- The stomach mixes and churns food together with gastric juices. Hydrochloric acid and the enzyme pepsin initiate protein digestion, and a minimal amount of fat digestion begins through the action of gastric lipase.
- The stomach periodically releases the partially digested food, referred to as chyme, into the small intestine.
- Most digestion and absorption of nutrients occurs in the small intestine.
- The gallbladder, pancreas, and liver are examples of accessory organs to the gastrointestinal tract.
- The gallbladder concentrates and stores bile and secretes it into the small intestine to assist with the digestion of fat.
- The pancreas manufactures and secretes digestive enzymes into the small intestine. Pancreatic amylase digests carbohydrates, pancreatic lipase digests fats, and proteases digest proteins. The pancreas also synthesizes two hormones that play a critical role in carbohydrate metabolism: insulin and glucagon.
- The lining of the small intestine has thousands of folds and fingerlike projections that increase the surface area more than 500 times, significantly increasing the absorptive capacity of the small intestine.
- The liver processes and stores all absorbed nutrients, alcohol, and drugs. The liver also synthesizes bile and regulates the metabolism of monosaccharides, fatty acids, and amino acids.
- The large intestine absorbs water, fatty acids, and electrolytes and moves feces to the rectum for elimination.
- The neuromuscular system involves coordination of the muscles, the central nervous system, and the enteric nervous system to move food along the gastrointestinal tract and to control all aspects of digestion, absorption, and elimination.
- Heartburn is caused by hydrochloric acid seeping backward from the stomach into the esophagus and burning its lining.
- Gastroesophageal reflux disease (GERD) is a more painful type of heartburn that occurs more than twice per week. GERD can cause bleeding, ulcers, and cancer of the esophagus.
- A peptic ulcer is an area in the stomach or duodenum that has been eroded away by hydrochloric acid and pepsin. A bacterium, *Helicobacter pylori*, is the most common cause of peptic ulcers. Prolonged use of nonsteroidal anti-inflammatory drugs (NSAIDs) can also cause peptic ulcers.
- A food allergy is an allergic reaction to food that is caused by an activation of the immune system. A food intolerance is gastrointestinal discomfort caused by foods that is not a result of an immune system reaction.
- Celiac disease is a genetic disorder characterized by a total intolerance to gluten. This disease causes damage to the lining of the small intestine, leading to malabsorption of nutrients.
- Inflammatory bowel disease includes Crohn's disease and ulcerative colitis that results in inflammation and swelling of the intestine.
- Irritable bowel syndrome is a disorder that interferes with normal functions of the colon, causing pain, diarrhea, and constipation.
- Diarrhea is the frequent (more than three times per day) elimination of loose, watery stools. Diarrhea should be treated promptly to avoid dehydration.
- Constipation is a condition in which no stools are passed for two or more days, or for a time considered abnormally long for the individual. Constipation can be relieved by medications, drinking plenty of water, exercising, and eating foods with ample dietary fibre.

*my*nutritionlab Go to MyNutritionLab at www.pearsoned.ca/mynutritionlab and enrich your understanding of nutrition! You'll find key animations, interactive exercises, access to My DietAnalysis, and much more.

REVIEW QUESTIONS

1. Which of the following represents the levels of organization in the human body?
   a. Cells, molecules, atoms, tissues, organs, systems
   b. Atoms, molecules, cells, organs, tissues, systems
   c. Atoms, molecules, cells, tissues, organs, systems
   d. Molecules, atoms, cells, tissues, organs, systems

2. Bile is a greenish fluid that
   a. is stored by the pancreas.
   b. is stored by the kidneys.
   c. denatures proteins.
   d. emulsifies fats.

3. The region of brain tissue that is responsible for prompting us to seek food is the
   a. pituitary gland.
   b. cephalic phase.
   c. hypothalamus.
   d. thalamus.

4. Heartburn is caused by
   a. seepage of gastric acid into the esophagus.
   b. seepage of gastric acid into the cardiac muscle.
   c. seepage of bile into the stomach.
   d. seepage of salivary amylase into the stomach.

5. Which of the following foods is likely to keep a person satiated for the longest time?
   a. A bean and cheese burrito
   b. A serving of full-fat ice cream
   c. A bowl of rice cereal in whole milk
   d. A tossed salad with oil and vinegar dressing

6. Early morning swim practices are hard on Mike, but they are important for the swim meet he has coming up next week. After completing the hour-long drill set, Mike's stomach is rumbling despite the breakfast he had before practice. Mike is hungry because of
   a. hunger, a psychological response.
   b. hunger, a physiologic response.
   c. appetite, a psychological response.
   d. appetite, a physiologic response.

7. Food is partially digested and churned in which organ?
   a. Large intestine
   b. Small intestine
   c. Stomach
   d. Mouth

8. Joyce is really excited to be on a weeklong cruise trip. Despite the lure of buffet-style meals every day, she's made a point of eating well during her vacation. At the breakfast buffet, Joyce surveys all the different types of entrees and sides she could choose from. The choices are endless! Everything looks so delicious! Since she knows that fruits and vegetables are rich in vitamins and minerals, Joyce approaches the fruit bar. She piles her plate with pineapple rings, honeydew chunks, grape clusters, kiwi slices, and a nice ripe banana. The bread section catches her eye and Joyce adds a whole-wheat bagel to her breakfast. Before returning to her seat to eat, she picks up a container of yogurt to accompany her fruit.

   At which point did Joyce undergo the cephalic phase of digestion?

   Her breakfast choice is high in vitamins and minerals. Where in the gastrointestinal system are these absorbed? Being on a trip, Joyce is at risk for traveller's diarrhea. What can she change in her breakfast to minimize her risk?

9. A person with celiac disease cannot tolerate foods containing or made from
   a. wheat, rye, and barley.
   b. seeds, nuts, and legumes.
   c. milk or milk products.
   d. phenylalanine.

10. Discuss some factors that can help prevent or relieve constipation.

11. Imagine that the lining of your small intestine were smooth, like the inside of a rubber tube. Would this design be efficient in performing the main function of this organ? Why or why not?

12. Why doesn't the acidic environment of the stomach cause it to digest itself?

13. After dinner, your roommate lies down to rest for a few minutes before studying. When he gets up, he complains of a sharp, burning pain in his chest. Offer a possible explanation for his pain.

CASE STUDY

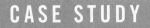

William is excited that his Grade 6 class is going on a trip to Ottawa to see the Parliament buildings and visit all the museums. At the last minute, however, William decides not to go because he is too embarrassed about his peanut allergy. Some girls in his class make fun of him for not being able to eat certain things, and he hates having to ask people not to eat peanut butter around him. Even worse, he is scared that the restaurants where they dine on the trip will not understand the severity of his condition and may accidentally contaminate his food with peanut products.

What strategy might William use to communicate his food allergy to servers at restaurants? What could he say to his classmates to give them a better understanding of why he cannot eat some foods? What other obstacles might William confront on a school trip because of his allergy?

WEB LINKS

www.ibsassociation.ca
Irritable Bowel Syndrome Association of Canada
A nonprofit organization dedicated to helping people who suffer from IBS through support groups, treatment, accurate information, and education.

www.cdhf.ca
Canadian Digestive Health Foundation
This website covers more than a dozen different digestive disorders, with information written by physicians.

www.badgut.com
Canadian Society of Intestinal Research
This great website has lots of information for people suffering from digestive disorders.

www.ccfc.ca
Crohn's and Colitis Foundation of Canada
Another consumer-oriented website, this one is especially helpful for families with members suffering from Crohn's disease and ulcerative colitis.

www.hc-sc.gc.ca/iyh-vsv/index_e.html
It's Your Health
Subscribe to this free bulletin from Health Canada that covers a wide range of health and safety topics, including diseases, lifestyle, and food.

http://digestive.niddk.nih.gov
National Digestive Diseases Information Clearinghouse (NDDIC)
Explore this site to learn more about diarrhea, celiac disease, irritable bowel syndrome (IBS), heartburn, and gastroesophageal reflux disease (GERD).

www.nlm.nih.gov/medlineplus
MEDLINE Plus Health Information
Search "food allergies" to obtain additional resources as well as the latest news about food allergies.

www.healthfinder.gov
Health Finder
Search this site to learn more about disorders related to digestion, absorption, and elimination.

Test Yourself Answers

1. **True** Sometimes you may have an appetite even though you are not hungry. These feelings are referred to as cravings and are associated with physical or emotional cues.

2. **False** Your brain, not your stomach, is the primary organ responsible for telling you when you are hungry.

3. **True** Although there are individual variations, the entire process of digestion and absorption of one meal usually takes about 24 hours.

4. **True** Most ulcers result from an infection of the bacterium *Helicobacter pylori* (*H. pylori*). Contrary to popular belief, ulcers are not caused by stress or food.

5. **False** Irritable bowel syndrome is a relatively common disease that affects approximately 6% of Canadians. The age at onset is typically around 20 years of age.

ific.org
International Food Information Council Foundation (IFIC)
Scroll down to "Food Safety Information" and click the link for "Food Allergies and Asthma" for additional information on food allergies.

www.foodallergy.org
The Food Allergy and Anaphylaxis Network (FAN)
Visit this site to learn more about common food allergens.

www.gfmall.com
Gluten-Free Mall
Find out where you can buy gluten-free products.

Should I Choose Products with Probiotics and Prebiotics?

New products are always appearing on supermarket shelves through the hard work of the evergrowing food industry. While shopping for milk and dairy products, you may notice new products containing probiotics and prebiotics. Are these items as beneficial as they claim to be? Or is this simply the newest nutrition myth?

Strangely enough, there is no legal definition for probiotics (Douglas and Saunders 2008). Moreover, the scientific community uses many different definitions for this one term. Generally, probiotics are live microorganisms that have beneficial health effects at sufficient quantities (Guarner and Schaafsma 1998). Probiotic yogurts, therefore, have added microorganisms. When you eat the yogurt, the microorganisms are alive and are expected to bring about the health benefits as indicated by the manufacturer.

Probiotics have been linked to a long list of potential health benefits (Douglas and Saunders 2008). They have been shown to protect against diarrhea and constipation in addition to enhancing immune function. Preliminary evidence links probiotics to the prevention of some cancers, heart disease, and allergies. More research is needed since the evidence for these potential health effects varies from study to study (World Health Organization 2001). Why is this?

Probiotics refer to many different microorganisms that are classified by their genus, species, and strain. Therefore, probiotics are not all the same and all variants do not have the same effects on human health (Douglas and Saunders 2008). Not surprisingly, studies that use different variants at different dosages will result in different results (Huff 2004). This has made it very difficult to study probiotics and impossible to set a recommended dosage for probiotics to receive the benefits (Douglas and Saunders 2008).

It is important to remember that to be effective, a minimum number of bacteria must be present in foods. Although the exact number of bacteria is not known, it is estimated that a daily dose of at least one billion to ten billion (or 1×10^9 to 1×10^{10}) bacteria are needed to be effective (Sanders et al. 1996). Since probiotics are live microorganisms, the food industry has had the challenge of keeping them alive through their product's shelf life. Production, storage, and quality control are all important factors in ensuring that the products live up to their claims (Clancy and Pang 2007). Microbes are known to keep better when refrigerated (Douglas and Saunders 2008). However, new products that use dried probiotics can keep at room temperature (World Health Organization 2001). In the act of drying, the microbes become dormant until rehydrated. In any case, it is important to check the expiry dates of the products to be sure the probiotics are still viable (Douglas and Saunders 2008). At this time, there are no Canadian standards for identifying the level of active bacteria in foods or supplements.

Despite the limited evidence backing manufacturer health claims, a growing number of consumers are choosing to buy probiotics (Huff 2004). This is not a surprise since these products are easily accessible and inexpensive (Douglas and Saunders 2008). Most consumers who choose probiotics are otherwise healthy people. They hope that the product will help maintain their health and protect them from illnesses (World Health Organization 2001). Unfortunately, there are no studies yet with solid evidence that probiotics can help maintain good health better than proper diet and exercise. Therefore, healthy consumers should not choose probiotics over eating well and exercising (World Health Organization 2001).

Probiotics are generally deemed safe for healthy individuals (Douglas and Saunders 2008). Historically, there have been no serious adverse effects in common probiotics, such as lactobacilli and bifidobacteria (World Health Organization 2001). Some probiotics have been consumed by humans for hundreds of years, and others have been found to be normal residents of the human gut (Saunders 2003). However, probiotics can have negative effects—there are documented cases

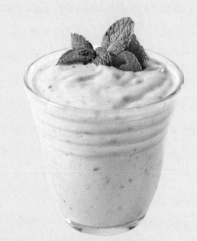

Probiotics can be found in fermented yogurt.

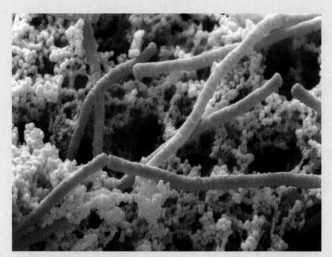

An electron micrograph of the bacteria *Lactobacillus* (pink), taken from yogurt with live active cultures.

of infection caused by probiotic intake in individuals with compromised health or underlying diseases (Saunders 2003). Therefore, it is important that these individuals take probiotics only under the supervision of a health care provider (Douglas and Saunders 2008).

What about prebiotics? What are they and how do they affect human health? Prebiotics are defined as indigestible food components that encourage the growth of specific microbes linked to health benefits (Douglas and Saunders 2008; Grajek et al. 2005). They are a class of carbohydrates that are fermentable yet are not easily digestible (Grajek et al. 2005). In short, they are fibres that ferment in the human gut. The end products from the fermentation process encourage the growth of microbes, such as probiotics (Douglas and Saunders 2008).

Our diets include many foods that contain fermentable fibres; however, these must not be confused with prebiotics. Not all fermentation end products enhance the activity of probiotics. Therefore, not all fermentable fibres are prebiotics (Lenoir-Wijnkoop et al. 2007).

Similar to probiotics, the consumption of 3 to 8 grams of prebiotics is linked to various positive health effects (Douglas and Saunders 2008). Prebiotics have been studied for preventive effects on colon cancer, improved calcium absorption, and enhanced immune function (Lenoir-Wijnkoop et al. 2007; Roberfroid 2000). Moreover, some studies have found evidence that prebiotics may reduce the risk of osteoporosis and atherosclerotic cardiovascular disease (Roberfroid 2000).

What about products that incorporate both probiotics and prebiotics? In combining the two, the result is symbiotic. The combination of both probiotics and prebiotics enhances the survival rate of the beneficial microbes. Longer-surviving microbes can therefore extend their effect beyond the upper gastrointestinal tract (Roberfroid 2000).

In the end, the research behind probiotics and prebiotics is mostly preliminary. There are currently no studies examining their long-term effectiveness. Product labels often do not identify the probiotics content and are not helpful to consumers trying to make an informed choice. Moreover, there is evidence that many of these products do not contain quantities of probiotics to sufficiently meet their health claims (Huff 2004).

Based on what you have just learned about probiotics, do you think products containing these bacteria should be consumed on a daily basis? Are you interested in adding probiotics to your diet? Do we really know enough about their role in human health to make broad-based recommendations for people? Do you think that the standards of the food and supplement industries need to be improved in regard to defining bacterial content and activity level before we can make national recommendations to consume foods that contain probiotics? How do you think food labels can be improved to assist consumers in identifying key aspects of probiotics-containing foods? As the number of probiotics-containing foods increases in the marketplace, these are just some of the questions that need to be answered to assist consumers in making healthful food choices.

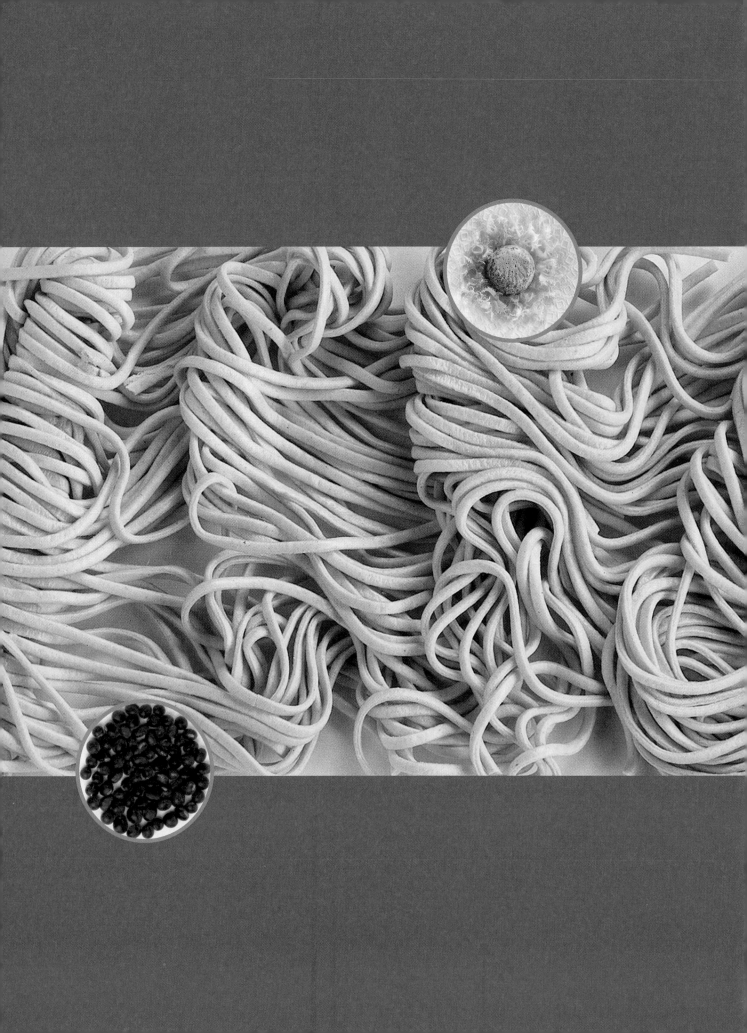

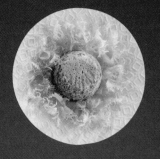

CHAPTER 4

Carbohydrates: Bountiful Sources of Energy and Nutrients

Test Yourself **True** or **False**

1. The terms *carbohydrate* and *sugar* mean the same thing. **T or F**

2. Diets high in sugar cause tooth decay, diabetes, and obesity. **T or F**

3. Our bodies have a difficult time digesting and absorbing carbohydrates, so we should consume a diet that is low in carbohydrates. **T or F**

4. Carbohydrates are the primary fuel source for our brain and body tissues. **T or F**

5. Alternative sweeteners, such as aspartame, are safe for us to consume. **T or F**

Test Yourself answers can be found at the end of the chapter.

Does the consumption of sugary foods, like soft drinks, lead to diabetes—or, for that matter, to obesity or any other disorder? Several popular diets—including the Zone Diet (Sears 1995), Sugar Busters (Steward et al. 1995), and Dr. Atkins' New Diet Revolution (Atkins 1992)—claim that carbohydrates are bad for your health and advocate reducing carbohydrate consumption and increasing protein and fat intake. Should we reduce our intake of carbohydrates? If you noticed that a friend regularly consumed four or five soft drinks a day, plus candy and other sweet snacks, would you say anything? Are carbohydrates a health menace, and is one type of carbohydrate as bad as another?

In this chapter, we explore the differences between simple and complex carbohydrates and learn why some carbohydrates are better than others. We also learn how the human body breaks down carbohydrates and uses them to maintain our health and to fuel our activity and exercise. Because carbohydrate metabolism sometimes does go wrong, we'll also discuss its relationship to some common health disorders.

MyDiet Analysis

www.mynutritionlab.com

carbohydrate One of the three classes of macronutrients; a compound made up of carbon, hydrogen, and oxygen that is derived from plants and provides energy.

glucose The most abundant sugar molecule; a monosaccharide generally found in combination with other sugars. The preferred source of energy for the brain and an important source of energy for all cells.

photosynthesis The process by which plants use sunlight to fuel a chemical reaction that combines carbon dioxide and hydrogen atoms from water into glucose, which is then stored in the plants' cells.

What Are Carbohydrates?

As we noted in Chapter 1, **carbohydrates** are one of the three classes of macronutrients. As such, they are an important energy source for the entire body and are the preferred energy source for red blood cells (erythrocytes) and nerve cells, including those of the brain. We will say more about their functions later in this chapter.

The term *carbohydrate* literally means "hydrated carbon." You know that water (H_2O) is made of hydrogen and oxygen and that when something is said to be *hydrated*, it contains water. Thus, the chemical abbreviation for carbohydrate (CHO) indicates the atoms it contains: **c**arbon, **h**ydrogen, and **o**xygen.

We obtain carbohydrates predominantly from plant foods, such as fruits, vegetables, and grains. Plants make the most abundant form of carbohydrate, called **glucose**, through a process called **photosynthesis**. During photosynthesis, the green pigment of plants, called *chlorophyll*, absorbs sunlight, which provides the energy needed to fuel the manufacture of glucose. As shown in Figure 4.1, the hydrogen atoms from water absorbed from the earth by the plants' roots are used with carbon dioxide present in the leaves to produce the carbohydrate glucose. Plants continually store glucose and use it to support their own growth. Then, when we eat plant foods, our bodies digest the carbohydrate and absorb and use the glucose.

> **Recap:** Carbohydrates are one of the three macronutrient classes that provide energy to our bodies. Carbohydrates contain carbon, hydrogen, and oxygen. Plants make one type of carbohydrate, glucose, through the process of photosynthesis.

Animations

• Carbohydrates

simple carbohydrate Commonly called simple sugar or just sugar; a monosaccharide or disaccharide, such as glucose.

monosaccharide The simplest of carbohydrates. Consists of one sugar molecule, the most common form of which is glucose.

disaccharide A carbohydrate compound consisting of two sugar molecules joined together.

What's the Difference Between Simple and Complex Carbohydrates?

Carbohydrates can be classified as *simple* or *complex*. Simple carbohydrates contain either one or two molecules of sugar, while complex carbohydrates contain hundreds to thousands of molecules of sugar joined together.

Simple Carbohydrates Include Monosaccharides and Disaccharides

Simple carbohydrates are commonly referred to as *sugars* or *simple sugars*. Three of these sugars are called **monosaccharides** because they consist of a single sugar molecule (*mono* meaning "one," and *saccharide* meaning "sugar"). The other three sugars are **disaccharides**, which consist of two molecules of sugar joined together (*di* meaning "two").

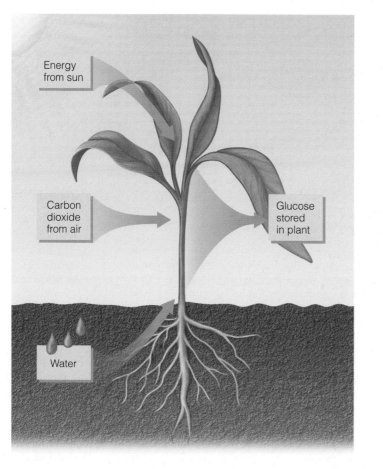

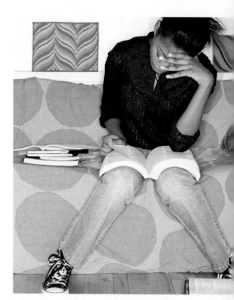

In our bodies, glucose is the preferred source of energy for the brain.

Figure 4.1 Plants make carbohydrates through the process of photosynthesis. Water, carbon dioxide, and energy from the sun are used to produce glucose.

Glucose, Fructose, and Galactose Are Monosaccharides

Glucose, *fructose*, and *galactose* are the three most common monosaccharides in our diet. Each of these monosaccharides contains six carbon atoms, twelve hydrogen atoms, and six oxygen atoms (Figure 4.2). Very slight differences in the structure of the molecules in these three monosaccharides cause major differences in their level of sweetness.

- Interactive Molecule: D-Glucose

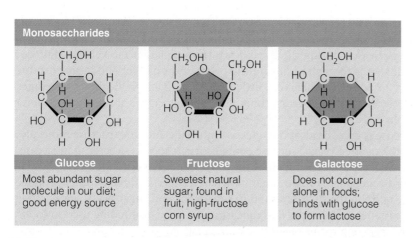

Figure 4.2 The three most common monosaccharides. Notice that all three monosaccharides contain identical atoms: six carbon, twelve hydrogen, and six oxygen. It is only the arrangement of these atoms that differs.

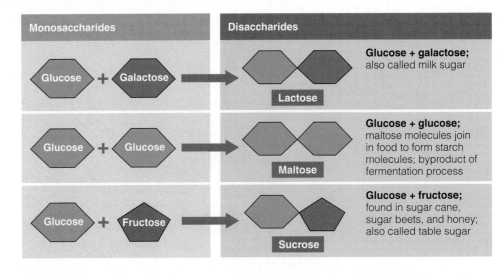

Figure 4.3 Galactose, glucose, and fructose join together to make the disaccharides lactose, maltose, and sucrose.

Given what you've just learned about how plants manufacture glucose, it probably won't surprise you to discover that glucose is the most abundant sugar molecule found in our diets and in our bodies. Glucose does not generally occur by itself in foods but attaches to other sugars to form disaccharides and complex carbohydrates. In our bodies, glucose is the preferred source of energy for the brain, and it is a very important source of energy for all cells.

Fructose, the sweetest natural sugar, occurs naturally in fruits and vegetables. Fructose is also called *levulose*, or *fruit sugar*. In many processed foods, it comes in the form of *high-fructose corn syrup*. This syrup is made from corn and is used to sweeten soft drinks, desserts, candies, and jellies.

Galactose does not occur alone in foods. It joins with glucose to create lactose, one of the three most common disaccharides.

Lactose, Maltose, and Sucrose Are Disaccharides

A disaccharide consists of two monosaccharides joined together in a condensation reaction. The three most common disaccharides found in foods are *lactose*, *maltose*, and *sucrose* (Figure 4.3). **Lactose** (also called *milk sugar*) consists of one glucose molecule and one galactose molecule. Interestingly, human breast milk has a higher amount of lactose than cow's milk, which makes human breast milk taste sweeter.

Maltose (also called *malt sugar*) consists of two molecules of glucose. It does not generally occur by itself in foods; rather, is bound together with other molecules and released during the breakdown of these larger molecules. Maltose is also the sugar that is fermented during the production of beer and liquor products. Contrary to popular belief, very little maltose remains in alcoholic beverages after the fermentation process; thus, alcoholic beverages are not good sources of carbohydrate.

Sucrose is composed of one glucose molecule and one fructose molecule and is called *table sugar*. Because sucrose contains fructose, it is sweeter than lactose or maltose. Sucrose provides much of the sweet taste found in honey, maple syrup, fruits, and vegetables. Brown sugar, powdered sugar, and many other products are made by refining the sucrose found in sugar cane and sugar beets. See the Highlight box to learn more about the different forms of sugar commonly used in foods. Are naturally occurring forms of sucrose more healthful than manufactured forms? The Nutrition Myth or Fact box on page 116 investigates the common belief that honey is more nutritious than table sugar.

fructose The sweetest natural sugar; a monosaccharide that occurs in fruits and vegetables. Also called levulose, or fruit sugar.

galactose A monosaccharide that joins with glucose to create lactose, one of the three most common disaccharides.

lactose Also called milk sugar, a disaccharide consisting of one glucose molecule and one galactose molecule. Found in milk, including human breast milk.

maltose A disaccharide consisting of two molecules of glucose. Does not generally occur independently in foods but results as a byproduct of digestion. Also called malt sugar.

sucrose A disaccharide composed of one glucose molecule and one fructose molecule. Sweeter than lactose or maltose. Also called table sugar.

> ▶ HIGHLIGHT

Forms of Sugar Commonly Used in Foods

- Brown sugar
- Concentrated fruit juice sweetener
- Confectioner's sugar
- Corn sweeteners
- Corn syrup
- Dextrose
- Fructose

- Galactose
- Glucose
- Granulated sugar
- High-fructose corn syrup
- Honey
- Invert sugar
- Lactose

- Levulose
- Maltose
- Mannitol
- Maple sugar
- Molasses
- Natural sweeteners
- Raw sugar

- Sorbitol
- Turbinado sugar
- White sugar
- Xylitol

Recap: Simple carbohydrates include monosaccharides and disaccharides. Glucose, fructose, and galactose are monosaccharides; lactose, maltose, and sucrose are disaccharides.

All Complex Carbohydrates Are Polysaccharides

Complex carbohydrates, the second major type of carbohydrate, generally consist of long chains of glucose molecules. The technical name for complex carbohydrates is **polysaccharides** (*poly* meaning "many"). They include starch, glycogen, and most fibres (Figure 4.4).

Starch Is a Polysaccharide Stored in Plants

Plants store glucose not as single molecules but as polysaccharides in the form of **starch**. Excellent food sources of starch include grains (wheat, rice, corn, oats, and barley), legumes (peas, beans, and lentils), and tubers (potatoes and yams). Our cells cannot use the complex starch molecules exactly as they occur in plants. Instead, our bodies must break them down into the monosaccharide glucose, from which we can then fuel our energy needs.

complex carbohydrate A nutrient compound, such as starch, glycogen, or fibre, consisting of long chains of glucose molecules.

polysaccharide A complex carbohydrate consisting of long chains of glucose.

starch A polysaccharide stored in plants; the storage form of glucose in plants.

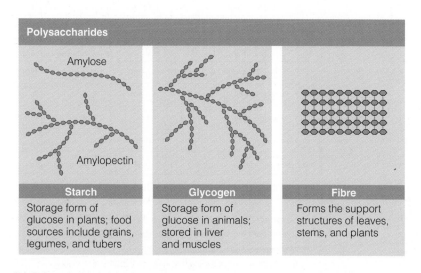

Polysaccharides		
Amylose / Amylopectin		
Starch	**Glycogen**	**Fibre**
Storage form of glucose in plants; food sources include grains, legumes, and tubers	Storage form of glucose in animals; stored in liver and muscles	Forms the support structures of leaves, stems, and plants

Figure 4.4 Polysaccharides, also referred to as complex carbohydrates, include starch, glycogen, and fibre.

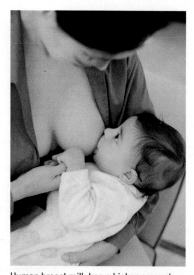

Human breast milk has a higher amount of lactose than cow's milk does, which makes human breast milk taste sweeter.

▶ **NUTRITION MYTH OR FACT**

Is Honey More Nutritious Than Table Sugar?

Liz's friend Tiffany is dedicated to eating healthful foods. She advises Liz to avoid sucrose and to eat foods that contain honey, molasses, or raw sugar. Like many people, Tiffany believes these sweeteners are more natural and nutritious than refined table sugar. How can Liz sort sugar fact from fiction?

Remember that sucrose consists of one glucose molecule and one fructose molecule joined together. From a chemical perspective, honey is almost identical to sucrose, since honey also contains glucose and fructose molecules in almost equal amounts. However, enzymes in bees' "honey stomachs" separate some of the glucose and fructose molecules, resulting in honey looking and tasting slightly different from sucrose. As you know, bees store honey in combs and fan it with their wings to reduce its moisture content. This also alters the appearance and texture of honey.

Honey does not contain any more nutrients than sucrose, so it is not a more healthful choice than sucrose. In fact, per tablespoon, honey has more calories (or energy) than table sugar. This is because the crystals in table sugar take up more space on a spoon than the liquid form of honey, so a tablespoon contains less sugar. However, some people argue that honey is sweeter, so you use less.

It is important to note that honey commonly contains bacteria that are not effectively destroyed by pasteurization and can cause fatal food poisoning in infants. The more mature digestive system of older children and adults is immune to the effects of these bacteria, but babies younger than 12 months should never be given honey.

Are raw sugar and molasses more healthful than table sugar? Actually, the raw sugar available in North America is not really raw. Truly raw sugar is made up of the first crystals obtained when sugar is processed. Sugar in this form contains dirt, parts of insects, and other byproducts that make it illegal to sell in North America. The raw sugar products in stores have actually gone through more than half of the same steps in the refining process used to make table sugar.

Molasses is the syrup that remains when sucrose is made from sugar cane. Molasses is darker and less sweet than table sugar. It does contain some iron, but this iron does not occur naturally. It is a contaminant from the machines that process the sugar cane!

Table 4.1 compares the nutrient content of white sugar, honey, molasses, and raw sugar. As you can see, none of them contains many nutrients that are important for health. This is why highly sweetened products are referred to as *empty calories*.

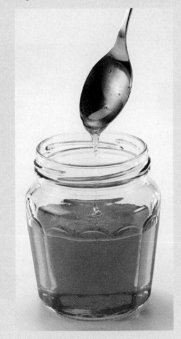

Table 4.1   Nutrient Comparison of Four Different Sugars

	Table Sugar	Honey	Blackstrap Molasses	Raw Sugar
Energy (kcal.)	48.8	63.8	47.0	48.8
Carbohydrate (grams)	12.6	17.3	12.2	12.6
Fat (grams)	0	0	0	0
Protein (grams)	0	0.06	0	0
Fibre (grams)	0	0.04	0	0
Vitamin C (mg)	0	0.11	0	0
Vitamin A (IU)	0	0	0	0
Thiamin (mg)	0	0	0.007	0
Riboflavin (mg)	0.003	0.008	0.01	0.003
Folate (μgrams)	0	0.42	0.20	0
Calcium (mg)	0.042	1.26	172.0	0.042
Iron (mg)	0	0.088	3.5	0
Sodium (mg)	0	0.84	11.0	0
Potassium (mg)	0.25	10.9	498.4	0.25

Source: U.S. Department of Agriculture, Agricultural Research Service. USDA National Nutrient Database for Standard Reference, Release 16, 2003, Nutrient Data Laboratory homepage, www.nal.usda.gov/fnic/foodcomp.
Note: Nutrient values are identified for 15 mL (1 Tbsp) of each product.

Our bodies easily digest most starches; however, some starch in plants is not digestible and is called *resistant*. When our intestinal bacteria try to digest resistant starch, a fatty acid called *butyrate* is produced. Consuming resistant starch may be beneficial because butyrate is suggested to reduce the risk of colon cancer (Topping and Clifton 2001). Legumes contain more resistant starch than do grains, fruits, or vegetables. This quality, plus their high protein and fibre content, makes legumes a healthful food.

Glycogen Is a Polysaccharide Stored by Animals

Glycogen is the storage form of glucose for animals, including humans. Very little glycogen exists in food; thus, glycogen is not a dietary source of carbohydrate. We can break down glycogen very quickly into glucose when we need it for energy. We store glycogen in our muscles and liver; the storage and use of glycogen is discussed in more detail on page 119.

Fibre Is a Polysaccharide That Gives Plants Their Structure

There are currently a number of definitions of fibre. For example, the Food and Nutrition Board of the U.S. Institute of Medicine has proposed three distinctions: *dietary fibre*, *functional fibre*, and *total fibre* (Institute of Medicine 2002). **Dietary fibre** is the indigestible parts of plants that form the support structures of leaves, stems, and seeds (see Figure 4.4). In a sense, you can think of dietary fibre as the plant's "skeleton." **Functional fibre** consists of indigestible forms of carbohydrates that are extracted from plants or manufactured in a laboratory and have known health benefits. Functional fibre is added to foods and is the form found in fibre supplements. **Total fibre** is the sum of dietary fibre and functional fibre.

Good food sources of dietary fibre include oat and wheat brans, oats, wheat, rye, barley, brown rice, seeds, legumes, fruits, and vegetables. Examples of functional fibre sources you might see on nutrition labels include cellulose, guar gum, pectin, and psyllium.

Like starch, fibre consists of long polysaccharide chains. Unlike with starch, however, the body does not easily break down the bonds that connect fibre molecules. This means that both dietary and functional fibres pass through the digestive system without being digested and absorbed. Bacteria in the intestine ferment some of the fibre, producing fatty acids. These fatty acids contribute small amounts of energy. Fibre offers many other health benefits, as we will see shortly (page 126).

Different Types of Fibres Have Different Physical Properties

Although the terms *dietary fibre*, *functional fibre*, and *total fibre* are the most recent scientific definitions, many people will describe fibre according to its physical properties—in particular, its solubility.

Soluble fibres are types of dietary and functional fibres that absorb water and swell to form gels. These gels can trap nutrients, such as glucose, and slow down their absorption into the blood. Food stays in the small intestine longer, and this is useful for people with diabetes and for people with irritable bowel syndrome who suffer from diarrhea (discussed in Chapter 3). Water-soluble fibres include naturally occurring pectins in fruit (apples, bananas, grapefruit, oranges, and strawberries), also sold commercially as thickeners for jams and jellies (e.g., Certo), and natural gums and mucilages found in oatmeal, oat bran, barley, and legumes.

Other fibres attract water, but they cling to it rather than absorbing it. **Insoluble fibre** helps the contents of the large intestine move more quickly through the body and can help to prevent constipation. These substances—lignin (found in vegetables), cellulose (in wheat), and hemicellulose (in cereals and vegetables)—give structure to plants. Lignin binds bile acids, which are needed for cholesterol absorption. By making bile acids less available for cholesterol absorption, some cholesterol is then carried out of the body and blood cholesterol levels can be lowered. Cellulose and

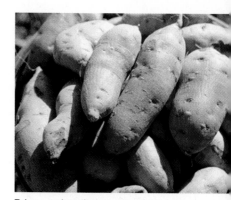

Tubers, such as these sweet potatoes, are excellent food sources of starch.

glycogen A polysaccharide stored in animals; the storage form of glucose in animals.

dietary fibre The indigestible carbohydrate parts of plants that form the support structures of leaves, stems, and seeds.

functional fibre The indigestible forms of carbohydrate that are extracted from plants or manufactured in a laboratory and have known health benefits.

total fibre The sum of dietary fibre and functional fibre.

soluble fibre Natural pectins, mucilages, and gums that absorb water and form gels. In humans, these substances slow down the movement of material through the small intestine.

insoluble fibre Components of plants that attract and cling to water. In humans, these substances speed up the movement of material through the large intestine.

hemicellulose add bulk to the fecal material (called the stool), which helps the walls of the intestine keep their muscle tone. These substances are partially fermented by bacteria that naturally reside in the colon. The fermentation produces small amounts of energy in the form of short-chain fatty acids and may help to convert toxic or cancer-causing compounds into harmless compounds.

Because both soluble and insoluble fibre need water to pass through the intestinal tract, it is important that we drink enough fluids. It also helps to increase fibre intakes gradually so the intestinal tract becomes accustomed to the physical properties of the fibre and bulky stools.

Recap: All complex carbohydrates are polysaccharides. They include starch, glycogen, and fibre. Starch is the storage form of glucose in plants, while glycogen is the storage form of glucose in animals. Fibre forms the support structures of plants; our bodies cannot digest fibre. Different types of fibres have different physical properties. Soluble fibres absorb water and swell to form gels, which slow down the movement of material through the intestinal tract. Insoluble fibres attract water and speed up the movement of material through the large intestine.

- Carbohydrate Digestion
- Carbohydrate Absorption

How Do Our Bodies Digest and Absorb Carbohydrates?

Because glucose is the form of sugar that our bodies use for energy, the primary goal of carbohydrate digestion is to break down polysaccharides and disaccharides into monosaccharides (glucose, fructose, and galactose). Fructose and galactose are then converted to glucose in the liver. Chapter 3 provided an overview of digestion of the three types of macronutrients, plus vitamins and minerals. Here, we focus specifically and in a bit more detail on the digestion and absorption of carbohydrates. Figure 4.5 provides a visual tour of carbohydrate digestion.

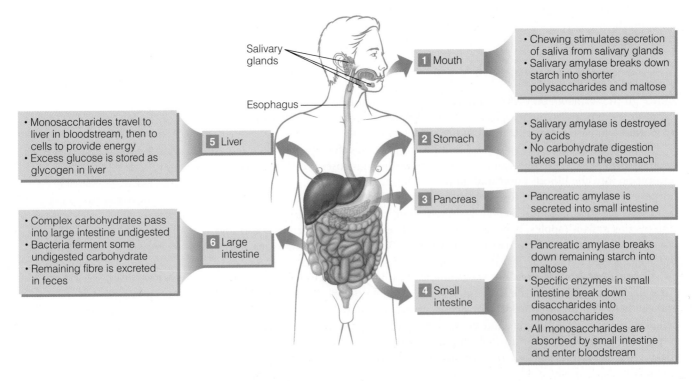

Figure 4.5 A review of carbohydrate digestion and absorption.

Digestion Breaks Down Most Carbohydrates into Monosaccharides

Carbohydrate digestion begins in the mouth (Figure 4.5, Step 1). As you saw in Chapter 3, the starch in the foods you eat mixes with your saliva during chewing. Saliva contains an enzyme called **salivary amylase**, which breaks starch into smaller particles and eventually into the disaccharide maltose. The next time you eat a piece of bread, notice that you can actually taste it becoming sweeter; this indicates the breakdown of starch into maltose. Disaccharides are not digested in the mouth.

As the bolus of food leaves the mouth and enters the stomach, all digestion of carbohydrates eventually ceases. This is because the acid in the stomach inactivates most of the salivary amylase enzyme (Figure 4.5, Step 2).

The majority of carbohydrate digestion occurs in the small intestine. As the contents of the stomach enter the small intestine, an enzyme called **pancreatic amylase** is secreted by the pancreas into the small intestine (Figure 4.5, Step 3). Pancreatic amylase continues to digest any remaining starch into maltose. Additional enzymes, found in the microvilli of the mucosal cells that line the intestinal tract, work to break down disaccharides into monosaccharides. Maltose is digested into glucose by the enzyme **maltase**. Sucrose is digested into glucose and fructose by the enzyme **sucrase**. The enzyme **lactase** digests lactose into glucose and galactose (Figure 4.5, Step 4). Notice that enzyme names are identifiable by the *-ase* suffix. All monosaccharides are then absorbed into the mucosal cells lining the small intestine, where they pass through and enter the bloodstream.

salivary amylase An enzyme in saliva that breaks starch into smaller particles and eventually into the disaccharide maltose.

pancreatic amylase An enzyme secreted by the pancreas into the small intestine that digests any remaining starch into maltose.

maltase A digestive enzyme that digests maltose into glucose.

sucrase A digestive enzyme that digests sucrose into glucose and fructose.

lactase A digestive enzyme that digests lactose into glucose and galactose.

The Liver Converts Monosaccharides into Glucose

Once the monosaccharides enter the bloodstream, they travel to the liver. Fructose and galactose are converted to glucose in the liver (Figure 4.5, Step 5). If needed immediately for energy, the liver releases glucose into the bloodstream, where it can travel to the cells to provide energy. If there is no immediate demand by the body for glucose, it is stored as glycogen in the liver and muscles. Enzymes in liver and muscle cells combine glucose molecules to form glycogen (an anabolic, or building, process) and break glycogen into glucose (a catabolic, or destructive, process), depending on our bodily needs. Our liver can store 70 grams (280 kcal or 1170 kJ) of glycogen, and our muscles can normally store about 120 grams (480 kcal or 2000 kJ) of glycogen. Between meals, our bodies draw on liver glycogen reserves to maintain blood glucose levels and support the needs of our cells, including those of our brain, spinal cord, and red blood cells (Figure 4.6).

The glycogen stored in our muscles provides energy to the muscles during intense exercise. Endurance athletes can increase their storage of muscle glycogen from two to four times the normal amount through a process called *glycogen*, or *carbohydrate, loading* (see Chapter 12). Any excess glucose is stored as glycogen in the liver and muscles and saved for such future energy needs as exercise.

Fibre Is Excreted from the Large Intestine

We do not possess enzymes that can break down fibre. Thus, fibre passes through the small intestine undigested and enters the large intestine, or colon. Once in the large intestine, bacteria ferment some previously undigested carbohydrates, causing the production of gas and a few fatty acids. Some of these fatty acids go back to the liver; others are used by the cells of the large intestine for energy. The fibre remaining in the colon adds bulk to our stools and is excreted in feces (Figure 4.5, Step 6). In this way, fibre assists in maintaining bowel regularity. The health benefits of fibre are discussed later in this chapter (page 126).

> **Recap:** Carbohydrate digestion starts in the mouth and continues in the small intestine. Glucose and other monosaccharides are absorbed into the bloodstream and travel to the liver, where non-glucose sugars are converted to glucose. Glucose is either used by the cells for energy or is converted to glycogen and stored in the liver and muscle for later use.

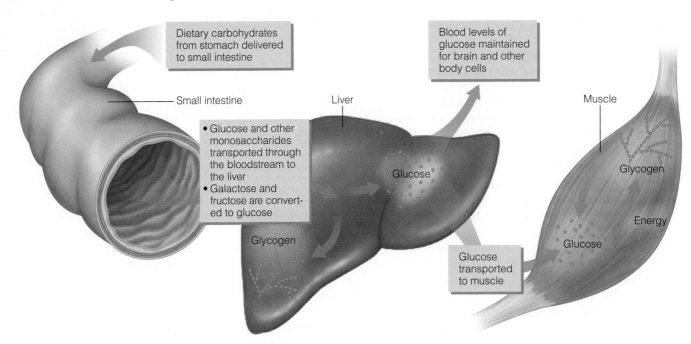

Figure 4.6 Glucose is stored as glycogen in both liver and muscle. The glycogen stored in the liver maintains blood glucose between meals; muscle glycogen provides immediate energy to the muscle during exercise.

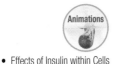

- Effects of Insulin within Cells
- Blood Glucose

insulin Hormone secreted by the beta cells of the pancreas in response to increased blood levels of glucose. Facilitates uptake of glucose by body cells.

glucagon Hormone secreted by the alpha cells of the pancreas in response to decreased blood levels of glucose. Causes breakdown of liver stores of glycogen into glucose.

Insulin and Glucagon Regulate the Level of Glucose in Our Blood

Our bodies regulate blood glucose levels within a fairly narrow range to provide adequate glucose to the brain and other cells. Two hormones, insulin and glucagon, assist the body with maintaining blood glucose. Specialized cells in the pancreas synthesize, store, and secrete both hormones.

When we eat a meal, our blood glucose level rises. But glucose in our blood cannot help the nerves, muscles, and other tissues function unless it can cross into them. Glucose molecules are too large to cross the cell membranes of our tissues independently. To get in, glucose needs assistance from the hormone **insulin**, which is secreted by the beta cells of the pancreas (Figure 4.7a). Insulin is transported in the blood to the cells of tissues throughout the body, where it stimulates special molecules located in the cell membrane to transport glucose into the cell. Insulin can be thought of as a key that opens the gates of the cell membrane and carries the glucose into the cell interior, where it can be used for energy. Insulin also stimulates the liver and muscles to take up glucose molecules and convert them to glycogen for storage.

When you have not eaten for some time, your blood glucose levels decline. This decrease in blood glucose stimulates the alpha cells of the pancreas to secrete another hormone, **glucagon** (Figure 4.7b). Glucagon acts in an opposite way to insulin: it causes the liver to convert its stored glycogen into glucose, which is then secreted into the bloodstream and transported to the cells for energy. Glucagon also assists in the breakdown of body proteins to amino acids so the liver can stimulate *gluconeogenesis*, or the production of new glucose from non-carbohydrate source, in this case certain amino acids.

Normally the effects of insulin and glucagon balance each other to maintain blood glucose within a healthy range. If this balance is altered, it can lead to such health conditions as diabetes (page 139) or hypoglycemia (page 144).

Recap: Two hormones, insulin and glucagon, are involved in regulating blood glucose. Insulin lowers blood glucose levels by facilitating the entry of glucose into cells. Glucagon raises blood glucose levels by stimulating gluconeogenesis and the breakdown of glycogen stored in the liver.

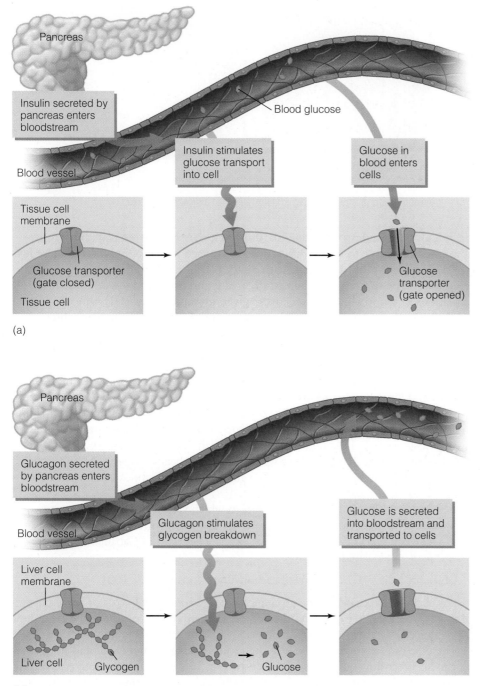

Figure 4.7 Regulation of blood glucose by the hormones insulin and glucagon. (a) When blood glucose levels increase after a meal, the pancreas secretes insulin. Insulin opens gates in the cell membrane to allow the passage of glucose into the cell. (b) When blood glucose levels are low, the pancreas secretes glucagon. Glucagon enters the liver cells, where it stimulates the breakdown of stored glycogen into glucose. This glucose is then released into the bloodstream.

The Glycemic Index Shows How Foods Affect Our Blood Glucose Levels

The **glycemic index** refers to the potential of foods to raise blood glucose levels. Dr. David Jenkins, Dr. Tom Wolever, and their research colleagues at St. Michael's Hospital in Toronto were the first to rank foods based on the degree to which they raised blood glucose and insulin levels. They used white bread as their standard and

Animations

• Regulation of Blood Sugar Levels by Insulin and Glycogen

glycemic index Rating of the potential of foods to raise blood glucose levels.

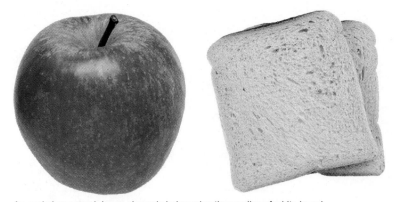

An apple has a much lower glycemic index value than a slice of white bread.

gave it a glycemic index (GI) value of 100. Then they conducted experiments to determine the degree to which different foods caused increases in blood glucose levels and the time it took, compared with a slice of white bread. Foods that were converted to glucose more slowly than white bread, and produced low to moderate fluctuations of blood glucose levels, were given glycemic index (GI) values of less than 100. Foods that were broken down into glucose more quickly than white bread, and caused sudden large increases in blood glucose, followed by large increases in insulin, were given glycemic index values greater than 100. Other researchers have assigned glycemic index values by using the glycemic effect of pure glucose as the reference, with a value of 100. Table 4.2 gives examples of high, medium, and low glycemic foods, using pure glucose as the reference.

Do any of these rankings surprise you? Most people assume that foods containing simple sugars have a higher glycemic index than starches, but this is not always the case. For instance, whole-grain cereals, such as bran flakes and Cheerios, are in the high glycemic index category, where we also find jelly beans, doughnuts, and frozen waffles. And apple juice and oranges fall in the low glycemic index category, where we find All-Bran and oatmeal cereals.

Research has examined both the extent to which various high-carbohydrate foods raise blood glucose levels—the *quality* of the carbohydrate, determined by the GI—and the *quantity* of carbohydrate eaten (Dietitians of Canada 2008). The *glycemic load* is calculated as follows:

Glycemic load = GI × grams of carbohydrate consumed ÷ 100

For example, to calculate the glycemic load of 250 mL (8 fl. oz.) of apple juice (GI = 42), you would first look up the number of grams of carbohydrate in this amount of apple juice (29 grams). The glycemic load would be 42 × 29 grams ÷ 100 = 12.2.

The type of carbohydrate, the way the food is prepared, and its fat and fibre content can all affect how quickly the body absorbs it. It is important to note that we eat most of our foods combined into a meal. In this case, the glycemic index of the total meal becomes more important than the ranking of each food.

Why do we care about the glycemic index? Foods or meals with a lower glycemic index are a better choice for someone with diabetes, for instance, because they will not trigger dramatic fluctuations in blood glucose. They may also reduce the risk of heart disease and colon cancer because they generally contain more fibre and help decrease fat levels in the blood. Recent studies have shown that people who eat lower glycemic index meals have higher levels of high-density lipoprotein, or HDL (which lowers their risk of heart disease), and their blood glucose values are more likely to be normal (Liu et al. 2001; Buyken et al. 2001). The easiest way to eat lower glycemic index foods and meals without having to look up the index is to consume such foods as beans and lentils; parboiled, or converted, rice; pasta; fresh vegetables; and whole wheat bread (stone-ground or containing whole grains).

Despite some encouraging research findings, the glycemic index remains controversial. Many nutrition researchers feel that the evidence supporting its health

Table 4.2 Selected High, Medium, and Low Glycemic Index (GI) Foods, Using Glucose as the Reference

Low GI (55 or less)* † Choose most often ✔✔✔	Medium GI (56–69)* † Choose more often ✔✔	High GI (70 or more)* † Choose less often ✔
Breads 100% stone ground whole wheat Heavy mixed grain Pumpernickel	**Breads** Whole wheat Rye Pita	**Breads** White bread Kaiser roll Bagel, white
Cereal All Bran™ Bran Buds with Psyllium™ Oat Bran™	**Cereal** Grapenuts™ Puffed wheat Oatmeal Oats Raisin Bran™ (Kellogg's)	**Cereal** Bran flakes Corn flakes Rice Krispies™
Grains Barley Bulgar Pasta/noodles Parboiled or converted rice	**Grains** Basmati rice Brown rice Couscous	**Grains** Short-grain rice

Other
 Sweet potato
 Yam
 Legumes: lentils, chickpeas,
     kidney beans, split peas, soy
     beans, baked beans
 Fruit and juices: apples, apple
     juice, bananas, oranges, pears
 Plain yoghurt
 Skim milk
	Other
	 Potato, new/white
	 Sweet corn
	 Pineapple
	 Raisins
	 Popcorn
	 Stoned Wheat Thins™
	 Ryvita™ (rye crisps)
	 Black bean soup
	 Green pea or split pea soup
		Other
		 Potato, baking (Russet)
		 Potatoes, boiled and mashed
		 French fries
		 Carrots, boiled
		 Parsnip, Rutabaga
		 Watermelon
		 Pretzels
		 Rice cakes
		 Soda crackers
		 Doughnuts

*expressed as a percentage of the value for glucose
†Canadian values where available

Source: Adapted from The Glycemic Index, Canadian Diabetes Association, www.diabetes.ca/files/GlycemicIndex_08.pdf, accessed Nov. 2008, Foster-Powell K, Holt SHA, Brand-Miller JC. International table of glycemic index and glycemic load values Am J Clin Nutr. 2002;76:5-76 and The Glycemic Index, The University of Sydney, Dec. 2005, www.glycemicindex.com, accessed Nov. 2008.

benefits is weak and that we do not know enough about the impact of low glycemic index foods on long-term health. They suggest that it may be prudent to focus on higher-fibre foods (especially cereal fibre) until more scientific studies can be conducted (Pi-Sunyer 2005). Some believe the glycemic index concept is too complex for people to apply to their daily lives. Other researchers insist that helping people to choose lower glycemic index foods is critical to the prevention and treatment of many chronic diseases.

In Australia, foods have a GI symbol and their GI value on their package labels. The government has set a national standard and developed a logo for foods that have been tested and confirmed as having a low glycemic index. To be able to carry the official Glycemic Index Tested logo, the foods must also meet specific criteria for energy (kilojoules), total and saturated fat, fibre, and sodium, so that they are consistent with the Dietary Guidelines for Australians. You can read more about this program at www.gisymbol.com.au.

> **Recap:** The glycemic index is a value that indicates the potential of foods to raise blood glucose and insulin levels. Foods with a high glycemic index cause sudden large increases in blood glucose and insulin, while foods with a low glycemic index cause low to moderate fluctuations in blood glucose. The glycemic load may be of greater value than the glycemic index alone because it takes into account the amount of the food eaten.

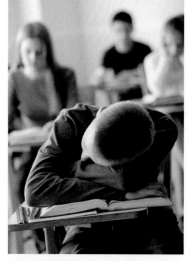

Our red blood cells can use only glucose and other monosaccharides, and our brain and other nervous tissues primarily rely on glucose. This is why you get tired, irritable, and shaky when you have not eaten for a prolonged period.

Why Do We Need Carbohydrates?

We have seen that carbohydrates are an important energy source for our bodies. Let's now learn more about this and discuss other functions of carbohydrates.

Carbohydrates Provide Energy

Carbohydrates, an excellent source of energy for all our cells, provide 4 kilocalories (17 kJ) of energy per gram. Some of our cells can also use fat and even protein for energy if necessary. However, our red blood cells can use only glucose and our brain and other nervous tissues primarily rely on glucose. This is why you get tired, irritable, and shaky when you have not eaten for a prolonged period.

Carbohydrates Fuel Daily Activity

Many popular diets—such as Dr. Atkins' New Diet Revolution and the Sugar Busters plan—are based on the idea that our bodies actually "prefer" to use fat and protein for energy. They claim that current carbohydrate recommendations are much higher than we really need.

In reality, the body relies on both carbohydrates and fat for energy. In fact, as shown in Figure 4.8, our bodies always use some combination of carbohydrates and fat to fuel daily activities.

Fat is the predominant energy source used by our bodies at rest and during low-intensity activities, such as sitting, standing, and walking. Even during rest, however, our brain cells and red blood cells still rely on glucose.

Carbohydrates Fuel Exercise

When we exercise, whether running, briskly walking, bicycling, or performing any other activity that causes us to breathe harder and sweat, we begin to use more glucose than fat. Fat breakdown is a slow process and requires oxygen, but we can break down glucose very quickly, with or without oxygen. Even during very intense

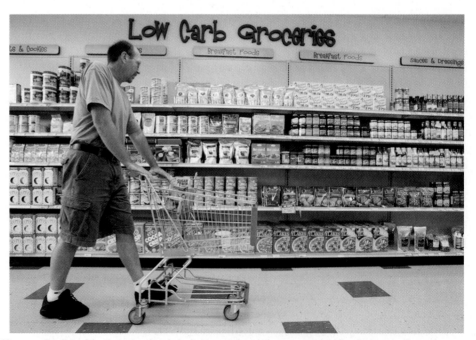

Many popular diets claim that current carbohydrate recommendations are much higher than we really need.

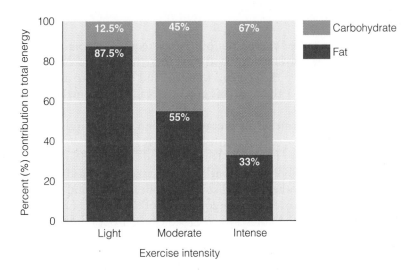

Figure 4.8 Amounts of carbohydrate and fat used during light, moderate, and intense exercise. (Adapted from J. A. Romijn, E. F. Coyle, L. S. Sidossis, A. Gastaldelli, J. F. Horowitz, E. Endert, and R. R. Wolfe, 1993, Regulation of endogenous fat and carbohydrate metabolism in relation to exercise intensity and duration, *Am. J. Physiol.* 265 [Endocrinol. Metab. 28]:E380–E391.)

exercise, when less oxygen is available, we can still break down glucose very quickly for energy. That's why when you are exercising at maximal effort, carbohydrates are providing almost 100% of the energy your body requires.

If you are physically active, it is important to eat enough carbohydrates to provide energy for your brain, red blood cells, and muscles. In Chapter 12, we discuss in more detail the carbohydrate recommendations for active people. In general, if you do not eat enough carbohydrate to support regular exercise, your body will have to rely upon fat and protein as alternative energy sources. When your carbohydrate intake is insufficient, body protein is used for energy (the consequences of which are discussed beginning on page 126). In addition, you will have to reduce your amount and intensity of exercise so that you can rely more on fat for energy. One advantage of becoming highly trained for endurance-type events such as marathons and triathlons is that our muscles are able to store more glycogen, which provides us with additional glucose we can use during exercise. (See Chapter 12 for more information on how exercise improves our use and storage of carbohydrates.)

Low Carbohydrate Intake Can Lead to Ketoacidosis

When we do not eat enough carbohydrate, the body must find other sources of energy. Although most of our body tissues can use fat and protein for energy, our brains prefer to use glucose. Thus, when our carbohydrate intake is inadequate, our body seeks an alternative source of fuel for the brain and begins to break down stored fat. This process, called **ketosis**, produces an alternative fuel called **ketones**.

Ketosis is an important mechanism for providing energy to the brain during situations of fasting, low carbohydrate intake, or vigorous exercise (Pan et al. 2000). However, ketones also suppress appetite and cause dehydration and acetone breath (the breath smells like nail polish remover). If inadequate carbohydrate intake continues for an extended period, the body will produce excessive amounts of ketones. Because many ketones are acids, high ketone levels cause the blood to become acidic, leading to a condition called **ketoacidosis**. The high acidity of the blood interferes with basic body functions, causes the loss of lean body mass, and damages many body tissues. People with untreated diabetes are at high risk for ketoacidosis, which can lead to coma and even death. (See page 140 for further details about diabetes.)

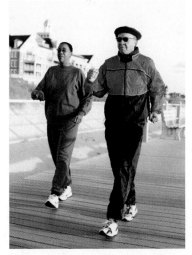

When we exercise, whether power walking or performing any other activity that causes us to breathe harder and sweat, we begin to use more glucose than fat.

ketosis The process by which the breakdown of fat during fasting results in the production of ketones.

ketones Substances produced during the breakdown of fat when carbohydrate intake is insufficient to meet energy needs. Provide an alternative energy source for the brain when glucose levels are low.

ketoacidosis A condition in which excessive ketones are present in the blood, causing the blood to become very acidic, which alters basic body functions and damages tissues. Untreated ketoacidosis can be fatal. This condition is found in individuals with untreated diabetes mellitus.

Carbohydrates Spare Protein

Some cells can rely on fat for energy, but other cells require glucose. If the diet does not provide enough carbohydrate, the body will make its own glucose from protein. This involves breaking down the proteins in blood and tissues into amino acids, then converting some of them to glucose. This process is called **gluconeogenesis** (or "generating new glucose").

When our body uses proteins for energy, the amino acids from these proteins cannot be used to make new cells, repair tissue damage, support our immune system, or perform any of their other functions. During periods of starvation or when eating a diet that is very low in carbohydrate, our body will take amino acids from the blood first, and then from other tissues like muscles, heart, liver, and kidneys. Using amino acids in this manner over a prolonged period of time can cause serious, possibly irreversible, damage to these organs. (See Chapter 6 for more details on using protein for energy.)

> **Recap:** Carbohydrates are an excellent energy source for us at rest and during exercise, and provide 4 kcal (17 kJ) of energy per gram. Carbohydrates are necessary in the diet to spare body proteins and prevent ketosis.

gluconeogenesis *The generation of glucose from the breakdown of proteins into amino acids.*

Complex Carbohydrates Have Health Benefits

The relationship among carbohydrates, heart disease, and obesity is the subject of considerable controversy. Proponents of low-carbohydrate diets claim that eating carbohydrates, not fat, makes you overweight. However, anyone who consumes extra energy, whether in the form of sugar, complex carbohydrates, protein, or fat, may eventually become obese. Studies indicate that overweight people tend to eat higher amounts of energy, including both sugar and fat, and they are not physically active enough to expend this extra energy. Thus, weight gain occurs.

Fat is more energy-dense than carbohydrate: it contains 9 kcal (37 kJ) per gram, while carbohydrate contains only 4 kcal (17 kJ) per gram. Thus, gram for gram, fat is twice as "fattening" as carbohydrate. In fact, eating complex carbohydrates that are high in fibre and other nutrients has been shown to reduce the overall risk for obesity, heart disease, and diabetes. Thus, all carbohydrates are not bad, and a small amount of simple carbohydrates can be included in a healthful diet. People who are very active and need more calories can eat more simple carbohydrates, while those who are older, less active, or overweight should limit their consumption and focus on complex carbohydrates.

• Diverticulosis and Fibre

Fibre Helps Us Stay Healthy

Although we cannot digest fibre, it is still an important substance in our diet. Research indicates that it helps us stay healthy and may prevent many digestive and chronic diseases. The potential benefits of fibre consumption include the following:

- May reduce the risk of colon cancer. Although there is still some controversy surrounding this issue, many researchers believe that fibre can bind cancer-causing substances and speed their elimination from the colon. However, recent studies of colon cancer and fibre have shown that this relationship is not as strong as previously thought.

- Helps prevent hemorrhoids, constipation, and other intestinal problems by keeping our stools moist and soft. Fibre gives intestinal muscles "something to push on" and makes it easier to eliminate stools.

- Reduces the risk of *diverticulosis*, a condition that is caused in part by trying to eliminate small, hard stools. A great deal of pressure must be generated in the

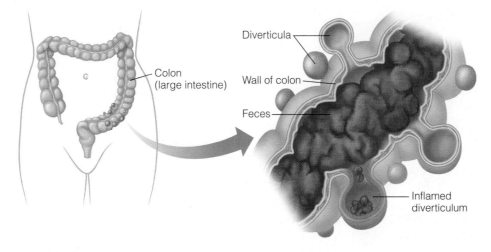

Figure 4.9 Diverticulosis occurs when bulging pockets form in the wall of the colon. These pockets can become infected and inflamed, causing a painful condition called diverticulitis.

large intestine to pass hard stools. This increased pressure weakens intestinal walls, causing them to bulge outward and form pockets (Figure 4.9). Feces and fibrous materials can be trapped in these pockets, which become infected and inflamed. This painful condition is called diverticulitis and is treated with antibiotics or surgery.

- May reduce the risk of heart disease by delaying or physically blocking the absorption of dietary cholesterol into the bloodstream. Fibre also contributes small amounts of fatty acids that may lower the amount of low-density lipoprotein (LDL) to healthful levels in our bodies.

- May enhance weight loss, as eating a diet high in soluble fibre causes a person to feel more full. Soluble fibre absorbs water, expands in our intestine, and slows the movement of food through the upper part of the digestive tract. This causes people to feel full longer.

- May lower the risk of type 2 diabetes. In slowing absorption, soluble fibre also slows the release of glucose into the blood. It thereby improves the body's regulation of insulin production and blood glucose levels.

- Promotes regular bowel movements. Insoluble fibre attracts and holds on to water in the intestine, speeding up intestinal activity and decreasing the transit time through the intestine.

Recap: Complex carbohydrates contain fibre and other nutrients that can reduce the risk for obesity, heart disease, and diabetes. Fibre may reduce the risk for colon cancer; helps prevent hemorrhoids, constipation, and diverticulosis; may reduce risk of heart disease; and may assist with weight loss.

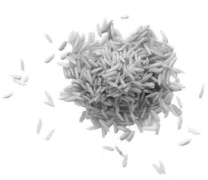

Brown rice is a good source of dietary fibre.

How Much Carbohydrate Should We Eat?

Carbohydrates are an important part of a balanced, healthy diet. The Recommended Dietary Allowance (RDA) for carbohydrate is based on the amount of glucose our brain uses (Institute of Medicine 2002). The current RDA for carbohydrate for adults 19 years of age and older is 130 grams of carbohydrate per day. It is important to emphasize that this RDA does not cover the amount of carbohydrate needed to support daily activities; it covers only the amount of carbohydrate needed to supply adequate glucose to the brain.

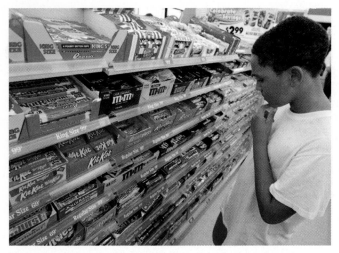

Foods with added sugars, like candy, have lower levels of vitamins and minerals than most foods that naturally contain simple sugars, such as fruit.

As introduced in Chapter 1, carbohydrates and the other macronutrients have been assigned an Acceptable Macronutrient Distribution Range (AMDR). This is the range of intake associated with a decreased risk of chronic diseases. The AMDR for carbohydrates is 45% to 65% of total energy intake, with added sugars providing 25% or less of total energy intake. Most health experts agree that the majority of the carbohydrates you eat each day should be complex—or whole grain and unprocessed—carbohydrates. As recommended in *Eating Well with Canada's Food Guide,* ensuring that at least half of your grain products are whole grain or multigrain and choosing vegetables and fruit more often than juice, will ensure that you get enough fibre and other complex carbohydrates in your diet. Keep in mind that fruits predominantly comprise simple sugar and contain little or no starch. They are healthful food choices, however, as they are good sources of vitamins, some minerals, and fibre, particularly if the skins are eaten.

> **Recap:** The RDA for carbohydrate is 130 grams per day; this amount is sufficient only to supply adequate glucose to the brain. The AMDR for carbohydrate is 45% to 65% of total energy intake. Added sugars should provide 25% or less of total energy intake.

Most Canadians Eat Too Many Simple Carbohydrates

Data from the 2004 Canadian Community Health Survey (CCHS v.2) show that, on average, Canadian adults get half of their energy (50.1%) from carbohydrates and children get 55.4% of their energy from carbohydrates. Both values are well within the AMDR of 45%–65% of total energy (Health Canada 2007a; Garriguet 2006). More adults than children and teens have carbohydrate intakes that fall below the AMDR. On average, 31.8% of men aged 19 and older, and 21.5% of women aged 19 and older had less than 45% of their total energy from carbohydrates.

Simple sugars account for approximately 25% of the carbohydrate calories (Statistics Canada 2003). Where does all this sugar come from? Some sugar comes from healthful food sources, such as fruit and milk. However, much of our simple sugar intake comes from *added sugars.* **Added sugars** include white sugar, brown sugar, honey, maple syrup, and corn sweeteners (dextrose, glucose syrup, and high fructose corn syrup) added to foods during processing or preparation (Canadian Sugar Institute 2006).

added sugars Sugars and syrups that are added to food during processing or preparation.

One common source of added sugars is regular soft drinks; Canadians drink an average of 100 litres per person per year (Canadian Institute for Health Information 2004). Consider that one 355 mL (12 fl. oz.) can of regular cola contains 38.5 grams of sugar, or almost 50 mL (10 tsp). If you drink the average amount, you are consuming about 11 320 grams of sugar—almost 15 litres (60 cups)—each year! Other common sources of added sugars include cookies, cakes, pies, fruit drinks, fruit punches, and candy.

Added sugars are not chemically different from naturally occurring sugars. However, foods and beverages with added sugars have lower levels of vitamins and minerals than most foods that naturally contain simple sugars. With these nutrient limitations in mind, it is recommended that our diets contain 25% or less of our total energy from added sugars. No accurate database of the amount of added sugars in foods is available, so the Canadian Community Health Survey (Health Canada 2007a) did not measure this in the nutrition component of the survey.

The Canadian Sugar Institute (2006) estimates that added sugars account for approximately 13% of our total energy intake and that this has been relatively constant over the past decade.

Simple Carbohydrates Are Blamed for Many Health Problems

Why do simple carbohydrates have such a bad reputation? First, they are known to cause tooth decay. Second, some people believe they cause hyperactivity in children. Third, eating a lot of simple carbohydrates could increase the levels of unhealthy lipids, or fats, in our blood, increasing our risk for heart disease. High intakes of simple carbohydrates have also been blamed for causing diabetes and obesity. Let's now learn the truth about these accusations related to simple carbohydrates.

Sugar Causes Tooth Decay

Simple carbohydrates do play a role in dental problems because the bacteria that cause tooth decay thrive on them. These bacteria produce acids that eat away at tooth enamel and can eventually cause cavities and gum disease (Figure 4.10). Eating sticky foods that adhere to teeth—such as caramels, crackers, sugary cereals, dried fruit, and licorice—and sipping sweetened beverages over a period of time increase the risk of tooth decay. This means that people shouldn't slowly sip pop or juice and that babies should not be put to sleep with a bottle unless it contains only water. As we have seen, even breast milk contains sugar, which can slowly drip onto the baby's gums. As a result, infants should not routinely be allowed to fall asleep at the breast.

   To reduce your risk for tooth decay, brush your teeth after each meal and especially after drinking sugary drinks and eating candy. Drinking fluoridated water and using a fluoride toothpaste also will help protect your teeth.

There Is No Link Between Sugar and Hyperactivity in Children

Although many people believe that eating sugar causes hyperactivity and other behavioural problems in children, there is little scientific evidence to support this claim. Some children actually become less active shortly after a high-sugar meal! However, it is important to emphasize that most studies of sugar and children's behaviour have only looked at the effects of sugar a few hours after ingestion. We know very little about the long-term effects of sugar intake on the behaviour of children. Behavioural and learning problems are complex issues, most likely caused by a multitude of factors. Because of this complexity, the Institute of Medicine (2002) has stated that overall, there currently does not appear to be enough evidence that eating too much sugar causes hyperactivity or other behavioural problems in children. Thus, it has not set a Tolerable Upper Intake Level for sugar.

High Sugar Intake Can Lead to Unhealthful Levels of Blood Lipids

There is research evidence suggesting that consuming a diet high in simple sugars, particularly fructose, can lead to unhealthful changes in blood lipids. You will learn more about blood lipids (including cholesterol and lipoproteins) in Chapter 5. Briefly, higher intakes of simple sugars are associated with increases in triglycerides (lipids in our blood) and LDLs, which are commonly referred to as "bad cholesterol." At the same time, high simple sugar intake appears to *decrease* our HDLs, which are protective and are often referred to as "good cholesterol" (Institute of Medicine 2002; Howard and Wylie-Rosett 2002). These changes are of concern, as increased levels of triglycerides and LDL and decreased levels of HDL are known risk factors for heart disease. However, there is not enough scientific evidence at the present time to state with

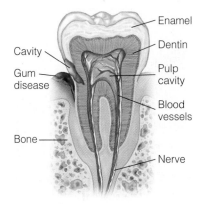

Figure 4.10 Eating simple carbohydrates can cause an increase in cavities and gum disease. This is because bacteria in the mouth consume simple carbohydrates present on the teeth and gums and produce acids, which eat away at these tissues.

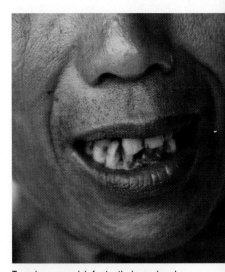

To reduce your risk for tooth decay, brush your teeth after each meal and especially after drinking sugary drinks and eating candy.

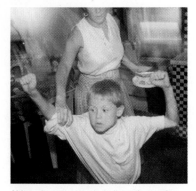

Although many people believe that eating sugar causes hyperactivity and other behavioural problems in children, there is little scientific evidence to support this claim.

confidence that eating a diet high in simple sugars causes heart disease. Based on our current knowledge, it is prudent for a person at risk for heart disease to eat a diet low in simple sugars.

High Sugar Intake Does Not Cause Diabetes but May Contribute to Obesity

There is no scientific evidence that eating a diet high in sugar causes diabetes. In fact, studies examining the relationship between sugar intake and type 2 diabetes report either no association between sugar intake and diabetes or a decreased risk of diabetes with increased sugar intake (Meyer et al. 2000; Colditz et al. 1992). However, people who have diabetes need to moderate their intake of sugar and closely monitor their blood glucose levels.

To date, there is no evidence to convincingly prove that sugar intake causes obesity; however, one study found that overweight children consumed more regular (not diet) soft drinks than did children of normal weight (Troiano et al. 2000). Another study found that for every extra sugared soft drink consumed by a child per day, the risk of obesity increases by 60% (Ludwig, Peterson, and Gortmaker 2001). We do know that if you consume more energy than you expend, you will gain weight. It makes intuitive sense that people who consume extra energy from high-sugar foods are at risk for obesity, just as people who consume extra energy from fat gain weight. In addition to the increased potential for obesity, another major concern about high-sugar diets is that they are often inadequate in nutrients critical to maintaining our health. Although we cannot state with certainty that consuming a high-sugar diet causes obesity, it is important to optimize your intake of nutrient-dense foods and limit added sugars. The relationship between soft drinks and obesity is highly controversial and discussed in more detail in the Nutrition Debate on page 150.

> **Recap:** Added sugars are sugars and syrups added to foods during processing or preparation. Our intake of added sugars should be 25% or less of our total energy intake each day. Sugar causes tooth decay but does not appear to cause hyperactivity in children. Higher intakes of simple sugars are associated with increases in triglycerides and low-density lipoproteins. Diets high in sugar can cause unhealthy changes in blood lipids but do not cause diabetes. The relationship between added sugars and obesity is controversial.

Most North Americans Eat Too Few Complex Carbohydrates

Do you get enough complex carbohydrates each day? Do you eat whole grains and legumes every day? Many people eat plenty of breads, pastas, and cereals, but most do not consistently choose whole-grain products. As we explained earlier, whole-grain foods have a lower glycemic index than simple carbohydrates; thus, they prompt a more gradual release of insulin and result in less severe fluctuations in blood levels of insulin and glucose. Whole-grain foods also provide more nutrients and fibre than foods made with enriched flour.

Table 4.3 defines terms commonly used on nutrition labels for breads and cereals. Read the label for the breads you eat—does it list *whole wheat flour* or just enriched *wheat flour*? Although most labels for breads and cereals list enriched wheat flour as the first ingredient, this term actually refers to enriched white flour, which is made when wheat flour is processed. Don't be fooled— becoming an educated consumer will help you select whole grains instead of processed foods.

We Need at Least 25 Grams of Fibre Daily

How much fibre do we need? The Adequate Intake for fibre is 25 grams per day for women and 38 grams per day for men (Institute of Medicine 2002), or 14 grams of

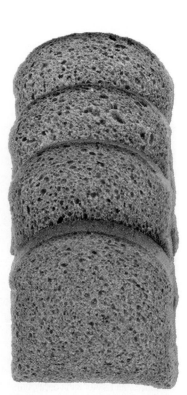

Whole-grain foods provide more nutrients and fibre than foods made with enriched white flour.

Table 4.3   Terms Used to Describe Grains and Cereals on Nutrition Labels

Term	Definition
Brown bread	Bread coloured by the use of whole wheat flour, graham flour, bran, molasses or caramel
Enriched white bread	Bread made using only enriched wheat flour; contains thiamin, riboflavin, niacin, folic acid, iron; may contain vitamin B_6, pantothenic acid, magnesium, calcium
Whole wheat bread	Bread containing not less than 60% whole wheat flour in relation to the total amount of flour used
Whole wheat flour or entire wheat flour	Bread containing not less than 95% of the natural constituents of the wheat berry
Graham flour	Flour with additional bran and other constituents of the wheat berry
Cracked wheat flour	Flour containing the natural constituents in the proportions found in the wheat used.

Source: Adapted from Canadian Food Inspection Agency. Guide to Food Labelling and Advertising, 9.8 Grain and Bakery Products, http://www.inspection.gc.ca/english/fssa/labeti/guide/ch9ae.shtml#9.8 accessed February 2008.

fibre for every 1000 Calories (4200 kJ) per day that a person eats. Average daily intakes of men and women aged 19 and over are 19.1 grams and 15.6 grams of fibre, respectively. Although fibre supplements are available, it is best to get fibre from food because foods contain additional nutrients, such as vitamins and minerals.

Eating the amounts of whole grains, vegetables, fruits, nuts, and legumes recommended in *Eating Well with Canada's Food Guide* for your sex and age category will ensure that you eat adequate fibre. Table 4.4 lists some common foods and their fibre content. Think about how you can design your own diet to include high-fibre foods.

It is also important to drink more water as you increase your fibre intake, since fibre binds with water to soften stools. Inadequate water intake with a high-fibre diet can actually result in hard, dry stools that are difficult to pass through the colon.

Can you eat too much fibre? Excessive fibre consumption can lead to such problems as intestinal gas, bloating, and constipation. Because fibre binds with water, it causes the body to eliminate more water, so a very high-fibre diet could result in dehydration. Since fibre binds many vitamins and minerals, a high-fibre diet can reduce our absorption of important nutrients, such as iron, zinc, and calcium. In children, some older adults, people with chronic illnesses, and other at-risk populations, extreme fibre intake can even lead to malnutrition—they feel full before they have eaten enough to provide adequate energy and nutrients. So although some societies are accustomed to a very high-fibre diet, many people in Canada find it difficult to tolerate more than 25 grams of fibre per day.

Shopper's Guide: Hunting for Complex Carbohydrates

Table 4.5 compares the food and fibre content of two diets, one rich in complex carbohydrates and the other high in simple carbohydrates. Here are some hints for selecting healthful carbohydrate sources:

- Select breads and cereals that are made with whole grains, such as wheat, oats, barley, and rye (make sure the label says "whole" before the word *grain*).
- Choose foods that have at least 2 or 3 grams of fibre per serving.

Table 4.4 Fibre Content of Common Foods

Food	Fibre Content (grams)
Breads and Cereals:	
Bagel, 1 each plain, 3 ½-inch diameter	2
French bread, 1 small slice	2
White bread, 1 slice	1
Pumpernickel bread, 1 small slice	2
Whole wheat bread, 1 slice	2
Oatmeal, quick, 250 mL (1 cup)	4
Cheerios, 250 mL (1 cup)	1
Corn Flakes, 300 mL (1 ¼ cup)	1
Lucky Charms, 250 mL (1 cup)	1
Fruits and Juices:	
Apple, 1 small, with peel	3
Apple juice, 250 mL (8 fl. oz.)	< 1
Blackberries, 250 mL (1 cup)	6
Banana, 1 medium	2
Orange, 1 small, peeled	3
Orange juice, 250 mL (8 fl. oz.), from concentrate	< 1
Pear, 1 medium, with skin	5
Vegetables:	
Asparagus, cooked, 6 spears	2
Broccoli, raw, chopped, 250 mL (1 cup)	3
Broccoli, cooked, chopped, 250 mL (1 cup)	5
Cabbage, raw, chopped, 250 mL (1 cup)	1
Collard greens, cooked, 125 mL (½ cup)	2
Corn, canned, whole kernel, 125 mL (½ cup)	6
Kale, cooked, 125 mL (½ cup)	1
Lettuce, iceberg, shredded, 250 mL (1 cup)	1
Legumes:	
Black beans, cooked, 125 mL (½ cup)	7
Lima beans, cooked, 125 mL (½ cup)	7
Navy beans, cooked, 125 mL (½ cup)	8
Kidney beans, cooked, 125 mL (½ cup)	8
Lentils, cooked,125 mL (½ cup)	5

Source: U.S. Department of Agriculture, Agricultural Research Service, USDA National Nutrient Database for Standard Reference, Release 16, 2004, Nutrient Data Laboratory homepage, www.nal.usda.gov/fnic/foodcomp. Values obtained from the USDA Nutrient Database for Standard Reference, Release 16.

Note: The Adequate Intake for fibre is 25 grams per day for women and 38 grams per day for men.

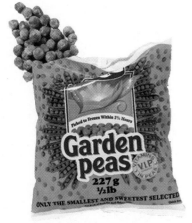

Frozen vegetables and fruits can be a nutritious alternative when fresh produce is not available.

- Buy fresh fruits and vegetables whenever possible. When appropriate, eat such foods as potatoes, apples, and pears with the skin left on.

- Frozen vegetables and fruits can be a nutritious alternative when fresh produce is not available. Check frozen selections to make sure there is no extra sugar or salt added.

- Be careful when buying canned fruits and vegetables, as many are high in sodium and added sugar. Foods that are packed in their own juice are more nutritious than those packed in syrup.

- Eat legumes frequently, every day if possible. Canned or fresh beans, peas, and lentils are excellent sources of complex carbohydrates, fibre, vitamins, and minerals. Add them to soups, casseroles, and other recipes—it is an easy way to eat more of them. If you are trying to consume less sodium, rinse canned beans to remove extra salt or choose low-sodium alternatives.

Table 4.5 Comparison of Two High-Carbohydrate Diets

High-Complex-Carbohydrate Diet	High-Simple-Carbohydrate Diet
Nutrient Analysis 2150 Calories (9000 kJ) 60% of energy from carbohydrates 22% of energy from fat 18% of energy from protein 38 grams of dietary fibre	**Nutrient Analysis** 4012 Calories (16 790 kJ) 60% of energy from carbohydrates 25% of energy from fat 15% of energy from protein 18.5 grams of dietary fibre
Breakfast 375 mL (1½ cups) Cheerios 250 mL (8 fl. oz.) skim milk 2 slices whole wheat toast with 15 mL (1 Tbsp) light margarine 1 medium banana 250 mL (8 fl. oz.) fresh orange juice	**Breakfast** 375 mL (1½ cups) Froot Loops cereal 250 mL (8 fl. oz.) skim milk 2 slices white toast with 15 mL (1 Tbsp) light margarine 250 mL (8 fl. oz.) fresh orange juice
Lunch 250 mL (8 fl. oz.) low-fat blueberry yogurt Tuna sandwich: 2 slices whole wheat bread 50 mL (¼ cup) tuna packed in water 5 mL (1 tsp) Dijon mustard 10 mL (2 tsp) low-fat mayonnaise 2 carrots, raw, with peel 250 mL (1 cup) raw cauliflower 15 mL (1 Tbsp) peppercorn ranch salad dressing (for dipping vegetables)	**Lunch** McDonald's Quarter Pounder, 1 sandwich 1 large order French fries 500 mL (16 fl. oz.) cola drink 30 jelly beans
(No Snack)	**Snack** 1 cinnamon raisin bagel 30 mL (2 Tbsp) cream cheese 250 mL (8 fl. oz.) low-fat strawberry yogurt
Dinner ½ chicken breast, roasted 250 mL (1 cup) cooked brown rice 250 mL (1 cup) cooked broccoli Spinach salad: 250 mL (1 cup) chopped spinach 1 hard-cooked egg without the yolk 2 slices lean bacon 3 cherry tomatoes 30 mL (2 Tbsp) creamy bacon salad dressing 2 baked apples (no sugar added)	**Dinner** 1 whole chicken breast, roasted 500 mL (2 cups) mixed green salad 30 mL (2 Tbsp) ranch salad dressing 1 serving macaroni and cheese 355 mL (12 fl. oz.) cola drink Cheesecake (⅛ of cake)
(No Snack)	**Late Night Snack** 500 mL (2 cups) gelatin dessert 3 raspberry oatmeal low-fat cookies

Try the Nutrition Label Activity (page 134) to learn how to recognize various carbohydrates on food labels. Armed with this knowledge, you are now ready to make more nutritious food choices.

Recap: The Adequate Intake for fibre is 25 grams per day for women and 38 grams per day for men. Many Canadians eat only half the fibre they need each day. Foods high in fibre and complex carbohydrates include whole grains and cereals, legumes, fruits, and vegetables. The more processed the food, the fewer complex carbohydrates it contains.

Recognizing Carbohydrates on the Label

Figure 4.11 shows labels for two breakfast cereals. Cereal A, on the left, is processed and sweetened, and Cereal B, on the right, is a whole-grain product with little added sugar.

- Check each label to locate the amount of total carbohydrate. For Cereal A, the total carbohydrate is 30 grams, and for Cereal B it is 22 grams for the same serving size.

- Look at the information listed as subgroups under Carbohydrate. The label for Cereal A shows that the cereal contains 1 gram of dietary fibre, 8 grams of sugars, and 21 grams of starch per serving.

- The label for Cereal B lists only the fibre (3 grams) and sugars (1 gram) per serving. In this case, the amount of

Nutrition Facts (A)
Serving 1 cup (30 g)

Amount	Cereal Only	With 1/2 cup 2% milk
Calories	120	180
		% Daily Value
Fat 0 g*	0%	4%
Saturated 0 g	0%	8%
+ Trans 0 g		
Cholesterol 0 g	0%	3%
Sodium 160 mg	7%	10%
Carbohydrate 30 g	10%	12%
Fibre 1 g	4%	4%
Sugars 8 g		
Starch 21 g		
Protein 3 g		
Vitamin A	0%	8%
Vitamin C	0%	0%
Calcium	10%	20%
Iron	30%	30%
Vitamin D	0%	25%
Thiamin	45%	50%
Riboflavin	35%	50%
Niacin	8%	15%
Vitamin B$_6$	10%	15%
Folate	10%	10%
Vitamin B$_{12}$	0%	25%
Pantothenate	6%	15%
Phosphorus	10%	20%
Magnesium	10%	15%
Zinc	6%	10%
*Amount in cereal		

(a) Sweetened Cereal

Nutrition Facts (B)
Serving 1 cup (30 g)

Amount	Cereal Only	With 1/2 cup 2% milk
Calories	120	180
		% Daily Value
Fat 2 g*	3%	7%
Saturated 0.4 g	2%	10%
+ Trans 0 g		
Cholesterol 0 g	0%	3%
Sodium 280 mg	12%	14%
Carbohydrate 22 g	7%	9%
Fibre 3 g	12%	12%
Sugars 1 g		
Starch		
Protein 4 g		
Vitamin A	0%	7%
Vitamin C	0%	0%
Calcium	9%	23%
Iron	30%	30%
Vitamin D	0%	25%
Thiamin	40%	44%
Riboflavin	2%	15%
Niacin	3%	8%
Vitamin B$_6$	13%	16%
Folate	8%	10%
Vitamin B$_{12}$	0%	23%
Pantothenate	12%	18%
Phosphorus	10%	20%
Magnesium	9%	16%
Zinc	8%	15%
*Amount in cereal		

(b) Whole-grain Cereal

Figure 4.11 Labels for two breakfast cereals: (a) sweetened cereal; (b) whole-grain cereal.

starch is the difference between the total carbohydrate and the sum of dietary fibre and sugars, or 22 grams — 4 grams = 18 grams of starch.

- Now look at the percentage values listed to the right of the Carbohydrate section (for cereal only, without milk). For the processed and sweetened Cereal A, the percentage contribution to the daily value for carbohydrate is 10%. For the whole-grain Cereal B, the percentage contribution to daily value for carbohydrate is 7%. This does not mean that 10% and 7%, respectively, of the Calories in Cereals A and B come from carbohydrates. Instead, this percentage refers to the daily values. For a person consuming a 2000 kcal (8400 kJ) diet, the recommended amount of carbohydrate each day is 300 grams. One serving of Cereal A contains 30 grams ÷ 300 grams, or 10% of the recommended amount, and 1 serving of Cereal B contains 22 grams ÷ 300 grams, or about 7% of the recommended amount of carbohydrates.
- To calculate the percentage of Calories that comes from carbohydrate, do the following:
  a. Calculate the Calories in the cereal that come from carbohydrate. Multiply the total grams of carbohydrate per serving by the energy value of carbohydrate:

  Cereal A: 30 grams of carbohydrate × 4 Calories (17 kJ) per gram = 120 kcal (510 kJ) from carbohydrate

  Cereal B: 22 grams of carbohydrate × 4 Calories (17 kJ) per gram = 88 kcal (370 kJ)

  b. Calculate the percent of Calories in the cereal that come from carbohydrate. Divide the Calories from carbohydrate by the total Calories for 1 serving:

  Cereal A: 120 kcal ÷ 130 kcal = 92% of kcal from carbohydrate

  Cereal B: 88 kcal ÷ 110 kcal = 80% of kcal from carbohydrate

Which cereal should you choose? Both cereals are good choices, with 30% of the daily value for iron, no trans fatty acids, little or no fat, and many B vitamins. Although the sweetened, more refined product (Cereal A) is enriched with more B vitamins, most people get adequate amounts of B vitamins from other food sources but need more dietary fibre in their diets. Therefore for most people, Cereal B is a better choice.

What's the Story on Alternative Sweeteners?

Most of us love sweets but want to avoid the extra calories and tooth decay that go along with eating simple sugars. Remember that all carbohydrates, including simple and complex, contain 4 kcal (17 kJ) of energy per gram. Because sweeteners, such as sucrose, fructose, honey, and brown sugar, contribute energy, they are called **nutritive sweeteners**.

Other nutritive sweeteners include the *sugar alcohols*; those approved for use in Canada are mannitol, sorbitol, isomalt, xylitol, lactitol, maltitol, and erythritol. Popular in sugar-free gums and mints, sugar alcohols are less sweet than sucrose (Figure 4.12). One major advantage is that they do not promote dental problems because they do not support the bacteria that cause tooth decay. However, eating large amounts of sugar alcohols can cause diarrhea, and, because they provide 2 to 4 kcal (8 to 17 kJ) of energy per gram, they are not calorie free.

nutritive sweeteners Sweeteners, such as sucrose, fructose, honey, and brown sugar, that contribute energy.

Alternative Sweeteners Are Non-Nutritive

A number of other products have been developed to sweeten foods without promoting tooth decay and weight gain. As these products provide little or no energy, they are called **non-nutritive**, or *alternative*, **sweeteners.**

non-nutritive sweeteners Also called alternative sweeteners; manufactured sweeteners that provide little or no energy.

Limited Use of Alternative Sweeteners Is Not Harmful

Contrary to popular belief, alternative sweeteners are safe for adults, children, and individuals with diabetes. It appears safe for pregnant women to consume some

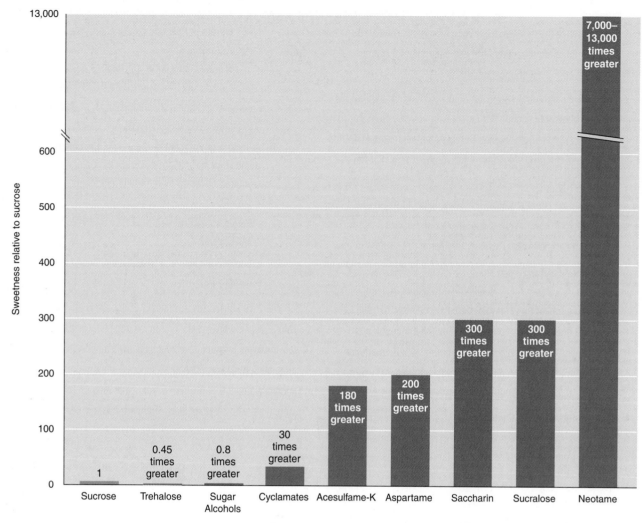

Figure 4.12 Relative sweetness of alternative sweeteners as compared to sucrose. (Adapted from M. Kroger, K. Meister, and R. Kava, Low-calorie Sweeteners and Other Sugar Substitutes: A Review of the Safety Issues, Comprehensive Reviews in *Food Science and Food Safety* Vol. 5 (2) © 2006 Institute of Food Technologists, Table 1, pg. 36)

acceptable daily intake (ADI) An estimate made by Health Canada of the amount of a non-nutritive sweetener that someone can consume each day over a lifetime without adverse effects.

alternative sweeteners in amounts within the Health Canada guidelines. The **acceptable daily intake (ADI)** is an estimate made by Health Canada of the amount of a sweetener that someone can consume each day over a lifetime without adverse effects. The estimates are based on studies conducted on laboratory animals, and they include a 100-fold safety factor. Table 4.6 lists the ADI of alternative sweeteners as set by Health Canada. It is important to emphasize that actual intake by humans is typically well below the ADI.

The major alternative sweeteners available on the Canadian market today are saccharin, cyclamates, acesulfame-K, aspartame, and sucralose. Four alternative sweeteners are categorized as *high-intensity sweeteners*: acesulfame-K, aspartame, sucralose, and neotame (see Figure 4.12).

Saccharin

Discovered in the late 1800s, *saccharin* is about 300 times as sweet as sucrose. Evidence suggesting that saccharin may cause bladder tumours in rats surfaced in the 1970s. Although subsequent research with humans did not support this finding, the U.S. Food and Drug Administration felt it was prudent to ban the sweetener. The saccharin ban met with tremendous pressure from consumers and the food industry,

Table 4.6   Acceptable Daily Intake (ADI) Levels of Alternative Sweeteners as Set By Health Canada

Sweetener	ADI (mg per kg body weight per day)
Saccharin*	5
Cyclamates*	11
Acesulfame-K	15
Aspartame	40
Sucralose	15
Neotame	2

*Not recommended for pregnant or breastfeeding women.

so the U.S. government placed a moratorium on the ban. More than 20 years of scientific research has shown that saccharin is not related to bladder cancer in humans. Based on this evidence, in May 2000 the National Toxicology Program of the U.S. government removed saccharin from its list of products that may cause cancer. Saccharin is used in foods and beverages and sold as a tabletop sweetener.

Saccharin was not banned in Canada, but it has only been available as a tabletop sweetener (called Hermesetas) through pharmacies. The label must carry a statement that "continued use of saccharin may be injurious to health, and the sweetener should not be used by pregnant women except on the advice of a physician" (CFIA 2004). Health Canada released a proposal in November 2006 to allow saccharin as a food additive in a variety of foods, including canned fruits, frozen desserts, liqueurs, soft drinks, and jams and jellies. If saccharin is relisted as an approved food additive, packaged foods will have to include saccharin in their ingredient list (Health Canada 2007b).

Cyclamate

Cylcamate was banned along with saccharin in the United States in 1969 because both were part of the same mixture that reportedly caused cancer in laboratory animals. Although saccharin was recently allowed again, the U.S. government is still considering the evidence for cyclamate (ADA 2004). It is used in more than 50 countries, including Canada, and is marketed under the names Sucaryl, Sugar Twin (yellow box), and Sweet'n Low as a tabletop sweetener. Cyclamate is 30 times as sweet as sucrose and does not increase blood glucose levels or provide any energy. There must be a statement on the label that the sweetener should be used only on the advice of a physician (CFIA 2004).

Acesulfame-K

Acesulfame-K (or acesulfame potassium) is a high-intensity sweetener marketed under the names Sunette and Sweet One. It is a calorie-free sweetener that is 175 times as sweet as sugar. It is used to sweeten gums, candies, gelatins, puddings, soft drinks, instant tea, coffee, and other beverages. The taste of acesulfame-K does not change when it is heated, so it can be used in cooking. The body does not metabolize acesulfame-K, so it is excreted unchanged by the kidneys and does not provide any energy. It is often found in combination with other sweeteners, such as aspartame.

Aspartame

Aspartame, also called Equal and NutraSweet, is one of the most popular alternative sweeteners currently found in foods and beverages—and also one of the most

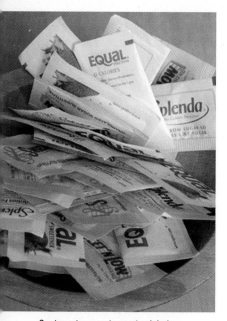

Contrary to recent reports claiming severe health consequences related to consumption of alternative sweeteners, major government health agencies believe that these products are safe for us to consume.

controversial. Aspartame is a high-intensity sweetener comprising two amino acids: phenylalanine and aspartic acid. When these amino acids are separate, one is bitter and the other has no flavour—but, joined together, they make a substance that is 200 times as sweet as sucrose. Although aspartame contains 4 kcal (17 kJ) of energy per gram, it is so sweet that only small amounts are necessary, thus it ends up contributing little or no energy. Because aspartame is made from amino acids, its taste is destroyed with heat (see Chapter 6); thus, it cannot be used in cooking.

Earlier concerns about the safety of aspartame were renewed in 2005 with a study published in the *European Journal of Oncology and Environmental Health Perspectives* by an Italian cancer research group (Soffritti et al. 2005). Unlike previous animal studies in which the animals were sacrificed at 110 weeks of age, this study allowed the animals to live until they died on their own; the last rat died at 159 weeks of age. Since cancers develop over time, the authors maintain that this allowed aspartame to fully demonstrate whether it has any link with cancer. Rats given aspartame had more lymphomas and leukemias compared with rats in the control groups, and the researchers hypothesized that this was likely related to the metabolism of methanol (from aspartame) to formaldehyde.

Both the Canadian and U.S. governments subsequently requested that the Italian researchers send them their data, and they re-reviewed all the available studies on aspartame. In 2007 the FDA issued a statement that "the data that were provided to FDA [from the Italian researchers] do not appear to support the aspartame-related findings reported by ERF (European Ramazzini Foundations)" (USFDA 2007). Health Canada is still studying the data, but says that its initial look at the data supports the conclusions of the European Food Safety Authority, which stated "on the basis of all the evidence currently available, that there is no need to further review the safety of aspartame nor to revise the previously established Acceptable Daily Intake" (Health Canada 2006).

Table 4.7 shows how many servings of aspartame-sweetened foods have to be consumed to exceed the ADI. Although eating less than the ADI is considered safe, note that children who consume many powdered drinks, diet pop, and other aspartame-flavoured products could potentially exceed this amount. Drinks sweetened with aspartame are extremely popular among children and teenagers, but they are very low in nutritional value and should not replace healthier beverages, such as milk, water, and fruit juice.

Some people should not consume aspartame at all: those with the disease *phenylketonuria (PKU)*. This is a genetic disorder that prevents the breakdown of the amino acid phenylalanine. Because the person with PKU cannot metabolize phenylalanine, it builds up in the tissues of the body and causes irreversible brain damage. In North America, all newborn babies are tested for PKU; those who have it are placed on a phenylalanine-limited diet. Some foods that are important sources of protein and other nutrients for growing children, such as meats and milk, contain phenylalanine. Thus, it is critical that children with PKU not waste what little phenylalanine they can consume on nutrient-poor products sweetened with aspartame.

Table 4.7   The Number of Servings That a 23 kg (50 lb.) Child and a 68 kg (150 lb.) Adult Would Have to Consume Each Day to Exceed the ADI for Aspartame

Food	23 kg (50 lb.) Child	68 kg (150 lb.) Adult
355 mL (12 fl. oz.) carbonated soft drink	7	20
250 mL (8 fl. oz.) powdered soft drink	11	34
125 mL (½ cup) gelatin dessert	14	42
Packets of tabletop sweetener	32	97

Source: Adapted from International Food Information Council, Food Safety and Nutrition Information. Sweeteners. Everything You Need to Know about Aspartame, 2001, http://ificinfo.health.org/brochure/aspartam.htm.

Sucralose

Sucralose is a high-intensity sweetener marketed under the brand name Splenda. It is made from sucrose, but chlorine atoms are substituted for the hydrogen and oxygen normally found in sucrose, and sucralose passes through the digestive tract unchanged, without contributing any energy. It is 600 times as sweet as sucrose and is stable when heated, so it can be used in cooking. It has been approved for use in many foods, including chewing gum, salad dressings, beverages, gelatin and pudding products, canned fruits, frozen dairy desserts, and baked goods. Safety studies have not shown sucralose to cause cancer or to have other adverse health effects. It is considered safe, even in large quantities.

Trehalose

In July 2005, the Canadian government approved *trehalose*, marketed by Cargill under the brand name Ascend, for use in Canada. Trehalose is a disaccharide made up of two glucose molecules joined together. Maltose is also two molecules of glucose joined together, but the two molecules of glucose are not in the same orientation—one is flipped upside down relative to the other. Unlike most of the other sweeteners, trehalose is only 45% as sweet as sucrose. And unlike maltose or sucrose, it does not enhance the growth of bacteria and dental caries. Trehalose is naturally present in mushrooms, honey, lobster, shrimp, and foods made with brewer's yeast, such as beer and bread.

Neotame

In July 2007, the sweetener *neotame* was approved for use in Canada as a high-intensity sweetener in a wide variety of beverages, breakfast cereals, desserts, bakery products, and fruit spreads (Government of Canada 2007). Neotame is an estimated 7000 to 13 000 times as sweet as sucrose and 30 to 40 times as sweet as aspartame. Like aspartame, it is composed of the amino acids aspartic acid and phenylalanine. However the amount of phenylalanine is small and it is considered safe for people with phenylketonuria.

> **Recap:** Alternative sweeteners can be used in place of sugar to sweeten foods. Most of these products do not promote tooth decay and contribute little or no energy. The alternative sweeteners approved for use in Canada are considered safe when eaten in amounts less than the acceptable daily intake. Some are not recommended for pregnant and breastfeeding women, however.

What Disorders Are Related to Carbohydrate Metabolism?

Health conditions that affect the body's ability to absorb or use carbohydrates include diabetes, hypoglycemia, and lactose intolerance.

Diabetes Mellitus: Impaired Regulation of Glucose

Diabetes mellitus is a chronic disease in which the body can no longer regulate glucose within normal limits, and blood glucose levels become dangerously high or fall dangerously low. It is imperative to detect and treat the disease as soon as possible because excessive fluctuation in blood glucose injures tissues throughout the body. If not controlled, diabetes can lead to blindness, seizures, kidney failure, nerve disease, amputations, stroke, and heart disease. In severe cases, it is fatal. The direct and indirect costs of diabetes in Canada are estimated to be $13.2 billion each year (Canadian Diabetes Association 2006). It is the seventh major cause of death in our country.

It is estimated that more than 2 million Canadians have diabetes (Canadian Diabetes Association 2006). Among those aged 20 and older, approximately 4.8% have been diagnosed with the condition.

diabetes mellitus A chronic disease in which the body can no longer regulate glucose levels in the blood.

The 1991 Aboriginal Peoples Survey, the latest data available, estimated that the rate is approximately 8.5% among First Nations peoples who live on reserves or Aboriginal settlements, 5.3% among First Nations peoples living off reserves, 5.5% among Métis, and 1.9% among Inuit people (Canadian Diabetes Association 2003, p. 3). Because most of these rates are so much higher and are increasing more quickly than the rates in the rest of the population, diabetes is considered an epidemic among Aboriginal Peoples. It is interesting to note that 50 years ago diabetes was virtually non-existent among Aboriginal populations.

There are two main forms of diabetes: type 1 and type 2. Some women develop a third form, *gestational diabetes*, during pregnancy; we will discuss this in more detail in Chapter 15.

In Type 1 Diabetes, the Body Does Not Produce Enough Insulin

type 1 diabetes A disorder in which the body cannot produce enough insulin.

Approximately 10% of people with diabetes have **type 1 diabetes**, in which the body cannot produce enough insulin. When they eat a meal and their blood glucose rises, the pancreas is unable to secrete sufficient insulin in response. Glucose levels soar, and the body tries to expel the excess glucose by excreting it in the urine. In fact, the medical term for the disease is *diabetes mellitus* (from the Greek *diabainein*, "to pass through," and Latin *mellitus*, "sweetened with honey"), and frequent urination is one of its warning signs (see Table 4.8 for other symptoms). If blood glucose levels are not controlled, a person with type 1 diabetes will become confused and lethargic and have trouble breathing. This is because their brains are not getting enough glucose to properly function. As discussed earlier, uncontrolled diabetes can lead to ketoacidosis; left untreated, the ultimate result is coma and death.

The cause of type 1 diabetes is unknown, but it may be an *autoimmune disease*. This means that the body's immune system attacks and destroys its own tissues, in this case the beta cells of the pancreas. It's thought that certain people inherit the tendency to develop abnormal antibodies that attack beta cells, but more research is needed.

Some recent research suggests that there may also be a link to viral infections or other environmental toxins. Of particular interest are infections caused by a group of non-polio enteroviruses called Coxsackie viruses (CDC 2000). Being exposed to these viruses early in life may trigger the abnormal antibody responses that damage the beta cells that manufacture insulin. Some researchers are looking at methods of measuring these antibodies and other substances that are indicators of autoimmune reactions.

Most cases of type 1 diabetes are diagnosed in adolescents around 10 to 14 years of age, although the disease can appear in younger children and adults. It occurs more often in families, so siblings and children of those with type 1 diabetes are at greater risk. There are no modifiable risk factors—that is, there are no risk factors that a person can control or alter to reduce his or her chances of getting type 1 diabetes.

The treatment for type 1 diabetes is daily insulin injections or the use of an insulin pump. Insulin is a hormone made of protein, so it would be digested in the

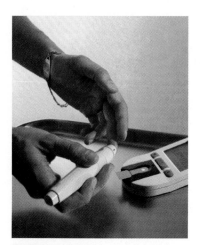

Monitoring blood glucose requires pricking the fingers several times each day and measuring the blood glucose by using a glucometer.

Table 4.8   Symptoms of Type 1 and Type 2 Diabetes

Type 1 Diabetes	Type 2 Diabetes*
Frequent urination	Any of the type 1 symptoms
Unusual thirst	Frequent infections
Extreme hunger	Blurred vision
Unusual weight loss	Cuts or bruises that are slow to heal
Extreme fatigue	Tingling or numbness in the hands or feet
Irritability	Recurring skin, gum, or bladder infections

Source: Adapted from the American Diabetes Association, Diabetes Symptoms, www.diabetes. org (accessed December 2003).

*Some people with type 2 diabetes experience no symptoms.

intestine if taken as a pill. Individuals with type 1 diabetes must monitor their blood glucose levels closely, by using a *glucometer*, and administer injections of insulin several times a day to maintain their blood glucose levels in a healthful range. The Highlight box on page 142 describes the long-term complications of diabetes.

In Type 2 Diabetes, Cells Become Less Responsive to Insulin

In **type 2 diabetes**, body cells become resistant, or less responsive to insulin. This type of diabetes develops progressively, meaning that the biological changes resulting in the disease occur over a long period. Type 2 diabetes accounts for 90% of the diabetes in the general population and most of the diabetes among Aboriginal Peoples.

In most cases, obesity is the trigger for a cascade of changes that eventually result in the disorder. Specifically, the cells of many obese people are less responsive to insulin, exhibiting a condition called *insulin insensitivity* (or insulin resistance). The pancreas attempts to compensate for this insensitivity by secreting more insulin. Over time, a person who is insulin insensitive will have to produce very high levels of insulin to use glucose for energy. Eventually the pancreas becomes incapable of secreting these excessive amounts, and the beta cells stop producing the hormone altogether. Thus, blood glucose levels may be elevated in a person with type 2 diabetes either (1) because of insulin insensitivity, (2) because the pancreas can no longer secrete enough insulin, or (3) because the pancreas has entirely stopped insulin production.

Many factors can cause type 2 diabetes. Genetics plays a role, so relatives of people with type 2 diabetes are at increased risk. Obesity and physical inactivity also increase the risk. Indeed, diabetes is thought to have become an epidemic because of a combination of our poor eating habits, sedentary lifestyles, increased obesity, and aging population. Most cases of type 2 diabetes develop after age 45, and type 2 diabetes in children was virtually unheard of until recently. Unfortunately, the disease is increasing dramatically among children and adolescents posing serious health consequences for them and their future children.

Type 2 diabetes can be treated in a variety of ways. Weight loss, healthy eating patterns, and regular exercise can control symptoms in some people. More severe cases may require oral medications. These drugs work in either of two ways: they improve body cells' sensitivity to insulin or reduce the amount of glucose the liver produces. If the pancreas of a person with type 2 diabetes can no longer secrete enough insulin, the patient must take daily injections of insulin just like a person with type 1 diabetes.

> **Recap:** Diabetes is a disease that results in dangerously high levels of blood glucose. Type 1 diabetes typically appears at a young age; the pancreas cannot secrete sufficient insulin so insulin injections are required. Type 2 diabetes develops over time and may be triggered by obesity: body cells are no longer sensitive to the effects of insulin or the pancreas no longer secretes sufficient insulin to meet body needs. Supplemental insulin may or may not be needed to treat type 2 diabetes. Diabetes increases the risk of dangerous complications, such as heart disease, blindness, kidney disease, and amputations. People with type 2 diabetes also must monitor their blood glucose levels closely.

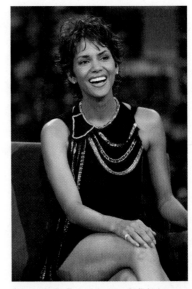

Actress Halle Berry has type 2 diabetes.

type 2 diabetes A progressive disorder in which body cells become less responsive to insulin.

What Is Prediabetes?

Prediabetes, or impaired fasting glucose, is a condition in which blood glucose levels are higher than normal but not high enough to be classified as full-blown diabetes. An estimated 4 million Canadians between the ages of 40 and 74 have impaired fasting glucose (Public Health Agency of Canada 2007).

After an overnight fast, most people have glucose levels between 3.9 mmol/L and 5.6 mmol/L. Type 2 diabetes is defined as a fasting plasma glucose level of 7.0 mmol/L or higher. Thus, when you consider these numbers, values above

▶ **HIGHLIGHT**

Diabetes Complications: The Long-Term Picture

Both type 1 and type 2 diabetes are associated with a number of serious complications over the longer term. Heart disease, for example, is common in many people with diabetes; genetics may have a role, and poorly controlled blood glucose levels do as well.

Arteries

Diabetes can cause blood vessel problems such as atherosclerosis (the buildup of plaque deposits in the blood vessels). This buildup can be particularly serious when it affects the coronary arteries, which supply your heart with blood. Also known as *macrovascular disease*, or large blood vessel disease, partial or total blockage of the coronary arteries can lead to a number of very serious complications, such as angina (chest pains) and heart attack. But research has found that people with diabetes are two to three times more likely to develop coronary artery disease (heart disease) compared to people without diabetes, and they also develop it 10 to 12 years earlier than people without diabetes.

Eyes

Microvascular disease, or small blood vessel disease, begins the process that can lead to partial and—if left untreated—total loss of vision. Retinopathy occurs when the small blood vessels in the retina, the light-sensitive inner lining at the back of the eye, become damaged as a result of high blood sugar levels. Damage to the eye may include hemorrhaging and the development of scar tissue. Good blood glucose control to prevent hyperglycemia, as well as good management of high blood pressure and abnormal blood lipids, can delay the progression of the disease. Laser therapy may be helpful in restoring partial vision in some people with some vision loss.

Nerves

Chronic high blood sugar can damage the nerves—a condition called neuropathy. Neuropathy can be "sensory"—nerve damage that affects the legs, arms, hands, chest or abdomen, resulting in a loss of sensa-

tion, pins and needles, tingling, or pain (and, in some cases, amputation). It can also be "autonomic" damage to the nerves that control the actions of a number of organs, including the bladder, stomach, intestine, and penis (for example, nerve damage can cause impotence). The best way to prevent neuropathy is to maintain lower blood glucose levels.

Kidneys

The kidneys filter out waste products from the blood into the urine. Chronic high blood sugar levels over time damage the filtering units in kidneys. The problem is that once the kidneys are damaged in this way, they cannot be repaired. Unfortunately, there may be no symptoms until the kidney damage (nephropathy) is quite advanced. It is estimated that 50% of people living with diabetes have chronic kidney (renal) disease, and therefore early screening for kidney disease and regular monitoring are important. Early treatment with medications and good blood glucose control can slow the progress of renal disease and slow the onset of end-stage renal disease. End-stage renal disease occurs when the kidneys function at only 10% or less of their capacity and requires dialysis or kidney transplants.

Ensuring Good Blood Sugar Control

Home monitoring of blood glucose with a glucometer gives the level of sugar in the blood at that exact moment. A simple blood test done by a doctor, called the glycosylated haemoglobin (HbA1c or A1C) test, shows the average blood sugar level over the past three months. It is a good indicator of overall diabetes control and a predictor of long-term complications. People with diabetes should ask their doctors for an HbA1c or A1C test every three to six months.

Source: Canadian Diabetes Association Clinical Practice Guidelines Expert Committee. Canadian Diabetes Association 2008 Clinical Practice Guidelines for the Prevention and Management of Diabetes in Canada. *Can J Diabetes.* 2008;32(suppl 1):S1–S201. Used with permission of the Canadian Diabetes Association, diabetes.ca

prediabetes A condition in which fasting blood glucose levels are above normal but below the level used to diagnose type 2 diabetes; also called impaired fasting glucose.

5.6 mmol/L and below 7.0 mmol/L fall just outside what is clinically defined as diabetes. When levels appear consistently within this outside range, bordering on diabetes, the term **prediabetes** is used.

For some people with slightly elevated glucose levels, lifestyle changes, such as healthy eating and regular moderate physical activity, may be all that is needed to get blood glucose levels back to normal. However, many people with prediabetes will eventually advance to type 2 diabetes. According to the Heart and Stroke Foundation,

> ▶ **HIGHLIGHT**

Dr. Timothy Kieffer: Leptin and Type 2 Diabetes

"Approximately 80% of those with type 2 diabetes are obese. However, when it comes to risk of diabetes, too little fat can be as bad as too much—why?"

This is a question that intrigues diabetes researcher Dr. Timothy Kieffer, a Professor in the Department of Cellular and Physiological Sciences and the Department of Surgery at the University of British Columbia. And he may have an answer.

Leptin (from the Greek word for "thin") is a protein hormone produced by the white adipose (fat) tissue in our bodies. Usually, the more body fat a person has, the more leptin he or she also has. Since leptin down-regulates appetite and increases energy expenditure, more leptin should logically help to keep a person's weight under control. Moreover, individuals prone to obesity and type 2 diabetes might be expected to have leptin deficiencies.

However, the majority of obese individuals with type 2 diabetes are not leptin deficient; instead, they have excess amounts circulating in their blood. Dr. Kieffer and his research team believe that these individuals are leptin resistant, in the same way that they are insulin resistant. Recall that in type 2 diabetes, the pancreas continues to produce insulin, but the cells have a reduced ability to use it. These individuals have hyperglycemia *and* hyperinsulinemia. Obese people with more adipose tissue do produce abundant amounts of leptin; yet it appears that the appetite centres in the hypothalamus are not adequately receiving the signals from leptin to down-regulate appetite and increase energy expenditure.

What about the remaining 20% of people with type 2 diabetes who are not obese? Interestingly, people who have too little body fat can also develop type 2 diabetes. Too little adipose tissue means too little leptin activity; these individuals have hyperglycemia, hyperinsulinemia, and leptin deficiency. Remarkably, leptin injections can completely treat the diabetes in these individuals.

Fat is very active tissue and also an endocrine organ, producing several hormones in addition to leptin. Too much fat and too little fat both have the same net effect—too little leptin activity and insulin resistance. In the case of leptin deficiency, restoring leptin levels can correct the insulin resistance and the diabetes.

What does this mean? It suggests that (1) fat plays a critical role in regulating glucose disposal in the body. Too much fat is bad as the body becomes leptin resistant and is unable to optimally use leptin. Too little fat is bad, as there is too little leptin activity. (2) Leptin appears to be a key hormone from fat that regulates glucose homeostasis (or glucose balance), perhaps by directly affecting the beta cells in the pancreas, which produce insulin as well as insulin-sensitive tissues (i.e., muscle, liver, fat).

The bottom line? Leptin may protect against diabetes, and having too little body fat or too much body fat compromises leptin activity. Dr. Kieffer and his team hope to learn more about leptin resistance and how insulin and leptin work together in the development of type 2 diabetes. Ultimately, he hopes to harness this knowledge to develop novel therapies for obesity and diabetes.

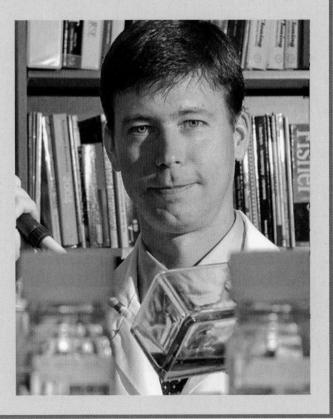

this is especially true for those who have prediabetes as part of the **metabolic syndrome**, meaning they also have higher blood pressure, higher blood levels of cholesterol and triglycerides, lower levels of HDL (the "good" cholesterol), and excess body fat around their waistline (Heart and Stroke Foundation of Canada 2007).

metabolic syndrome A syndrome characterized by high blood pressure, abnormal glucose and insulin levels, imbalance of blood fats, and large waistlines. It is strongly linked to diabetes and heart disease.

Lifestyle Choices Can Help Control or Prevent Diabetes

In general, people with diabetes should follow many of the same healthy eating guidelines recommended for those without diabetes. One difference is that people with diabetes may need to eat less carbohydrate and slightly more fat or protein to help regulate their blood glucose levels. Carbohydrates are still an important part of the diet, but nutritional recommendations must be developed separately based on individual responses to foods. In addition, people with diabetes should avoid alcoholic beverages, which can cause hypoglycemia (see below). The symptoms of alcohol intoxication and hypoglycemia are very similar. The person with diabetes and his or her companions may confuse these conditions; this can result in a potentially life-threatening situation.

Although there is no cure for type 2 diabetes, many cases could be prevented or their onset delayed. We cannot control our family history, but we can eat a balanced diet, exercise regularly, and maintain an appropriate body weight. Studies show that losing only 4.5 to 14 kg (10 to 30 lb.) can reduce or eliminate the symptoms of type 2 diabetes (ACSM 2000). In addition, moderate daily exercise may prevent the onset of type 2 diabetes more effectively than dietary changes alone (Pan et al. 1997). By selecting plenty of whole grains, legumes, vegetables, and fruits, and by staying active and maintaining a healthy body weight, our risk for diabetes should remain low.

> **Recap:** Lifestyle plays an important role in controlling diabetes. Many cases of prediabetes and type 2 diabetes could be prevented or delayed with a balanced diet, regular exercise, and the achievement and maintenance of a healthy body weight.

Hypoglycemia: Low Blood Glucose

hypoglycemia A condition marked by blood glucose levels that are below normal levels.

In **hypoglycemia**, blood glucose falls to lower-than-normal levels (Figure 4.13). One cause of hypoglycemia is excessive production of insulin, which lowers blood glucose too far. People with diabetes can develop hypoglycemia if they inject too much insulin or when they exercise and fail to eat enough carbohydrates. Two types of hypoglycemia can develop in people who do not have diabetes: reactive and fasting.

Reactive hypoglycemia occurs when the pancreas secretes too much insulin after a high-carbohydrate meal. The symptoms of reactive hypoglycemia usually appear about one to three hours after the meal and include nervousness, shakiness, anxiety, sweating, irritability, headache, weakness, and rapid or irregular heartbeat. Although many people believe they experience these symptoms, true hypoglycemia is rare. A person diagnosed with reactive hypoglycemia must eat smaller meals more frequently to level out blood insulin and glucose levels.

Fasting hypoglycemia occurs when the body continues to produce too much insulin, even when someone has not eaten. This condition is usually caused by

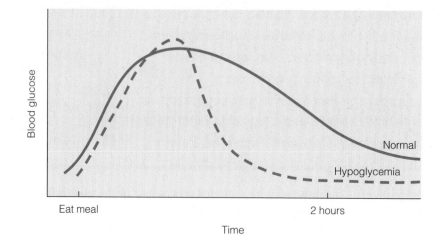

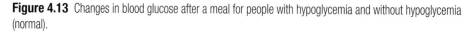

Figure 4.13 Changes in blood glucose after a meal for people with hypoglycemia and without hypoglycemia (normal).

another medical condition, such as cancer, liver infection, alcohol-induced liver disease, or a tumour in the pancreas.

> **Recap:** Hypoglycemia refers to lower-than-normal blood glucose levels. Reactive hypoglycemia occurs when the pancreas secretes too much insulin after a high-carbohydrate meal. Fasting hypoglycemia occurs when the body continues to produce too much insulin even when someone has not eaten.

Lactose Intolerance: Inability to Digest Lactose

Sometimes our bodies do not produce enough of the enzymes necessary to digest carbohydrates before they reach the colon. A common example is **lactose intolerance**, in which the body does not produce sufficient amounts of the enzyme lactase in the small intestine and therefore cannot fully digest foods containing lactose. Lactose intolerance should not be confused with a milk allergy. People who are allergic to milk experience an immune reaction to the proteins found in cow's milk. Symptoms of milk allergy include skin reactions, such as hives and rashes; intestinal distress, such as nausea, vomiting, cramping, and diarrhea; and respiratory symptoms, such as wheezing, a runny nose, and itchy and watery eyes. In severe cases, anaphylactic shock can occur.

lactose intolerance A disorder in which the body does not produce sufficient lactase enzyme and therefore cannot digest foods that contain lactose, such as cow's milk and fresh cheese.

Symptoms of lactose intolerance include intestinal gas, bloating, cramping, nausea, diarrhea, and discomfort. Although some infants are born with lactose intolerance, it is more common to see lactase enzyme activity decrease after two years of age. In fact, it is estimated that up to 70% of the world's adult population lose some ability to digest lactose as they age. Lactose intolerance is more common among non-Caucasian populations.

Not everyone experiences lactose intolerance to the same extent. Some people can digest small amounts of dairy products, while others cannot tolerate any. Suarez et al. (1998) found that many people who reported being lactose intolerant were able to consume multiple small servings of dairy products without symptoms, which enabled them to meet their calcium requirements. Thus, it is not necessary for them to avoid all dairy products; they may simply need to eat smaller amounts and experiment to find foods that do not cause intestinal distress.

It is important that people with lactose intolerance, regardless of age, find foods that can supply enough calcium for normal growth, development, and maintenance of bones. Many can tolerate specially formulated milk products that are low in lactose, while others take pills or use drops that contain the lactase enzyme when they eat

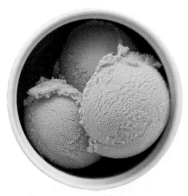

Milk products, such as ice cream, may be hard to digest for people who are lactose intolerant.

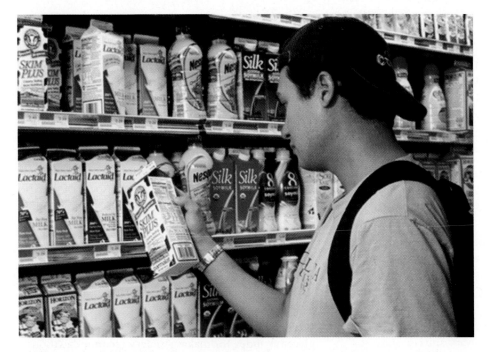

There are many products available on the market today that contain the lactase enzyme or are low in lactose. These products are developed for people with lactose intolerance.

dairy products. Calcium-fortified soy milk and orange juice are substitutes for cow's milk. Some lactose-intolerant people can also digest yogurt and aged cheese, as the bacteria or moulds used to ferment these products break down the lactose during processing or in the aging process.

How can you tell if you are lactose intolerant? Many people discover that they have problems digesting dairy products by trial and error. Because intestinal gas, bloating, and diarrhea may indicate other health problems too, you should consult a physician to determine the cause.

Tests for lactose intolerance include drinking a lactose-rich liquid and testing blood glucose levels over a two-hour period. If you do not produce the normal amount of glucose, you are unable to digest the lactose present. Another test involves measuring hydrogen levels in the breath, as lactose-intolerant people breathe out more hydrogen when they drink a beverage that contains lactose.

Recap: Lactose intolerance results from the inability to digest lactose because of insufficient amounts of lactase. Symptoms include intestinal gas, bloating, cramping, diarrhea, and nausea. Lactose intolerance commonly occurs in non-Caucasian populations. The extent of lactose intolerance varies from mild to severe. Many people with lactose intolerance can consume small quantities of dairy products and don't need to eliminate dairy products completely from their diets.

CHAPTER SUMMARY

- Carbohydrates contain carbon, hydrogen, and oxygen. Plants make the carbohydrate glucose during photosynthesis.

- Simple sugars include monosaccharides and disaccharides. The three primary monosaccharides are glucose, fructose, and galactose.

- Two monosaccharides joined together are called a disaccharide. Glucose and fructose join to make sucrose, glucose and glucose join to make maltose, and glucose and galactose join to make lactose.

- Starches are polysaccharides, and they are the storage form of glucose in plants.

- Glycogen is the storage form of glucose in humans. Glycogen is stored in the liver and in muscles. Liver glycogen provides glucose to help us maintain blood glucose levels, while muscle glycogen is used for energy during exercise.

- Dietary fibre is the indigestible parts of plants, while functional fibre is the indigestible forms of carbohydrate extracted from plants or manufactured in the laboratory. Fibre may reduce the risk of many diseases and digestive illnesses.

- Carbohydrate digestion starts in the mouth, where chewing and an enzyme called salivary amylase start breaking down the carbohydrates in food.

- Digestion continues in the small intestine. Specific enzymes are secreted to break starches into smaller monosaccharides and disaccharides. As disaccharides pass through the intestinal cells, they are digested into monosaccharides.

- Glucose and other monosaccharides are absorbed into the bloodstream and travel to the liver, where fructose and galactose are converted to glucose.

- Glucose is transported in the bloodstream to the cells, where it is either used for energy or stored in the liver or muscle as glycogen.

- Insulin and glucagon are hormones secreted by the pancreas in response to changes in blood glucose.

- Insulin is secreted when blood glucose increases sufficiently, and it assists with the transport of glucose into cells.

- Glucagon is secreted when blood glucose levels are low, and it assists with the conversion of glycogen to glucose and with gluconeogenesis.

- The glycemic index is a value that indicates how much a food increases blood glucose levels. High glycemic foods can trigger detrimental increases in blood glucose for people with diabetes. The usefulness of the glycemic index for making dietary recommendations is controversial.

- The glycemic load is a value that indicates the effects on blood glucose that result from the quality and quantity of carbohydrate consumed.

- All cells can use glucose for energy. The red blood cells, brain, and central nervous system prefer to use glucose exclusively for energy.

- Using glucose for energy helps spare body proteins, and glucose is an important fuel for the body during exercise. Exercising regularly trains our muscles to become more efficient at using both glucose and fat for energy.

- Fibre helps us maintain the healthy elimination of waste products. Eating adequate fibre may reduce the risk of colon cancer, type 2 diabetes, obesity, heart disease, hemorrhoids, and diverticulosis.

- The Acceptable Macronutrient Distribution Range for carbohydrate is 45% to 65% of total energy intake. Added sugars should provide 25% or less of total energy.

- High added-sugar intake can cause tooth decay and elevate triglyceride and low-density lipoprotein levels in the blood, and may contribute to obesity, but does not appear to cause hyperactivity in children.

- The Adequate Intake for fibre is 25 grams per day for women and 38 grams per day for men, or 14 grams of fibre for every 1000 Calories (4200 kJ) of energy consumed.

- Foods high in complex carbohydrates include whole grains and cereals, legumes, fruits, and vegetables.

- Alternative sweeteners are added to some foods because they sweeten foods without promoting tooth decay and add few or no calories to foods.

- Sugar alcohols, saccharin, acesulfame-K, aspartame, cyclamates, trehalose, sucralose, and neotame are examples of alternative sweeteners used in foods and beverages. Acesulfame-K, aspartame, sucralose, and neotame are classified as high-intensity sweeteners.

- All alternative sweeteners approved for use in Canada are felt to be safe when eaten at levels at or below the acceptable daily intake levels defined by Health Canada.

- Diabetes is caused by insufficient insulin or by the cells becoming resistant or insensitive to insulin. Diabetes causes dangerously high blood glucose levels. There are two primary types of diabetes: type 1 and type 2.

- Prediabetes, or impaired fasting blood glucose, is a condition in which blood glucose levels are higher than normal but not high enough to be classified as full-blown diabetes.

- Hypoglycemia is defined as lower-than-normal blood glucose levels. There are two types: reactive and fasting. Reactive hypoglycemia occurs when too much insulin is secreted after a high-carbohydrate meal; fasting hypoglycemia occurs when blood glucose drops even though no food has been eaten.

- Lactose intolerance results from an insufficient amount of the lactase enzyme. Symptoms include intestinal gas, bloating, cramping, diarrhea, and discomfort.

mynutritionlab   Go to MyNutritionLab at www.pearsoned.ca/mynutritionlab and enrich your understanding of nutrition! You'll find key animations, interactive exercises, access to My DietAnalysis, and much more.

REVIEW QUESTIONS   Quizzes

1. The glycemic index rates
   a. the acceptable amount of alternative sweeteners to consume in one day.
   b. the potential of foods to raise blood glucose and insulin levels.
   c. the risk of a given food for causing diabetes.
   d. the ratio of soluble to insoluble fibre in a complex carbohydrate.

2. Carbohydrates contain
   a. carbon, nitrogen, and water.
   b. carbonic acid and a sugar alcohol.
   c. hydrated sugar.
   d. carbon, hydrogen, and oxygen.

3. A1C is a blood test that measures
   a. the level of blood glucose at the time of the test.
   b. how much glucose has been in the bloodstream over the past three months.
   c. blood cholesterol levels.
   d. the rise in blood insulin levels after eating a particular food.

4. Glucose, fructose, and galactose are
   a. monosaccharides.
   b. disaccharides.
   c. polysaccharides.
   d. complex carbohydrates.

5. Aspartame should not be consumed by people who have
   a. phenylketonuria.
   b. type 1 diabetes.
   c. lactose intolerance.
   d. diverticulosis.

6. A drop in blood glucose levels stimulates the release of
   a. insulin.
   b. ketones.
   c. glucagon.
   d. gastric acid.

7. Which two monosaccharides join to form the disaccharide lactose?
   a. Glucose + glucose
   b. Glucose + galactose
   c. Galactose + fructose
   d. Fructose + glucose

8. Which of the following is a characteristic of insoluble fibre?
   a. Is able to absorb water
   b. Slows nutrient absorption in the blood
   c. Forms a gel
   d. Speeds up movement of contents in the large intestine

9. Which one of the following statements is *not* correct?
   a. Sugar causes tooth decay
   b. Eating sugar does not lead to hyperactivity in children
   c. Sugar causes diabetes
   d. High sugar may increase triglyceride levels

10. Choose the correct statement about people with lactose intolerance:
    a. They have a milk allergy
    b. They must avoid all dairy products
    c. Bloating and cramping are common symptoms they experience
    d. They produce sufficient amounts of the enzyme lactase

11. The process of breaking down proteins into amino acids and converting them to glucose is called
    a. Gluconeogenesis.
    b. Ketoacidosis.
    c. Photosynthesis.
    d. Glycolysis.

12. Compare and contrast the actions of soluble fibre and insoluble fibre in the small intestine.

13. Identify at least four ways in which fibre helps us maintain a healthy digestive system.

14. Explain why complex carbohydrates are a superior food choice to simple carbohydrates.

15. Defend the statement that obesity can trigger type 2 diabetes.

16. While eating lunch with your friends at the cafeteria, you notice that your friend Sonomi has ordered plain spaghetti, a piece of bread, a glass of apple juice, and some pudding for dessert. Another friend, Matthieu, informs Sonomi that her lunch is very unhealthy because it's basically a tray full of sugar. Sonomi disagrees and says that pasta is nothing like sugar, and she and Matthieu continue to argue for the rest of lunch. Is Matthieu or Sonomi correct? After learning about carbohydrate digestion, how would you explain what happens to Sonomi's meal once it enters her body? Is Sonomi's meal balanced? If not, what is she missing and what would you suggest that she add to her lunch tray?

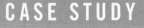

CASE STUDY

Cory, a 24-year old sedentary male, recently visited his physician complaining of increased thirst, increased hunger, fatigue, and increased urination. He has been diagnosed with prediabetes, meaning that his blood glucose is higher than normal but it is lower than the diabetes range. This puts him at risk for developing type 2 diabetes and heart disease.

a. What modifiable risk factors should Cory focus on to lessen his chance of developing type 2 diabetes?

b. Type 2 diabetes generally leads to elevated blood glucose levels. To help Cory understand the body's regulation of glucose in the blood, explain the relationship between the two hormones involved: insulin and glucagon.

c. The glycemic index (GI) ranks carbohydrate-rich foods by how much they raise blood glucose levels compared with glucose or white bread. Explain why consuming low GI foods, as opposed to high GI foods, would be beneficial for Cory. List several examples of low GI foods.

d. Cory questions whether dramatically decreasing his carbohydrate intake will help prevent type 2 diabetes. Knowing the importance of carbohydrates, explain to Cory several benefits of maintaining an adequate level of carbohydrates in his diet.

e. One of Cory's favourite foods is pasta. One serving (250 mL or 1 cup) of whole wheat spaghetti contains 37 grams of total carbohydrates.

- If this serving of pasta contains 1 gram of sugar and 30 grams of starches, how much fibre is present?
- Knowing that the Adequate Intake for dietary fibre is 38 grams per day for men, calculate the percentage of daily fibre Cory is getting from the pasta.
- Explain the potential benefits of Cory including fibre in his diet.

Test Yourself Answers

1. **False** The term *carbohydrate* refers to both simple and complex carbohydrates. The term *sugar* refers to the simple carbohydrates, monosaccharides and disaccharides.

2. **False** Diets high in sugar do cause tooth decay. Whether high-sugar diets cause obesity is still controversial. There is no evidence that diets high in sugar cause diabetes.

3. **False** Because carbohydrates are an important energy source for our bodies, we are generally able to digest and absorb carbohydrates easily. People with such health conditions as diabetes and hypoglycemia, however, experience challenges with carbohydrate absorption and metabolism.

4. **True** Our brains and red blood cells rely almost exclusively on glucose for energy, and our body tissues use glucose for energy both at rest and during exercise.

5. **True** Contrary to recent reports claiming severe health consequences related to consumption of alternative sweeteners, major health agencies have determined that these products are safe for most of us to consume in limited quantities.

WEB LINKS

www.diabetes.ca
Canadian Diabetes Association
This is an excellent website with all kinds of information about risk factors for diabetes, diabetes management, the glycemic index, and research that is being funded in Canada.

www.healthyeatingisinstore.ca
Healthy Eating Is in Store for You
This website, developed by the Canadian Diabetes Association and Dietitians of Canada, has information sheets for people with diabetes and frequently asked questions about food labels and sugar claims.

www.eatright.org
American Dietetic Association
Visit this website to learn more about diabetes, low- and high-carbohydrates diets, and general healthful eating habits.

ific.org
International Food Information Council Foundation (IFIC)
Search this site to find out more about sugars and low-calorie sweeteners.

www.cda-adc.ca
Canadian Dental Association
Go to this site to learn more about tooth decay as well as other oral health topics.

www.diabetes.org
American Diabetes Association
Find out more about the nutritional needs of people living with diabetes.

www2.niddk.nih.gov
National Institute of Diabetes and Digestive and Kidney Diseases (NIDDK)
Learn more about diabetes, including treatment, complications, U.S. statistics, clinical trials, and recent research.

Can Reducing Sugar Intake Be the Answer to Obesity?

Almost every day in the news we see headlines about obesity: "More Canadians Overweight!" "The Fattening of North America," "Obesity Is a National Epidemic!" These headlines accurately reflect the state of weight in Canada and the United States. Over the past 30 years, obesity rates have increased dramatically for both adults and children. Obesity has become public health enemy number one, as many chronic diseases, such as type 2 diabetes, heart disease, high blood pressure, and arthritis, go hand in hand with obesity.

Of particular concern are the rising obesity rates in children. It is estimated that the rate of overweight and obesity in Canadian children aged 2 to 17 years has doubled in the past 25 years (Statistics Canada 2005). Why should we concern ourselves with fighting obesity in children? First, it is well established that the treatment of existing obesity is extremely challenging, and our greatest hope of combating this disease is through prevention. Most agree that prevention should start with children at a very early age. Second, approximately 30% of children who are obese will remain obese as adults, potentially suffering the health problems that can accompany this disease. Young children are now experiencing type 2 diabetes, high blood pressure, and high cholesterol at increasingly younger ages, only compounding the devastating effects of these illnesses as they get older. We have reached the point where serious action must be immediately taken to curb the already growing crisis.

How can we prevent obesity? This is a difficult question to answer. One way is to better understand the factors that contribute to obesity and then take actions to alter these factors. We know of many factors that contribute to overweight and obesity. These include genetic influences, lack of adequate physical activity, and eating foods that are high in fat, added sugar, and energy. Although it is easy to blame our genetics, they cannot be held entirely responsible for the rapid rise in obesity that has occurred over the past 30 years. Our genetic makeup takes thousands of years to change; thus,

humans who lived 50 or 100 years ago have essentially the same genetic makeup as humans who live now. The fact that obesity rates have risen so dramatically in recent years illustrates that we need to look more closely at how our lifestyles have changed over this same period to truly understand the factors causing obesity.

One factor that has recently come to the forefront of nutrition research and policy making is the contribution of added sugars to overweight and obesity in children. As discussed earlier in this chapter, there is still much disagreement about whether added sugar does cause, and how much it might contribute to, obesity. Many health professionals are beginning to draw attention to the potential role of added sugars, specifically non-diet soft drinks, in rising obesity rates. Recent U.S. studies of soft drink consumption in children show that girls and boys ages 6 to 11 years drank about twice as many soft drinks in 1998 as compared with 1977, and consumption of milk over this same time period dropped by about 30% (Wilkinson Enns, Mickle, and Goldman 2002). Equally alarming is the finding that one fourth of a group of adolescents studied were heavy consumers of sugared soft drinks, drinking at least 770 mL (26 fl. oz.) of pop each day.

This intake is equivalent to almost 400 extra kcal (1680 kJ) each day, and these individuals consumed more calories from all foods than other adolescents and drank fewer nutrient-dense beverages, such as milk and fruit juice (Harnack, Stang, and Story 1999).

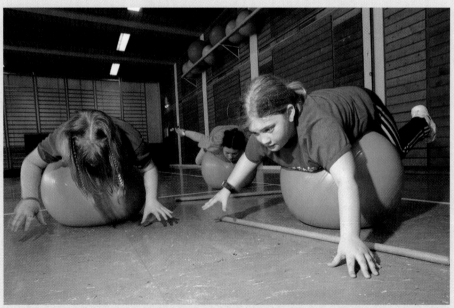

It is estimated that the rate of overweight in children has increased approximately 100% since the mid-1970s.

One report suggests that for each extra non-diet soft drink that children drink each day, the risk of obesity increases by 60% (Ludwig, Peterson, and Gortmaker 2001). Another harmful effect of soft drinks is that they tend to replace milk in the diet of adolescents, and this affects calcium intake (Whiting et al. 2001). This is especially harmful during childhood and adolescence, when bones are still growing.

With all this alarming information, you would expect dramatic changes in soft drink consumption around the country. However, this is not the case. Powerful influences are at work not only to maintain, but to increase soft drink consumption around the world. Dr. Marion Nestle highlights these influences in her book *Food Politics: How the Food Industry Influences Nutrition and Health* (Nestle 2002). Some of these influences include

- large increases in advertising by pop companies, with an emphasis on targeting young children;

- exclusive contracts between soft drink companies and schools, providing much-needed revenues to inadequate school budgets; and

- the competition between pop and other foods high in added sugar with nutritious foods served at schools, with children preferring high-sugar foods to those served through school nutrition programs.

The allegations brought against schools and the soft drink industry are strong. Many people feel that our schools have sold out our children's health for the sake of sports equipment. School food service programs are expected to be self-supporting, and they cannot compete against soft drinks, chips, and candy; thus, food service programs claim that school support of soft drinks and other junk foods undermines their programs and, in turn, our children's health. Soft drink companies are under attack for pushing non-nutritious foods to children. They are also accused of putting profits and brand loyalty ahead of our children's health.

Both schools and soft drink companies are quick to defend themselves. As adequate funding for public schools is waning from provincial and federal governments, schools are desperate to find sources of revenue to provide materials and programs to children. Thus, school administrators feel justified in accepting lucrative contracts from soft drink companies to support educational efforts. Soft drink companies argue that soft drinks and other snack foods can be part of a nutritious diet and that there is no evidence to prove that soft drinks cause obesity. In a society of capitalism, they believe that they have every right to maximize profits.

The Ontario government stepped into this debate recently and endorsed a set of recommendations from the Dietitians of Canada (2004) for changes to the snacks and beverages available in school vending machines. The new policy set out by the Ontario Ministry of Education directs school boards to "restrict the sale of all food and beverage items in elementary school vending machines to those that are healthy and nutritious" (Ontario Ministry of Education 2004). Water, 100% fruit juice, and lower-fat and non-fat milks are the recommended beverages, while fruit, fruit cups, and some crackers, cookies, pretzels, popcorn, and granola bars (depending upon their specific nutrient contents) are recommended snacks. Immediately following this announcement in Ontario, the B.C. government announced it will ban "junk food" in school vending machines.

This issue is extremely complex, and no easy solution is in sight. How do you feel about this issue? Should reducing soft drink consumption be up to individuals? Should schools and our government play a central role in controlling the types of foods served in schools? Should soft drink companies be allowed to pay large sums of money to schools in exchange for exclusive beverage contracts? Is there even enough evidence to suggest that soft drinks and other foods high in added sugars are linked with obesity? As this controversy grows, it is more likely that average citizens will be asked to take a stand on this issue.

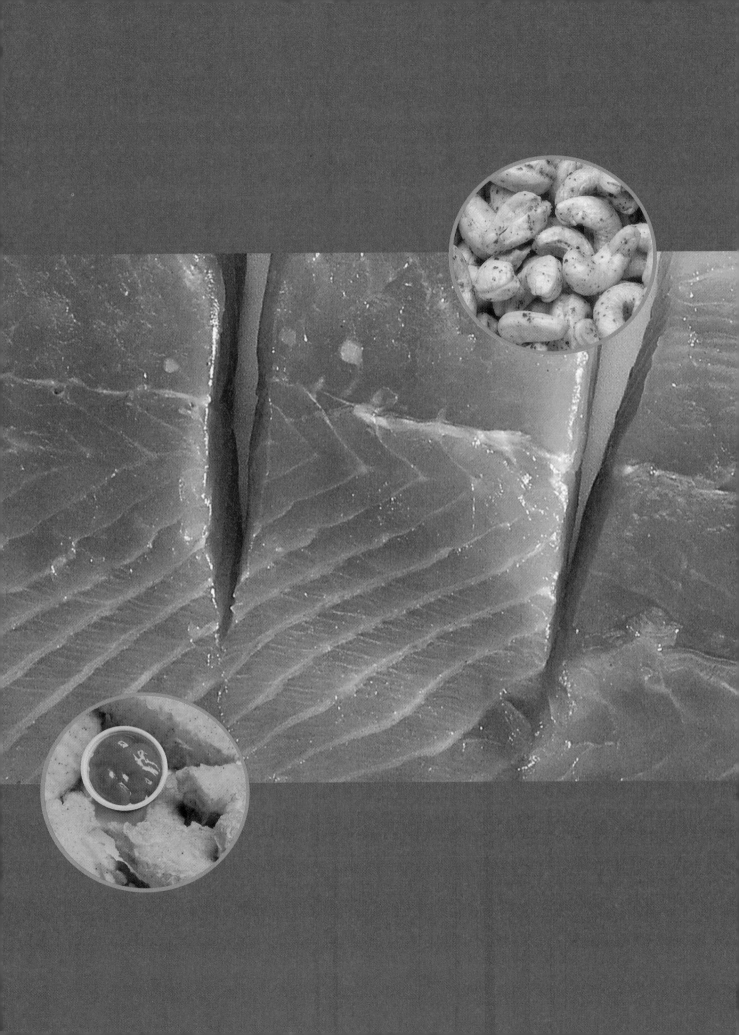

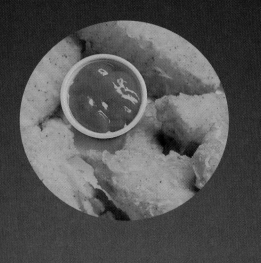

Lipids: Essential Energy-Supplying Nutrients

CHAPTER OBJECTIVES

After reading this chapter you will be able to:

1. Describe the three types of lipids found in foods, pp. 154–160.

2. Discuss how the level of saturation affects the shape and form of fatty acids, pp. 156–159.

3. Identify the primary difference between a *cis* fatty acid and a *trans* fatty acid, p. 158.

4. Describe the steps involved in fat digestion, pp. 161–165

5. Describe three functions of fat in our bodies, pp. 165–169.

6. Define the recommended dietary intakes for total fat, saturated fat, and the two essential fatty acids, pp. 171–172.

7. Describe the role of dietary fat in the development of cardiovascular disease, pp. 181–187.

8. Identify and describe the functions of four blood lipoproteins, p. 184.

Test Yourself True or False

1. Fat is unhealthful, and we should eat as little as possible in our diets. **T or F**

2. Reduced-fat and fat-free foods usually contain less than half the calories of full-fat versions of the same foods. **T or F**

3. Fat is an important fuel source during rest and exercise. **T or F**

4. Fried foods are relatively nutritious as long as vegetable shortening is used to fry the foods. **T or F**

5. Exercising regularly and eating a diet that is relatively low in fat and high in fruits, vegetables, and whole grains and can help reduce our risk for cardiovascular disease. **T or F**

Test Yourself answers can be found at the end of the chapter.

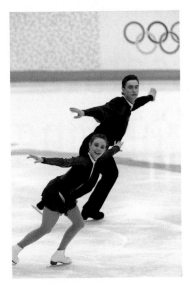

Sergei Grinkov, here skating with his partner and wife, Ekaterina Gordeeva, died of a heart attack at the age of 28.

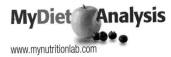

www.mynutritionlab.com

lipids A diverse group of organic substances that are insoluble in water; lipids include triglycerides, phospholipids, and sterols.

• Fats in Food

triglyceride A molecule consisting of three fatty acids attached to a three-carbon glycerol backbone.

fatty acids Long chains of carbon atoms bound to each other as well as to hydrogen atoms.

glycerol An alcohol composed of three carbon atoms; it is the backbone of a triglyceride molecule.

The world was stunned in the fall of 1995 when 28-year-old skater Sergei Grinkov, a two-time Olympic gold medallist, collapsed and died of a fatal heart attack while training in Lake Placid, New York. An autopsy revealed that Grinkov's coronary arteries were as severely clogged as those of a 70-year-old with established heart disease. Although his widow reported that he had never complained of chest pain or shortness of breath, his family history revealed one very important clue: his father had died of a heart attack at age 52.

What causes a heart attack, and how can you calculate your risk? Can a high-fat diet cause heart disease, and can a low-fat diet prevent it? When was the last time you heard anything good about dietary fat? If your best friend's father had died of a heart attack at age 44 and you noticed your friend regularly eating high-fat meals, would you say anything about it? If so, what would you say?

Although some people think of dietary fat as something to be avoided, a certain amount of fat is absolutely essential for good health. In this chapter, we'll discuss the function of fat in the human body and help you distinguish between beneficial and harmful types of dietary fat. You'll also assess how much fat you need in your diet and learn about the role of dietary fat in the development of heart disease and other disorders.

What Are Lipids?

Lipids are a large and diverse group of substances that are distinguished by the fact that they are insoluble in water. Think of a salad dressing made with vinegar and olive oil—a lipid. Shaking the bottle disperses the oil but doesn't dissolve it: that's why it separates back out again so quickly. Lipids are found in all sorts of living things, from bacteria to plants to human beings. In fact, their presence on your skin explains why you can't clean your face with water alone: you need some type of soap to break down the insoluble lipids before you can wash them away. In this chapter, we focus on the small group of lipids that are found in foods.

Lipids Come in Different Forms

There are many different types of lipids in our body and in our diet. For example, butter and olive oil are two different types of lipids. Fats, like butter, are solid at room temperature, while oils, such as olive oil, are liquid at room temperature.

Three Types of Lipids Are Present in Foods

Three types of lipids are commonly found in foods: triglycerides, phospholipids, and sterols. Let's take a look at each.

Triglycerides Are the Most Common Food-Based Lipid

Most of the fat we eat (95%) is in the form of triglycerides, which is the same way most of the fat in our body is stored. As reflected in the prefix *tri*, a **triglyceride** is a molecule consisting of three fatty acids attached to a *three*-carbon glycerol backbone. **Fatty acids** are long chains of carbon atoms bound to each other as well as to hydrogen atoms. They are acids because they contain an acid group (carboxyl group) at one end of their chain.

Glycerol, the backbone of a triglyceride molecule, is an alcohol composed of three carbon atoms. The carboxyl (COOH) end of a fatty acid attaches to the OH group of the glycerol, releasing one molecule of water (H_2O) (Figure 5.1a).

Triglycerides Are Classified by Their Length, Saturation, and Shape

To understand why we want more of some fats than others, we need to know more about their properties and how they work in our body. In general, triglycerides can

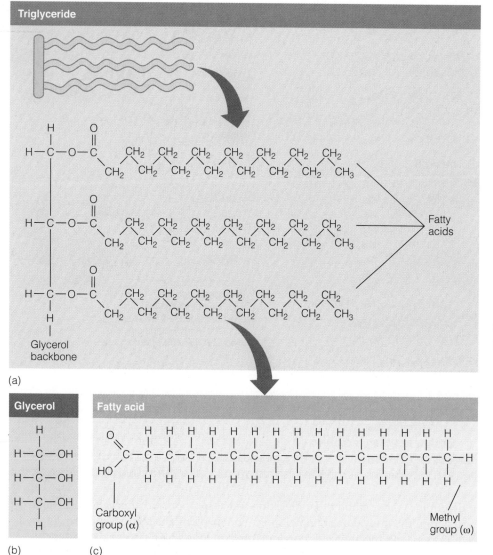

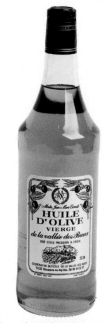

Some fats, such as olive oil, are liquid at room temperature.

Figure 5.1 (a) A triglyceride consists of three fatty acids attached to a three-carbon glycerol backbone. (b) Structure of glycerol. (c) Structure of a fatty acid showing the carboxyl carbon (α) and the methyl carbon (ω) ends.

(Source: The Science of Nutrition, by J.L. Thompson, M.M. Manore, and L.A. Vaughan, © Pearson Education, Inc., publishing as Pearson Benjamin Cummings, p. 177. Used by permission of Pearson Education, Inc.)

be classified by their chain length (number of carbons in each fatty acid), by their level of saturation (how much hydrogen, H, is attached to each carbon atom in the fatty acid chain), and their shape, which is determined in some cases by how they are commercially processed. All these factors influence how we use the triglyceride within our bodies.

Chain Length The fatty acids attached to the glycerol backbone can vary in the number of carbons they contain, referred to as their *chain length:*

- **Short-chain fatty acids** are usually fewer than six carbon atoms in length.
- **Medium-chain fatty acids** are six to twelve carbons in length.
- **Long-chain fatty acids** are 14 or more carbons in length.

The carbons of a fatty acid can be numbered beginning with the carbon of the carboxyl end (COOH), which is designated the α-carbon (that is, the alpha or first carbon), or from the carbon of the last methyl group (CH₃), called the ω-carbon (the omega or last carbon) (see Figure 5.1c). Fatty acid chain length is important because

short-chain fatty acids Fatty acids fewer than six carbon atoms in length.
medium-chain fatty acids Fatty acids that are six to twelve carbon atoms in length.
long-chain fatty acids Fatty acids that are 14 or more carbon atoms in length.

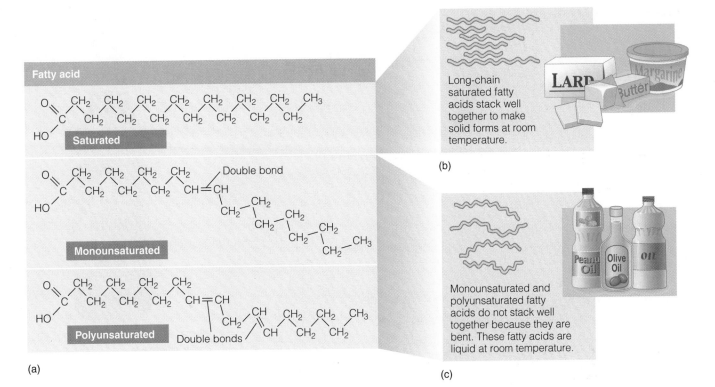

Fatty acid

Saturated

Monounsaturated

Double bond

Polyunsaturated   Double bonds

(a)

Long-chain saturated fatty acids stack well together to make solid forms at room temperature.

(b)

Monounsaturated and polyunsaturated fatty acids do not stack well together because they are bent. These fatty acids are liquid at room temperature.

(c)

Figure 5.2 Examples of levels of saturation among fatty acids and how these levels of saturation affect the shape of fatty acids. (a) Saturated fatty acids are saturated with hydrogen, meaning they have no carbons bonded together with a double bond. Monounsaturated fatty acids contain two carbons bound by one double bond. Polyunsaturated fatty acids have more than one double bond linking carbon atoms. (b) Saturated fats have straight fatty acids packed tightly together and are usually solid at room temperature. (c) Unsaturated fats have kinked fatty acids at the area of the double bond, preventing them from packing tightly together; they are liquid at room temperature.

saturated fatty acids (SFAs) Fatty acids that have no carbons joined together with a double bond; these types of fatty acids are generally solid at room temperature.

monounsaturated fatty acids (MUFAs) Fatty acids that have two carbons in the chain bound to each other with one double bond; these types of fatty acids are generally liquid at room temperature.

polyunsaturated fatty acids (PUFAs) Fatty acids that have more than one double bond in the chain; these types of fatty acids are generally liquid at room temperature.

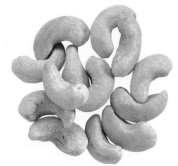

Cashew nuts are high in monounsaturated fatty acids.

it determines the method of fat digestion and absorption and affects how fats function within the body. For example, short- and medium-chain fatty acids are digested, transported, and metabolized more quickly than long-chain fatty acids. In general, long-chain fatty acids are more abundant in nature, and thus more abundant in our diet, than short- or medium-chain fatty acids. We will discuss digestion and absorption of fats in more detail shortly.

Level of Saturation Triglycerides can also vary by the types of bonds found in the fatty acids. If a fatty acid has no carbons bonded together with a double bond, it is referred to as a **saturated fatty acid (SFA)** (Figure 5.2a). This is because every carbon atom in the chain is *saturated* with hydrogen: each has the maximum amount of hydrogen bound to it. Some foods that are high in saturated fatty acids are coconut oil, palm kernel oil, butter, cream, whole milk, and beef fat.

If two carbon atoms are bound to each other with a double bond, one hydrogen atom is excluded. This lack of hydrogen at *one* part of the molecule results in a fat that is referred to as *monounsaturated* (recall from Chapter 4 that the prefix *mono-* means one). A monounsaturated molecule is shown in Figure 5.2b. **Monounsaturated fatty acids (MUFAs)** are usually liquid at room temperature. Foods that are high in monounsaturated fatty acids are olive oil, canola oil, and cashew nuts.

If the fat molecules have *more than one* double bond, they contain even less hydrogen and are referred to as **polyunsaturated fatty acids (PUFAs)** (see Figure 5.2c). Polyunsaturated fatty acids are also liquid at room temperature and include soybean, sunflower, safflower, and corn oils.

Scientists use an abbreviated system to describe fatty acids—a ratio of the number of carbons to the number of double bonds. For example, the saturated (no double bonds) 18-carbon fatty acid would be written as 18:0; this is stearic acid, and it is

Table 5.1   Major Sources of Dietary Fatty Acids

Food	Distribution of Fatty Acids by Type				
	% of total kcal from fat	% total fat kcal as EFA	% total fat kcal as SFA	% total fat kcal as MUFA	% total fat kcal as PUFA
Butter	100%	4%	65%	31%	4%
Milk, whole (3.3% fat)	49%	4%	63%	33%	4%
Milk, 2% fat	40%	4%	66%	30%	4%
Milk, 1% fat	17%	< 1%	68%	32%	< 1%
Beef, ground (16% fat)	54%	4%	45%	51%	4%
Chicken, breast skinless roasted	19%	13%	33%	41%	25%
Turkey, boneless	26%	28%	32%	25%	35%
Tuna, water-packed	6%	39%	32%	22%	46%
Tuna, oil-packed	37%	36%	21%	40%	39%
Salmon, Chinook	33%	16%	25%	48%	24%
Egg, large	62%	13%	37%	46%	16%
Canola oil	100%	30%	7%	59%	30%
Safflower oil	100%	74%	9%	12%	74%
Corn oil	100%	60%	13%	25%	60%
Corn oil margarine (tub)	100%	37%	20%	26%	37%
Sesame oil	100%	42%	14%	41%	42%
Olive oil	100%	10%	14%	74%	10%
Salmon oil (fish oil)	100%	34%	20%	29%	40%
Cottonseed oil	100%	50%	26%	20%	52%
Palm kernel oil	100%	2%	82%	11%	2%
Coconut oil	100%	2%	87%	6%	2%
Walnuts	86%	63%	10%	23%	64%
Cashew nuts	72%	17%	20%	59%	17%

Source: Data from Food Processor, Version 7.01 (ESHA Research, Salem, OR).
Note: EFA (essential fatty acid), SFA (saturated fatty acid), MUFA (monounsaturated fatty acid), and PUFA (polyunsaturated fatty acid).

found in most animal fats. The monounsaturated (one double bond) 18-carbon fatty acid called oleic acid would be written as 18:1; it is found in olive and canola oils. The polyunsaturated (more than one double bond) 18-carbon fatty acid with two double bonds is linoleic acid (18:2). It is an essential fatty acid found in soybean, sunflower, safflower, and corn oils. Another essential fatty acid is alpha-linolenic acid (18:3), a polyunsaturated 18-carbon fatty acid with three double bonds. Good food sources are soybean, canola, and flaxseed oils and walnuts. Essential fatty acids will be discussed in more detail later in this chapter.

Foods vary in the types of fatty acids they contain. For example, animal fats provide approximately 40% to 60% of their energy from saturated fats, while plant fats provide 80% to 90% of their energy from monounsaturated and polyunsaturated fats (Table 5.1). You will notice that canola oil is listed as being high in both MUFAs and PUFAs. Most oils are a combination of fats, making them a good source of more than one type of fat. There are some exceptions, however. Notice that only 20% to 30% of the fat in cooked skinless chicken breast, turkey, and fish is saturated and 70% to 80% is monounsaturated or polyunsaturated. Conversely, the short-chain, plant-based

Nutrition Facts
Valeur nutritive

Per 125 g   par 125 g

Amount Teneur	% Daily Value % valeur quotidienne
Calories / Calories 110	
Fat / Lipides 1.5 g	2 %
Saturated / saturés 0.5 g + Trans / trans 0 g	3 %
Polyunsaturated / polyinsaturés 0.4 g	
Omega-6 / oméga-6 0.1 g	
Omega-3 / oméga-3 0.3 g	

In 2003 Health Canada ruled that trans fatty acids, or trans fat, must be listed on Nutrition Facts labels for conventional foods and some dietary supplements. Research studies show that diets high in trans fatty acids can increase the risk of cardiovascular disease.

palm kernel oil and coconut oil are extremely saturated. Diets higher in plant foods will usually be lower in saturated fats than diets high in animal products. The impact that various types of fatty acids have on health will be discussed later in this chapter (beginning on page 166).

Shape Have you ever noticed how many toothpicks are packed into a small box? A hundred or more! But if you were to break a bunch of toothpicks into V shapes anywhere along their length, how many could you then fit into the same box? It would be very few because the bent toothpicks would jumble together, taking up much more space. Molecules of saturated fat are like straight toothpicks: they have no double carbon bonds and always form straight, rigid chains. As they have no kinks, these chains can pack together tightly (Figure 5.2b). That is why saturated fats, such as the fat in meats, are usually solid at room temperature.

In contrast, each double carbon bond of unsaturated fats gives them a kink along their length (Figure 5.2c). This means that they are unable to pack together tightly—for example, to form a stick of butter—and instead are liquid at room temperature. In addition, unsaturated fatty acids can occur in either a *cis* or a *trans* shape. The prefix *cis* means things are located on the same side or near each other, while *trans* is a prefix that denotes across or opposite. These terms describe the positioning of the hydrogen atoms around the double carbon bond as follows:

- A *cis* fatty acid has both hydrogen atoms located on the same side of the double bond (Figure 5.3a), thus the prefix *cis*. This positioning gives the cis molecule a pronounced kink at the double carbon bond. We typically find the cis fatty acids in nature and thus in foods like olive oil.

- In contrast, in a *trans* fatty acid the hydrogen atoms are attached on diagonally opposite sides of the double carbon bond (Figure 5.3b). This positioning makes trans fatty acids fats straighter and more rigid, just like saturated fats.

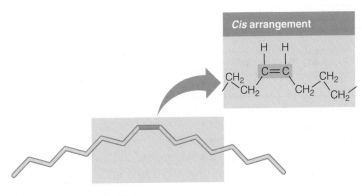

(a) Cis polyunsaturated fatty acid

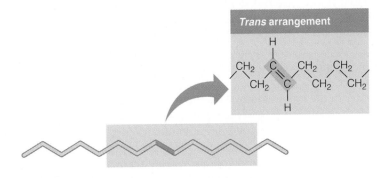

(b) Trans polyunsaturated fatty acid

Figure 5.3 Structure of (a) a *cis* and (b) a *trans* polyunsaturated fatty acid. Cis fatty acids are kinked at the area of the double bond; trans fatty acids are straight at the area of the double bond.

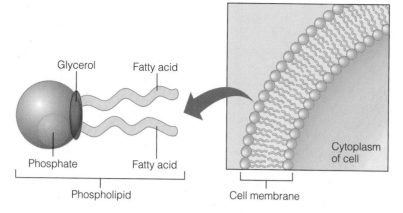

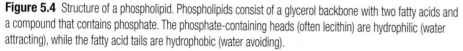

Figure 5.4 Structure of a phospholipid. Phospholipids consist of a glycerol backbone with two fatty acids and a compound that contains phosphate. The phosphate-containing heads (often lecithin) are hydrophilic (water attracting), while the fatty acid tails are hydrophobic (water avoiding).

Although a limited amount of trans fatty acids (2% to 6% of total fat) are naturally found in cow's milk, beef, and lamb (Health Canada 2007b), in the majority of trans oils, such as corn or safflower oil, hydrogen is added to the fatty acids during **hydrogenation**. In this process, some of the double bonds found in the monounsaturated and polyunsaturated fatty acids in the oil are broken and additional hydrogen is inserted at diagonally opposite sides of the double bonds. This process straightens out the molecules, making the liquid fat more solid at room temperature—and also more saturated. Thus, corn oil margarine is a partially hydrogenated fat made from corn oil. Margarines that are hydrogenated have more trans fatty acids than butter. The hydrogenation of fats helps foods containing these fats, such as cakes, cookies, and crackers, to resist spoilage from oxygen (rancidity). However, some of the unsaturated bonds are modified and result in the production of trans fatty acids.

Does the straight, rigid shape of the saturated and trans fats we eat have any effect on our health? Absolutely! Research over the last two decades has shown that diets high in saturated fatty acids increase blood cholesterol and our risk of heart disease.

We now know that trans fatty acids appear to function much like saturated fatty acids in our diet: both trans and saturated fatty acids raise blood cholesterol levels and appear to change cell membrane function. Most health professionals feel that diets high in trans fatty acids can increase the risk of cardiovascular disease, similar to diets high in saturated fat. Because of the concerns related to trans fatty acid consumption and heart disease, manufacturers are required to list the amount of trans fatty acids per serving on the food label. Many food manufacturers have begun producing products free of trans fatty acids, and they clearly state this claim on the label. We will talk more about trans fatty acids later in this chapter (page xx).

Phospholipids Combine Lipids with Phosphate

Along with the triglycerides just discussed, we also find phospholipids and sterols in the foods we eat. **Phospholipids** consist of a glycerol backbone with fatty acids attached at the first and second carbons and another compound that contains phosphate attached at the third carbon (Figure 5.4). This addition of a phosphate compound makes phospholipids soluble in water, a property that enables phospholipids to emulsify and assist in transporting fats in our bloodstream. We discuss this concept in more detail later in this chapter (page xx). The phospholipids are unique in that they have a hydrophobic (water-avoiding) end, which is their fatty acid tail, and a hydrophilic (water-attracting) end, which is their phosphate head.

Sterols Have a Ring Structure

Sterols are also a type of lipid found in foods and in the body, but their multiple-ring structure is quite different from that of triglycerides (Figure 5.5a). Sterols are found in both plant and animal foods, and they are produced by the body. Plant sterols are

hydrogenation The process of adding hydrogen to unsaturated fatty acids, making them more saturated and thereby more solid at room temperature.

phospholipids A type of lipid with a glycerol backbone to which are attached two fatty acids and another compound that contains phosphate; unlike other lipids, phospholipids are soluble in water.

sterols A type of lipid found in foods and in the body that has a ring structure; cholesterol is the most common sterol that occurs in our diets. Plant sterols block the absorption of cholesterol.

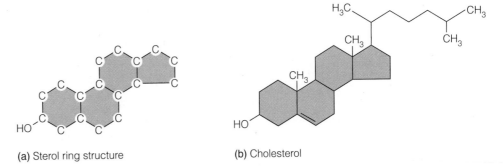

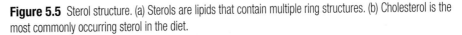

(a) Sterol ring structure   (b) Cholesterol

Figure 5.5 Sterol structure. (a) Sterols are lipids that contain multiple ring structures. (b) Cholesterol is the most commonly occurring sterol in the diet.

naturally found in small amounts in the cell membranes of fruits, vegetables, nuts, seeds, grains, and legumes; soybean oil is a particularly rich source. Plant sterols appear to block the absorption of dietary cholesterol in the small intestine, and their potential health benefits have been studied for more than 50 years (Klingberg et al. 2008). It was believed that people don't typically consume enough plant sterols each day to significantly lower their blood cholesterol levels, so sterols in the form of esters have been added to high-fat food products, such as margarine and mayonnaise. Research suggests that these added sterol esters reduce blood levels of total cholesterol 5% to 13%, and blood levels of LDL cholesterol 5% to 24% (Lau, Journoud, and Jones 2005), without adverse effects on HDL cholesterol. (LDL and HDL cholesterol are explained in more detail on pp. 181–184.) More recent research suggests that plant sterols consumed naturally as plant foods in a typical diet may be sufficient to reduce blood levels of cholesterol in people with high levels (Klingberg et al. 2008). The United States Food and Drug Administration (FDA) permits foods with added plant sterol esters to claim that consuming these foods "may reduce the risk of heart disease" and that they "can reduce cholesterol levels" (IFICF 2003). Canada does not permit the sale of products with added plant sterols.

Cholesterol is the most common sterol and is found only in animals. Products like vegetable oils and peanut butter that are derived from plants are sometimes labelled "cholesterol free"—a misleading claim, since plants don't contain cholesterol. Because cholesterol is a type of lipid, it is found in the fatty parts of meats and poultry, in egg yolks, in milk fat, and in products made from milk, such as butter and cheese. Low- or reduced-fat cheese, milk, and meats contain less cholesterol. In humans, the liver synthesizes cholesterol and normally adjusts its production according to the amount of cholesterol consumed. If we ate no cholesterol, our livers would normally increase their cholesterol production to meet our bodies' needs. Conversely, on days when we consume large amounts of cholesterol, our bodies should cut back on cholesterol synthesis. In some people, this regulating mechanism fails and blood cholesterol levels remain high.

This continuous production of cholesterol is vital to our health because cholesterol is part of every cell membrane, where it works in conjunction with fatty acids to help maintain cell membrane integrity. It is particularly plentiful in the neural cells that make up our brain, spinal cord, and nerves. The body also uses cholesterol to synthesize several important sterol compounds, including sex hormones (estrogen, androgen, and progesterone), adrenal hormones, and vitamin D. Thus, despite cholesterol's bad reputation, it is absolutely essential to human health.

Recap: Lipids are essential for health. There are three types of lipids typically found in foods: triglycerides, phospholipids, and sterols. Triglycerides are the most common lipid found in food. A triglyceride is made up of glycerol and three fatty acids. These fatty acids can be classified based on chain length, level of saturation, and shape. Phospholipids combine two fatty acids and a glycerol backbone with a phosphate group, making them soluble in water. Sterols have a multiple ring structure; cholesterol is the most commonly occurring sterol in our diets and is found only in animal products.

How Does Our Body Break Down Lipids?

Because lipids are not soluble in water, they cannot enter our bloodstream easily from the digestive tract. Thus, fats must be digested, absorbed, and transported within the body differently from carbohydrates and proteins, which are water-soluble substances.

The digestion and absorption of dietary fat were discussed in Chapter 3, but we briefly review the process here (Figure 5.6). Dietary fats usually come mixed with other foods, which we chew and then swallow. Salivary enzymes have a limited role in the breakdown of fats, so most fat reaches the stomach intact (Figure 5.6, Step 1). The primary role of the stomach in fat digestion is to mix and break up the fat into smaller pieces or droplets. Some digestion takes place in the stomach when gastric lipase is released. Because they are not soluble in water, these fat droplets typically float on top of the watery digestive juices in the stomach until they are passed into the small intestine (Figure 5.6, Step 2).

The Gallbladder, Liver, and Pancreas Assist in Lipid Digestion

Because lipids are not soluble in water, their digestion requires the help of digestive enzymes from the pancreas and bile from the gallbladder. Recall from Chapter 3 that the gallbladder is a sac attached to the underside of the liver and the pancreas is an oblong-shaped organ sitting below the stomach. Both have a duct connecting them to the small intestine. As fat enters the small intestine, the cells of the intestinal wall respond by secreting the hormone cholecystokinin (CCK). This hormone acts on the gallbladder, causing it to contract and release bile (Figure 5.6, Step 3) into the common bile duct, which leads to the duodenum (the first part of the small intestine). Cholecystokinin also slows down the motility (movement) in the gastrointestinal tract. Secretin, another hormone released from the cells of the intestinal wall, also plays a role in gallbladder contraction.

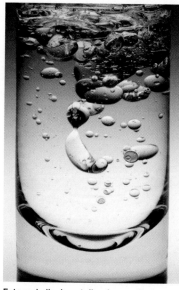

Fats and oils do not dissolve readily in water.

Animations

- Fat Digestion
- Emulsification of Fat

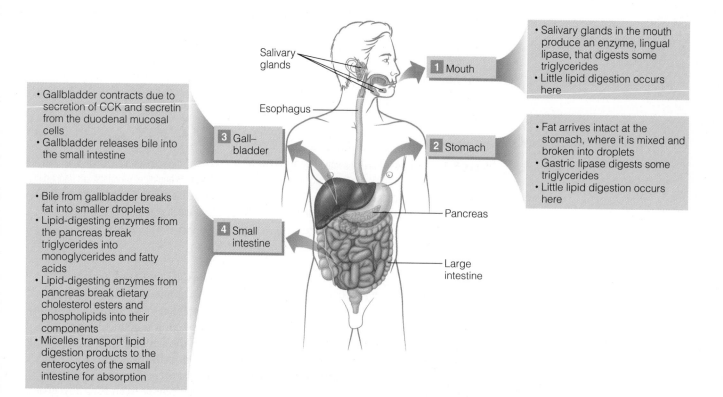

- Salivary glands
- Esophagus
- **3** Gall-bladder
- **4** Small intestine
- **1** Mouth
- **2** Stomach
- Pancreas
- Large intestine

- Salivary glands in the mouth produce an enzyme, lingual lipase, that digests some triglycerides
- Little lipid digestion occurs here

- Fat arrives intact at the stomach, where it is mixed and broken into droplets
- Gastric lipase digests some triglycerides
- Little lipid digestion occurs here

- Gallbladder contracts due to secretion of CCK and secretin from the duodenal mucosal cells
- Gallbladder releases bile into the small intestine

- Bile from gallbladder breaks fat into smaller droplets
- Lipid-digesting enzymes from the pancreas break triglycerides into monoglycerides and fatty acids
- Lipid-digesting enzymes from pancreas break dietary cholesterol esters and phospholipids into their components
- Micelles transport lipid digestion products to the enterocytes of the small intestine for absorption

Figure 5.6 The process of lipid digestion.

(*Source: The Science of Nutrition,* by J.L. Thompson, M.M. Manore, and L.A. Vaughan, © Pearson Education, Inc., publishing as Pearson Benjamin Cummings, p. 186. Used by permission of Pearson Education, Inc.)

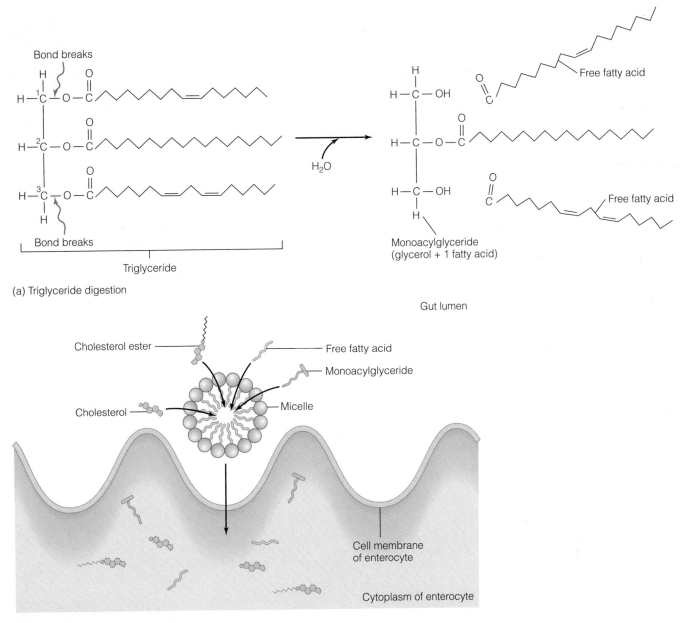

(a) Triglyceride digestion

(b) Micelle transport into enterocyte

Figure 5.7 Lipid digestion and absorption. (a) In the presence of enzymes, triglycerides are broken down into fatty acids and monoglycerides. (b) These products, along with free cholesterol and other products, are trapped in the micelle, a spherical compound made up of bile salts and phospholipids. The micelle then transports these lipid digestion products to the intestinal mucosal cells, and these products are then absorbed into the cell.

(*Source: The Science of Nutrition,* by J.L. Thompson, M.M. Manore, and L.A. Vaughan, © Pearson Education, Inc., publishing as Pearson Benjamin Cummings, p. 177. Used by permission of Pearson Education, Inc.)

Bile is produced in the liver and is sent to the gallbladder, where it is concentrated and stored until needed. Bile is composed mainly of bile salts made from cholesterol, lecithins, and other phsopholipids, and electrolytes (for example, sodium, potassium, chloride, and calcium). You can think of bile acting much like soap, breaking up the fat into smaller and smaller droplets. At the same time, lipid-digesting enzymes produced in the pancreas travel through the pancreatic duct into the small intestine. Once bile has broken the fat into small droplets, these pancreatic enzymes (called pancreatic lipases) take over, breaking the fatty acids away from their glycerol backbones. Each triglyceride molecule is broken down into two free fatty acids and one *monoglyceride,* a glycerol molecule with one fatty acid still attached (Figure 5.7a).

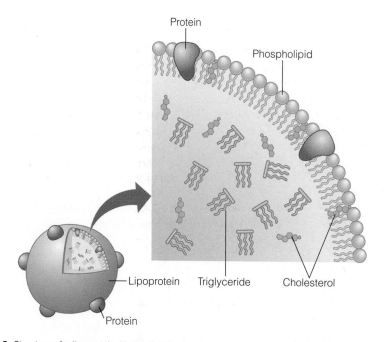

Figure 5.8 Structure of a lipoprotein. Notice that the fat clusters in the centre of the molecule and the phospholipids, which are water soluble, form the outside of the sphere. This enables lipoproteins to emulsify fat (i.e., keep it dispersed and soluble in water) and to transport fats in the lymph and bloodstream.

Absorption of Lipids Occurs Primarily in the Small Intestine

The majority of fat absorption occurs in the mucosal lining of the small intestine with the help of micelles (Figure 5.7b). A **micelle** is a spherical compound made up of bile and phospholipids that can trap the free fatty acids and the monoglycerides. Because the micelles are water soluble, they can transport the lipids to the mucosal cells for absorption. How do the absorbed lipids get into the bloodstream? Because fats do not mix with water, most fats cannot be transported freely in the bloodstream.

To solve this problem, the longer-chain fatty acids and monoglycerides are reformulated back into triglycerides in the mucosal cells of the intestinal wall. They are packaged with proteins and phospholipids into transport vessels called lipoproteins. A **lipoprotein** is a spherical compound in which the fat clusters in the centre and phospholipids and proteins form the outside of the sphere (Figure 5.8).

The specific lipoprotein produced in the mucosal cell to transport the longer-chain fatty acids and monoglycerides from a meal is called a **chylomicron**. This unique compound is now soluble in water because phospholipids and proteins are water soluble. Like micelles, the chylomicrons are vehicles that can keep fat soluble so that it can be transported outside the gastrointestinal tract. The chylomicrons are then released into the lymphatic system and travel through the lymph until they reach the thoracic duct near the heart, where they enter the bloodstream. Thus, the chylomicrons bypass the liver at first and carry the triglycerides through the bloodstream directly to the body's cells to be used for energy or stored as fat. In this way, dietary fat finally arrives in your blood.

As noted earlier, short- and medium-chain fatty acids (those fewer than 14 carbons in length) can be transported in the body more readily than long-chain fatty acids. When short- and medium-chain fatty acids are digested and transported to the mucosal cells of the small intestine, they do not have to be re-formed into triglycerides and incorporated into chylomicrons (Figure 5.9). Instead, they can enter the bloodstream bound to either a transport protein or a phospholipid. For this reason, shorter-chain fatty acids get into the system more quickly than long-chain fatty acids.

Animations

• Lipid Absorption

micelle A spherical compound made up of bile and phospholipids; traps and transports free fatty acids, monoglycerides, and free cholesterol to the mucosal cells lining the small intestine.

lipoprotein A spherical compound in which fat clusters in the centre and phospholipids and proteins form the outside of the sphere.
chylomicron A lipoprotein produced in the mucosal cells lining the intestine; transports dietary fat from a meal out of the intestinal tract into the lymphatic system.

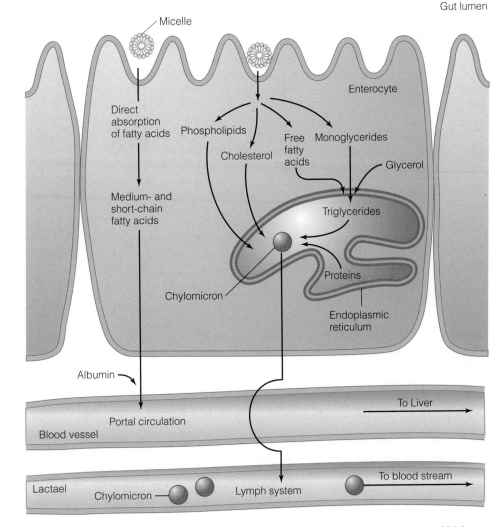

Figure 5.9 The reassembly of the lipid components (for example, triglycerides) into a chylomicron, which is released into the lymph stream and then into the bloodstream at the thoracic duct (at the heart). Short- and medium-chain fatty acids pass directly into the blood stream and go to the liver.

(*Source: The Science of Nutrition,* by J.L. Thompson, M.M. Manore, and L.A. Vaughan, © Pearson Education, Inc., publishing as Pearson Benjamin Cummings, p. 177. Used by permission of Pearson Education, Inc.)

Triglycerides Are Stored in Adipose Tissues for Later Use

The chylomicrons, which are filled with the dietary triglycerides you just ate, now begin to circulate through the blood looking for a place to deliver their load. There are three primary fates of these dietary triglycerides:

1. They can immediately be taken up and used as a source of energy for the cells, especially by the muscle cells.
2. They can be used to make lipid-containing compounds in the body.
3. They can be stored in the muscle or adipose tissue for later use.

How do the triglycerides get out of the chylomicrons and into the cell? This process occurs with the help of an enzyme called **lipoprotein lipase**, or LPL, which sits on the outside surface of our adipose cells. LPL comes in contact with the chylomicrons when they touch the surface of the adipose cell. As a result of this contact, LPL breaks apart the triglycerides in the core of the chylomicrons. This process results in the movement of individual fatty acids from within the core of the chylomicrons and out into the adipose cell. If the cell needs the fat for energy, these fatty acids will be quickly transported into the mitochondria and used as fuel. If the body doesn't need the fatty acids for immediate energy, the cell can re-create the

lipoprotein lipase An enzyme that sits on the outside of cells and breaks apart triglycerides so that their fatty acids can be removed and taken up by the cell.

triglycerides and store them for later use. The primary storage site for this extra energy is the adipose cell, shown in Figure 5.10. However, if you are physically active, your body will preferentially store this extra fat in the muscle tissue first, so the next time you go out for a run, the fat is readily available to the cell for energy. Thus, people who engage in physical activity are more likely to have extra fat stored in the muscle tissue and to have less adipose tissue—something many of us would prefer. Of course, fat stored in the adipose tissue can also be used for energy during exercise, but it must be broken down first and then transported to the muscle cells.

> **Recap:** Lipid digestion begins when triglycerides are broken into droplets by bile. Pancreatic lipases subsequently digest the triglycerides into two free fatty acids and one monoglyceride. These end products of digestion, as well as other lipids, are then transported into the intestinal mucosal cells with the help of micelles. Once inside the mucosal cells, triglycerides are re-formed and packaged into lipoproteins called chylomicrons. Their outer layer is made up of proteins and phospholipids, which allows them to travel in the blood. Dietary fat, in the form of triglycerides, is transported by the chylomicrons to cells within the body that need energy. Triglycerides stored in the muscle tissue are used as a source of energy during physical activity. Excess triglycerides are stored in the adipose tissue and can be used whenever the body needs energy.

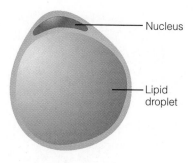

Figure 5.10 Diagram of an adipose cell.

(*Source: The Science of Nutrition*, by J.L. Thompson, M.M. Manore, and L.A. Vaughan, © Pearson Education, Inc., publishing as Pearson Benjamin Cummings, p. 177. Used by permission of Pearson Education, Inc.)

Why Do We Need Lipids?

Lipids, in the form of dietary fat, provide energy and help our bodies perform essential physiologic functions.

Lipids Provide Energy

Dietary fat is a primary source of energy because fat has more than twice the energy per gram as carbohydrate or protein. Fat provides 9 kcal (37 kJ) per gram, while carbohydrate and protein provide only 4 kcal (17 kJ) per gram. This means that fat is much more energy dense. For example, 15 mL (1 Tbsp) of butter or oil contains approximately 100 kcal (420 kJ), while it takes approximately 625 mL (2 1/2 cups) of steamed broccoli or 1 slice of whole wheat bread to provide 100 kcal (420 kJ) from these foods.

Lipids Are a Major Fuel Source When We Are at Rest

At rest, we are able to deliver plenty of oxygen to our cells so that metabolic functions can occur. Just as a candle needs oxygen for the flame to continue burning, our cells need oxygen to use fat for energy. Thus, approximately 30% to 70% of the energy used at rest by the muscles and organs comes from lipids (Jebb et al. 1996). The exact amount of energy coming from lipids at rest will depend on how much fat you are eating in your diet, how physically active you are, and whether you are gaining or losing weight. If you are dieting, more fat will be used for energy than if you are gaining weight. During times of weight gain, more of the fat consumed in the diet is stored in the adipose tissue, and the body uses more dietary protein and carbohydrate as fuel sources at rest.

Lipids Fuel Physical Activity

Lipids are the major energy source during physical activity, and one of the best ways to lose body fat is to exercise and reduce energy intake. During exercise, fat can be mobilized from any of the following sources: muscle tissue, adipose tissue, blood lipoproteins, and any dietary fat consumed during exercise. A number of hormonal changes signal the body to break down stored energy to fuel the working muscles. The hormonal responses, and the amount and source of the fat used, depend on

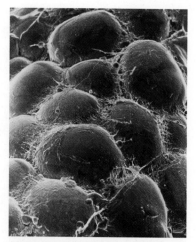

Adipose tissue. During times of weight gain, excess fat consumed in the diet is stored in the adipose tissue.

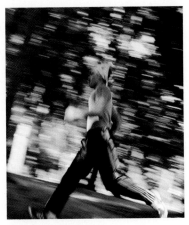

Lipids provide energy.

your level of fitness; the type, intensity, and duration of the exercise; and how well-fed you are before you exercise.

For example, adrenaline stimulates the breakdown of stored fat. Blood levels of adrenaline rise dramatically within seconds of beginning exercise, and this action activates additional hormones within the fat cell to begin breaking down fat. Adrenaline also signals the pancreas to *decrease* insulin production. This is important, because insulin inhibits fat breakdown. Thus, when the need for fat as an energy source is high, blood insulin levels are typically low. As you might guess, blood insulin levels are high when we are eating, because during this time our need for getting energy from stored fat is low and the need for fat storage is high.

Once fatty acids are released from the adipose cell, they travel in the blood attached to a protein, *albumin,* to the muscles where they enter the mitochondria and use oxygen to produce adenosine triphosphate (ATP), which is the cell's energy source. If you are physically fit, you burn fat more easily by delivering more oxygen to your muscles. In addition, you can exercise longer when you are fit. Since the body has only a limited supply of stored carbohydrate as glycogen in muscle tissue, the longer you exercise, the more fat you use for energy. This point is illustrated in Figure 5.11. In this example, an individual is running for four hours at a moderate intensity. As the muscle glycogen levels become depleted, the body relies on fat from the adipose tissue as a fuel source.

Body Fat Stores Energy for Later Use

Our body stores extra energy in the form of body fat, which then can be used for energy at rest, during exercise, or during periods of low energy intake. Having a readily available energy source in the form of fat allows the body to always have access to energy even when we choose not to eat (or are unable to eat), when we are exercising, and while we are sleeping. Our bodies have little stored carbohydrate—only enough to last about one to two days—and there is no place that our body can store extra protein. We cannot consider our muscles and organs as a place where extra protein is stored! For these reasons, the fat stored in our adipose and muscle tissues is necessary to fuel the body between meals. Although we do not want too much stored adipose tissue, some fat storage is essential to protect our health.

essential fatty acids (EFA) Fatty acids that must be consumed in the diet because they cannot be made by our bodies. The two essential fatty acids are linoleic acid and alpha-linolenic acid.

linoleic acid An essential fatty acid found in vegetable and nut oils; an omega-6 fatty acid.

Lipids Provide Essential Fatty Acids

Dietary fat provides the **essential fatty acids (EFA)** needed to make a number of important biological compounds. (Information on the EFA content of various foods is given in Table 5.1, page 159.) Essential fatty acids are called essential because they must be consumed in the diet and cannot be made in our bodies. The two essential fatty acids are linoleic acid and alpha-linolenic acid (Figure 5.12).

Linoleic Acid

Linoleic acid (18:2), an omega-6 fatty acid, is found in vegetable and nut oils, such as sunflower, safflower, corn, soy, and peanut oil. If you eat lots of vegetables, or use vegetable oil–based margarines or vegetable oils, you are probably getting adequate amounts of this essential fatty acid in your diet. Linoleic acid is converted in the body to arachidonic acid (20:4), which is a precursor to a number of important biological compounds that regulate body functions, such as blood clotting and blood pressure. The omega-6 class of fatty acids has the first double bond at the sixth carbon from the methyl (CH_3) end (see Figure 5.12).

The longer you exercise, the more fat you use for energy. Cyclists in long-distance races use fat stores for energy.

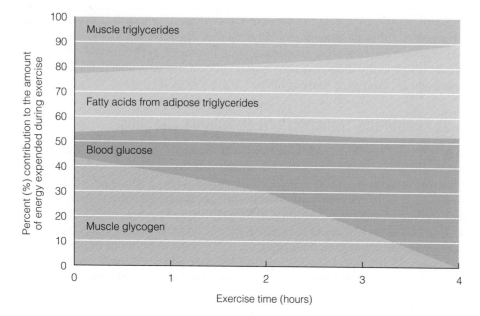

Figure 5.11 Various sources of energy used during exercise. As a person exercises for a prolonged time, fatty acids from adipose cells contribute relatively more energy than do carbohydrates stored in the muscle or circulating in our blood (Coyle 1995).

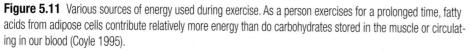

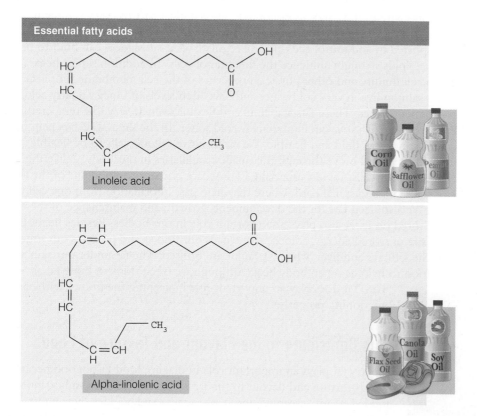

Figure 5.12 The two essential fatty acids: linoleic acid (omega-6 fatty acid) and alpha-linolenic acid (omega-3 fatty acid).

Alpha-Linolenic Acid

The second essential fatty acid is **alpha-linolenic acid** (18:3), an omega-3 fatty acid. The omega-3 class of fatty acids has the first double bond at the third carbon from the methyl (CH$_3$) end (see Figure 5.12). This fatty acid is found primarily in leafy green vegetables, flaxseeds and flaxseed oil, soy oil and soy foods, canola oil, walnuts, seafood, and fish oils.

alpha-linolenic acid An essential fatty acid found in leafy green vegetables, flaxseed oil, soy oil, fish oil, fish products, and "omega-3 eggs"; an omega-3 fatty acid.

North Americans appear to get adequate amounts of omega-6 fatty acids, probably because of the large amount of salad dressings, vegetable oils, margarine, and mayonnaise we eat; however, our consumption of omega-3 fatty acids is more variable and can be low in the diets of people who do not eat fish or walnuts, drink soy milk, or use soybean, canola, or flaxseed oil.

Lipids Enable the Transport of Fat-Soluble Vitamins

Lipids transport the fat-soluble vitamins (A, D, E, and K) needed by our bodies for many essential metabolic functions. For example, vitamin A is especially important for normal vision and gives you the ability to see at night. Vitamin D is important for regulating blood calcium and phosphorus concentrations within normal ranges, which indirectly helps maintain bone health. If vitamin D is low, blood calcium levels will drop below normal, and the body will draw calcium from the bones to maintain blood levels. Vitamin E functions primarily as an antioxidant in our bodies and keeps cell membranes healthy by preventing oxidation of body fats. Finally, vitamin K is important for proteins involved in blood clotting and bone health. We discuss these vitamins in detail in Chapters 8 and 9.

Lipids Help Maintain Cell Function and Provide Protection to the Body

Lipids, especially PUFAs and phospholipids, are a critical part of every cell membrane, where they help to maintain membrane integrity, determine what substances are transported in and out of the cell, and regulate what substances can bind to the cell. Thus, lipids strongly influence the function of cells. In addition, lipids help maintain cell fluidity and other physical properties of the cell membrane. For example, wild salmon live in very cold water and have high levels of omega-3 fatty acids in their cell membranes. These fats stay fluid and flexible even at very low temperatures, which allows the fish to swim in extremely cold water. In the same way, fats help our cell membranes stay fluid and flexible. We want our red blood cells to be flexible enough to bend and move through the smallest capillaries in our body, delivering oxygen to all our cells. Lipids, especially PUFAs, are primary components of the tissues of the brain and spinal cord, where they help pass information from one cell to another. We also need fats for the development, growth, and maintenance of these tissues. Stored body fat also plays an important role in our bodies. Besides being the primary site of stored energy, adipose tissue pads our bodies and protects our organs, such as the kidneys and liver, when we fall or are bruised. The fat under our skin acts as insulation to help us retain body heat. Although we often think of body fat as "bad," it does play an important role in keeping the body healthy and functioning properly.

Fats Contribute to the Flavour and Texture of Foods

Dietary fat plays an important role in making food taste good because it adds texture and flavour to foods. Fat makes salad dressings smooth and ice cream "creamy," and it gives cakes and cookies their moist, tender texture. Canadians like fat so much that many of us eat fried foods, such as french fries, on a daily basis.

Fats Help Us to Feel Satiated

Fats in foods contribute to making us feel satiated after a meal. Two factors probably contribute to this effect: first, fat has a much higher energy density than carbohydrate or protein. For example, a pat of butter weighing 5 grams will contain 35 kcal (145 kJ); 5 grams of an

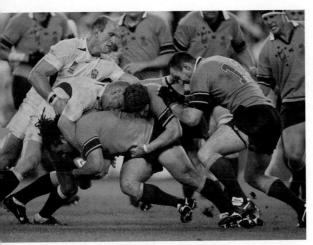

Adipose tissue pads our body and protects our organs when we fall or are bruised.

apple contains only 3 kcal (13 kJ). So for every gram of fat you consume, you get 2.25 times the amount of energy that you get with the same number of grams consumed in protein or carbohydrate.

Second, lipids take longer to digest and absorb than protein or carbohydrate because more steps are involved in the digestion process, which may make you feel fuller for a longer time because energy is slowly being released into your body.

Conversely, you can eat more fat in a meal without feeling overly full because fat is generally compact in its size. Going back to our apple and butter example, one medium apple weighs 117 grams (approximately 4 oz.) and has 70 kcal (290 kJ), but the same number of calories of butter—two pats—would hardly make you feel full! Looked at another way, an amount of butter weighing the same number of grams as a medium apple would contain 840 kcal (3510 kJ)!

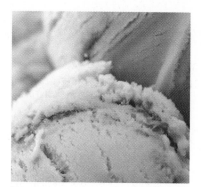

Fat adds texture and flavour to foods.

> **Recap:** Dietary lipids play a number of important roles within the body. (1) They provide more than twice the energy of protein and carbohydrate, at 9 kcal (37 kJ) per gram, and provide the majority of energy required at rest. Lipids are also a major fuel source during exercise, especially endurance exercise. (2) Dietary fats provide essential fatty acids (linoleic and alpha-linolenic acid). (3) Dietary fats help transport the fat-soluble vitamins into the body. (4) Dietary fats help regulate cell function and maintain membrane integrity. (5) Stored body fat in the adipose tissue helps protect vital organs and pad the body. (6) Fats contribute to the flavour and texture of foods and the satiety we feel after a meal.

When Are Lipids Harmful?

Like many things, a little can be good, but a lot can be harmful. We have just discussed why lipids are an essential part of a good diet and necessary for health, but too much fat, regardless of the type, can be damaging to our bodies.

Eating Too Much of Certain Fats Can Lead to Disease

As mentioned earlier, diets high in saturated and trans fatty acids increase our risk of cardiovascular disease. It is also well documented that diets that are high in fat, regardless of the type of fat, are high in calories and can contribute to weight gain and obesity. Thus, our goal is to select the right amount and types of fats to include in our diet.

Fats Limit the Shelf Life of Foods

Fats make food taste good. This is one reason most of our fast foods and convenience foods are high in fat and why they are so popular. Unfortunately, all fats are susceptible to oxidation, which causes them to smell or taste rancid or stale. When foods high in fat, such as cookies, chips, margarines, and salad dressings, are exposed to oxygen and become stale or rancid, their shelf life is shortened. Polyunsaturated fats, with two or more double bonds, are unstable and particularly prone to oxidation. Saturated fats, with no double bonds, are more resistant to oxidation and rancidity. Naturally occurring unprocessed fats are also more stable. This may be because they have naturally occurring antioxidants.

Manufacturers can deal with oxidation in three ways. First, they can package foods in airtight containers to prevent the food from being exposed to oxygen. Higher-fat products often need to be protected from the light and refrigerated as well to prevent spoilage. But this gets expensive and isn't practical for many foods. A second solution is to add preservatives and antioxidants to products high in fat to extend their shelf life. Vitamin E is often added to high-fat foods, such as margarines, because it acts as an antioxidant. Last, manufacturers have the option of adding hydrogen atoms to reduce the amount of unsaturation and make the product more resistant to oxygen. Most products are only partially hydrogenated so that some of

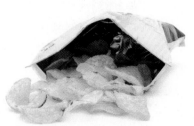

Potato chips are packaged in air-tight and opaque bags to prevent oxidation and spoilage.

▶ HIGHLIGHT

Is There an Alternative to Trans Fatty Acids?

Since Health Canada's release of new labelling regulations in 2003, food manufacturers have taken on the challenge of creating products that can be labelled as "trans fat free." One possible strategy is to replace all trans fat found in processed food products (chips, cookies, etc.) with a healthier alternative that mimics the functional properties of a trans fatty acid.

Dr. Alejandro Marangoni, University of Guelph

Dr. Alejandro Marangoni of the Department of Food Science at the University of Guelph and his international research team have developed a solid fat product with similar functional properties to trans fatty acids but none of the detrimental effects related to cardiovascular risk.

Marangoni explains, "There will always be people who consume junk food; the aim is to create healthier alternatives with the same eating qualities, taste, and value. For example, an individual can consume over 25% of their daily fat requirements in one store-bought muffin alone, most of it being unhealthy saturated and trans fats. By eliminating trans fats and reducing saturates in the muffin but maintaining similar qualities, such as taste, an individual can still enjoy the food without the potentially harmful side effects."

What is the secret to this "healthier" fat? It is a simple oil, water, monoglyceride, and fatty acid mixture that functions as a solid fat at room temperature, is spreadable, and can withstand high baking and heating temperatures. The mixture is run through a machine called a Roto-Stator, which uses shear force to mix the two phases (oil and water) and produce monoglyceride vesicles filled with oil (or microencapsulated) surrounded by water. The result is "a solid crystalline structure, which gives a lot of resistance. Eventually the crystals will pack together enough to squeeze the water out, forming a gel (or Coagel) which is solid at room temperature."

Not only can this trans fat–free gel replace the fats found in spreads and other processed foods, Dr. Marangoni has also shown that the gel can lower triglyceride and free fatty acid levels in the blood after eating, which in turn results in lower insulin levels (Marangoni et al. 2007).

"We gave a sample of individuals 60 g of the monoglyceride gel to eat and saw a decrease in serum triglycerides and free fatty

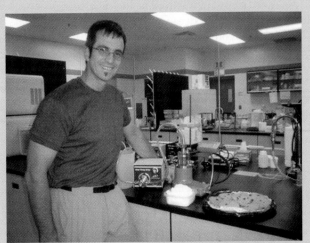

Dr. Marangoni is pictured here with the Roto-stator, a machine that uses shear force to mix the oil and water phases together to produce a solid fat made of 40% water. The fat can then be used in baking to produce trans fat–free products, like cookies and muffins.

acids after consumption" explains Dr. Marangoni. "Glucose levels remained the same but we saw a decrease in insulin resistance." This controlled release of lipids in the body combined with the regulation of insulin may potentially lower the risks of type 2 diabetes.

Dr. Marangoni and his team have been approached by *Tasty Collections*, a company that distributes products to brand-name chains, such as A&P and Wal-Mart, to produce a 2 oz. cookie made with their trans fat alternative. Dr. Marangoni goes on to say that "with the addition of our trans fat–free gel, the following claims are permitted on the cookie's packaging: (1) trans fat free, (2) low in saturated fats, (3) a source of omega-3 fatty acids, and (4) the health claim 'A healthy diet low in saturated and trans fats can reduce the risk of heart disease.'" Other Canadian and European manufacturers are interested in incorporating this trans fat alternative in candy bars and processed breakfast foods geared toward children aged 6 to 12.

Dr. Marangoni cautions that there are technical issues that need to be addressed, such as the ability to produce vast amounts of the gel in large-scale production. "However, we are almost there!" he says.

the double bonds remain and the desired consistency (solid versus fluid) of the product can be controlled. One disadvantage of the hydrogenation process is that trans fatty acids are formed, and, as discussed earlier, these behave like saturated fat in the human body. Consumers need to understand that all three options have disadvantages and, at present, there is no ideal way of limiting oxidation and extending the shelf life of high-fat foods. See the Highlight box to learn about one scientist's efforts to create an alternative to trans fats.

> **Recap:** The dietary fats we eat can either contribute to health or increase our risk of disease. Selecting the right amount and type of lipids in your diet is important for improving health. Because lipids added to foods can be oxidized and become rancid, foods high in polyunsaturated fat can quickly spoil. Manufacturers add preservatives or partially hydrogenate foods high in fat to increase their shelf life.

How Much Dietary Fat Should We Eat?

Without a doubt, most people think dietary fat is bad! How many people have you heard say they are trying to dramatically reduce fat in their diet? Yet, because fat plays such an important role in keeping our bodies healthy, we must eat diets providing a moderate amount of energy from fat. But what, exactly, is a moderate amount? And what foods contain the most nutritious fats? We'll explore these questions here.

Dietary Reference Intake for Total Fat

The Acceptable Macronutrient Distribution Range (AMDR) for fat is 20% to 35% of total energy (Institute of Medicine 2002). This recommendation is based on evidence that higher intakes of fat increase the risk of obesity and its complications, especially heart disease, but that diets too low in fat and too high in carbohydrate can also increase the risk of heart disease if they cause blood triglycerides to rise (Institute of Medicine 2002). We are also advised to keep our intake of saturated and trans fats low to reduce our risk of heart disease.

Because dietary carbohydrates are needed to replenish glycogen stores, athletes and other physically active people are advised to consume less fat and more carbohydrate than sedentary people do. Specifically, it is recommended that athletes consume 20% to 25% of their total energy from fat, 55% to 60% of energy from carbohydrate, and 12% to 15% of energy from protein (Manore, Barr, and Butterfield 2000). This level of fat intake represents approximately 45 to 55 grams per day of fat for an athlete consuming 2000 kcal (8400 kJ), and 78 to 97 grams per day of fat for an athlete consuming 3500 kcal (14 700 kJ).

Although many people trying to lose weight consume less than 20% of their energy from fat, this practice may do more harm than good, especially if they are also limiting energy intake (eating fewer than 1500 kcal [6280 kJ] per day). Research suggests that very low-fat diets, or those with less than 15% of energy from fat, do not provide additional health or performance benefits over moderate-fat diets and are usually very difficult to follow (Lichenstein and Van Horn 1998). In fact, most people find they feel better, are more successful in weight maintenance, and are less preoccupied with food if they keep their fat intakes at 20% to 25% of energy intake. Additionally, people attempting to reduce their dietary fat frequently eliminate food groups, such as meat, dairy, eggs, and nuts. Unfortunately, eliminating these food groups also eliminates potential sources of protein and many essential vitamins and minerals important for good health and maintaining an active lifestyle. Diets extremely low in fat may also be deficient in essential fatty acids.

Dietary Reference Intakes for Essential Fatty Acids

For the first time, DRIs for the two essential fatty acids were set in 2002 (Institute of Medicine 2002). The Adequate Intake (AI) for linoleic acid is 14 to 17 grams per

day for adult men and 11 to 12 grams per day for women 19 years and older, whereas the AI for alpha-linolenic acid is 1.6 grams per day for adult men and 1.1 grams per day for adult women. Using the typical energy intakes for adult men and women, this translates into an AMDR of 5% to 10% of energy for linoleic acid and 0.6% to 1.2% for alpha-linolenic acid. For example, an individual consuming 2000 kcal (8400 kJ) per day should consume about 11 to 22 grams of linoleic acid (omega-6) and about 1.3 to 2.6 grams per day of alpha-linolenic acid (omega-3).

Most Canadians Eat Within the Recommended Amount of Fat but Eat the Wrong Types

For almost 20 years, health professionals have been advising Canadians to eat less fat, and it appears that Canadians have cut back on both energy and fat. Data from the 1970 Nutrition Canada survey suggested that Canadians were consuming about 40% of their calories from fat, while new data from the 2004 Canadian Community Health Survey (Health Canada 2007b) suggest that 30% to 31% of calories were from fat, as shown in Table 5.2.

Of the dietary fat we eat, saturated and trans fats are most highly correlated with an increased risk of heart disease because they increase blood cholesterol levels by altering the way cholesterol is removed from the blood. The recommendation is to keep intakes of saturated fat as low as possible (Institute of Medicine 2002); unfortunately, our average intake of saturated fats is 10% of energy (Health Canada 2007b). The Institute of Medicine (2002) also recommends that we keep our intake of trans fatty acids to an absolute minimum. Determining the actual amount of trans fatty acids consumed in North America has been hindered by the lack of an accurate and comprehensive database of foods containing trans fatty acids. This is partly because many food manufacturers and fast-food companies are in the midst of reformulating their food items to reduce the trans fat content. Health Canada's research suggests that Canadians eat, on average, 8.4 grams of trans fatty acids per day, or roughly 10% of their total fat intake (Health Canada 2005).

> **Recap:** The Acceptable Macronutrient Distribution Range (AMDR) for total fat is 20% to 35% of total energy. The Adequate Intake (AI) for linoleic acid is 14 to 17 grams per day for adult men and 11 to 12 grams per day for adult women. The AI for alpha-linolenic acid is 1.6 grams per day for adult men and 1.1 grams per day for adult women. Because saturated and trans fatty acids can increase the risk of heart disease, health professionals recommend that we keep our intake of saturated fat as low as possible and reduce our intake of trans fatty acids to the absolute minimum.

Table 5.2   Comparison of Average Daily Energy Intake and Percentage of Total Energy from Fat, by Age Group and Sex, Canada (excluding territories): 1972 and 2004

	1972	1972	2004	2004
Age and Sex Group	**Average Energy Intake (kcal)**	**% of Total Energy from Fat**	**Average Energy Intake**	**% of Total Energy from Fat**
20 to 39 Male	3 374	41	2 660	31.0
20 to 39 Female	2 001	40	1 899	31.2
40 to 64 Male	2 671	40	2 345	31.7
40 to 64 Female	1 726	39	1 757	31.8
65 or older Male	2 056	39	1 948	31.0
65 or older Female	1 530	37	1 544	30.5

Source: Adapted from Statistics Canada publication Health Reports, Catalogue 82-003, Vol. 18, No. 2, May 2007, page 19, http://www.stat-can.ca/english/freepub/82-003-XIE/82-003-XIE2006006.pdf

Shopper's Guide: Food Sources of Fat

The last time you popped a frozen dinner into the microwave, did you stop and read the Nutrition Facts table on the box? If you had, you might have been shocked to learn how much saturated and trans fat was in the meal. As we discuss here, many processed foods are hidden sources of fat, especially saturated and trans fat. In contrast, many whole foods, such as oils and nuts, are rich sources of the healthful fats our bodies need.

Visible Versus Invisible Fats

We not only eat many high-fat foods but also commonly add fat to our foods to improve their taste. There is nothing like cream in our coffee or real butter on our pancakes. These added fats, such as oils, butter, cream, shortening, margarine, or dressings (such as mayonnaise and salad dressings) are called **visible fats** because we can easily see that we are adding them to our food.

When we add fat to foods, we know how much we are adding and what kind. When fat is added in the preparation of a casserole or a fast-food burger and fries, we are less aware of how much or what type of fat is used. In fact, unless we read food labels carefully, we might not be aware that a food contains any fat at all. We call fats in prepared and processed foods **invisible fats** because they are hidden within the food. Their invisibility often tricks us into choosing them over more nutritious foods. For example, a slice of yellow cake is much higher in fat (40% of total energy) than a slice of angel food cake (1% of total energy). Yet many consumers just assume the fat content of these foods are the same, since they are both cake. For most of us, the majority of the fat in our diets comes from invisible fat. Foods that can be high in invisible fats are baked goods, regular-fat dairy products, processed meats or meats that are not trimmed, and most convenience and fast foods, such as hamburgers, hot dogs, chips, ice cream, french fries, and other fried foods.

Because high-fat diets have been associated with obesity, many people have tried to reduce their total fat intake. Food manufacturers have been more than happy to provide consumers with low-fat alternatives to their favourite foods. However, these lower-fat foods may not always have fewer kilocalories. Read the Highlight box on page 176 and Table 5.3 to learn how to be a better consumer of reduced-fat foods.

visible fats Fat we can see in our foods or see added to foods, such as butter, margarine, cream, shortening, salad dressings, chicken skin, and untrimmed fat on meat.

invisible fats Fats that are hidden in foods, such as the fats found in baked goods, regular-fat dairy products, marbling in meat, and fried foods.

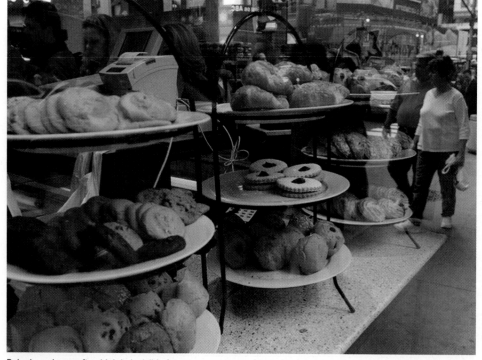

Baked goods are often high in invisible fats.

▶ **HIGHLIGHT**

Low-Fat, Reduced-Fat, Non-Fat . . . What's the Difference?

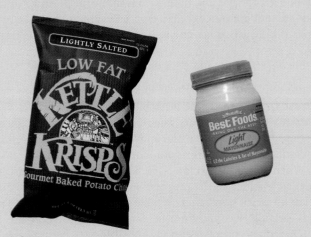

Although most of us love high-fat foods, we also know that eating too much fat isn't good for our health or our waistlines. Because of this concern, food manufacturers have produced a host of modified-fat foods—so you can have your cake and eat it too!

In Table 5.3, we list a number of full-fat foods with their lower-fat alternatives. These products, if incorporated in the diet on a regular basis, can significantly reduce the amount of fat consumed but may or may not reduce the amount of energy consumed. For example, drinking skim milk (86 kcal or 360 kJ and < 0.5 grams fat per serving) instead of whole milk (150 kcal or 630 kJ and 8.2 grams fat per serving) will dramatically reduce both fat and energy intake. However, eating Oreo's 25% less fat cookies (three cookies have 130 kcal and 5 grams of fat) instead of regular Oreos (three cookies have 160 kcal and 7 grams of fat) will have little impact on your energy and fat intakes.

Thus, if you think that eating fat-free foods means you're not getting any Calories and can eat all you want without gaining weight,

you're mistaken. The reduced fat is often replaced with added carbohydrate, as with the Oreos example, resulting in a very similar total energy intake. Thus, if you want to reduce both the amount of fat and the energy you consume, you must read the labels of modified-fat foods carefully before you buy.

Table 5.3   Comparison of Full-Fat, Reduced-Fat, and Low-Fat Foods

Product	Serving Size	Energy (kcal)	Protein (g)	Carbohydrate (g)	Fat (g)
Milk, whole (3.3% fat)	250 mL (8 fl. oz.)	150	8.0	11.4	8.2
Milk, 2% fat	250 mL (8 fl. oz.)	121	8.1	11.7	4.7
Milk, 1% fat	250 mL (8 fl. oz.)	102	8.0	11.7	2.6
Milk, skim (non-fat)	250 mL (8 fl. oz.)	86	8.4	11.9	0.5
Cheese, cheddar regular	30 g (1 oz.)	111	7.1	0.5	9.1
Cheese, cheddar low-fat	30 g (1 oz.)	81	9.1	0.0	5.1
Mayonnaise, regular	15 mL (1 Tbsp)	100	0.0	0.0	11.0
Mayonnaise, light	15 mL (1 Tbsp)	50	0.0	1.0	5.0
Mayonnaise, fat-free	15 mL (1 Tbsp)	10	0.0	2.0	0.0
Margarine, regular corn oil	15 mL (1 Tbsp)	100	0.0	0.0	11.0
Margarine, reduced-fat	15 mL (1 Tbsp)	60	0.0	0.0	7.0
Peanut butter, regular	15 mL (1 Tbsp)	95	4.1	3.1	8.2
Peanut butter, reduced-fat	15 mL (1 Tbsp)	81	4.4	5.2	5.4
Cream cheese, soft regular	15 mL (1 Tbsp)	50	1.0	0.5	5.0
Cream cheese, soft light	15 mL (1 Tbsp)	35	1.5	1.0	2.5
Crackers, Wheat Thins Original	18 crackers	158	2.3	21.4	6.8
Crackers, Wheat Thins 33% less fat	18 crackers	120	2.0	21.0	4.0
Cookies, Oreos regular	3 cookies	160	2.0	23.0	7.0
Cookies, Oreos 25% less fat	3 cookies	130	2.0	25.0	5.0
Cookies, Fig Newtons regular	3 cookies	210	3.0	30.0	4.5
Breakfast bars, regular	1 bar	140	2.0	27.0	2.8

Source: Data from Food Processor, Version 7.01 (ESHA Research, Salem, OR).

Food Sources of Beneficial Fats

You may have read about the health benefits of omega-3 fatty acids. Two of these fatty acids, **eicosapentaenoic acid** or **EPA** (20:5) and **docosahexaenoic acid** or **DHA** (22:6), are necessary for the synthesis of a number of regulatory compounds in the body. Research indicates that DHA in particular is critical for the proper development of the brain and the eyes during pregnancy and through the first year of life. During adulthood, EPA and DHA tend to reduce inflammatory responses in the body, reduce blood clotting and plasma triglyceride levels, and thereby may lower a person's risk of death from a heart attack. Recent epidemiological studies suggest that higher levels of omega-3 fatty acids may be associated with a slower rate of cognitive decline as people age and may reduce the risk of macular degeneration, a common cause of blindness (see Chapter 8 for further discussion).

Because the body converts only small amounts of alpha-linolenic acid to EPA and DHA, we should include pre-formed sources of these fatty acids in our diets. Fish and fish oils are the best dietary sources of EPA and DHA. Consumers who don't like the taste of fish can buy milk, yogurt, cheese, bread, eggs, orange juice, and other products with added omega-3 fatty acids. Some of these may only contain ALA, not EPA and DHA, and thus will not be a suitable replacement for fish. Check to see the source of omega-3.

The recommendation in *Eating Well with Canada's Food Guide* (Health Canada 2007a) is to eat at least 2 *Food Guide* servings (75 grams each, for a total of 150 grams) a week of fish. Higher-fat fish, such as char, herring, mackerel, rainbow trout, salmon, and sardines, are specifically mentioned as good choices. Table 5.4 shows the amounts of EPA and DHA that would be obtained from eating 150 grams of cooked fish a week and the same amounts averaged over 7 days in the week, for an estimated daily amount.

We often get conflicting messages about eating fish. Nutritionists encourage people to eat more fish for its high-quality protein, heart-healthy fats, and important vitamins (such as vitamin D) and minerals (such as selenium). As shown in Table 5.4, fatty fish, such as mackerel, salmon, and herring, are particularly rich sources of EPA and DHA, but all seafood, even lower-fat choices like cod and shrimp, are sources of these omega-3 fatty acids. However, government agencies may issue warnings about the levels of persistent organochlorine contaminants (such as dioxins and PCBs), which accumulate in the fatty tissues of fish, and heavy metals, particularly mercury, which accumulate in their flesh.

Provincial agencies monitor the levels of contaminants in various fish species from various lakes, rivers, and shoreline locations and issue advice on eating sport-caught fish. For example, the Sport Fish Contaminant Monitoring Program provides the basis on which the Ontario Ministry of the Environment issues the *Guide to Eating Ontario Sport Fish* every other year. Specific advice is directed toward women of childbearing years and children under the age of 15, since high levels of contaminants, such as PCBs and mercury, can have adverse health effects, especially neurological effects, for these groups. In general, predatory species, such as shark; large, long-lived fish, such as sturgeon; and bottom-feeders, such as carp, are best eaten less often, since they tend to have larger accumulations of contaminants in their bodies. Smaller "pan" sport fish, such as yellow perch, white perch, rock bass, brook trout, black crappie, white crappie, bluegill, and sunfish are generally safer choices for people eating sport-caught fish.

In 2007, Health Canada analyzed the available mercury data and issued revised guidelines for consuming retail fish. Predatory fish tend to accumulate higher levels of mercury and therefore should be eaten less often by young children and women who are or may become pregnant or are breastfeeding. These fish species include fresh or frozen tuna, shark, swordfish, marlin, orange

eicosapentaenoic acid (EPA) A very long chain PUFA (20:5) found pre-formed in fish and fish oils. EPA and DHA appear to reduce our risk of death from a heart attack.

docosahexaenoic acid (DHA) A very long chain PUFA (22:6); critical for proper development of the central nervous system and the retina of the eyes. Found pre-formed in fish and fish oils.

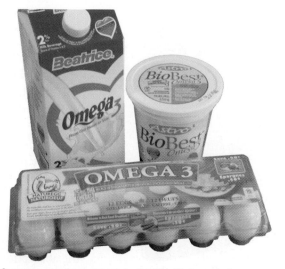

Consumers can buy many products with added omega-3 fatty acids.

Table 5.4   Estimated EPA + DHA Content of 150 Grams Selected Fish Species

Fish (150 grams per week)	EPA + DHA (grams per week)	EPA + DHA (averaged as mg per day)
Herring, Pacific	3.15 g	450 mg
Salmon, Atlantic	3.00 g	429 mg
Mackerel, Pacific and Jack	2.70 g	386 mg
Salmon, Sockeye, canned	2.10 g	300 mg
Mackerel, Atlantic	1.80 g	257 mg
Trout, Rainbow	1.65 g	236 mg
Sole	0.75 g	107 mg
Light tuna, canned	0.45 g	64 mg
Shrimp	0.45 g	64 mg
Cod	0.45 g	64 mg
Haddock	0.30 g	43 mg

Source: U.S. Department of Agriculture, Agricultural Research Service, 2005, USDA National Nutrient Database for Standard Reference, Release 18, Nutrient Data Laboratory Home Page, www.ars.usda.gov/ba/bhnrc/ndl.

roughy, and escolar (sometimes called snake mackerel or oilfish). The recommended amounts of these fish follow:

- 150 grams per week for the general population; 150 grams is 2 *Food Guide* servings of 75 grams, 2 1/2 oz., 125 mL, or 1/2 cup each
- 150 grams per month for women who are or may become pregnant or are breastfeeding
- 125 grams per month for children 5–11 years old
- 75 grams per month for children 1–4 years old

Most canned tuna products tend to use smaller species, such as skipjack, yellowfin, and tongol, which have less mercury than fresh or frozen tuna. The exception is canned albacore tuna, a large species that can accumulate considerable amounts of mercury. Thus people who frequently eat canned albacore or white tuna may be exposed to unacceptably high levels of mercury. Similar to the advice on predatory fish above, Health Canada has recommended limits for canned albacore tuna, as follows:

- 300 g per week (4 *Food Guide* servings) for women who are or may become pregnant, or are breastfeeding
- 150 g per week (2 *Food Guide* servings) for children 5–11 years old
- 75 g per week (1 *Food Guide* serving) for children 1–4 years old

Health Canada (2007c) notes that "the advice does not apply to canned light tuna, nor does it apply to Canadians outside of the specified groups."

Fat Replacers

One way to lower the fat content of foods, such as chips, muffins, cakes, and cookies, is by replacing the fat in a food with a *fat replacer*. Snack foods have been the primary target for fat replacers, since it is more difficult to eliminate the fat from these types of products without dramatically changing the taste. The challenge in replacing fat in foods is to ensure that the fat-soluble vitamins A, D, E, and K, and other fat-soluble compounds, such as carotenoids, will remain in the foods and that the absorption of these vitamins won't be compromised.

There are three main types of fat replacers—carbohydrate based, protein based, and fat based—as shown in Table 5.5.

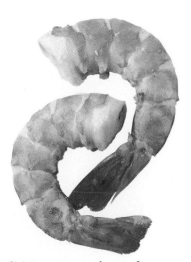

Shrimp are a source of omega-3 fatty acids.

Table 5.5   Common Fat Replacers

Types of Fat Replacers	Names of Common Fat Replacers	Description	Foods That May Contain Fat Replacers
Carbohydrate-based fat replacers that provide energy	Dextrins Maltodextrins Modified food starch	Bland, nonsweet carbohydrates made from hydrolyzed starches that can mimic the texture and mouth feel of fat due to their gel-like structure. Provides 1 to 4 Calories (4 to 17 kJ) per gram. Can completely replace or partially replace the fat in food.	Salad dressings Puddings Spreads Dairy products Frozen desserts
	Oatrim (Beta-Trim™, NutrimX)	A beta-glucan (type of soluble fibre) derived from oat fibre. Provides 4 Calories (17 kJ) per gram. Can replace fat and add the additional cholesterol-lowering benefit of oat bran.	Baked goods Fillings and frostings Frozen desserts Dairy beverages Cheese Salad dressings Processed meats Confections
Carbohydrate-based fat replacers that provide negligible energy (dietary fibres)	Z-Trim	A noncaloric, bland mix of insoluble fibre made from the crushed hulls of corn, oats, and rice.	Baked goods Burgers Hot dogs Cheese Ice cream Yogurt
	Polydextrose	A nonsweet starch polymer made from food-grade dextrose and small amounts of sorbitol and citric acid. Polydextrose passes through the body largely undigested, with only 5% to 10% digested, and provides only 1 Calorie (4 kJ) per gram. Can replace up to one-half the fat in a product.	Baked goods Chewing gums Confections Salad dressings Frozen dairy desserts Gelatins Puddings
	Gum	Gums are a type of dietary fibre that mimics the functional properties of fat when water is used to replace fat in foods. Gums are not digested in the small intestine so add few Calories to the products made with them.	Salad dressings Desserts Processed meats
Protein-based fat replacers	Microparticulated protein (Simplesse)	Made from milk or egg white proteins, water, sugar, pectin, and citric acid. Supplies 1 to 2 Calories (4 to 8 kJ) per gram.	Baked goods Butter Cheese Mayonnaise spreads Salad dressings Sour cream
	Dairy-Lo™	Manufactured by Parmalat Canada for use in ice cream. Made of 100% whey protein.	Ice cream
Fat-based fat replacers	Olestra (Olean)	Only available in the United States. Made by binding sucrose with 6 to 8 long-chain fatty acids. Olestra is not sweet, has the appearance, taste, texture and mouth feel of fat, and can be used in fried, cooked, and baked products. Because it is not digested, it is calorie-free, but it may reduce the absorption of fat-soluble vitamins. Foods made with olestra have vitamins A, D, E, and K added, but not carotenoids.	Chips Crackers

Source: Calorie Control Council, 5775 Peachtree-Dunwoody Road, Building G, Suite 500, Atlanta, GA 30342, www.caloriecontrol.org.

▶ **NUTRITION LABEL ACTIVITY**

How to Choose a Healthy Margarine

There are so many different types of margarines on the market, how do you choose one that is good for you? The Nutrition Facts panel and ingredient list below are from a regular margarine (versus ones on the market that are labelled "light," "salt free," or "added olive oil").

Ingredients: Canola and sunflower oils 74%, water, modified palm and palm kernel oils 6%, salt 1.8%, whey protein concentrate 1.4%, soy lecithin 0.2%, vegetable monoglycerides, potassium sorbate, vegetable colour, artificial flavour, citric acid, vitamin A palmitate, vitamin D3, alpha-tocopherol acetate.

First, notice that the serving size is 2 teaspoons (10 grams), or 10 mL. Of the 8 grams of fat in this serving, only 1 gram is saturated, and there are no trans fatty acids in the product. Look at the ingredient list and you'll see that 6% of the margarine (by weight) is from modified palm and palm kernel oils, whereas approximately three quarters of the margarine is canola and sunflower oils. Modified palm and palm kernel oils are contributing to the saturated fat content. Canola oil is high in both monounsaturated and polyunsaturated fatty acids, and sunflower oil is high in polyunsaturated fatty acids. Since these are the main ingredients in the margarine, they account for the high amounts of monounsaturated (3.5 grams of the total 8 grams) and polyunsaturated (2.5 grams of the total 8 grams) fatty acids. No hydrogenated or partially hydrogenated vegetable oils or shortenings are found on the ingredient list; therefore, the canola and sunflower oils used in making this margarine were not hydrogenated (i.e., had hydrogen atoms added to the double bonds) and this product does not contain trans fats.

Remember that margarines are made from plant oils, which do not contain cholesterol or dietary fibre. Although some whey (milk) protein concentrate is added to mimic the consistency and flavour of butter, the amount is so small that it does not contribute to the % daily value for protein. The fat-soluble vitamins A, D, and E are also added.

Is this margarine a good choice? Yes. It is non-hydrogenated, low in saturated fat, and contains no trans fats. "Light" margarines will generally have water listed as the first ingredient, may contain gelatin to help stabilize the product, and often have half the energy of regular margarine. Because they contain so much water (e.g., 58%) they don't melt smoothly and are not generally recommended for baking and frying but can be good choices for table spreads.

Nutrition Facts per 2 tsp (10 g) serving		
Energy	**70 Calories**	**%DV***
Total Fat	8 g	12%
Saturated	1 g	1%
+ Trans 0 g		
Polyunsaturated	2.5 g	
Omega-6	2.0 g	
Omega-3	0.4 g	
Monounsaturated	3.5 g	
Cholesterol	0 mg	0%
Sodium	70 mg	3%
Total Carbohydrate	0 g	0%
Dietary Fibre	0 g	0%
Sugars	0 g	
Protein	0 g	
Vitamin A		10%
Vitamin B		0%
Calcium		0%
Iron		0%
Vitamin D		30%
Vitamin E		15%
* Based on a 2000-Calorie diet		

The carbohydrate-based fat replacers include processed starches and fibres; they hold water and thus mimic fat by providing bulk, viscosity, and a smooth mouth feel. Fruit purées, with their naturally occurring fibre and pectin, can be good replacements for fats; they also provide natural antioxidants. Oatrim and Z-Trim may be listed on ingredient lists as hydrolyzed oat or corn flour. These products can be used in processed meats, pasteurized cheeses, non-dairy creamers, and baked and frozen goods.

Protein-based fat replacers can be simple products, like gelatin or egg whites, that give bulk and a smooth mouth feel, or highly processed microparticulated whey protein products, such as Simplesse, which provides good flavour and creaminess with only one third of the Calories of fat. These fat replacers can't be used in frying but

work well in ice cream, margarine, and salad dressings. Sometimes the protein-based fat replacers are blended with gums or food starches.

Fat-based fat replacers are generally emulsifiers or triglycerides with altered structures that are able to withstand the high temperatures of frying. Typically, these fat replacers are not hydrolyzed (digested) by the body, so they provide little or no energy.

Olestra (brand name Olean) is a fat-based fat replacer developed by Procter & Gamble. Technically called a sucrose polyester, it is composed of sucrose and triglycerides, with bonds that can't be digested in the intestine. The molecules are too large to be absorbed, and olestra passes unchanged through the digestive tract. Procter & Gamble reportedly spent 25 years and $200 million to develop this product, the first of its kind that is able to withstand frying temperatures. However, olestra has two properties that make it controversial. First, it can act as a laxative in some people, causing loose stools and diarrhea. Second, it carries carotenoids and fat-soluble vitamins from other foods in the digestive tract along with it and out of the body. Manufacturers in the United States are required to fortify the fat replacer with the four fat-soluble vitamins but not with carotenoids. Until recently, potato chips and other snack foods in the United States containing olestra were required to carry warnings on their packaging of possible "abdominal cramping" and "loose stools." The Food and Drug Administration (FDA) decided in 2003 that these warnings were no longer necessary on the labels. To date, the United States is the only country in the world that has approved olestra for use as a fat replacer. Health Canada reviewed the scientific background studies for olestra in 2000 and decided it would not allow the product to be used in Canada.

Since fat replacers are new to the market, the effect they have on total fat intake and the reduction of obesity and cardiovascular disease has not yet been determined. Thus, the benefit of their use for most people is still controversial.

> **Recap:** Visible fats are foods, such as margarine and salad dressing, that can be easily recognized as containing fat. Invisible fats are those fats added to our food during the manufacturing or cooking process, so we are unaware of how much fat was added. In general, we want to switch to healthier sources of fats without increasing our total fat intake. For example, use olive and canola oil in place of butter and margarine, select fish more often instead of high-fat meats (hot dogs, hamburgers, sausage), and choose reduced-fat dairy products when possible. Fat replacers are those substances used to replace the typical fats found in foods to reduce the amount of fat in the food.

What Health Problems Are Related to Fat Intake or Metabolism?

There appears to be a generally held assumption that if you eat fat-free or low-fat foods you will lose weight and prevent chronic diseases. Certainly, we know that high-fat diets, especially those high in saturated and trans fatty acids, can contribute to chronic diseases, including heart disease and cancer; however, as we have explored in this chapter, unsaturated fatty acids do not have this negative effect and are essential to good health. Thus, a sensible health goal would be to eat the appropriate amounts and types of fat.

Fats Can Protect Against or Promote Cardiovascular Disease

Cardiovascular disease is a general term used to refer to any abnormal condition involving dysfunction of the heart and blood vessels. A common form of this disease occurs when blood vessels supplying the heart (the *coronary arteries*) become blocked or constricted; such blockage reduces blood flow to the heart or brain and can result in a heart attack or a stroke. According to a 2003 report released by Health Canada's Centre for Chronic Disease Prevention and Control, the Canadian Cardiovascular Society, and the Heart and Stroke Foundation of Canada, cardiovascular diseases are the underlying cause of death for one third of Canadians. One

cardiovascular disease A general term that refers to abnormal conditions involving the heart and blood vessels; cardiovascular disease can result in heart attack or stroke.

quarter of people over 70 years of age have cardiovascular disease, but many people are diagnosed in their 40s and 50s. The rates across Canada vary: Newfoundland and Labrador has the highest rates of death from ischemic heart disease, heart attacks (acute myocardial infarction), stroke (cerebrovascular disease), and all forms of cardiovascular disease combined. In general, northern areas of Canada have lower mortality rates from cardiovascular diseases (except congestive heart failure) than the country's southern parts. On average, more men die from ischemic heart disease and heart attacks (acute myocardial infarction), and more women die from congestive heart failure and stroke (cerebrovascular disease).

Risk Factors for Cardiovascular Disease

Over the last two decades, researchers have identified a number of factors that contribute to an increased risk for cardiovascular disease. The following is a brief description of each of these major risk factors, many of which have a dietary component (Hahn and Heath 1998).

- Overweight—Being overweight is associated with higher rates of death from cardiovascular disease. The risk is due primarily to a greater occurrence of high blood pressure, abnormal blood lipids (discussed in more detail on page 181), and higher rates of diabetes in overweight individuals. In general, an overweight condition develops from an energy imbalance from eating too much and exercising too little (see Chapter 11).

- Physical inactivity—Numerous research studies have shown that physical activity can reduce your risk of cardiovascular disease by improving several risk factors, including improved blood lipid levels, lower resting blood pressure, lower body fat and weight, and improved blood glucose levels both at rest and after eating.

- Smoking—Research indicates that smokers have a 70% greater chance of developing cardiovascular disease than non-smokers. Without question, smoking cessation or never starting initially is one of the best ways to reduce your risk of cardiovascular disease. People who stop smoking live longer than those who continue to smoke, and a 15-year cessation period will reduce your risk factors for cardiovascular disease to those of a non-smoker.

- High blood pressure—High blood pressure stresses the heart and increases the chance that blockage or rupture of a blood vessel will occur. Elevated blood pressure is associated with a number of factors, including dietary factors (e.g., high sodium intakes or low potassium intakes, high caffeine intake), elevated blood lipid levels, obesity, smoking, diabetes mellitus, and physical inactivity.

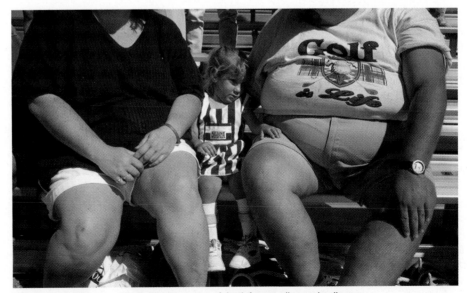

Being overweight is associated with higher rates of death from cardiovascular disease.

• Diabetes—As discussed in Chapter 4, in many individuals with type 2 diabetes, the condition is directly related to being overweight or obese, which is also associated with abnormal blood lipids and high blood pressure. The risk for cardiovascular disease is three times as high in women with diabetes and two times as high in men with diabetes compared with individuals without diabetes.

In addition to these lifestyle or modifiable risk factors, there are three important non-modifiable risk factors that people have no control over: age, family history of cardiovascular diseases, and gender. Visit the Heart and Stroke Foundation of Canada's website and take the Risk Assessment test to find out more about your personal risk factors: www.heartandstroke.com.

The Role of Dietary Fats in Cardiovascular Disease

• Lipoproteins

As you recall from our discussion of fat metabolism, fats are transported in the blood by lipoproteins made up of a lipid centre and a protein outer coat. These lipoproteins are soluble in our blood, so they are commonly called *blood lipids*. At various times, whether eating or fasting, our blood contains a different mix of various types of these blood lipids. Research indicates that high intakes of saturated and trans fatty acids negatively alter the blood lipid assessment measures associated with heart disease. These blood lipid assessment measures are total blood cholesterol and the cholesterol found in very low density lipoproteins (VLDLs) and low-density lipoproteins (LDLs). Conversely, omega-3 fatty acids decrease our risk of heart disease in a number of ways, one of which is by increasing high-density lipoproteins (HDLs) (Harris 1997). We will talk about each of these blood lipid assessment measures, or lipoproteins, and explain how they are linked to heart disease risk.

We have already discussed that high blood cholesterol increases the risk of heart disease. The question is, how? Much of this blood cholesterol is packaged in the LDLs that circulate in the blood. Normally, cells that need the cholesterol take up these lipoproteins; however, diets high in saturated fat *decrease* the removal of these lipoproteins by the cells. Failure to remove the LDLs from the blood results in their continued circulation in the blood. The more cholesterol circulating in the blood, the greater the risk that some of it will adhere to the walls of the blood vessels. As more and more cholesterol builds up, it forms a fatty patch, or *plaque*, that eventually blocks the artery (Figure 5.13). Because high blood levels of LDL cholesterol increase your risk of heart disease, it is often labelled the "bad cholesterol."

For some individuals, the level of dietary cholesterol eaten can also influence blood cholesterol levels. As you learned earlier, we consume cholesterol in our diet and make it in our body. Normally, as the dietary level of cholesterol increases, the body decreases the amount of cholesterol it makes, which keeps the body's level of

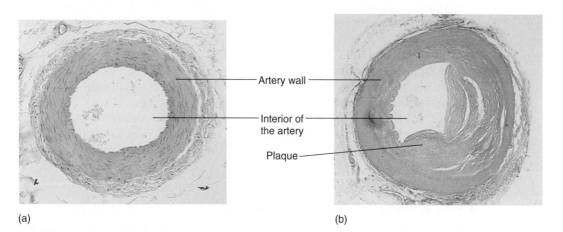

(a)   (b)

Artery wall

Interior of the artery

Plaque

Figure 5.13 These light micrographs show a cross section of (a) a normal artery containing little cholesterol-rich plaque and allowing adequate blood flow through the heart, and (b) an artery that is partially blocked with cholesterol-rich plaque, which can lead to a heart attack.

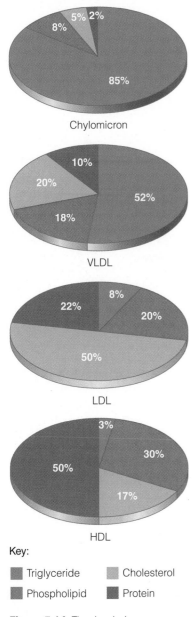

Key:
- ■ Triglyceride
- ■ Cholesterol
- ■ Phospholipid
- ■ Protein

Figure 5.14 The chemical components of various lipoproteins. Notice that chylomicrons contain the highest proportion of triglycerides, making them the least dense, while high-density lipoproteins (HDL) have the highest proportion of protein, making them the densest.

cholesterol constant. Unfortunately, this feedback mechanism does not work well in everyone. For some individuals, eating dietary cholesterol doesn't decrease the amount of cholesterol produced in the body, and their total body cholesterol levels rise. This also increases the levels of cholesterol in the blood. These individuals benefit from reducing their intake of dietary cholesterol. Although this appears somewhat complicated, both dietary cholesterol and saturated fats are found in animal foods; thus, by limiting your intake of animal products or selecting low-fat animal products you will reduce your intake of both saturated fat and cholesterol.

HDLs are small lipoproteins that circulate in the blood, picking up cholesterol and returning it to the liver. The liver takes up the HDLs and the cholesterol they carry, effectively removing it from the circulatory system. The liver then uses this cholesterol to make the bile required for the digestion of fats in the small intestine. High levels of HDL cholesterol are therefore associated with a lower risk of coronary artery disease. That's why HDL cholesterol is often referred to as the "good cholesterol." There is some evidence that eating a diet high in omega-3 fatty acids and participating in regular physical exercise can modestly *increase* HDL cholesterol levels.

High blood triglyceride levels can also increase your risk of heart disease. Triglycerides are primarily transported in chylomicrons and VLDLs. Normally, chylomicrons, which transport dietary triglycerides, are low in the blood except after a meal. Therefore, we are most concerned about the triglycerides transported in the VLDLs, which are made primarily in the liver and intestines and are filled with endogenous triglycerides (triglycerides made in the body). Diets high in fat, simple sugars, and extra energy can increase the production of endogenous VLDLs, while diets high in omega-3 fatty acids can help reduce the production of endogenous triglycerides and VLDLs. In addition, exercise can reduce VLDLs because the fat produced in the body is quickly used for energy instead of remaining to circulate in the blood.

Figure 5.14 graphically shows the amount of triglycerides, phospholipids, cholesterol, and protein found in each of these lipoproteins. Table 5.6 contains a brief description and overview of the functions of the various blood lipoproteins. Finally, refer to the Highlight box on page 186 to gain more insight into understanding your blood lipid levels.

We have known for a long time that saturated fats increase our blood levels of total cholesterol and LDL cholesterol and increase our risk of heart disease. Because saturated fat is found primarily in the fats of animal products, we can easily reduce our intake of saturated fats by eating low-fat dairy and meat products. Vegetable oils can be converted to high-saturated-fat spreads through the hydrogenation of the fatty acids in these oils. Once the oil has been converted to a hard spread (e.g., corn oil to corn oil margarine), the level of saturated fat dramatically increases, as does the level of trans fatty acids. Thus, to reduce the saturated fats in our diets, we must eat fewer high-fat animal products and hydrogenated vegetable products.

Although saturated fat increases the risk of heart disease by increasing blood LDL cholesterol levels, recent research indicates that trans fatty acids both increase blood LDL cholesterol levels and reduce blood HDL cholesterol levels (Health Canada, 2007b). Food labels in Canada must list the trans fatty acid content for conventional foods and some dietary supplements; unfortunately, foods intended for children under the age of 2 years are not required to declare their trans fat content. (See the Nutrition Debate at the end of this chapter for more discussion on this topic.)

As well, in June 2007 Health Canada endorsed the recommendations of the Trans Fat Task Force, which included the Heart and Stroke Foundation of Canada and other stakeholders, and called upon the food and restaurant industries to "limit the trans fat content:

- of vegetable oils and soft margarines to 2% of the total fat content; and
- for all other foods to 5% of the total fat content." (Health Canada 2007b)

It established a Trans Fat Monitoring Program to track the progress of the food and restaurant industries over the next two years. The second report, released July 2008, shows that most fast-food restaurants and retailers have made good progress

Table 5.6   Descriptions and Functions of the Various Blood Lipoproteins

Lipoprotein	Description	Primary Function
Chylomicrons	Formed in the gut after a meal, these lipoproteins are released into the lymph system and then into the blood Largest of the lipoproteins, with the lowest density After triglycerides are removed from this lipoprotein, a chylomicron remnant remains and is taken up by the liver	Transports dietary fat into the blood and transports it to the tissues of the body
Very low-density lipoproteins (VLDLs)	Formed in the liver (80% of production) and the intestine (20% of production)	Transports endogenous lipids, especially triglycerides, to the various tissues of the body
Low-density lipoproteins (LDLs)	Formed in the blood from VLDL Transformation from VLDL to LDL occurs as the triglycerides are removed from the VLDL	Transports cholesterol to the cells of the body
High-density lipoproteins (HDLs)	Synthesized in the liver and released into the blood Move in the blood through the body, picking up free cholesterol	Transports cholesterol from tissues back to the liver

toward meeting these recommendations by lowering trans fats and not replacing them with equally harmful saturated fats, and by reformulating other products (Health Canada 2008).

Fast-food outlets and family restaurants are not required to provide nutrition facts for any of their foods at the present time in Canada. Read food labels and use the following guidelines to help reduce your intake of trans fatty acids (Wootan, Lieberman, and Rosoesky 1996):

- Limit your intake of foods that contain "vegetable shortening" or "partially hydrogenated" oil.

- Avoid deep-fried foods, especially those from fast-food restaurants that reuse vegetable shortening to fry their foods.

- If you use margarine, buy tubs rather than sticks. Look for margarines that contain no trans fatty acids. Use olive or canola oil instead of margarine or shortening whenever possible.

Lifestyle Changes Can Prevent or Reduce Cardiovascular Disease

Diet and exercise interventions aimed at reducing the risk of cardiovascular disease centre on reducing high levels of triglycerides and LDL cholesterol while raising HDL cholesterol. The Centers for Disease Control and Prevention (CDC) (Hahn and Heath 1998) and the Expert Panel on Detection, Evaluation, and Treatment of High Blood Cholesterol in Adults (APT III) (NIH 2001) have made the following dietary and lifestyle recommendations to improve blood lipid levels and reduce the risk of cardiovascular disease:

- Maintain total fat intake to within 20% to 35% of energy (Institute of Medicine 2002), and keep intake of saturated and trans fatty acids low. Polyunsaturated fats (e.g., soy and canola oil) can comprise up to 10% of total energy intake, while monounsaturated fats (e.g., olive oil) can comprise up to 20% of total energy intake. For some people, a lower fat intake may help to maintain a healthy body weight.

▶ **HIGHLIGHT**

Blood Lipid Levels: Know Your Numbers!

"One of the most important steps you can take to reduce your risk of heart disease is to know your 'numbers'—that is, your blood lipid values. However, cholesterol testing isn't necessary for everyone of all ages. Canadian guidelines released in 2003 recommend that you have your blood cholesterol tested if you

1. are male and over 40 years of age,

2. are female and over 50 years of age,

3. are female and post-menopause,

4. have heart disease,

5. have diabetes,

6. have high blood pressure,

7. have a waist measuring more than 102 cm (40 in.) for men and more than 88 cm (35 in.) for women,

8. smoke,

9. or have a strong family history of heart disease" (Heart and Stroke Foundation of Canada 2005).

If you fall into one of the above categories, your doctor might begin by testing your total LDL ("bad") and HDL ("good") cholesterol levels. Record these values. In this way you can know your own blood levels and keep track of your risk for heart disease.

How are your blood lipids actually measured? Generally, you want blood lipid levels described in Table 5.7, however, the more risk factors you have for heart disease or stroke, the lower your target levels should be. "When deciding the 'right' target levels for you, your doctor will take into account factors that increase your risk of heart disease and stroke, such as your age, sex, blood pressure, and whether you have diabetes or stroke. If any of your cholesterol levels are outside the 'right' target level for you, your doctor will discuss lifestyle changes and may prescribe medication to keep your levels in balance" (Heart and Stroke Foundation of Canada 2005).

In Canada, the results of the cholesterol tests are given in millimoles per litre (mmol/L), but in the United States, the results are expressed in milligrams per decilitre (mg/dL); these values are shown in brackets in Table 5.7 below.

Table 5.7   Blood Lipid Values for Those at Moderate Risk of Developing Heart Disease or Stroke

Blood Lipid	Suggested Target Levels
Total cholesterol	Less than 5.2 mmol/L (200 mg/dL)
LDL cholesterol	Less than 3.5 mmol/L (about 130 mg/dL)
HDL cholesterol	Greater than 1.0 mmol/L for men and 1.2 mmol/L for women (about 40 mg/dL)
Total cholesterol: HDL cholesterol ratio	Less than 5.0
Triglycerides	Less than 1.7 mmol/L

Source: Heart and Stroke Foundation of Canada, *Living with Cholesterol: Cholesterol and Healthy Living.* © Reproduced with the permission of the Heart and Stroke Foundation of Canada, 2008. www.heartandstroke.ca

- Decrease dietary saturated fat to less than 7% of total energy intake. Decrease cholesterol intake to less than 300 mg per day, and keep trans fatty acid intake low. Lowering the intakes of these fats will lower your LDL cholesterol level. Replace saturated fat (e.g., butter, margarine, vegetable shortening, or lard) with more healthful cooking oils, such as olive or canola oil.

- Increase dietary intakes of whole grains, fruits, and vegetables so that total dietary fibre is 20 to 30 grams per day, with 10 to 25 grams per day coming from fibre sources, such as oat bran, legumes, and fruits. Foods high in fibre decrease blood LDL cholesterol levels.

- Maintain blood glucose and insulin concentrations within normal ranges. High blood glucose levels are associated with high blood triglycerides. Consume whole foods (such as whole wheat breads and cereals, whole fruits and vegetables, beans, peas and lentils), and select low-saturated-fat meats and dairy products while limiting your intake of high-sugar and high-fat foods (e.g., cookies, high-sugar drinks and snacks, candy, fried foods, and convenience and fast foods).

- Eat throughout the day (e.g., smaller meals and snacks) instead of eating most of your calories in the evening before bed.

- Maintain an active lifestyle. Exercise most days of the week for 30 to 60 minutes if possible. Exercise will increase HDL cholesterol while lowering blood triglyceride levels. Exercise also helps maintain a healthy body weight and a lower blood pressure and reduces your risk for diabetes.

- Maintain a healthy body weight. Blood lipids and glucose levels typically improve when obese individuals lose weight and engage in regular physical activity.

The impact of diet on reducing the risk of cardiovascular disease was clearly demonstrated in the Dietary Approaches to Stop Hypertension (DASH) study, which is discussed in detail in Chapter 2. Although this study focused on dietary interventions to reduce hypertension (high blood pressure), the results of the study showed that eating the DASH way could dramatically improve blood lipids and lower blood pressure. The DASH diet includes high intakes of fruits, vegetables, whole grains, low-fat dairy products, poultry, fish, and nuts and reduced intakes of fats, red meat, sweets, and sugar-containing beverages. Combining the DASH dietary approach with an active lifestyle significantly reduces the risk of cardiovascular disease.

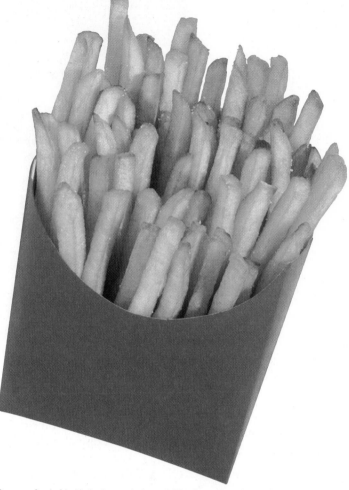

Because foods fried in hydrogenated vegetable oils, such as french fries, are high in trans fatty acids, these types of foods should be limited in our diet.

Does a High-Fat Diet Cause Cancer?

Cancer develops as a result of a poorly understood interaction between the environment and genetic factors. In addition, most cancers take years to develop, so examining the impact of diet on cancer development can be a long and difficult process. Diet and lifestyle are two of the most important environmental factors that have been identified in the development of cancer (Kim 2001, 573–589). Of the dietary factors, dietary fat intake and the development of cancer have been extensively researched. There appears to be a weak relationship between type and amount of fat consumed and increased risk for breast cancer (Willett 1999, 1243–1253). Early research showed an association between animal fat intake and increased risk for colon cancer, while more recent research indicates that the association is between factors other than fat that are found in red meat. Because we now know that physical activity can reduce the risk of colon cancer, earlier diet and colon cancer studies that did not control for this factor are now being questioned.

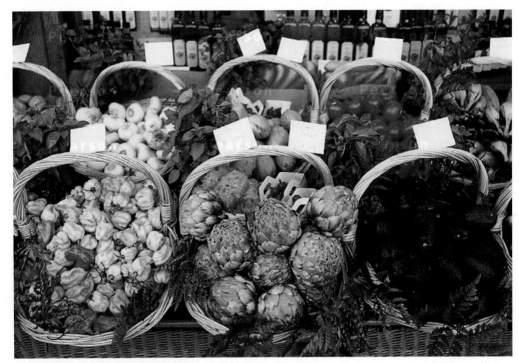

Fruits and vegetables can reduce your risk for cardiovascular disease.

Recap: The types of fats we select to eat can significantly affect our health and risk of disease. Saturated and trans fatty acids increase our risk of heart disease, while omega-3 fatty acids can reduce our risk. Other risk factors for heart disease include being overweight, being physically inactive, smoking, having high blood pressure, and having diabetes. High levels of LDL cholesterol and low levels of HDL cholesterol increase our risk of heart disease. Selecting appropriate types of fat in the diet may also reduce the risk of some cancers, especially prostate cancer.

CHAPTER SUMMARY

- Fats and oils are forms of a larger and more diverse group of substances called lipids; most lipids are insoluble in water.

- The three types of lipids commonly found in foods are triglycerides, phospholipids, and sterols.

- Most of the fat we eat is in the form of triglycerides; a triglyceride is a molecule that contains three fatty acids attached to a glycerol backbone.

- The various fatty acids in triglycerides are classified based on chain length, level of saturation, and shape.

- Short-chain fatty acids are usually fewer than six carbon atoms in length; medium-chain fatty acids are six to twelve carbons in length, and long-chain fatty acids are 14 or more carbons in length.

- Saturated fatty acids have no carbons attached together with a double bond, which means that every carbon atom in the fatty acid chain is saturated with hydrogen.

- Monounsaturated fatty acids contain one double bond between two carbon atoms; monounsaturated fatty acids are usually liquid at room temperature.

- Polyunsaturated fatty acids contain more than one double bond between carbon atoms, and these fatty acids are also liquid at room temperature.

- Saturated fats are straight in shape, allowing the fatty acid chains to pack tightly together and making them solid at room temperature.

- Unsaturated fats (those with one or more double bonds in their fatty acid chains) have a kink along their length,

which prevents them from packing tightly together and results in their being liquid at room temperature.

- A cis fatty acid has hydrogen atoms located on the same side of the double bond in an unsaturated fatty acid. This cis positioning produces a kink in the unsaturated fatty acid and is the shape found in naturally occurring fatty acids.

- A trans fatty acid has hydrogen atoms located on opposite sides of the double carbon bond. This positioning causes trans fatty acids to be straighter and more rigid, like saturated fats. This trans positioning results when oils are hydrogenated during food processing.

- Phospholipids consist of a glycerol backbone with two fatty acids and a phosphate group; phospholipids are soluble in water and assist with transporting fats in the bloodstream.

- Sterols have a ring structure; cholesterol is the most common sterol in our diets.

- The majority of fat digestion and absorption occurs in the small intestine. Fat is broken into smaller components by bile, which is produced by the liver and stored in the gallbladder.

- Because fats are not soluble in water, triglycerides are packaged into lipoproteins before being released into the bloodstream for transport to the cells.

- Dietary fat is primarily used either as an energy source for the cells or to make lipid-containing compounds in the body, or it is stored in the muscle and adipose tissue as triglyceride for later use.

- Fats are a primary energy source during rest and exercise, are our major source of stored energy, provide essential fatty acids, enable the transport of fat-soluble vitamins, help maintain cell function, provide protection for body organs, contribute to the texture and flavour of foods, and help us feel satiated after a meal.

- The AMDR for fat is 20% to 35% of total energy. Our intake of saturated fats and trans fatty acids should be kept to a minimum.

- For the essential fatty acids, 5% to 10% of energy intake should be in the form of linoleic acid and 0.6% to 1.2% as alpha-linolenic acid.

- Visible fats are those we can easily see, such as butter, cream, shortening, oils, dressings, poultry skin, and fat on the edge of meats.

- Invisible fats are those hidden in foods and include fats found in cakes, cookies, marbling in meat, regular-fat dairy products, and fried foods.

- Diets high in saturated fat and trans fatty acids can increase our risk for cardiovascular disease. Other risk factors for cardiovascular disease are overweight or obesity, physical inactivity, smoking, high blood pressure, and diabetes.

- High levels of circulating low-density lipoproteins, or LDLs, increase total blood cholesterol and the formation of plaque on arterial walls, leading to an increased risk for cardiovascular disease. This is why LDLs are sometimes called the "bad" cholesterol.

- High levels of circulating high-density lipoproteins, or HDLs, reduce our blood cholesterol level and our risk for cardiovascular disease. This is why HDLs are sometimes called the "good" cholesterol.

mynutritionlab   Go to MyNutritionLab at www.pearsoned.ca/mynutritionlab and enrich your understanding of nutrition! You'll find key animations, interactive exercises, access to My DietAnalysis, and much more.

REVIEW QUESTIONS

Quizzes

1. Omega-3 fatty acids are
   a. a form of trans fatty acids.
   b. metabolized in the body to arachidonic acid.
   c. synthesized in the liver and small intestine.
   d. found in flaxseeds, soy milk, and fish.
2. One of the most sensible ways to reduce body fat is to
   a. limit intake of fat to less than 15% of total energy consumed.
   b. exercise regularly.
   c. avoid all consumption of trans fatty acids.
   d. restrict total energy intake to 1200 kcal (5000 kJ) per day.
3. Fats in chylomicrons are taken up by cells with the help of
   a. lipoprotein lipase.
   b. micelles.
   c. sterols.
   d. pancreatic enzymes.

4. The risk of heart disease is reduced in people who have high blood levels of
   a. triglycerides.
   b. very low density lipoproteins.
   c. low-density lipoproteins.
   d. high-density lipoproteins.

5. Triglycerides with one double bond on each fatty acid molecule are referred to as
   a. monounsaturated fats.
   b. hydrogenated fats.
   c. saturated fats.
   d. sterols.

6. Choose the incorrect statement:
   a. Most of the fat in our body is stored in the form of triglycerides
   b. Phospholipids aid in transporting fats in our bloodstream
   c. Sterols are lipids containing a single ring structure
   d. In the small intestine, plant sterols appear to block dietary cholesterol absorption

7. Select the correct statement regarding fat digestion:
   a. Bile is stored in the liver
   b. Digestion primarily occurs in the stomach
   c. Bile breaks fat into small droplets
   d. The triglyceride molecule is broken down into one free fatty acid and two diglycerides

8. Which one of the following is strongly associated with an increase in blood cholesterol?
   a. High-density lipoproteins
   b. Low-density lipoproteins
   c. Dietary cholesterol
   d. Free fatty acids

9. Explain how the straight, rigid shape of the saturated and trans fatty acids we eat affects our health.

10. You have volunteered to participate in a walk-a-thon to raise money for a local charity. You have been training for several weeks, and the event is now two days away. An athlete friend of yours advises you to "load up on carbohydrates" today and tomorrow and says you should avoid eating any foods that contain fat during the day of the walk-a-thon. Do you take this advice? Why or why not?

11. Your father is feeling down after an appointment with his doctor. He tells you that his "blood test didn't turn out so good." He then adds, "My doctor told me I can't eat any of my favourite foods anymore. He says red meat and butter have too much fat. I guess I'll have to switch to cottage cheese and margarine!" What type of blood test do you think your father had? How would you respond to his intention to switch to cottage cheese and margarine? Finally, suggest a non-dietary lifestyle choice that might improve his health.

12. Your friend Maria has determined that she needs to consume about 2000 Calories (8400 kJ) per day to maintain her healthy weight. Create a chart for Maria showing the recommended maximum number of Calories she should consume in each of the following forms: unsaturated fat, saturated fat, linoleic acid, alpha-linolenic acid, and trans fatty acids.

CASE STUDY

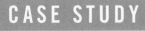

Let's meet Kyle, a 23-year-old university student and varsity soccer player. Currently, Kyle's BMI (see Chapter 11 for a detailed discussion of Body Mass Index) places him within the "overweight" category leading to increased health risks. Kyle and one of his housemates have decided to make an effort to lose weight. Kyle has decided his primary weight-loss goal is to dramatically decrease the amount of fat in his diet. However, what he may not realize is that fat plays an important role in good health, and a very low-fat diet can be unhealthy. It is important

for Kyle to realize the differences between "good" fats and "bad" fats.

Kyle's Typical Daily Intake
- Breakfast: 250 mL orange juice, 3 eggs, 3 slices of bacon
- Mid-morning snack: 1 energy bar
- Lunch: 1 foot-long steak and cheese sub with mayonnaise and butter, 500 mL orange juice
- Mid-afternoon snack: 2 chocolate chip cookies, 1 medium banana, 1 medium coffee with cream and sugar

- Dinner: Stir fry: broccoli, carrots, red pepper, and cashews fried in shortening, 2 pieces of beer-battered cod, 2 large baked potatoes, 250 mL 2% milk
- Evening snack: 2 cups macaroni and cheese

a. There are three levels of saturation for fatty acids: saturated, monounsaturated, and polyunsaturated. Discuss the health implications of saturated fats and identify two sources in Kyle's diet. How could Kyle reduce his consumption of saturated fats?

b. Kyle has decided one diet change he would like to make is to substitute margarine for butter. However, some margarines undergo hydrogenation, which results in trans fatty acids. Explain what Kyle should look for on margarine labels to make a healthy choice.

c. Although decreasing fat intake plays a role in helping Kyle to lose weight, can you think of additional dietary changes he could make to improve his diet?

d. Distinguish between the two essential fatty acids: linoleic acid and alpha-linoleic acid. How can Kyle incorporate them into his diet?

e. List several drawbacks of very low fat diets (< 15% energy from fat) compared with moderate-fat diets (20%–35% energy from fat).

f. List three functions of fat that might motivate Kyle to maintain a moderate-fat diet rather than a very low fat diet.

Test Yourself Answers

1. **False** Eating too much fat, or too much of unhealthy fats, such as saturated and trans fatty acids, can increase our risk for diseases, such as cardiovascular disease and obesity. However, fat is an important part of a nutritious diet, and we need to consume a certain minimum amount to provide adequate levels of essential fatty acids and fat-soluble vitamins.

2. **False** A comparison of reduced-fat and fat-free foods with their full-fat versions shows that some lower-fat versions, such as skim milk and fat-free mayonnaise, have significantly fewer calories, whereas others, such as some fat-free baked goods, have only slightly reduced calories.

3. **True** Fat is our primary source of energy, both at rest and during low-intensity exercise. Fat is also an important fuel source during prolonged exercise.

4. **False** Even foods fried in vegetable shortening can be unhealthy because they are higher in trans fatty acids. In addition, fried foods are high in fat and energy and can contribute to overweight and obesity.

5. **True** Other lifestyle changes that can reduce our risk for cardiovascular disease include not smoking and maintaining a healthy body weight.

WEB LINKS

www.fcpmc.com/issues/transfat/index.html
Food and Consumer Products of Canada
Look at the trans fat issue from the perspective of food manufacturers.

www.heartandstroke.com
Heart and Stroke Foundation of Canada
Visit this website and find out more about your personal risk factors for cardiovascular disease and stroke.

www.hc-sc.gc.ca/fn-an/securit/chem-chim/environ/mercur/cons-adv-etud-eng.php
Health Canada
Check out Health Canada's website for the latest information on mercury in fish.

www.nih.gov
The National Institutes of Health (NIH), U.S. Department of Health and Human Services
Search this site to learn more about dietary fats and the DASH diet (Dietary Approaches to Stop Hypertension).

www.nlm.nih.gov/medlineplus
MEDLINE Plus Health Information
Search "fats" or "lipids" to obtain additional resources and the latest news on dietary lipids, heart diseases, and cholesterol.

www.hsph.harvard.edu/nutritionsource
The Nutrition Source: Knowledge for Healthy Eating Harvard University's Department of Nutrition
Go to this site and click on Fats & Cholesterol to find out how fat can be part of a healthful diet.

http://ific.org/nutrition/fats/index.cfm
International Food Information Council Foundation
Access this site to find out more about fats and dietary fat replacers.

Should All Foods Be Labelled for Their Trans Fatty Acid Content?

Trans fatty acids (TFA, or trans fat) have been a subject of discussion and ongoing research over the past decade. Health Canada's research suggests that Canadians eat, on average, 8.4 grams of trans fatty acids per day, or roughly 10% of their total fat intake (Health Canada 2005). Concerned about rising intakes of trans fat in the Canadian diet, Health Canada issued new labelling regulations in 2003 that force food companies to report the trans fat content on the Nutrition Facts panel of packaged foods. In spite of the federal government's step in the right direction, however, labels for trans fat are not required on food products intended for infants under the age of 2 or for restaurant and fast food items.

Dr. Bruce Holub, University of Guelph

"I think it's inexcusable that baby foods would be exempt," says Canadian researcher Dr. Bruce Holub, Professor Emeritus in the Department of Human Biology and Nutritional Sciences at the University of Guelph. Dr. Holub has spent much of his time identifying the amount of trans fat in common food items and has been actively trying to put pressure on the Canadian government to adopt trans fat labelling on *all* product labels.

"While we're not worrying necessarily about babies getting heart disease—although heart disease starts early in life—trans fats have effects independent of the heart disease story. . . . Trans can reduce the conversion efficiency of alpha-linolenic [acid] to DHA—which is already compromised—as can high omega-6." Our bodies can convert some alpha-linolenic acid to DHA, an omega-3 fatty acid with important health benefits. Holub goes on to note, "Studies in humans show that our conversion efficiencies range from non-detectable in males to 7% to 8% conversion in women. Babies convert less than 1%."

Why is the fact that trans fat compromises an already negligible conversion of alpha-linolenic acid to DHA a concern? Nutrition research has confirmed that omega-3 fatty acids play a major role in the development of the brain and retina during fetal development and in the first year of life.

Dr. Holub's most recent "trans-watching" work reveals that formulated products, such as baby biscuits and some infant cereals, contain vegetable shortening and partially hydrogenated vegetable oil. As a result, a substantial portion of the total fat in these products is trans fats. He has also found that one of the highest dietary sources of trans fat in the North American food supply is breast milk, with quantities directly proportional to a mother's dietary intake of trans fat. He feels strongly that the current trans labelling situation in Canada must be partly to blame.

In the late 1980s, Health Canada introduced a rule that allowed companies to claim that a food was "cholesterol free" if it was low in saturated fat. In an interview with the *National Post*, Dr. Holub explained that this move prompted the companies to switch to trans fats and slap "cholesterol-free" labels on everything from cookies to potato chips. He went on to say, "As a result, we're now eating trans fat in cholesterol-free peanut butter, cholesterol-free cookies and bakery products and french fries and snack foods and doughnuts." It will be very important to ensure that, as industry moves to reduce or eliminate trans fats from products, it does not go in the reverse direction and add back saturated fat (Innis 2004).

Trans fats are worse than the saturated fats found in animal products because they contribute to both the buildup of LDL cholesterol and the destruction of the "good" HDL cholesterol. "Gram for gram, trans fatty acids are many times worse than saturated fat," Dr. Holub says. In fact, his research has shown that trans fats can be five to ten times worse than saturated fat, though trans fats are present in foods in much smaller quantities.

He suggests that along with consumer education on trans fats, trans fats should be measured and labelled in milligrams, rather than grams, to help consumers recognize harmful amounts of trans relative to saturated fat and cholesterol. "When you put saturated and trans in the same box [on the Nutrition Facts table], you'll imply that trans is about as bad as saturates. To me, that's misleading, potentially, to the consumer who thinks they're about the same thing." Dr. Holub feels, "Many moms unknowingly are exposing their babies to very high levels of trans because [the moms] are eating foods labelled 'cholesterol free' and 'low in saturated fat.' . . . She's trying to do good things for herself and her baby. Unfortunately, this trans is running about 7% to 8% to 10% of the breast milk fat because the women are eating 8 to 10 grams of trans fats [a day] during pregnancy and lactation."

Although Dr. Holub applauds the fact that the Canadian labelling standards for "trans-free" products are much stricter than those used in the United States (0.2 grams versus 0.5 grams), he feels the exemption of trans fat labelling on products geared toward those under the age of 2 makes it extremely difficult for parents to make the best dietary choices for their children.

In addition to his work with baby biscuits and infant cereals, Dr. Holub is also closely monitoring the trans fat content of processed and fast-food products. He notes that various snack foods, including crackers, croissants, cookies, and potato chips, often contain up to 25% to 50% of the total fat as trans fat. Many, but not all, brand-name products—including cake and pancake mixes, frozen breakfast waffles, and fast foods, including doughnuts, french fries, breaded meats, and fish fillets— are also high in trans fats.

Despite the fact that foods from restaurants and fast-food chains are among the leading sources of trans fat in the Canadian diet, no nutrition labelling is required. Dr. Holub feels strongly that consumers should know that they are consuming anywhere from 3 to 5 grams of trans fat in a single fast-food item.

How do you feel about this issue? Do you think that consumers will change their eating behaviours if the amounts of trans and saturated fats in fast foods and restaurant foods are disclosed on fast-food containers and restaurant menus? And should the Nutrition Facts table on foods intended for children less than 2 years of age include a breakdown of the types of fats and the amounts in a single serving?

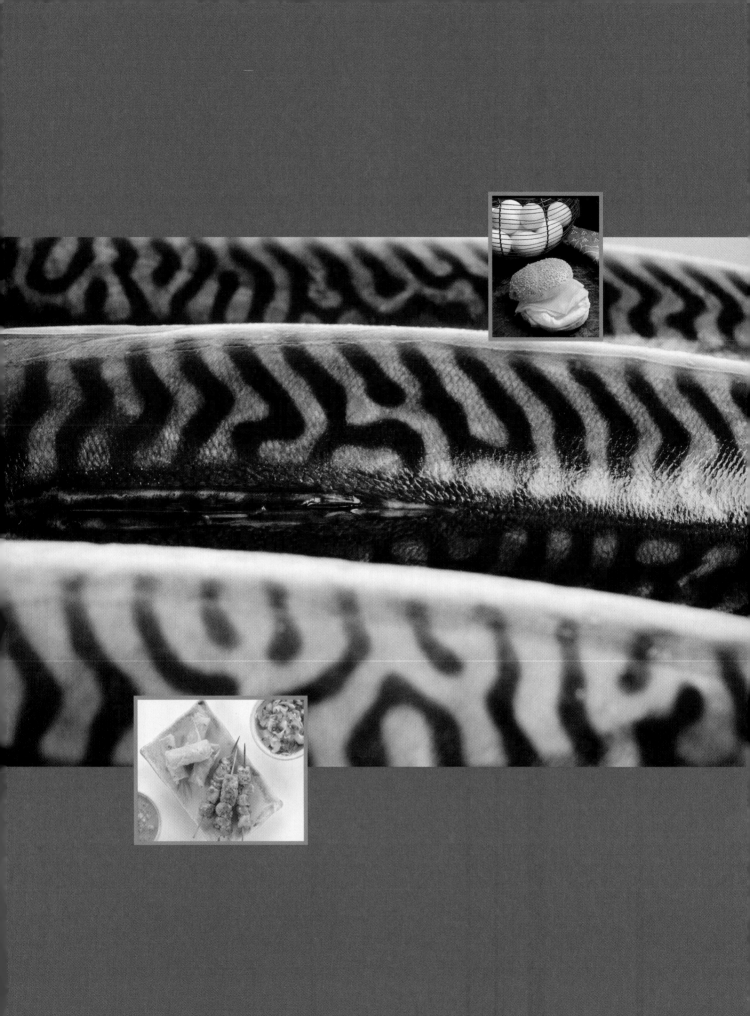

CHAPTER 6

Proteins: Crucial Components of All Body Tissues

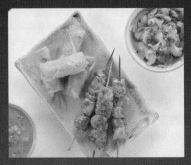

Test Yourself True or False

1. Protein is a primary source of energy for our bodies. **T or F**

2. We must consume amino acid supplements to build muscle tissue. **T or F**

3. Our protein needs are calculated based on our body weight. **T or F**

4. Vegetarian diets are inadequate in protein. **T or F**

5. Most people in Canada consume enough protein to meet their needs. **T or F**

Test Yourself answers can be found at the end of the chapter.

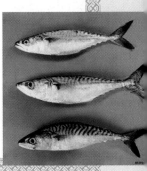

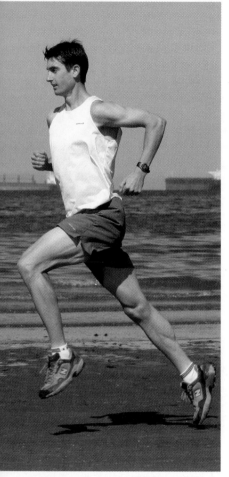

Ironman Brendan Brazier follows a vegan diet.

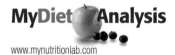

www.mynutritionlab.com

proteins Large, complex molecules made up of amino acids and found as essential components of all living cells.

What do North Vancouver's Ironman triathlete Brendan Brazier, former Canadian Olympic men's figure skater Gary Beacom, and four-time Mr. Universe bodybuilder Bill Pearl have in common? They are all vegetarians! Olympic track icon Carl Lewis states: "A person does not need protein from meat to be a successful athlete . . . my best year of track competition was the first year I ate a vegan diet." We don't have statistics on the number of vegetarian athletes in North America, but an estimated 4% of Canadian adults follow vegetarian diets.

What is a protein, and what makes it so different from carbohydrates and fats? How much protein do you really need, and do you get enough in your daily diet? What exactly is a vegetarian anyway? Do you qualify? If so, how do you plan your diet to include sufficient protein, especially if you play competitive sports? Are there real advantages to eating meat, or is plant protein just as good?

It seems as if everybody has an opinion about protein, both how much you should consume and from what sources. In this chapter, we address these and other questions to clarify the importance of protein in the diet and dispel common myths about this crucial nutrient.

What Are Proteins?

Proteins are large, complex molecules found in the cells of all living things. Although proteins are best known as a part of our muscle mass, they are, in fact, critical components of all tissues of the human body, including bones, blood, and hormones. As *enzymes*, proteins function in metabolism. As *antibodies*, proteins are fundamental to a healthy immune system. Without adequate proteins, the body cannot maintain its balance of fluids or its ratio of acids to bases. Although our bodies prefer to use carbohydrates and fats for energy, proteins do provide energy in certain circumstances. All these functions of proteins will be discussed in this chapter.

How Do Proteins Differ from Carbohydrates and Fats?

As we saw in Chapter 1, proteins are one of the three macronutrients and are found in a wide variety of foods. Our bodies are able to manufacture, or synthesize, proteins, carbohydrates, and fats. But unlike carbohydrates and fats, our genetic material, or DNA, dictates the structure of each protein molecule. We'll explore how our body synthesizes proteins and the role that DNA plays in this process shortly.

Another key difference between proteins and the other macronutrients lies in their chemical makeup. In addition to the carbon, hydrogen, and oxygen also found in carbohydrates and fats, proteins contain a special form of nitrogen that our bodies can readily use. This nitrogen is found in amino acids, which are the building blocks of proteins. By eating proteins found in plants and animals, we are able to break down these proteins into their respective amino acid components and use the nitrogen for many important body processes. Carbohydrates and fats cannot provide this critical form of nitrogen.

> **Recap:** Proteins are critical components of all tissues of the human body. Like carbohydrates and fats, they contain carbon, hydrogen, and oxygen. Unlike the other macronutrients, they contain nitrogen and their structure is dictated by DNA.

• Protein Building Blocks

amino acids Nitrogen-containing molecules that combine to form proteins.

The Building Blocks of Proteins Are Amino Acids

The proteins in our bodies are made of building blocks called **amino acids**, molecules composed of a central carbon atom connected to four other groups: an amine group, an acid group, a hydrogen atom, and a side chain (Figure 6.1a). The word *amine* means "nitrogen containing," and nitrogen is indeed the essential component of the amine portion of the molecule.

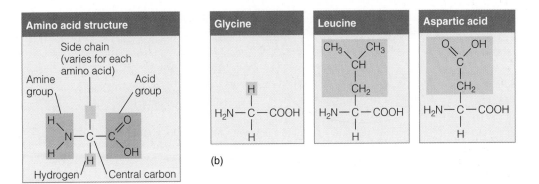

Figure 6.1 Structure of an amino acid. (a) All amino acids contain five parts: a central carbon atom, an amine group around the atom that contains nitrogen, an acid group, a hydrogen atom, and a side chain. (b) Only the side chain differs for each of the 20 amino acids, giving each its unique properties.

The singular term *protein* is misleading, as there are potentially an infinite number of unique types of proteins in living organisms. Most of the proteins in our bodies are made from combinations of just 20 amino acids, identified in Table 6.1. By combining a few dozen to more than 300 copies of these 20 amino acids in various sequences, our bodies form an estimated 10 000 to 50 000 unique proteins.

As shown in Figure 6.1(b), the portion of the amino acid that makes each one unique is its side chain. The amine group, acid group, and carbon and hydrogen atoms do not vary. Variations in the structure of the side chain give each amino acid its distinct properties.

We Must Obtain Essential Amino Acids from Food

Of the 20 amino acids in our bodies, 9 are classified as essential. This does not mean that they are more important than the 11 non-essential amino acids. Instead, an **essential amino acid** is one that our bodies cannot produce at all or cannot produce in sufficient quantities to meet our physiologic needs. Thus, we must obtain an essential amino acid from our food. Without the proper amount of essential amino acids in our bodies, we lose our ability to make the proteins and other nitrogen-containing compounds we need.

essential amino acids Amino acids not produced by the body that must be obtained from food.

Table 6.1   Amino Acids of the Human Body

Essential Amino Acids	Non-Essential Amino Acids
These amino acids must be consumed in the diet.	These amino acids can be manufactured by the body.
Histidine	Alanine
Isoleucine	Arginine
Leucine	Asparagine
Lysine	Aspartic acid
Methionine	Cysteine
Phenylalanine	Glutamic acid
Threonine	Glutamine
Tryptophan	Glycine
Valine	Proline
	Serine
	Tyrosine

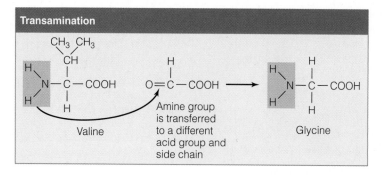

Figure 6.2 Transamination. Our bodies can make non-essential amino acids by transferring the amine group from an essential amino acid to a different acid group and side chain.

• Deamination / Transamination

non-essential amino acids Amino acids that can be manufactured by the body in sufficient quantities and therefore do not need to be consumed regularly in our diet.

transamination The process of transferring the amine group from one amino acid to another to manufacture a new amino acid.

Our Body Can Make Non-Essential Amino Acids

Non-essential amino acids are just as important to our bodies as essential amino acids, but our bodies can make them in sufficient quantities so we do not need to consume them in our diet. We make non-essential amino acids by transferring the nitrogen-containing group from an essential amino acid to a different acid group and side chain. The process of transferring the amine group from one amino acid to another acid group and side chain is called **transamination** and is shown in Figure 6.2. The acid groups and side chains can be donated by amino acids, or they can be made from the breakdown products of carbohydrates and fats. Thus, by combining parts of different amino acids, the necessary non-essential amino acid can be made.

Under some conditions, a non-essential amino acid can become an essential amino acid. In this case, the amino acid is called a *conditionally essential amino acid.* Consider what occurs in the disease known as phenylketonuria (PKU). As discussed in Chapter 4, someone with PKU cannot metabolize phenylalanine (an essential amino acid). Normally, the body uses phenylalanine to produce the non-essential amino acid tyrosine, so the inability to metabolize phenylalanine results in failure to make tyrosine. If PKU is not diagnosed immediately after birth, it results in irreversible brain damage. In this situation, tyrosine becomes a conditionally essential amino acid that must be provided by the diet.

> **Recap:** The building blocks of proteins are amino acids. The amine group of the amino acid contains nitrogen. The portion of the amino acid that changes, giving each amino acid its distinct identity, is the side chain. The body cannot make essential amino acids so we must obtain them from our diet. Our body can make non-essential amino acids from parts of other amino acids, carbohydrates, and fats.

• Protein Structure

How Are Proteins Made?

As we have stated, our bodies can synthesize proteins by selecting the needed amino acids from the pool of all amino acids available at any given time. Let's look more closely at how this occurs.

Amino Acids Bond to Form a Variety of Peptides

peptide bonds Unique types of chemical bonds in which the amine group of one amino acid binds to the acid group of another to manufacture dipeptides and all larger peptide molecules.

Figure 6.3 shows that when two amino acids join together, the amine group of one binds to the acid group of another in a unique type of chemical bond called a **peptide bond**. In the process, a molecule of water is released as a byproduct.

Two amino acids joined together form a *dipeptide,* and three amino acids joined together are called a *tripeptide.* The term *oligopeptide* is used to identify a

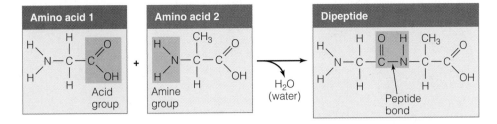

Figure 6.3 Amino acid bonding. Two amino acids join together to form a dipeptide. By combining multiple amino acids, proteins are made.

string of four to nine amino acids, while a *polypeptide* is ten or more amino acids bonded together. As a polypeptide chain grows longer, it begins to fold into any of a variety of complex shapes that give proteins their sophisticated structure and functions.

Genes Regulate Amino Acid Binding

Our genetic makeup, or heredity, determines the sequence of the amino acids for each individual protein molecule. Each of us is unique because we inherited a specific genetic code from our parents. Each person's specific genes lead to minute differences in amino acid sequences, which in turn lead to slight differences in body proteins. These differences in proteins result in the unique physical and physiologic characteristics each one of us possesses.

As mentioned earlier, DNA dictates the structure of each protein our body synthesizes. Figure 6.4 shows how this process occurs. **Gene expression** is a term used to refer to the process of using a gene in a cell to make a protein. A gene is a segment of DNA that serves as a template for the structure of a protein. As proteins are manufactured at the site of ribosomes in the cytoplasm, and DNA never leaves the nucleus, a special molecule is needed to copy, or transcribe, the information from DNA and carry it to the ribosome. This is the job of *messenger RNA* (*messenger ribonucleic acid*, or *mRNA*); during **transcription**, mRNA copies the genetic information from DNA in the nucleus and carries it to the ribosomes in the cytoplasm. Once this genetic information is at the ribosome, **translation** occurs: genetic information from the mRNA is translated into a growing chain of amino acids that are bonded together to make a specific protein.

Although the DNA for making every protein in our bodies is contained within each cell nucleus, not all genes are expressed and each cell does not make every type of protein. For example, each cell contains the DNA to manufacture the hormone insulin; however, only the cells of the pancreas express the insulin gene, so they are the only cells that can produce insulin. Our physiologic needs alter gene expression, as do various nutrients. For instance, a cut in the skin that causes bleeding leads to the production of various proteins that clot the blood. If we consume more dietary iron than we need, the gene for ferritin (a protein that stores iron) is expressed so that we can store this excess iron. Our genetic makeup and how appropriately we express our genes are important factors in our health.

gene expression The process of using a gene to make a protein.

transcription The process through which messenger RNA copies genetic information from DNA in the nucleus.

translation The process that occurs when the genetic information carried by messenger RNA is translated into a chain of amino acids at the ribosome.

Amino Acid Binding and Attraction Determine Shape

The different amino acids in a polypeptide chain possess unique chemical characteristics that cause the chain to twist and turn into various specific shapes. The shape of each protein is also determined by how each amino acid is attracted to, or repelled by, the surrounding fluid and other amino acids. Some side chains of amino acids carry electrical charges that attract water. Others have neutral charges that repel water.

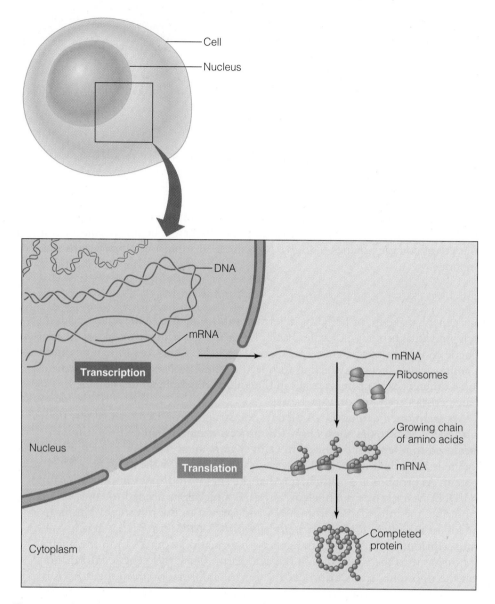

Figure 6.4 Gene expression. Messenger RNA (mRNA) transcribes the genetic information from DNA in the nucleus and carries it to the ribosomes in the cytoplasm. At the ribosome, this genetic information is translated into a chain of amino acids that eventually make a protein.

• Protein Function

Protein Shape Determines Function

The three-dimensional shape of a protein is critically important because it determines that protein's function in the body. For example, the proteins that form tendons are much longer than they are wide. Tendons are connective tissues that attach bone to muscle, and their long, rod-like structure provides strong, fibrous connections. In contrast, the proteins that form red blood cells are globular in shape, and they result in the red blood cells being shaped like flattened discs with depressed centres, similar to a miniature doughnut (Figure 6.5). This structure and the flexibility of the proteins in the red blood cells permit them to change shape and flow freely through even the tiniest capillaries to deliver oxygen and still return to their original shape.

Proteins can uncoil and lose their shape when they are exposed to heat, acids, bases, heavy metals, alcohol, and other damaging substances. The term used to describe this permanent change in the shape of proteins is **denaturation**. When a protein is denatured, its function is also lost. Examples of protein denaturation that we can see are the stiffening of egg whites when they are whipped, the curdling of

denaturation A change in the shape of a protein caused by heat, acids, bases, heavy metals, alcohol, or other substances; results in protein losing its ability to function.

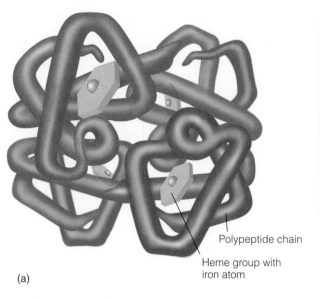

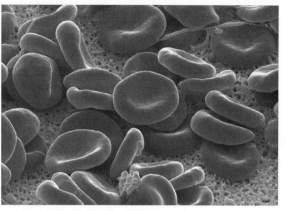

Polypeptide chain

Heme group with
iron atom

(a)

(b)

Figure 6.5 Protein shape determines function. (a) Hemoglobin, the protein that forms red blood cells, is globular in shape. (b) The globular shape of hemoglobin results in red blood cells being shaped like flattened discs.

milk when lemon juice or another acid is added, and the solidifying of eggs as they cook. Denaturation also occurs when we digest proteins.

> **Recap:** Amino acids bind together to form proteins. Genes regulate the amino acid sequence, and thus the structure, of all proteins. The shape of a protein determines its function. When a protein is denatured by damaging substances, such as heat and acids, it loses its shape and its function.

Protein Synthesis Can Be Limited by Missing Amino Acids

Animations

- Overview of Protein Synthesis
- Protein Synthesis

For protein synthesis to occur, all essential amino acids must be available to the cell. If this is not the case, the amino acid that is missing or in the smallest supply is called the **limiting amino acid**. Without the proper combination and quantity of essential amino acids, protein synthesis slows to the point at which proteins cannot be generated. For instance, the protein hemoglobin contains the essential amino acid histidine. If we do not consume enough histidine, it becomes the limiting amino acid in hemoglobin production. As no other amino acid can be substituted, our body becomes unable to make adequate hemoglobin, and we lose the ability to transport oxygen to our cells. Our cells cannot function and will eventually die if they do not receive adequate oxygen. Inadequate energy consumption also limits protein synthesis. If not enough energy is available from our diets, our bodies will use any accessible proteins for energy, thus preventing them from being used to build new proteins.

limiting amino acid The essential amino acid that is missing or in the smallest supply in the amino acid pool and is thus responsible for slowing or halting protein synthesis.

A protein that does not contain all the essential amino acids in sufficient quantities to support growth and health is called an **incomplete** (or *low-quality*) **protein**. Proteins that have all nine essential amino acids are considered **complete** (or *high-quality*) **proteins**. The most complete protein sources are from animal sources and include egg whites, ground beef, chicken, tuna and other fish, and milk. Soybeans are the only complete source of vegetable protein. In general, the typical Canadian diet is very high in complete proteins, as we eat proteins from a variety of food sources.

incomplete proteins Proteins that do not contain all the essential amino acids in sufficient amounts to support growth and health.

complete proteins Proteins that contain all nine essential amino acids. Proteins from animal sources are complete proteins. Soybeans are the only complete source of plant protein.

Protein Synthesis Can Be Enhanced by Mutual Supplementation

Many people believe that we must consume meat or dairy products to obtain complete proteins. Not true! Consider a meal of beans and rice. Beans are low in the essential amino acids methionine and tryptophan but have adequate amounts of isoleucine and

Table 6.2   Complementary Food Combinations: Turning Incomplete Proteins into Complete Proteins

Food	Limiting Amino Acid	Foods High in Limiting Amino Acid	Complementary Food Combination
Legumes	Methionine and cysteine	Grains, nuts, and seeds	Rice and lentils Red beans and rice Rice and black-eyed peas Hummus (chickpeas and sesame seeds)
Grains	Lysine	Legumes	Peanut butter and bread Barley and lentil soup Corn tortilla and beans
Vegetables	Lysine, methionine, cysteine	Legumes (lysine), grains, nuts, and seeds (methionine and cysteine)	Tofu and broccoli with almonds Spinach salad with pine nuts and kidney beans

mutual supplementation The process of combining two or more incomplete protein sources to make a complete protein.

complementary proteins Two or more foods that together contain all nine essential amino acids necessary for a complete protein. It is not necessary to eat complementary foods at the same meal.

pepsin An enzyme in the stomach that begins the breakdown of proteins into shorter polypeptide chains and single amino acids.

lysine. Rice is low in essential isoleucine and lysine but contains sufficient methionine and tryptophan. By combining beans and rice, a complete protein source is created.

Mutual supplementation is the process of combining two or more incomplete protein sources to make a complete protein, and the two foods involved are called complementary foods; these foods provide **complementary proteins** (Table 6.2) that, when combined, provide all nine essential amino acids. It is not necessary to eat these foods at the same meal. We maintain a free pool of amino acids in the blood; these amino acids come from food and sloughed-off cells. When we eat one complementary protein, its amino acids join those in the free amino acid pool. These free amino acids can then combine to synthesize complete proteins as long as the amount of amino acids present meets the requirements for a particular protein. However, it is wise to eat complementary-protein foods during the same day, as partially completed proteins cannot be stored and saved for a later time. Mutual supplementation is important for people who eat vegetarian diets, particularly if they consume no animal products whatsoever.

> **Recap:** When a particular amino acid is limiting, protein synthesis cannot occur. A complete protein provides all nine essential amino acids. Mutual supplementation combines two complementary protein sources to make a complete protein.

Animations

• Protein Digestion

How Do Our Bodies Break Down Dietary Protein?

Our bodies do not directly use proteins from the foods we eat to make the proteins we need. Dietary proteins are first digested and broken into smaller particles, such as amino acids, dipeptides, and tripeptides, so that they can be absorbed and transported to the cells. In this section, we will review how proteins are digested and absorbed. As you read about each step in this process, refer to Figure 6.6 for a visual tour through the digestive system.

Stomach Acids and Enzymes Break Proteins into Short Polypeptides

Virtually no enzymatic digestion of proteins occurs in the mouth. As shown in Step 1 in Figure 6.6, proteins in food are chewed, crushed, and moistened with saliva to ease swallowing and to increase the surface area of the protein for more efficient digestion. No further digestive action on proteins occurs in the mouth.

When proteins reach the stomach, they are broken apart by *hydrochloric acid* (Figure 6.6, Step 2). Hydrochloric acid denatures the strands of protein and converts the inactive enzyme, *pepsinogen,* into its active form, **pepsin**. Although pepsin is a

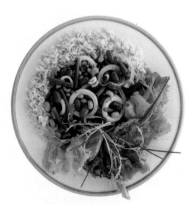

This dish of beans, rice, and vegetables is an example of mutual supplementation.

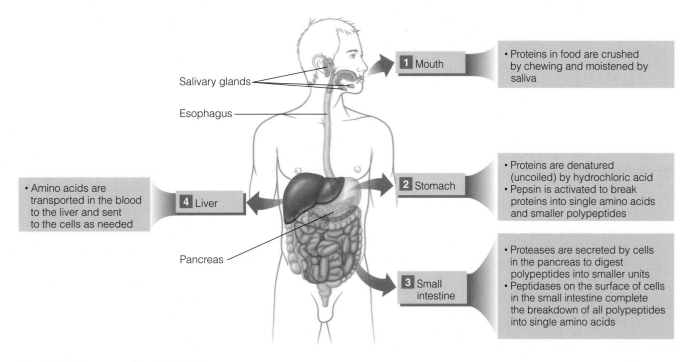

Salivary glands

Esophagus

1 Mouth

• Proteins in food are crushed by chewing and moistened by saliva

Pancreas

2 Stomach

• Proteins are denatured (uncoiled) by hydrochloric acid
• Pepsin is activated to break proteins into single amino acids and smaller polypeptides

4 Liver

• Amino acids are transported in the blood to the liver and sent to the cells as needed

3 Small intestine

• Proteases are secreted by cells in the pancreas to digest polypeptides into smaller units
• Peptidases on the surface of cells in the small intestine complete the breakdown of all polypeptides into single amino acids

Figure 6.6 The process of protein digestion.

• Protein Absorption

protein, it is not denatured by the acid in the stomach because it has evolved to work optimally in an acidic environment. Pepsin begins breaking proteins into single amino acids and shorter polypeptides that then travel to the small intestine for further digestion.

Enzymes in the Small Intestine Break Polypeptides into Single Amino Acids

The shorter polypeptides and single amino acids are part of a mixture of partially digested food and strongly acidic digestive juices called chyme. This acidic mix enters the opening of the small intestine in tiny amounts by means of the opening and closing of the pyloric sphincter. By controlling the release of the chyme into the small intestine, the pyloric sphincter can prevent the acid mixture from damaging the tissues lining the small intestine. It also helps prevent the mixture from flowing backward, from the small intestine back up into the stomach.

The pepsin, which was activated in the strongly acidic juices of the stomach, is rendered inactive in the neutral pH of the small intestine. The pancreas begins to secrete other enzymes called proteases. **Proteases** hydrolyze the peptide bonds, splitting the polypeptides into oligopeptides, tripeptides, dipeptides, and free amino acids (Figure 6.6, Step 3).

A second set of enzymes secreted from the intestinal cells then completes the digestion process. **Peptidases** split apart most of the oligopeptides, tripeptides, and dipeptides into single amino acids for absorption. Any remaining dipeptides and tripeptides then enter the cells in the intestinal wall, where they are digested to single amino acids. The single amino acids enter into the bloodstream, where they travel to the liver and on to cells throughout our bodies as needed (Figure 6.6, Step 4). Because the peptidases, proteases, and pepsin are proteins, they also become denatured and are ultimately digested.

An important fact to remember is that the cells of the small intestine have different sites that specialize in transporting certain types of amino acids, dipeptides, and tripeptides. When very large doses of single amino acids are taken on an empty stomach, there is the potential of similar amino acids competing for the same absorption sites. When we consume too much of one kind, it can block the absorption of other amino acids. Some nutritionists believe that this is why it is not beneficial to consume

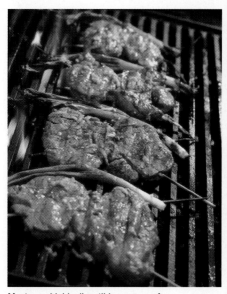

Meats are highly digestible sources of dietary protein.

proteases A set of enzymes secreted by cells in the pancreas that hydrolyze (break apart) the peptide bonds in shorter polypeptides, splitting them into oligopeptides, tripeptides, dipeptides, and free amino acids.

peptidases A set of enzymes on the surface of intestinal cells that hydrolyze peptide bonds in oligopeptides, tripeptides, and dipeptides, splitting them into single amino acids for absorption.

individual amino acid supplements. In reality, people rarely take very large doses of single amino acids on an empty stomach. The primary reason people should not take single amino acids is that the amount taken is usually so small that they don't have any beneficial effect.

Protein Digestibility Affects Protein Quality

Earlier in this chapter, we discussed how foods differ in the quality of their protein. The amount of essential amino acids is one factor in determining quality—the more essential amino acids a food contains, the more proteins are available to the body. Foods with more essential amino acids are therefore considered to have better-quality protein than foods with fewer essential amino acids.

Another aspect of protein quality is digestibility, or how completely our bodies can digest a protein and absorb the amino acids. Proteins from eggs, fish, meat, dairy products, and other animal foods are highly digestible, as are many soy products. We can absorb more than 90% of these proteins. Legumes are also highly digestible (about 80%). Grains and many vegetable proteins are less digestible, ranging from 60% to 90%.

protein digestibility–corrected amino acid score (PDCAAS) A measurement of protein quality that considers the balance of essential amino acids as well as the digestibility of the protein in the food.

The **protein digestibility–corrected amino acid score (PDCAAS)** is a measurement of protein quality that considers the balance of essential amino acids, as well as the digestibility of the protein in the food. To calculate the PDCAAS, the amount of each essential amino acid is first calculated in milligrams per gram of the protein. These amounts are then compared with the amounts in a reference protein, which has been calculated from the amino acid requirements of a preschool-age child. The most limiting essential amino acid determines the protein's *amino acid score*. The amino acid score is then multiplied by a digestibility factor based on fecal digestibility measured in studies of rats. The maximum PDCAAS value allowed is 100%, so the calculated values for the milk protein casein (121) and egg white protein (118), the highest-quality proteins, have been reduced to 100. The PDCAAS for beef, soy, and wheat are 92, 91, and 42, respectively (Schaafsma 2000).

Some scientists have recently questioned the use of a reference protein based on data obtained many years ago from amino acid balance studies using 2-year-old children, as well as the measurement of digestibility using fecal values that don't account for losses of amino acids in the small intestine. They have also argued against truncating PDCAAS to 100% (Schaafsma 2000). However, the PDCAAS is widely used and is still the method that the Food and Agriculture Organization (FAO) of the United Nations and the World Health Organization (WHO) jointly recommend for assessing protein quality in human diets.

Other measures of protein quality include the protein efficiency ratio and net protein utilization. The *protein efficiency ratio* assesses protein quality by comparing the weight gained by a laboratory animal consuming a test protein with the weight gained by a laboratory animal consuming an equivalent amount of a reference, or standardized, protein. *Net protein utilization* is a process that compares the amount of nitrogen retained in our bodies with the amount of nitrogen we consume in our diets. The more nitrogen we retain, the higher the quality of the protein we have consumed.

These measures of protein quality are useful when determining the quality of protein available to populations of people. However, these measures are not practical or useful for individual diet planning.

Recap: In the stomach, hydrochloric acid denatures (uncoils) proteins and converts pepsinogen to pepsin; pepsin breaks proteins into smaller polypeptides and individual amino acids. In the small intestine, proteases break polypeptides into smaller fragments and single amino acids. The cells in the wall of the small intestine break the smaller peptide fragments into single amino acids, which are then transported in the bloodstream to the liver for distribution to cells.

Why Do We Need Proteins?

The functions of proteins in the body are so numerous that only a few can be described in detail in this chapter. Note that proteins function most effectively when we also consume adequate amounts of energy as carbohydrates and fat. When there is not enough energy available, the body uses proteins as an energy source, limiting their availability for the functions described below.

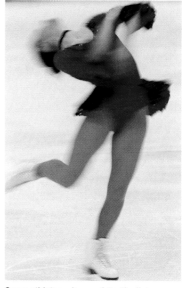

Some athletes who persistently diet are at risk for low protein intake.

Proteins Contribute to Cell Growth, Repair, and Maintenance

The proteins in our body are dynamic, meaning that they are constantly being broken down, repaired, and replaced. When proteins are broken down, many amino acids are recycled into new proteins. Think about all of the new proteins that are needed to allow an embryo to develop and grow. In this case, an entirely new human body is being made! In fact, a newborn baby has more than ten trillion body cells.

Even in the mature adult, our cells are constantly turning over, meaning old cells are broken down and parts are used to create new cells. In addition, cellular damage that occurs must be repaired to maintain our health. Our red blood cells live for only three to four months, and then are replaced by new cells that are produced in our bone marrow. The cells lining our intestinal tract are replaced every three to six days. The old intestinal cells are treated just like the proteins in food; they are digested and the amino acids are absorbed back into the body. The constant turnover of proteins from our diet is essential for such cell growth, repair, and maintenance.

Proteins also provide the frameworks for most of the body's structures. The protein collagen provides the structure to which mineral crystals adhere when bones or teeth are being formed. Proteins also are key components of muscles, membranes, organs, skin, and connective tissues, such as tendons, ligaments, and scars.

Proteins Act as Enzymes and Hormones

Enzymes are proteins that speed up chemical reactions, without being changed by the chemical reaction themselves. Enzymes can act to bind substances together or break them apart and can transform one substance into another. Figure 6.7 shows how an enzyme can bind two substances together.

Animations

- Enzymes
- How Enzymes Work

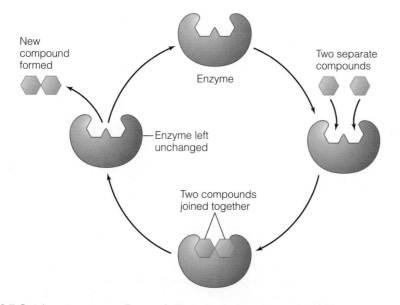

New compound formed

Enzyme

Two separate compounds

Enzyme left unchanged

Two compounds joined together

Figure 6.7 Proteins act as enzymes. Enzymes facilitate chemical reactions, such as joining two compounds together.

Each cell contains thousands of enzymes that facilitate specific cellular reactions. For example, the enzyme phosphofructokinase (PFK) increases carbohydrate metabolism during physical exercise. This enzyme is critical to driving the rate at which we break down glucose and use it for energy during exercise. Without PFK, we would be unable to generate energy at a fast enough rate to allow us to be physically active.

Hormones are substances that act as chemical messengers in the body. Some hormones are made from amino acids, while others are made from lipids (refer to Chapter 5). Hormones are stored in various glands in the body, which release them in response to changes in the body's environment. They then act on the body's organs and tissues to restore the body to normal conditions.

Insulin, a hormone made from amino acids, plays an important role in regulating blood concentrations of glucose. Although glucose is an important source of energy for body cells, high blood levels can damage cells. When you digest a meal, the breakdown of the carbohydrates raises your blood glucose levels, which stimulates your pancreas to increase its production and release of insulin. Insulin acts on cell membranes to speed up the transport of glucose into the cells and return blood glucose levels to normal.

Other examples of amino acid–containing hormones are glucagon, which responds to conditions of low blood glucose, and thyroid hormone, which helps control our resting metabolic rate.

Proteins Help Maintain Fluid and Electrolyte Balance

Electrolytes are electrically charged particles that assist in maintaining fluid balance. For our bodies to function properly, fluids and electrolytes must be maintained at healthy levels inside and outside cells and within blood vessels. Proteins attract fluids, and the proteins that are in the bloodstream, in the cells, and in the spaces surrounding the cells work together to keep fluids moving across these spaces in the proper quantities to maintain fluid balance and blood pressure. When protein intake is inadequate or deficient, the concentration of proteins in the bloodstream is insufficient to draw fluid from the tissues and across the blood vessel walls; fluid then collects in the tissues, causing **edema**. In addition to being uncomfortable, edema can lead to serious medical problems.

Sodium (Na^+) and potassium (K^+) are examples of common electrolytes. Under normal conditions, Na^+ is more concentrated outside the cell, and K^+ is more concentrated inside the cell. This proper balance of Na^+ and K^+ is accomplished by the action of **transport proteins** located within the cell membrane. Figure 6.8 shows how these transport proteins work to pump Na^+ outside and K^+ inside the cell. Conduction of nerve signals and contraction of muscles depends on a proper balance of electrolytes. If protein intake is inadequate or deficient, we lose our ability to maintain these functions, resulting in potentially fatal changes in the rhythm of the

edema A disorder in which fluids build up in the tissue spaces of the body, causing fluid imbalances and a swollen appearance.

transport proteins Protein molecules that help to transport substances throughout the body and across cell membranes.

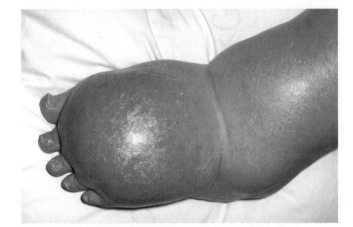

Edema can result from deficient protein intake. This foot with edema is swollen due to fluid imbalance.

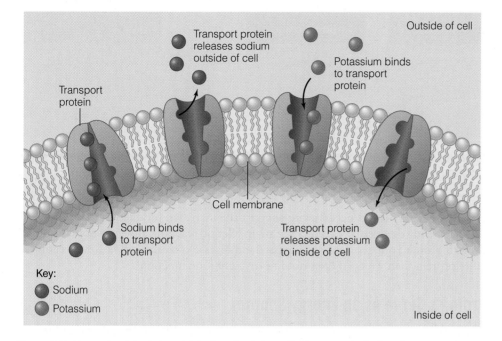

Figure 6.8 Transport proteins help maintain electrolyte balance. Transport proteins in the cell membrane pick up potassium and sodium and transport them across the cell membrane.

heart. Other consequences of chronically low protein intakes include muscle weakness and spasms, kidney failure, and, if conditions are severe enough, death.

Proteins Help Maintain Acid–Base Balance

The body's cellular processes result in the constant production of acids and bases. These substances are transported in the blood to be excreted through the kidneys and the lungs. The human body maintains very tight control over the **pH**, or the acid–base balance of the blood. The body goes into a state called **acidosis** when the blood becomes too acidic. **Alkalosis** results if the blood becomes too basic. Both acidosis and alkalosis can be caused by respiratory or metabolic problems. Acidosis and alkalosis can cause coma and death by denaturing body proteins.

Proteins can be excellent **buffers**, meaning they help maintain proper acid–base balance. Acids contain hydrogen ions, which are positively charged. The side chains of proteins have negative charges that attract the hydrogen ions and neutralize their detrimental effects on the body. Proteins can release the hydrogen ions when the blood becomes too basic. By buffering acids and bases, proteins maintain acid–base balance and blood pH.

Proteins Help Maintain a Strong Immune System

Antibodies are special proteins that are critical components of the immune system. When a foreign substance attacks the body, the immune system produces antibodies to defend against it. Bacteria, viruses, toxins, and allergens (substances that cause allergic reactions) are examples of antigens that can trigger antibody production. (An *antigen* is any substance—but typically a protein—that our bodies recognize as foreign and that triggers an immune response.)

Each antibody is designed to destroy a specific invader. When that substance invades the body, antibodies are produced to attack and destroy the specific antigen. Once antibodies have been made, the body remembers this process and can respond faster the next time that particular invader appears. *Immunity* refers to the development of the molecular memory to produce antibodies quickly on subsequent invasions.

pH Stands for percentage of hydrogen. It is a measure of the acidity—or level of hydrogen—of any solution, including human blood.

acidosis A disorder in which the blood becomes acidic; that is, the level of hydrogen in the blood is excessive. It can be caused by respiratory or metabolic problems.

alkalosis A disorder in which the blood becomes basic; that is, the level of hydrogen in the blood is deficient. It can be caused by respiratory or metabolic problems.

buffers Proteins that help maintain proper acid–base balance by attaching to, or releasing, hydrogen ions as conditions change in the body.

antibodies Defensive proteins of the immune system. Their production is prompted by the presence of bacteria, viruses, toxins, and allergens.

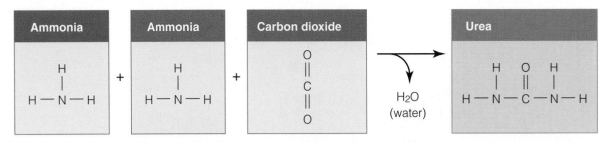

Figure 6.9 To make ammonia less toxic before it enters the bloodstream, it is combined in the liver with carbon dioxide to produce urea.

Adequate protein is necessary to support the increased production of antibodies that occurs in response to a cold, a flu, or an allergic reaction. If we do not consume enough protein, our resistance to illnesses and disease is weakened; however, eating more protein than we need does not improve immune function.

- Deamination / Transamination
- Nitrogen Balance

deamination The process by which an amine group is removed from an amino acid. The nitrogen is then transported in a special form to the kidneys for excretion in the urine, while the carbon skeleton is metabolized for energy or used to make other compounds.

Proteins Serve As an Energy Source

The body's primary energy sources are carbohydrate and fat. Remember that both carbohydrate and fat have specialized storage forms that can be used for energy— carbohydrate as glycogen and fat as triglycerides. Proteins do not have a specialized storage form for energy; when proteins need to be used for energy, they are taken from the blood and body tissues, such as the liver and skeletal muscle. In healthy people, proteins contribute very little to energy needs. Because we are efficient at recycling amino acids, protein needs are relatively low compared with carbohydrate and fat.

When there are more amino acids than needed, the liver removes them from the blood and cleaves off the nitrogen-containing amino (or amine) group in a process called deamination. **Deamination** results in two products: ammonia (NH_3), which is highly toxic to the liver, and a carbon skeleton that is missing the amino group. The liver detoxifies the ammonia before sending it into the bloodstream by combining it with carbon dioxide to form urea (Figure 6.9). The urea then enters the bloodstream and travels to the kidneys to be excreted from the body.

The carbon skeleton that remains after deamination contains hydrogen, oxygen, and, of course, carbon. The body can metabolize (break down) this component further to acetyl CoA, which is then used for energy or converted to fatty acids and sent to the body's fat tissues. Alternatively, the liver can add another nitrogen-containing amino group to make a non-essential amino acid. Most amino acids can be used to make glucose and are termed *glucogenic or gluconeogenic.* This is a critical process during times of low carbohydrate intake or starvation. Fat cannot be converted to glucose, but body proteins can be broken down and converted into glucose to provide needed energy to the brain and red blood cells.

To protect the proteins in our body tissues, it is important that we regularly eat enough carbohydrate and fat to meet our energy needs. We also need to consume enough dietary protein to perform the required work without using up the proteins that already are playing an active role in our bodies. Unfortunately, our body cannot store excess dietary protein. As a consequence, eating too much protein results in the removal and excretion of the nitrogen in the urine and the use of the remaining components for energy.

Recap: Proteins serve many important functions, including (1) enabling growth, repair, and maintenance of body tissues; (2) acting as enzymes and hormones; (3) maintaining fluid and electrolyte balance; (4) maintaining acid–base balance; (5) making antibodies, which strengthen our immune system; and (6) providing energy when carbohydrate and fat intake are inadequate. Proteins function best when we also consume adequate amounts of energy as carbohydrate and fat.

How Much Protein Should We Eat?

Many people worry that they are not getting enough protein in their diets. In fact, one of the most common concerns among active people and athletes is that their diets are deficient in protein (see the Nutrition Myth or Fact box for a discussion of this topic). This concern about dietary protein is generally unnecessary, as we get more than enough protein from the various plant and animal foods we consume.

Recommended Dietary Allowance (RDA) for Protein

How much protein should we eat? The RDA for sedentary people is 0.8 gram per kilogram of body weight per day. The Acceptable Macronutrient Distribution Range (AMDR) for protein is 10%–35% of total energy intake. Protein needs are higher for children, adolescents, and pregnant or lactating women because more protein is needed during times of growth and development (see Chapters 15 and 16 for details on protein needs during these portions of the life cycle). Protein needs can also be higher for active people and for vegetarians. Table 6.3 lists the daily recommendations for protein for a variety of lifestyles.

How can we convert this recommendation into total grams of protein for the day? In the You Do the Math box, let's calculate Matthew's RDA for protein.

Is it possible for Matthew to eat this much protein each day? It may surprise you to discover that many Canadians eat 1.5 times the RDA for protein without any effort! In the following sections, we describe the average protein intake in Canada, review foods that are good sources of protein, and give an example of calculating your daily protein intake. We will also look at potential risks of high-protein diets.

> ▶ **NUTRITION MYTH OR FACT**
>
> ## Athletes Need More Protein Than Inactive People
>
> At one time it was believed that the Recommended Dietary Allowance (RDA) for protein, which is 0.8 gram/kilogram body weight, was sufficient for both inactive people and athletes. Recent studies, however, show that athletes' protein needs are higher. Why do athletes need more protein? Regular exercise increases the transport of oxygen to body tissues, requiring changes in the oxygen-carrying capacity of the blood. To carry more oxygen, we need to produce more of the protein that carries oxygen in the blood (i.e., hemoglobin). During intense exercise, we use a small amount of protein directly for energy. We also use protein to make glucose to maintain adequate blood glucose levels and to prevent hypoglycemia (low blood glucose) during exercise. Regular exercise stimulates tissue growth and causes tissue damage, which must be repaired by additional proteins.
>
> Strength athletes (such as bodybuilders and weightlifters) need 1.8 to 2 times as much protein as the current RDA, while endurance athletes (such as distance runners and triathletes) need 1.5 to 1.75 times as much protein as the current RDA (Lemon 2000). Later in this chapter we will calculate the protein needs for inactive and active people.
>
> Does this mean you should add more protein to your diet? Not necessarily. Most Canadians, including inactive people and athletes, already consume more than the RDA for protein. Thus, taking amino acid and protein supplements is not necessary. In fact, eating more protein does not cause muscles to become bigger or stronger, and taking individual amino acid supplements can actually reduce protein production. Only regular strength training can achieve the goal of bigger and stronger muscles. For healthy individuals, evidence does not support eating more than two times the RDA for protein to increase strength, build muscle, or improve athletic performance. By eating a balanced diet and consuming a variety of foods, both inactive and active people can easily meet their protein requirements.

Table 6.3   Recommended Daily Protein Intakes

Group	Protein Intake (grams per kilogram* body weight)
Most adults[1]	0.8
Nonvegetarian endurance athletes[2]	1.2 to 1.4
Nonvegetarian strength athletes[2]	1.6 to 1.7
Vegetarian endurance athletes[2]	1.3 to 1.5
Vegetarian strength athletes[2]	1.7 to 1.8

Source: [1]Food and Nutrition Board, Institute of Medicine, *Dietary Reference Intakes for Energy, Carbohydrate, Fiber, Fat, Fatty Acids, Cholesterol, Protein, and Amino Acids (Macronutrients)*, Washington, DC: National Academies Press, 2002, 465–608.
[2] American College of Sports Medicine, American Dietetic Association, and Dietitians of Canada, Joint Position Statement, Nutrition and athletic performance, 2001, *Med. Sci. Sports Exerc.* 32:2130–45.
*To convert body weight to kilograms, divide weight in pounds by 2.2: Weight (pounds) ÷ 2.2 = Weight (kilograms)
Weight (kilograms) × protein recommendation (grams/kilograms body weight/day) = protein intake (grams/day)

Most Canadians Meet or Exceed the RDA for Protein

The 2004 Canadian Community Health Survey (Health Canada 2007) results show that the average protein intake among adults is 16.8%, well within the AMDR of 10%–35%. Very few people fell below or above this range of protein intakes, suggesting that almost all Canadians have average protein intakes that meet current dietary recommendations.

What are the typical protein intakes of active people? Table 6.4 reviews the self-reported protein intake of athletes participating in a variety of sports (Manore and Thompson 2000). As you can see, the protein intake ranges from 1.1 to 3.1 grams per kilogram body weight per day and accounts for 13% to 36% of the total daily energy intake in these active individuals. However,

▶ YOU DO THE MATH

Calculating Your Protein Needs

Matthew wants to know how much protein he needs each day. Off season, he works out three times a week at a gym and practises basketball with friends every Friday night. He is not a vegetarian. Although Matthew exercises regularly, he does not qualify as an endurance athlete or as a strength athlete. At this level of physical activity, Matthew's RDA for protein probably ranges from 0.8 to 1.0 grams per kg body weight per day (see Table 6.3). To calculate the total number of grams of protein Matthew should eat each day,

1. Convert Matthew's weight from pounds to kilograms. Matthew currently weighs 200 pounds. To convert this value to kilograms, divide by 2.2: (200 pounds) ÷ (2.2 pounds/kg) = 91 kg.

2. Multiply Matthew's weight in kilograms by his RDA for protein:

$$(91 \text{ kg}) \times (0.8 \text{ grams/kg}) = 72.8 \text{ grams of protein per day}$$

$$(91 \text{ kg}) \times (1.0 \text{ grams/kg}) = 91 \text{ grams of protein per day}$$

What happens during basketball season, when Matthew practises or has games five to six days a week? This will probably raise his protein needs to approximately 1.0 to 1.2 grams per kg body weight per day. How much more protein should he eat?

$$91 \text{ kg} \times 1.2 \text{ grams/kg} = 109.2 \text{ grams of protein per day.}$$

Now calculate your recommended protein intake based upon your activity level.

Table 6.4   Self-Reported Protein Intakes of Athletes

Sport Type	Gender	Protein Intake (gram/kilogram body weight/day)	Protein Intake (% total Calories)
Football	M	1.5	15.0
Weightlifting	M	1.9	18.0
Soccer	M	2.2	14.4
Triathlon	M	2.0	13.0
Marathon running	M	2.0	14.5
Distance running	M	1.6	12.8
	F	1.1	14.1
Ultradistance running	M	1.4	16.7
	F	1.2	15.1
Bodybuilding	M	2.7–3.1	22.5–37.7
	F	1.9–2.7	22.6–35.8

Source: Adapted by permission from M. Manore and J. Thompson, *Sport Nutrition for Health and Performance,* Champaign, IL: Human Kinetics, 2000, 118.

certain groups of athletes are at risk for low protein intakes. Athletes who consume inadequate energy and limit food choices, such as distance runners, figure skaters, female gymnasts, and wrestlers who are dieting, are all at risk for low protein intakes. Unlike people who consume adequate energy, individuals who are restricting their total energy intake (kcal) need to pay close attention to their protein intake.

> **Recap:** The RDA for protein for most adults who are not pregnant, not lactating, and not vegetarians is 0.8 grams per kilogram body weight. Children, pregnant women, nursing mothers, vegetarians, and active people need slightly more. Most people who have enough energy and carbohydrates in their diets have no problem meeting their RDA for protein.

Too Much Dietary Protein Can Be Harmful

High protein intake may increase the risk of some health problems. Three health conditions that have received particular attention are heart disease, bone loss, and kidney disease.

High Protein Intake Is Associated with High Cholesterol

High-protein diets comprising predominantly animal sources are associated with higher blood cholesterol levels. This is probably due to the saturated fat in animal products, which is known to increase blood cholesterol levels and the risk of heart disease. One study showed that people with heart disease improved their health when they ate a diet that was high in whole grains, fruits, and vegetables and met the RDA for protein (Fleming 2000). However, some of the people in this study chose to eat a high-protein diet, and their risk factors worsened. In addition, vegetarians have been shown to have a greatly reduced risk of heart disease (Fraser 1999) and lower rates of death from heart disease (Key et al. 1999).

High Protein Intake May Contribute to Bone Loss

How might a high-protein diet lead to bone loss? Until recently, nutritionists have been concerned about high-protein diets because they increase calcium excretion. This may be because animal products contain more of the sulphur amino acids (methionine and cysteine). Metabolizing these amino acids makes the blood more acidic, and calcium is pulled from the bone to buffer these acids. Although eating more protein can cause you to excrete more calcium, it is very controversial whether high protein intakes actually cause bone loss. We do know that eating too little protein causes bone loss, which increases the risk of fractures and osteoporosis. Higher intakes of animal and soy protein have been shown to protect bone in middle-aged and older women (Munger, Cerhan, and Chiu 1999; Alekel et al. 2000). There does not appear to be enough direct evidence at this time to show that higher protein intakes cause bone loss in healthy people.

High Protein Intake Can Increase the Risk for Kidney Disease

A third risk associated with high protein intakes is kidney disease. People who are susceptible to kidney disease, such as those with diabetes mellitus, may benefit from a lower-protein diet (Kontessis et al. 1995). There is no evidence, however, that eating more protein causes kidney disease in healthy people who are not susceptible to this condition. In fact, one study found that athletes consuming up to 2.8 grams of protein per kilogram body weight per day experienced no unhealthy changes in kidney function (Poortmans and Dellalieux 2000). Experts agree that eating no more than 2 grams of protein per kilogram body weight each day is safe for healthy people.

It is important for people who consume a lot of protein to drink more water. This is because eating more protein increases protein metabolism and urea production. As we mentioned earlier, urea is a waste product that forms when nitrogen is removed during amino acid metabolism. Adequate fluid is needed to flush excess urea from the kidneys. This is particularly important for athletes, who need more fluid because of higher sweat losses.

Shopper's Guide: Good Food Sources of Protein

Table 6.5 compares the protein content of a variety of foods. In general, good sources of protein include meats, poultry, seafood, dairy products and eggs, soy products, legumes, whole grains, and nuts. Although most people are aware that meats are an excellent source of protein, many people are surprised to learn that the quality of the protein in some legumes is almost equal to that of meat.

Legumes include kidney beans, pinto beans, black beans, soybeans, garbanzo beans (or chickpeas), lentils, green peas, black-eyed peas, and lima beans. Interestingly, the quality of soybean protein is almost identical to that of meat, and the protein quality of other legumes is relatively high. In addition to being excellent sources of protein, legumes are high in fibre, iron, calcium, and many of the B vitamins. They are also low in saturated fat and cholesterol.

Legumes are not nutritionally complete, however, as they do not contain vitamins B_{12}, C, or A and are deficient in methionine, an essential amino acid. Eating legumes regularly, including foods made from soybeans, may help reduce the risk of heart disease by lowering blood cholesterol levels. Diets high in legumes and soy products are also associated with lower rates of some cancers.

Fruits and many vegetables are not particularly high in protein; however, these foods provide fibre and many vitamins and minerals and are excellent sources of carbohydrates. Thus, eating these foods can help provide the carbohydrates and energy that our bodies need so that we can spare protein for use in building and maintaining

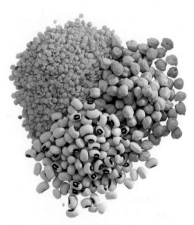

The quality of the protein in some legumes, such as these black-eyed peas, lentils, and chickpeas, is almost equal to that of meat.

Table 6.5 Protein Content of Commonly Consumed Foods

Food	Serving Size	Protein (g)	Food	Serving Size	Protein (g)
Beef:			*Beans:*		
Ground, lean, baked (16% fat)	100 g (3.5 oz.)	24	Refried	125 mL (½ cup)	7
Corned beef, brisket, cooked	100 g (3.5 oz.)	18	Kidney, red	125 mL (½ cup)	9
Prime rib, broiled (½-in. trim)	100 g (3.5 oz.)	21	Black	125 mL (½ cup)	8
Top sirloin, broiled (¼-in. trim)	100 g (3.5 oz.)	27	Pork and beans, canned	125 mL (½ cup)	7
Poultry:			*Nuts:*		
Chicken breast, broiled, no skin	90 g (3.0 oz.)	25	Peanuts, dry roasted	30 g (1 oz.)	7
Chicken thigh, barbecued (BBQ) no skin	60 g (2.2 oz.)	14	Peanut butter, creamy	30 mL (2 Tbsp)	8
Chicken drumstick, BBQ, with skin	70 g (2.5 oz.)	16	Almonds, blanched	30 g (1 oz.)	6
Turkey dark meat, roasted, no skin	100 g (3.5 oz.)	29	Sunflower seeds	60 mL (¼ cup)	7
Seafood:			Pecan halves	30 g (1 oz.)	5
Cod, steamed	100 g (3.5 oz.)	22	*Cereals, Grains, and Breads:*		
Salmon, chinook, baked	100 g (3.5 oz.)	26	Barley, cooked	250 mL (1 cup)	4
Shrimp, steamed	100 g (3.5 oz.)	21	Oatmeal, quick cooking	250 mL (1 cup)	6
Oysters, boiled	100 g (3.5 oz.)	19	Cheerios	250 mL (1 cup)	3
Tuna, in water, drained	100 g (3.5 oz.)	29	Corn Bran	250 mL (1 cup)	2
Pork:			Grape Nuts	125 mL (½ cup)	7
			Raisin Bran	250 mL (1 cup)	5
Pork loin chop, broiled	100 g (3.5 oz.)	24	Brown rice, cooked	250 mL (1 cup)	5
Spareribs, cooked, with bone	100 g (3.5 oz.)	29	Whole wheat bread	1 slice	2
Ham, roasted, lean	100 g (3.5 oz.)	21	Rye bread	1 slice	2
Dairy:			Bagel, 3½-in. diameter	1 each	7
Whole milk (3.3% fat)	250 mL (8 fl. oz.)	8	*Vegetables:*		
1% milk	250 mL (8 fl. oz.)	8	Carrots, raw (7.5 × 1⅛ in.)	1 each	1
Skim milk	250 mL (8 fl. oz.)	8	Asparagus, boiled	6 spears	2
Low-fat yogurt	250 mL (8 fl. oz.)	13	Green beans, cooked	125 mL (½ cup)	1
Cheddar cheese, processed	30 g (1 oz.)	6	Broccoli, raw, chopped	125 mL (½ cup)	1
Swiss cheese	30 g (1 oz.)	6	Spinach, raw, chopped	1 cup	2
Cottage cheese, low-fat (2%)	250 mL (1 cup)	31			
Soy Products:					
Tofu	125 mL (½ cup)	10			
Tempeh, cooked	100 g (3.3 oz.)	18			
Soy milk beverage	250 mL (1 cup)	7			

Source: Values obtained from U. S. Department of Agriculture (USDA), Nutrient Database for Standard Reference, www.nal.usda.gov/fnic/cgi-bin/nut_search.pl (accessed July 2003).

our bodies rather than using it for energy. Try the Nutrition Label Activity to determine how much protein you typically eat.

Recap: Eating too much protein from animal sources high in saturated fat may increase your risk for heart disease and kidney disease, if you are already at risk for these diseases. Good sources of protein include meats, eggs, dairy products, soy products, legumes, and seafood.

Can a Vegetarian Diet Provide Adequate Protein?

Vegetarianism is the practice of restricting the diet to foods of vegetable origin, including fruits, grains, and nuts. Results from a 2002 survey suggest that approximately 4% of Canadian adults (900 000 people) follow vegetarian diets. Many

vegetarianism The practice of restricting the diet to foods of plant origin, including vegetables, fruits, grains, and nuts.

▶ **NUTRITION LABEL ACTIVITY**

How Much Protein Do You Eat?

Matthew wants to know if his diet contains enough protein. To calculate his protein intake, he records in a food diary all the foods that he eats for three days. The foods Matthew consumed for one of his three days are listed below on the left, and the protein content of those foods is listed on the right. He recorded the protein content listed on the Nutrition Facts table for those foods with labels. For products without labels, he used the nutrient analysis program that came with this book.

There are also websites you can use at no cost. The Canadian Nutrient File, produced by Health Canada and the Canadian Food Inspection Agency, can be found at www.hc-sc.gc.ca/fn-an/nutrition/fiche-nutri-data/index_e.html. The U.S. Department of Agriculture's website can be found at www.ars.usda.gov/main/site_main.htm?modecode= 12–35–45–00.

As calculated in the You Do the Math box on page 208, Matthew's RDA is 72.8 to 91 grams of protein. He is consuming 2.2 to 2.7 times that amount! You can see that he does not need to use amino acid or protein supplements, since he has more than adequate amounts of protein to build lean tissue.

Now calculate your own protein intake using food labels and the nutrient analysis program included with this book. Do you obtain more protein from animal or plant sources? If you consume mostly plant sources, are you eating soy products and complementary foods throughout the day? If you eat animal-based products on a regular basis, notice how much protein you consume from even small servings of meat and dairy products.

Foods Consumed	Protein Content (g)
Breakfast:	
Coffee (500 mL/16 fl. oz.) with 30 mL (2 Tbsp) half & half cream	1
Bagel (13 cm/5 in.)	10
Cream cheese (30 mL/2 Tbsp)	2
Mid-morning snack:	
Cola beverage (500 mL/16 fl. oz.)	0
Low-fat strawberry yogurt (250 mL/1 cup)	10
Snackwells Apple Cinnamon Bars (37 g each; 2 bars eaten)	2
Lunch:	
Ham and cheese sandwich:	
Whole wheat bread (2 slices)	4
Mayonnaise (30 mL/2 Tbsp)	1
Lean ham (100 g/4 oz.)	24
Swiss cheese (50 g/2 oz.)	16
Iceberg lettuce (2 leaves)	0.5
Sliced tomato (3 slices)	0.5
Banana (1 large)	1
Triscuit crackers (20 crackers)	7
Bottled water (20 fl. oz.)	0
Dinner:	
Double cheeseburger:	
Lean ground beef (200 g/8 oz. cooked)	64
Processed cheddar cheese (1 slice)	6
Bun with sesame seeds (1 large)	6
Ketchup (30 mL/2 Tbsp)	1
Mustard (15 mL/1 Tbsp)	1
Shredded lettuce (125 mL/1/2 cup)	0.5
Sliced tomato (3 slices)	0.5
French fries (30 strips, each 6 to 8 cm/2 to 3 in.)	6
Milk, 1% fat (500 mL/16 fl. oz.)	16
Chocolate chip cookies (4 cookies, each 8 cm/3 in.)	3
Evening snack:	
Cheerios (500 mL/2 cups)	6
Milk, 1% fat (250 mL/8 fl. oz.)	8
Total Protein Intake for the Day:	**197 grams**

vegetarians are college and university students; moving away from home and taking responsibility for their own eating habits appears to influence some young adults to try it as a lifestyle choice.

Types of Vegetarian Diets

There are almost as many types of vegetarian diets as there are vegetarians. Some people who consider themselves vegetarians regularly eat poultry and fish. Others avoid the flesh of animals but consume eggs, milk, and cheese liberally. Still others

Table 6.6   Terms and Definitions of a Vegetarian Diet

Type of Diet	Foods Consumed	Comments
Semivegetarian (also called partial vegetarian)	Vegetables, grains, nuts, fruits, legumes; sometimes seafood, poultry, eggs, and dairy products	Typically excludes or limits red meat; may also avoid other meats
Lacto-ovo-pesco-vegetarian	Similar to a semivegetarian but excludes poultry	*Pesco* means fish
Lacto-ovo-vegetarian	Vegetables, grains, nuts, fruits, legumes, dairy products (*lacto*) and eggs (*ovo*)	Excludes animal flesh and seafood
Lactovegetarian	Similar to a lacto-ovo-vegetarian but excludes eggs	Relies on milk and cheese for animal sources of protein
Ovovegetarian	Vegetables, grains, nuts, fruits, legumes, and eggs	Excludes dairy, flesh, and seafood products
Vegan (also called strict vegetarian)	Only plant-based foods (vegetables, grains, nuts, seeds, fruits, legumes)	May not provide adequate vitamin B_{12}, zinc, iron, or calcium
Macrobiotic diet	Vegan-type diet; becomes progressively more strict until almost all foods are eliminated. At the extreme, only brown rice and small amounts of water or herbal tea are consumed.	Taken to the extreme, can cause malnutrition and death
Fruitarian	Only raw or dried fruit, seeds, nuts, honey, and vegetable oil	Very restrictive diet; deficient in protein, calcium, zinc, iron, vitamin B_{12}, riboflavin, and other nutrients

strictly avoid all products of animal origin, including milk and eggs, and even byproducts, such as candies and puddings made with gelatin.

Table 6.6 identifies the various types of vegetarian diets, ranging from the most inclusive to the most restrictive. Notice that the more restrictive the diet the more challenging it becomes to achieve an adequate protein intake.

Why Do People Become Vegetarians?

When discussing vegetarianism, one of the most often asked questions is why people would make this food choice. The most common responses are included here.

Religious, Ethical, and Food-Safety Reasons

Some make the choice for religious or spiritual reasons. Several religions prohibit or restrict the consumption of animal flesh; however, generalizations can be misleading. For example, while certain sects within Hinduism forbid the consumption of meat, perusing the menu at any Indian restaurant will reveal that many other Hindus regularly consume small quantities of meat, poultry, and fish. Many Buddhists are vegetarians, as are some Christians, including Seventh-day Adventists.

Many vegetarians are guided by their personal philosophy to choose vegetarianism. These people feel that it is morally and ethically wrong to consume animals and any products from animals (such as dairy

Many vegetarians consume milk, cheese, and legumes as sources of dietary protein.

or egg products) because they view the practices in the modern animal industries as inhumane. They may consume milk and eggs but choose to purchase them only from family farms where animals are treated humanely.

One recent concern surrounding beef is mad cow disease. However, food-borne illness outbreaks are far more common in produce than in meat, and vegetarians have had to face scares about salmonella in tomatoes and *E. coli* O157:H7 in packaged spinach recently in the United States and Canada. See Chapter 14 for a review of mad cow disease and food-borne illness.

Ecological Benefits

Many people choose vegetarianism because of their concerns about the effect of meat industries on the global environment. Because of the high demand for meat in developed nations, meat production has evolved from small family farming operations into the larger system of agribusiness. Critics of agribusiness are concerned with the environmental damages that agribusiness can cause. When animals are raised on smaller farms or allowed to range freely, they consume grass, crop wastes, and scraps recycled from the kitchen, which is an efficient means of using food sources that humans do not consume. The waste produced by these animals can be used for fertilizer and fuel.

Critics of agribusiness point out that animals raised in huge farm operations eat large quantities of grain that humans could consume. Water use can also be tremendous—it takes an estimated 1630 litres (430 gallons) of water to produce 0.45 kg (1 lb.) of pork. This is in contrast to the 572 litres (151 gallons) of water it takes to produce 0.45 kg (1 lb.) of wheat. Housing large numbers of animals in close quarters has also led to increased use of antibiotics, which raises concerns about the possibility of antibiotic residues in meat. Some people are concerned about the use of hormones that promote growth in the dairy cattle and beef industries, as well.

Other concerns are related to the waste produced from livestock operations and greenhouse gas emissions. Although much of the livestock waste is used as fertilizer, some of it can run off and pollute neighbouring streams, rivers, and lakes. Environment Canada has estimated that 10% of the total emissions of greenhouse gases (nitrous oxide, methane, and carbon dioxide) in Canada come from the agricultural sector. Nitrous oxide comes mainly from the handling and storage of manure and commercial fertilizers, while methane comes primarily from the beef industry and livestock manure.

Internationally, it is believed that millions of hectares of rain forests have been destroyed to provide grazing land for livestock and that the loss of these rain forests has been a major contributor to global warming. Beef imported from Central and South America, primarily Nicaragua, accounted for 10% of all beef imports in 1990 and 2.6% of the beef consumed by Canadians.

In response to these concerns for the environment, the Canadian Cattlemen's Association provides fact sheets and information about its industry's practices at www.cattle.ca/cca%20home.htm. They point out that most of the grain fed to livestock is unfit for human consumption and much of the land used for grazing is not suitable for crops. The Canadian Cattlemen's Association is part of the Greenhouse Gas Mitigation Program, in partnership with Agriculture and Agri-Food Canada, the Soil Conservation Council, Canadian Pork Council, and Dairy Farmers of Canada. The Greenhouse Gas Mitigation Program is trying to reduce greenhouse gas emissions from agriculture by better soil, nutrient, and livestock management practices.

The environmental damage caused by raising livestock is the result not only of how the animals are raised but also of the large number of animals produced. People are currently tending to reduce their consumption of animal products so that the overall demand for meat is considerably lessened. In addition to the environmental benefits, eating less meat may also reduce our risk for chronic diseases, such as heart disease and some cancers.

Health Benefits

Still others practise vegetarianism because of its health benefits. Research over several years has consistently shown that a varied and balanced vegetarian diet can reduce the risk of many chronic diseases. Health benefits include (Messina and Messina 1996)

- Reduced intake of fat and total energy, which reduces the risk for obesity. This may in turn lower a person's risk of type 2 diabetes.

- Lower blood pressure, which may be due to a higher intake of fruits and vegetables. People who eat vegetarian diets tend to be non-smokers, to drink little or no alcohol, and to exercise more regularly, which are also factors known to reduce blood pressure and help maintain a healthy body weight.

- Reduced risk of heart disease, which may be due to lower saturated fat intake and a higher consumption of *antioxidants* that are found in plant-based foods. Antioxidants, discussed in detail in Chapter 8, are substances that can protect our cells from damage. They are abundant in fruits and vegetables.

- Fewer digestive problems, such as constipation and diverticular disease, most likely due to the higher fibre content of vegetarian diets. Diverticular disease or diverticulosis, discussed in Chapter 4, occurs when the wall of the colon (large intestine) develops small pockets on the outside that can trap fecal material and become inflamed.

- Reduced risk of some cancers. Research shows that vegetarians may have lower rates of cancer, particularly colon cancer (Phillips and Snowdon 1983). Many components of a vegetarian diet could contribute to reducing cancer risks, including higher fibre and antioxidant intakes, lower dietary fat intake, lower consumption of **carcinogens** (cancer-causing agents) that are formed when cooking meat, and higher consumption of soy protein, which may have anticancer properties (Messina 1999).

- Reduced risk of kidney disease, kidney stones, and gallstones. The lower protein contents of vegetarian diets, plus the higher intake of legumes and vegetable proteins, such as soy, may be protective against these conditions.

carcinogens Cancer-causing agents, such as certain pesticides, industrial chemicals, and pollutants.

What Are the Challenges of a Vegetarian Diet?

Although a vegetarian diet can be healthful, it also presents many challenges. By limiting consumption of flesh and dairy products, there is the potential for inadequate intakes of certain nutrients. Table 6.7 lists the nutrients that can be deficient in a vegan-type diet plan and describes good non-animal sources that can provide these nutrients.

Vegetarians who consume dairy or egg products obtain these nutrients more easily. However, it is important for vegetarians and non-vegetarians to consume a varied and adequate diet. Research indicates that a sign of disordered eating in some female athletes is the switch to a vegetarian diet (Benson, Englebert-Fenton, and Eisenman 1996). Instead of eating a healthy variety of non-animal foods, people with disordered eating problems may use vegetarianism as an excuse to restrict many foods from their diets.

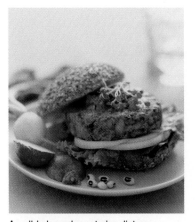

A well-balanced vegetarian diet can provide adequate protein.

Table 6.7   Nutrients of Concern in a Vegan Diet

Nutrient	Functions	Nonmeat/Nondairy Food Sources
Vitamin B_{12}	Assists with DNA synthesis; protection and growth of nerve fibres	Vitamin B_{12} fortified cereals, yeast, and soy products and other meat analogues; vitamin B_{12} supplements
Vitamin D	Promotes bone growth	Vitamin D fortified cereals, margarines, and soy products; adequate exposure to sunlight; supplementation may be necessary for those who do not get adequate exposure to sunlight
Riboflavin (vitamin B_2)	Promotes release of energy; supports normal vision and skin health	Whole and enriched grains, green leafy vegetables, mushrooms, beans, nuts, and seeds
Iron	Assists with oxygen transport; involved in making amino acids and hormones	Whole-grain products, prune juice, dried fruits, beans, nuts, seeds, and leafy vegetables such as spinach
Calcium	Maintains bone health; assists with muscle contraction, blood pressure, and nerve transmission	Fortified soy milk and tofu, almonds, dry beans, leafy vegetables, calcium-fortified juices, and fortified breakfast cereals
Zinc	Assists with DNA and RNA synthesis, immune function, and growth	Whole-grain products, wheat germ, beans, nuts, and seeds

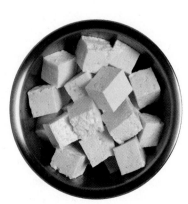

Beans, nuts, seeds, eggs, or meat substitutes are good sources of protein for vegetarians.

Can a vegetarian diet provide enough protein? Since high-quality protein sources are quite easy to obtain in developed countries, a well-balanced vegetarian diet can provide adequate protein. In fact, Dietitians of Canada (2003) endorses an appropriately planned vegetarian diet as healthful, nutritionally adequate, and providing many benefits in reducing and preventing various diseases. As you can see, the emphasis is on a *balanced* and *adequate* vegetarian diet; thus, it is important for vegetarians to consume soy products, eat complementary proteins, and obtain enough energy from other macronutrients to spare protein from being used as an energy source. Although the digestibility of a vegetarian diet is potentially lower than an animal-based diet, there is no separate protein recommendation for vegetarians who consume complementary plant proteins (Institute of Medicine 2002, 465–608).

Recap: A balanced vegetarian diet may reduce the risk of obesity, type 2 diabetes, heart disease, digestive problems, some cancers, kidney disease, kidney stones, and gallstones. Although varied vegetarian diets can provide enough protein, vitamins, and minerals, vegans who consume no animal products do need to supplement their diet with good sources of vitamin B_{12}, vitamin D, riboflavin, iron, calcium, and zinc.

What Disorders Are Related to Protein Intake or Metabolism?

As we have seen, consuming inadequate protein can result in severe illness and death. Typically, this occurs when people do not consume enough total energy.

Protein-Energy Malnutrition Can Lead to Debility and Death

protein-energy malnutrition A disorder caused by inadequate consumption of protein energy and other nutrients. It is characterized by severe wasting.

When a person consumes too little protein and energy, the result is **protein-energy malnutrition (PEM)**—the most serious nutrition problem in the world today, particularly when it is combined with infectious and parasitic diseases that cause diarrhea. Diarrhea causes food to pass through the GI tract quickly, which means that nutrients may not be absorbed, and parasites cause chronic internal blood loss. Infections, such as gastroenteritis and measles, common in children, can also cause poor appetite (WHO 2000). The World Bank (2005) estimates that approximately one third of children in developing countries have their growth stunted or are underweight because of a lack of protein and energy. Further complicating matters, mineral and vitamin deficiencies, such as iron deficiency anemia and vitamin A deficiency (discussed in Chapters 8 and 10), and severe, life-threatening electrolyte imbalances (Chapter 7) often accompany protein-energy malnutrition.

As you learned earlier, if we don't consume adequate protein, our immune system is weakened and we become more susceptible to infections and diseases. This is especially true in the case of AIDS, in which a weakened immune system makes adults more susceptible to the virus that causes the disease to develop (World Bank 2005). In addition, malnutrition is thought to reduce the effectiveness of antiretroviral drugs used to treat AIDS.

Research suggests that the most severe effects of malnutrition occur in the growing unborn child and during the first two years of life (World Bank 2005). At these times of rapid brain growth, malnutrition can lead to lower intelligence in children—and this is irreversible. It creates a cycle of poverty and malnutrition: a population has a less productive work force, the economy remains poor, and poverty and malnutrition continue (World Bank 2005). Two conditions historically associated with PEM are marasmus and kwashiorkor.

Marasmus: Wasting and Stunting

Marasmus is PEM that results from grossly inadequate intakes of protein, energy, and other nutrients. Essentially, people with marasmus slowly starve to death. It is most common in infants and toddlers (6 to 16 months of age) who are living in impoverished conditions. These children are fed diluted cereal drinks that are inadequate in energy, protein, and most nutrients. People suffering from marasmus have the look of "skin and bones," as their body fat and tissues are wasting. Those with marasmus often have loose skin hanging down around the buttocks, usually referred

marasmus A form of protein-energy malnutrition that results from grossly inadequate intakes of protein, energy, and other nutrients.

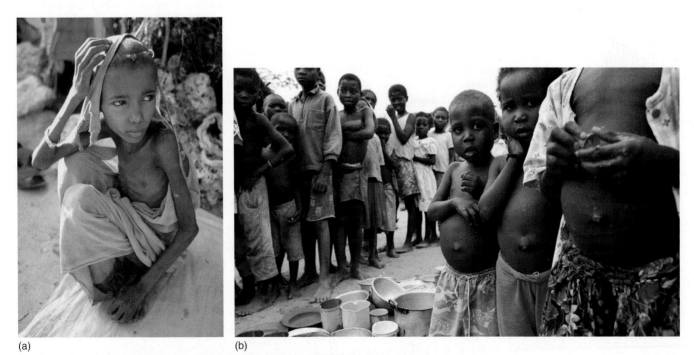

(a)   (b)

Two forms of protein-energy malnutrition are (a) marasmus and (b) kwashiorkor.

to as "baggy pants" (WHO 2000). Marasmus is also known as the "dry" form of PEM because of the thin, desiccated appearance of its victims (Merck Manuals 2005). Consequences of marasmus include

- wasting and weakening of muscles, including the heart muscle;
- stunted brain development and learning impairment;
- depressed metabolism and little insulation from body fat, causing a dangerously low body temperature;
- stunted physical growth and development;
- deterioration of the intestinal lining, which further inhibits absorption of nutrients;
- iron deficiency anemia (abnormally low levels of hemoglobin in the blood);
- severely weakened immune system;
- fluid and electrolyte imbalances.

If marasmus is left untreated, death from dehydration, heart failure, or infection will result. Handling marasmus involves carefully correcting fluid and electrolyte imbalances through IV treatment. Hypokalemia, hypocalcemia, hypophosphatemia, and hypomagnesemia (low blood levels of potassium, calcium, phosphate, and magnesium, respectively) are the common types of electrolyte imbalances (Merck Manuals 2005). Protein and carbohydrates are given once the body's condition has stabilized. Fat is introduced much later, as the protein levels in the blood must improve to the point where they can carry fat so it can be safely metabolized by the body.

Kwashiorkor: PEM plus Infection

kwashiorkor A form of protein-energy malnutrition that is typically seen in developing countries in infants and toddlers who are weaned early because of the birth of a subsequent child. Denied breast milk, they are fed a cereal diet that provides adequate energy but inadequate protein.

Kwashiorkor often occurs in developing countries where infants are weaned early due to the arrival of a subsequent baby. In fact, the word *kwashiorkor* loosely translates into "displaced child" or "first child–second child." This PEM is typically seen in young children (1 to 3 years of age) who no longer drink breast milk. Instead, they often are fed a low-protein, starchy cereal. Unlike marasmus, kwashiorkor often develops quickly in combination with an infection and causes the person to look swollen, particularly in the belly. This can further exacerbate the problem, as caregivers can misinterpret this symptom as a sign that the child is well-fed and full. Further, the children don't seem hungry, and it can be difficult to persuade them to eat (WHO 2000). The swelling in the belly, known as edema, is due to the low protein content of the blood being inadequate to keep fluids from seeping into tissue spaces and electrolyte imbalances. Part of the swelling may also be the result of an enlarged, fatty liver. As you will recall from Chapter 5, when fat is absorbed it travels to the liver where it is packaged with protein as lipoproteins for transport in the blood to all parts of the body. Without protein to manufacture lipoproteins, the fat isn't transported out of the liver and begins to accumulate there, resulting in a fatty liver. Because of this fluid swelling, kwashiorkor is also known as the "wet" form of PEM. Other symptoms of kwashiorkor include

- some weight loss and muscle wasting, with some retention of body fat;
- retarded growth and development but less severe than that seen with marasmus;
- edema, which results in extreme distension of the belly and is caused by fluid and electrolyte imbalances;
- fatty degeneration of the liver;
- loss of appetite, sadness, irritability, apathy;
- development of sores and other skin problems; skin pigmentation changes;
- dry, brittle hair that changes colour, straightens, and falls out easily.

Kwashiorkor can be reversed if adequate protein and energy are given in time and underlying infections are effectively treated. Because of their severely weakened immune systems, many individuals with kwashiorkor die from diseases they contract in their weakened state. Of those who are treated, many return home to the same impoverished conditions, only to develop this deficiency once again.

Marasmic Kwashiorkor Results in Both Wasting and Edema

In many cases, a malnourished person will be suffering from both the wasting aspect of marasmus and the swollen belly characteristic of kwashiorkor. The symptoms of this condition will be a combination of marasmus and kwashiorkor, though children with marasmic kwashiorkor have slightly more body fat than those suffering from marasmus alone (Merck Manuals 2005).

Many people think that only children in developing countries suffer from these diseases. PEM occurs in all countries, however, and affects both children and adults. Adults will have muscle wasting, weakness, and edema, and will show signs of mental changes. In Canada, poor people living in inner cities and isolated rural areas are most affected. Others at risk include older adults, the homeless, people with eating disorders, those addicted to alcohol and drugs, and individuals with wasting diseases, such as AIDS and cancer. In 2002, 164 people in Canada died from an unspecified form of PEM (Statistics Canada 2002). Malnutrition can and does occur here, despite the country producing more than enough food.

Disorders Related to Genetic Abnormalities

Numerous disorders are caused by defects in our DNA, or genetic material. A few of these disorders include phenylketonuria (discussed on p. 196), sickle cell anemia, and cystic fibrosis.

Sickle cell anemia is an inherited disorder of the red blood cells in which a single amino acid present in hemoglobin is changed. As shown in Figure 6.5 (page 199), normal

sickle cell anemia A genetic disorder that causes red blood cells to be sickle or crescent shaped. These cells cannot travel smoothly through blood vessels, causing cell breakage and anemia.

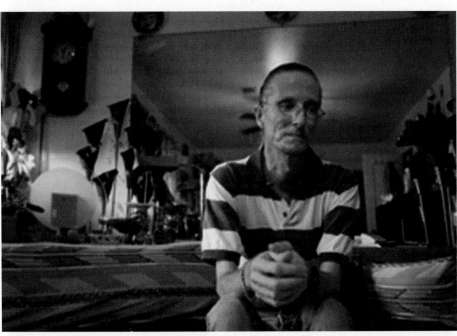

Protein-energy malnutrition occurs in several populations in Canada, including those with such wasting diseases as AIDS and cancer.

cystic fibrosis A genetic disorder that causes an alteration in chloride transport, leading to the production of thick, sticky mucus that causes life-threatening respiratory and digestive problems.

hemoglobin is globular in shape, which results in red blood cells having a round, doughnut-like shape. The genetic alteration that occurs with sickle cell anemia causes the red blood cells to be shaped like a sickle, or a crescent. Sickled red blood cells are hard and sticky and so cannot flow smoothly through small blood vessels. These cells get clogged in the vessels and break apart, damaging the cells and causing anemia. This disease occurs in any person who inherits the sickle cell gene from both parents.

Cystic fibrosis is an inherited disease that primarily affects the respiratory system and digestive tract. Cystic fibrosis is caused by an abnormal protein that prevents the normal passage of chloride into and out of certain cells. This alteration in chloride transport causes cells to secrete thick, sticky mucus. The linings of the lungs and pancreas are particularly affected, causing breathing difficulties, lung infections, and digestion problems that lead to nutrient deficiencies. Symptoms include wheezing, coughing, and stunted growth. The severity of this disease varies greatly among those who suffer from it; some individuals with cystic fibrosis live relatively normal lives, while others are seriously debilitated and die in childhood.

Recap: Protein-energy malnutrition (PEM) with wasting and stunting is known as marasmus. PEM with infections is known as kwashiorkor. These diseases primarily affect impoverished children in developing nations. However, residents of developed countries are also at risk, especially older adults, the homeless, people with eating disorders, alcoholics, drug addicts, and people with AIDS, cancer, and other wasting diseases. Genetic disorders that cause protein abnormalities include phenylketonuria, sickle cell anemia, and cystic fibrosis.

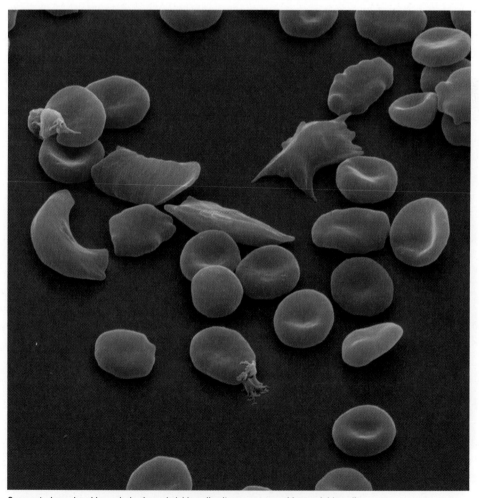

Crescent-shaped and irregularly shaped sickle cells sit among normal hemoglobin cells.

► **HIGHLIGHT**

Global Nutrition: Malnutrition in Developing Countries

More than half (or 54%) of all deaths in children younger than 5 years of age in developing nations are due to malnutrition (Wegman 2001). Seventy percent of all childhood deaths in developing countries result from malnutrition, pneumonia, diarrhea, measles, or malaria. It is important to emphasize that malnutrition interacts with these other illnesses and diseases, leading to much higher death rates. Millions of people in developing countries suffer from chronic malnutrition. Factors contributing to global malnutrition include the following:

1. Famine, resulting from drought, flood, pests, war, and political sanctions that limit the importation of adequate food.
2. Population growth that has outpaced food production.
3. Deforestation, which has led to erosion and the devastation of critical water supplies.
4. Air pollution that has damaged crops, reduced food production, and poisoned water supplies.
5. Climatic changes, particularly global warming trends, have been suggested to cause heat waves and lower rainfall. Both of these changes can reduce soil moisture, impair pollination of certain crops, slow crop growth, and weaken disease resistance of crops.
6. Decreases in water supply, which reduce crop yield.
7. Unmitigated deterioration of land and water resources will eventually limit the number of animals that can be supported as potential food sources. Overgrazing and poor land management lead to rangeland deterioration, and pollution and overfishing have significantly reduced the availability of many fish, including various species of shark, sturgeon, halibut, and grouper (Musick et al. 2000).

These events eventually affect all people of the world, including those in wealthier countries. It is very important to consider global malnutrition as a crisis that affects us all. The causes of global malnutrition are diverse and complex, and it will take the efforts of all nations and people working together to prevent it.

CHAPTER SUMMARY

- Proteins are large, complex molecules that are critical components of all tissues, including blood, bone, and hormones.

- Unlike carbohydrates and fat, the structure of proteins is dictated by DNA and proteins contain nitrogen.

- Amino acids are the building blocks of proteins; they comprise an amine group, an acid group, a hydrogen atom, and a unique side chain.

- There are 20 amino acids in our bodies: 9 are essential amino acids, meaning that our bodies cannot produce them and we must obtain them from food; 11 are non-essential, meaning our bodies can make them so they do not need to be consumed in the diet.

- Our genetic makeup determines the sequence of amino acids in our proteins. Gene expression refers to using a gene in a cell to make a protein.

- The three-dimensional shape of proteins determines their function in the body.

- When proteins are exposed to damaging substances, such as heat, acids, bases, and alcohol, they are denatured, meaning they lose their shape and function.

- A limiting amino acid is one that is missing or in limited supply, preventing the adequate synthesis of proteins.

- Mutual supplementation is the process of combining two incomplete protein sources to make a complete protein. The two foods involved in this process are called complementary proteins.

- Most digestion of protein occurs in the small intestine.

- Protein digestibility affects its quality, with proteins that are more digestible being of higher quality. Animal sources, soy protein, and legumes are highly digestible forms of protein.

- Proteins are needed to promote cell growth, repair, and maintenance. They act as enzymes and hormones; help maintain the balance of fluids, electrolytes, acids, and bases; and support healthy immune function.

►

CHAPTER SUMMARY

- The RDA for protein for sedentary people is 0.8 grams of protein per kilogram of body weight per day; the AMDR for protein is 10%–35% of total energy intake.

- Most people in Canada have average protein intakes that fall within the AMDR.

- High protein intakes from animal sources high in saturated fat may be harmful and can lead to increased blood cholesterol levels, increased calcium excretion, and increased risk for kidney disease in people who are susceptible to kidney problems.

- Good sources of protein include meat, poultry, fish, dairy products, eggs, legumes, whole grains, and nuts.

- There are many forms of vegetarianism: lacto-ovo-vegetarians eat plant foods plus eggs and dairy products; vegans are considered strict vegetarians and consume only plant foods.

- Consuming a well-planned vegetarian diet may reduce the risk of obesity, heart disease, type 2 diabetes, and some forms of cancer.

- Vegans may need to supplement their diet with vitamins B_{12} and D, riboflavin, iron, calcium, and zinc.

- Marasmus and kwashiorkor are two forms of protein-energy malnutrition that result from grossly inadequate energy and protein intake.

- Phenylketonuria is a genetic disease in which the person cannot break down the amino acid phenylalanine. The buildup of phenylalanine and its byproducts leads to brain damage.

- Sickle cell anemia is a genetic disorder of the red blood cells. Because of an alteration of one amino acid in hemoglobin, the red blood cells become sickle shaped and cannot travel smoothly through blood vessels, thereby causing cell breakage and subsequent anemia.

- Cystic fibrosis is a genetic disease that causes an alteration in chloride transport that leads to the production of thick, sticky mucus. This mucus causes serious respiratory and digestive problems, which lead to variable levels of debilitation and, in some cases, premature death.

mynutritionlab Go to MyNutritionLab at www.pearsoned.ca/mynutritionlab and enrich your understanding of nutrition! You'll find key animations, interactive exercises, access to My DietAnalysis, and much more.

REVIEW QUESTIONS

Quizzes

1. The process of combining peanut butter and whole wheat bread to make a complete protein is called
   a. deamination.
   b. vegetarianism.
   c. transamination.
   d. mutual supplementation.

2. Which of the following meals is an example of a vegan diet?
   a. Rice, pinto beans, acorn squash, soy butter, and almond milk
   b. Veggie dog, bun, and a banana blended with yogurt
   c. Brown rice and green tea
   d. Egg salad on whole wheat toast, broccoli, carrot sticks, and soy milk

3. The substance that breaks down polypeptides in the small intestine is called
   a. hydrochloric acid.
   b. pepsin.
   c. protease.
   d. ketones.

4. The portion of an amino acid that contains nitrogen is called the
   a. side chain.
   b. amine group.
   c. acid group.
   d. nitrate cluster.

5. Proteins contain
   a. carbon, oxygen, and nitrogen.
   b. oxygen and hydrogen.
   c. carbon, oxygen, hydrogen, and nitrogen.
   d. carbon, oxygen, and hydrogen.

6. Which of the following is *not* characteristic of marasmus?
   a. Wasted and weakened muscles
   b. Stunted physical growth
   c. Edema
   d. Low body temperature

7. Which one of the following statements about proteins in *not* correct?
   a. When denatured, function is lost.
   b. Amino acids are the building blocks of proteins.
   c. Most enzymatic digestion occurs in the mouth.
   d. Proteins act as enzymes and hormones.

8. Choose the correct statement about amino acids.
   a. There are 11 essential and 9 non-essential amino acids.
   b. A non-essential amino acid can never become an essential amino acid.
   c. An oligopeptide refers to a string of ten or more amino acids.
   d. Amino acid bonding and attraction determine protein shape.

9. Derek, a moderately active male weighing 70 kg, consumes about 61 grams of protein per day. How many grams of protein per kilogram of body weight is Derek consuming?
   a. 1.37
   b. 1.15
   c. 0.87
   d. 0.80

10. Explain the relationship between inadequate protein intake and the swollen bellies of children with kwashiorkor.

11. Explain the relationship between excessive protein intake and an increased risk for kidney disease.

12. Identify six ways in which proteins are indispensable to human functioning.

13. Create a healthful one-day diet plan for an active 20-year-old lacto-ovo-vegetarian.

14. Draw a sketch showing how amino acids bond to form proteins.

15. You're over at your friend Stuart's house for dinner. You notice that his mother is looking better than ever—she seems so lean and fit! You ask him what she's been doing lately, and he tells you that she has been on a high-protein diet for the past two months. When you sit down at the dinner table, there are no breads or potatoes to go with the steak. Instead of vegetables, there are scrambled eggs, dripping with butter. For dessert, there's ice cream piled with nuts. Stuart's mother comments on how she never feels hungry anymore. You think about all the pasta and bread you eat, and realize that you're often hungry between meals. Could it be that carbohydrates really are the enemy?

    For many years, using high-protein diets for weight loss has been a major controversy. Popular diets, such as the Atkins Diet, the Zone Diet, and the Sugar Busters, plan support the use of high-protein—or low-carbohydrate—meals to lose weight. After reading the Nutrition Debate at the end of this chapter, what do you think of this kind of diet? Do you think Stuart's mother is safe using this diet? Would your opinion change if you found out she has high LDL cholesterol and a family history of heart disease? What advice might you give Stuart's mother about adapting her diet?

16. Haley is the star of your school's basketball team. She is muscular and fit and always seems to have endless energy. You learn that she is a passionate vegan and never consumes any meat or dairy products. Your friend Rabyah, another avid athlete, refuses to believe that Haley doesn't eat meat. Rabyah says she always craves meat after a hard workout and argues that animal protein is what fuels muscles.

    Is meat truly essential in an athlete's diet? Are the claims Rabyah makes about the role of meat really valid? Given what you know about the nature of plant and animal proteins, how would you explain to Rabyah that a vegetarian or vegan diet can be healthy?

CASE STUDY

Stephanie, a 22-year-old college student studying nutrition, has recently become very interested in vegetarianism. Learning the various health benefits has sparked her interest. However, Stephanie is concerned she will not be able to consume adequate amounts of certain nutrients. Stephanie is an endurance female athlete weighing 59 kg (130 pounds). Completing the following questions will let you help Stephanie to see that when a vegetarian diet is planned appropriately, it can be healthful and nutritionally adequate.

a. Over the years, research has consistently shown benefits to adopting a vegetarian diet. List three benefits you feel would be important for Stephanie to know.

b. A primary concern of the vegetarian diet is inadequate protein intake since the most complete protein sources are from animal sources.

   Explain mutual supplementation and its importance to Stephanie regarding initiation of a vegetarian diet. Include discussion of incomplete and complete proteins in your answer.

There are various types of vegetarian diets. Which ones include some foods from animal sources?

What is the only complete source of vegetable protein? What other foods are good sources of protein?

c. Stephanie is unsure of how much protein she actually requires in her diet. Refer to the Recommended Dietary Allowance (RDA) for protein to calculate how much protein Stephanie should be consuming per day.

Assume that Stephanie has not yet begun a vegetarian diet.

Now assume that Stephanie has begun a vegetarian diet.

Why do active individuals generally require a diet higher in protein than sedentary individuals?

WEB LINKS

www.nal.usda.gov/fnic/pubs/bibs/gen/vegetarian.pdf
Food and Nutrition Information Center: Vegetarian Nutrition Resource List
This is an up-to-date list of reliable websites, magazines, newsletters, and books that vegetarian consumers will find useful and interesting. Topics include vegetarianism through the lifecycle and vegetarianism for athletes.

www.cattle.ca/cca%20home.htm
Canadian Cattlemen's Association
Visit this site to learn more about the industry's involvement in the Green House Gas Mitigation Program, mad cow disease, and other issues.

www.oxfam.ca
Oxfam Canada
Oxfam Canada is a non-profit international development organization formed in 1963 to support community programs in food security, health, nutrition, and democratic development, with an emphasis on working with women. Visit this site to see their work in developing countries.

www.worldbank.org/nutrition
World Bank
Visit this site to learn about programs developed by the World Bank to alleviate hunger and low birth weights in the developing world. Check out the Nutrition Toolkit they use for these programs.

www.eatright.org
American Dietetic Association
Search for vegetarian diets to learn how to plan healthful meat-free meals.

www.aphis.usda.gov
Animal and Plant Health Inspection Service
Select Hot Issues or search for "Bovine Spongiform Encephalopathy (BSE)" to learn more about mad cow disease.

www.vrg.org
The Vegetarian Resource Group
Obtain vegetarian and vegan news, recipes, information, and additional links.

www.cdc.gov
Centers for Disease Control and Prevention
Click on Health Topics A-Z to learn more about *E. coli*.

www.who.int/nutrition/en
World Health Organization Nutrition Site
Visit this site to find out more about the worldwide magnitude of protein-energy malnutrition and the diseases that can result from inadequate intakes of protein, energy-yielding carbohydrates and fats, and various additional nutrients.

www.nlm.nih.gov/medlineplus
MEDLINE Plus Health Information
Search for "sickle cell anemia" and "cystic fibrosis" to obtain additional resources and the latest news about these inherited diseases.

Test Yourself Answers

1. **False** Although protein can be used for energy in certain circumstances, fats and carbohydrates are the primary sources of energy for our bodies.

2. **False** There is no evidence that consuming amino acid supplements assists in building muscle tissue. Exercising muscles, specifically using weight training, is the stimulus needed to build muscle tissue.

3. **True** The larger a person's body, the more protein that individual needs to maintain normal function.

4. **False** Vegetarian diets can meet and even exceed an individual's protein needs, assuming that adequate energy-yielding macronutrients, a variety of protein sources, and complementary protein sources are consumed.

5. **True** Most people in Canada have protein intakes that provide 10%–35% of their total energy intake.

High-Protein Diets—Are They the Key to Weight Loss?

High-protein diets have been popular over the last 40 years. Very low-energy, high-protein programs (200 to 400 kcal or 840 to 1680 kJ per day, 1.5 grams of protein per kilogram body weight) were highly popular in the 1970s. Many of these diets consisted of low-quality protein, however, and at least 58 people died from heart problems while following them. As a result of these deaths, we now know that these extreme diets are only appropriate for severely obese people and must include high-quality protein sources. Supervision by a qualified physician is critical when following this type of diet plan.

Proponents of high-protein diets claim that you can eat your favourite foods and still lose weight. Is this possible? Chapter 11 provides a detailed explanation of weight loss. The key to weight loss is eating less energy than you expend. If you eat more energy than you expend, you can gain weight. Thus, any type of diet, even high-protein diets, must contain fewer calories than a person expends to result in weight loss.

It is important to recognize that high-protein diets are synonymous with low-carbohydrate diets, since high-protein foods typically replace those high in carbohydrates. In addition, many high-protein diets are also high in fat. It is well established that reducing carbohydrate intake causes the body to break down its stored carbohydrate (or glycogen) in the liver and muscle; this is necessary to maintain blood glucose levels and provide energy to the brain. As water is stored along with glycogen, using stored carbohydrate for energy results in the loss of water from the body, which registers on the scale as rapid weight loss. In addition, the deamination of excess protein results in an increased production of urea, and urea is a diuretic.

There are many supporters of high-protein diets, particularly people supporting the Atkins Diet. A highly controversial article in support of the Atkins Diet was published in the *New York Times Magazine* (Taubes 2002). In this article, the Atkins Diet is touted as the most effective program for weight loss. Supporters of this diet emphasize that eating a high-carbohydrate diet (including potatoes, white bread, pasta, and refined sugars) has caused obesity. Supporters emphasize that not only does the Atkins Diet result in substantial weight loss, but it does not cause unhealthy changes in blood cholesterol despite its high saturated fat content.

In 2005, a dietitian with the Dr. Robert C. Atkins Foundation wrote an article entitled "Low-Carbohydrate Diets, Pro: Time to Rethink Our Current Strategies" (Bloch 2005). She argues that, given the $75 billion a year spent in the United States on obesity-related illnesses, such as diabetes, insulin resistance, hypertension, high blood lipids, and arthritis, physicians should be open to trying other means of helping people achieve healthy weights when traditional low-Calorie, low-fat diet approaches have failed. She states, "The controlled-carbohydrate regimen could be a viable alternative dietary approach for weight management used by clinicians managing patients who are failing with conventional approaches" (p. 3).

In the same journal, Robert F. Kushner wrote a counterbalancing article entitled "Low-Carbohydrate Diets, Con: The Mythical Phoenix or Credible Science?" in which he systematically debunks the six most common claims made by fans of very low-carbohydrate diets (Kushner 2005):

1. Calories don't count. Not so, according to Dr. Kushner, who maintains that many meticulous metabolic experiments have shown that the law of conservation of energy (energy balance = energy intake equivalent to energy expenditure) holds true.

2. Obesity is caused by the composition of the diet. At present, no studies definitively prove that equal-Calorie diets with different proportions of fat and carbohydrates result in different amounts of weight lost over the longer term.

3. Carbohydrate (meaning refined sugar) is the metabolic "poison." On the contrary, we know that some carbohydrates—dietary fibre and low glycemic index foods—are beneficial in slowing down the rate at which glucose enters the bloodstream after a meal. They also prevent some dietary cholesterol from being absorbed in the intestine.

4. Excess carbohydrate is converted to fat. This is true; however, excess dietary fat and protein can also be converted to fatty acids and sent to adipose tissue for storage. The basic rule still holds: if energy intake exceeds energy needs and energy expenditure, you gain weight!

5. Carbohydrate (meaning simple carbohydrates, or sugar) leads to insulin resistance. While the causes of insulin resistance are not well understood, scientists believe that high-fat diets contribute to the development of insulin resistance and diets high

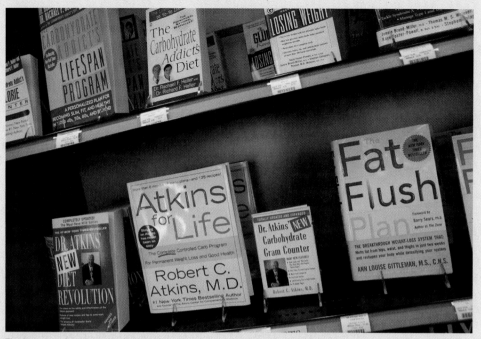

The long-term health implications of high-protein diets are unknown at this time.

in complex-carbohydrates and fibre may improve insulin sensitivity.

6.   Carbohydrate-restricted diets are effective and safe. To date, there have been no long-term studies of these diets, so we don't know if they are effective and safe.

What Is the Scientific Evidence?

What do the findings from recent scientific studies tell us? In a study published in the prestigious *New England Journal of Medicine* in 2008, researchers randomly assigned 322 moderately obese people, including people with type 2 diabetes and heart disease, to one of three diets: low fat, restricted energy; Mediterranean, restricted energy; or low carbohydrate, non-restricted energy (Shai et al. 2008). More than 95% of the participants were still following their diet at 1 year, and 84.6% continued to follow their diet for 2 years. This is the longest dietary trial of this type to date, and the participants were monitored closely for ketones in their urine, changes in blood glucose and insulin levels, and changes in their blood lipid profiles.

Participants lost their greatest amounts of weight in the first six months, and then all groups regained some weight and weight stabilized by about 12 months. Among the 272 participants who finished the trial, the average amount of weight loss was 3.3 kg for the low-fat group, 4.6 kg for the Mediterranean Diet group, and 5.5 kg for the low-carbohydrate group. Levels of HDL-cholesterol continued to improve over the 2-year period in all groups, but the most favourable levels were seen in the group following the low-carbohydrate diet. The group following the Mediterranean Diet had the

highest intakes of monounsaturated fats, and this may explain the favourable changes seen in insulin and glucose levels among these participants. The authors concluded that "Mediterranean and low-carbohydrate diets may be effective alternatives to low-fat diets. The more favourable effects on lipids (with the low-carbohydrate diet) and on glycemic control (with the Mediterranean Diet) suggest that personal preferences and metabolic considerations might inform individualized tailoring of dietary interventions" (p. 229).

Similar findings were published by Yancy and colleagues (2004) and Volek et al. (2004). Both studies were carefully done randomized controlled trials. Yancy et al. used participants with unhealthy blood lipid profiles and followed them for six months, while Volek et al. used participants with normal levels of blood lipids and put them on diets lasting just four weeks. In both studies, participants in the low-carbohydrate groups lost more weight, on average, than those on the low-fat diets. Those who had unhealthy blood lipid levels experienced positive changes, and those who had normal blood lipids experienced beneficial changes to their insulin levels and insulin resistance when following the low-carbohydrate diets.

The findings from these three careful studies were a surprise to many health professionals, who had been arguing that the high-fat content of low-carbohydrate diets might increase the risk of heart disease for some people. Instead, the evidence suggested that people with insulin resistance, diabetes, and unhealthy levels of blood lipids might benefit, at least in the short term. We don't know, though, whether these findings were simply because people lost weight or whether the composition of the diet was the key factor.

Are There Any Risks?

No studies to date have looked at the possible drawbacks of consuming large amounts of protein among people who have various forms of kidney disease or kidney problems as a result of diabetes. Large amounts of protein can place a stress on already vulnerable kidneys, and might lead to kidney stones in some people. Although these diets may result in short-term weight loss and improved insulin sensitivity, this needs to be weighed against the possible negative effects on kidney function.

Another consideration is the low amounts of dietary fibre in low-carbohydrate diets. Studies have shown that people with high blood cholesterol or high blood glucose levels benefit when they follow high-fibre diets. Dietary fibre is important for a healthy gastrointestinal tract, slows down the absorption of glucose into the bloodstream, and may help the body get rid of some cholesterol in the stools.

Although studies using moderately overweight and obese participants have not shown any worrisome side effects of low-carbohydrate diets on blood lipids, there still is concern about the long-term effects of consuming diets that are high in animal products, and therefore also high in saturated fats, on heart health. If it is true that the body is burning saturated fat for energy while people are following low-carbohydrate diets, does this continue over the longer term? If so, are there any adverse effects?

The Bottom Line

Although it may sound trite, the bottom line is that much more research is needed with different types of populations and for longer periods before scientists can determine whether low-carbohydrate, high-protein, and high-fat diets are effective in helping people lose weight and keep it off and are safe for people who may be at risk for heart disease and diabetes. Shai and colleagues (2008) had few women in their trial and noted that women tended to do better on the Mediterranean Diet in their study (p. 238). They called for more research exploring possible sex differences in weight loss, particularly leptin levels.

The results to date suggest that people with type 2 diabetes or insulin resistance may benefit from following a low-carbohydrate diet or a Mediterranean Diet for short periods. For these people, losing even small amounts of weight can sometimes greatly improve their control over blood insulin levels. Anyone with diabetes needs to consult with a physician or dietitian before trying these diets, though, to make sure that his or her diabetes medications or insulin are properly adjusted for the amount of carbohydrate in the diet. Carefully planning a diet so the amount of saturated fat is as low as possible is also advisable.

Should you adopt a high-protein diet? Each of us must decide on the type of diet to consume based on our own needs, preferences, health risks, and lifestyle. Based on what we currently know, the healthiest weight loss plans are those that are moderately reduced in energy intake and contain ample fruits, vegetables, and whole grains; adequate carbohydrate and protein; moderate amounts of total fat; and relatively low amounts of saturated fat. It is also important to choose a food plan that you can follow throughout your lifetime. By researching the benefits and risks of various diet plans, you can make an educated decision about the type of diet that will work best to maintain a healthful weight and muscle mass and provide enough energy and nutrients to maintain your lifestyle and your long-term health.

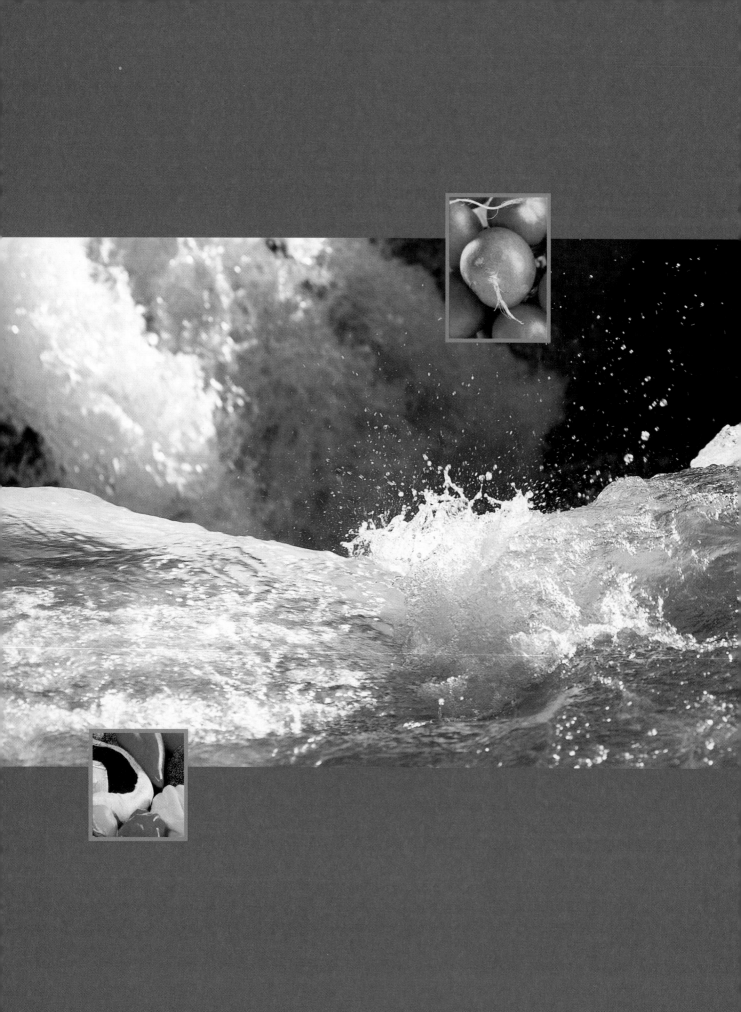

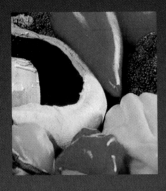

CHAPTER 7

Nutrients Involved in Fluid and Electrolyte Balance

CHAPTER OBJECTIVES

After reading this chapter you will be able to:

1. Identify four nutrients that function as electrolytes in our bodies, pp. 232–233.

2. Discuss three functions of water in our bodies, pp. 233–234.

3. Describe how electrolytes assist in the regulation of fluid balance, pp. 236–239.

4. Discuss the physical changes that occur to trigger our thirst mechanism, p. 237.

5. Describe the avenues of fluid intake and excretion in our bodies, pp. 237–238.

6. Define hyponatremia and identify factors that can cause this condition, p. 246.

7. Identify four symptoms of dehydration, pp. 251–252.

8. Define hypertension and list three ways we can change our lifestyle to reduce hypertension, pp. 253–254.

Test Yourself True or False

1. About 50% to 70% of our body weight is made up of water. **T or F**

2. Most of the sodium consumed by Canadians is added to foods during cooking and at the table. **T or F**

3. Drinking until we are no longer thirsty always ensures that we are properly hydrated. **T or F**

4. Although persistent vomiting is uncomfortable, it does not have any long-term adverse effects on our health. **T or F**

5. Eating a high-sodium diet causes high blood pressure in most individuals. **T or F**

Test Yourself answers can be found at the end of the chapter.

In April of 2002, Cynthia Lucero, a healthy 28-year-old woman who had just completed her doctoral dissertation, was running the Boston Marathon. Although not a professional athlete, Cynthia was running in her second marathon, and, in the words of her coach, she had been "diligent" in her training. While her parents, who had travelled from Ecuador, waited at the finish line, friends in the crowd watched as Cynthia steadily completed kilometre after kilometre, drinking large amounts of fluid as she progressed through the course. They described her as looking strong as she jogged Heartbreak Hill, about ten kilometres (six miles) from the finish. But then she began to falter. One of her friends ran to her side and asked if she was okay. Cynthia replied that she felt dehydrated and rubber-legged, and then she fell to the pavement. She was rushed to nearby Brigham and Women's Hospital, but by the time she got there, she was in an irreversible coma. The official cause of her death was *hyponatremia*, commonly called low blood sodium. Among marathon runners seeking medical treatment after a race, as many as 10% show signs of this condition.

What is hyponatremia, and are you at risk? Even if you don't run marathons, do you or any of your friends play sports, exercise, or work a physically demanding job in hot weather? If so, do you drink sports drinks or just plain water? If at the start of football practice on a hot, humid afternoon, a friend confided to you that he had been on a drinking binge the night before, would you know how to advise him? Should you tell his coach, and why?

In this chapter, we explore the role of fluids and electrolytes in keeping our bodies properly hydrated and maintaining the functions of our nerves and muscles. We also discuss how we maintain blood pressure and take a look at some disorders that occur when our fluids and electrolytes are out of balance.

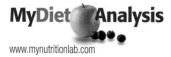

www.mynutritionlab.com

fluid A substance composed of molecules that move past one another freely. Fluids are characterized by their ability to conform to the shape of whatever container holds them.

• Intracellular and Extracellular Fluid

What Are Fluids and Electrolytes, and What Are Their Functions?

Of course you know that orange juice, blood, and shampoo are all fluids, but what makes them so? A **fluid** is characterized by its ability to move freely and changeably, adapting to the shape of the container that holds it. This might not seem very important, but as you'll learn in this chapter, the fluid composition of your cells and tissues is critical to your body's ability to function.

Body Fluid Is the Liquid Portion of Our Cells and Tissues

Between about 50% and 70% of a healthy adult's body weight is fluid. When we cut a finger, we can see some of this fluid dripping out as blood, but that can't account for such a large percentage. So where is all this fluid hiding?

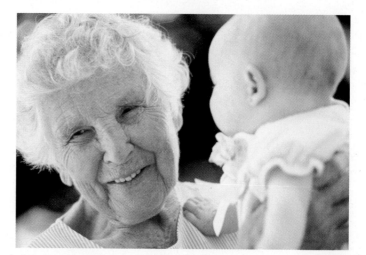

As we age, our body water content decreases: approximately 75% of an infant's body weight is comprised of water, while an elderly adult's is only 50% (or less).

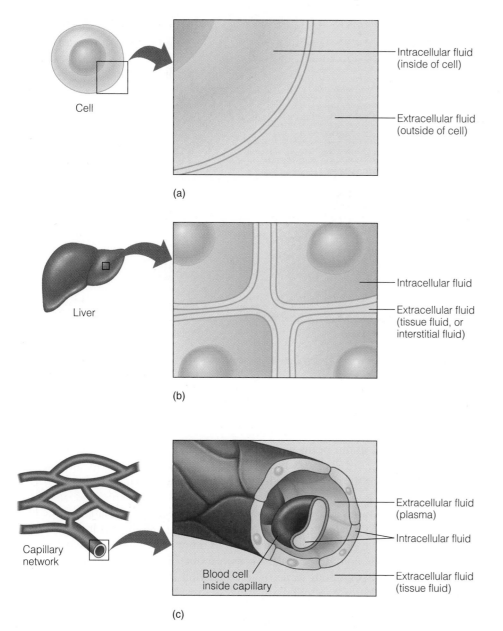

Figure 7.1 Intracellular fluid is contained within the cells that make up our body tissues. Extracellular fluid is external to cells. Tissue fluid is external to tissue cells, and plasma is external to blood cells.

About two thirds of our body fluid is held within the walls of our cells and is therefore called **intracellular fluid** (Figure 7.1a). Every cell in our body contains fluid. When our cells lose their fluid, they quickly shrink and die. Conversely, when cells take in too much fluid, they swell and burst. This is why appropriate fluid balance—which we'll discuss throughout this chapter—is so critical to life.

The remaining third of our body fluid is referred to as **extracellular fluid** because it flows outside our cells (see Figure 7.1a). There are three types of extracellular fluid:

1. *Tissue fluid* (sometimes called *interstitial fluid*) flows between the cells that make up a particular tissue or organ, such as muscle fibres or the liver (Figure 7.1b).

2. *Plasma* is the extracellular fluid that causes your blood to drip. It is the liquid portion of blood, and it carries the red blood cells through our vessels like a river carrying ships to distant regions (Figure 7.1c).

intracellular fluid The fluid held at any given time within the walls of the body's cells.

extracellular fluid The fluid outside the body's cells, either in the body's tissues; as the liquid portion of blood, called plasma; or as digestive juices.

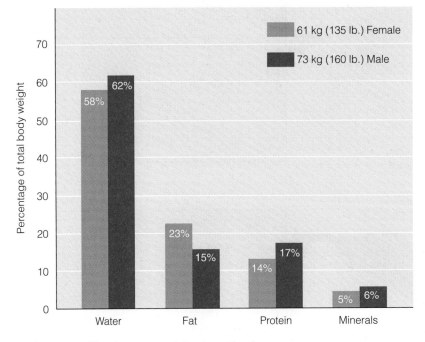

Figure 7.2 Body composition of an average adult male and female.

3. *Digestive juices* secreted by cells in the pancreas, stomach, and small intestine are also extracellular fluids.

Not every tissue in our body contains the same amount of fluid. Lean tissues, such as muscle, are more than 70% fluid, whereas fat tissue is only between 10% and 20% fluid. This is not surprising considering the hydrophobic nature of lipid cells, which we discussed in Chapter 5.

Body fluid also varies according to gender and age. Figure 7.2 compares the body composition of a 73 kg (160 lb.) adult male and a 61 kg (135 lb.) adult female. As you can see, males have more lean tissue and thus more body fluid than females. Our total amount of body fluid decreases as we age. About 75% of an infant's body weight is water, whereas the total body water of an older adult is generally less than 50% of body weight. This decrease in total body water is a result of the loss of lean tissue that occurs as we age.

- Structure of Water
- Interactive Molecule: Water

Body Fluid Is Composed of Water and Dissolved Substances Called Electrolytes

As you know, pure water is made up of molecules consisting of two hydrogen atoms bound to one oxygen atom (H_2O). You might think that such pure water would be ideal, but if our cell and tissue fluids contained only pure water, we would quickly die. Instead, within our body fluids are a variety of dissolved substances (called *solutes*) critical to life. These include four major minerals: sodium, potassium, chloride, and phosphorus. We consume these minerals in compounds called *salts,* especially table salt, which is made of sodium and chloride.

These mineral salts are called **electrolytes**, because when they dissolve in water, the two component minerals separate and form electrically charged particles called **ions**, which are capable of carrying an electrical current. The electrical charge is the spark that stimulates nerves and causes muscles to contract, so electrolytes are critical to body functioning.

If you've ever jump-started a car, you know that electrical charges can be either positive or negative. Of the four major minerals just mentioned, sodium (Na^+) and potassium (K^+) are positively charged, whereas chloride (Cl^-) and phosphorus (in the

electrolyte A substance that disassociates in solution into positively and negatively charged ions and is thus capable of carrying an electrical current.

ion Any electrically charged particle, either positively or negatively charged.

form of hydrogen phosphate, or HPO_4^{2-}) are negatively charged. In the intracellular fluid, potassium and phosphate are the predominant electrolytes. In contrast, in the extracellular fluid, sodium and chloride predominate. There is a slight difference in electrical charge on either side of the cell's membrane, which is needed for the cell to perform its normal functions.

Fluids Serve Many Critical Functions

Animations

• Water Balance

Water not only quenches our thirst but also performs a number of functions that are critical to supporting life.

Fluids Dissolve and Transport Substances

Water is involved in almost all chemical reactions of our bodies. It is an excellent **solvent**, which means it is capable of dissolving (i.e., mixing with and breaking apart) a wide variety of substances. Since blood plasma and the interior of blood cells are mostly water, blood is an excellent vehicle for transporting these dissolved substances, or solutes, throughout our body. All water-soluble substances—such as amino acids, glucose, water-soluble vitamins, minerals, and medications—are readily transported via the bloodstream. In contrast, fats do not dissolve in water. To overcome this chemical incompatibility, fatty substances, such as cholesterol and fat-soluble vitamins, are either attached to or surrounded by water-soluble proteins so they, too, can be transported in the blood to the cells.

solvent A substance that is capable of mixing with and breaking apart a variety of compounds. Water is an excellent solvent.

Fluids Account for Blood Volume

Blood volume is the amount of fluid in blood. As you might expect, appropriate fluid levels are essential to maintaining healthy blood volume. When blood volume rises, blood pressure increases; when blood volume decreases, blood pressure decreases. High blood pressure is an important risk factor for heart disease and stroke, whereas low blood pressure can cause us to feel tired, lethargic, confused, and dizzy, or even to faint. The heart, blood vessels, certain blood proteins, and kidneys work together to regulate blood volume and blood pressure in a fairly complex process that we will not describe here. We discuss high blood pressure (called *hypertension*) in the disorders section at the end of this chapter.

blood volume The amount of fluid in blood.

Fluids Help Maintain Body Temperature

Just as overheating is disastrous to a car engine, so can a high internal temperature cause our bodies to stop functioning. Fluids are vital to our ability to maintain body temperature within a safe range. Two factors account for the ability of fluids to keep us cool. First, water has a relatively high heat capacity. In other words, it takes a lot of external energy to raise its temperature. Since our bodies contain a lot of water, it takes sustained high heat to increase our body temperature. Thus, the water content of our bodies protects us from high environmental temperatures.

Second, body fluids are our primary coolant. When we need to release heat from the body, we increase the flow of blood from our warm body core to the vessels lying just under the skin. This action transports the heat from the core of the body out to the periphery, where it can be released from the skin. When we are hot, the sweat glands secrete more sweat. As this sweat evaporates off the skin's surface, heat is released and the skin and underlying blood are cooled (Figure 7.3). This cooler blood flows back to the body's core and reduces internal body temperature.

Fluids Protect and Lubricate Our Tissues

Water is a major part of the fluids that protect our organs and tissues from injury. The cerebrospinal fluid that surrounds the brain and spinal column protects these vital tissues from damage, and a fetus in a mother's womb is protected by amniotic fluid. Body fluids also act as lubricants. Synovial fluid secreted by membranes

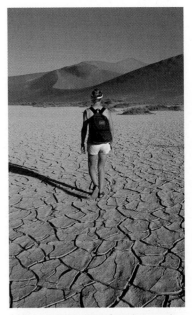

A hiker must consume adequate amounts of water to prevent heat illness in hot and dry environments.

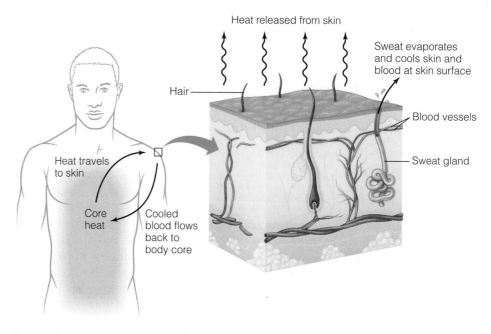

Figure 7.3 Evaporative cooling occurs when heat is transported from the body core through the bloodstream to the surface of the skin. The water evaporates into the air and carries away heat. This cools the blood, which circulates back to the body core, reducing body temperature.

surrounding our joints acts as a lubricant for smooth joint motion, and tears cleanse and lubricate our eyes. Our saliva moistens the food we eat, which helps us to effectively swallow and transport food to the stomach. The fluid-filled mucus lining the walls of our stomach and intestines facilitates the smooth movement of food and nutrients through our digestive tract, and the pleural fluid covering our lungs allows their friction-free expansion and retraction behind our chest wall.

> **Recap:** Our body fluid consists of water plus a variety of dissolved substances, including electrically charged minerals called electrolytes. Water serves many important functions in our bodies, including dissolving and transporting substances, accounting for blood volume, regulating body temperature, and cushioning and lubricating body organs and tissues.

Electrolytes Support Many Body Functions

Now that you know why fluid is so essential to our bodies' functioning, you are ready to explore the critical role of the minerals within it.

Electrolytes Help Regulate Fluid Balance

• Electrolytes in Water Balance

Our cell membranes are *permeable* to water. This means that water flows easily through them. Our cells have no control over this flow of water and thus cannot actively control the overall balance of fluid between the intracellular and extracellular compartments by directly regulating water flow. In contrast, our cell membranes are *not* freely permeable to electrolytes. Sodium, potassium, and the other electrolytes stay where they are, either inside or outside a cell, unless they are actively transported elsewhere by special proteins. So how do electrolytes help our cells maintain their fluid balance? To answer this question, we need to review a bit of chemistry.

Imagine that you have a special filter that has the same properties as our cell membranes; in other words, this filter is freely permeable to water but not permeable to electrolytes. Now imagine that you insert this filter into a glass of pure distilled water to divide the glass into two separate chambers (Figure 7.4a). The levels of water on either side of the filter would, of course, be identical, since it is freely permeable

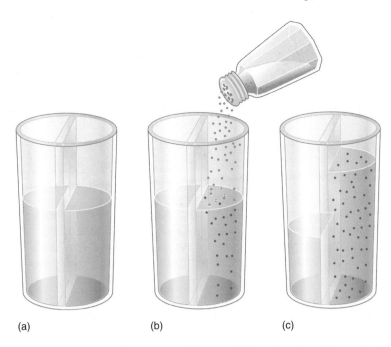

(a)   (b)   (c)

Figure 7.4 Osmosis. (a) A filter that is freely permeable to water is placed in a glass of pure water. (b) Salt is added to only one side of the glass. (c) Drawn by the high concentration of electrolytes, pure water flows to the salt-water side of the filter. This flow of water into the concentrated solution will continue until the concentrations of electrolytes on both sides of the membrane are equal.

to water. Now imagine that you add a teaspoon (5 mL) of salt (which contains the electrolytes sodium and chloride) to the water on one side of the filter only (Figure 7.4b). You would see the water on the "pure water" side of the glass suddenly begin to flow through the filter to the "salt water" side of the glass (Figure 7.4c). Why would this mysterious movement of water occur? The answer is that water always moves from areas where solutes, such as sodium and chloride, are poorly concentrated to areas where they are highly concentrated. To put it another way, electrolytes *draw* water toward areas where they are concentrated. This movement of water toward solutes continues until the concentrations of solutes are equal on both sides of the cell membrane.

Water follows the movement of electrolytes; this action provides a means to control movement of fluid into and out of the cells. Our cells can regulate the balance of fluids between their internal and extracellular environments by using special transport proteins to actively pump electrolytes across their membranes. An example of how transport proteins pump sodium and potassium across the cell membrane was illustrated in Chapter 6 (Figure 6.8). By maintaining the appropriate movement of electrolytes into and out of the cell, the proper balance of fluid and electrolytes is maintained between the intracellular and extracellular compartments (Figure 7.5a). If the concentration of electrolytes is much higher inside the cells than outside them, water will flow into the cells in such large amounts that the cells can burst (Figure 7.5b). Conversely, if the extracellular environment contains too high a concentration of electrolytes, water flows out of the cells, and they can dry up (Figure 7.5c).

Certain illnesses can threaten this delicate balance of fluid inside and outside of the cells. You may have heard of someone being hospitalized because of excessive diarrhea and vomiting. When this happens, the body loses a great deal of fluid from the intestinal tract and extracellular compartment. This heavy fluid loss causes the extracellular electrolyte concentration to become very high. In response, a great deal of intracellular fluid leaves the cells to try to balance this extracellular fluid loss. This imbalance in fluid and electrolytes changes the flow of electrical impulses through the heart, causing an irregular heart rate that can eventually lead to death if left untreated.

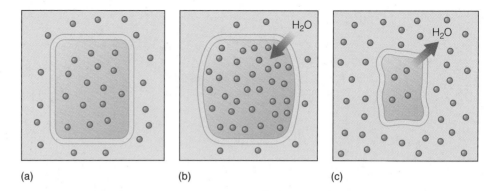

(a)   (b)   (c)

Figure 7.5 The health of our body's cells depends on maintaining the proper balance of fluids and electrolytes on either side of the cell membrane. (a) The concentrations of electrolytes are the same on either side of the cell membrane. (b) The concentration of electrolytes is much greater inside the cell, drawing water into the cell and making it swell. (c) The concentration of electrolytes is much greater outside the cell, drawing water out of the cell and making it shrink.

Food poisoning and eating disorders involving repeated vomiting and diarrhea can also result in death because of these life-threatening fluid and electrolyte imbalances.

Electrolytes Enable Our Nerves to Respond to Stimuli

In addition to their role in maintaining fluid balance, electrolytes are critical in enabling our nerves to respond to stimuli. Nerve impulses are initiated at the membrane of a nerve cell because of a change in the degree of electrical charge. Changes occur that allow an influx of sodium into the cell, causing the cell to become slightly less negatively charged. This is called *depolarization*. If enough sodium enters the cell, the change in electrical charge triggers an *action potential*, an electrical signal that is propagated along nerve and muscle cells. Once this signal is complete, the cells return to their normal electrical state through the release of potassium to the outside of the cell. This return of the cell to its initial electrical state is termed *repolarization*. As you can see, both sodium and potassium play critical roles in ensuring that nerve impulses are generated in response to a variety of stimuli.

Electrolytes Signal Our Muscles to Contract

Our muscles contract through a series of complex physiologic changes that we will not describe in detail here. Simply stated, our muscles are stimulated to contract in response to stimulation of nerve cells. As described above, sodium and potassium play a key role in the generation of nerve impulses, or electrical signals. When a muscle fibre is stimulated by an electrical signal, changes occur in the cell membrane that lead to an increased flow of calcium into the muscle from the extracellular space. This release of calcium into the muscle provides the stimulus for muscle contraction. Our muscles can relax after a contraction once the electrical signal is complete and calcium has been pumped out of the muscle cell.

> **Recap:** Electrolytes help regulate fluid balance by controlling the movement of fluid into and out of cells. Electrolytes, specifically sodium and potassium, play a key role in generating nerve impulses in response to stimuli. Calcium is an electrolyte that stimulates muscle contraction.

How Do Our Bodies Maintain Fluid Balance?

We maintain the proper balance of fluid in our bodies by a series of mechanisms that prompt us to drink and retain fluid when we are dehydrated and to excrete fluid as urine when we consume more than we need.

Our Thirst Mechanism Prompts Us to Drink Fluids

Imagine that, at lunch, you ate a ham sandwich and a bag of salted potato chips. Now it's almost time for your afternoon seminar to end, and suddenly you are very thirsty. The last five minutes of class are a torment, and when the instructor ends the session you dash to the nearest drinking fountain. What happened here? What prompted you suddenly to feel so thirsty?

Our body's command centre for fluid intake is a cluster of nerve cells in a part of the brain called the *hypothalamus*. It is this group of cells, collectively referred to as the **thirst mechanism**, that causes you to consciously desire fluids. Our thirst mechanism prompts us to feel thirsty when it is stimulated by any of the following:

- Increased concentration of salt and other dissolved substances in our blood. Remember that ham sandwich and those potato chips? Both these foods are salty, and eating them causes the release of high concentrations of sodium into our blood.

- A reduction in blood volume and blood pressure. This can occur when fluids are lost because of profuse sweating, blood loss, vomiting, or diarrhea, or simply when fluid intake is too low.

- Dryness in the tissues of the mouth and throat. Tissue dryness reflects a lower amount of fluid in the bloodstream, which causes a reduced production of saliva.

Once the hypothalamus detects such changes, it stimulates the release of a hormone that signals the kidneys to reduce urine flow and return more water to the bloodstream. The kidneys also secrete an enzyme that triggers blood vessels throughout our body to constrict. This helps us to retain water. Water is drawn out of the salivary glands in our mouths in an attempt to further dilute the concentration of substances in our blood; this causes our mouth and throat to become dry. Together, these mechanisms allow us to prevent a further loss of body fluid and help avoid dehydration.

Although our thirst mechanism can trigger us to drink more water, this mechanism alone is not always sufficient: we tend to drink until we are no longer thirsty, but the amount of fluid we consume may not be enough to achieve fluid balance. This is particularly true when we lose body water rapidly, such as during intense exercise in the heat. Because our thirst mechanism has some limitations, it is important that you drink regularly throughout the day and not wait to drink until you become thirsty, especially if you are active. Because our thirst mechanism becomes less sensitive as we age, older people can fail to drink adequate amounts of fluid and thus are at high risk for dehydration. For this reason, older adults should be careful to drink fluids on a regular basis throughout the day. Finally, infants are also at increased risk for dehydration. A large proportion of an infant's body weight is water, so they need to drink a relatively large amount of fluid for their body size. For the same reason, fluid loss from diarrhea and vomiting are also more serious for infants.

thirst mechanism A cluster of nerve cells in the hypothalamus that stimulate our conscious desire to drink fluids in response to an increase in the concentration of salt in our blood or a decrease in blood pressure and blood volume.

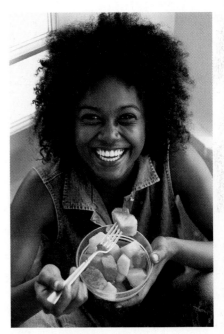

Fruits and vegetables are delicious sources of water.

We Gain Fluids by Consuming Beverages and Foods and Through Metabolism

We obtain the fluid we need each day from three primary sources: beverages, foods, and the production of metabolic water by our bodies. Of course, you know that beverages are mostly water, but it isn't as easy to see the water content in the foods we eat. For example, iceberg lettuce is almost 99% water, and even bacon contains a small amount of water. Table 7.1 lists the water content of commonly consumed beverages and foods.

Metabolic water is the water formed from our body's metabolic reactions. In the breakdown of fat, carbohydrate, and protein, adenosine triphosphate (ATP)—the cell's basic energy source—and water are produced. The water that is formed during metabolic reactions contributes about 10% to 14% of the water we need each day.

metabolic water The water formed as a byproduct of our body's metabolic reactions.

Table 7.1   Water Content of Common Beverages and Foods

	100%	90%–99%	80%–89%	60%–79%	40%–59%	20%–39%	10%–19%	1%–9%[1]
Beverages	Water Plain tea Soda water Diet soft drinks	Gatorade Clear broth Tomato juice Skim milk	Sugar-sweetened soft drinks Fruit juices 2% milk					
Fruits		Grapefruit Strawberry Tomato	Apple	Banana Avocado			Raisins	
Vegetables		Cabbage Lettuce Celery Cucumber Broccoli Squash	Carrots	Baked potato Mashed potato Boiled yams				
Eggs/Dairy			Egg whites Yogurt		Egg yolk Cream cheese Mozzarella cheese	Cheddar cheese		
Meats[2] and Alternatives				Lean steak Shrimp Pork chop Turkey Lean ham Salmon Cooked lentils	Sausage Chicken Hot dog		Bacon	
Grain Products				Cooked spaghetti	Pancakes Waffles	Bread Bagel Cooked oatmeal	Cooked rice	Ready-to-eat cereals
Oils/Fats				Low-calorie mayonnaise	Diet margarine		Butter Margarine Regular mayonnaise	
Other		Sugar-free gelatin	Yellow mustard	Instant pudding Ketchup		Cake Maple syrup Preserves		Peanut butter Popcorn Pretzels

Source: U.S. Department of Agriculture, USDA Nutrient Database for Standard Reference, Release 13, Nutrient Data Laboratory homepage, 1999, www.nal.usda.gov/fnic/foodcomp (accessed February 2002).

[1] Cooking oils, meat fats, shortening, and white sugar have 0% water content.

[2] Value is for cooked meat.

We Lose Fluids Through Urine, Sweat, Exhalation, and Feces

Our kidneys are constantly helping to maintain fluid balance by either excreting or retaining the fluid we consume. We excrete most of our water through the kidneys in the form of urine. When we consume more water than we need, the kidneys process this excess fluid and excrete it in the form of dilute urine.

During times when we need to conserve body water, the sodium concentration of our extracellular fluid increases. Special cells in the hypothalamus of the brain sense this increase in sodium levels and cause hormones to be secreted that signal the kidneys to reabsorb water instead of excreting it.

Our kidneys also respond to massive changes in fluid balance and blood pressure, such as those that occur when someone suffers a large loss of blood. Major blood loss causes a significant drop in blood pressure. This drop in blood pressure signals the kidneys to retain more water and reduce urine output. In addition, the kidneys excrete certain enzymes and hormones that cause constriction of the peripheral blood vessels and also allow for the retention of water and sodium. Since water follows sodium, retaining sodium in the kidneys also helps retain water. The sodium and water can then be absorbed back into the bloodstream and cause an increase in blood volume and blood pressure.

Water is lost from our skin in the form of sweat and from our lungs during breathing. We refer to this type of water loss as **insensible water loss**. Our sweat glands produce more sweat during exercise or when we are in a hot environment. The evaporation of sweat from our skin releases heat, which cools our skin and reduces our core temperature. Under normal resting conditions, our insensible water loss is less than 1 litre of fluid each day; during heavy exercise or in hot weather, we can lose up to 2 litres of water per hour through insensible water loss.

We excrete a relatively small amount of water in our feces. Under normal conditions, we lose only about 150 to 200 mL (5 to 7 fl. oz.) of water each day in our feces. Our gastrointestinal tract typically reabsorbs much of the large amounts of fluids that pass through it each day. However, when someone suffers from extreme diarrhea because of illness or from consuming excess laxatives, water loss in the feces can be as high as several litres per day.

In addition to these four avenues of regular fluid loss, certain situations can cause a significant loss of fluid from our bodies:

- Illnesses that involve fever, coughing, vomiting, diarrhea, and a runny nose significantly increase fluid loss. This is why doctors advise people to drink plenty of fluids when they are ill.

- Traumatic injury, internal hemorrhaging, blood donation, and surgery also increase loss of fluid because of the blood loss involved.

- Exercise increases fluid loss via sweat and respiration: although urine production typically decreases during exercise, fluid losses increase through the skin and lungs.

- Environmental conditions that increase fluid loss include high altitudes, cold and hot temperatures, and low humidity, such as in a desert or flying in an airplane. The water content of the environment is much lower at high altitude, in an airplane, and in the desert. Thus, water from our body more easily evaporates into the dry environment. We also breathe faster at higher altitudes because of the lower oxygen pressure, which results in greater fluid loss via the lungs. We sweat more in the heat, thus losing more water. Cold temperatures can trigger hormonal changes that result in an increased fluid loss.

- Pregnancy increases fluid loss from the mother because fluids are continually diverted to the fetus and amniotic fluid.

- Breastfeeding requires a tremendous increase in fluid intake to make up for the loss of fluid in breast milk.

- Consumption of **diuretics**—substances that increase fluid loss via the urine—can result in dangerously excessive fluid loss. Diuretics include certain prescription medications, alcohol, and caffeine-containing beverages, such as coffee, cola, and tea. Many over-the-counter weight loss remedies are really just diuretics.

Recap: We maintain healthy fluid levels in our body by balancing intake with excretion. Primary sources of fluids include water and other beverages, foods, and the production of metabolic water in the body. Fluid losses occur through urination, sweating, our feces, and evaporation from our lungs.

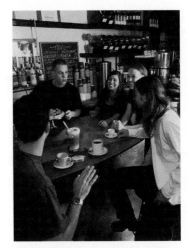

Drinking beverages that contain alcohol or caffeine causes an increase in water loss, as these drinks are diuretics.

insensible water loss The loss of water from the skin in the form of sweat and from the lungs during breathing.

diuretic A substance that increases fluid loss via the urine. Common diuretics include coffee, tea, cola, and other caffeine-containing beverages, as well as prescription medications for high blood pressure and other disorders.

Table 7.2   Functions, Recommended Intakes, and Toxicity and Deficiency Symptoms of Primary Electrolytes

Nutrient	Primary Functions	Recommended Intake	Toxicity Symptoms	Deficiency Symptoms
Sodium	Major positively charged electrolyte in extracellular fluid Maintains proper acid–base balance Assists with transmission of nerve signals Aids muscle contraction Assists in the absorption of glucose and other nutrients	1.5 g/day[1]	Water retention High blood pressure May increase loss of calcium in urine	Muscle cramps Loss of appetite Dizziness Fatigue Nausea Vomiting Mental confusion
Potassium	Major positively charged electrolyte in intracellular fluid Regulates contraction of muscles Regulates transmission of nerve impulses Assists in maintaining healthy blood pressure levels	4.7 g/day[1]	Muscle weakness Vomiting Irregular heartbeat	Muscle weakness Muscle paralysis Mental confusion
Chloride	Assists with maintaining fluid balance Aids in preparing food for digestion (as HCl) Helps kill bacteria Assists in the transmission of nerve impulses	2.3 g/day[1]	Vomiting	Dangerous changes in pH Irregular heartbeat
Phosphorus	Major negatively charged electrolyte in intracellular fluid Maintains proper fluid balance Plays critical role in bone formation Component of ATP, which provides energy for our bodies Helps regulate biochemical reactions Major part of genetic materials (DNA, RNA) A component in cell membranes, LDL	700 mg/day[2]	Muscle spasms Convulsions Low blood calcium levels	Muscle weakness Bone pain Dizziness

[1]Adequate Intake (AI)
[2]RDA

A Profile of Nutrients Involved in Hydration and Neuromuscular Function

Nutrients that assist us in maintaining hydration and neuromuscular function include water and the minerals sodium, potassium, chloride, and phosphorus. As discussed in Chapter 1, these minerals are classified as *major minerals,* as the body needs more than 100 mg of each of these minerals per day. Table 7.2 reviews the primary functions of each of these minerals. As you can see, they play many roles in the body. Calcium and magnesium also function as electrolytes and influence our body's fluid balance and neuromuscular function. However, because of their critical importance to bone health, they are discussed in Chapter 9.

Water

Water is essential for life. Although we can live weeks without food, we can only survive one to two days without water, depending on environmental temperature.

We do not have the capacity to store water, so we must continuously replace the water we lose each day.

How Much Water Should We Drink?

Our need for water varies greatly depending upon our age, body size, health status, physical activity level, and exposure to environmental conditions. It is important to pay attention to how much our need for water changes under various conditions so that dehydration can be avoided.

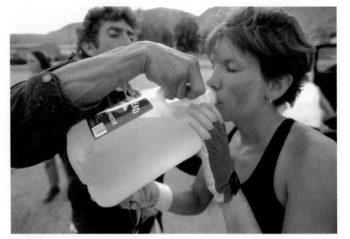

Vigorous exercise causes significant water loss that must be replenished to optimize performance and health.

Recommended Intake   Fluid requirements are very individualized. For example, a highly active male athlete training in a hot environment may require up to 10 litres of fluid per day to maintain healthy fluid balance, while an inactive, petite woman who lives in a mild climate and works in a temperature-controlled office building may only require about 3 litres of fluid per day. The DRI for adult men aged 19 to 50 years is 3.7 litres of total water per day. This includes approximately 3.0 litres (or 13 cups) as total beverages, which includes drinking water (Institute of Medicine 2004). The DRI for adult women aged 19 to 50 is 2.7 litres of total water per day. This includes about 2.2 litres (or 9 cups) as total beverages, which includes drinking water (Institute of Medicine 2004).

Figure 7.6 shows the amount and sources of water intake and output for a woman expending 2500 kcal (10 500 kJ) per day. Based on current recommendations, this woman needs about 2700 mL of water per day:

- Water from metabolism provides 300 to 400 mL of water.

- The foods she eats provide her with an additional 1000 mL of water each day.

- The beverages she drinks provide the remainder of water needed, which is equal to 1300 mL to 1400 mL.

An 8-fluid-ounce glass of water is equal to 240 mL. In this example, the woman would need to drink five to six glasses of fluid to meet her needs. You can now see why drinking eight glasses of fluid each day is recommended for most

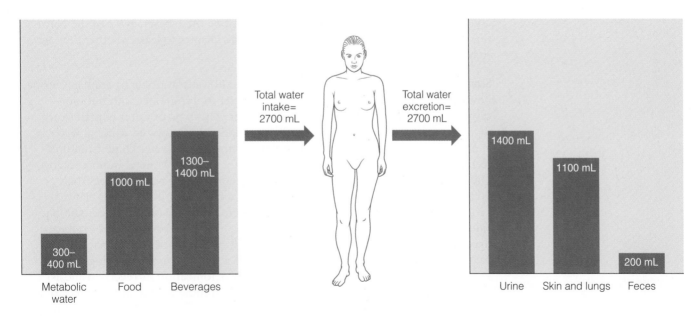

Figure 7.6 Amount and sources of water intake and output for a woman expending 2500 kcal (10 500 kJ) per day.

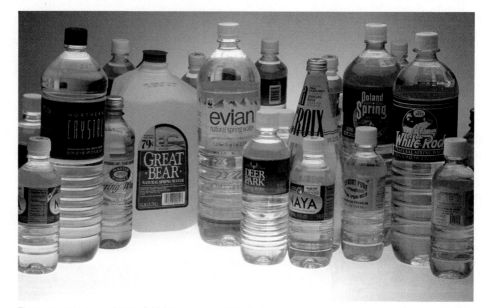

There are numerous varieties of drinking water available to consumers.

people. Drinking this amount will provide you with enough fluid to maintain proper fluid balance. Remember that this recommendation of eight glasses of fluid each day is a general guideline. You may need to drink a different amount to meet your fluid needs.

Athletes or people who are active, especially those working in very hot environments, may require more fluid than the current recommendations. The amount of sweat lost during exercise is very individualized and depends on body size, exercise intensity, environmental temperature, and humidity. We do know that some people can lose as much as 1.8 kg (4 lb.) of fluid per hour as sweat (ACSM 1996)! Thus, these individuals need to drink more to replace the fluid they lose. One litre of sweat contains about 1 gram of sodium (ACSM 2000); we also lose some potassium and small amounts of minerals, such as iron and calcium, in sweat.

Because of these fluid and electrolyte losses during exercise, some athletes drink sport beverages instead of plain water to help them maintain fluid balance. Recently, sport beverages have also become popular with recreationally active people and non-athletes. Is it really necessary for people to consume these beverages? See the Nutrition Debate on sport beverages at the end of this chapter to learn whether they are right for you.

Sources of Drinking Water   There are so many types of water available to drink in Canada, how can we distinguish among them? If we prefer to drink water with bubbles—carbonation—we can choose carbonated water. This type of water contains carbon dioxide gas that either occurs naturally or is added to the water. Mineral water is another beverage option. Both mineral water and spring water come from protected underground sources (not a public water supply). Mineral water contains 500 mg per litre or more dissolved solids, whereas spring water has less than 500 mg per litre of dissolved solids (Health Canada 2007). Although many people prefer the unique taste of mineral water, a number of brands contain high amounts of sodium and should be avoided by people who are trying to reduce their sodium intake. When mineral or spring water is not treated to remove bacteria, it can be labelled as "natural mineral water" or "natural spring water." Distilled water and bottled water produced by deionization or reverse osmosis contain no more than 10 mg per litre of dissolved minerals and are referred to as purified water.

▶ NUTRITION MYTH OR FACT

Bottled Water Is No Safer Than Tap Water

Bottled water has become increasingly popular over the past 20 years. Canadians drink an average of 47 litres of bottled water per person per year (International Council of Bottled Water Associations n.d.). Many people prefer the taste of bottled water to that of tap water. Some people also feel that bottled water is safer than tap water. Is this true?

The water we drink in Canada generally comes from two sources: surface water and ground water. Surface water comes from lakes, rivers, and reservoirs. Common contaminants of surface water include runoff from highways, pesticides, animal wastes, and industrial wastes. Ground water comes from underground rock formations called aquifers. About 26% of Canadians, mostly people who live in rural areas or small towns, rely on ground water pumped from wells (Natural Resources Canada 2004). Hazardous substances leaking from waste sites, dumps, landfills, and oil and gas pipelines can contaminate ground water.

Health Canada sets out strict standards for water quality to ensure our water is safe to drink. Most of the 4000 municipal water treatment plants in Canada use chlorine to kill contaminants. Ultraviolet light (irradiation) or ozonation can also be used to treat and purify water.

The tragedy in Walkerton, Ontario, highlights the importance of properly monitoring and treating municipal water supplies for hazardous chemicals and organic contaminants. In May 2000, heavy rain washed animal waste from a local farm into a town well, contaminating the town's water supply with *E. coli* 0157:H7 and other bacteria. The proper chlorination procedures hadn't been followed, and 7 people died while 2000 others became ill, some with kidney failure.

Bottled water is considered a food and is regulated under Canada's Food and Drugs Act and monitored by federal inspectors from the Canadian Food Inspection Agency. Most bottling plants use an ozone treatment instead of chlorine to disinfect water, and many people feel this process leaves the water tasting better than tap water treated with chlorine.

In Canada, labels must indicate how the bottled water has been treated—carbonated, demineralized, distilled, filtered, and so on—and must give the location and source of the water. Although bottled water may taste better than tap water, there is no evidence that it is safer to drink. Bottled water (except spring or mineral water) may come directly from the tap! Some types of bottled water may contain more minerals than tap water, but there are no other additional nutritional benefits in drinking bottled water.

Health Canada has the following advice for consumers of bottled water:

- Don't refill old bottles—buy new ones.
- Look on the label for the best-before date.
- Look for the chemical analysis (the declaration of minerals).
- Look for the type of treatment (ozonated, etc.).
- Don't keep bottled water past its two-year shelf life.
- Don't share bottles.
- Always refrigerate opened bottles.

In addition, Health Canada recommends that you look for bottles that have no-spill caps, to make sure that water is not spilled and air does not enter the bottled water, and avoid bottles with broken seals (Health Canada 2007).

For more information on drinking water safety, go to Health Canada's website at www.hc-sc.gc.ca/ewh-semt/water-eau/drink-potab/index_e.html.

Source: Adapted from Health Canada, Questions and Answers on Bottled Water, www.hc-sc.gc.ca/fn-an/securit/facts-faits/faqs_bottle_water-eau_embouteillee_e.html (accessed July 2008).

One of the major changes in the beverage industry over the past 20 years has been the marketing of bottled water. The meteoric rise in bottled water production and consumption is most likely because of the convenience of drinking bottled water, the health messages related to drinking more water, and the public's fears related to the safety of tap water. Is bottled water safer than tap water? Refer to the Nutrition Myth or Fact box on bottled water to find the answer to this question.

What Happens If We Drink Too Much Water?

Drinking too much water and becoming overhydrated is very rare, but it can occur. Some individuals suffering from certain forms of mental illness have an uncontrollable urge to consume large quantities of water. If these individuals have healthy kidneys, this condition generally does not lead to major health problems because their kidneys are able to process this excess water. Certain illnesses can cause increases in levels of a hormone that stimulates reabsorption of water by the kidneys. When this occurs, overhydration and dilution of sodium result. Dilution of sodium, also called *hyponatremia,* causes headaches, confusion, seizures, and coma. Hyponatremia is discussed in more detail in the next section.

What Happens If We Don't Drink Enough Water?

Dehydration results when we do not drink enough water. Fluid loss is one of the leading causes of death around the world, with infants and older adult individuals being particularly affected. Dehydration is generally due to some form of illness or gastrointestinal infection that causes diarrhea and vomiting. When these occur over a prolonged time, fluid loss is excessive and dehydration results, leading to impaired physical and mental function and even death if not treated quickly. The impact of dehydration on our health is discussed in detail on page 251.

- Interactive Molecule: Sodium Chloride

Sodium

Many people think of salt when they hear the word *sodium,* but the terms shouldn't be used interchangeably. Salt, or sodium chloride (its chemical name), is about 40% sodium and 60% chloride by weight. One teaspoon (5 mL) of salt weighs 5 grams and contains about 2300 mg of sodium (IFICF 2005).

Over the past 20 years, researchers have linked high sodium intakes to an increased risk for high blood pressure. Because of this link, many people have come to believe that sodium is harmful to the body. This simply is not true: in reality, sodium is an essential nutrient that our body needs to function optimally.

Functions of Sodium

Sodium has a variety of functions. As discussed earlier in this chapter, it is the major positively charged electrolyte in the extracellular fluid. Its exchange with potassium across cell membranes allows our cells to maintain proper fluid balance, blood pressure, and acid–base balance.

Sodium also assists with the transmission of nerve signals and aids in muscle contraction. To review, the release of sodium from inside to outside the cell stimulates the spread of nerve signals to nervous tissue and muscles. The stimulation of muscles by nerve impulses provides the impetus for muscle contraction.

Finally, sodium assists in the absorption of certain nutrients, such as glucose. Glucose cannot be passively absorbed into the cell through the cell membrane. Cells transport glucose via the process of active transport, which involves assistance from a sodium-potassium pump. This pump works by acting as a carrier protein that transports glucose through the cell membrane.

How Much Sodium Should We Consume?

Many people are concerned with consuming too much sodium in the diet, as they believe it causes high blood pressure and bloating. Although this concern is warranted for certain individuals, sodium is an important nutrient that is necessary for maintaining health.

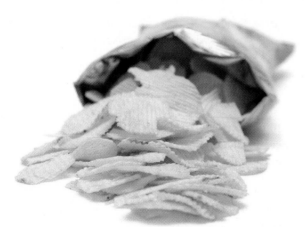

Many popular snack foods are high in sodium.

▶ **HIGHLIGHT**

Functions of Common Sodium-Containing Ingredients

Sodium-containing ingredients of foods serve a variety of important functions. Here are examples of just a few:

- Sodium benzoate: a preservative that prevents growth of yeasts and bacteria; used in acidic foods such as fruit juices, jams, relishes, and beverages.
- Sodium bicarbonate (baking soda): used as a leavening agent; helps to release carbon dioxide in baked goods during baking to increase volume and tenderness.
- Sodium caseinate: used as a thickener and binder in coffee whiteners, non-dairy whipped toppings, processed meats, and desserts.

- Sodium propionate: used as a preservative and mould inhibitor in baked goods, cheese, confections and frostings, gelatin, pudding, jams and jellies, meat products, and soft candy.
- Sodium nitrite or nitrate: a curing agent used to preserve foods and prevent growth of bacteria that cause spoilage and food-borne illness.
- Monosodium glutamate (MSG): a flavour enhancer.

Source: International Food Information Council Foundation, IFIC Review: Sodium in Food and Health, January 2005, www.ific.org/publications/reviews/sodiumir.cfm (accessed March 2005). © Reprinted from the International Food Information Council Foundation, 2005.

Recommended Dietary Intake for Sodium The AI for sodium is 1.5 g per day (1500 mg per day or 65 mmol per day) for adult men and women aged 19 to 50 years (Institute of Medicine 2004). The Tolerable Upper Intake Level (UL) is 2.3 g per day (2300 mg or 100 mmol). Data from the 2004 Canadian Community Health Survey showed that on average, Canadians consume 3092 mg of sodium daily, well above the UL (Garriguet 2007). Among young adults aged 19 to 30, 98.8% of males and 76.3% of female had usual sodium intakes above the UL. In fact, for every age and gender category from 1 year of age onward, at least 77% of the group exceeded the UL. From age 9 onward, males had significantly higher usual sodium intakes than females. Sodium consumption also varied by province, with intakes highest in Quebec and British Columbia, and lowest in Ontario.

Shopper's Guide: Good Food Sources of Sodium An estimated 77% of the sodium we consume comes from processed foods, 6% comes from salt added at the table, and 5% comes from salt added during cooking (IFICF 2005). The remaining 12% is found naturally in milk, meat, poultry, shellfish, vegetables, bottled water, and tap water.

Although about 90% of the sodium added during food processing is in the form of sodium chloride (salt), 10% comes from other sodium-containing compounds added for flavour, food safety, or preservation. See the Highlight box on the functions of common sodium-containing ingredients.

Table 7.3 shows foods that are high in sodium and gives lower-sodium alternatives. Are you surprised to see the sodium content of these food items? When eating processed foods, such as canned soups, vegetable juices, and prepackaged rice and pasta dishes, remember to look for labels with the words *low sodium.*

What Happens If We Consume Too Much Sodium?

High blood pressure is more common in people who consume high-sodium diets. This strong relationship between high-sodium diets and high blood pressure has prompted many health organizations to recommend low sodium intakes. Whether high-sodium diets actually cause high blood pressure is unclear and controversial; this controversy is discussed on page 253. In addition, there are other less controversial reasons to consume no more than the recommended amount of sodium each day. Eating excess sodium can cause an increased excretion of calcium in some people,

Table 7.3   High-Sodium Foods and Lower-Sodium Alternatives

High-Sodium Food	Portion	Sodium	Lower-Sodium Food	Portion	Sodium
Dill pickle	1 large, 10 cm (4 in.)	1731 mg (75 mmol)*	Low-sodium dill pickle	1 large, 10 cm (4 in.)	23 mg (1 mmol)*
Ham, cured, roasted	90 g (3 oz.)	1023 mg (44 mmol)	Pork, loin roast	90 g (3 oz.)	54 mg (2.3 mmol)
Tomato juice, regular	250 mL (1 cup)	877 mg (38 mmol)	Tomato juice, lower sodium	250 mL (1 cup)	24 mg (1 mmol)
Canned cream-style corn	250 mL (1 cup)	730 mg (32 mmol)	Cooked corn, fresh or frozen	250 mL (1 cup)	28 mg (1.2 mmol)
Tomato soup, canned	250 mL (1 cup)	695 mg (30 mmol)	Tomato soup, canned, lower sodium	250 mL (1 cup)	480 mg (21 mmol)
Potato chips, salted	25 g (1 oz.)	168 mg (7.3 mmol)	Baked potato, unsalted	1 medium	14 mg (0.6 mmol)
Saltine crackers	4 crackers	156 mg (6.8 mmol)	Saltine crackers, unsalted	4 crackers	100 mg (4.3 mmol)

Source: U.S. Department of Agriculture, USDA Nutrient Database for Standard Reference, Release 13, Nutrient Data Laboratory Home Page, 1999, www.ars.usda.gov/main/site_main.htm?modecode=12354500 (accessed February 2002).
*1 mmol = 23 mg sodium

which in turn may increase the risk for bone loss; however, the extent to which excess sodium intake affects bone health is also the subject of controversy (Cohen and Roe 2000). Consuming excess sodium also causes bloating, as water is pulled from inside the cells into the extracellular space in an attempt to dilute the excess sodium.

hypernatremia A condition in which blood sodium levels are dangerously high.

Hypernatremia refers to an abnormally high blood sodium concentration (clinically defined as greater than 145 millimoles [mmol] per litre of blood). It is usually caused by a rapid intake of high amounts of sodium, such as when a shipwrecked sailor drinks seawater. Eating too much sodium does not usually cause hypernatremia in a healthy person, as the kidneys are able to excrete excess sodium and avoid hypernatremia. But people with congestive heart failure or kidney disease are not able to excrete sodium effectively, making them more prone to the condition. Hypernatremia is dangerous because it causes an abnormally high blood volume, leading to edema (swelling) of our tissues and raising blood pressure to unhealthy levels.

What Happens If We Don't Consume Enough Sodium?

hyponatremia A condition in which blood sodium levels are dangerously low.

Because our dietary sodium intake is so high in North America, deficiencies are extremely rare, except in individuals who sweat heavily or consume little or no sodium in the diet. Nevertheless, certain conditions can cause dangerously low blood sodium levels. **Hyponatremia**, or low blood sodium levels (clinically defined as less than 136 milliequivalent per litre of blood), can occur in active people who drink large volumes of water and fail to replace sodium. This is discussed in the Highlight box on hyponatremia. Severe diarrhea, vomiting, or excessive prolonged sweating can also cause hyponatremia. Symptoms include headaches, dizziness, fatigue, nausea, vomiting, and muscle cramps. If hyponatremia is left untreated, it can lead to seizures, coma, and death. Treatment for hyponatremia includes replacement of the lost minerals by consuming liquids and foods high in sodium and other minerals. It may be necessary to administer electrolyte-rich solutions intravenously if the person has lost consciousness or is not able to consume beverages and foods by mouth.

> ▶ **HIGHLIGHT**

Can Water Be Too Much of a Good Thing? Hyponatremia in Marathon Runners

At the beginning of this chapter, we described the death of marathon runner Cynthia Lucero. Her case is only one of several that have gained attention in recent years. How can seemingly healthy, highly fit individuals competing in marathons collapse and even die during or after a race? One common issue faced by these athletes is maintaining a proper balance of fluid and electrolytes during the race. It is well known that people participating in distance events, such as marathons (42.2 km or 26.2 miles), need to drink enough fluid to ensure proper fluid balance. Recent research has shown that some runners drink too much water and develop hyponatremia, or abnormally low blood sodium levels.

A study examined marathon runners who were treated for hyponatremia after a race (Davis et al. 2001). The major contributing factors appeared to be a longer race time and drinking large amounts of water during the race. Experts speculate that less experienced athletes run more slowly, increasing the total time that they are competing; at the same time, they consume very large amounts of water to avoid potential dehydration. The longer these individuals run, the more water they drink and the more diluted their blood sodium levels become. About half the hyponatremic runners in these studies had to be hospitalized.

A recent study of long-distance triathletes (competing in running, swimming, and cycling) found that about 18% of these athletes suffered from hyponatremia, but only one third of these individuals had symptoms that required medical care (Speedy et al. 1999). Thus, other individuals competing in long-distance events or activities are also at risk for this disorder. Hyponatremia is a dangerous and potentially fatal condition that can be prevented. Drinking sport beverages, which contain electrolytes, and moderating fluid intake during marathons and other long-distance activities can help prevent the occurrence of hyponatremia.

Recap: Sodium is the primary positively charged electrolyte in the extracellular fluid. It works to maintain fluid balance and blood pressure, assists in acid–base balance and transmission of nerve signals, aids muscle contraction, and assists in the absorption of some nutrients. The Adequate Intake (AI) for sodium is 1.5 g/day. Deficiencies are rare, since the typical North American diet is high in sodium. In some studies, excessive sodium intake has been related to high blood pressure, bloating, and loss of bone density.

Potassium

As we discussed previously, potassium is the major positively charged electrolyte in the intracellular fluid. It is a major constituent of all living cells and is found in both plants and animals.

Functions of Potassium

Potassium and sodium work together to maintain proper fluid balance. In addition to its role in maintaining fluid balance, potassium plays a major role in regulating the contraction of muscles and transmission of nerve impulses, and it assists in maintaining blood pressure. In contrast to a high-sodium diet, eating a diet high in potassium actually helps maintain a lower blood pressure.

How Much Potassium Should We Consume?

Potassium is found in abundance in many fresh foods. We can reduce our risk for high blood pressure by consuming adequate potassium in our diet. Natural forms of potassium, such as in fruits and vegetables, reduce bone loss.

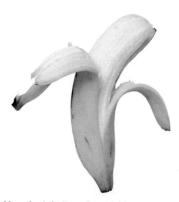

Many fresh fruits and vegetables are excellent sources of potassium and help reduce bone loss.

Table 7.4   Potassium Content of Common Foods

Food	Serving Size	Potassium
Potato, baked, flesh and skin	1 medium	721 mg (18 mmol)*
Non-fat yogurt, plain	250 mL (1 cup)	579 mg (14.5 mmol)
Banana	1 large	554 mg (13.9 mmol)
Tomato juice	250 mL (1 cup)	535 mg (13.4 mmol)
Halibut, cooked	90 g (3 oz.)	490 mg (12.3 mmol)
Orange juice, from concentrate	250 mL (1 cup)	473 mg (11.8 mmol)
Milk, 1% fat	250 mL (1 cup)	443 mg (11.1 mmol)
Cantaloupe	1/4 of medium melon	426 mg (10.7 mmol)
Spinach, raw	250 mL (1 cup)	167 mg (4.2 mmol)

Source: U.S. Department of Agriculture, USDA Nutrient Database for Standard Reference, Release 13, Nutrient Data Laboratory homepage, 1999, www.nal.usda.gov/fnic/foodcomp (accessed February 2002).
*1 mmol = 40 mg potassium

Recommended Dietary Intake for Potassium   The AI for potassium for adult men and women aged 19 to 50 years is 4.7 g/day (4700 mg/day or 120 mmol/day) (Institute of Medicine 2004).

Shopper's Guide: Good Food Sources of Potassium   Processing foods generally increases their amount of sodium and decreases their amount of potassium. Thus, the best sources of potassium include fresh foods, particularly fresh fruits and vegetables. Table 7.4 identifies foods that are high in potassium. You can optimize your potassium intake and reduce your sodium intake by avoiding processed foods and eating more fresh fruits, vegetables, and whole grains. Most salt substitutes are made from potassium chloride, and these products contain relatively high amounts of potassium.

What Happens If We Consume Too Much Potassium?

People with healthy kidneys are able to excrete excess potassium effectively. However, people with kidney disease are not able to regulate their blood potassium levels. **Hyperkalemia**, or high blood potassium levels (clinically defined as greater than 5 mmol per litre of blood), occurs when potassium is not excreted efficiently from the body. Because of potassium's role in cardiac muscle contraction, severe hyperkalemia can alter the normal rhythm of the heart, resulting in heart attack and death. People with kidney failure must monitor their potassium intake very carefully to prevent complications from hyperkalemia. Individuals at risk for hyperkalemia should avoid consuming salt substitutes, as these products are high in potassium.

What Happens If We Don't Consume Enough Potassium?

Because potassium is widespread in many foods, a dietary potassium deficiency is rare. However, potassium deficiency is not uncommon among people who have serious medical disorders. Kidney disease, diabetic acidosis, and other illnesses can lead to potassium deficiency.

In addition, people with high blood pressure who are prescribed diuretic medications to treat their disease are at risk for potassium deficiency. As we noted earlier, diuretics promote the excretion of fluid as urine through the kidneys. Some diuretics also increase the body's excretion of potassium. People who are taking diuretic medications should have their blood potassium monitored regularly and should eat foods that are high in potassium to prevent **hypokalemia**, or low blood potassium levels (clinically defined as less than 3.8 mmol per litre of blood). This is not a universal recommendation however, because some diuretics are specially formulated

hyperkalemia A condition in which blood potassium levels are dangerously high.

hypokalemia A condition in which blood potassium levels are dangerously low.

to spare potassium, and people taking this class of diuretic should not increase their dietary potassium above recommended levels.

Extreme dehydration, vomiting, and diarrhea can also cause hypokalemia. People who abuse alcohol or laxatives can also suffer from hypokalemia. Symptoms include confusion, loss of appetite, and muscle weakness. Severe cases of hypokalemia result in fatal changes in heart rate; many deaths attributed to extreme dehydration or an eating disorder are caused by abnormal heart rhythms resulting from hypokalemia.

> **Recap:** Potassium is the major positively charged electrolyte inside the cell. It regulates fluid balance, blood pressure, and muscle contraction, and it helps in the transmission of nerve impulses. Potassium is found in abundance in fresh foods, particularly fruits, vegetables, and meats. Both hyperkalemia, or excessive blood potassium, and hypokalemia, or low blood potassium, can result in heart failure and death.

Chloride

Chloride should not be confused with *chlorine,* which is a poisonous gas used to kill bacteria and other germs in our water supply. Chloride is a negatively charged ion that we obtain almost exclusively in our diets from consuming sodium chloride, or table salt.

Functions of Chloride

Coupled with sodium in the extracellular fluid, chloride assists with the maintenance of fluid balance. Chloride is also a part of hydrochloric acid (HCl) in the stomach, which aids in preparing food for further digestion (see Chapter 3). Chloride works with the white blood cells of our body during an immune response to help kill bacteria, and it assists in the transmission of nerve impulses.

How Much Chloride Should We Consume?

The AI for chloride for adult men and women aged 19 to 50 years is 2.3 grams per day (2300 mg per day or 65 mmol per day) (Institute of Medicine 2004). As chloride is coupled with sodium to form table salt, our primary dietary source of chloride is salt in our foods. Chloride is also found in some fruits and vegetables.

What Happens If We Consume Too Much Chloride?

As we consume virtually all of our dietary chloride in the form of sodium chloride, consuming excess amounts of this mineral over a prolonged period leads to hypertension in salt-sensitive individuals (people whose blood pressure increases when they eat high-sodium foods). There is no other known toxicity symptom for chloride (National Research Council 1989).

What Happens If We Don't Consume Enough Chloride?

Most people consume more than enough chloride. Even when a person consumes a low-sodium diet, chloride intake is usually adequate.

A chloride deficiency can occur, however, during conditions of severe dehydration and frequent vomiting. This occurs often in people with eating disorders who regularly vomit to rid their bodies of unwanted calories.

> **Recap:** Chloride is the major negatively charged electrolyte outside the cell. It assists with maintaining fluid balance and aids digestion of food. It also helps our immune system fight infection and assists in the transmission of nerve impulses. Our main dietary source of chloride is sodium chloride. Excess consumption of chloride can lead to hypertension in salt-sensitive individuals. Chloride deficiencies are rare but can occur during severe dehydration and frequent vomiting.

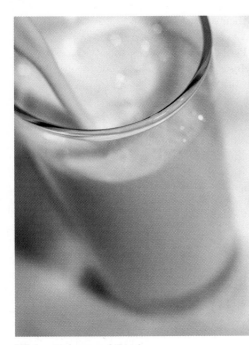

Milk is a good source of phosphorus.

Phosphorus

Phosphorus is the major intracellular negatively charged electrolyte. In our bodies, phosphorus is most commonly found combined with oxygen in the form of phosphate, PO_4^{3-}. Phosphorus is an essential constituent of all cells and is found in both plants and animals.

Functions of Phosphorus

Phosphorus works with potassium inside the cell to maintain proper fluid balance. It also plays a critical role in bone formation, as it is a part of the mineral complex of bone (see Chapter 9). Indeed, about 85% of our body's phosphorus is stored in our bones.

As a primary component of adenosine triphosphate (ATP), phosphorus plays a key role in creating energy for our bodies. It also helps regulate many biochemical reactions by activating and deactivating enzymes. Phosphorus is a part of our genetic materials, including deoxyribonucleic acid (DNA) and ribonucleic acid (RNA), and it is a component in cell membranes (as phospholipids) and part of the lipoproteins, such as low-density lipoprotein (LDL) and high-density lipoprotein (HDL).

How Much Phosphorus Should We Consume?

The RDA for phosphorus is 700 mg (22.6 mmol) per day (Institute of Medicine 2004). Phosphorus is widespread in many foods and is found in high amounts in foods that contain protein. Milk, meats, and eggs are good sources of phosphorus, and phosphorus deficiency is rare in North America. Table 7.5 shows the phosphorus content of various foods.

Table 7.5   Phosphorus Content of Common Foods

Food	Serving Size	Phosphorus
Cheese, cheddar	90 g (3 oz.)	435 mg (14.0 mmol)*
Cheese, provolone	90 g (3 oz.)	423 mg (13.6 mmol)
Non-fat yogurt, plain	250 mL (1 cup)	356 mg (11.5 mmol)
Lentils, cooked	250 mL (1 cup)	356 mg (11.5 mmol)
Chicken, white meat, cooked	250 mL (1 cup)	323 mg (10.4 mmol)
All-Bran cereal	125 mL (1/2 cup)	294 mg (9.5 mmol)
Chicken, dark meat, roasted	250 mL (1 cup)	250 mg (8.1 mmol)
Milk, skim	250 mL (1 cup)	247 mg (8.0 mmol)
Milk, 1% fat	250 mL (1 cup)	245 mg (7.9 mmol)
Milk, 2% fat	250 mL (1 cup)	245 mg (7.9 mmol)
Black beans, cooked	250 mL (1 cup)	241 mg (7.8 mmol)
Tofu, calcium processed	125 mL (½ cup)	239 mg (7.7 mmol)
Ground beef, extra lean, broiled	90 g (3 oz.)	137 mg (4.4 mmol)
Almonds	24 almonds (30g/1 oz.)	134 mg (4.3 mmol)
Pancakes, made from mix	1 pancake	127 mg (4.1 mmol)
Soy milk	250 mL (1 cup)	120 mg (3.9 mmol)
Peanut butter, smooth style	30 mL (2 Tbsp)	118 mg (3.8 mmol)

Source: U.S. Department of Agriculture, USDA Nutrient Database for Standard Reference, Release 13, Nutrient Data Laboratory homepage, 1999, www.ars.usda.gov/main/site_main.htm?modecode=12354500 (accessed February 2002).
*1 mmol = 31 mg phosphorus

It is important to note that we absorb the phosphorus from animal sources more readily than from plant sources. The phosphorus in plant foods, such as beans, cereals, and nuts, is found in the form of **phytic acid**, a plant storage form of phosphorus. Our bodies do not produce enzymes that can break down phytic acid, but we are still able to absorb up to 50% of the phosphorus found in plant foods because other foods and the bacteria in our large intestines can break down phytic acid. Cola soft drinks are another source of phosphorus in our diet. Phosphate salts are a common additive to foods. The phosphorus content of packaged mixes (such as pancakes mixes) and refrigerated cookie dough is high.

phytic acid The form of phosphorus stored in plants.

What Happens If We Consume Too Much Phosphorus?

People suffering from kidney disease and people taking too many vitamin D supplements or too many aluminum-containing antacids can suffer from high blood phosphorus levels. Severely high levels of blood phosphorus cause muscle spasms and convulsions.

What Happens If We Don't Consume Enough Phosphorus?

As mentioned previously, deficiencies of phosphorus are rare. People who may suffer from low phosphorus levels include premature infants, older adults with poor diets, and people who abuse alcohol. People with vitamin D deficiency, hyperparathyroidism (oversecretion of parathyroid hormone), and those who overuse antacids that bind with phosphorus may also have low blood phosphorus levels. The symptoms of phosphorus deficiency include bone pain, muscle weakness, and dizziness.

> **Recap:** Phosphorus is the major negatively charged electrolyte inside of the cell. It helps maintain fluid balance and bone health. It also assists us in making energy available and in regulating chemical reactions, and it is a primary component of our genetic materials. The RDA for phosphorus is 700 mg (22.6 mmol) per day, and it is commonly found in high-protein foods. Excess phosphorus can lead to muscle spasms and convulsion, while phosphorus deficiencies are rare.

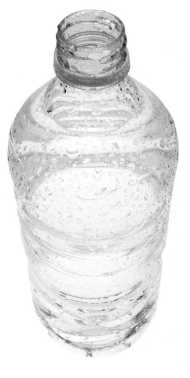

What Disorders Are Related to Fluid and Electrolyte Imbalances?

There are a number of serious, and potentially fatal, disorders resulting from the imbalance of fluid and electrolytes in our bodies. Let's review some of these now.

Dehydration

Dehydration is a serious health problem that results when fluid excretion exceeds fluid intake. It is classified in terms of the percentage of weight loss that is exclusively due to the loss of fluid. Dehydration commonly occurs as a result of heavy exercise or exposure to high environmental temperatures because rapid weight loss is always due to losses of body water through increased sweating and breathing. However, older adults and infants can get dehydrated even when inactive, as their risk for dehydration is much higher than that of healthy young and middle-aged adults. In older adults it is because they have a lower total amount of body water, and their thirst mechanism is less effective than that of a younger person; they are therefore less likely to meet their higher fluid needs. Infants excrete urine at a higher rate, cannot express when they are thirsty, and have a greater ratio of body surface area to body core, causing them to respond more dramatically to heat and cold and to lose more body water than an older person.

As indicated in Table 7.6, relatively small losses in body water, equal to a 1% to 2% change in body weight, result in symptoms, such as thirst, discomfort, and loss of

dehydration Depletion of body fluid that results when fluid excretion exceeds fluid intake.

Table 7.6 Percentages of Body Fluid Loss Correlated with Weight Loss and Symptoms

% Body Water Loss	Weight Lost If You Weigh 73 kg (160 lbs)	Weight Lost If You Weigh 59 kg (130 lbs)	Symptoms
1–2	0.7–1.5 kg (1.6–3.2 lb.)	0.6–1.2 kg (1.3–2.6 lb.)	Strong thirst, loss of appetite, feeling uncomfortable
3–5	2.2–3.6 kg (4.8–8.0 lb.)	1.8–3.0 kg (3.9–6.5 lb.)	Dry mouth, reduced urine output, greater difficulty working and concentrating, flushed skin, tingling extremities, impatience, sleepiness, nausea, emotional instability
6–8	4.4–5.8 kg (9.6–12.8 lb.)	3.5–4.7 kg (7.8–10.4 lb.)	Increased body temperature that doesn't decrease, increased heart rate and breathing rate, dizzy, difficulty breathing, slurred speech, mental confusion, muscle weakness, blue lips
9–11	6.5–8.0 kg (14.4–17.6 lb.)	5.3–6.5 kg (11.7–14.3 lb.)	Muscle spasms, delirium, swollen tongue, poor balance and circulation, kidney failure, decreased blood volume and blood pressure

Figure 7.7 Urine colour chart. Colour variations indicate levels of hydration.

Adequate hydration

Minor dehydration

Severe dehydration

heatstroke A potentially fatal response to high temperature characterized by failure of the body's heat-regulating mechanisms. Symptoms include rapid pulse; reduced sweating; hot, dry skin; high temperature; headache; weakness; and sudden loss of consciousness. Commonly called sunstroke.

appetite. For a person weighing 73 kg (160 lb.), these symptoms occur after a rapid loss of 0.7 to 1.5 kg (1.6 to 3.2 lb.). More severe water losses, equal to 3% to 5% of body weight, result in symptoms that include sleepiness, nausea, flushed skin, and problems with mental concentration. Severe losses of body water, greater than 8% of body weight, equal to about 5.9 kg (13 lb.) of water for someone weighing 73 kg (160 lb.), can result in delirium, coma, and death. Thus, a rapid loss of body fluid leads to a dangerous increase in body temperature, kidney failure, and eventual death.

We discussed earlier the importance of fluid replacement when you are exercising. How can you tell whether you are drinking enough fluid before, during, and after your exercise sessions? First, you can measure your body weight before and after each session. If you weighed in at 73 kg (160 lb.) before basketball practice and immediately afterward you weigh 72 kg (158 lb.), then you have lost approximately 1 kg or 2 lb. of body weight. This is equal to 1.3% of your body weight prior to practice. As you can see in Table 7.6, you are most likely feeling strong thirst, diminished appetite, and you may even feel generally uncomfortable. Your goal is to consume enough water and other fluids to bring your body weight back to 73 kg (160 lb.) before your next exercise session.

A simpler method of monitoring your fluid levels is to observe the colour of your urine (Figure 7.7). If you are properly hydrated, your urine should be clear to pale yellow in colour, similar to diluted lemonade. Urine that is medium to dark yellow in colour, similar to apple juice, indicates an inadequate fluid intake. Very dark or brown-coloured urine, like the colour of a cola beverage, is a sign of severe dehydration and indicates potential muscle breakdown and kidney damage. People should strive to maintain a urine colour that is clear or pale yellow.

Heatstroke

Athletes who work out in hot weather are particularly vulnerable to dangerous fluid loss. In August 2001, 27-year-old National Football League all-star player Korey Stringer died of complications from **heatstroke** after working out in a hot and humid environment. Heatstroke is a potentially fatal heat illness characterized by failure of the body's heat-regulating mechanisms. Symptoms include a rapid pulse, hot and dry skin, a high temperature, and loss of consciousness. As illustrated in the Korey Stringer case, heatstroke can be fatal. Despite his access to ample fluid and excellent medical assistance, Stringer's body core temperature rose to 42°C, or 108°F. It appears that a combination of dehydration, heat, humidity, protective clothing and headgear, and Stringer's large body size (1.9 m, 150 kg, or 6'4", 330 pounds) contributed to his death. Although there were suspicions that ephedra, a stimulant used by many athletes, also played a part, no evidence was found to support this.

Our ability to sweat is extremely limited in a humid environment, and large individuals with a great deal of muscle mass produce a lot of body heat. In addition, people who have excess body fat have an extra layer of insulation that makes it even more difficult to dissipate body heat at rest and during exercise.

Similar deaths have occurred in the past with college, university, and high school football players. These deaths prompted national attention and resulted in strict guidelines encouraging regular fluid breaks and cancelling events or changing the time of the event to avoid high heat and humidity. In addition, people who are active in a hot environment should stop exercising if they feel dizzy, light-headed, disoriented, or nauseated. Injury and death through heat illnesses can be avoided by maintaining a healthy fluid balance before, during, and after exercise.

Water Intoxication

Is it possible to drink too much water? **Overhydration**, or *water intoxication*, can occur but it is rare. It generally only occurs in people with health problems that cause the kidneys to retain too much water, causing overhydration and hyponatremia, which were discussed earlier.

Hypertension

One of the major chronic diseases in Canada is high blood pressure, which health care professionals refer to as **hypertension**. Approximately one in five adults has hypertension, and it is estimated that 42% of those adults are not aware that they have it (Heart and Stroke Foundation of Canada 2008). This is because there are often no symptoms with hypertension itself. However, high blood pressure increases a person's risk for many other serious conditions, such as heart disease, stroke, and kidney disease. In fact, the most important risk factor for stroke is high blood pressure, and Canadians suffer 40 000 to 50 000 strokes each year (Health Canada 2006). Approximately 15 000 people die from strokes each year; 59% of stroke deaths are in women.

A person with hypertension is unable to maintain blood pressure in a healthy range. We measure blood pressure in two phases, systolic and diastolic. *Systolic blood pressure* represents the pressure exerted in our arteries at the moment that the heart contracts, sending blood into our blood vessels. *Diastolic blood pressure* represents the pressure in our arteries between contractions, when our heart is relaxed. You can also think of diastolic blood pressure as the resistance in our arteries that our heart must pump against every time it beats. We measure blood pressure in millimetres of mercury (mm Hg). Optimal systolic blood pressure is *lower than* 120 mm Hg, while optimal diastolic blood pressure is *lower than* 80 mm Hg. Prehypertension is defined as a systolic blood pressure between 120 and 139 mm Hg or a diastolic blood pressure between 80 and 89 mm Hg. You would be diagnosed with hypertension if your systolic blood pressure was greater than or equal to 140 mm Hg or your diastolic blood pressure was greater than or equal to 90 mm Hg when measured in a doctor's office, or 135/85 mm Hg when measured at home (CHEP 2008). People with diabetes or kidney disease should aim for a blood pressure measurement lower than 130/80 mm Hg (CHEP 2008).

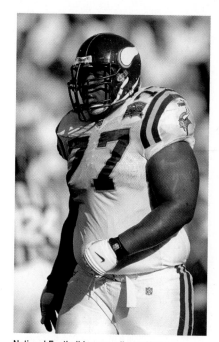

National Football League all-star Korey Stringer died in 2001 as a result of heatstroke.

overhydration Dilution of body fluid. It results when water intake or retention is excessive.

hypertension A chronic condition characterized by above-average blood pressure readings; specifically, systolic blood pressure of more than 140 mm Hg or diastolic blood pressure of more than 90 mm Hg (140/90 mm Hg) when measured in a doctor's office or higher than 135/85 mm Hg when measured at home.

What Causes Hypertension?

What causes hypertension? For about 95% of people who have it, the causes are unknown. This type is referred to as *primary* or *essential hypertension*. For the other 5% of people with hypertension, causes may include kidney disease, sleep apnea (a sleep disorder that affects breathing), and sensitivity to salt.

What Can Be Done to Reduce Hypertension?

Although we don't know what causes most cases of hypertension, the 2008 public recommendations by the Canadian Hypertension Education Program, in partnership with the Canadian Hypertension Society, Heart and Stroke Foundation of Canada, and Blood Pressure Canada, focus on preventing hypertension as follows (CHEP 2008):

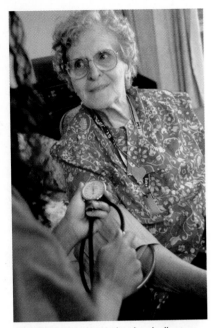

Hypertension is a major chronic disease in Canada, affecting one in five adults.

- Be physically active for 30 to 60 minutes on most days of the week. Try walking, biking, swimming, cross-country skiing, or any other physical activity that you enjoy. Remember that even a little bit of physical activity is better than no activity at all.

- Choose the following more often: vegetables, fruit, low-fat dairy products, whole grains, and lean meat, fish, and poultry. Limit fast foods, canned foods, or foods that are bought prepared or those that are high in salt, sugar, and saturated or trans fat.

- Eat less salt. In general, the more processed a food is, the higher the salt content. Try not to add salt to your cooking and remove the saltshaker from the table.

If you drink alcohol, limit the amount to one to two drinks a day or fewer. A regular-sized bottle or can of beer, 45 mL (1.5 oz.) of hard liquor, or a regular-sized glass of wine are all equal to a single alcoholic drink.

If you are overweight, losing about 5 kg (10 lbs.) will lower your blood pressure, and reducing your weight to within a healthy range will lower your blood pressure even more.

It is important to stop smoking if you have high blood pressure. Smoking increases the risk of development of heart problems and other diseases. Living and working places that are smoke-free are also important.

The Heart and Stroke Foundation of Canada and the Canadian Hypertension Education Program looked at research examining the effects of weight loss, moderate physical activity, a DASH-type diet, and reduced sodium intakes on high blood pressure. On average, hypertensive Canadians who followed a healthy diet or exercised at least three times a week showed the greatest reductions in blood pressure (Table 7.7).

Table 7.7   Impact of Lifestyle Therapies on Blood Pressure in Hypertensive Adults

Lifestyle Change	Average Decrease in	
	Systolic Blood Pressure (mm Hg)	Diastolic Blood Pressure (mm Hg)
DASH-type diet	−1.4	−5.5
Exercising 30 to 45 minutes, 3 times a week	−0.4	−7.5
Losing 4.5 kg (about 10 lb.)	−7.2	−5.9
Reducing salt consumption by 100 mmol a day	−4.8	−2.5
Reducing alcohol consumption by 2.7 drinks a day*	−4.6	−2.3

Source: Lifestyle changes to manage your high blood pressure. http://www.heartandstroke.com/site/c.ikIQLcMWJtE/b.4091465/k.DD27/Lifestyle_changes_to_manage_your_high_blood_pressure.htm © Reproduced with the permission of the Heart and Stroke Foundation of Canada, 2008. www.heartandstroke.ca.
*1 drink = 1 bottle (350mL) of beer (5% alcohol), 5 oz. (150mL) of wine (12% alcohol), or 1 1/2 oz. (50mL) of liquor (40% alcohol).

We have recently learned, however, that not everyone with hypertension is sensitive to sodium. Unfortunately, it is impossible to know who is sensitive to sodium, as there is not an easy test for sodium sensitivity. Because lowering sodium intake does not reduce blood pressure in all people with hypertension, there is significant debate over whether everyone can benefit from eating a lower-sodium diet. The Canadian Hypertension Education Program (CHEP 2008) estimates that 30% of Canadians are **salt sensitive** and recommends that all people should read food package labels and avoid foods that are high in sodium, but it doesn't suggest that individuals with normal blood pressure need to follow low-sodium diets (Touyz et al. 2004). Canadian recommendations for the control of hypertension suggest that people with hypertension should keep their sodium intake at 1500 to 2300 mg per day and that people with normal blood pressure who have a high risk of developing hypertension (e.g., those who are salt sensitive or have a strong family history of hypertension) should do the same (Touyz et al. 2004).

salt sensitive Those whose blood pressure increases when sodium intake is high.

In contrast to sodium, other minerals, such as calcium, magnesium, and potassium, have been shown to help reduce hypertension. As discussed in Chapter 2, the DASH (Dietary Approaches to Stop Hypertension) diet is an eating plan that is high in these minerals, moderately low in sodium, low in saturated fat, and includes 10 servings of fruits and vegetables each day. The DASH diet has been shown to significantly reduce blood pressure in people with and without hypertension, with even greater reductions occurring in a lower-sodium version of the DASH diet (Appel et al. 1997; Sacks et al. 2001). Thus, eating a nutritious diet that contains plenty of fruits, vegetables, whole grains, and low-fat dairy products has been proven to reduce blood pressure levels.

In the DASH-Sodium Trial, one group of people with hypertension followed the DASH diet while a control group followed a typical U.S. diet that was restricted to 1500 mg (65 mmol) of sodium. One of the key findings was that lower sodium intakes, combined with higher intakes of calcium, magnesium, and potassium in the DASH diet, produced an additive effect on lowering blood pressure (Sacks et al. 2001). As well, people following the DASH diet with 1500 mg of sodium a day met their other nutrient requirements, whereas people following the control diet often did not. This is nicely illustrated in Table 7.8.

For some individuals, lifestyle changes are not completely effective in normalizing hypertension. When this is the case, a variety of medications can be prescribed to bring a person's blood pressure into the normal range. Individuals taking medications to control blood pressure should also continue to practise the healthy lifestyle changes listed earlier in this section, as these changes will continue to benefit their long-term health.

Hypertension is called "the silent killer," because often there are no obvious symptoms of this disease. The Canadian Hypertension Education Program (CHEP 2008) estimates that 90% of Canadians will experience hypertension at some point in their lifetime and recommends that everyone have their blood pressure checked at least once every two years. Tragically, many people with hypertension fail to take their prescribed medication because they do not feel sick. Many of these people eventually suffer the consequences of their actions by experiencing a heart attack or stroke.

Neuropsychiatric Disorders

Electrolyte imbalances can cause changes in nervous function that result in psychiatric disorders. Low levels of magnesium, hypokalemia, and chronic hyponatremia can be associated with conditions of apathy and depression. High blood levels of calcium can also cause depression. A variety of electrolyte imbalances can cause confusion, delirium, and psychosis, including hyponatremia, excessive blood calcium, and low blood calcium. Electrolyte disorders can also impair cognitive function, diminishing a person's capacity to think, concentrate, solve problems, and remember information.

Table 7.8   Calculated Nutrient Profiles of the DASH and the Typical American (Control) Diets at 1.5 g (65 mmol) Sodium Intake

Nutrient	DASH Diet	Typical U.S. (Control) Diet	RDA or AI[a]
Protein, g	94.3	74.5	56
Protein, % kcal	18.0	14.3	10–35
Carbohydrate, g	306	256	130
Carbohydrate, % kcal	58.5	49.0	45–65
Total fat, g	63.1	87.1	–
Total fat, % kcal	27.2	37.6	20–35
Saturated fat, g	14.4	35.7	–
Saturated fat, % kcal	6.2	15.4	ALAP[b]
Monounsaturated fat, g	25.0	28.5	–
Monounsaturated fat, % kcal	11.2	12.3	–
Polyunsaturated fat, g	18.1	16.4	18.6[c]
Polyunsaturated fat, % kcal	7.8	7.1	5.5–11[d]
Cholesterol, mg	128	272	ALAP
Total dietary fibre, g	29.9	10.8	29.4[e]
Potassium, g	4.5	1.7	4.7
Magnesium, g	0.50	0.17	0.32
Calcium, g	1260	453	1000
Zinc, mg	12.1	7.7	11
Thiamin, mg	1.7	1.4	1.2
Riboflavin, mg	2.1	1.4	1.3
Niacin, mg	24.1	22.6	16
Vitamin B_6, mg	2.8	1.4	1.3
Vitamin B_{12}, μg	3.8	3.1	2.4
Vitamin C, mg	300	143	90
Vitamin E, mg d-alpha-tocopherol equivalents	14.0	7.9	15

Source: Adapted from Shirley R. Craddick, MHA, RD, The DASH diet and blood pressure, 2003, *Current Atherosclerosis Reports,* 5(6):484–491. © 2005 by Current Science, Inc. Reprinted with permission of Current Science, Inc.
[a]Average of recommended intake for young adult men and women; RDA = Recommended Dietary Allowance; AI = Adequate Intake
[b]As low as possible (ALAP) while consuming a nutritionally adequate diet
[c]AI for men for n-3 fatty acids = 1.6 g; for n-6 fatty acids = 17 g; total = 18.6 g
[d]n-3 fatty acids = 0.5–1.0% of kcal; n-6 fatty acids = 5–10% of kcal
[e]Amount listed is based on 14 g dietary fibre per 1000 kcal

Muscle Disorders

Muscle function is altered by electrolyte imbalances because of the changes in nervous system function that occur with these imbalances. Seizures are an example of a muscle disorder that can occur with electrolyte imbalances. **Seizures** are uncontrollable muscle spasms that may be localized to one area of the body, such as the face, or can violently shake a person's entire body. Some people lose consciousness during seizures, while others may experience hallucinations, flashbacks, or emotional

seizures Uncontrollable muscle spasms caused by increased nervous system excitability that can result from electrolyte imbalances.

outbursts. Severe seizures can result in bone fractures, loss of bowel and bladder control, and severe biting of the tongue.

Muscle cramps are involuntary, spasmodic, and painful muscle contractions that last for many seconds or even minutes. Hypernatremia that occurs with dehydration is known to cause cramps, as are other electrolyte imbalances. Muscle weakness and paralysis can also occur with various electrolyte imbalances, such as hypokalemia, hyperkalemia, and low blood phosphorus levels.

muscle cramps Involuntary, spasmodic, and painful muscle contractions that last for many seconds or even minutes; electrolyte imbalances are often the cause of muscle cramps.

Recap: Dehydration, heatstroke, and even death can occur when water loss exceeds water intake. Since our thirst mechanism is not always sufficient, it is important to drink water regularly throughout the day to promote adequate fluid intake. High blood pressure is a major chronic illness in Canada; it can be controlled by losing weight, increasing physical activity, decreasing alcohol intake, and making specific dietary changes. Electrolyte imbalances can lead to neuropsychiatric disorders, such as depression, delirium, and psychosis; they can also lead to muscle disorders, such as seizures and muscle cramps.

CHAPTER SUMMARY

- Between 50% and 70% of a healthy adult's body weight is fluid. Two thirds of this fluid is intracellular fluid, and the remainder is extracellular fluid.

- Electrolytes are electrically charged particles found in body fluid that assist in maintaining fluid balance and the normal functioning of cells and the nervous system.

- Water acts as a solvent in our bodies, provides protection and lubrication for our organs and tissues, and acts to maintain blood volume, body temperature, and blood pressure.

- The three primary sources of fluid intake are beverages, foods, and metabolic water produced by our bodies.

- The three primary avenues of fluid excretion are urine, insensible water loss (via sweat and exhalation), and feces.

- Conditions that significantly increase water loss from our bodies include fever, vomiting, diarrhea, hemorrhage, blood donation, heavy exercise, and exposure to heat, cold, and altitude.

- Fluid intake needs are highly variable and depend upon body size, age, physical activity, health status, and environmental conditions.

- Drinking too much water can lead to overhydration and hyponatremia, or dilution of blood sodium, whereas drinking too little water leads to dehydration, one of the leading causes of death around the world.

- Sodium assists in maintaining fluid balance, blood pressure, nervous function, and muscle contraction.

- Consuming excess sodium can cause high blood pressure or hypernatremia. Sodium deficiencies are rare, but hyponatremia can occur from excessive fluid intake not accompanied by adequate sodium intake.

- Potassium assists in maintaining fluid balance, healthy blood pressure, transmission of nerve impulses, and muscle function.

- Hyperkalemia is excess blood potassium, which occurs through kidney disease or malfunction. Hypokalemia is low blood potassium and can occur as a result of kidney disease, of diabetic acidosis, and through the use of some diuretic medications.

- Chloride assists in maintaining fluid balance, normal nerve transmission, and the digestion of food via the action of HCl.

- Excessive chloride intake occurs with excessive sodium intake, leading to hypertension in salt-sensitive people. Chloride deficiency is rare but can occur with prolonged dehydration and vomiting.

- Phosphorus assists in maintaining fluid balance and transferring energy via ATP. It is also a component of bone, phospholipids, genetic material, and lipoproteins.

- High blood phosphorus levels can occur with kidney disease and when individuals consume too many vitamin D supplements or phosphorus-containing antacids.

- Phosphorus deficiencies are rare but can occur with vitamin D deficiency and in premature infants or people with poor diets.

CHAPTER SUMMARY

- Dehydration occurs when water excretion exceeds water intake. Individuals at risk include the older adults, infants, people exercising heavily for prolonged periods in the heat, and individuals suffering from prolonged vomiting and diarrhea.

- Heatstroke occurs when the body's core temperature rises above 37.8°C, or 100°F. Heatstroke can lead to death if left untreated.

- Overhydration, or water intoxication, is a rare condition caused by consuming too much water. Hyponatremia can also result from water intoxication.

- Hypertension, or high blood pressure, increases the risk for heart disease, stroke, and kidney disease. Consuming excess sodium is associated with hypertension in some people.

- Electrolyte imbalances can cause neuropsychiatric disorders, such as apathy, depression, confusion, and psychosis. These imbalances can also cause seizures, muscle cramps, muscle weakness, and paralysis.

mynutritionlab Go to MyNutritionLab at www.pearsoned.ca/mynutritionlab and enrich your understanding of nutrition! You'll find key animations, interactive exercises, access to My DietAnalysis, and much more.

REVIEW QUESTIONS

Quizzes

1. Which of the following is a characteristic of potassium?
   a. It is the major positively charged electrolyte in the extracellular fluid
   b. It can be found in fresh fruits and vegetables
   c. It is a critical component of the mineral complex of bone
   d. It is the major negatively charged electrolyte in the extracellular fluid

2. Which of the following people probably has the greatest percentage of bodily fluid?
   a. A female adult who is slightly overweight and vomits nightly after eating dinner
   b. An elderly male of average weight who has low blood pressure
   c. An overweight football player who has just completed a practice session in high heat
   d. A healthy infant of average weight

3. Plasma is one example of
   a. extracellular fluid.
   b. intracellular fluid.
   c. tissue fluid.
   d. metabolic water.

4. Which of the following is true of the cell membrane?
   a. It is freely permeable to most solutes except fats
   b. It is freely permeable to water and all solutes
   c. Is freely permeable only to fats
   d. It is freely permeable to water but impermeable to solutes

5. Which of the following lifestyle changes has been shown to reduce hypertension in all people?
   a. Consuming a low-sodium diet
   b. Losing weight if overweight
   c. Getting at least eight hours of sleep nightly.
   d. Consuming at least two glasses of red wine daily

6. What are diuretics?
   a. Substances that increase urine output and therefore increase fluid loss
   b. Medications that control blood pressure in people with hypertension
   c. Substances that cause vomiting and increase fluid loss
   d. Substances that are used to purify water for drinking

7. Which of the following statements about blood pressure is correct?
   a. Hypertension is diagnosed when an individual's blood pressure in a doctor's office is 130/85 mm Hg
   b. A person with diabetes needs to keep his or her blood pressure lower than 130/80 mm Hg
   c. The causes of 50% of hypertension cases are not known
   d. Most hypertension is caused by excess sodium intake

8. Which one of the following foods contains the most sodium per serving?
   a. Roast pork
   b. Baked salmon
   c. Baked ham
   d. Roast chicken

9. Which one of the following foods is the best source of potassium?
   a. French fries
   b. White bread
   c. Cola soft drinks
   d. Baked potato

10. Hypertension is the most important risk factor for
    a. obesity
    b. stroke
    c. type 2 diabetes
    d. liver disease

11. Explain why chronic diarrhea in a young child can lead to death from abnormal heart rhythms.

12. After winning a cross-country relay race, you and your teammates celebrate with a trip to the local pub for a few beers. That evening, you feel shaky and disoriented, and you have a "pins and needles" feeling in your hands and feet. What could be going on that is contributing to these feelings?

13. For lunch today, your choices are (a) chicken soup, a ham sandwich, and a can of tomato juice; or (b) potato salad, a tuna sandwich, and a bottle of mineral water. You have hockey practice in mid-afternoon. Which lunch should you choose, and why?

14. Your cousin, who is breastfeeding her 3-month-old daughter, confesses to you that she has resorted to taking over-the-counter weight loss pills to help her lose the weight she gained during pregnancy. What would you advise her?

15. It is winter in Manitoba, and Cheyenne is freezing cold. She remembers her gym teacher's advice to drink 10 cups of fluid a day, so she makes sure to stop by the coffee shop and grab a skim milk latte on her walk to and from school and at lunchtime. She also has a cup of warm apple cider during her spare period and refills her water bottle several times throughout the day. At dinner she guzzles a couple of glasses of cranberry juice, and before bedtime she enjoys a big mug of tea to warm up. Cheyenne is excited that she's followed her teacher's advice—but she could do without having to go the bathroom so much.

   Is the advice Cheyenne received sound? Does every person have the same fluid requirement? Do you think that Cheyenne is making the best choices of fluids? Why does she have to use the bathroom so often? After learning about hydration, what suggestions would you give her to improve her fluid intake?

CASE STUDY

Michel works in a winery in the Okanagan, where the temperatures reach 35°C (95°F) during the growing season. He's used to working in the fields in these temperatures and drinks lots of water, but lately he's been complaining of feeling weak and sick to his stomach. He says, "It's probably just my high blood pressure acting up again."
a. What do you think might be wrong with Michel?
b. If you learned that he was following a low-sodium diet prescribed to manage his high blood pressure, would this information argue for or against your theory, and why?
c. What would you advise Michel to do differently in the fields tomorrow?

Test Yourself Answers

1. **True** Between approximately 50% and 70% of our body weight consists of water.

2. **False** About three quarters of the sodium we consume comes from processed foods.

3. **False** Our thirst mechanism signals that we need to replenish fluids, but it is not sufficient to ensure we are completely hydrated.

4. **False** Persistent vomiting can lead to long-term health consequences and even death.

5. **False** We do not know the cause of high blood pressure in most people. A high-sodium diet can cause high blood pressure in people who are sensitive to sodium.

WEB LINKS

www.hypertension.ca
Canadian Hypertension Society
Click on Canadian Hypertension Education Program (CHEP) for information about hypertension, taking your own blood pressure, and buying a blood pressure monitor.

www.phac-aspc.gc.ca/ccdpc-cpcmc
Centre for Chronic Disease Prevention and Control, Health Canada
Click on What are Chronic Diseases? to find out about hypertension, heart disease, and stroke in Canada.

www.heartandstroke.com
Heart and Stroke Foundation of Canada
Go to the Blood Pressure Action Plan to learn the most effective ways to lower your blood pressure.

www.hc-sc.gc.ca/ewh-semt/water-eau/drink-potab/guide/
Health Canada
Visit this website for information on drinking water safety in Canada.

www.bottledwaterweb.com
Bottled Water Web
Find current and accurate information about bottled water.

www.mayoclinic.com
MayoClinic.com
Search for "hyponatremia" to learn more about this potentially fatal condition.

www.nlm.nih.gov/medlineplus
MEDLINE Plus Health Information
Search for "dehydration" and "heat stroke" to obtain additional resources and the latest news about the dangers of these heat-related illnesses.

www.nhlbi.nih.gov
National Heart, Lung, and Blood Institute
Go to this site to learn more about heart and vascular diseases, including how to prevent high blood pressure and hypertension.

www.nih.gov
The National Institutes of Health (NIH)
Search this site to learn more about the DASH (Dietary Approaches to Stop Hypertension) diet.

Sport Beverages: Help or Hype?

Once considered specialty items used exclusively by elite athletes, sport beverages have become popular everyday beverage choices for both active and sedentary people. The market has become so lucrative that many of the large soft drink companies now produce these drinks. This surge in popularity of sport beverages leads us to ask three important questions:

- Do these beverages benefit highly active athletes?

- Do these beverages benefit recreationally active people?

- Do non-athletes need to consume sport beverages?

The first question is relatively easy to answer. Sport beverages were originally developed to meet the unique fluid, electrolyte, and carbohydrate needs of competitive athletes. As you learned in this chapter, highly active people need to replenish both fluids and electrolytes to avoid either dehydration or hyponatremia. Sport beverages can especially benefit athletes who exercise in the heat and are thus at an even greater risk for loss of water, electrolytes, and carbohydrates through respiration and sweat. The carbohydrates in sport beverages provide critical fuel during relatively intense (more than 60% of maximal effort) exercise bouts lasting more than one hour. Thus, endurance athletes are able to exercise longer, maintain a higher intensity, and improve performance times when they drink a sport beverage during exercise (Manore and Thompson 2000). Sport beverages may help athletes consume more energy than they could by eating solid foods and drinking water alone. Some athletes, such as endurance bicyclists, train or compete for six to eight hours each day on a regular basis. It is virtually impossible for these athletes to consume enough solid foods to support this intense level of exercise.

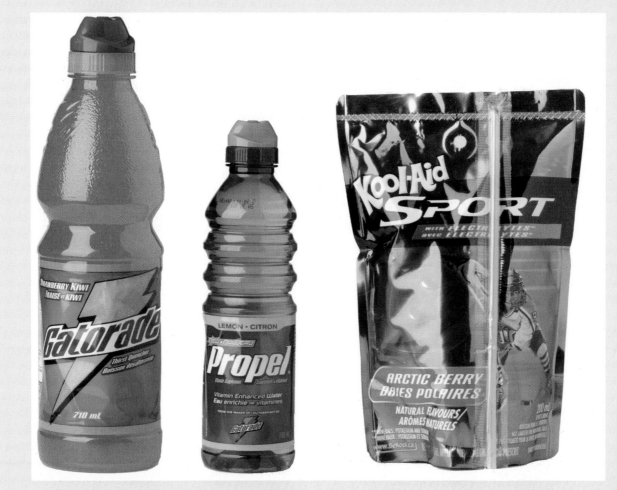

Do recreationally active people need to consume sport beverages? Most probably do not, but if they exercise for periods longer than one hour at more than 60% maximal effort, they can benefit from consuming the carbohydrate and electrolytes in sport beverages during exercise. Laboratory studies have shown that healthy people who are active but not elite athletes are able to exercise longer in high temperatures when they consume sport beverages (Bilzon, Allsopp, and Williams 2000; Galloway and Maughan 2000). These beverages can also be beneficial when exercising in an indoor environment, since often the temperature in indoor areas is relatively high and results in a large volume of fluid being lost during the activity.

It is not always easy to determine whether someone should consume a sport beverage. However, keep in mind that these beverages were originally formulated for people who exercise. Whether these beverages are needed depends on the duration and intensity of exercise, the environmental conditions, and the characteristics of the individual. Here are some situations in which drinking a sport beverage is appropriate (Manore and Thompson 2000):

- Before exercise where dehydration can occur, especially if someone is already dehydrated prior to exercise.

- During exercise or physical work in high heat or high humidity, or if someone has recently had diarrhea or vomiting; it may also be appropriate for someone who is not accustomed to activity in the heat.

- During exercise at high altitude and in cold environments; these conditions increase fluid and electrolyte losses.

- After exercise for rapid rehydration or between exercise bouts when it is difficult to consume food, such as between multiple soccer matches during a tournament.

- During long-duration exercise when blood glucose levels get low. For bouts of continuous, vigorous exercise lasting longer than 60 minutes, sport beverages may be needed, both to maintain energy levels and to provide the fluid necessary to prevent dehydration.

- During exercise in people who may have poor glycogen stores prior to exercise or who are not well fed because of illness or the inability to eat enough solid food prior to exercise.

Interestingly, sport beverages have become very popular with people who do little or no regular exercise. Are there any benefits or negative consequences for inactive or lightly active people who regularly consume these drinks? There does not appear to be any evidence that people who do not exercise derive any benefits from consuming sport beverages. Even if these individuals live in a hot environment, they should be able to replenish the fluid and electrolytes they lose during sweating by drinking water and other beverages and eating a normal diet.

Negative consequences could result when inactive people drink sport beverages. The primary consequence is weight gain, which could lead to obesity. As you can see in Table 7.9, sport beverages contain not only fluid and electrolytes but also energy. Drinking 375 mL (12 fl. oz.) of Gatorade adds 90 kcal (380 kJ) to a person's daily energy intake. Many inactive people consume two to three times this amount each day, which contributes an additional 180 to 270 kcal (750 to 1130 kJ)

Table 7.9 Nutrient Content of Sport Beverages and Other Common Beverages*

Beverage	Energy kcal (kJ)	Carbohydrate (g)	Sodium (mg)	Potassium (mg)
Cola, regular	153 (640)	39	15	4
Ginger ale	124 (520)	32	26	4
Beer, regular	146 (610)	9	18	89
Gatorade	90 (380)	22.5	144	39
Beer, light	99 (420)	< 1	1	5
Coffee, brewed	7.5 (30)	1.5	7.5	192
Cola, diet	4 (17)	< 1	21	0
Tea, brewed	3 (13)	< 1	7	88
Water, bottled	0 (0)	0	2	0
Water, tap	0 (0)	0	7	0

*Amounts compared are 375 mL (12 fl. oz.)

of energy to their diet. An inactive person has much lower energy needs than someone who is physically active. As with any other food, sport beverages could contribute to excess energy consumption, especially if these drinks are consumed in addition to alcoholic beverages and sugared drinks. With obesity rates at an all-time high, it is important that we attempt to consume only the foods and beverages necessary to support our health. Recent research at the dental school in Baltimore suggests that sports drinks can be worse for your teeth than regular soft drinks (Picard 2005). The acidity of these drinks lowers the pH level in the mouth, causing the dental enamel to break down. Food additives, such as phosphoric acid, citric acid, malic acid, and tartaric acid, are added to some beverages, such as Snapple, Coca-Cola, Pepsi, Red Bull, Gatorade, and Powerade. The study's principal investigator found, "The enamel damage caused by non-cola and sports beverages was three to 11 times greater than cola-based drinks, with energy drinks and bottled lemonades causing the most harm to dental enamel."

Sport beverages are not designed to be consumed by inactive people, and they do not contribute to the overall health of inactive or lightly active people. What do you think—are there any reasons why an inactive person might benefit from drinking sport beverages, or should these drinks be used exclusively by athletes and highly active people?

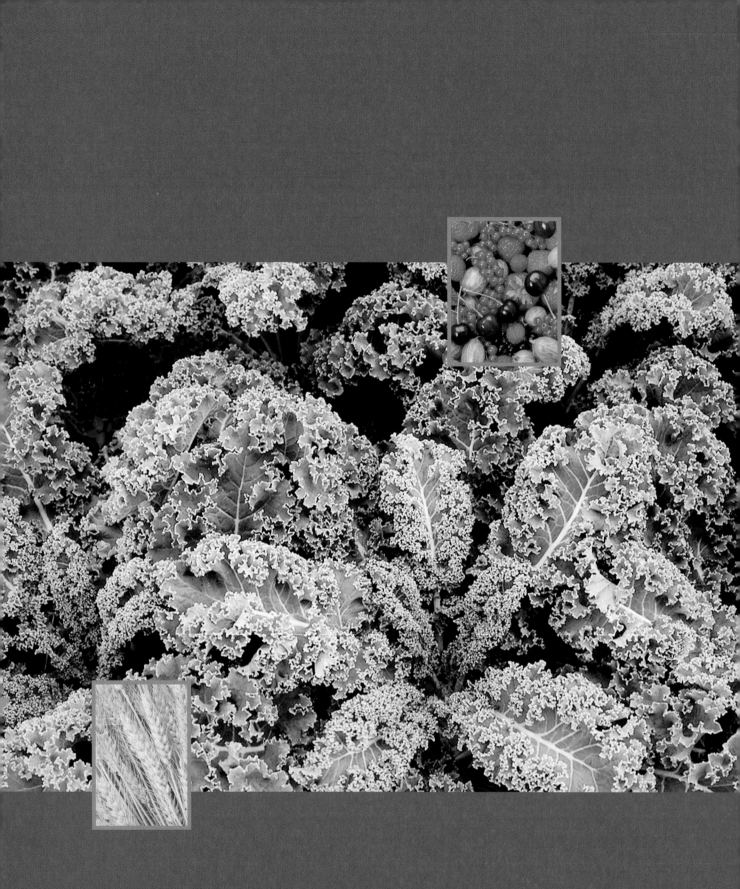

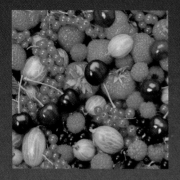

CHAPTER 8

Nutrients That May Function As Antioxidants

CHAPTER OBJECTIVES

After reading this chapter you will be able to:

1. Define free radicals and discuss how they can damage cells, pp. 267–269.

2. Describe how antioxidants protect our cells from the oxidative damage caused by free radicals, p. 270.

3. Identify two minerals and three vitamins with antioxidant properties, pp. 271–288.

4. Identify three antioxidant enzyme systems and describe how they help fight oxidative damage, p. 270.

5. Identify food sources that are high in nutrients with antioxidant properties, pp. 272–279.

6. Describe the relationship between antioxidant nutrients and cancer, pp. 283–289.

7. Define phytochemicals and describe their relationship with cancer, pp. 294–295.

8. Discuss how consuming nutrients with antioxidant properties can reduce our risk for cardiovascular disease, pp. 295–296.

Test Yourself True or False

1. Consuming antioxidant nutrients can help cure cancer. T or F

2. Taking vitamin C supplements does not reduce our risk of suffering from the common cold. T or F

3. The word *natural* on a supplement container means that the product is safe. T or F

4. We cannot consume enough antioxidant nutrients in our diets, so we should take supplements containing these nutrients. T or F

5. Some diseases associated with aging may be prevented by consuming antioxidants. T or F

Test Yourself answers can be found at the end of the chapter.

Baseball greats Eric Davis and Darryl Strawberry have a special bond that goes beyond their childhood friendship and amiable rivalry in the major leagues. At the height of their careers, each began experiencing the same symptoms: extreme weight loss, debilitating fatigue, rectal bleeding, and severe abdominal pain. Davis was diagnosed in the spring of 1997, and Strawberry's diagnosis came in the fall of 1998—both had colon cancer. But wait a minute! Doesn't colon cancer only strike elderly people of European ancestry? Davis says, "It's not a white disease. It's not a young, it's not an old. It's a deadly disease."

What exactly is colon cancer anyway? Does any aspect of your lifestyle increase your risk? Can a poor diet cause cancer, and can a healthful diet prevent it? What are antioxidants, and why do some people claim they fight cancer? If your health food store was promoting an antioxidant supplement, would you buy it?

It isn't easy to sort fact from fiction when it comes to antioxidants. Fitness and health magazines, supplement companies, and even food manufacturers tout their benefits. In contrast, some researchers claim that antioxidants do not give any added protection from diseases and in some cases may even be harmful. In this chapter, you will learn what antioxidants are and how they work in our bodies. We will also profile the antioxidant nutrients and discuss their relationship to health. Finally, you'll learn about the role antioxidants may play in preventing cancer and heart disease and in slowing the aging process.

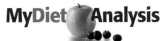

www.mynutritionlab.com

antioxidant A compound that has the ability to prevent the damage caused by oxidation.

atom A discrete, irreducible unit of matter. It is the smallest unit of an element and is identical to all other atoms of that element.

nucleus The positively charged central core of an atom. It is made up of two types of particles—protons and neutrons—bound tightly together. The nucleus of an atom contains essentially all of its atomic mass.

electron A negatively charged particle attracted to the nucleus of an atom.

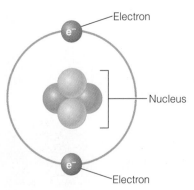

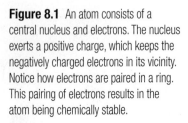

Figure 8.1 An atom consists of a central nucleus and electrons. The nucleus exerts a positive charge, which keeps the negatively charged electrons in its vicinity. Notice how electrons are paired in a ring. This pairing of electrons results in the atom being chemically stable.

What Are Antioxidants, and How Do Our Bodies Use Them?

Antioxidants are compounds that protect our cells from the damage caused by oxidation. *Anti* means "against," and antioxidants work *against,* or *prevent,* oxidation. Before we can go further in our discussion of antioxidants, we need to learn what oxidation is and how it does damage.

Oxidation Is a Chemical Reaction in Which Atoms Lose Electrons

A review of some basic chemistry will help us understand the process of oxidation.

Molecules Are Composed of Atoms

Molecules are the smallest *physical unit* of an element or a compound. They consist of one or more of the same atoms in an element (e.g., hydrogen gas, or H_2) and two or more different atoms in a compound (such as water, H_2O). Our bodies are constantly breaking down molecules of food and air into their component atoms, and then rearranging these freed atoms to build the different types of molecules our body needs. But what, really, are atoms? Simply put, an **atom** is a small but *unique* unit of matter. Elements, such as carbon or hydrogen, are unique because their atoms are unique. Every atom of carbon, for example, is identical to every other atom of carbon. The same is true for hydrogen and for every other element of matter. All the matter in the universe breaks down into just 92 elements, each consisting of one unique type of atom. Even more surprisingly, just six elements make up 99% of the matter in our bodies.

Atoms Are Composed of Particles

During the twentieth century, physicists learned how to split atoms into even smaller particles. As you can see in Figure 8.1, their research revealed that all atoms have a central core, called a **nucleus,** which is positively charged. Around this nucleus are one or more **electrons,** which are negatively charged. The opposite attraction between the positive nucleus and the negative electrons keeps an atom together by making the atom stable, so that its electrons remain with it and do not veer off toward other atoms.

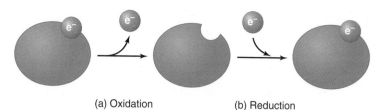

(a) Oxidation   (b) Reduction

Figure 8.2 The exchange reaction. Exchange reactions consist of two parts. (a) During oxidation, molecules lose electrons. (b) In the second part of the reaction, molecules gain electrons, which is called reduction.

During Metabolism, Atoms Exchange Electrons

As you recall from Chapter 3, the process by which our bodies break down and build up molecules is called *metabolism*. During metabolism, atoms may lose electrons (Figure 8.2a). We call this loss of electrons **oxidation**, because it is usually fuelled by oxygen. Atoms are capable of gaining electrons during metabolism as well. We call this process *reduction* (Figure 8.2b). This loss and gain of electrons typically results in an even exchange of electrons. Scientists call this loss and gain of electrons an *exchange reaction*.

> **Recap:** An atom is a small and unique unit of matter having a nucleus and electrons. Atoms exist together with other atoms as molecules. During metabolism, molecules break apart and their atoms lose electrons; this process is usually fuelled by oxygen and is called oxidation.

oxidation A chemical reaction in which molecules of a substance may be broken down into their component atoms. During oxidation, the atoms involved lose electrons.

Animations

• Free Radical Formation

free radical A highly unstable atom with an unpaired electron in its outermost shell.

Oxidation Sometimes Results in the Formation of Free Radicals

Stable atoms have an even number of electrons in pairs at successive distances (called *shells*) from the nucleus. When a stable atom loses an electron during oxidation, it is left with an odd number of electrons in its outermost shell. In other words, it now has an *unpaired electron*. In most exchange reactions, unpaired electrons immediately pair up with other unpaired electrons, making newly stabilized atoms, but in rare cases, atoms with unpaired electrons in their outermost shell remain unpaired. Such atoms are highly unstable and are called **free radicals**. Examples of free radicals include superoxide (O_2^-), hydroxyl radical (OH), and nitric oxide (NO).

Energy Metabolism Involves Oxidation and Gives Rise to Free Radicals

Free radicals are formed as a byproduct of many of our bodies' fundamental physiologic processes. Although some free radicals are a necessary part of our bodily functions, others cause serious damage to our cells and other body components. Let's look at the most common way free radicals are created.

Our bodies use oxygen and hydrogen to generate the energy (ATP) that is needed by the body (Figure 8.3). We are constantly inhaling air into our bodies, thereby providing the oxygen needed to fuel this reaction. At the same time, we generate the necessary hydrogen as a result of digesting food. As shown in Figure 8.4, occasionally during metabolism, oxygen accepts a single electron that was released during this process. When it does so, the newly unstable oxygen molecule becomes a free radical because of the added unpaired electron.

Other Factors Can Also Cause Free Radical Formation

Free radicals are also formed from other metabolic processes, such as when our immune systems fight infections. Other factors that cause free radical formation include pollution, overexposure to the sun, toxic substances, radiation exposure, tobacco smoke, and asbestos. Continual exposure to these factors leads to uncontrollable free radical formation.

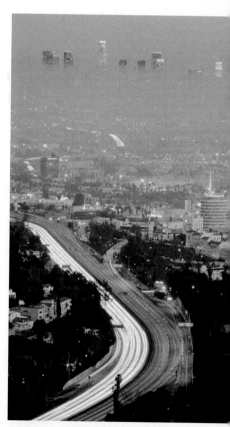

Exposure to pollution from car exhaust and industrial waste increases our production of free radicals.

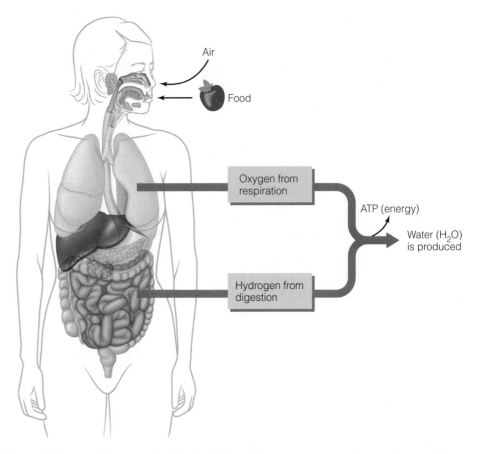

Figure 8.3 Oxygen (O) is consumed by inhaling air. Through the process of metabolizing food, hydrogen (H) is produced. As these substances undergo exchange reactions during metabolism, electrons are freed to contribute their energy to the production of ATP, which occurs throughout the body at the cellular level. The hydrogen and oxygen then recombine to form water (H_2O).

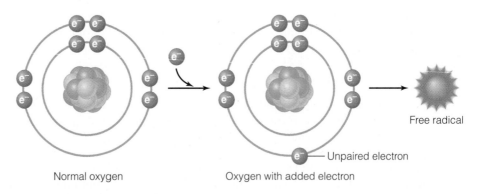

Figure 8.4 Normally, an oxygen molecule contains eight electrons. Occasionally oxygen will accept an unpaired electron during the oxidation process. This acceptance of a single electron causes oxygen to become an unstable molecule called a free radical.

Free Radicals Can Destabilize Other Molecules and Damage Our Cells

Why are we concerned with the formation of free radicals? Simply put, it is because of their destabilizing power. If you were to think of paired electrons as a married couple, a free radical would be an extremely seductive outsider. Its unpaired electron exerts a powerful attraction toward all stable molecules around it. In an attempt to

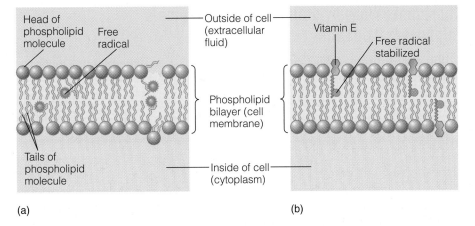

Head of phospholipid molecule

Free radical

Tails of phospholipid molecule

Outside of cell (extracellular fluid)

Vitamin E

Free radical stabilized

Phospholipid bilayer (cell membrane)

Inside of cell (cytoplasm)

(a)   (b)

Figure 8.5 (a) The formation of free radicals in the lipid portion of our cell membranes can cause a dangerous chain reaction that damages the integrity of the membrane and can cause cell death. (b) Vitamin E is stored in the lipid portion of our cell membranes. By donating an electron to free radicals, it protects the lipid molecules in our cell membranes from themselves being oxidized and stops the chain reaction of oxidative damage.

stabilize itself, a free radical will "steal" an electron from stable compounds, in turn generating more unstable free radicals. This is a dangerous chain reaction, since the free radicals generated can damage or destroy our cells.

One of the most significant sites of free radical damage is the cell membrane. As shown in Figure 8.5(a), free radicals that form within the lipid layer of cell membranes steal electrons from these stable lipid molecules. When the lipid molecules, which are hydrophobic, are destroyed, they no longer repel water. With the cell membrane's integrity lost, the ability to regulate the movement of fluids and nutrients into and out of the cell is also lost. This loss of cell integrity causes damage to the cell and to all systems affected by this cell.

Other sites of free radical damage include low-density lipoproteins (LDLs), cell proteins, and our genetic material (DNA, or deoxyribonucleic acid). Damage to these sites disrupts the transport of substances into and out of cells, alters protein function, and can disrupt cell function because of defective DNA. These changes may increase our risk for heart disease and cancer and can cause our cells to die prematurely.

Not surprisingly, many diseases are linked with free radical production:

- cancer
- heart disease
- diabetes
- arthritis
- cataracts
- kidney disease
- Alzheimer's disease
- Parkinson's disease

Recap: Free radicals are formed during oxidation when a stable atom loses or gains an electron and this electron remains unpaired. Free radicals can be produced when ATP is formed, when our immune system fights infections, and when we are exposed to pollution, toxic substances, radiation, the sun, and tobacco smoke. Free radicals are highly unstable entities that cause the production of more free radicals. They can damage our LDLs, cell proteins, and DNA and are associated with many diseases, including heart disease, cancer, and diabetes.

Antioxidants Work by Stabilizing Free Radicals or Opposing Oxidation

In 2000, the Institute of Medicine published a fairly strict definition of a dietary antioxidant:

> A dietary antioxidant is a substance in foods that significantly decreases the adverse effects of reactive species, such as reactive oxygen and nitrogen species, on normal physiological function in humans. (p. 42)

In other words, it must be established that, first, free radicals have adverse effects on a particular disease and, second, antioxidants are capable of reducing the risk of that disease. In addition, the antioxidant activity must be clearly present in humans, as well as in vitro.

How do our bodies fight free radicals and repair the damage they cause? Dietary antioxidants perform in one of two ways:

1. Certain antioxidant vitamins work independently by donating their electrons or hydrogen molecules to free radicals to stabilize them and reduce the damage caused by oxidation (Figure 8.5b).

2. Certain minerals function within complex antioxidant enzyme systems that convert free radicals to less damaging substances that are then excreted by our bodies. The minerals selenium, copper, iron, zinc, and manganese act as **cofactors**, or helpers, that are needed to allow enzyme systems to function properly. These minerals activate enzyme systems, such as superoxide dismutase, catalase, and glutathione peroxidase.
   - Superoxide dismutase converts free radicals to less damaging substances, such as hydrogen peroxide.
   - Catalase removes hydrogen peroxide from our bodies by converting it to water and oxygen.
   - Glutathione peroxidase also removes hydrogen peroxide from our bodies and stops the production of free radicals in lipids.

Antioxidant enzyme systems also work to break down fatty acids that have become oxidized and to destroy the free radicals that caused the oxidized fatty acids. In addition to the antioxidant vitamins and antioxidant enzyme systems, other dietary compounds that do not function as antioxidants, such as phytochemicals, can help stabilize free radicals and prevent damage to cells and tissues.

In summary, free radical formation is generally kept safely under control by the protective antioxidant systems in our body. When our natural antioxidant defences are not sufficient, free radical damage can be quite significant.

cofactor A compound that is needed to allow enzymes to function properly.

Recap: Antioxidant vitamins donate electrons or hydrogen atoms to free radicals to stabilize them and reduce oxidative damage. Antioxidant minerals are part of antioxidant enzyme systems that convert free radicals to less damaging substances, which our bodies then excrete. Other compounds stabilize free radicals, which prevent them from damaging cells and tissues. Selenium, copper, iron, zinc, and manganese act as cofactors for the antioxidant enzyme systems, allowing the enzymes to function properly. Superoxide dismutase, catalase, and glutathione peroxidase are examples of antioxidant enzymes.

A Profile of Nutrients That May Function as Antioxidants

Our bodies can form some antioxidants, but most are consumed in our diet. Nutrients that appear to have antioxidant properties or are part of our protective antioxidant enzyme systems include vitamins E, C, and A, beta-carotene (a precursor to vitamin A), and the mineral selenium. The minerals copper, iron, zinc, and manganese play a peripheral role in fighting oxidation and are briefly introduced in this chapter. Let's review each of these nutrients now and learn more about their functions in the body.

Vitamin E

As reviewed in Chapter 1, vitamin E is one of the fat-soluble vitamins, which means that dietary fats carry it from our intestines through the lymph system and eventually transport it to our cells. As you remember, our bodies store the fat-soluble vitamins. The liver serves as a storage site for vitamins A and D, and about 90% of the vitamin E in our bodies is stored in our adipose tissue. The remaining vitamin E is found in cell membranes.

Vitamin E includes several different forms of compounds called **tocotrienols** and **tocopherols**. The tocotrienol compounds do not appear to play an active role in our bodies. The tocopherol compounds are the biologically active forms of vitamin E in our bodies. Four different tocopherol compounds have been discovered: alpha, beta, gamma, and delta. Of these, the most active, or potent, vitamin E compound found in food and supplements is *alpha-tocopherol* (Figure 8.6). The RDA for vitamin E is expressed as alpha-tocopherol in milligrams per day (α-tocopherol, mg per day). Food labels and vitamin and mineral supplements may express vitamin E in units of alpha-tocopherol equivalents (α-TE), as milligrams, and as International Units (IU). For conversion purposes, 1 α-TE is equal to 1 mg of active vitamin E. In supplements, 1 IU is equal to 0.67 mg α-TE if the vitamin E in the supplement is from natural sources.

If synthetic vitamin E is used in the supplement, 1 IU is equal to 0.45 mg α-TE. The synthetic form of vitamin E used in fortified foods and supplements is sometimes found on labels as dl-α-tocopheryl acetate, and the natural form of vitamin E and its esters are sometimes labelled as d-α-tocopherol.

Functions of Vitamin E

Vitamin E is different from most nutrients because it has no known role in metabolism. Its primary function is as an antioxidant. As described earlier in this chapter, this means that vitamin E donates an electron to free radicals, stabilizing them and preventing them from destabilizing other molecules. Once vitamin E is oxidized, it is either excreted from the body or recycled back into active vitamin E through the help of other antioxidant nutrients, such as vitamin C.

tocotrienol A form of vitamin E that does not play an important biological role in our bodies.

tocopherol The active form of vitamin E in our bodies. Alpha-tocopherols are the forms used to establish human vitamin E requirements.

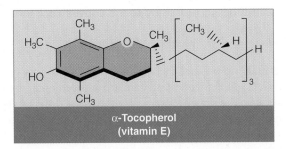

Figure 8.6 The chemical structure of alpha-tocopherol.

Because vitamin E is prevalent in our adipose tissues and cell membranes, its action specifically protects *polyunsaturated fatty acids* (PUFAs) and other fatty components of our cells and cell membranes from being oxidized (see Figure 8.5b). Vitamin E also protects our low-density lipoproteins (LDLs) from being oxidized, which lowers our risk for heart disease. (The relationship between antioxidants and heart disease is reviewed later in this chapter.) In addition to protecting our PUFAs and LDLs, vitamin E protects the membranes of our red blood cells from oxidation, reducing our risk of anemia, and plays a critical role in protecting the cells of our lungs, which are constantly exposed to oxygen and the potentially damaging effects of oxidation.

Vitamin E serves many other roles essential to human health. Vitamin E is critical for normal fetal and early childhood development of nerves and muscles, as well as for maintenance of their functions. It enhances our immune function by protecting white blood cells and other components of our immune system, thereby helping to defend our bodies against illness and disease. Vitamin E also improves the absorption of vitamin A if the dietary intake of vitamin A is low. A full list of the functions, requirements, and toxicity and deficiency symptoms associated with vitamin E is provided in Table 8.1.

How Much Vitamin E Should We Consume?

Considering the importance of vitamin E to our health, you might think that you need to consume a huge amount daily. In fact, the RDA is modest and the food sources plentiful.

Recommended Dietary Allowance for Vitamin E   The RDA for vitamin E for men and women is 15 mg (35 μmol) alpha-tocopherol per day. The Tolerable Upper Intake Level (UL) is 1000 mg alpha-tocopherol per day. Remember that one of the primary roles of vitamin E is to protect PUFAs from oxidation. Thus, our need for vitamin E increases as we eat more oils and other foods that contain PUFAs. Fortunately these foods also contain vitamin E, so we typically consume enough vitamin E within them to protect their PUFAs from oxidation.

Shopper's Guide: Good Food Sources of Vitamin E   Vitamin E is very widespread in the foods we eat. Much of the vitamin E that we consume comes from vegetable oils and the products made from them (Figure 8.7). Safflower oil, sunflower oil, canola oil, and soybean oil are good sources of vitamin E. Mayonnaise and salad dressings made from these oils also contain vitamin E. Nuts, seeds, and some vegetables also contribute vitamin E to our diet. Although no single fruit or vegetable contains very high amounts of vitamin E, eating 7 to 10 servings of fruits and vegetables each day will help ensure adequate intake of this nutrient. Cereals in Canada are not fortified with vitamin E, but other grain products contribute modest amounts of vitamin E to our diet. Wheat germ and soybeans are also good sources of vitamin E. Animal and dairy products are poor sources of vitamin E.

Vitamin E is destroyed by exposure to oxygen, metals, ultraviolet light, and high temperatures. Although raw (uncooked) vegetable oils contain vitamin E, heating these oils destroys vitamin E. Thus, foods that are deep-fried and processed contain little vitamin E. This includes most fast foods and convenience foods.

What Happens If We Consume Too Much Vitamin E?

Vitamin E toxicity is uncommon, and there is little evidence to support significant health problems with vitamin E supplementation. Standard supplemental doses (1 to 18 times the RDA) are not associated with any adverse health effects. Interestingly, it appears that taking even much higher doses of vitamin E may be safe. Daily intakes of up to 800 mg alpha-tocopherol (or about 53 times the RDA) are known to be tolerable.

As with any nutrient, however, it is important to exercise caution when supplementing. Some individuals do report side effects, such as nausea, intestinal distress, and diarrhea, with vitamin E supplementation. Certain medications interact negatively

Table 8.1   Functions, Recommended Intakes, and Toxicity and Deficiency Symptoms of Substances with Antioxidant Properties

Antioxidant	Primary Functions	Recommended Intake	Deficiency Symptoms/ Adverse Effects	Tolerable Upper Intake Level	Toxicity Symptoms/ Side Effects
Vitamin E (fat-soluble)	Protects cell membranes from oxidation Protects polyunsaturated fatty acids (PUFAs) from oxidation Protects vitamin A from oxidation Protects white blood cells and enhances immune function Improves absorption of vitamin A	RDA: Men = 15 mg alpha-tocopherol Women = 15 mg alpha-tocopherol (35 µmol)	Red blood cell hemolysis Anemia Impairment of nerve transmission Muscle weakness and degeneration Leg cramps Difficulty walking Fibrocystic breast disease	UL: 1000 mg (2325 µmol)	Inhibition of blood clotting Increased risk of hemorrhagic stroke Intestinal discomfort
Vitamin C (water-soluble)	Antioxidant in extracellular fluid and lungs Regenerates oxidized vitamin E Reduces formation of nitrosamines in stomach Assists with collagen synthesis Enhances immune function Assists in the synthesis of hormones, neurotransmitters, and DNA Enhances absorption of iron	RDA: Men = 90 mg Women = 75 mg Smokers = 35 mg more per day than RDA	Scurvy Bleeding gums Loose teeth Weakness Hemorrhaging of hair follicles Poor wound healing Swollen ankles and wrists Diarrhea Bone pain and fractures Depression Anemia	UL: 2000 mg	Nausea and diarrhea Nosebleeds Abdominal cramps Increased oxidative damage Increased formation of kidney stones in those with kidney disease
Beta-carotene* (fat-soluble provitamin for vitamin A)	Protects cell membranes and LDLs from oxidation Enhances immune system Protects skin from sun's ultraviolet rays Protects eyes from oxidative damage	None at this time	Unknown	None	Carotenosis or carotenoderma (yellowing of skin)
Vitamin A ** (fat-soluble)	Necessary for our ability to adjust to changes in light Protects colour vision Cell differentiation Necessary for sperm production in men and fertilization in women Contributes to healthy bone growth	RDA: Men = 900 µg RAE Women = 700 µg RAE	Night blindness Xerophthalmia, which leads to permanent blindness Impaired immunity and increased risk of illness and infection Inability to reproduce Failure of normal growth	UL: 3000 µg (preformed only)	Spontaneous abortions and birth defects in fetus of pregnant women Loss of appetite Blurred vision Hair loss Abdominal pain, nausea, diarrhea Liver and nervous system damage
Selenium (trace mineral)	Part of glutathione peroxidase, an antioxidant enzyme Indirectly spares vitamin E from oxidation Assists in production of thyroid hormone Assists in maintaining immune function	RDA: Men = 55 µg Women = 55 µg	Keshan disease: a specific form of heart disease Kashin-Beck disease: deforming arthritis Impaired immune function Increased risk of viral infections Infertility Depression, hostility Muscle pain and wasting	UL: 400 µg	Brittle hair and nails Skin rashes Vomiting, nausea Weakness Cirrhosis of liver

*Beta-carotene does not meet the Institute of Medicine (2000) definition of an antioxidant because antioxidant activity in humans has not been conclusively established.

**Vitamin A is still under investigation as a potential antioxidant.

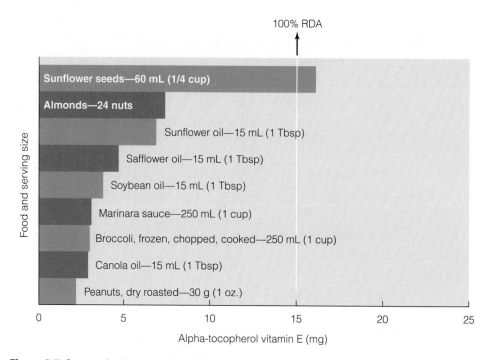

100% RDA

Sunflower seeds—60 mL (1/4 cup)

Almonds—24 nuts

Sunflower oil—15 mL (1 Tbsp)

Safflower oil—15 mL (1 Tbsp)

Soybean oil—15 mL (1 Tbsp)

Marinara sauce—250 mL (1 cup)

Broccoli, frozen, chopped, cooked—250 mL (1 cup)

Canola oil—15 mL (1 Tbsp)

Peanuts, dry roasted—30 g (1 oz.)

Food and serving size

0　　5　　10　　15　　20　　25

Alpha-tocopherol vitamin E (mg)

Figure 8.7 Common food sources of vitamin E. The RDA for vitamin E is 15 mg alpha-tocopherol per day for men and women. (Data from U.S. Department of Agriculture, Agricultural Research Service, USDA Nutrient Database for Standard Reference, Release 15, 2002, Nutrient Data Laboratory homepage, www.nal.usda.gov/fnic/foodcomp, accessed August 2002.)

with vitamin E. The most important of these are the *anticoagulants*, substances that stop blood from clotting excessively. Aspirin is an anticoagulant, as is the prescription drug Coumadin. Vitamin E supplements can augment the action of these substances, causing uncontrollable bleeding. In addition, new evidence suggests that in some people, long-term use of standard vitamin E supplements may cause hemorrhaging in the brain, leading to a type of stroke called *hemorrhagic stroke*.

What Happens If We Don't Consume Enough Vitamin E?

True vitamin E deficiencies are uncommon in humans. This is primarily because vitamin E is fat-soluble, which allows us to store ample amounts in our fatty tissues. Thus, we typically have adequate amounts of vitamin E available even when our diet is low in this nutrient. Although we have no comparable Canadian data, results from the third U.S. National Health and Nutrition Examination Survey (NHANES) show that 27% to 41% of Americans have low blood levels of vitamin E. This puts these individuals at risk for cardiovascular disease (Ford and Sowell 1999).

Despite the rarity of vitamin E deficiencies, they do occur. One vitamin E deficiency symptom is *erythrocyte hemolysis*, or the rupturing (*lysis*) of red blood cells (*erythrocytes*). The rupturing of our red blood cells leads to *anemia*, a condition in which our red blood cells cannot carry and transport enough oxygen to our tissues, leading to fatigue, weakness, and a diminished ability to perform physical and mental work. We discuss anemia in more detail in Chapter 10. Premature babies can suffer from vitamin E–deficiency anemia; if born too early, the infant does not receive vitamin E from its mother, since the transfer of this vitamin from mother to baby occurs during the last few weeks of the pregnancy.

Other symptoms of vitamin E deficiency include loss of muscle coordination and reflexes, leading to impairments in vision, speech, and movement. As you might expect, vitamin E deficiency can also impair immune function, especially if accompanied by low body stores of the mineral selenium.

In adults, vitamin E deficiencies are usually caused by diseases, particularly diseases that cause malabsorption of fat, such as those that affect the liver, gallbladder, and pancreas. As reviewed in Chapter 3, the liver makes bile, which is necessary for the absorption of fat. The bile travels to the gallbladder, where it is concentrated and stored. The gallbladder delivers the bile into our intestines, where it facilitates digestion of fat. The pancreas makes fat-digesting enzymes. Thus, when the liver, gallbladder, or pancreas are not functioning properly, fat and the fat-soluble vitamins, including vitamin E, cannot be absorbed, leading to their deficiency.

> **Recap:** Vitamin E protects our cell membranes from oxidation, enhances immune function, and improves our absorption of vitamin A if dietary intake is low. The RDA for vitamin E is 15 mg alpha-tocopherol per day for men and women. Vitamin E is found primarily in vegetable oils and nuts. Toxicity is uncommon, but taking very high doses can cause excessive bleeding. Deficiency is rare, but symptoms include anemia and impaired vision, speech, and movement.

Vitamin C

Vitamin C is a water-soluble vitamin. We must therefore consume it on a regular basis, since any excess is excreted (primarily in our urine) rather than stored. There are two active forms of vitamin C: ascorbic acid and dehydroascorbic acid (Figure 8.8). Interestingly, most animals can make their own vitamin C from glucose. All primates, including humans, and guinea pigs and fruit bats, however, cannot synthesize their own vitamin C and must consume it in the diet.

Functions of Vitamin C

Vitamin C is probably most well known for its role in preventing scurvy, a disease that ravaged sailors on long sea voyages centuries ago. It was characterized by bleeding tissues, especially of the gums, and over half of the deaths that occurred at sea were attributable to scurvy. During these long voyages, the crew ate all the fruits and vegetables early in the trip, and then had only grain and animal products available until they reached land to resupply. In 1740 in England, Dr. James Lind discovered that citrus fruits could prevent scurvy. This is due to their high vitamin C content. Fifty years after the discovery of the link between citrus fruits and prevention of scurvy, the British Navy finally required all ships to provide daily lemon juice rations for each sailor to prevent the onset of scurvy. A century later, sailors were given lime juice rations, earning them the nickname "limeys." It wasn't until 1930 that vitamin C was discovered and identified as a nutrient.

One important role of vitamin C is to assist in the synthesis of **collagen**. Collagen, a protein, is a critical component of all connective tissues in our bodies, including bone, teeth, skin, tendons, and blood vessels. Collagen assists in preventing bruises, and it ensures proper wound healing, as it is a part of scar tissue and a component of the tissue that mends broken bones. Without adequate vitamin C, our bodies cannot form collagen, and tissue hemorrhage, or bleeding, is a major symptom of vitamin C deficiency.

Vitamin C also acts as an antioxidant. Like vitamin E, it donates electrons to free radicals, thus preventing the damage of cells and tissues. Since it is water-soluble, vitamin C primarily acts as an antioxidant in the extracellular fluid. Vitamin C acts as an important antioxidant in the lungs, protecting us from the damage caused by ozone and cigarette smoke. Vitamin C also regenerates vitamin E by donating an electron after it has been oxidized. This enables vitamin E to continue to protect our cell membranes and other tissues. In the stomach, vitamin C reduces the formation of *nitrosamines,* cancer-causing agents found in such foods as cured and processed meats. We discuss the role of vitamin C and other antioxidants in preventing some forms of cancer later in this chapter (page 293).

collagen A protein found in all connective tissues in our body.

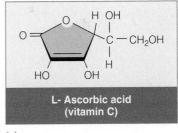

**L- Ascorbic acid
(vitamin C)**

(a)

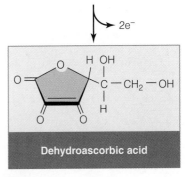

Dehydroascorbic acid

(b)

Figure 8.8 Chemical structure of (a) L-ascorbic acid and (b) dehydroascorbic acid.

▶ **NUTRITION MYTH OR FACT**

Can Vitamin C Prevent the Common Cold?

What happens when you feel a cold coming on? If you are like many people, you will drink a lot of orange juice or take vitamin C supplements to ward off a cold. Do these tactics really help prevent a cold?

It is well known that vitamin C is important for a healthy immune system. A vitamin C deficiency can seriously weaken our immune cells' ability to detect and destroy invading microbes, increasing our susceptibility to many diseases and illnesses—including the common cold. Many people have taken vitamin C supplements to prevent the common cold, basing their behaviour on its actions of enhancing our immune function. Interestingly, scientific studies do not support this precaution.

A recent review of many of the studies of vitamin C and the common cold found that people taking vitamin C experienced as

many colds as people who took a placebo (Hemila 1997). The amount of vitamin C taken in these studies was quite high, at least 1000 mg per day (more than 10 times the RDA). Thus, despite their popularity, vitamin C supplements do not appear to enhance our ability to fight the common cold.

Consuming a healthy diet that includes excellent sources of vitamin C will assist us with maintaining a strong immune system, but vitamin C supplements do not appear to be effective in enhancing the immune system of an already well-nourished individual. So next time you feel yourself getting a cold, you may want to think twice before taking extra vitamin C.

Vitamin C also enhances our immune response, protecting us from illness and infection. But contrary to popular belief, it is not a miracle cure (see the accompanying Nutrition Myth or Fact box on vitamin C, above). Vitamin C also assists in the synthesis of DNA, neurotransmitters, such as serotonin (which helps regulate mood), and various hormones. Vitamin C helps ensure that appropriate levels of thyroxine, a hormone produced by the thyroid gland, are produced to support our basal metabolic rate and to maintain body temperature.

Vitamin C also enhances the absorption of iron. It is recommended that people with low iron stores consume vitamin C–rich foods along with iron sources to improve absorption. For people with high iron stores, this practice can be dangerous and lead to iron toxicity (discussed on page 366). Refer to Table 8.1 for a review of the functions, requirements, and toxicity and deficiency symptoms associated with vitamin C.

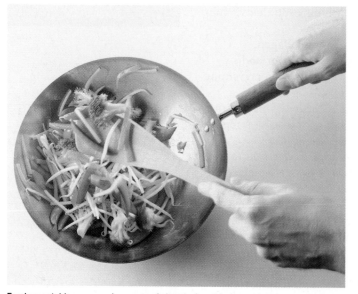

Fresh vegetables are good sources of vitamin C and beta-carotene.

How Much Vitamin C Should We Consume?

Although popular opinion suggests our need for vitamin C is high, we really only require amounts that are easily obtained when we eat the number of servings of fruits and vegetables recommended by *Canada's Food Guide.*

Recommended Dietary Allowance for Vitamin C   The RDA for vitamin C is 90 mg per day for men and 75 mg per day for women. The Tolerable Upper Intake Level (UL) is 2000 mg (2 grams) per day for adults. Smoking increases a person's need for vitamin C. Thus, the RDA for smokers is 35 mg more per day than for non-smokers. This equals 125 mg per day for men and 110 mg per day for women.

Shopper's Guide: Good Food Sources of Vitamin C   Fruits and vegetables are the best sources of vitamin C. Because heat and oxygen destroy vitamin C, fresh sources of these

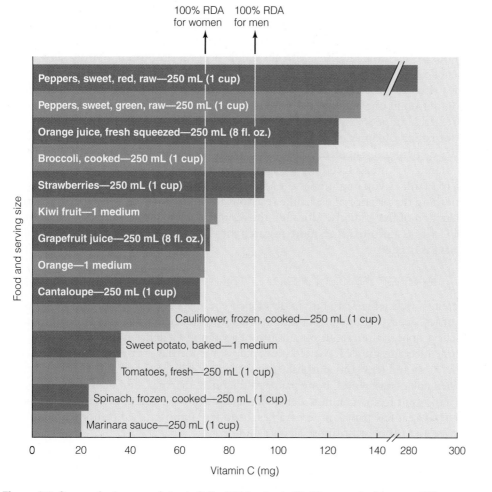

Figure 8.9 Common food sources of vitamin C. The RDA for vitamin C is 90 mg per day for men and 75 mg per day for women.

(Data from U.S. Department of Agriculture, Agricultural Research Service, USDA Nutrient Database for Standard Reference, Release 15, 2002, Nutrient Data Laboratory homepage, www.ars.usda.gov/main/site_main.htm?modecode=12354500, accessed August 2002.)

foods have the highest content of vitamin C. Cooking foods, especially boiling them, leaches their vitamin C, which is then lost when we strain them. Some research has also suggested that microwaving vegetables may destroy large amounts of antioxidants, such as vitamin C (Puuponen-Pimiä et al. 2003). Forms of cooking that are least likely to compromise the vitamin C content of foods include steaming and stir-frying.

As indicated in Figure 8.9, many fruits and vegetables are high in vitamin C. Citrus fruits (such as oranges, lemons, and limes), potatoes, strawberries, tomatoes, kiwi fruit, broccoli, spinach and other leafy greens, cabbage, green and red peppers, and cauliflower are excellent sources of vitamin C. Fortified beverages and cereals are also sources of vitamin C. Dairy foods, meats, root vegetables, and unfortified cereals and grains provide little or no vitamin C. Remember that a serving of vegetables is 125 mL (1/2 cup) of cooked or 250 mL (1 cup) of raw vegetables or 125 mL (4 fl. oz.) of vegetable juice, while a serving of fruit is one medium fruit, 125 mL (1/2 cup) of chopped or canned fruit or 125 mL (4 fl. oz.) of fruit juice.

What Happens If We Consume Too Much Vitamin C?

Because vitamin C is water soluble, we usually excrete any excess. Consuming excess amounts in food sources does not lead to toxicity, and only supplements can lead to toxic doses. Doses of a nutrient that are 10 or more times as large as the recommended amount are referred to as **megadoses**. Taking megadoses of vitamin C is not

megadose A dose of a nutrient that is 10 or more times as large as the recommended amount.

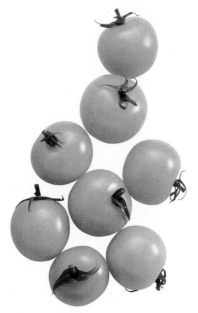

Many fruits, like these yellow tomatoes, are high in vitamin C.

pro-oxidant A nutrient that promotes oxidation and oxidative cell and tissue damage.

fatally harmful. However, side effects of doses exceeding 2000 mg (2 grams) per day for a prolonged period include nausea, diarrhea, nosebleeds, and abdominal cramps.

In rare instances, consuming even moderately excessive doses of vitamin C can be harmful. As mentioned earlier, vitamin C enhances the absorption of iron. This action is beneficial to people who need to increase iron absorption. It can be harmful, however, to people with a disease called *hemochromatosis,* which causes an excess accumulation of iron in our bodies. Such iron toxicity can damage our tissues and lead to a heart attack. In people who have kidney disease, taking excess vitamin C can lead to the formation of kidney stones. This does not appear to occur in healthy individuals. Critics of vitamin C supplementation claim that taking the supplemental form of the vitamin is "unbalanced" nutrition and leads vitamin C to act as a pro-oxidant. A **pro-oxidant**, as you might guess, is a nutrient that promotes oxidation. It does this by pushing the balance of exchange reactions toward oxidation, which promotes the production of free radicals. Although the results of a few studies suggested that vitamin C acts as a pro-oxidant, more research into the pathological significance of this in humans is needed.

What Happens If We Don't Consume Enough Vitamin C?

Vitamin C deficiencies are rare in developed countries but can occur in developing countries. Scurvy is the most common vitamin C deficiency disease. The symptoms of scurvy appear after about one month of a vitamin C–deficient diet. Symptoms include bleeding gums, loose teeth, weakness, hemorrhages around the hair follicles of the arms and legs (tiny purplish spots called petechiae), wounds that fail to heal, swollen ankles and wrists, bone pain and fractures, diarrhea, and depression. Anemia can also result from vitamin C deficiency. People most at risk of deficiencies include those who eat few fruits and vegetables, including impoverished or homebound individuals, and people who abuse alcohol and drugs.

> **Recap:** Vitamin C scavenges free radicals and regenerates vitamin E after it has been oxidized. Vitamin C prevents scurvy and assists in the synthesis of collagen, hormones, neurotransmitters, and DNA. Vitamin C also enhances iron absorption. The RDA for vitamin C is 90 mg per day for men and 75 mg per day for women. Many fruits and vegetables are high in vitamin C. Toxicity is uncommon; symptoms include nausea, diarrhea, and nosebleeds. Deficiency symptoms include scurvy, anemia, diarrhea, and depression.

Beta-Carotene

provitamin An inactive form of a vitamin that the body can convert to an active form. An example is beta-carotene.

Although beta-carotene is not considered an essential nutrient, it is a *provitamin* found in many fruits and vegetables. **Provitamins** are inactive forms of vitamins that the body cannot use until they are converted to their active form. Our bodies convert beta-carotene to the active form of vitamin A, or *retinol;* thus, beta-carotene is a precursor of retinol. It takes 2 units of beta-carotene to make 1 unit of active vitamin A.

carotenoids Fat-soluble plant pigments that the body stores in the liver and adipose tissues. The body is able to convert certain carotenoids to vitamin A.

Beta-carotene is classified as a **carotenoid**, one of a group of plant pigments that are the basis for the red, orange, and deep yellow colours of many fruits and vegetables. (Even dark green leafy vegetables contain plenty of carotenoids, but the green pigment, chlorophyll, masks their colour!) Although more than 600 carotenoids are found in nature, only about 50 are found in the typical human diet. The six most common carotenoids found in human blood are alpha-carotene, beta-carotene, cryptoxanthin, lutein, lycopene, and zeaxanthin. Notice, however, that our bodies can convert only alpha-carotene, beta-carotene, and beta-cryptoxanthin to retinol. These are referred to as provitamin A carotenoids. We are just beginning to learn more about how carotenoids function in our body and how they may affect our health. Most of our discussion will focus on beta-carotene, as the majority of research on carotenoids to date has focused on this substance.

Functions of Beta-Carotene

Beta-carotene and some other carotenoids are known to have antioxidant properties in vitro, but it is not clear whether the antioxidant activity also occurs in humans. Therefore, strictly speaking beta-carotene and other carotenoids are not antioxidants. Like vitamin E, beta-carotene is fat soluble and fights the harmful effects of oxidation in the lipid portions of our cell membranes and in our LDLs; but, compared with vitamin E, beta-carotene is a relatively weak antioxidant. In fact, other carotenoids, such as lycopene and lutein, may be stronger antioxidants than beta-carotene. Research is currently being conducted to elucidate how many carotenoids are found in foods and which ones are effective antioxidants.

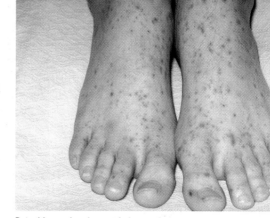
Petechiae and corkscrew hair seen in scurvy

Carotenoids play other important roles in our bodies. Specifically, they

- enhance our immune system and boost our ability to fight illness and disease;

- protect our skin from the damage caused by the sun's ultraviolet rays;

- protect our eyes from damage, preventing or delaying age-related vision impairment.

Carotenoids are also associated with a decreased risk of certain types of cancer. We discuss the roles of carotenoids and other antioxidants in cancer later in this chapter. Refer to Table 8.1 for a review of beta-carotene's functions and requirements.

How Much Beta-Carotene Should We Consume?

Although there is evidence in the research laboratory that beta-carotene is an antioxidant, its importance to health is not known. Therefore, no formal DRI for beta-carotene has been determined.

Recommended Dietary Allowance for Beta-Carotene   Nutritionists do not consider beta-carotene and other carotenoids to be essential nutrients, as they play no known essential roles in our body and are not associated with any deficiency symptoms. Thus, no RDA for these compounds has been established. It has been suggested that consuming 6 to 10 mg of beta-carotene per day from food sources can increase its levels in our blood to amounts that may reduce our risks for some diseases, such as cancer and heart disease (Burri 1997). Supplements containing beta-carotene have become very popular, and supplementation studies have prescribed doses of 15 to 30 mg of beta-carotene. Refer to the accompanying Nutrition Myth or Fact box on beta-carotene, page 281, to learn more about how supplementation with this compound may affect your risk for cancer.

Shopper's Guide: Good Food Sources of Beta-Carotene   Fruits and vegetables that are red, orange, yellow, and deep green are generally high in beta-carotene and other carotenoids, such as lutein and lycopene. Tomatoes, carrots, cantaloupe, sweet potatoes, apricots, leafy greens such as kale and spinach, and pumpkin are good sources of beta-carotene. Eating the recommended number of fruits and vegetables each day ensures an adequate intake of beta-carotene and other carotenoids. Also, because of its colour, beta-carotene is used as a natural colouring agent for many foods, including margarine, cereal, cake mixes, gelatins, and soft drinks. However, these foods are not significant sources of beta-carotene. Figure 8.10 identifies common foods that are high in beta-carotene.

We generally absorb only between 20% and 40% of the carotenoids present in the foods we eat. In contrast to vitamins E and C, heating foods high in carotenoids improves our ability to digest and absorb these compounds. Carotenoids are bound in the cells of plants, and the process of lightly cooking these plants breaks chemical bonds

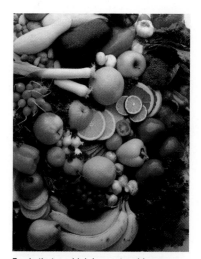
Foods that are high in carotenoids are easy to recognize by their bright colours.

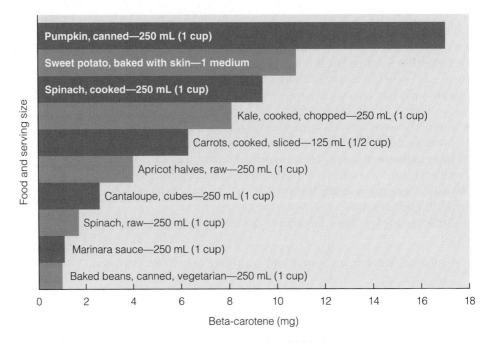

Figure 8.10 Common food sources of beta-carotene. There is no RDA for beta-carotene.

(Data from U.S. Department of Agriculture, Agricultural Research Service, USDA–NCC Carotenoid Database for U.S. Foods, 1998, Nutrient Data Laboratory homepage, www.ars.usda.gov/main/site_main.htm?modecode=12354500, accessed August 2002.)

and can rupture cell walls, which humans don't digest. These actions result in more of the carotenoids being released from the plant. For instance, 100 grams of raw carrots contains approximately 7.3 mg of beta-carotene, while the same amount of cooked carrots contains approximately 8.0 mg (U.S. Department of Agriculture 1998).

What Happens If We Consume Too Much Beta-Carotene?

Consuming large amounts of beta-carotene or other carotenoids in foods does not appear to cause toxic symptoms. However, your skin can turn yellow or orange if you consume large amounts of foods that are high in beta-carotene. This condition is referred to as *carotenosis* or *carotenoderma*, and it appears to be both reversible and harmless. Taking beta-carotene supplements is not generally recommended, as we can get adequate amounts of this nutrient by eating more fruits and vegetables.

What Happens If We Don't Consume Enough Beta-Carotene?

There are no known deficiency symptoms of beta-carotene or other carotenoids apart from beta-carotene's function as a precursor for vitamin A. Although studies have shown that eating foods high in carotenoids is associated with reduced risks of diseases, such as heart disease and cancer, taking carotenoid supplements is not linked with any health benefits, and in some cases may be harmful, as illustrated in the Nutrition Myth or Fact box concerning beta-carotene supplements and cancer rates.

> **Recap:** Beta-carotene is a carotenoid and a provitamin of vitamin A. It protects the lipid portions of our cell membranes and LDL cholesterol from oxidative damage. It also enhances our immune function and protects our vision. There is no RDA for beta-carotene. Orange, red, and deep green fruits and vegetables are good sources of beta-carotene. There are no known toxicity or deficiency symptoms, but yellowing of the skin can occur if too much beta-carotene is consumed.

▶ **NUTRITION MYTH OR FACT**

Beta-Carotene Supplements May Increase the Risk of Cancer

Beta-carotene is one of many carotenoids known to have antioxidant properties. Because there is substantial evidence that people eating foods high in antioxidants have lower rates of cancer, large-scale studies are being conducted to determine if taking antioxidant supplements can decrease our risk for cancer. One such study is the Alpha-Tocopherol Beta-Carotene (ATBC) Cancer Prevention Study (Albanes et al. 1995).

The ATBC Cancer Prevention Study was conducted in Finland from 1985 to 1993. The primary purpose of this study was to determine the effects of beta-carotene and vitamin E supplements on the rates of lung cancer and other forms of cancer. The study focused on the benefit of these antioxidants on a group of male smokers, who are considered to be at high risk for lung and other cancers. Almost 30 000 men between the ages of 50 and 69 participated in the study. The participants were given daily either a beta-carotene supplement, a vitamin E supplement, a supplement containing both beta-carotene and vitamin E, or a placebo.

The average time people participated in this study was six years. Contrary to what was expected, the male smokers who took beta-carotene supplements experienced an increased number of deaths during the study. More men in this group died of lung cancer, heart disease, and stroke. There was also a trend in this group for higher rates of prostate and stomach cancers. This negative effect appeared to be particularly strong in men who had a higher alcohol intake.

The reasons why beta-carotene increased lung cancer risk in this population are not clear. It is possible that the supplementation period was too brief to benefit these high-risk individuals, although studies of shorter duration have found beneficial effects. There may be other components in foods besides beta-carotene that are protective against cancer, making supplementation with an isolated nutrient ineffective. In any case, the results of this study suggest that for certain people, supplementation with beta-carotene may be harmful. There is still much to learn about how people of differing risk levels respond to antioxidant supplementation.

Vitamin A

Vitamin A is a fat-soluble vitamin. We store about 90% of the vitamin A we absorb in our liver, with the remainder stored in our adipose tissue, kidneys, and lungs. Because fat-soluble vitamins cannot dissolve in our blood, they require proteins that can bind with and transport them through the bloodstream to target tissues and cells. *Retinol-binding protein* is one such carrier protein for vitamin A. Retinol-binding protein carries retinol from the liver to the cells that require it. Chylomicrons may also transport vitamin A.

There are three active forms of vitamin A in our bodies: **retinol** is the alcohol form; **retinal** is the aldehyde form; and **retinoic acid** is the acid form. These three forms are collectively referred to as the *retinoids* (Figure 8.11). Remember from the previous section that beta-carotene is a precursor to vitamin A. When we eat foods with beta-carotene, it is converted to retinol in the wall of our small intestine.

The unit of expression for vitamin A is retinol activity equivalents (RAE). You may still see the expression *retinol equivalents* (RE) or International Units (IU) for vitamin A on food labels or dietary supplements. The conversions to RAE from various forms of retinol and from the units IU and RE are as follows:

- 1 RAE = 1 microgram (μg) retinol
- 1 RAE = 12 μg beta-carotene
- 1 RAE = 24 μg alpha-carotene or beta-cryptoxanthin
- 1 RAE = 1 RE (usually, but not always)
- 1 RAE = 3.3 IU

Animations

• Vitamin A and the Visual Cycle

retinol An active alcohol form of vitamin A that plays an important role in healthy vision and immune function.

retinal An active aldehyde form of vitamin A that plays an important role in healthy vision and immune function.

retinoic acid An active acid form of vitamin A that plays an important role in cell growth and immune function.

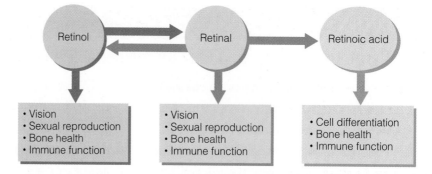

Figure 8.11 The three active forms of vitamin A in our bodies are retinol, retinal, and retinoic acid. Retinol and retinal can be converted interchangeably; retinoic acid is formed from retinal, and this process is irreversible. Each form of vitamin A contributes to many of our bodily processes.

- Vitamin A and the Epithelial Tissue

Functions of Vitamin A

The known functions of vitamin A are numerous, and researchers speculate that many are still to be discovered.

Vitamin A Acts as an Antioxidant Limited research indicates that vitamin A may act as an antioxidant (Livrea et al. 1995; Gutteridge and Halliwell 1994). Like vitamins E and C, it appears to scavenge free radicals and protect our LDLs from oxidation. As you might expect, adequate vitamin A levels in the blood are associated with lower risks of some forms of cancer and heart disease. However, the role of vitamin A as an antioxidant is not strongly established and is still under investigation.

Vitamin A Is Essential to Sight Vitamin A's most critical role in our bodies is certainly in the maintenance of healthy vision. Specifically, vitamin A affects our sight in two ways: it enables us to react to changes in the brightness of light, and it enables us to distinguish between different wavelengths of light—in other words, to see different colours. Let's take a closer look at this process.

Light enters our eyes through the cornea, travels through the lens, and then hits the **retina**, which is a delicate membrane lining the back of the inner eyeball (see Figure 8.12). You might already have guessed how *retinal* got its name: it is found in—and integral to—the retina. When light hits the retina, retinal is used to effect a chemical transformation in the light-sensitive *rod cells*, causing the transmission of a signal to the brain that is interpreted as a black and white image. This process goes on continually, allowing our eyes to adjust moment to moment to subtle changes in our surroundings or in the level of light. At the same time, the *cone cells* of the retina, which are only effective in bright light, use retinal to interpret different wavelengths of light as different colours.

In summary, our abilities to adjust to dim light, recover from a bright flash of light, and see in colour are all critically dependent on adequate levels of retinal in our eyes.

Vitamin A Contributes to Cell Differentiation Another important role of vitamin A is its contribution to **cell differentiation,** the process by which cells mature into highly specialized cells that perform unique functions. Obviously, this process is critical to the development of healthy organs and effectively functioning body systems. Vitamin A affects cell differentiation through its ability to turn on or turn off the genes that code for specific proteins that control various functions in cells. In this way, the retinoids, or active forms of vitamin A, can control the amounts of proteins that are made, and thus the activities within cells that determine how immature cells will mature and which type of specific functions they will have. As an example of cell differentiation, let's look at the development of the mucus-producing cells in our epithelial tissues. Epithelial tissues include our skin and the protective linings of the lungs, vagina, intestines, stomach, bladder, urinary tract, and eyes. The mucus that epithelial tissues produce lubricates the tissue and helps us to propel microbes, dust particles, foods, or fluids out of

retina The delicate, light-sensitive membrane lining the inner eyeball and connected to the optic nerve. It contains retinal.

cell differentiation The process by which immature, undifferentiated stem cells develop into highly specialized functional cells of discrete organs and tissues.

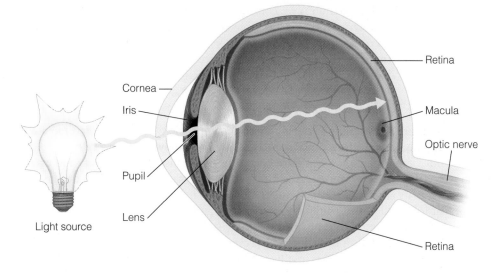

Figure 8.12 Vitamin A is necessary to maintain healthy vision. Light enters the eye through the cornea, travels through the lens, and hits the retina located in the back of the eye. The light reacts with the retinal stored in the retina, which allows us to see black and white images.

our body tissues (e.g., when we cough up secretions or empty our bladder). When vitamin A levels are insufficient, the epithelial cells fail to differentiate appropriately, and we lose these protective barriers against infection and irritants. Vitamin A is also critical to the differentiation of specialized immune cells called *T-lymphocytes*, or *T-cells*, which help us fight infections. You can now see why vitamin A deficiency can lead to a breakdown of our immune responses and to infections and other disorders of the lungs and respiratory tract, urinary tract, vagina, and eyes.

Other Functions of Vitamin A   Vitamin A is involved in reproduction. Although its exact role is unclear, it appears necessary for sperm production in men and for fertilization to occur in women. Vitamin A also regulates a gene that controls the production of an enzyme in liver cells that enables the liver to make glucose.

Two popular treatments for acne contain derivatives of vitamin A. Retin-A, or tretinoin, is a treatment applied to the skin. Accutane is taken orally. These medications should be used carefully and only under the supervision of a licensed physician. Although they are relatively less toxic forms of vitamin A, they can cause birth defects in the developing fetus if used while a woman is pregnant and can lead to other toxicity problems in some individuals. It is recommended that these medications be stopped at least two years prior to conceiving. Interestingly, vitamin A itself has no effect on acne; thus, vitamin A supplements are not recommended in its treatment. See Table 8.1 for the functions, requirements, and toxicity and deficiency symptoms associated with vitamin A.

How Much Vitamin A Should We Consume?

Vitamin A toxicity can occur readily because it is a fat-soluble vitamin, so it is important to consume only the amount recommended, as it is known to be safe.

Recommended Dietary Intake for Vitamin A   The RDA for vitamin A is 900 µg (RAE) per day for men and 700 µg (RAE) per day for women. (See p. 281 for converting carotenes to RAE.) The UL is 3000 µg (RAE) per day of preformed vitamin A in women (including those pregnant and lactating) and men.

Shopper's Guide: Good Food Sources of Vitamin A   We consume vitamin A from both animal and plant sources. About half of the vitamin A in our diets is the pre-formed vitamin A found in animal foods, such as beef liver, chicken liver, eggs, and whole-fat dairy products. Vitamin A is also found in fortified reduced-fat milks and margarine (Figure 8.13).

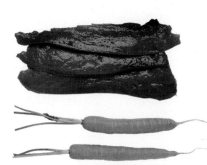
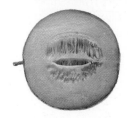

Liver, carrots, and cantaloupe all contain pre-formed vitamin A, or beta-carotene, that can be converted to vitamin A in our bodies.

The other half of the vitamin A we consume comes from foods high in beta-carotene and other carotenoids that can be converted to vitamin A. As discussed earlier in this chapter, dark green, orange, red, and deep yellow fruits and vegetables are good sources of beta-carotene, and thus of vitamin A. Carrots, spinach, mango, cantaloupe, and tomato juice are excellent sources of vitamin A because they contain beta-carotene.

What Happens If We Consume Too Much Vitamin A?

The retinoid forms of vitamin A are highly toxic, and toxicity symptoms develop after consuming only three to four times the RDA. Toxicity rarely results from food sources, but vitamin A supplements are known to have caused severe illness and even death. Consuming excess vitamin A while pregnant can cause serious birth defects and spontaneous abortions. Other toxicity symptoms include loss of appetite, blurred vision, hair loss, abdominal pain, nausea, diarrhea, and damage to the liver and nervous system. If caught in time, many of these symptoms are reversible once vitamin A supplementation is stopped. However, permanent damage can occur to the liver, eyes, and other organs. Because liver contains such a high amount of vitamin A, children and pregnant women should not consume liver on a daily or weekly basis.

What Happens If We Don't Consume Enough Vitamin A?

night blindness A vitamin A–deficiency disorder that results in the loss of the ability to see in dim light.

Night blindness is a condition caused by vitamin A deficiency. It results in the inability to adjust to dim light and can also result in the failure to regain sight quickly after a bright flash of light. As we discussed earlier, since the cone cells of the retina process colours, colour blindness can also result from a vitamin A deficiency.

How severe a problem is night blindness? Although less common among people of developed nations, vitamin A deficiency is a severe public health concern in low-income nations. Refer to the Highlight box "Global Nutrition" for a more complete discussion of this health issue.

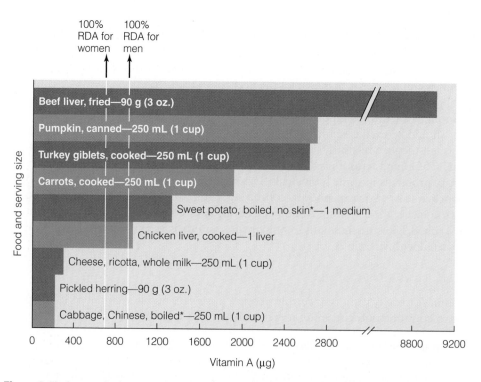

Figure 8.13 Common food sources of vitamin A. The RDA for vitamin A is 900 µg RAE per day for men and 700 µg RAE per day for women.

(Data from U.S. Department of Agriculture, Agricultural Research Service, USDA Nutrient Database for Standard Reference, Release 15, 2002, Nutrient Data Laboratory homepage, www.ars.usda.gov/main/site_main.htm?modecode=12354500, accessed August 2002.)

* These values are converted from carotene to µg vitamin A. See p. 281 for conversions to RAEs.

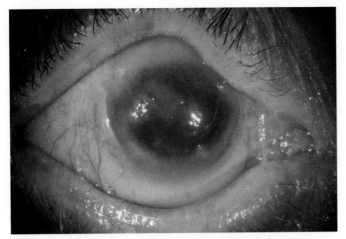

Xerophthalmia in a child. The hardening of the cornea can cause irreversible blindness.

If vitamin A deficiency progresses, it can result in irreversible blindness through hardening of the cornea (the transparent membrane covering the front of the eye), a condition called *xerophthalmia*. The prefix of this word, *xero*, comes from a Greek word meaning "dry." Lack of vitamin A causes the epithelial cells of the cornea to lose their ability to produce mucus, causing the eye to become very dry. This leaves the cornea susceptible to damage, infection, and hardening. Once the cornea hardens, the resulting blindness is irreversible. This is why it is critical to catch vitamin A deficiency in its early stages and treat it with either the regular consumption of fruits and vegetables that contain beta-carotene or with vitamin A supplementation.

Other deficiency symptoms include impaired immunity, increased risk of illness and infections, reproductive system disorders, and failure of normal growth. Individuals who are at risk for vitamin A deficiency include older adults with poor diets, young children with inadequate vegetable and fruit intakes, and alcoholics. Any condition that results in fat malabsorption can also lead to vitamin A deficiency. Children with cystic fibrosis; individuals with diseases of the liver, pancreas, or gallbladder; and people who consume large amounts of the fat substitute olestra are at risk for vitamin A deficiency.

> **Recap:** The role of vitamin A as an antioxidant is still under investigation. Vitamin A is critical for maintaining our vision. It is also necessary for cell differentiation, reproduction, and growth. The RDA for vitamin A is 900 μg (RAE) per day for men and 700 μg (RAE) per day for women. Animal livers, dairy products, and eggs are good animal sources of vitamin A; dark green, red, orange, and deep yellow fruits and vegetables are high in beta-carotene, which is used to synthesize vitamin A. Supplementation can be dangerous, as toxicity is reached at levels of only three to four times the RDA. Toxicity symptoms include birth defects, spontaneous abortions, blurred vision, and liver damage. Deficiency symptoms include night blindness, impaired immune function, and growth failure.

Selenium

Selenium is a trace mineral, and it is found in varying amounts in soil. As reviewed in Chapter 1, trace minerals are needed by our bodies in amounts less than 100 mg per day. Keep in mind that, although we need only minute amounts of trace minerals, they are just as important to our health as the vitamins and the major minerals.

Functions of Selenium

It is only recently that we have learned about the critical role of selenium as a nutrient in human health. In 1979, Chinese scientists reported an association between a heart

▶ **HIGHLIGHT**

Global Nutrition: Combating Vitamin A Deficiency Around the World

Vitamin A deficiency and its resultant illness, night blindness, is a major health concern in developing nations. Approximately 118 nations are affected, particularly African and Southeast Asian countries. According to the World Health Organization (WHO 2002), between 100 and 140 million children suffer from vitamin A deficiency. Of the children affected, 250 000 to 500 000 become permanently blinded every year. At least half of these children will die within one year of losing their sight. Death is due to infections and illnesses, including measles and diarrhea, that are easily treated in wealthier countries.

Vitamin A deficiency is also a tragedy for pregnant women in these countries. These women suffer from night blindness, are more likely to transmit HIV to their child if HIV-positive, and run a greater risk of maternal mortality.

What is being done to combat this tragedy? WHO has partnered with the United Nations International Children's Emergency Fund (UNICEF), the Canadian International Development Agency, the U.S. Agency for International Development, and the Micronutrient Initiative to bring the Vitamin A Global Initiative into high-risk countries. This initiative provides support to deliver vitamin A supplements through immunization programs.

Providing high-dose vitamin A supplements has reduced overall mortality by 23%, and it has reduced mortality from measles by 50%.

Although this is an important short-term solution, longer-term interventions include

- encouraging breastfeeding, since breast milk is a critical source of vitamin A for infants;
- fortifying with vitamin A the food sources that are readily available to high-risk groups;
- assisting in the development and maintenance of home and community gardens that provide a diverse supply of vitamin A–rich fruits and vegetables.

Significant progress has been made in the fight against vitamin A deficiency and night blindness. Despite this progress, there are still too many people suffering from this preventable disorder. A recent study of children in Bangladesh found that although the rate of night blindness in preschool children is decreasing, a significant number of children and pregnant women still show low serum retinol levels (Ahmed 1999). Children in Ethiopia also show alarmingly high rates of night blindness and low serum retinol levels (Haider and Demissie 1999). These findings illustrate that many people are still at risk for vitamin A deficiency and that the supplementation programs already employed must be strengthened with the intervention strategies listed above.

Keshan disease A heart disorder caused by selenium deficiency. It was first identified in children in the Keshan province of China.

disorder called **Keshan disease** and selenium deficiency. This disease occurs in children in the Keshan province of China, where the soil is depleted of selenium. The scientists found that Keshan disease can be prevented with selenium supplementation.

The selenium in our bodies is contained in proteins, or more specifically, amino acids. Two amino acid derivatives contain the majority of selenium in our bodies: *selenomethionine* is the storage form for selenium, while *selenocysteine* is the active form of selenium.

Selenium is a critical component of the antioxidant system, functioning as part of the glutathione peroxidase enzyme system mentioned earlier (page 270). Thus, selenium helps spare vitamin E and prevents oxidative damage to our cell membranes.

Selenium is also needed for the production of *thyroxine*, or thyroid hormone. By this action, selenium is involved in the maintenance of our basal metabolism and body temperature. Selenium appears to play a role in immune function, and poor selenium status is associated with higher rates of some forms of cancer. The functions, requirements, and toxicity and deficiency symptoms associated with selenium are listed in Table 8.1.

How Much Selenium Should We Consume?

Selenium content is highly variable in our foods. As it is a trace mineral, we need only minute amounts to maintain health.

Recommended Dietary Allowance for Selenium The RDA for selenium is 55 µg per day for both men and women. The UL is 400 µg per day.

Shopper's Guide: Good Food Sources of Selenium Selenium is present in both plant and animal food sources but in variable amounts. Because it is stored in the tissues of animals, selenium is found in reliably consistent amounts in animal foods. Organ meats, such as liver and kidney, pork, and seafood are particularly good sources of selenium (see Figure 8.14).

In contrast, the amount of selenium in plants is dependent upon the selenium content of the soil in which the plant is grown. Thus, the amount of selenium in the fruits and vegetables you eat can vary widely depending on the part of the world in which the plant is grown. Many companies marketing selenium supplements warn that the agricultural soils in North America are depleted of selenium and inform us that we need to take selenium supplements. In reality, the selenium content of soil varies greatly across North America, and because we obtain our food from a variety of geographic locations, few people suffer from selenium deficiency. This is especially true for people who eat even small quantities of meat or seafood. As indicated in Figure 8.14, nuts, wheat, and seafood are particularly rich sources of selenium.

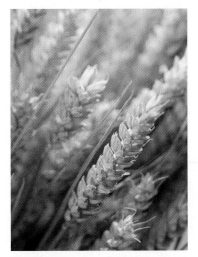

Wheat is a rich source of selenium.

What Happens If We Consume Too Much Selenium?

Selenium toxicity does not result from eating foods high in selenium. However, supplementation with selenium can cause toxicity. Toxicity symptoms include brittle hair and nails, which can eventually break and fall off. Other symptoms of toxicity include skin rashes, vomiting, nausea, weakness, and cirrhosis of the liver.

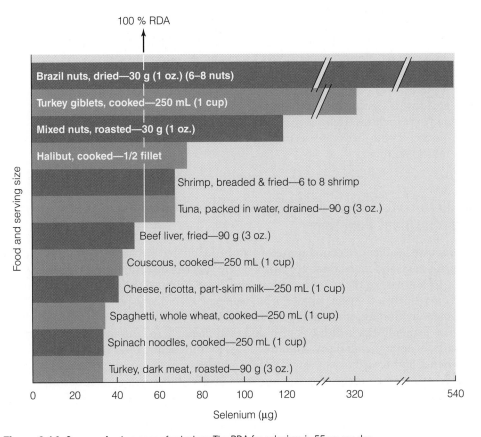

Figure 8.14 Common food sources of selenium. The RDA for selenium is 55 µg per day.

(Data from U.S. Department of Agriculture, Agricultural Research Service, USDA Nutrient Database for Standard Reference, Release 15, 2002, Nutrient Data Laboratory homepage, www.ars.usda.gov/main/site_main.htm?modecode=12354500, accessed August 2002.)

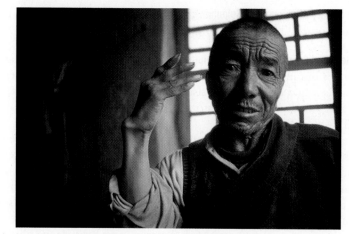

Selenium deficiency can lead to a deforming arthritis called Kashin-Beck disease.

What Happens If We Don't Consume Enough Selenium?

As discussed previously, selenium deficiency is associated with a special form of heart disease called Keshan disease. Selenium deficiency does not cause the disease, but selenium is necessary to help the immune system effectively fight the virus that causes the disease. Another deficiency disease is *Kashin-Beck disease,* a deforming arthritis found in selenium-depleted areas in China and in Tibet. Other deficiency symptoms include impaired immune responses, increased risk of viral infections, infertility, depression, hostility, impaired cognitive function, and muscle pain and wasting.

> **Recap:** Selenium is part of the glutathione peroxidase enzyme system. It indirectly spares vitamin E from oxidative damage, and it assists with immune function and the production of thyroid hormone. The RDA for selenium is 55 µg per day for men and women. Organ meats, pork, and seafood are good sources of selenium, as are nuts and wheat. The selenium content of plants is dependent upon the amount of selenium in the soil in which they are grown. Toxicity symptoms include brittle hair and nails, vomiting, nausea, and liver cirrhosis. Deficiency symptoms and side effects include Keshan disease, Kashin-Beck disease, impaired immune function, infertility, and muscle wasting.

Copper, Iron, Zinc, and Manganese Play a Peripheral Role in Antioxidant Function

As discussed earlier, there are numerous antioxidant enzyme systems in our bodies. Copper, zinc, and manganese are a part of the superoxide dismutase enzyme complex. Iron is part of the structure of catalase. In addition to their role in protecting us from oxidative damage, copper, iron, manganese, and zinc play major roles in the optimal functioning of many other enzymes in our bodies. Copper, iron, and zinc help us maintain the health of our blood, and manganese is an important cofactor in carbohydrate metabolism. The functions, requirements, food sources, and deficiency and toxicity symptoms of these nutrients are discussed in detail in Chapter 10, which focuses on the nutrients involved in energy metabolism and blood formation.

> **Recap:** Copper, zinc, and manganese are cofactors for the superoxide dismutase antioxidant enzyme system. Iron is a cofactor for the catalase antioxidant enzyme. These minerals play critical roles in blood health and energy metabolism.

What Disorders Are Related to Oxidation?

Through your experiences, you may have found that there are a plethora of claims related to the functions of antioxidants. These claims include the slowing of aging and age-related diseases and the prevention of cancer and heart disease. In opposition to these claims is some evidence that taking antioxidant supplements may be harmful for certain people (refer back to the Nutrition Myth or Fact box on beta-carotene, page 281). In this section, we will review what is currently known about the role of antioxidant nutrients in cancer, heart disease, and aging.

Cancer

Before we explore how antioxidants affect our risk for cancer, let's take a closer look at precisely what cancer is and how it spreads. **Cancer** is actually a group of diseases that are all characterized by cells that grow "out of control." By this we mean that cancer cells reproduce spontaneously and independently, and they are not inhibited by the boundaries of tissues and organs. Thus, they can aggressively invade tissues and organs far away from those in which they originally formed.

Most forms of cancer result in one or more **tumours**, which are newly formed masses of cells that are immature and may have no physiologic function. Although the word *tumour* sounds frightening, it is important to note that not every tumour is *malignant,* or cancerous. Many are *benign* (not harmful to us) and are made up of cells that will not spread widely.

Figure 8.15 shows how changes to normal cells prompt a series of other changes that can progress into cancer. There are three primary steps of cancer development: initiation, promotion, and progression.

1. *Initiation*—The initiation of cancer occurs when a cell's DNA is *mutated* (or changed). This mutation causes permanent changes in the cell.

2. *Promotion*—During this phase, the genetically altered cell is stimulated to repeatedly divide. The mutated DNA is locked into each new cell's genetic instructions. Since the enzymes that normally work to repair damaged cells cannot detect alterations in the DNA, the cells can continue to divide uninhibited.

3. *Progression*—During this phase, the cancerous cells grow out of control and invade surrounding tissues. These cells then *metastasize* (spread) to other sites of the body. In the early stages of progression, our immune system can sometimes detect these cancerous cells and destroy them. However, if the cells continue to grow, they develop into malignant tumours, and cancer results.

Genetic, Lifestyle, and Environmental Factors Can Increase Our Risk for Cancer

Cancer is the second leading cause of death in Canada. The Canadian Cancer Society estimates that there will be 166 400 new cases of cancer in 2008 and 73 800 cancer deaths. Based on the current number of new cases each year, 39% of women and 45% of men will develop cancer at some point during their lifetime (Canadian Cancer Society 2008). Are you and your loved ones at risk? The answer depends on several factors, including your family history of cancer, your exposure to environmental agents, and various lifestyle factors.

The Canadian Cancer Society estimates that 50% of cancers are preventable and advises consumers to follow its "Seven Steps to Health" (see Highlight, page 291). Five important factors are considered modifiable risk factors:

- *Tobacco use*—About 30% of all cancers and more than 85% of all lung cancers in Canada are attributed to tobacco use. More than 4000 compounds have been identified in tobacco and tobacco smoke, and more than 40 of these compounds are **carcinogens**, or substances that can cause cancer. Lung cancer is the leading

- Events in the Development of Cancer

cancer A group of diseases characterized by cells that reproduce spontaneously and independently and may invade other tissues and organs.

tumour Any newly formed mass of cells that are less differentiated than normal cells. Tumours can be benign (not harmful to us) or malignant (cancerous).

carcinogens Any substances capable of causing the cellular mutations that lead to cancer.

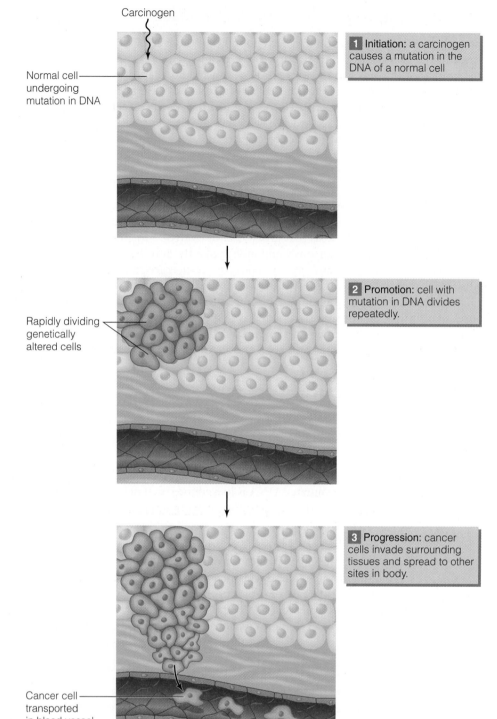

Carcinogen

Normal cell undergoing mutation in DNA

1 Initiation: a carcinogen causes a mutation in the DNA of a normal cell

Rapidly dividing genetically altered cells

2 Promotion: cell with mutation in DNA divides repeatedly.

3 Progression: cancer cells invade surrounding tissues and spread to other sites in body.

Cancer cell transported in blood vessel

Figure 8.15 Cancer cells develop as a result of a genetic mutation in the DNA of a normal cell. The mutated cell replicates uncontrollably, eventually resulting in a tumour. If not destroyed or removed, the cancerous tumour metastasizes and spreads to other parts of the body.

cause of cancer death in men and women in Canada (Canadian Cancer Society 2008). Smoking also increases your risk of developing cancers of the mouth, throat, larynx, cervix, pancreas, esophagus, colon, rectum, kidney, and bladder and can cause heart disease, stroke, and emphysema. People who don't smoke but are exposed to second-hand smoke are also at risk for cancer and other lung diseases. Each year in Canada, an estimated 1000 non-smokers die from exposure to second-hand smoke (Canadian Cancer Society 2008).

▶ **HIGHLIGHT**

Canadian Cancer Society's Seven Steps to Health

1. Be a nonsmoker and avoid second-hand smoke.
2. Eat 5 to 10 servings of vegetables and fruit a day. Choose high-fibre, lower-fat foods. If you drink alcohol, limit your intake to one to two drinks a day.
   - For a healthy diet, balance your daily meals with foods from the four food groups described in *Eating Well with Canada's Food Guide.*
3. Be physically active on a regular basis: this will also help you maintain a healthy body weight.
4. Protect yourself and your family from the sun.*
   - Check your skin regularly and report any changes to your doctor.
   - Avoid tanning parlours and sunlamps: they're not safe.
   - Keep babies under one year old out of direct sun.
   - When you are in the sun, always remember SLIP, SLAP, SLOP.
     - SLIP on clothing to cover your arms and legs.
     - SLAP on a wide-brimmed hat.
     - SLOP on sunscreen (SPF 15 or higher).
5. Follow cancer screening guidelines. One way to detect cancer early is to have regular screening tests.
   - For women, discuss mammography, Pap tests, and breast exams with a health professional.
   - For men, discuss testicular exams and prostate screening with a health professional.
   - Both men and women should also discuss screening for colon and rectal cancers.

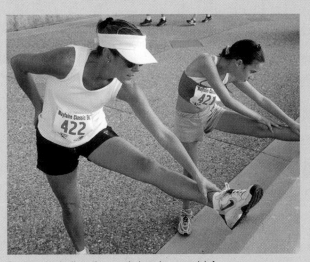

Staying physically active may help reduce our risk for some cancers.

6. Visit your doctor or dentist if you notice any change in your normal state of health (for example, sores that don't heal, a cough that goes on for more than two weeks, or a change in bowel habits).
7. Follow health and safety instructions at home and at work when using, storing, and disposing of hazardous materials. Health Canada and Environment Canada have guidelines for handling cancer-causing substances.

* Note that some exposure to the sun is needed for normal vitamin D synthesis in the skin. See Chapter 9 for the role of vitamin D in bone health.

Source: Canadian Cancer Society, Seven Steps to Health, www.cancer.ca (updated 2007; accessed May 2008). Adapted with permission of the Canadian Cancer Society, 2008.

- *Exposure to the sun*—Skin cancer is the most commonly diagnosed cancer in Canada. And most cases of skin cancer are linked to exposure to the sun. The ultraviolet (UV) rays of the sun can damage the DNA of your skin cells and increase your risk for skin cancer, even if you do not get sunburned. Skin cancer includes the non-melanoma (basal cell and squamous cell) cancers and melanoma, the latter of which is the most deadly. Skin cancer can be cured if caught early. Wearing a sunscreen with at least a 15 SPF (sun protection factor) and protective clothing, and avoiding the sun between 11 a.m. and 4 p.m. can help lower your risk for skin cancer. If you are going to be outside for most of the day, choose a sunscreen with at least a 30 SPF and that has "broad spectrum" or "protects against both UVA and UVB ultraviolet rays" on the label (Canadian Cancer Society 2008).

- *Nutrition*—Researchers estimate that 30% to 35% of all cancers may be prevented by eating a healthy diet, being physically active, and having a healthy

Table 8.2   Nutritional Factors That Can Influence Our Risk for Cancer

Factors That May Increase Cancer Risk	Factors That May Be Protective Against Cancer*	Factors Falsely Claimed to Cause Cancer
Heterocyclic amines in cooked meat: carcinogenic chemicals formed when meat is cooked at high temperatures, such as during broiling, barbecuing, and frying.	Antioxidants: includes vitamins E, C, A, beta-carotene and other carotenoids, and minerals, such as selenium. Supplementation with individual antioxidants does not show consistent benefits.	Fluoridated water: studies conducted over the past 40 years show no association between drinking fluoridated water and increased cancer risk.
Nitrates in drinking water: a carcinogenic chemical found in fertilizers that is proven to increase the risk of non-Hodgkin's lymphoma. People drinking contaminated tap water in agricultural areas may be at risk.	Dietary fibre: some studies show reduced risks for esophagus, colon, and rectal cancer with increased fibre intake, although findings are not consistent.	Food additives: it is estimated that more than 15 000 substances are added to our foods during growth, processing, and packaging. To date, there is no evidence that food additives contribute significantly to cancer risk.
Nitrites and nitrates: compounds found in cured meats, such as sausage, ham, bacon, and some lunch meats. These compounds bind with amino acids to form nitrosamines, which are potent carcinogens linked to stomach cancer.	Phytoestrogens: compounds found in soy-based foods and some vegetables and grains that may decrease the risk for breast, endometrial, and prostate cancers.	
Obesity: appears to increase the risk of cancers of the breast (postmenopause), colon, prostate, endometrium (the lining of the uterus), kidney, gallbladder, liver, pancreas, rectum, and esophagus (World Cancer Research Fund/AICR 2007). The exact link between obesity and increased cancer risk is not clear but may be linked with hormonal changes that occur with having excess body fat.	Coffee: some researchers suggest that foods and beverages containing phenols may be more important antioxidants than vitamins because they are found in larger amounts in the North American diet. Coffee is high in phenolic acids and in a recent study was shown to contribute, on average, 31% of the antioxidants in a typical North American diet.	
High-fat diet: has been associated with increased risk of many cancers, including prostate and breast. However, not all studies support this association.	Tea: like coffee, tea contains phenolic acids, which are the major antioxidants in the North American diet. In 2007 Health Canada approved three health claims for tea: tea is a "source of antioxidants for the maintenance of good health"; "increases alertness" and "helps to maintain and/or support cardiovascular health."	
Alcohol: use is linked with an increased risk of cancers of the esophagus, pharynx, and mouth. Alcohol use may also increase the risk for cancers of the liver, breast, colon, and rectum (World Cancer Research Fund/AICR 2007). Alcohol may impair the cell's ability to repair damaged DNA, increasing the possibility of cancer initiation.	Omega-3 fatty acids: includes alpha-linolenic acid, eicosapentaenoic acid (EPA), and docosahexaenoic acid (DHA). These fatty acids are found in fish and fish oils. Consuming foods high in omega-3 fatty acids is associated with reduced rates of colon and rectal cancers.	

Source: Information gathered from the American Cancer Society (www.cancer.org, accessed July 2002), the National Cancer Institute (www.cancer.gov, accessed July 2002), and P. Greenwald, C. K. Clifford, and J. A. Milner, Diet and cancer prevention, 2001, *European Journal of Cancer*, 37:948–965.

* Eating a diet high in whole grains, fruits, and vegetables: such a diet is associated with lower cancer risks.

body weight (Canadian Cancer Society 2008) (see Table 8.2). Eating more vegetables and fruit has been shown to reduce the risk for cancers of the esophagus, mouth, stomach, colon, rectum, lung, and prostate, and it may also reduce the risk for breast cancer in premenopausal women (Zhang et al. 1999). Nutritional factors that may be protective against cancer include antioxidants, dietary fibre, and phytochemicals, which are chemicals in plants that may provide significant health benefits (discussed in detail on page 294).

- *Environmental and occupational exposures*—These include such things as cigarette and cigar smoke, chemicals in our food and water supply, sun exposure, infectious diseases, radiation, and chemicals in the workplace. Proven carcinogens found in various workplaces include benzene, asbestos, vinyl chloride, arsenic, coal tars, radon, wood dust, and aflatoxins (produced by moulds in agricultural products, such as peanuts). Only two forms of radiation have been linked to cancer: ionizing and ultraviolet. Ionizing radiation sources include x-rays, gamma rays, cosmic rays, radon, and particles given off by radioactive materials. Our primary source of ultraviolet rays is from the sun.

- *Level of physical activity*—Studies conducted over the past 10 years have shown a possible link between lower cancer risk and higher levels of physical activity. A recent review of these studies has found that higher levels of leisure and occupational physical activity are associated with a 20% to 30% reduction in our overall risk for cancer (Thune and Furberg 2001). Exercise was found to have to a clear protective effect specifically for breast and colon cancers. Furthermore, the intensity of physical activity appears to be important, as the reduction in risk was found only for moderate or vigorous intensity activity. At this time, we don't know how exercise reduces the overall risk for cancer or for certain types of cancer. Suggested mechanisms include (1) improved circulation; (2) increased ventilation and shortened bowel transit time, which reduces the time our lungs and bowels are exposed to potential carcinogens; (3) maintenance of healthier body weights; (4) improved immune function; (5) modulation of sex hormones, such as estrogen and testosterone, which could reduce the risk of breast, endometrial, ovarian, testicular, and prostate cancers; and (6) enhanced repair of damaged DNA. None of these mechanisms have been sufficiently studied to allow us to draw any firm conclusions about how physical activity may protect against cancer.

Antioxidants Play a Role in Preventing Cancer

There is a large and growing body of evidence that antioxidants play an important role in cancer prevention. How do antioxidants work to reduce our risk for cancer? Some proposed mechanisms include

- enhancing our immune system, which assists in the destruction and removal of precancerous cells from our bodies;

- inhibiting the growth of cancer cells and tumours;

- preventing oxidative damage to our cells' DNA by scavenging free radicals and stopping the formation and subsequent chain reaction of oxidized molecules.

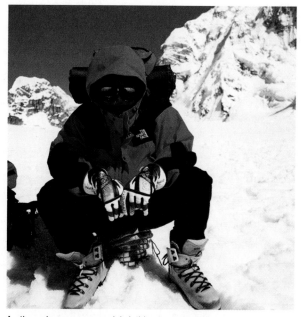

Although very few studies show benefits of individual antioxidant nutrients, such as vitamins E, C, beta-carotene, and selenium, eating whole foods that are high in these nutrients—especially fruits, vegetables, and whole grains—is consistently shown to be associated with decreased cancer risk (Greenwald, Clifford, and Milner 2001). Additional studies show that populations eating diets low in antioxidant nutrients have a higher risk for cancer. These studies show a strong association between eating whole foods high in antioxidants and lower cancer risk, but they do not prove cause and effect. Nutrition experts agree that there are important interactions between antioxidant nutrients and other substances in foods, such as fibre and phytochemicals, which work together to reduce the risk for many types of cancers. Studies are now being conducted to determine whether eating foods high in antioxidants directly causes lower rates of cancer.

The link between taking antioxidant supplements and reducing cancer risk is not very clear. Laboratory animal and test tube studies show that the individual nutrients reviewed in this

Arctic explorers wear special clothing to protect themselves from the cold, as well as the high levels of ultraviolet rays from the sun.

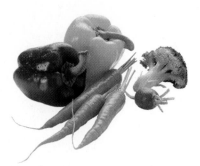

Eating more fruits and vegetables has been shown to reduce the risk of several cancers.

chapter act as antioxidants in various situations. However, supplementation studies in humans do not consistently show benefits of taking antioxidant supplements in the prevention of cancer and other diseases. For example, in the Alpha-Tocopherol Beta-Carotene Cancer Prevention Study discussed earlier in the Nutrition Myth or Fact box (Albanes et al. 1995), supplementation with vitamin E resulted in a lower risk for cancers of the prostate, colon, and rectum, but was related to more cancers of the stomach. In this same study, beta-carotene supplements increased risk for cancers of the lung, prostate, and stomach in current and former smokers (Heinonen et al. 1998). In the Nutritional Prevention of Cancer Trial (Clark et al. 1998), selenium supplementation was found to reduce the risk of prostate, colon, and lung cancers, but it did not reduce the risk of non-melanoma skin cancers. The Linxian intervention trials, named for the region of China where the studies were conducted, found that a supplement containing beta-carotene, vitamin E, and selenium reduced mortality from overall cancer, specifically reducing the risk for cancers of the esophagus and stomach (Blot et al. 1995).

Why do antioxidant supplements appear to work in some studies and for some cancers but not in others? The human body is very complex, as is the development and progression of the numerous forms of cancer. People differ substantially in their susceptibility for cancer and in their response to protective factors and to cancer-causing agents. These complexities cloud the relationship between nutrition and cancer. It is impossible to control all factors that may increase our risk for cancer in any research study. Thus, there are many unknown factors that can affect study outcomes. It has also been speculated that antioxidants taken in supplemental form may act as pro-oxidants in some situations, but consuming antioxidants in the form of food may provide these nutrients in a more balanced state. Current recommendations are to meet nutrient need through diet alone; supplements are not recommended for cancer prevention (AICR 2007). Refer to the Nutrition Debate at the end of the chapter to gain a better understanding of situations that may warrant vitamin and mineral supplementation.

Phytochemicals Contribute to Cancer Prevention

phytochemicals Chemicals found in plants (*phyto* is from the Greek word for plant), such as pigments and other substances, that have biological activity in the body.

Phytochemicals are naturally occurring chemicals in plants that are biologically active in the body. Phytochemicals are found in abundance in fruits, vegetables, whole grains, legumes, seeds, soy products, garlic, onion, and green and black teas. Table 8.3 lists many of the phytochemicals that are linked to cancer prevention.

Table 8.3 Food Sources of Various Phytochemicals

Phytochemical	Example	Food Sources
Carotenoids	Alpha-carotene, beta-carotene, lycopene, lutein	Yellow-red, red, orange, and deep green vegetables and fruit, such as carrots, cantaloupe, sweet potatoes, apricots, kale, spinach, pumpkin, and tomatoes
Glucosinolates, isothiocyanates, indoles	Glucobrassicin, indole-3-carbinol	Cruciferous vegetables, such as broccoli, cabbage, cauliflower, and Brussels sprouts
Organosulphur compounds	Diallyl sulphide, allyl methyl trisulphide, dithiolthiones	Allium vegetables, including onion and garlic, and cruciferous vegetables, such as broccoli, cabbage, cauliflower, and Brussels sprouts
Polyphenols	Flavonoids and phenolic acids	Apple skins, berries, broccoli, citrus fruit, red wine, black and green tea
Phytoestrogens	Isoflavones, lignans	Soybeans and soy-based foods, vegetables, rye

Source: Adapted from P. Greenwald C. K. Clifford, and J. A. Milner, Diet and cancer prevention, 2002, *European Journal of Cancer* 37:948–965. Copyright © 2001, with permission from Elsevier.

Phytochemicals have been studied in the laboratory, and they exhibit clear cancer-prevention properties under this condition. At this time, our knowledge of phytochemicals and their effect on cancer in humans is in its infancy. We do not know the specific phytochemical content of most foods, and a marker (or markers) of phytochemical intake in humans has not yet been discovered. Progress is being made in this area of research, however. There is growing evidence that phytochemicals, such as lycopene (found in tomato products), organosulphur compounds (found in garlic, onions, and cruciferous vegetables), flavonoids (found in fruits, vegetables, tea, and red wine), and phytoestrogens (found in whole grains, vegetables, and soy products) may reduce the risk for some forms of cancer (Greenwald et al. 2001). Future studies will provide insight into how phytochemicals work to reduce our risk for cancer, how these substances work in conjunction with other nutrients to improve health, and whether supplementing our diets with phytochemicals is protective against chronic diseases.

> **Recap:** Cancer is a group of diseases in which genetically mutated cells grow out of control. Tobacco use, sun exposure, nutritional factors, radiation and chemical exposures, and low physical activity levels are related to a higher risk for some cancers. Eating foods high in antioxidants is associated with lower rates of cancer, but studies of antioxidant supplements and cancer are equivocal. Phytochemicals are recently discovered substances in plants that may reduce our risk for cancer.

Cardiovascular Disease

The details of *cardiovascular disease* (*CVD*) and its relationship to cholesterol and lipoproteins were presented in Chapter 5. A brief review of CVD is presented in this section, and an explanation is provided on how antioxidants may reduce our risk for CVD.

CVD is the leading cause of death for adults in Canada, but the rates of heart disease and stroke have declined 50% over the past 20 years (Heart and Stroke Foundation of Canada 2008). CVD encompasses all diseases of the heart and blood vessels, including coronary heart disease, hypertension (or high blood pressure), and atherosclerosis (or hardening of the arteries). The two primary manifestations of CVD are heart attack and stroke. In 2004, 31% of the deaths among men of all ages were linked to CVD; among women, the figure was 33%. Health Canada has estimated that CVD costs the Canadian economy $6818 million in direct health care and $11 655 million in indirect costs each year (Heart and Stroke Foundation 2003).

Remember that the major risks for CVD are

- smoking;
- hypertension (high blood pressure);
- high blood levels of low-density lipoprotein (LDL) cholesterol;
- obesity;
- sedentary lifestyle.

Other risk factors include a low level of high-density lipoprotein (HDL) cholesterol, impaired glucose tolerance or diabetes, family history (CVD in males younger than 55 years of age and females younger than 65 years of age), being a male older than 45 years of age, and menopause in women. Although we cannot alter our gender, family history, or age, we can change our nutrition and physical activity habits to reduce our risk for CVD.

Research has recently identified a risk factor for CVD that may be even more important than elevated cholesterol levels. This risk factor is a condition called *low-grade inflammation* (de Ferranti and Rifai 2002). This condition weakens the plaque in the blood vessels, making it more fragile. You may remember from Chapter 5 that plaque is the fatty material that builds on the inside of our arteries and causes hardening of the arteries. As the plaque becomes more fragile, it is more likely to burst and break away from the sides of our arteries. It may then form a blood clot that closes off

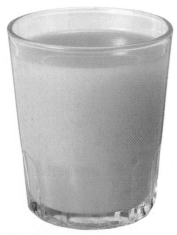

Folate, found in orange juice, can help reduce the risk of CVD.

the vessels of the heart or brain, leading to a heart attack or stroke, respectively. The marker in our bodies that indicates the degree of inflammation is C-reactive protein. Having higher levels of C-reactive protein increases our risk for a heart attack even if we do not have elevated cholesterol levels. For people with high levels of C-reactive protein and cholesterol, their risk of a heart attack is almost nine times as high as that of someone with normal cholesterol and C-reactive protein levels. These findings have prompted the medical community to develop standards for testing C-reactive protein along with cholesterol as a test for CVD risk.

How can antioxidants decrease our risk for CVD? There is growing evidence that certain antioxidants, specifically vitamin E and lycopene, work in a variety of ways that reduce the damage to our vessels, which in turn reduces our risk of a heart attack or stroke. Some of the ways these nutrients decrease our risk for CVD include

- *Scavenging free radicals*—This action prevents oxidative damage to the LDLs. Remember from Chapter 5 that oxidized LDL particles stimulate the buildup of plaque in the blood vessel walls.

- *Reducing low-grade inflammation*—This action can prevent the rupture of plaque in the blood vessels, thus preventing the release of clots that can cause a heart attack or stroke.

- *Reducing blood coagulation and the formation of clots*—Vitamin E has known anticoagulant properties. This means that it acts to prevent excessive thickening and clotting of the blood, preventing the formation of clots that can block blood vessels.

As with the research conducted on cancer, the studies of antioxidants and CVD show inconsistent results. Two large-scale surveys conducted in the United States show that men and women who eat more fruits and vegetables have a significantly reduced risk of CVD (Joshipura et al. 2001; Liu et al. 2001). However, few intervention studies have been conducted to determine the effect of antioxidant supplements on risk for CVD. Vitamin E was found to lower the number of heart disease deaths in smokers in the Alpha-Tocopherol Beta-Carotene Cancer Prevention Study (The ATBC Study Group 1994) but had no overall effect on the risk of stroke. In the HOPE study (The HOPE Investigators 2000), vitamin E had no impact on the risk for CVD in people who are at high risk for heart attack and stroke. The Women's Health Study showed no benefit of vitamin E on cardiovascular events or mortality. The American Heart Association does not recommend vitamin E supplements to reduce CVD risk; there is the possibility that vitamin E supplements are associated with increased mortality (AHA 2006).

It is important to note that there are other compounds (besides antioxidants) that are found in fruits, vegetables, and whole grains that can reduce our risk for CVD. For instance, soluble fibre has been shown to reduce elevated LDL cholesterol and total cholesterol. The most successful effects have been found in people eating oatmeal and oat bran cereals. Dietary fibre in general has been shown to reduce blood pressure, lower total cholesterol levels, and improve blood glucose and insulin levels. Folate, a B vitamin, is found in fortified cereals, green leafy vegetables, bananas, legumes, and orange juice. Folate is known to reduce homocysteine levels in the blood, and a high concentration of homocysteine in the blood is thought to be a risk factor for CVD. A recent study from the Netherlands showed that individuals who drank more than three cups of black tea (which is high in flavonoids) had a lower rate of heart attacks than non-tea drinkers (Geleijnse et al. 2002). Thus, it appears that there are a plethora of nutrients and other components in fruits, vegetables, and whole-grain foods that may be protective against CVD.

Recap: Cardiovascular disease (CVD) is the leading cause of death in Canada. Risk factors for CVD include smoking, hypertension, high LDL cholesterol, obesity, and a sedentary lifestyle. Antioxidants may help reduce our risk for heart disease by preventing oxidative damage to LDL cholesterol, reducing inflammation in our blood vessels, and reducing the formation of blood clots.

Vision Impairment and Other Results of Aging

In most Eastern and non-industrialized cultures, aging is viewed as a natural and desirable process that begins with conception and ends with death. The aged are respected and valued for their wisdom and experience and are often the decision makers in their communities. In contrast, for centuries, many people in Western countries have searched to find an elixir of eternal youth. Today, researchers continue this search, developing skin creams, supplements, botulism toxin injections, and new techniques of plastic surgery to conceal or fight the effects of aging. Despite these efforts, aging is inevitable.

Antioxidant supplements have received a great deal of attention as potential substances to reverse the effects of aging. This is because the process of aging is associated with increased oxidative damage and reduced activity of antioxidant enzymes in most body tissues. Despite this link between antioxidants and aging, there is no scientific evidence to support the contention that taking antioxidant supplements can prolong our lives.

However, we know that our ability to digest, absorb, and metabolize many nutrients is impaired as we age (refer to Chapter 16 for more detailed information on aging). These nutritional limitations have prompted some experts to suggest that specific RDAs be increased for adults according to new, narrower age brackets, such as 51 to 60 years, 61 to 70 years, 71 to 80 years, and 81 to 90 years. Currently, the RDAs are defined for adults 51 to 70 years and 71 years and older. A great deal more will be learned about optimal nutrition for older adults over the next decade as people live longer and we learn more about how our nutritional needs change as we age.

There are some diseases associated with aging that may be preventable by consuming antioxidants. Two of these diseases are *macular degeneration* and *cataracts*, both of which impair vision in older adults.

Macular degeneration is the leading cause of legal blindness among Canadians 60 years and older. The macula is the central part of the retina (Figure 8.16a), and it is responsible for our central vision and our ability to see details. When a person has macular degeneration, he or she loses the ability to see details, such as small print, small objects, and facial features. Objects seem to fade or disappear, straight lines or edges appear wavy or curved, and the ability to read standard print type is lost (Figure 8.16b). Macular degeneration does not affect our peripheral vision.

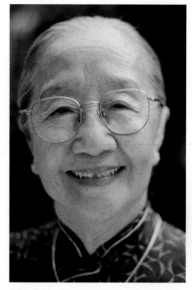

Aging is a natural and inevitable process of life.

macular degeneration A vision disorder caused by deterioration of the central portion of the retina and marked by loss or distortion of the central field of vision.

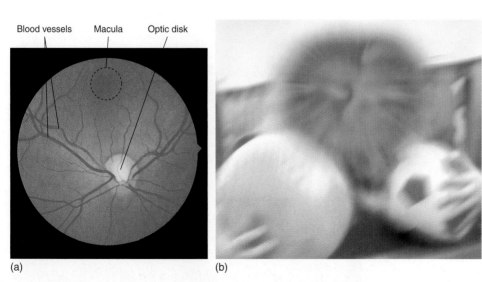

(a)   (b)

Figure 8.16 Macular degeneration is the leading cause of blindness in adults age 60 years and older. (a) The macula is the central part of the retina that allows us to see details and small print. (b) This simulation of the vision loss typical in patients with macular degeneration illustrates the loss of central vision.

(Source: National Eye Institute, National Institutes of Health, November 2003, Photos, Images, and Videos, Ref # EDS05, www.nei.nih.gov/photo/search/ref_num.asp?ref=EDS05&Submit=Go (accessed February 2004).

There is no known cure for macular degeneration. The causes of this disease are unknown, but proposed causes include

- lack of nutrients to the retina, including antioxidant nutrients;
- poor circulation in the retina;
- untreated health problems that cause undue pressure to the eye, such as high blood pressure; other health problems, such as high cholesterol and diabetes may degenerate the macula over time;
- excessive exposure to ultraviolet rays;
- genetic susceptibility.

cataract A damaged portion of the eye's lens, which causes cloudiness that impairs vision.

A **cataract** is a damaged portion of the eye's lens (Figure 8.17a), the portion of the eye through which we focus entering light. Cataracts cause cloudiness in the lens that impairs vision (Figure 8.17b). People with cataracts have a very difficult time seeing in bright light; for instance, they see halos around lights, glare, and scattering of light. Having cataracts also impairs a person's ability to adjust from dark to bright light. It is estimated that 15% of the blindness in Canada is attributable to cataracts.

Cataracts can be treated with surgery. As with macular degeneration, the causes of cataracts are unknown. However, some possible causes of cataracts include

- free radical damage caused by exposure to oxygen, ultraviolet light, and x-rays;
- inflammation caused by some eye diseases;
- use of certain drugs, such as corticosteroids;
- complications of diabetes.

Current research findings are showing some promise of reducing the risk for macular degeneration and cataracts through the use of antioxidant supplements. A recent study conducted with individuals who had early signs of macular degeneration found that consuming an antioxidant supplement reduced the progression of this disease (Age-Related Eye Disease Study Research Group 2001a). Earlier studies have also shown that higher blood levels of antioxidants and consuming more antioxidants in the diet are associated with a lower risk of macular degeneration (Delcourt et al. 1999;

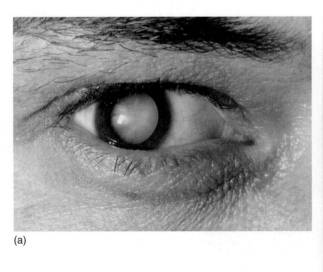

(a)

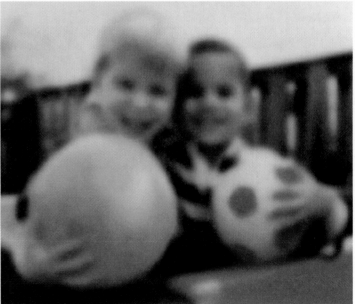

(b)

Figure 8.17 A cataract from a clouded lens (a) and the visual field (b). Source: National Eye Institute, National Institutes of Health, November 2003, Photos, Images, and Videos, Ref # EDS03, www.nei.nih.gov/photo/search/ref_num.asp?ref=EDS03&Submit=Go (accessed February 2004).

West et al. 1994). The effects of antioxidant supplements and cataracts are mixed, with some studies showing a reduced rate of cataract development in people taking antioxidant supplements or having higher blood levels of antioxidants (Chylack et al. 2002; Gale et al. 2001), but other studies showing no benefit of antioxidants (Age-Related Eye Disease Study Research Group 2001b).

At this time, it is not possible to reach a conclusion regarding the effectiveness of antioxidant supplements to prevent these two diseases of aging. However, there is enough evidence that consuming a healthful diet that includes fruits, vegetables, and whole grains is associated with improved quality of life as we age.

> **Recap:** There is no evidence that antioxidants can reverse or prevent aging in humans or significantly prolong our lives. Macular degeneration and cataracts are two diseases of vision that are associated with aging. Antioxidant nutrients have been found to reduce the risk of these diseases in some studies.

CHAPTER SUMMARY

- Antioxidants are compounds that protect our cells from oxidative damage.

- Free radicals are produced under many situations, including when our body generates ATP, when our immune system fights infection, and when we are exposed to environmental toxins, such as pollution, overexposure to the sun, radiation, and tobacco smoke.

- Free radicals are dangerous because they can damage the lipid portion of our cell membranes, destroying the integrity of our cell membranes. Free radicals also damage LDLs, cell proteins, and DNA.

- Antioxidant vitamins donate their electrons or hydrogen molecules to free radicals to neutralize them. Antioxidant minerals are cofactors in antioxidant enzyme systems, which convert free radicals to less damaging substances that our body excretes.

- Vitamin E is an antioxidant that protects the fatty components of cell membranes from oxidation. It also protects LDLs, vitamin A, and our lungs from oxidative damage. Other functions of vitamin E are the development of nerves and muscles, enhancement of the immune function, and improvement of the absorption of vitamin A if intake of vitamin A is low.

- Vitamin C is an antioxidant that is oxidized by free radicals and prevents the damage of cells and tissues. Vitamin C also regenerates vitamin E after it has been oxidized. Other functions of vitamin C include helping the synthesis of collagen, various hormones, neurotransmitters, and DNA; enhancing immune function; and increasing the absorption of iron.

- Beta-carotene is 1 of about 600 carotenoids identified to date. Beta-carotene is a provitamin, or precursor, to vitamin A, meaning it is an inactive form of vitamin A that is converted to vitamin A in the body.

- Beta-carotene appears to have some antioxidant activity by protecting the lipid portions of our membranes and the LDL cholesterol from oxidative damage. Other functions of beta-carotene include enhancing our immune system, protecting our skin from sun damage, and protecting our eyes from oxidative damage. The carotenoids may help reduce our risk for some forms of cancer.

- Vitamin A is a fat-soluble vitamin. The three active forms of vitamin A are retinol, retinal, and retinoic acid. Beta-carotene is converted to vitamin A in our small intestine.

- Vitamin A is extremely important for healthy vision. It ensures our ability to adjust to changes in the brightness of light, and it also helps us maintain colour vision. Vitamin A may also act as an antioxidant, as it protects LDL cholesterol from oxidative damage, but this needs to be confirmed. Other functions of vitamin A include assistance in cell differentiation, sexual reproduction, and proper bone growth.

- Selenium is a trace mineral. Selenium is part of the structure of glutathione peroxidases, a family of antioxidant enzymes. These enzymes break down fatty acids that have become oxidized, which indirectly spares vitamin E from oxidation and helps prevent oxidative damage to our cell membranes and fatty tissues. Other functions of selenium include assisting in the production of thyroid hormone and enhancing immune function.

CHAPTER SUMMARY

- Copper, iron, zinc, and manganese are minerals that act as cofactors for antioxidant enzyme systems. Cofactors are necessary to allow enzymes to function properly. Copper, zinc, and manganese are part of the superoxide dismutase complex, while iron is part of catalase. These minerals also play critical roles in energy metabolism and blood formation.

- Antioxidants play a role in cancer prevention. Eating foods high in antioxidants results in lower rates of some cancers, but supplementing with antioxidants has been linked to an increased risk of cancer in some situations.

- Phytochemicals are naturally occurring components in food that may reduce our risk for diseases. Phytochemicals are found in fruits, vegetables, nuts, seeds, whole grains, soy products, garlic, onion, and tea. The impact of phytochemicals on reducing our risk for cancer is still under investigation.

- Antioxidants may help reduce our risk for CVD by scavenging free radicals and preventing oxidative damage to LDL cholesterol, reducing low-grade inflammation (which in turn prevents the rupture of plaque in our blood vessels), and preventing the formation of blood clots.

- Antioxidants may help prevent two age-related diseases of vision: macular degeneration and cataracts. Macular degeneration causes us to lose the ability to see details, small print, and facial features. A cataract is a damaged portion of the eye's lens. This damage leads to cloudiness and impairs vision. Cataracts impair our ability to adjust from dark to bright light. Antioxidant supplements have been found to reduce the risk for macular degeneration and cataracts in some studies.

mynutritionlab Go to MyNutritionLab at www.pearsoned.ca/mynutritionlab and enrich your understanding of nutrition! You'll find key animations, interactive exercises, access to My DietAnalysis, and much more.

REVIEW QUESTIONS

Quizzes

1. Which of the following is a characteristic of vitamin E?
   a. It enhances the absorption of iron
   b. It can be manufactured from beta-carotene
   c. It is a critical component of the glutathione peroxidase system
   d. It is destroyed by exposure to high heat

2. Oxidation is best described as a process in which
   a. a carcinogen causes a mutation in a stem cell's DNA.
   b. an atom loses an electron.
   c. an element loses an atom of oxygen.
   d. a compound loses a molecule of water.

3. Which of the following disorders is linked with the production of free radicals?
   a. Cardiovascular disease
   b. Carotenosis
   c. Ulcers
   d. Malaria

4. Which of the following are known carcinogens?
   a. Phytochemicals
   b. Antioxidants
   c. Carotenoids
   d. Nitrates

5. Taking daily doses of three to four times the RDA of which of the following nutrients may cause toxicity?
   a. Vitamin A
   b. Vitamin C
   c. Vitamin E
   d. Selenium

6. Which best describes the danger of free radicals?
   a. They impair eye sight
   b. They destabilize our cells
   c. They cause hemorrhaging
   d. They are associated with Kashin-Beck disease

7. Vitamin C helps regenerate
   a. vitamin A.
   b. vitamin E.
   c. beta-carotene.
   d. selenium.

8. Which is not a good source of selenium?
   a. Pork
   b. Seafood
   c. Nuts
   d. Legumes

9. Elena has had a heart attack in the past and her doctor has since prescribed her Aspirin. She has turned a new leaf since her attack and is doing much better now with daily exercise in addition to proper nutrition. In being more health conscious, Elena has thought about taking vitamin supplements and asks her health care provider for advice. Which vitamin supplement should Elena be careful with?

10. Natalie and William are welcoming their first child in four months. Being a doting husband, William has tirelessly run to the grocery store every time Natalie has had a craving. For the past two weeks, she has been craving fried beef liver and pumpkin puree almost every day. Should William be worried? What toxicity symptoms should he be looking for?

11. Explain how free radicals damage cell membranes and lead to cell death.

12. Describe the process by which cancer occurs, beginning with initiation and ending with metastasis of the cancer to widespread body tissues.

13. Explain why people taking anticoagulants should avoid vitamin E supplementation.

14. Discuss the contribution of trace minerals, such as selenium, to the prevention of oxidation.

15. Explain how vitamin E reduces our risk for heart disease.

CASE STUDY

Breast Cancer Awareness Month is always a tough time for Sylvie because it brings back painful memories of her mother's struggle with this disease. Despite this, Sylvie believes that she is at no greater risk for developing cancer. She reasons that she makes sure to eat a piece of fruit or a vegetable at each meal and she eats red meat only two or three times a week. She doesn't smoke or drink, and she gets lots of sunshine and exercise because she works outside all day.

a. What lifestyle factors reduce Sylvie's risk of cancer?
b. What factors increase her risk?
c. What do you think of Sylvie's diet?
d. What might you suggest she change about her lifestyle to help reduce her risk of developing cancer?

Test Yourself Answers

1. **False** Currently, there is no known dietary cure for cancer. However, eating a diet that is plentiful in fruits and vegetables, and exercising regularly, may help reduce our risk for some forms of cancer.

2. **True** Overall, the research on vitamin C and colds does not show strong evidence that taking vitamin C supplements reduces our risk of suffering from the common cold.

3. **False** Some natural sources of calcium, for example, contain lead and other substances that are harmful.

4. **False** By eating at least 5 servings of fruits and vegetables each day, we can consume enough antioxidants in our diets.

5. **True** Consuming antioxidants may reduce the risk of macular degeneration and cataracts.

WEB LINKS

www.cancer.ca
The Canadian Cancer Society
Click on Prevention for more information on ways you can reduce your risk of cancer. To learn about different types of cancers, click on About Cancer. For descriptions of cancer research underway in Canada, click on Cancer Research.

www.heartandstroke.com
Heart and Stroke Foundation of Canada
Find out about your own personal risk profile by taking the Heart and Stroke Risk Assessment. This profile will also provide a free, confidential, customized action plan for healthy living.

www.cnib.ca
The Canadian National Institute for the Blind
Find out more about common causes of vision loss in Canada, and the support services available.

www.ffb.ca
The Foundation Fighting Blindness—Canada
Learn more about age-related macular degeneration.

http://healthycanadians.ca/pr-rp/billC-51_e.html
Natural Health Products Directorate, Health Products and Food Branch, Health Canada
Visit this site to learn more about the federal government regulations for natural health products.

www.who.int/topics/en
World Health Organization (WHO)
Click on Health Topics and select "deficiency diseases" to find out more about vitamin A deficiency around the world.

www.nei.nih.gov
National Eye Institute
Visit this site to find out more about how macular degeneration and cataracts can impair vision.

www.fda.gov
U.S. Food and Drug Administration (FDA)
Select Dietary Supplements from the pull-down menu for more information on how to make informed decisions and evaluate information related to dietary supplements.

www.nal.usda.gov/fnic
The Food and Nutrition Information Center (FNIC)
Click the Dietary Supplements button to obtain information on vitamin and mineral supplements, including consumer reports and industry regulations.

http://ods.od.nih.gov
Office of Dietary Supplements
Go to this site to obtain current research results and reliable information about dietary supplements.

Vitamin and Mineral Supplementation: Necessity or Waste?

Ben has type 2 diabetes and high blood cholesterol and is worried about his health. He attended a nutrition seminar in which the health benefits of various vitamin and mineral supplements were touted. After attending this seminar, Ben was convinced that he needed to take a series of supplements that contain more than 200% of the RDA for many vitamins and minerals. After a few months of taking these supplements on a daily basis, Ben started to experience headaches, nausea, diarrhea, and tingling in his hands and feet. Although Ben was not an expert in nutrition, he suspected that he might be experiencing side effects related to nutrient toxicity. He decided to talk to his doctor about the supplements he was taking to determine if they could be causing his symptoms.

Ben's story is not unique. More than half of Canadian consumers surveyed report that they use vitamins, minerals, herbal products, or homeopathic medicines on a regular basis.

Why do so many people take dietary supplements? Many people believe they cannot consume adequate nutrients in their diet, and they take a supplement as extra nutritional insurance. Others have been advised by their health care provider to take a supplement because of a health condition. There are people, like Ben, who believe that certain supplements can be used to treat illness or disease. There are also people who believe supplements are necessary to enhance their physical looks or athletic performance.

Although many people believe taking dietary supplements benefits their health, this is not always the case. Who should be taking supplements? This question is not simple. Before deciding whether you may benefit from taking dietary supplements, a review of the definition of dietary supplements and their regulation is necessary to gain a more complete understanding of how these products are marketed and regulated for safety.

Dietary Supplements Include Vitamins, Minerals, and Other Products

In Canada, dietary supplements are included in a new class of substances called natural health products (NHPs). A natural health product (Health Canada 2003) is defined as

- a plant or plant material, an alga, a bacterium, a fungus, or non-human animal material;

- an extract or isolate of the above;
- any of the following vitamins: biotin, niacin, pantothenic acid, riboflavin, thiamin, vitamin A, vitamin B_6, vitamin B_{12}, vitamin C, vitamin D, vitamin E;
- an amino acid;
- an essential fatty acid;
- a synthetic duplicate of any of the above;
- a mineral;
- a probiotic (e.g., *Lactobacillus acidophilus*).

The definition includes herbal remedies, homeopathic medicines, and traditional medicines (e.g., medicines used by Aboriginal healers or in Chinese traditional medicine). Natural health products are usually sold in capsule, pill, tablet, liquid, or bulk form (such as certain herbs that have no food purpose) without prescriptions, and are primarily taken for medicinal reasons, rather than to satisfy hunger or thirst or nourishment needs. In this way, NHPs are more similar to drugs than to foods.

How Are Dietary Supplements Regulated?

Before 2004, NHPs were sold either as drugs with drug information numbers (DINs) or as food. If they were sold as food, they were not permitted to carry health claims and often had no safety information provided on their labels.

On January 1, 2004, the Natural Health Products Regulations came into effect as part of Canada's revised Food and Drugs Act. For the first time ever, the manufacturing, packaging, labelling, storage, importation, distribution, and sale of NHPs are now under the control of federal regulations and are required to meet the same standards of quality and safety as drugs. This means that there are standards for product licensing, reporting of "adverse reactions," site licensing, good manufacturing practices, clinical trials involving human subjects, and labelling and packaging.

The purpose of these strict regulations is to ensure that Canadians can readily obtain NHPs that are known to be safe, effective, and of high quality. The NHP regulations are administered by the Natural Health Products Directorate, which is part of the Health Products and Food Branch under Health Canada. During the first year under the new regulations, more than 150 naturopathic remedies were approved.

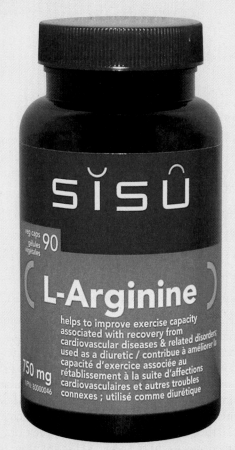

L-Arginine, produced by Sisu Inc., has a naturopathic product number (NPN), indicating it has been approved by Health Canada.

Two examples, both manufactured by Sisu Inc. of Burnaby, B.C., are

- *L-Lysine,* which helps reduce the recurrence, severity and healing time of cold sores. NPN: 80000036;

- *L-Arginine,* which helps improve exercise capacity when recovering from cardiovascular diseases and similar conditions. NPN: 80000046.

Federal advertising regulations also require that any advertising on the label must be truthful and not misleading and that advertisers must have adequate substantiation of all product claims before disseminating the advertisement. Any products not meeting these labelling and advertising guidelines can be removed from the market.

How Can We Protect Ourselves from Fraudulent or Dangerous Supplements?

Although many of the supplement products sold today are safe, many products are not. In addition, some companies are less than forthright about the true content of ingredients in their supplements. How can we avoid purchasing fraudulent or dangerous supplements? Consumers can do the following to protect themselves from fraudulent or dangerous supplements (U.S. FDA 1998):

1. Look for a drug identification number (DIN), a naturopathic product number (NPN), or a homeopathic medicine number (DIN-HM). These indicate that the manufacturer followed the standards established for purity, strength, quality, packaging, labelling, and acceptable length of storage.

2. Consider buying recognized brands of supplements. Although not guaranteed, products made by nationally recognized companies are more likely to have well-established manufacturing standards.

3. Do not assume that the word *natural* on the label means that the product is safe. Arsenic, lead, and mercury are all natural substances that can kill you if consumed in large enough quantities.

4. Do not hesitate to contact a company about how it makes its products. Reputable companies have nothing to hide and are more than happy to inform their customers about the safety and quality of their products.

Many supplements are also sold today over the internet. Dancho and Manore (2001) suggest six criteria that can be used to evaluate dietary supplement websites. Keep these criteria in mind each time you consider buying a dietary supplement over the Web:

1. What is the purpose of the site? Is the website trying to sell a product or educate the consumer? Keep in mind that the primary purpose of supplement companies is to make money. Look for sites that provide educational information about a specific nutrient or product and don't just focus on selling the products.

2. Does the site contain accurate information? Accuracy of the information on the website is the most difficult thing for a consumer to determine. Testimonials (claims by athletes or other famous people) are *not* reliable and accurate; claims supported by scientific research are most desirable. If what the company claims about its product sounds too good to be true, it probably is.

3. Does the site contain reputable references? References should be from articles published in peer-reviewed scientific journals. The reference should be complete and contain author names, title of article, journal title, date, volume, and page numbers. This information allows the consumer to check original research for the validity of a company's claims about its product. Be cautious of sites that refer to claims that are proven by research studies but fail to provide a complete reference.

4. Who owns or sponsors the site? Full disclosure regarding sponsorship and possible sources of bias

or conflict of interest should be included in the site's information.

5. Who wrote the information? Websites should clearly identify the author of the article and include the credentials of the author. Recognized experts include individuals with relevant health-related credentials, such as RD, PhD, MD, or MSc. Keep in mind that this person is responsible for the information posted in the article but may not be the creator of the website.

6. Is the information current and updated regularly? As information about supplements changes regularly, websites should be updated regularly, and the date should be clearly posted. All websites should also include contact information to allow consumers to ask questions about the information posted.

For more information on how to make informed decisions and evaluate information related to dietary supplements, go to the Natural Health Products Directorate at www.hc-sc.gc.ca/ahc-asc/branch-dirgen/hpfb-dgpsa/nhpd-dpsn/index-eng.php. Other websites that contain reliable information about dietary supplements include the National Institutes of Health (NIH) Office of Dietary Supplements at http://ods.od.nih.gov, and the Food and Nutrition Information Center (FNIC) at www.nal.usda.gov/fnic/.

Dietary Supplements Can Be Both Helpful and Harmful

As mentioned earlier in this debate, it is not always easy to determine who should take dietary supplements. Our nutritional needs change throughout our lifespan, and some of us may need to take supplements at certain times for various conditions. For instance, some athletes can benefit from consuming foods formulated to provide carbohydrate and other nutrients necessary to support intense exercise. Women at risk for osteoporosis may benefit from taking calcium and vitamin D supplements. Dietary supplements include hundreds of thousands of products sold for many purposes, and it is impossible to discuss here all of the various situations in which these supplements may be needed. To simplify this discussion, let's focus on describing who may or may not benefit from taking vitamin and mineral supplements.

Who Might Benefit from Taking Vitamin and Mineral Supplements?

Contrary to what some people believe, the Canadian food supply is not void of nutrients, and all people do not need to supplement all the time. In fact, we now know that foods contain a diverse combination of compounds that are critical to our health, and vitamin

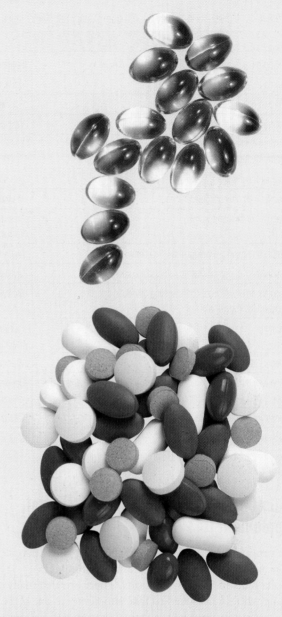

Always research supplements and supplement manufacturers before purchasing.

and mineral supplements do not contain the same amount or variety of substances found in foods. Thus, dietary supplements are not substitutes for whole foods.

However, there are certain individuals who may benefit from taking vitamin and mineral supplements. Table 8.4 lists various individuals who may benefit from supplementation. It is important to remember that analyzing your total diet is an important first step in determining whether you might need to take a vitamin and mineral supplement. It is always a good idea to check with your health care provider or a registered dietitian (RD) before taking any supplements, as supplements can interfere with some prescription and over-the-counter medications.

Table 8.4   Individuals Who May Benefit from Dietary Supplementation

Example of Individual	Specific Supplements That May Help
Newborns	Routinely given a single dose of vitamin K at birth
Infants	Depends on condition; may need iron or other nutrients, vitamin D for breastfed infants
Children not drinking fluoridated water	Fluoride supplements
Children on strict vegetarian diets	Vitamin B_{12}, iron, zinc, vitamin D (if not exposed to sunlight)
Children with poor eating habits or overweight children on an energy-restricted diet	Multivitamin-mineral supplement that does not exceed the RDA for the nutrients it contains
Pregnant teenagers	Iron and folic acid; other nutrients may be necessary if diet is very poor
Women who may become pregnant	Multivitamin or multivitamin-mineral supplement that contains 0.4 mg of folic acid
Pregnant or lactating women	Multivitamin-mineral supplement that contains iron, folic acid, zinc, copper, calcium, vitamin B_6, vitamin C, vitamin D
People on prolonged weight-reduction diets	Multivitamin-mineral supplement
People recovering from serious illness or surgery	Multivitamin-mineral supplement
People with HIV/AIDS or other wasting diseases; people addicted to drugs or alcohol	Multivitamin-mineral supplement or single-nutrient supplements
Women	Calcium supplements: women need to consume 1000 to 1300 mg of calcium per day through food, and supplements may also be necessary
People eating a vegan diet	Vitamin B_{12}, riboflavin, calcium, vitamin D, iron, and zinc
People who have had portions of the intestinal tract removed; people who have a malabsorptive disease	Depends upon the exact condition; may include various fat-soluble and/or water-soluble vitamins and other nutrients.
People with lactose intolerance	Calcium supplements, vitamin D
Older adults	Multivitamin-mineral supplement, vitamin B_{12}, vitamin D

When Can Taking a Vitamin and Mineral Supplement Be Harmful?

You can see from Table 8.4 that there are many people who can benefit from taking vitamin and mineral supplements in certain situations. There are also many people who do not need to take supplements but do so anyway. Instances in which taking vitamin and mineral supplements are unnecessary or harmful include the following:

1. Providing fluoride supplements to children who already drink fluoridated water.

2. Taking supplements in the belief that they will cure a disease, such as cancer, diabetes, or heart disease.

3. Taking supplements with certain medications. For instance, people who take the blood-thinning drug Coumadin should not take vitamin E supplements, as this can cause excessive bleeding. People who take Aspirin daily should check with their physician before taking vitamin E supplements, as Aspirin also thins the blood.

4. Taking non-prescribed supplements if you have liver or kidney diseases. Physicians may prescribe vitamin and mineral supplements for their patients because many nutrients are lost during treatment for these diseases. However, these individuals cannot properly metabolize certain supplements and should not take any that are not prescribed by their physician because of a high risk for toxicity.

5. Taking beta-carotene supplements if you are a smoker. As already mentioned, there is evidence that beta-carotene supplementation increases the risk of lung and other cancers in smokers.

6. Taking vitamins and minerals in an attempt to improve physical appearance or athletic performance. There is no evidence that vitamin and mineral supplements enhance appearance or athletic performance in healthy adults who consume a varied diet with adequate energy.

7. Taking supplements to increase your energy level. Vitamin and mineral supplements do not provide energy, because they do not contain fat, carbohydrate, or protein. Although many vitamins and minerals are necessary for us to produce energy, taking dietary supplements in place of eating food will not provide us with the energy necessary to live a healthy and productive life.

8. Taking single-nutrient supplements, unless a qualified health care practitioner prescribes a single-nutrient supplement for a diagnosed medical condition (for example, prescribing iron supplements for someone with anemia). These products contain very high amounts of the given nutrient, and taking these types of products can quickly lead to toxicity.

The research literature reveals two opposing views on the use of vitamin and mineral supplements. Some argue that, with a few exceptions, most people will probably not benefit from taking multivitamins every day (e.g., Bender 2002; Wooltorton 2003). This view holds that most Western diets are adequate and vitamin deficiencies are uncommon. Further, the evidence that extra amounts of vitamins and minerals can prevent chronic diseases is not consistent, and too much of some nutrients, such as beta-carotene, can be harmful to some people (in this case, smokers).

Other scientists argue that all adults would benefit from a daily multivitamin, and some groups, such as older adults, should take two multivitamin pills each day (e.g., Josefson 2002; Fairfield and Fletcher 2002).

The ideal nutritional strategy for optimizing health is to eat a healthful diet that contains a variety of foods. This way, you will not need to take vitamin and mineral supplements. However, some people may still need to take supplements despite their best efforts. If you do supplement your diet, select a supplement that contains no more than 100% of the recommended levels for the nutrients it contains. Avoid taking single-nutrient supplements unless advised by your health care practitioner. Finally, avoid taking supplements that contain substances that are known to cause illness or injuries. Some of these substances are listed in Table 8.5.

Table 8.5 Ingredients Found in Supplements That Are Associated with Illnesses and Injuries

Ingredient	Potential Risks
Herbal Ingredients	
Chaparral	Liver disease
Comfrey	Obstruction of blood flow to liver, possible death
Slimming/dieter's teas	Nausea, diarrhea, vomiting, stomach cramps, constipation, fainting, possible death
Ephedra (also known as ma huang, Chinese ephedra, and epitonin)	High blood pressure, irregular heart beat, nerve damage, insomnia, tremors, headaches, seizures, heart attack, stroke, possible death
Germander	Liver disease, possible death
Lobelia	Breathing problems, excessive sweating, rapid heart beat, low blood pressure, coma, possible death
Magnolia-Stephania preparation	Kidney disease, can lead to permanent kidney failure
Willow bark	Reye's syndrome (a potentially fatal disease that can occur when children take Aspirin), allergic reaction in adults
Wormwood	Numbness of legs and arms, loss of intellectual processing, delirium, paralysis
Vitamins and Essential Minerals	
Vitamin A (excessive amounts)	Birth defects, bone abnormalities, severe liver disease
Vitamin B_6 (when taking more than 100 mg per day)	Loss of balance, injuries to nerves that alter our touch sensation
Niacin (when taking slow-release doses of 500 mg or more per day, or when taking immediate-release doses of 750 mg or more per day)	Stomach pain, nausea, vomiting, bloating, cramping, diarrhea, liver disease, damage to the muscles, eyes, and heart
Selenium (when taking 800 to 1000 micrograms per day)	Tissue damage
Other Ingredients	
Germanium (a non-essential mineral)	Kidney damage, possible death
L-tryptophan (an amino acid)	Eosinophilia-myalgia syndrome (a potentially fatal blood disorder that causes high fever, joint and muscle pain, swelling of legs and arms, skin rash, and weakness)

Source: U.S. Food and Drug Administration, Supplements associated with illnesses and injuries, 1998, *FDA Consumer Magazine*, September/October, www.fda.gov/fdac/features/1998/dietchrt.html (accessed August 2002).

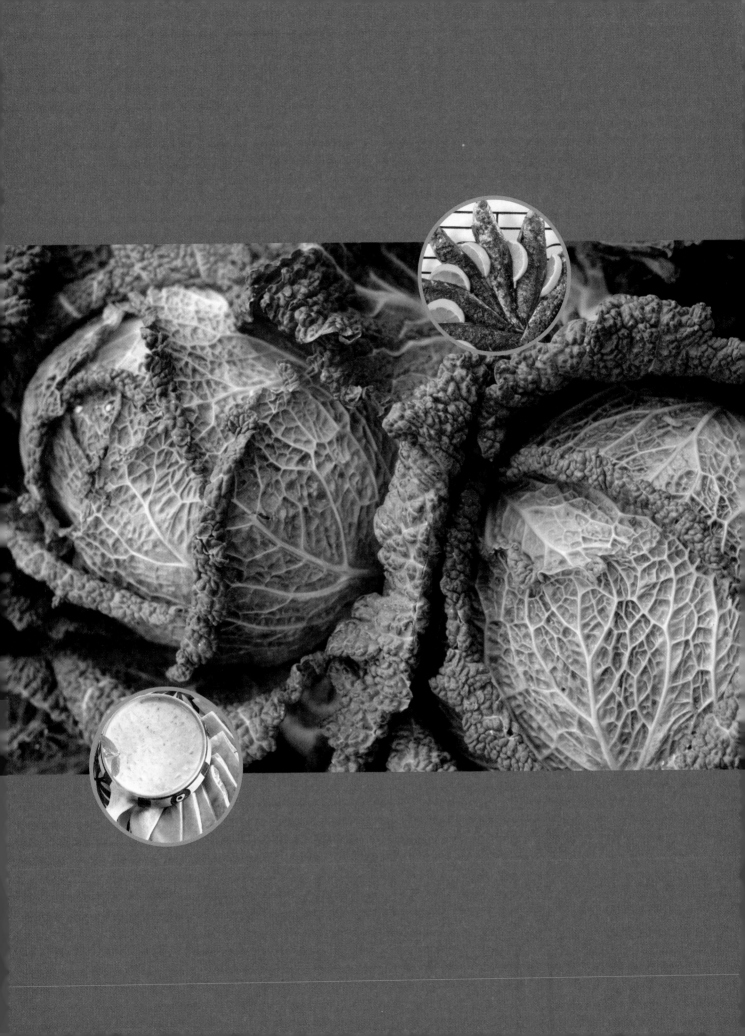

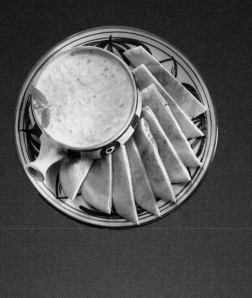

CHAPTER 9

Nutrients Involved in Bone Health

CHAPTER OBJECTIVES

After reading this chapter you will be able to:

1. Describe the differences between cortical bone and trabecular bone, p. 311.

2. Discuss the processes of bone growth, modelling, and remodelling, pp. 312–313.

3. Describe three methods used to measure bone density, pp. 314–315.

4. Describe the roles of two vitamins and three minerals in maintaining bone health, pp. 315–336.

5. Identify foods that are good sources of calcium, pp. 318–336.

6. Describe three potential reasons why consumption of soft drinks may be detrimental to bone health, pp. 332, 346–347.

7. Define osteoporosis, and discuss how it affects a person's health, p. 337.

8. Describe three factors that influence our risk for osteoporosis, pp. 337–390.

Test Yourself True or False

1. Most people are unable to consume enough calcium in their diets; therefore, they must take calcium supplements. **T or F**

2. Osteoporosis is a disease that affects only elderly women. **T or F**

3. We are capable of making vitamin D within our bodies by using energy obtained from exposure to sunlight. **T or F**

4. In addition to most dairy products, many green leafy vegetables are good sources of calcium. **T or F**

5. Cigarette smoking increases a person's risk for osteoporosis. **T or F**

Test Yourself answers can be found at the end of the chapter.

As a young woman, Erika Goodman leapt across the stage in leading roles with the Joffrey Ballet, one of the premier dance companies in the world. Now in her mid-fifties, she cannot cross a room without assistance. Goodman has a disease called *osteoporosis*, which means "porous bone." As you might suspect, the less dense the bone, the more likely it is to break; indeed, osteoporosis can cause bones to break during even minor weight-bearing activities, such as carrying groceries. In advanced cases, bones in the hip and spine can fracture spontaneously, merely from the effort of holding the body erect.

If you are age 20 or older, your bones are already at or close to their peak density. But just how dense are your bones, and what changes can you make right now, no matter what your age, to keep them as strong as possible? What foods build bone? Are there foods that break it down? In this chapter, we discuss the nutrients and lifestyle factors that play a critical role in maintaining bone health.

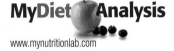

www.mynutritionlab.com

How Does the Body Maintain Bone Health?

Contrary to what most people think, the skeleton is not an inactive collection of bones that simply holds the body together. Bones are living organs that contain several tissues, including bone tissue, nerves, cartilage, and connective tissue. Blood vessels supply nutrients to bone to support its activities. Bones have many important functions in our bodies, some of which might surprise you (Table 9.1). For instance, did you know that most of your red blood cells are formed deep within your bones?

Given the importance of bones, it is critical that we maintain their health. Bone health is achieved through complex interactions among nutrients, hormones, and genetic and environmental factors. To better understand these interactions, we first need to learn about how bone structure and the constant activity of bone tissue influence bone health throughout our lifetime.

Bone Composition and Structure Provide Strength and Flexibility

We tend to think of bones as rigid, but if they were, how could we twist and jump our way through a basketball game or carry an armload of books up a flight of stairs? Our bones need to be both strong and flexible so they can resist the compression, stretching, and twisting that occur in our daily activities. Fortunately, the composition of bone is ideally suited for its complex job: about 65% of bone tissue is made up of an assortment of minerals (mostly calcium and phosphorus) that provide hardness, but the remaining 35% is a mixture of organic substances that provide strength, durability, and flexibility. The most important of these substances is a fibrous protein called collagen. You might be surprised to learn that collagen fibres are actually stronger than steel fibres of similar size. Within our bones, the minerals form tiny crystals (called *hydroxyapatite*) that cluster around the collagen fibres.

Table 9.1   Functions of Bone in the Human Body

Functions Related to Structure and Support	Functions Related to Metabolic Processes
Bones provide physical support for our organs and body segments.	Bone tissue acts as a storage reservoir for many minerals, including calcium, phosphorus, and fluoride. The body draws upon such deposits when these minerals are needed for various body processes; however, this can reduce bone mass.
Bones protect our vital organs; for example, the rib cage protects our lungs, the skull protects our brain, and the vertebrae in our spine protect our spinal cord.	
Bones provide support for muscles that allow movement—muscles attach to bones via tendons, and we are able to move all of our joints because of the connections between our muscles and our bones	Most of the blood cells needed by our bodies are produced in the marrow of our bones.

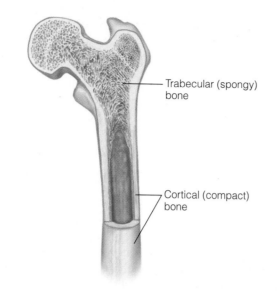

Trabecular (spongy) bone

Cortical (compact) bone

Figure 9.1 The structure of bone. Notice the difference in density between the trabecular (spongy) bone and the cortical (compact) bone.

This design enables bones to bear our weight while responding to our demands for movement.

Bone strength and flexibility are also affected by bone structure. If you examine a bone very closely, you will notice two distinct types of tissue (Figure 9.1): cortical bone and trabecular bone. **Cortical bone**, which is also called *compact bone,* is very dense. It makes up approximately 80% of our skeleton. The outer surface of all bones is cortical; plus many small bones of the body, such as the bones of the wrists, hands, and feet, are made entirely of cortical bone. Although cortical bone looks solid to the naked eye, it actually contains many microscopic openings that serve as passageways for blood vessels and nerves.

In contrast, **trabecular bone** makes up only 20% of our skeleton. It is found within the ends of the long bones (such as the bones of the arms and legs), inside the spinal vertebrae, inside the flat bones (breastbone, ribs, and most bones of the skull), and inside the bones of the pelvis. Trabecular bone is sometimes referred to as *spongy* (or *cancellous) bone* because to the naked eye it looks like a sponge, with no clear organization. The microscope reveals that trabecular bone is in fact aligned in a precise network of columns that protects the bone from extreme stress. You can think of trabecular bone as the scaffolding of the inside of the bone, as it supports the outer cortical bone much like the interior scaffolding of a building supports its outer walls.

Cortical and trabecular bone also differ in their rate of turnover; that is, in how quickly the bone tissue is broken down and replenished. Trabecular bone has a faster turnover rate than cortical bone, meaning that more of the trabecular bone is being broken down and replenished at any given time as compared with cortical bone. This makes trabecular bone more sensitive to changes in hormones and nutritional factors, and we can more easily detect a loss of trabecular bone than we can of cortical bone. It also accounts for the much higher rate of age-related fractures in the spine and pelvis (including the hip)—all of which contain a significant amount of trabecular bone. Let's now investigate how bone turnover, or the constant activity of bone, influences our bone health.

Recap: Bones are organs that contain metabolically active tissues composed primarily of minerals and a fibrous protein called collagen. We have two types of bone: cortical and trabecular. Cortical bone is dense and composes about 80% of our bone. Trabecular bone is porous in nature and composes about 20% of our bone. Trabecular bone is more sensitive to hormonal and nutritional factors and turns over more rapidly than cortical bone.

cortical bone (compact bone) A dense bone tissue that makes up the outer surface of all bones, as well as the entirety of most small bones of the body.

trabecular bone (spongy or cancellous bone) A porous bone tissue that makes up only 20% of our skeleton and is found within the ends of the long bones, inside the spinal vertebrae, inside the flat bones (breastbone, ribs, and most bones of the skull) and inside the bones of the pelvis.

The Constant Activity of Bone Tissue Promotes Bone Health

Our bones develop through a series of three processes: bone growth, bone modelling, and bone remodelling (Figure 9.2). Bone growth and modelling begin during the early months of fetal life when our skeleton is forming and continue through infancy, childhood, and adolescence. As a result of this constant activity, the shape and size of our bones is well defined by the time we reach puberty. Bone remodelling predominates during adulthood; this process helps us to maintain a healthy skeleton as we age.

Bone Growth and Modelling Determine the Size and Shape of Our Bones

Through the process of *bone growth,* the size of our bones increases. The first period of rapid bone growth is from birth to age 2, but growth continues in spurts throughout childhood and into adolescence. Most girls reach their adult height by age 14, and boys generally reach adult height by age 17 (Ball and Bindler 2003). In the later decades of life, some loss in height usually occurs because of decreased bone density in the spine, as will be discussed shortly.

Bone modelling is the process by which the shape of our bones is determined, from the round "pebble" bones that make up our wrists, to the uniquely shaped bones of our face, to the long bones of our arms and legs. Although our bones stop growing in length by the time we are 18 to 21 years of age, bones can still increase in thickness if they are stressed by excessive or repetitive exercise, such as weight training, or by being overweight or obese.

Bone Remodelling Maintains a Balance Between Breakdown and Repair

bone density The degree of compactness of bone tissue, reflecting the strength of the bones. Peak bone density is the point at which a bone is strongest.

Although the shape and size of our bones do not significantly change after puberty, our **bone density**, or the strength of our bones, continues to develop into early adulthood. *Peak bone density* is the point at which our bones are strongest because they are at their highest density. Recent research has shown that peak bone density occurs earlier than previously thought. Whiting and colleagues (2004) measured peak bone mass accrual in a sample of 59 boys and 53 girls. On average this occurred at age 14 for boys and 12.5 years for girls. Before we reach adulthood, our bodies have reached peak bone mass, and we can no longer significantly add to our bone density. In our twenties and thirties, our bone density remains relatively stable, but by age 40, it begins its irreversible decline.

remodelling The two-step process by which bone tissue is recycled; includes the breakdown of existing bone and the formation of new bone.

Although our bones cannot increase their peak density after our twenties, bone tissue still remains very active throughout adulthood. To preserve bone density to the extent possible, our bodies attempt to achieve a balance between the breakdown of older bone tissue and the formation of new bone tissue. Thus, our bone mass is regularly recycled in a process called **remodelling**. We also use remodelling to repair bone that has been broken or damaged and to strengthen bone regions that are exposed to higher physical stress. The process of remodelling involves two steps: the breakdown of existing bone and the formation of new bone.

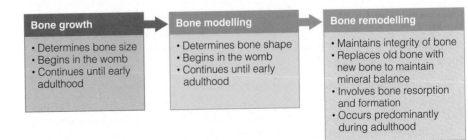

Figure 9.2 Bone develops through three processes: bone growth, bone modelling, and bone remodelling.

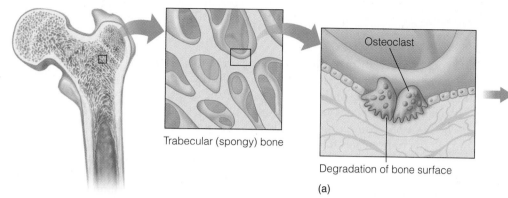

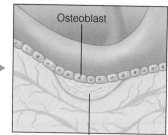

Trabecular (spongy) bone

Osteoclast

Degradation of bone surface

(a)

Osteoblast

New bone

(b)

Figure 9.3 Bone remodelling involves resorption and formation. (a) Osteoclasts erode the bone surface by degrading its components, including calcium, other minerals, and collagen; these components are then transported to the bloodstream. (b) Osteoblasts work to build new bone by filling the pit formed by the resorption process with new bone.

Bone is broken down through a process referred to as **resorption** (Figure 9.3a). During resorption, cells called **osteoclasts** erode the bone surface by secreting enzymes and acids that dig grooves into the bone matrix. Their ruffled surface also acts much like a scrubbing brush to assist in the erosion process. But why would we ever want to break down our bones? One of the primary reasons is to release calcium into our bloodstream. As discussed in more detail later in this chapter, calcium is critical for many physiologic processes, and our bone is an important source of calcium needed to support these processes. We also want to break down bone when we fracture (or break) a bone and need to repair it. Breaking down the damaged bone at the injury site smoothes the rough edges created by the break. We may also break down bone in areas away from the damaged site to obtain the minerals, or raw materials, that are needed to repair the damage caused by the break. Regardless of the reason, once bone is broken down, the resulting products of this breakdown process are transported into the bloodstream and utilized for various body functions.

New bone is formed through the action of cells called **osteoblasts**, or "bone builders" (see Figure 9.3b). These cells work to synthesize new bone matrix by laying down the collagen-containing organic component of bone. Within this substance, the hydroxyapatite crystallizes and packs together to create new bone where it is needed.

In young healthy adults, the processes of bone resorption and formation are equal, so that just as much bone is broken down as is built, resulting in bone mass being maintained. Around 40 years of age, bone resorption begins to occur more rapidly than bone formation, and this imbalance results in an overall loss in bone density. Because this affects the vertebrae of the spine, we also tend to lose height as we age. As we discuss shortly, achieving a high peak bone mass through proper nutrition and exercise when we are young provides us with a stronger skeleton before we begin to lose bone as we age, and it can be protective against the debilitating effects of osteoporosis.

Recap: The three types of bone activity are growth, modelling, and remodelling. Our bones reach their peak bone mass by our late teenage years and into our twenties; bone mass begins to decline around age 40. Bone is constantly being recycled through a process called remodelling. Remodelling of bone involves the resorption of bone through the action of osteoclasts and the formation of bone through the action of osteoblasts.

How Do We Assess Bone Health?

Until relatively recently, we had no way to measure the health of bone tissue. Over the past 30 years, however, technological advancements have led to the development of a number of affordable methods for measuring bone health.

resorption The process by which the surface of bone is broken down by cells called osteoclasts.

osteoclasts Cells that erode the surface of bones by secreting enzymes and acids that dig grooves into the bone matrix.

osteoblasts Cells that prompt the formation of new bone matrix by laying down the collagen-containing component of bone that is then mineralized.

Dual Energy X-Ray Absorptiometry Provides a Measure of Bone Density

dual energy x-ray absorptiometry (DXA or DEXA) Currently the most accurate tool for measuring bone density.

Dual energy x-ray absorptiometry, also referred to as DXA (or DEXA), is considered the most accurate assessment tool for measuring bone density. This method can measure the density of the bone mass over the entire body. Special software is also available that provides an estimation of percentage body fat.

The DXA procedure is simple, painless, safe, and non-invasive. The person participating in the test remains fully clothed but must remove all jewellery or other metal objects. The participant lies quietly on a table, and bone density is assessed through the use of a very low level of x-ray. The test takes less than 15 minutes for a scan of the hip and lower spine, while a whole-body scan takes about 30 minutes. The level of radiation exposure during a DXA test is much lower than the exposure during a dental x-ray.

T-score A comparison of an individual's bone density to the average peak bone density of a 30-year-old healthy adult of the same sex and race. If bone density is normal, the T-score will be between +1 and −1.

DXA is a very important tool to determine a person's risk for osteoporosis. Once someone's bone mineral density is determined, his or her number is compared with the average peak bone density of a 30-year-old healthy adult of the same sex and race. Doctors use this comparison, which is known as the **T-score**, to assess the risk of fracture and determine whether or not this person has osteoporosis. A negative T-score indicates lower than normal bone mass. For instance, if the T-score is between −1 and −2.5, this person has osteopenia, which is characterized by low bone mass, and is at an increased risk for fractures. If the T-score is more negative than −2.5, this person has osteoporosis. If bone density is normal, the T-score will range between +1 and −1 of the 30-year-old healthy adult value. A T-score above +1 indicates better than normal bone mass, and is desirable.

DXA tests are generally recommended for postmenopausal women because they are at highest risk for osteoporosis and fracture. Men and younger women may also be recommended for a DXA test if they have significant risk factors for osteoporosis (see page 337).

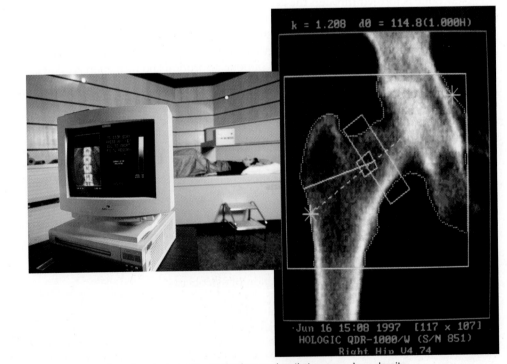

Dual energy x-ray absorptiometry is a safe and simple procedure that assesses bone density.

Recap: Dual energy x-ray absorptiometry (DXA or DEXA) is the gold standard measurement of bone mass. It is a simple, safe, and painless procedure. DXA can measure bone mass throughout the entire body. The results of a DXA include a T-score, which is a comparison of your bone density with that of a 30-year-old healthy adult of the same sex and race. A T-score between +1 and –1 is normal; a score between –1 and –2.5 indicates poor bone density; and a score more negative than –2.5 indicates osteoporosis.

Other Bone Density Measurement Tools

Three other technologies have been developed to measure bone density. The quantitative ultrasound technique uses sound waves to measure the density of bone in the heel, shin, and kneecap. Peripheral dual energy x-ray absorptiometry, or pDXA, is a form of DXA that measures bone density in the peripheral regions of our bodies, including the wrist, heel, or finger. Single energy x-ray absorptiometry is a method that measures bone density at the wrist or heel. These technologies are frequently used at health fairs because the machines are portable and provide scores faster than the traditional DXA. If your results from these tests indicate low bone density, you should contact your physician to schedule a DXA to determine the bone density status of your hip and spine or your full body.

Recap: Quantitative ultrasound, peripheral dual energy x-ray absorptiometry, and single energy x-ray absorptiometry are other methods that can be used to measure bone density. These methods typically measure the bone density of peripheral sites such as the heel, wrist, or finger.

A Profile of Nutrients That Maintain Bone Health

Calcium is the most recognized nutrient associated with bone health; however, vitamins D and K, phosphorus, magnesium, and fluoride are also essential for strong bones. Let's now learn more about these nutrients and their functions in our bodies.

Calcium

Remember from Chapter 1 that major minerals are those required in our diet in amounts greater than 100 mg per day. Calcium is by far the most abundant major mineral in our body, composing about 2% of our entire body weight! Not surprisingly, it plays many critical roles in maintaining overall function and health.

Functions of Calcium

One of the primary roles of calcium is to provide structure to our bones and teeth. About 99% of the calcium found in our bodies is stored in our bones. As discussed earlier in this chapter, calcium and phosphorus crystallize to form hydroxyapatite. These crystals pack themselves tightly together and build up on the collagen foundation of bone. This combination of crystals and collagen provides both the characteristic hardness of bone and the flexibility needed to support various activities. Thus, one major role of calcium is to form and maintain bones and teeth.

The remaining 1% of calcium in our bodies is found in the blood and soft tissues. Calcium is alkaline, or basic, and because of this property it plays a critical role in assisting with acid–base balance. We cannot survive for long if our blood calcium level rises above or falls below a very narrow range; therefore, our bodies maintain the appropriate blood calcium level at all costs. This means that if we do not consume

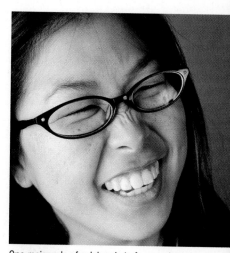

One major role of calcium is to form and maintain bones and teeth.

or absorb enough calcium from our diet, osteoclasts will erode our bones so that calcium can be released into our blood. Thus, the skeleton not only provides physical support to our bodies, but it also acts as a storehouse for calcium to assist in the regulation of blood calcium. However, we need to consume enough calcium in our diet to make sure it balances the calcium we take from our bones so that we can maintain a healthy bone density.

Calcium is also critical for the normal transmission of nerve impulses. Calcium flows into nerve cells and stimulates the release of molecules called neurotransmitters, which transfer the nerve impulses from one nerve cell (neuron) to another. Without adequate calcium, our nerves' ability to transmit messages is inhibited. Not surprisingly, when blood calcium levels fall dangerously low, a person can experience convulsions.

A fourth role of calcium is to assist in muscle contraction. Our muscles are relaxed when calcium levels in the muscle are low. Contraction of our muscles is stimulated by calcium flowing into the muscle cell; conversely, our muscles relax when calcium is pumped back outside the muscle cell. If calcium levels are inadequate, normal muscle contraction and relaxation is inhibited, and the person may suffer from twitching and spasms. This problem affects the function not only of skeletal muscles, but also of heart muscle and can cause heart failure.

Other roles of calcium include the maintenance of healthy blood pressure, the initiation of blood clotting, and the regulation of various hormones and enzymes. A summary of the functions, recommended intakes, and toxicity and deficiency symptoms associated with calcium is provided in Table 9.2.

How Much Calcium Should We Consume?

Much attention has recently been given to the fact that many people, particularly women, do not consume enough calcium to maintain bone health.

Recommended Dietary Intake for Calcium   Calcium requirements, and thus recommended intakes, vary according to age and gender. There are no RDA values for calcium. The Adequate Intake (AI) value for adult men and women aged 19 to 50 years is 1000 mg of calcium per day. Data from the 2004 Canadian Community Health Survey, cycle 2.2 (Statistics Canada 2007) indicate that on average, women aged 19 years and older consume 793 mg of calcium per day, and men consume 931 mg daily. For men and women older than 50 years of age, the AI increases to 1200 mg of calcium per day; however, estimated intakes are much lower, with Canadian men consuming an average of 832 mg and women an average of 740 mg daily. The AI for boys and girls aged 15 to 18 years is even higher, being 1300 mg per day; on average, boys meet the AI, while average intakes are just 917 mg among girls. The upper level (UL) for calcium is 2500 mg (2.5 grams) for all age and gender groups.

bioavailability The degree to which our bodies can absorb and use any given nutrient.

The term **bioavailability** refers to the degree to which our bodies can absorb and use any given nutrient. The bioavailability of calcium depends in part upon our age and our need for calcium. For example, infants and children can absorb more than 60% of the calcium they consume, as calcium needs are very high during these stages of life. In addition, pregnant and lactating women can absorb about 50% of dietary calcium. In contrast, healthy young adults only absorb about 30% of the calcium consumed in the diet. When our calcium needs are high, the body can generally increase its absorption of calcium from the small intestine. Although older adults have a high need for calcium, the ability to absorb calcium diminishes as we age and can be as low as 25%. Our reduced ability to absorb calcium as we age is primarily due to changes in absorption capacity from the small intestine. This change in calcium absorption with aging was taken into account when calcium recommendations were determined.

The bioavailability of calcium also depends on how much calcium we consume throughout the day or at any one time. When our diets are generally high in calcium,

Table 9.2   Nutrients Essential to Bone Health

Nutrient	Primary Functions	Recommended Intake	Toxicity Symptoms or Related Diseases	Deficiency Symptoms or Related Diseases
Calcium (major mineral)	Primary component of bone and foot structure Helps maintain optimal acid–base balance Maintains normal nerve transmission Supports muscle contraction and relaxation Regulates blood pressure, blood clotting, and various hormones and enzymes	Adequate Intake (AI): Men and women aged 19 to 50 years = 1000 mg/day Men and women aged > 50 years = 1200 mg/day	Potential mineral imbalances; calcium can interfere with absorption of iron, zinc, and magnesium; shock; kidney failure; fatigue; mental confusion	Osteoporosis—bone fractures; convulsions and muscle spasms; heart failure
Vitamin D (fat-soluble vitamin)	Aids calcium absorption Regulates blood calcium levels Maintains bone health Cell differentiation	AI*: Men and women aged 19 to 50 = 5 µg/day Men and women aged 50 to 70 = 10 µg/day Men and women aged > 70 = 15 µg/day	Hypercalcemia, including weakness, loss of appetite, diarrhea, mental confusion, vomiting, excessive urine output, extreme thirst, and formation of calcium deposits in kidney, liver, and heart Increased bone loss	Rickets (in children), leading to bone weakness and deformities Osteomalacia (in adults), leading to bone weakness and increased rate of fractures Osteoporosis, leading to increased rate of fractures
Vitamin K (fat-soluble vitamin)	Serves as a coenzyme during production of specific proteins that assist in blood coagulation and bone metabolism	AI: Men = 120 µg/day Women = 90 µg/day	No known side effects or toxicity symptoms from consuming excess vitamin K	Reduced ability to form blood clots, leading to excessive bleeding and easy bruising Effect on bone health is controversial
Phosphorus (major mineral)	Part of hydroxyapatite crystals, which are the mineral complex of bone Assists in maintaining fluid balance Primary component of ATP Helps activate and inactivate enzymes Component of DNA and RNA Component of cell membranes and lipoproteins	Recommended Dietary Allowance (RDA): Men and women = 700 mg/day	High blood phosphorus levels, causing muscle spasms and convulsions	Low blood phosphorus levels, causing dizziness, bone pain, muscle weakness, and muscle damage
Magnesium (major mineral)	An essential component of bone tissue Influences formation of hydroxyapatite crystals and bone growth Cofactor for more than 300 enzyme systems, including ATP, DNA, and protein synthesis, vitamin D metabolism and action Supports muscle contraction and blood clotting	RDA: Men aged 19 to 30 = 400 mg/day Men aged > 30 = 420 mg/day Women aged 19 to 30 = 310 mg/day Women aged > 30 = 320 mg/day	No known toxicity symptoms of consuming excess in diet Toxicity from pharmacological use includes diarrhea, nausea, abdominal cramps; in severe cases, massive dehydration, cardiac arrest, and death can result	Hypomagnesemia, resulting in low blood calcium levels, muscle cramps, spasms or seizures, nausea, weakness, irritability, and confusion Chronic diseases, such as heart disease, high blood pressure, osteoporosis, and type 2 diabetes
Fluoride (trace mineral)	Maintains health of teeth and bones Protects teeth against dental caries Stimulates new bone growth	Adequate Intake (AI): Men = 4 mg/day Women = 3 mg/day	Dental fluorosis, which causes staining and pitting of teeth Skeletal fluorosis, which ranges from mild to severe; causes joint pain and stiffness, and in extreme cases can cause crippling, wasting of muscles, and osteoporosis of the extremities	High occurrence of dental caries and tooth decay Low fluoride intakes may also be associated with lower bone density

* Based on the assumption that a person does not get adequate sun exposure.

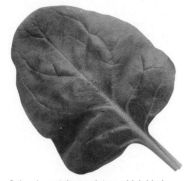

Spinach contains oxalates, which bind calcium and inhibit calcium absorption.

our absorption of calcium is reduced. In addition, our bodies cannot absorb more than 500 mg of calcium at any one time, and as the amount of calcium in a single meal or supplement goes up, the fraction that we absorb goes down. This explains why it is critical to consume calcium-rich foods throughout the day, rather than relying on a single high-dose supplement. Conversely, when dietary intake of calcium is low, we increase our absorption of calcium.

Dietary factors can also affect our absorption of calcium. Binding factors, such as phytates and oxalates, occur naturally in some calcium-rich seeds, nuts, grains, and vegetables, such as spinach and Swiss chard. Such factors bind to some of the calcium in these foods and prevent their absorption from the intestine. Additionally, consuming calcium at the same time as iron, zinc, magnesium, or phosphorus has the potential to interfere with the absorption and utilization of all of these minerals. Despite these potential interactions, the Institute of Medicine (1997) concluded that, at the present time, there is not sufficient evidence to suggest that these interactions cause deficiencies of calcium or other minerals in healthy individuals. However, there are people who are vulnerable to mineral deficiencies, such as older adults or people consuming very low mineral intakes, and more research needs to be done in these populations to determine the health risks associated with interactions between calcium and other minerals.

Finally, because vitamin D is necessary for the absorption of calcium, lack of vitamin D severely limits the bioavailability of calcium. We discuss this and other contributions of vitamin D to bone health shortly (page 322).

Shopper's Guide: Good Food Sources of Calcium   Dairy products are the most common sources of calcium in the Canadian diet. Skim milk, low-fat cheeses, and non-fat yogurt are excellent sources of calcium, and they are low in fat and energy (Figure 9.4).

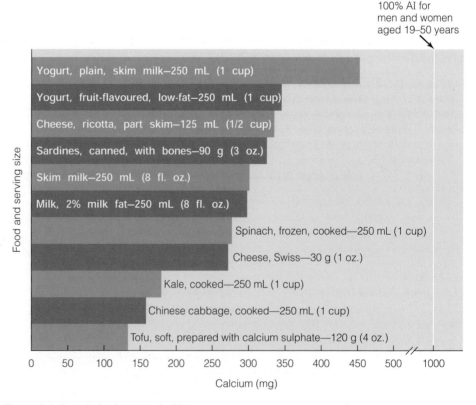

Figure 9.4 Common food sources of calcium.

Note: This figure does not account for bioavailability.

(Nutrient data from U.S. Department of Agriculture, Agricultural Research Service, USDA Nutrient Database for Standard Reference, Release 15, 2002, Nutrient Data Laboratory homepage, www.ars.usda.gov/main/site_main.htm?modecode=12354500, accessed May 2003.)

Ice cream, regular cheese, and whole milk also contain a relatively high amount of calcium, but these foods should be eaten in moderation because of their high fat and energy content. Cottage cheese is one dairy product that is a relatively poor source of calcium, as the processing of this food removes a great deal of the calcium. One cup or 250 mL of low-fat cottage cheese contains approximately 150 mg of calcium, while the same serving of low-fat milk contains almost 300 mg.

Other good sources of calcium are green leafy vegetables, such as kale, turnip greens, broccoli, cauliflower, green cabbage, Brussels sprouts, and Chinese cabbage (bok choy). The bioavailability of the calcium in these vegetables is relatively high compared to spinach, as these vegetables contain low levels of oxalates. Many packaged foods are now available fortified with calcium. For example, you can buy calcium-fortified orange juice, and soy milk and tofu processed with calcium. Some dairies have even boosted the amount of calcium in their brand of milk. When you are selecting foods that are good sources of calcium, it is important to remember that we do not absorb 100% of the calcium contained in our foods. For example, although a serving of milk contains approximately 300 mg of calcium, we do not actually absorb this entire amount into our bodies. To learn more about how calcium absorption rates vary for select foods, see the Nutrition Label Activity on page 320.

Natural soy milk is a poor source of calcium; however, some brands are fortified with calcium and vitamin D, so check the Nutrition Facts panel on product containers. The distinguished bone researcher Dr. Robert Heaney cautions that the amount of calcium added to a product isn't necessarily the amount you consume, as the added calcium salts do not disperse evenly in soy beverages and tend to settle at the bottom of the container. Heaney and Rafferty (2006) tested eight brands of fortified soy milks, and in six of the eight products, even vigorous shaking did not re-disperse the calcium well enough to get rid of the sediment at the bottom of the container. One product did not even have 20% of the calcium stated on the label when a serving was poured into a glass, despite vigorous shaking. The researchers note that "there are obvious technical problems that manufacturers must overcome if they are to provide a calcium-fortified product that delivers anything remotely approaching the labelled content" (p. 1753).

In general, meats and fish are not good sources of calcium. An exception is canned fish with bones (for example, sardines or salmon), providing you eat the bones. Fruits (except dried figs) and non-fortified grain products are also poor sources of calcium.

Although there are many foods in the Canadian diet that are good sources of calcium, many people do not consume adequate amounts because they consume few dairy-based foods. At particular risk are women and young girls. If you do not consume enough dietary calcium, you will probably benefit from taking calcium supplements. Refer to the Highlight box on page 321 to learn how to choose a calcium supplement that is right for you.

What Happens If We Consume Too Much Calcium?

In general, consuming too much calcium in the diet does not lead to significant toxicity symptoms in healthy individuals. Much of the excess calcium we consume is not absorbed from the intestine but instead is excreted in our feces. However, excessive intake of calcium from supplements can lead to health problems. As mentioned earlier, one concern with consuming too much calcium is that it can lead to various mineral imbalances because calcium interferes with the absorption of other minerals, including iron, zinc, and magnesium. This interference may only be of major concern in individuals vulnerable to mineral imbalance, such as older adults and people who consume very low amounts of minerals in their diets.

In the Women's Health Initiative Calcium and Vitamin D trial, more than 36 000 postmenopausal women were given calcium (1000 mg of elemental calcium as calcium carbonate) and vitamin D (400 IU) supplements in an effort to

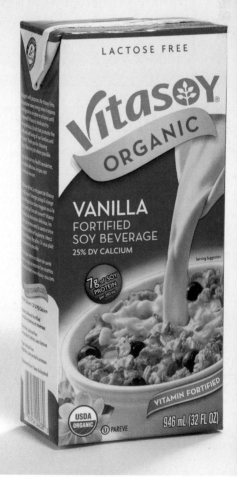

Some soy milks are fortified with calcium and vitamin D. Be sure to shake the containers well to make sure the calcium doesn't settle as sediment on the bottom of the container.

▶ **NUTRITION LABEL ACTIVITY**

How Much Calcium Am I Really Consuming?

As you have learned in this chapter, we do not absorb 100% of the calcium contained in the foods we eat. This is particularly true for individuals who eat a diet predominated by foods that are high in fibre, oxalates, and phytates, such as whole grains and certain vegetables. Thus, it is important to understand how the rate of calcium absorption differs for various foods as you plan a diet that contains adequate calcium to optimize bone health.

How do you determine the amount of calcium you are absorbing from various foods? Unfortunately, the absorption rate of calcium has not been determined for most foods. However, estimates have been established for a variety of common foods that are considered good sources of calcium. The table below shows some of these foods, their calcium content per 250 mL serving, the calcium absorption rate, and the estimated amount of calcium absorbed from each food.

As you can see from this table, many dairy products have a similar calcium absorption rate, just more than 30%. Interestingly, many green leafy vegetables have a higher absorption rate of around 60%; however, because a serving of these foods contains typically much less calcium than dairy foods, you would have to eat more servings of vegetables to get the same amount of calcium as you would from a standard serving of dairy foods. Note the relatively low calcium absorption rate for spinach, even though it contains a relatively high amount of calcium.

Remember that the DRIs for calcium already account for these differences in absorption rate. Thus, the 300 mg of calcium in a glass of milk counts as 300 mg toward your daily calcium goal. In general, you can trust that dairy products, such as milk, yogurt and cheese (but not cottage cheese) are good, absorbable sources of calcium, as are some dark green leafy vegetables. Other good sources of calcium with good absorption rates include calcium-fortified orange juice and tofu processed with calcium (Keller, Lanou, and Barnard 2002).

Food	Serving Size	Calcium per Serving (mg)[1]	Absorption Rate (%)[2]	Estimated Amount of Calcium Absorbed (mg)
Yogurt, plain skim milk	250 mL (1 cup)	452	32	145
2% milk	250 mL (8 fl. oz.)	298	32	95
Skim milk	250 mL (8 fl. oz.)	301	32	95
Kale, cooked	250 mL (1 cup)	179	59	106
Broccoli, frozen, chopped, cooked	250 mL (1 cup)	61	61	37
Spinach, frozen, cooked	250 mL (1 cup)	290	5	15

[1] *Source:* U.S. Department of Agriculture, Agricultural Research Service, USDA Nutrient Database for Standard Reference, Release 15, 2002, Nutrient Data Laboratory homepage, - www.nal.usda.gov/fnic/foodcomp (accessed May 2003).
[2] *Sources:* C. M. Weaver, W. R. Proulx, and R. Heaney, Choices for achieving adequate dietary calcium with a vegetarian diet, 1999, *American Journal of Clinical Nutrition* 70(suppl.):543S–548S; C. M. Weaver and K. L. Plawecki, Dietary calcium: Adequacy of a vegetarian diet, 1994, *American Journal of Clinical Nutrition* 59(suppl.):1238S–1241S.

reduce postmenopausal bone loss and prevent factures (Jackson et al. 2006). The results showed that the women receiving the supplements had slightly greater bone density at their hips and lower rates of hip fractures compared with the women who received a placebo pill. However, the group receiving the supplements had higher rates of kidney stones compared with the placebo group. More studies need to be done to determine the relationship between calcium and vitamin D supplementation and kidney stones.

Various diseases and metabolic disorders can alter our ability to regulate blood calcium. **Hypercalcemia** is a condition in which our blood calcium levels reach abnormally high concentrations. Hypercalcemia can be caused by cancer and also by the overproduction of a hormone called **parathyroid hormone (PTH)**. PTH

hypercalcemia A condition marked by an abnormally high concentration of calcium in the blood.

parathyroid hormone (PTH) A hormone that helps to regulate blood calcium levels.

▶ **HIGHLIGHT**

Calcium Supplements: Which Ones Are Best?

We know that calcium is a critical nutrient for bone health. Ideally, people should try to consume the recommended amount of calcium in their daily diet. But for vegans and people who avoid dairy products, it may be difficult to get sufficient calcium from the diet. Small or inactive people who eat less to maintain a healthy weight may not be able to consume enough food to provide adequate calcium, and older adults may need more calcium than they can obtain in their normal diets. In these circumstances, calcium supplements may be warranted.

There are an abundance of calcium supplements available to consumers, but which one is best? Most supplements come in the form of calcium carbonate, calcium citrate, calcium lactate, or calcium phosphate. Our bodies are able to absorb about 30% of the calcium from these various forms. Calcium citrate malate, which is the form of calcium used in fortified juices, is slightly more absorbable at 35%. Many antacids are also good sources of calcium, and it appears these are safe to take as long as you only consume enough to get the recommended level of calcium.

What is the most cost-effective form of calcium? In general, supplements that contain calcium carbonate tend to have more calcium per pill than other types. Thus, you are getting more calcium for your money when you buy this type. However, be sure to read the label of any calcium supplement you are considering taking to determine just how much calcium it contains. Some very expensive calcium supplements, such as coral calcium, do not contain a lot of calcium per pill, and you could be wasting your money. Coral calcium is advertised as being more absorbable than regular calcium supplements and having special curative properties, including reversing cancer (Barrett 2004). However, it is simply calcium carbonate and some samples have been contaminated with lead. The curative claims have not been substantiated and have been prohibited by the U.S. Federal Trade Commission (Barrett 2004).

Chelated forms of calcium supplements are sometimes touted as the best supplements available. Chelate refers to a claw-shaped protein that protects the calcium. Chelated calcium is easier to absorb, as the chelate protects the calcium from inhibitors, such as phytates and oxalates, that can bind with calcium in our intestine and make it harder to absorb. However, chelated calcium products are typically much more expensive and improve the absorption of calcium only by about 5% to 10%.

The lead content of calcium supplements is an important public health concern. Calcium supplements made from "natural" sources, such as oyster shell, bone meal, and dolomite (a type of rock containing calcium magnesium carbonate), are known to be higher in lead. In fact, many of these products can contain dangerously high levels of lead and should be avoided. We have typically considered calcium supplements that include refined sources of calcium carbonate to be very low in lead. However, a study conducted on 22 calcium supplements found that 8 (or 36%) of the supplements tested were unacceptably high in lead; this was true for oyster shell supplements and refined calcium carbonate (Ross, Szabo, and Tebbett 2000). Shockingly, the supplement with the highest lead content was a popular, nationally recognized brand-name supplement! How can we avoid taking supplements that contain too much lead? Unfortunately, the lead content of supplements is not reported on the label. However, there are some supplements available that claim to be lead-free; in the study by Ross et al. (2000), the supplements claiming to be lead-free were found to have no detectable levels of lead. In addition, most supplements not made from oyster shell and other natural products are generally very low in lead.

How should we take our supplements? Recall that too much calcium from supplements can interfere with the body's absorption of iron, magnesium, phosphorus, and zinc and lead to mineral imbalances. So taking a calcium supplement along with a multivitamin and mineral supplement is not a good idea. Remember that our bodies cannot absorb more than 500 mg of calcium at any given time. Thus, taking a supplement that contains 1000 mg will be no more effective than one that contains 500 mg calcium. If at all possible, try to consume calcium supplements in small doses throughout the day. In addition, we absorb calcium better with meals, as the calcium stays in our intestinal tract longer during a meal and more calcium can be absorbed. However, it is better to take one calcium supplement outside of meals than to do nothing. By consuming foods high in calcium every day, we can minimize our need for calcium supplements. When we cannot consume enough calcium in our diets, there are many inexpensive, safe, and effective supplements available. The best supplement for you is the one you can tolerate, is affordable, and is readily available when you need it.

stimulates the osteoclasts to break down bone and release more calcium into the bloodstream. Symptoms of hypercalcemia include fatigue, muscle and joint aches, abdominal pain, constipation, and mental confusion. Severe hypercalcemia can lead to kidney failure, coma, irregular heartbeats, and possibly death.

What Happens If We Don't Consume Enough Calcium?

There are no short-term symptoms associated with consuming too little calcium. Even when we do not consume enough dietary calcium, our bodies continue to tightly regulate blood calcium levels by taking the calcium from bone. The long-term repercussion of inadequate calcium intake is osteoporosis. This disease is discussed in more detail beginning on page 337.

Hypocalcemia is a term that describes an abnormally low level of calcium in the blood. Hypocalcemia does not result from consuming too little dietary calcium, but is caused by various diseases. Some of the causes of hypocalcemia include kidney disease, vitamin D deficiency, and diseases that inhibit the production of PTH. Symptoms of hypocalcemia include muscle spasms and convulsions.

hypocalcemia A condition characterized by an abnormally low concentration of calcium in the blood.

> **Recap:** Calcium is the most abundant mineral in our bodies. It is a significant component of our bones. Blood calcium is maintained within a very narrow range, and we use our bone calcium to maintain normal blood calcium if dietary intake is inadequate. Calcium is necessary for normal nerve and muscle function. The AI for calcium is 1000 mg per day for adults aged 19 to 50; the AI increases to 1200 mg per day for older adults and is 1300 mg per day for adolescents. Dairy products, canned fish with bones, and some green leafy vegetables are good sources of calcium. The most common long-term effect of inadequate calcium consumption is osteoporosis. Hypercalcemia causes muscle and joint aches and mental confusion, while hypocalcemia causes muscle spasms and convulsions.

Animations

- Activation of Vitamin D
- Calcium Metabolism

Vitamin D

Vitamin D is like other fat-soluble vitamins in that we store excess amounts in the liver and adipose tissue. But vitamin D is different from other nutrients in two ways. First, vitamin D does not always need to come from the diet. This is because our bodies can synthesize vitamin D by using energy from exposure to sunlight. However, when we do not get enough sunlight, we must consume vitamin D in our diet. Second, in addition to being a nutrient, vitamin D is considered a *hormone* because it is made in one part of the body yet regulates various activities in other parts of the body.

Figure 9.5 illustrates how our body makes vitamin D by converting a cholesterol compound in our skin to the active form of vitamin D that we need to function properly. When the ultraviolet rays of the sun hit our skin, they react with 7-dehydrocholesterol. This cholesterol compound is converted into a precursor of vitamin D called previtamin D_3, which is converted to cholecalciferol (vitamin D_3). It travels to the liver where it is converted to calcidiol (also called 25-hydroxyvitamin D), the circulating form of the vitamin. Although this is not the active form of vitamin D, it is easily measured in the blood and therefore used to estimate a person's vitamin D status (IFIC 2007). Calcidiol travels to the kidney, where it may be converted into **calcitriol** (also called **1,25-dihydroxyvitamin D**), which is considered the primary active form of vitamin D in our bodies. Calcitriol made by the kidneys is found in the blood and acts in the intestine and bone to promote calcium metabolism. Calcitriol made by other cells in the brain, breast, prostate, pancreas, and colon acts locally to promote calcium metabolism. This discovery may help to explain the emerging evidence of the role of vitamin D in some cancers and autoimmune and infectious diseases (IFIC 2007).

calcitriol (1,25-dihydroxyvitamin D) The primary active form of vitamin D in the body.

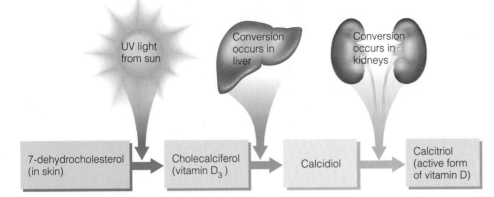

Figure 9.5 The process of converting sunlight into vitamin D in our skin. When the ultraviolet rays of the sun hit our skin, they react with 7-dehydrocholesterol. This compound is converted to an inactive form of vitamin D also called previtamin D$_3$. Previtamin D$_3$ is converted to cholecalciferol (vitamin D$_3$), which travels to the liver, where it is converted to calcidiol (25-hydroxyvitamin D, the circulating form of vitamin D). Calcidiol travels to the kidney, where it may be converted into calcitriol (1,25-dihydroxyvitamin D), which is considered the primary active form of vitamin D in our bodies.

Functions of Vitamin D

Vitamin D (as calcitriol), PTH, and another hormone called *calcitonin* all work together continuously to regulate blood calcium levels, which in turn maintains bone health. They do this by regulating the absorption of calcium and phosphorus from the small intestine, causing more to be absorbed when our needs for them are higher and less when our needs are lower. Vitamin D regulates calcium and phosphorus absorption by controlling genes that code for intestinal calcium transport proteins. In other words, vitamin D can "turn on" the genes that code for proteins to transport calcium across the intestinal wall; more transport proteins means that more calcium can move from the lumen of the intestine into the bloodstream. They also decrease or increase blood calcium levels by signalling the kidneys to excrete more or less calcium in our urine. Finally, vitamin D affects gene expression in bone cells and works with PTH to stimulate osteoclasts to break down bone when calcium is needed elsewhere in the body.

Vitamin D is also necessary for the normal calcification of bone; this means it assists the process by which minerals, such as calcium and phosphorus are crystallized. Similar to vitamin A, vitamin D appears to play a role in cell differentiation in various tissues. A review of the bone-related functions, recommended intakes, and toxicity and deficiency symptoms associated with vitamin D is provided in Table 9.2 (page 317).

Vitamin D may play some role in decreasing the formation of some cancerous tumours, as it can prevent certain types of cells from growing out of control. A study by Lappe and colleagues, published in the *American Journal of Clinical Nutrition* in 2007, caused a great deal of excitement. This randomized, double-blind, placebo-controlled trial followed approximately 1200 postmenopausal women for 4 years to determine the effects of a placebo, a calcium supplement (1400–1500 mg), and a combined calcium and vitamin D supplement with 1100 International Units (IU) of vitamin D. The results showed that the group receiving vitamin D and calcium had a 60% to 80% lower risk of all cancers compared with the placebo. However, since this trial was conducted to examine fractures and cancer was a secondary outcome, additional clinical trials are required to examine vitamin D supplements and cancer risk.

Other research suggests that vitamin D deficiency may play a role in cardiovascular disease, multiple sclerosis, and rheumatoid arthritis (IFIC 2007). Several European studies have found that infants receiving vitamin D supplements had significantly

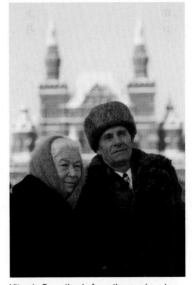

Vitamin D synthesis from the sun is not possible during most of the winter months for people living in high latitudes. Therefore, many people around the world, such as this couple in Russia, need to consume vitamin D in their diets, particularly during the winter.

Table 9.3   Factors Affecting Sunlight-Mediated Synthesis of Vitamin D in the Skin

Factors That Enhance Synthesis of Vitamin D	Factors That Inhibit Synthesis of Vitamin D
Season—Most vitamin D produced during summer months, particularly June and July	Season—Winter months (October through April) result in little or no vitamin D production
Latitude—Locations closer to the equator get more sunlight throughout the year	Latitude—Locations that are north of 40°N and south of 40°S get inadequate sun
Time of day—Generally between the hours of 10 a.m. and 3 p.m. (dependent upon latitude and time of year)	Time of day—Early morning, late afternoon, and evening hours
Age—Younger age	Age—Older age, particularly elderly (because of reduced skin thickness with age)
Limited or no use of sunscreen	Use of sunscreen with SPF 8 or greater
Sunny weather	Cloudy weather or air pollution (smog)
Exposed skin	Clothing or dark skin pigmentation
Light skin colour	Glass and plastics—Windows or other barriers made of glass or plastic (such as Plexiglas) block the sun's rays

lower risks of developing type 1 diabetes. Studies have used vitamin D supplements of 10 µg (400 IU) up to the UL of 50 µg (2000 IU), and this has prompted health professionals to call for a review of the 1997 Institute of Medicine DRI recommendations for vitamin D.

How Much Vitamin D Should We Consume?

If your exposure to the sun is adequate, then you do not need to consume any vitamin D in your diet. How do you know whether or not you are getting enough sun?

Recommended Dietary Intake for Vitamin D   As with calcium, there is no RDA for vitamin D. The AI is based on the assumption that an individual does not get adequate sun exposure. Of the many factors that affect our ability to synthesize vitamin D from sunlight, latitude and time of year are most significant (Table 9.3). Individuals living in very sunny climates relatively close to the equator, such as the southern United States and Mexico, may synthesize enough vitamin D from the sun to meet their needs throughout the year—as long as they spend time outdoors. However, vitamin D synthesis from the sun is not possible during most of the winter months for people living in places located at a latitude of more than 40°N or more than 40°S. This is because at these latitudes the sun never rises high enough in the sky during the winter to provide the direct sunlight needed. The 40°N latitude runs across the United States from northern Pennsylvania in the east to northern California in the west. Researchers in the Canadian Multicentre Osteoporosis Study (CaMos) have collected data on the bone health and vitamin D status of more than 9000 Canadians in nine regions across the country. Results from a sample of 188 men and women in Calgary showed that 34% of participants had low levels of vitamin D (vitamin D insufficiency) in at least one season of the year, most commonly fall or winter (Rucker et al. 2002). Calgary is said to have more hours of sunshine than any other Canadian city; however, at 51°N latitude, the sun's ultraviolet rays are not strong enough to produce sufficient vitamin D3 (cholecalciferol) in the skin of many people. Thus, Canadians cannot rely on sun exposure for vitamin D synthesis from October to April, and an adequate intake of vitamin D from diet and supplements becomes essential during those months.

Other factors influencing vitamin D synthesis include the time of day, skin pigmentation, and level of exposure. More vitamin D can be synthesized when the sun's rays are strongest, generally between 10 a.m. and 3 p.m. (Holick 2004). On overcast

▶ **HIGHLIGHT**

Dr. Stanley Zlotkin: Preventing Rickets

"Every penny counts!" We've all heard this age-old adage, but nowhere does it ring truer than in the case of providing nutritional supplements to impoverished children in developing countries. It may seem hard to believe, but just 3 cents a day can supply a child with a dose of micronutrients capable of preventing a host of debilitating diseases.

Although warding off these illnesses is no small task, these precious micronutrients are in fact delivered in tiny packages—no bigger than a sugar packet! This landmark creation is the brainchild of Dr. Stanley Zlotkin of the Hospital for Sick Children and University of Toronto. It is known as Supplefer Sprinkles, and it has the potential to purge developing countries of preventable diseases that severely diminish countless children's quality of life every day.

Although designed primarily for the purpose of treating and preventing anemia, Sprinkles has also had a profound effect on the prevention of rickets. Caused by a vitamin D deficiency, rickets is especially prevalent in poorer countries that have little exposure to sunlight during winter months. Mongolia is one country that perfectly fits this description, and when you factor in the lack of knowledge about this disease, it is no mystery why one third of Mongolian children have rickets (Bell 2004). Dr. Zlotkin has worked with World Vision Mongolia to distribute Sprinkles to the most vulnerable age group: 6 months to 3 years of age. After the age of 3, rickets cannot be completely reversed, but vitamin D in doses greater than the Adequate Intake is beneficial.

Some northern parts of Canada don't receive great amounts of sunlight in the winter months, so you may be wondering why rickets is not prevalent in our country. Here, milk is fortified with vitamin D to ensure that children receive enough of this crucial vitamin, but this was not always the case. In fact, according to Dr. Zlotkin, "In the 1930s, severe rickets was probably the single most frequent reason for a child to be admitted to Toronto's Hospital for Sick Children."

Providing micronutrient supplements to children in developing countries is not a new venture, but product design and unclear instructions have hindered past efforts. Before the introduction of Sprinkles, anemia was primarily prevented by giving an iron-fortified syrup to young children, who cannot swallow pills. This concoction,

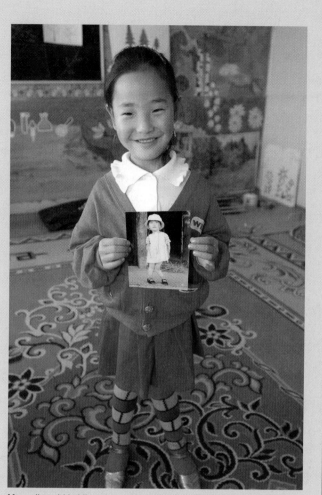

Mongolian girl holding photo of herself before treatment for rickets

however, stained teeth, tasted bad, often caused diarrhea, and lacked understandable instructions, sometimes leading to inadequate or dangerously high amounts being ingested (Bell 2004).

In developing Sprinkles, Dr. Zlotkin and his team had to address these issues to produce a product that could realistically be used by all families. To eliminate the tooth discolouration and bad taste, the iron in Sprinkles is encapsulated, a concept that has long been used to disguise the unpleasant taste of many medications (Zlotkin et al. 2001).

Encapsulation, in this case with soy lipid, prevents the oxidation process that is the culprit in altering the taste and colour of food (Zlotkin et al. 2001). To reduce the likelihood of insufficient quantities or accidental overdose, the brilliant idea of distributing micronutrients

(Continued)

in a single-serving sachet was put into action. Another matter that had to be attended to was the addition of some type of filler to bring the micronutrient mixture up to the 0.5 g minimum weight required to be packaged. Maltodextrin was decided to be the best candidate for this job. Ensuring that Sprinkles met the religious dietary requirements of Muslims (halal) and Jews (kosher) as well as developing a three-layer packaging system that could withstand the humidity of tropical environments were other considerations made while developing this product.

In 2000, Dr. Zlotkin and the H. J. Heinz Company of Pittsburgh, Pennsylvania, established a private–public partnership to help overcome obstacles associated with production of the tiny sachets of micronutrients. The actual cost per packet of Sprinkles varies according to how much is ordered, where it is produced, and the composition of the packet—it can range from US$0.015 to US$0.035.

The result of this long and careful development process is a convenient sachet filled with a fine powder that parents and guardians can easily sprinkle into their children's food without confusion or disagreeable side effects. Perhaps the most advantageous aspect of Sprinkles is how easy it is to address specific concerns in different countries. Any micronutrient can be added to a Sprinkles sachet, so the mixture can be revamped to include particular micronutrients that would benefit countries at elevated risk for certain diseases. For example, in Mongolia, the sachets include iron, ascorbic acid (to enhance iron absorption), zinc, vitamin A, folic acid, and vitamin D (Arthur and Zlotkin 2002). This short list of micronutrients belies the tremendous impact Sprinkles has had on this country: the incidence of vitamin D–related rickets in Mongolian children aged 6 months to 3 years has been reduced by 10% since the introduction of Sprinkles.

The remarkable success of Sprinkles so far is only the beginning. According to Dr. Zlotkin, "The long-term goal is to make Sprinkles available to populations in need throughout the world to help control the significant public health problem of anemia. Sprinkles for pregnant women and lactating mothers are currently being developed, and it is hoped that they will contribute to reducing the prevalence of anemia in this population group. The other long-term goal is to ensure sustainable methods of distribution in a country and to ensure that the most vulnerable people have access to them."

More than 10 million sachets of Sprinkles were distributed between 1997 and 2004, and this number will likely climb in the years to come as Dr. Zlotkin's vision is realized. Another exciting area of research that Dr. Zlotkin is pursuing is the effect of double-fortified table salt. It is clear that Dr. Stanley Zlotkin has had and will continue to make a huge impact on nutrition around the world.

Dr. Zlotkin is a professor in the departments of paediatrics, nutritional sciences, and public health sciences at the University of Toronto, senior scientist in the Research Institute of the Hospital for Sick Children, and head of the Division of Gastroenterology, Hepatology and Nutrition at the Hospital for Sick Children.

coenzyme An organic compound that combines with an inactive enzyme to form an active enzyme.

bone metabolism. A **coenzyme** is an organic compound that combines with an inactive enzyme to form an active enzyme. In the case of vitamin K, it assists in the production of *prothrombin*, a protein that plays a critical role in the clotting of our blood. It also assists in the production of *osteocalcin*, a protein that is associated with bone turnover. A summary of the functions, recommended intakes, and toxicity and deficiency symptoms associated with vitamin K is provided in Table 9.2 (page 317).

How Much Vitamin K Should We Consume?

We can obtain vitamin K from our diets, and we also produce vitamin K in our large intestine. These two sources of vitamin K usually provide adequate amounts of this nutrient to maintain health.

Recommended Dietary Intake for Vitamin K There is no RDA for vitamin K. AI recommendations for adult men and adult women are 120 µg per day and 90 µg per day, respectively. No Tolerable Upper Intake Level (UL) has been set for vitamin K.

Shopper's Guide: Good Food Sources of Vitamin K Only a few foods contribute substantially to our dietary intake of vitamin K. Green leafy vegetables including spinach, turnip greens, and leaf lettuce are good sources, as are broccoli, Brussels sprouts, and cabbage. Vegetable oils, such as soybean oil and canola oil, are also good sources of vitamin K. Figure 9.7 identifies the µg per serving for these foods.

What Happens If We Consume Too Much Vitamin K?

Based on our present knowledge, for healthy individuals there appear to be no side effects associated with consuming large amounts of vitamin K (Institute of Medicine 2002). This appears to be true for both supplements and food sources.

What Happens If We Don't Consume Enough Vitamin K?

Vitamin K deficiency is associated with a reduced ability to form blood clots, leading to excessive bleeding; however, primary vitamin K deficiency is rare in humans.

People with diseases that cause malabsorption of fat, such as celiac disease, Crohn's disease, and cystic fibrosis, can suffer from a secondary deficiency of vitamin K. Newborns are typically given an injection of vitamin K at birth, as they lack the intestinal bacteria necessary to produce this nutrient.

The impact of vitamin K deficiency on bone health is controversial. A recent study of vitamin K intake and risk of hip fractures found that women who consumed the least amount of vitamin K had a higher risk of bone fractures than women who consumed relatively more vitamin K (Feskanich et al. 1999). Despite the results of this study, there is not enough scientific evidence to support the contention that vitamin K deficiency leads to osteoporosis (Institute of Medicine 2002). In fact, there is no significant impact on overall bone density in people who take anticoagulant medications that result in a relative state of vitamin K deficiency.

Recap: Vitamin K is a fat-soluble vitamin and coenzyme that is important for blood clotting and bone metabolism. We obtain vitamin K largely from bacteria in the large intestine. The AIs for adult men and adult women are 120 µg per day and 90 µg per day, respectively. Green leafy vegetables and vegetable oils contain vitamin K. There are no known toxicity symptoms for vitamin K in healthy individuals. Vitamin K deficiency is rare and may lead to excessive bleeding.

Green leafy vegetables, including Brussels sprouts and turnip greens, are good sources of vitamin K.

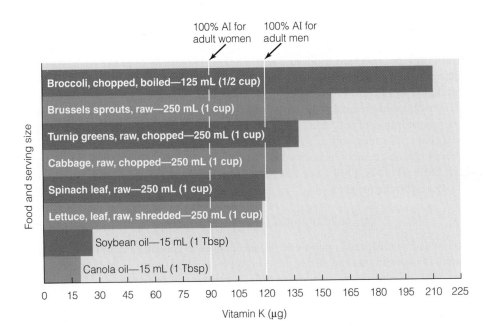

Figure 9.7 Common food sources of vitamin K.
(Nutrient data from U.S. Department of Agriculture, Agricultural Research Service, USDA Nutrient Database for Standard Reference, Release 15, 2002, Nutrient Data Laboratory homepage, www.ars.usda.gov/main/site_main.htm?modecode=12354500, accessed May 2003.)

Phosphorus

As discussed in Chapter 7, phosphorus is the major intracellular, negatively charged electrolyte. In our bodies, phosphorus is most commonly found combined with oxygen in the form of phosphate (or PO_4^{3-}). Phosphorus is an essential constituent of all cells and is found in both plants and animals.

Functions of Phosphorus

Phosphorus plays a critical role in bone formation, as it is a part of the mineral complex of bone. As discussed earlier in this chapter, calcium and phosphorus crystallize to form hydroxyapatite crystals, which provide the hardness to bone. About 85% of our bodies' phosphorus is stored in our bones, with the rest stored in soft tissues, such as muscles and organs.

The role of phosphorus in maintaining proper fluid balance was discussed in detail in Chapter 7. Phosphorus is also a primary component of adenosine triphosphate (ATP), the energy molecule that fuels body functions. It helps activate and deactivate enzymes, is a component of the genetic material in the nuclei of our cells (including both DNA and RNA), and is a component of our cell membranes and lipoproteins. A summary of the functions, recommended intakes, and toxicity and deficiency symptoms associated with phosphorus is provided in Table 9.2 (page 317).

How Much Phosphorus Should We Consume?

The details of phosphorus recommendations, food sources, and deficiency and toxicity symptoms were discussed in Chapter 7. A brief review is provided here.

Recommended Dietary Intake for Phosphorus The RDA for phosphorus for adults is 700 mg per day (Institute of Medicine 1997). Because the average North American adult consumes about twice this amount each day, phosphorus deficiencies are rare.

Shopper's Guide: Good Food Sources of Phosphorus Phosphorus is widespread in many foods and is found in high amounts in foods that contain protein. Milk, meats, and eggs are good sources. Refer to Table 7.5 for a review of the phosphorus content of various foods.

Phosphorus is found as a food additive in many processed foods, where it enhances smoothness, binding, and moisture retention. In the form of phosphoric acid, it is also a major component of cola soft drinks. Our society has increased its consumption of processed foods and soft drinks substantially over the past 20 years, resulting in an estimated 10% to 15% increase in phosphorus consumption (Institute of Medicine 1997).

Nutrition and medical professionals have become increasingly concerned that the heavy consumption of soft drinks may be detrimental to bone health. Studies have shown that consuming soft drinks is associated with reduced bone mass or an increased risk of fractures in both youth and adults (Wyshak et al. 1989; Wyshak and Frisch 1994; Wyshak 2000). See the Nutrition Debate at the end of this chapter to learn more about this issue.

What Happens If We Consume Too Much Phosphorus?

As discussed in Chapter 7, people with kidney disease and those who take too many vitamin D supplements can suffer from high blood phosphorus levels; severely high levels of blood phosphorus can cause muscle spasms and convulsions.

What Happens If We Don't Consume Enough Phosphorus?

Phosphorus deficiencies are rare but can occur in people who abuse alcohol, in premature infants, and in older adults with poor diets. People with vitamin D deficiency or hyperparathyroidism (oversecretion of parathyroid hormone) and those who overuse aluminum-containing antacids that bind with phosphorus may also have low blood phosphorus levels. Phosphorus deficiency symptoms include muscle weakness, bone pain, and dizziness.

> **Recap:** Phosphorus is the major negatively charged electrolyte inside the cell. It helps maintain fluid balance and bone health. It also assists in regulating chemical reactions, and it is a primary component of ATP, DNA, and RNA. The RDA for phosphorus for adults is 700 mg per day, and it is commonly found in high-protein foods. Excess phosphorus can lead to muscle spasms and convulsion, while phosphorus deficiencies are rare.

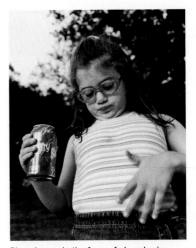

Phosphorus, in the form of phosphoric acid, is a major component of cola soft drinks.

Magnesium

Magnesium is a major mineral. Our total body magnesium content is approximately 25 grams. About 50% to 60% of the magnesium in our bodies is found in our bones, with the rest located in our soft tissues.

Functions of Magnesium

Magnesium is one of the minerals that make up the structure of bone. It is also important in the regulation of bone and mineral status. Specifically, magnesium influences the formation of hydroxyapatite crystals through its regulation of calcium balance and its interactions with vitamin D and parathyroid hormone.

Magnesium is a critical *cofactor* for more than 300 enzyme systems. A cofactor is a compound that is needed for an enzyme to be active. As discussed earlier in this book, a coenzyme is an organic compound that combines with an enzyme to make it active. The term *cofactor* refers to both organic compounds (coenzymes) and inorganic compounds (such as minerals) that combine with enzymes to make them active. Magnesium is necessary for the production of ATP, and it plays an important role in DNA and protein synthesis. Magnesium supports normal vitamin D metabolism and action and is necessary for normal muscle contraction and blood clotting. A review of the functions, recommended intakes, and toxicity and deficiency symptoms associated with magnesium is provided in Table 9.2 (page 317).

How Much Magnesium Should We Consume?

As magnesium is found in a wide variety of foods, people who are adequately nourished generally consume adequate magnesium in their diets.

Recommended Dietary Intake for Magnesium   The RDA for magnesium changes across age groups and genders. For adult men 19 to 30 years of age, the RDA for magnesium is 400 mg per day; the RDA increases to 420 mg per day for men 31 years of age and older. For adult women 19 to 30 years of age, the RDA for magnesium is 310 mg per day; this value increases to 320 mg per day for women 31 years of age and older. There is no UL for magnesium for food and water; the UL for magnesium from pharmacological sources is 350 mg per day.

Shopper's Guide: Good Food Sources of Magnesium   Magnesium is found in green leafy vegetables, such as spinach. It is also found in whole grains, seeds, and nuts. Other good food sources of magnesium include seafood, beans, and some dairy products. Figure 9.8 shows many foods that are good sources of magnesium. Refined and processed foods are low in magnesium.

The magnesium content of drinking water varies considerably. The harder the water, the higher its content of magnesium. This large variability in the magnesium content of water makes it impossible to estimate how much our drinking water may contribute to the magnesium content of our diets.

The ability of our small intestine to absorb magnesium is reduced when we consume diets that are very high in fibre and phytates because these substances bind with

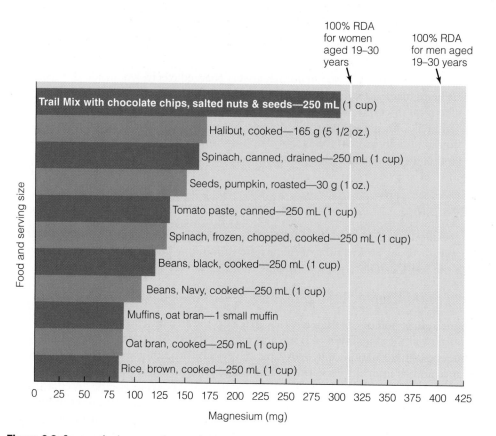

Figure 9.8 Common food sources of magnesium.
(Nutrient data from U.S. Department of Agriculture, Agricultural Research Service, USDA Nutrient Database for Standard Reference, Release 15, 2002, Nutrient Data Laboratory homepage, www.ars.usda.gov/main/site_main.htm?modecode=12354500, accessed May 2003.)

magnesium. Beans, seeds, nuts, and whole grains are high in both fibre and phytates. Our absorption of magnesium should be sufficient if we consume the recommended amount of fibre each day (20 to 35 grams per day). In contrast, higher dietary protein intakes enhance the absorption and retention of magnesium.

What Happens If We Consume Too Much Magnesium?

There are no known toxicity symptoms related to consuming excess magnesium in the diet. The toxicity symptoms that result from pharmacological use of magnesium include diarrhea, nausea, and abdominal cramps.

In extreme cases, large doses can result in acid–base imbalances, massive dehydration, cardiac arrest, and death. High blood magnesium levels, or **hypermagnesemia**, occur in individuals with impaired kidney function who consume large amounts of non-dietary magnesium, such as antacids. Side effects include impairment of nerve, muscle, and heart function.

What Happens If We Don't Consume Enough Magnesium?

Hypomagnesemia, or low blood magnesium, results from magnesium deficiency. This condition may result from kidney disease, chronic diarrhea, or chronic alcohol abuse. Older adults seem to be at particularly high risk of low dietary intakes of magnesium because they have a reduced appetite and blunted senses of taste and smell. In addition, some older adults face challenges related to shopping and preparing meals that contain foods high in magnesium, and their ability to absorb magnesium is reduced.

Low blood calcium levels are a side effect of hypomagnesemia. Other symptoms of magnesium deficiency include muscle cramps, spasms or seizures, nausea, weakness,

hypermagnesemia A condition marked by an abnormally high concentration of magnesium in the blood.

hypomagnesemia A condition characterized by an abnormally low concentration of magnesium in the blood.

irritability, and confusion. Considering magnesium's role in bone formation, it is not surprising that long-term magnesium deficiency is associated with osteoporosis. Magnesium deficiency is also associated with other chronic diseases, including heart disease, high blood pressure, and type 2 diabetes (Institute of Medicine 1997).

> **Recap:** Magnesium is a major mineral found in fresh foods, including spinach, nuts, seeds, whole grains, milk, and meats. Magnesium is important for bone health, energy production and muscle function. The RDA for magnesium is a function of age and gender. Hypermagnesemia can result in diarrhea, muscle cramps, and cardiac arrest. Hypomagnesemia causes hypocalcemia, muscle cramps, spasms, and weakness. Magnesium deficiencies are also associated with osteoporosis, heart disease, high blood pressure, and type 2 diabetes.

Trail mix with chocolate chips, salted nuts, and seeds is one common food source of magnesium.

Fluoride

Fluoride is the ionic form of the element fluorine, and it is also a trace mineral. As discussed in Chapter 1, trace minerals are minerals that our body needs in amounts of less than 100 mg per day; the amount of trace minerals found in our bodies is less than 5 grams. About 99% of the fluoride in our bodies is stored in our teeth and bones.

Functions of Fluoride

Fluoride assists in the development and maintenance of our teeth and bones. During the development of both our baby and permanent teeth, fluoride combines with calcium and phosphorus to form **fluorapatite**, which is more resistant to destruction by acids and bacteria than hydroxyapatite. Thus, teeth that have been treated with fluoride are more protected against the acids that cause dental caries (cavities) than teeth that have not been treated. Fluoride also stimulates new bone growth, and it is currently being researched as a potential treatment for osteoporosis. A review of the functions, recommended intakes, and toxicity and deficiency symptoms associated with fluoride is provided in Table 9.2 (page 317).

fluorapatite A mineral compound in human teeth that contains fluoride, calcium, and phosphorus and is more resistant to destruction by acids and bacteria than hydroxyapatite.

How Much Fluoride Should We Consume?

Most Canadians get adequate amounts of fluoride every day through dental products, foods we eat that naturally contain fluoride in trace amounts, foods made with fluoridated water, and fluoridated water supplies. Health Canada, the Canadian Public Health Association, the Canadian Dental Association, the Canadian Medical Association, and the World Health Organization recommend the addition of fluoride to municipal drinking water to prevent tooth decay. About 40% of Canadians live in communities with fluoridated water (Health Canada 2008b). Health Canada allows a maximum concentration of 1.5 mg fluoride per litre of water, and the Federal-Provincial–Territorial Committee on Drinking Water recommends 0.8 to 1.0 mg/L. Health Canada convened an expert panel on fluoride in January 2007 to review the latest science on the safety and efficacy of water fluoridation. The panel's findings were released in April 2008 and include the recommendation to slightly reduce the concentration of fluoride to 0.7 mg/L in drinking water (Health Canada 2008a).

Fluoride is absorbed directly into the teeth and gums, and can also be absorbed from the gastrointestinal tract once it is ingested. Because young children have a tendency to swallow toothpaste and mouth rinses, Health Canada has labelling requirements for dental products that contain fluoride (Health Canada 2008b). The expert panel has also recommended that toothpastes with lower concentrations of fluoride be available to children in Canada, as they are in other countries (Health Canada 2008a).

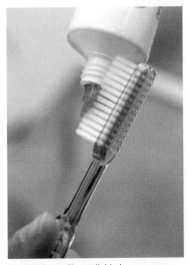

Fluoride is readily available in many communities in Canada through fluoridated water and dental products.

Recommended Dietary Intake for Fluoride   There is no RDA for fluoride. The AI for fluoride for children aged 4 to 8 years is 1 mg per day; this value increases to 2 mg per day for boys and girls aged 9 to 13 years. The AI for boys and girls aged 14 to 18 years is 3 mg per day. The AI for adults is 4 mg per day for adult men and 3 mg per day for adult women. The UL for fluoride is 2.2 mg per day for children aged 4 to 8 years; the UL for everyone older than 8 years of age is 10 mg per day.

Shopper's Guide: Good Food Sources of Fluoride   The two primary sources of fluoride are fluoridated dental products and fluoridated water. People who live in communities that do not have fluoridated water consume fluoride through beverages that contain fluoridated water and through fluoridated dental products. Toothpastes and mouthwashes that contain fluoride are widely marketed and used by the majority of consumers in North America, and these products can contribute as much if not more fluoride to our diets than fluoridated water. Most bottled waters do not contain fluoride.

What Happens If We Consume Too Much Fluoride?

fluorosis A condition marked by staining and pitting of the teeth; caused by an abnormally high intake of fluoride.

Consuming too much fluoride increases the protein content of tooth enamel, resulting in a condition called dental **fluorosis**. Because increased protein makes the enamel more porous, the teeth become stained and pitted. Teeth seem to be at highest risk for fluorosis during the first 6 or 7 years of life. Mild fluorosis generally causes white patches on the teeth, and it has no effect on tooth function. Moderate and severe fluorosis cause greater discolouration of the teeth, and there may be tooth pain that affects chewing but no other adverse effect on tooth function (Health Canada 2008b).

To prevent dental fluorosis in young children, Health Canada (2008b) advises against giving fluoride supplements and fluoridated mouthwash to children whose permanent teeth have not yet appeared (usually at about the age of 6 or 7 years). The availability of fluoride from a variety of sources (municipal water supplies, foods and beverages, dental products) means that most young children receive enough fluoride without the need for additional supplements. Excess consumption of fluoride can also cause fluorosis of our skeleton. Mild skeletal fluorosis results in an increased bone mass and stiffness and pain in the joints. Moderate and severe skeletal fluorosis can be crippling, leading to severe joint pain and stiffness, abnormal hardening of the bones in the pelvis and vertebrae, osteoporosis in the extremities, and wasting of the muscles. Severe skeletal fluorosis is an extremely rare progressive but not life-threatening condition (Institute of Medicine 1997).

What Happens If We Don't Consume Enough Fluoride?

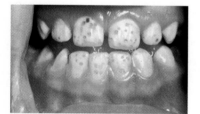

Consuming too much fluoride causes fluorosis, leading to staining and pitting of the teeth.

The primary result of fluoride deficiency is dental caries. Adequate fluoride intake appears necessary at an early age and throughout our adult life to reduce our risk for tooth decay. Inadequate fluoride intake may also be associated with lower bone density, but there is not enough research currently available to support the widespread use of fluoride to prevent osteoporosis. Studies are currently being done to determine the role fluoride might play in reducing our risk for osteoporosis and fractures.

Recap: Fluoride is a trace mineral whose primary function is to support the health of teeth and bones. The AI for fluoride is 4 and 3 mg per day for adult men and women, respectively. Primary sources of fluoride are fluoridated dental products and fluoridated water. Fluoride toxicity causes fluorosis of the teeth and skeleton, while fluoride deficiency causes an increase in tooth decay.

What Disorders Can Result from Poor Bone Health?

Of the many disorders associated with poor bone health, the most prevalent in North America is osteoporosis. In addition to osteoporosis, a few other disorders related to poor bone health are introduced in this section.

Osteoporosis

Osteoporosis is a disease characterized by low bone mass and deterioration of bone tissue, leading to enhanced bone fragility and increased fracture risk. The bone tissue of a person with osteoporosis is more porous and thinner than that of a person with healthy bone. These structural changes weaken the bone, leading to a significantly reduced ability of the bone to bear weight.

As mentioned earlier in this chapter, the hip and the vertebrae of the spinal column are common sites of osteoporosis; thus, it is not surprising that osteoporosis is the single most important cause of fractures of the hip and spine in older adults. These fractures are extremely painful and can be debilitating, with many individuals requiring nursing home care. In addition, they cause an increased risk of infection and other related illnesses that can lead to premature death. Osteoporosis Canada (2007b) notes that there are an estimated 25 000 hip fractures in Canada each year, and 70% of these are associated with osteoporosis. As many as 20% of people who suffer hip fractures die, and among those who survive, half will have some type of permanent disability. Canada spends an estimated $1.3 billion annually to treat osteoporosis and osteoporosis-related fractures (Osteoporosis Canada 2007b). Osteoporosis of the spine also causes a generalized loss of height and can be disfiguring: gradual compression fractures in the vertebrae of the upper back lead to a shortening and hunching of the spine, commonly referred to as *dowager's hump.*

Unfortunately, osteoporosis is a common disease: worldwide, one in three women and one in eight men are affected (International Osteoporosis Foundation 2003). In Canada, findings from the Canadian Multicentre Osteoporosis Study (CaMos) showed that 16% of women and 7% of men aged 50 and above had osteoporosis, and 10% of study participants in this age group had spinal fractures (CaMos 2004). Women in the 25- to 45-year age category who used oral contraceptives were found to have lower bone mineral density compared to women who didn't use oral contraceptives. Factors that influence our risk for osteoporosis include age, gender, genetics, nutrition, certain medications, and physical activity (Table 9.4). Let's review these factors and discuss how we can change our lifestyle to reduce our risk for osteoporosis.

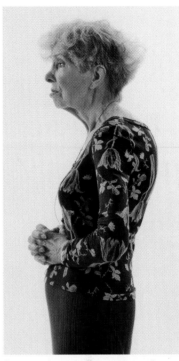

Osteoporosis can lead to a compression of vertebrae in the spine called a dowager's hump.

osteoporosis A disease characterized by low bone mass and deterioration of bone tissue, leading to increased bone fragility and fracture risk.

The Impact of Aging on Osteoporosis Risk

As discussed previously in this chapter, bone density declines as we age. Low bone mass and osteoporosis are therefore significant health concerns for both older men and women. By the year 2041 an estimated 25% of the Canadian population will be over the age of 65. The incidences of osteoporosis and low bone mass are expected to dramatically rise as people live longer (Osteoporosis Canada 2007d).

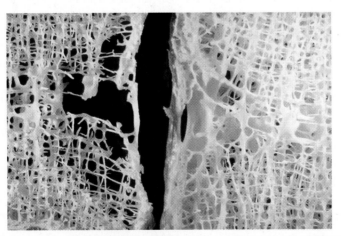

The vertebrae of a person with osteoporosis (left) are thinner and more collapsed than the vertebrae of a healthy person, in which the bone is denser and more uniform (right).

Table 9.4   Risk Factors for Osteoporosis

Modifiable Risk Factors	Non-Modifiable Risk Factors
Smoking	Older age (elderly)
Low body weight	Caucasian or Asian race
Low calcium intake	History of fractures as an adult
Low sun exposure	Family history of osteoporosis
Alcohol abuse	Female
History of amenorrhea (failure to menstruate) in women with inadequate nutrition	History of amenorrhea (failure to menstruate) in women with no recognizable cause
Estrogen deficiency (females)	
Testosterone deficiency (males)	
Repeated falls	
Sedentary lifestyle	
Certain medications (e.g., cortisone, prednisone, and anti-convulsants)	

Source: Table adapted from J. L. Milott, S. S. Green, and M. M. Schapira, Osteoporosis: Evaluation and treatment, 2000, *Complementary Therapies in Medicine,* 26:183–189. Copyright © 2000 American Society of Contemporary Medicine and Surgery. Reprinted with permission.

Hormonal changes that occur with aging have a significant impact on bone loss. Average bone loss approximates 0.3% to 0.5% per year after 30 years of age; however, during menopause in women, levels of the hormone estrogen decrease dramatically and cause bone loss to increase to 2% to 5% per year during the first five years of menopause (Osteoporosis Canada 2007b). Both estrogen and testosterone play important roles in promoting the deposition of new bone and limiting the activity of osteoclasts. Thus, men can also suffer from osteoporosis caused by age-related decreases in testosterone. In addition, reduced levels of physical activity in older people and a decreased ability to metabolize vitamin D with age exacerbate the hormone-related bone loss.

Gender and Genetics Affect Osteoporosis Risk

Osteoporosis disproportionately affects women: 16% of Canadian women aged 50 years and older have osteoporosis, compared with 7% of Canadian men (CaMos 2004). There are three primary reasons for this:

- Adult women have a lower absolute bone density than men. From birth through puberty, bone mass is the same in girls as in boys. But during puberty, bone mass increases more in boys, probably because of their prolonged period of accelerated growth. Thus, when bone loss begins around age 40, women have less bone stored in their skeletons than men. Since a woman's skeleton is already less dense, the loss of bone that occurs with aging causes osteoporosis sooner and to a greater extent in women than in men.

- As we have discussed, the hormonal changes that occur in men as they age do not have as dramatic an effect on bone density as those for women. The hormones in oral contraceptives may also have an effect on bone density. The CaMos study (2004) found that women in the 25- to 45-year age category who used oral contraceptives had lower bone density than women who didn't use oral contraceptives.

- Women live longer than men, and since risk increases with age, more elderly women suffer from this disease.

Secondary factors that are gender-specific include social pressure on girls to be extremely thin. Extreme dieting is particularly harmful in adolescence, when bone mass is building and adequate consumption of calcium and other nutrients is critical. In many girls, weight loss causes both a loss of estrogen and reduced weight-bearing stress on the bones. In contrast, boys experience pressure to bulk up, typically by lifting weights. This puts healthful stress on the bones, resulting in increased density.

Some individuals have a family history of osteoporosis, which increases their risk for this disease. Particularly at risk are Caucasian women of low body weight who have a first-degree relative (mother or sister) with osteoporosis. Asian women are also at higher risk than other non-Caucasian groups. Although we cannot change our gender or genetics, we can modify various lifestyle factors that affect our risk for osteoporosis.

Smoking and Poor Nutrition Increase Osteoporosis Risk

Cigarette smoking is known to decrease bone density because of its negative effects on hormones that affect bone formation and resorption; thus, cigarette smoking increases our risk for osteoporosis and resulting fractures.

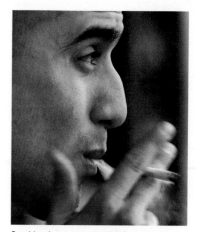

Smoking increases our risk for osteoporosis and resulting fractures.

Chronic alcoholism is detrimental to bone health and is associated with high rates of fractures. In contrast, numerous research studies have shown that bone density is higher in people who are *moderate* drinkers (Laitinen, Valimaki, and Keto 1991; Feskanich et al. 1999; Holbrook and Barrett-Connor 1993; Felson et al. 1995; Rapuri et al. 2000). Despite the fact that moderate alcohol intake may be protective for our bone, the dangers of alcohol abuse on overall health warrant caution in making any dietary recommendations. As is consistent with the alcohol recommendations related to heart disease, it is recommended that people should not start drinking if they are non-drinkers, and people who do drink should not consume more than two drinks per day.

Some researchers consider excess caffeine consumption to be detrimental to bone health. Caffeine is known to increase calcium loss in our urine, at least over a brief period. Younger people are able to compensate for this calcium loss by increasing absorption of calcium from the intestine. However, older people are not always capable of compensating to the same degree. Although the findings have been inconsistent, recent research now indicates that the relative amounts of caffeine and calcium consumed are critical factors affecting bone health. In general, older adult women do not appear to be at risk for increased bone loss if they consume adequate amounts of calcium and moderate amounts of caffeine (two cups of coffee, four cups of tea, or six 355 mL cans of caffeine-containing soft drinks per day) (Massey 2001). Older adult women who consume high levels of caffeine (more than three cups of coffee per day) have much higher rates of bone loss than women with low intakes (Rapuri et al. 2001). Thus, it appears important to bone health that we moderate our caffeine intake and ensure adequate consumption of calcium in our diets.

The effect of high dietary protein intake on bone health is controversial. Although it is well established that high protein intakes increase calcium loss, protein is a critical component of bone tissue and is necessary for bone health. High protein intakes have been shown to have both a negative and a positive impact on bone health. Similar to caffeine, the key to this mystery appears to be adequate calcium intake. Older adults taking calcium and vitamin D supplements and eating higher-protein diets were able to significantly increase bone mass over a three-year period, while those eating more protein and not taking supplements lost bone mass over this same time period (Dawson-Hughes and Harris 2002). Low protein intakes are also associated with bone loss and increased risk for osteoporosis and fractures in older adults. Thus, there appears to be an interaction between dietary calcium and protein, in that adequate amounts of each nutrient are needed together to support bone health.

As you've learned, a multitude of nutrients play critical roles in maintaining bone health. Of these nutrients, calcium and vitamin D have received the most attention regarding their role in the prevention of osteoporosis. Research studies conducted with older individuals have shown that their risk of bone fractures is reduced by taking calcium and vitamin D supplements. We know that if people do not consume enough of these two nutrients over a prolonged period, their bone density is lower and they have a higher risk of bone fractures. Because our bones reach peak density when we are young, it is very important that children and adolescents consume a high-quality diet that contains the proper balance of calcium, vitamin D, protein, and other nutrients to allow for optimal bone growth. Young adults also require a proper balance of these nutrients to maintain bone mass. In older adults, diets rich in calcium and vitamin D, and moderate in caffeine and alcohol, can help minimize bone loss.

In addition to their role in reducing our risk for heart disease and cancer, diets high in vegetables and fruits are also associated with improved bone health (Tucker et al. 1999; Tucker et al. 2002). This is most likely due to the fact that vegetables and fruits are good sources of nutrients that play a role in bone and collagen health, including magnesium, vitamin C, and vitamin K.

The Impact of Physical Activity on Osteoporosis Risk

Regular exercise is highly protective against bone loss and osteoporosis. Athletes are consistently shown to have denser bones than non-athletes, and regular participation in weight-bearing exercises, such as walking, jogging, tennis, and strength training, can help us increase and maintain our bone mass. When we exercise, our muscles contract and pull on our bones; this stresses our bone tissue in a way that stimulates increases in bone density. In addition, carrying our weight during activities, such as walking and jogging, stresses the bones of our legs, hips, and lower back, resulting in a healthier bone mass in these areas. It appears that people of all ages can improve and maintain bone health by consistent physical activity.

Can exercise ever be detrimental to bone health? Yes, when the body is not receiving the nutrients it needs to rebuild the hydoxyapatite and collagen broken down in response to physical activity. Thus, active people who are chronically malnourished, including people who are impoverished and those who suffer from eating disorders, are at increased fracture risk. Research has confirmed this association among nutrition, physical activity, and bone loss in the **female athlete triad**, a condition characterized by the coexistence of three (or a *triad* of) disorders in some athletic females: an eating disorder, amenorrhea, and osteoporosis. In the female athlete triad, inadequate food intake and regular strenuous exercise together result in a state of severe energy drain that causes a multitude of hormonal changes that affect menstrual function, including a reduction in estrogen production. These hormonal changes can result in the complete loss of menstrual function, called *amenorrhea*. As you have learned, estrogen is also important to maintaining healthy bone in women, so the loss of estrogen can lead to osteoporosis in young women. The female athlete triad is discussed in more detail in Chapter 13.

female athlete triad A condition characterized by the coexistence of three disorders in some athletic females: an eating disorder, amenorrhea, and osteoporosis.

Cancer Treatment and Bone Loss

Bone resorption (by osteoclasts) may outpace bone formation (by osteoblasts) when hormone levels are reduced, such as when estrogen levels drop during menopause in women. Hormonal changes are also part of some cancers, or they may be caused by some cancer treatments. Many breast cancers are associated with estrogen, for example, and cancer treatments may involve the use of drugs to reduce estrogen production. These treatments then lead to bone loss and the potential for bones to fracture. Similarly, androgen deprivation therapy (ADT) may be used to treat prostate cancer in men, however it increases the risk of osteoporosis. Health professionals are being encouraged to consider the longer-term consequences of cancer treatment on bone remodelling and bone health, since osteoporosis is often not diagnosed until bone fractures occur (Osteoporosis Canada 2007a). Some guidelines suggest regular DXA bone mineral density screening for men receiving ADT for prostate cancer, and for pre- and postmenopausal women who have received breast cancer therapy. It's estimated that only 3% to 32% of high-risk cancer patients currently have their bone mineral densities assessed. The use of bisphosphonates, discussed in the next section, is also encouraged to prevent bone loss in women receiving breast cancer treatment (Osteoporosis Canada 2007a).

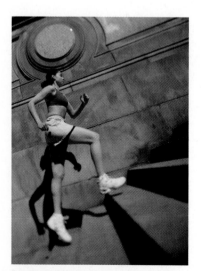

Regular weight-bearing exercises, such as jogging, can help us increase and maintain our bone mass.

Treatments for Osteoporosis

Although there is no cure for osteoporosis, a variety of treatments can slow, stabilize, and even reverse bone loss. First, individuals with osteoporosis are encouraged to consume adequate calcium and vitamin D and to exercise regularly. Studies have shown that the most effective exercise programs include weight-bearing exercises, such as jogging, stair climbing, and resistance training (South-Pal 2001).

Estrogen replacement therapy (ERT) and *hormone replacement therapy (HRT)* can be used for the prevention of osteoporosis in women. There are many brand names associated with these drugs, including Premarin and Prempro. ERT reduces bone loss, increases bone density, and reduces the risk of hip and spinal fractures. One major drawback of ERT is that taking estrogen alone increases a woman's risk for endometrial cancer, which is a cancer of the lining of the uterus. HRT combines estrogen with a hormone called progestin, greatly reducing the risk of endometrial cancer. Side effects of both ERT and HRT include breast tenderness, changes in mood, vaginal bleeding, and an increased risk for gallbladder disease.

Until recently, it was believed that HRT protected women against heart disease. A recent study found that one type of HRT actually increases a woman's risk for heart disease, stroke, and breast cancer. As a result, hundreds of thousands of women have recently quit taking HRT as a means to prevent or treat osteoporosis. However, there were positive health outcomes for those women taking HRT. The number of hip, spine, and other osteoporosis-related fractures was reduced, as was the risk of colorectal cancer. In general, the health risks associated with taking HRT are relatively low, and women need to weigh the benefits of reducing fracture risk with the increased risks of breast cancer and heart disease when considering HRT as an option for preventing or treating low bone density and osteoporosis.

In addition, several **anti-resorptive** medications are available; such medications slow or stop bone resorption but do not affect bone formation. This results in an overall reduction or cessation in the rate of bone loss in people with osteoporosis.

Alendronate (brand name Fosamax), etidronate (brand name Didrocal), and risedronate (brand name Actonel) are bisphosphonates, a class of drugs approved for the prevention and treatment of osteoporosis. These drugs decrease bone loss, increase bone density, and reduce the risk of spinal and non-spinal fractures. Side effects are not common and include abdominal or musculoskeletal pain, nausea, diarrhea, constipation, gas, heartburn, and irritation of the esophagus. These drugs must be taken in the morning on an empty stomach, at least 30 minutes before eating, drinking, or taking any other medications, and must be taken with 250 mL (8 fl. oz.) of water and no other liquid. In addition, the person taking these drugs must stay upright during the 30 minutes following drug administration. Health Canada recently approved a new bisphosphonate, Zoledronic acid (brand name Aclasta), which is given by a 15-minute intravenous infusion once a year. This new medication has been shown to cut the risk of spinal fractures and hip fractures by 70% and 41%, respectively (Osteoporosis Canada 2007c). It is estimated that from 40% to 60% of patients taking weekly or daily doses of bisphosphonates don't take their medications regularly, and a once-yearly medication may help to solve this problem.

Raloxifene (brand name Evista) is a selective estrogen-receptor modulator that was developed to mimic the beneficial effects of estrogen without the potential risks and is used for the prevention and treatment of osteoporosis. It increases bone mass and reduces the risk of spinal fractures while apparently reducing the risk of some forms of breast cancer. It may even reduce the risk of heart disease and stroke in women who have a high risk for these diseases. Side effects are not common and include hot flashes and the formation of blood clots in the veins.

Calcitonin (brand name Miacalcin) is a hormone that occurs naturally in our bodies and assists in the regulation of calcium and in bone metabolism. When used in the treatment of osteoporosis, calcitonin slows bone loss, increases the bone density of the spine, and reduces the risk for spinal fractures. Calcitonin is a protein; thus, it cannot be taken orally or it would be digested in our intestinal tract. It therefore must be

anti-resorptive Characterized by an ability to slow or stop bone resorption without affecting bone formation. Anti-resorptive medications are used to reduce the rate of bone loss in people with osteoporosis.

injected or inhaled through a nasal spray. Side effects of injected calcitonin include allergic reactions, flushing of the face and hands, skin rash, increased need to urinate, and nausea. Side effects of nasal calcitonin include nasal irritation, bloody nose, headaches, and backaches.

Recap: Osteoporosis is a major disease of concern for older adults. Osteoporosis increases our risk for fractures and premature death from subsequent illness. Factors that increase our risk for osteoporosis include genetics, being female, being of the Caucasian or Asian race, cigarette smoking, alcohol abuse, sedentary lifestyle, such medications as cortisone, prednisone, and anti-convulsants, and diets low in calcium and vitamin D. Certain hormone-related cancers and cancer therapies may increase bone loss. Medications are available for the prevention and treatment of osteoporosis. The newer drugs include bisphosphonates, calcitonin, and selective estrogen-receptor modulators. As various side effects are associated with each of these medications, patients must work closely with their physician to decide which is most appropriate.

CHAPTER SUMMARY

- Bones are organs that are dynamic and constantly active, building new bone and breaking down old bone.

- Bone develops through three processes: growth, modelling, and remodelling. Bone size is determined during growth, bone shape is determined during modelling and remodelling, and bone remodelling also affects the density of bone.

- Bone health can be assessed by measuring bone density. Dual energy x-ray absorptiometry (DXA) is the most accurate tool for measuring bone density. A score between +1 and −1 indicates normal bone density; scores above +1 are desirable.

- Calcium is a major mineral that is an integral component of bones and teeth. Calcium levels are constant in our blood at all times; calcium is also necessary for normal nerve transmission, muscle contraction, healthy blood pressure, and blood clotting.

- The AI for calcium is 1000 mg per day for adult men and women aged 19 to 50 years, and 1200 mg per day for adult men and women older than 50 years of age. The UL is 2500 mg per day for all age groups.

- Consuming excess calcium can lead to mineral imbalance, while consuming inadequate calcium can cause osteoporosis.

- Vitamin D is a fat-soluble vitamin that we can produce from the cholesterol in our skin by using the energy from sunlight. Vitamin D regulates absorption of calcium and phosphorus from our intestines, regulates blood calcium levels, and helps us maintain bone health.

- The AI for vitamin D is 5 μg (200 IU) per day for adult men and women aged 19 to 50 years; the AI increases to 10 μg (400 IU) per day for men and women aged 51 to 70 years, and to 15 μg (600 IU) per day for adults over the age of 70 years. The UL is 50 μg (2000 IU) per day for all age groups.

- Hypercalcemia results from consuming too much vitamin D, causing weakness, loss of appetite, diarrhea, vomiting, and muscle and joint aches. Vitamin D deficiency leads to soft bones that don't have sufficient mineralization, causing rickets in children or osteomalacia and osteoporosis in adults.

- Vitamin K is a fat-soluble vitamin that we obtain in the diet; it is also produced in our large intestine by normal bacteria. Vitamin K serves as a coenzyme for blood clotting and bone metabolism.

- The AI for vitamin K is 120 μg per day for men and 90 μg per day for women.

- There are no side effects of excess vitamin K intake for healthy individuals; vitamin K deficiency is rare and leads to excessive bleeding.

- Phosphorus is a major mineral that is an important part of the structure of bone; phosphorus is also a component of ATP, DNA, RNA, cell membranes, and lipoproteins.

- The RDA for phosphorus is 700 mg per day for all adults.

- Consuming too much phosphorus causes high blood phosphorus levels, leading to muscle spasms and convulsions; phosphorus deficiencies are rare and cause dizziness, bone pain, and muscle damage.

- Magnesium is a major mineral that is part of the structure of bone, influences the formation of hydroxyapatite crystals and bone health through its regulation of calcium balance and the actions of vitamin D and parathyroid hormone, and is a cofactor for more than 300 enzyme systems.

- The RDA for magnesium is 400 mg for men aged 19 to 30 years of age; 420 mg for men older than 30 years of age; 310 mg per day for women aged 19 to 30 years of age; and 320 mg per day for women older than 30 years of age.

- There are no known toxicity symptoms of consuming excess magnesium in the diet, though pharmacological excesses can result in such problems as diarrhea, cramping, dehydration, and cardiac arrest. Hypomagnesemia results from magnesium deficiency, resulting in low blood calcium levels, muscle cramps, seizures, confusion, and increased risk of some chronic diseases, such as heart disease and type 2 diabetes.

- Fluoride is a trace mineral that strengthens our teeth and bones and reduces our risk for dental caries.

- The AI for fluoride is 4 mg per day for men and 3 mg per day for women.

- Consuming too much fluoride causes fluorosis of the teeth and bones. Consuming too little fluoride increases our risk for dental caries and tooth decay and can weaken bones.

- Osteoporosis is a major bone disease in Canada, affecting 16% of women and 7% of men over the age of 50.

- Osteoporosis leads to increased risk of bone fractures and premature disability and death because of subsequent illness.

- Factors that increase our risk for osteoporosis include increased age, being female, being of the Caucasian or Asian race, cigarette smoking, alcohol abuse, low calcium and vitamin D intakes, certain medications, and a sedentary lifestyle.

mynutritionlab Go to MyNutritionLab at www.pearsoned.ca/mynutritionlab and enrich your understanding of nutrition! You'll find key animations, interactive exercises, access to My DietAnalysis, and much more.

REVIEW QUESTIONS

Quizzes

1. Hydroxyapatite crystals are predominantly made up of
   a. calcium and phosphorus.
   b. hydrogen, oxygen, and titanium.
   c. calcium and vitamin D.
   d. calcium and magnesium.

2. On a DXA test, a T-score of –0.5 indicates that the patient
   a. has osteoporosis.
   b. is at greater risk of fractures than an average, healthy person of the same age, sex, and race.
   c. has normal bone density as compared with an average, healthy 30-year-old of the same age, sex, and race.
   d. has slightly lower bone density than an average, healthy person of the same age, sex, and race.

3. Which of the following statements about trabecular bone is true?
   a. It accounts for about 80% of our skeleton
   b. It forms the core of almost all the bones of our skeleton
   c. It is also called compact bone
   d. It provides the scaffolding for cortical bone

4. Which of the following individuals is most likely to require vitamin D supplements?
   a. A dark-skinned child living and playing outdoors in Hawaii
   b. A fair-skinned construction worker living in Florida
   c. A fair-skinned retired teacher living in a nursing home in northern Manitoba
   d. A dark-skinned postal worker walking a route in California

5. Calcium is necessary for several body functions, including
   a. demineralization of bone, nerve transmission, and immune responses.
   b. cartilage structure, nerve transmission, and muscle contraction.
   c. structure of bone, nerve, and muscle tissue, immune responses, and muscle contraction.
   d. structure of bone, nerve transmission, and muscle contraction.

6. We can get vitamin D toxicity symptoms from
   a. too much exposure to the sun.
   b. eating too many milk products, including yogurt and cheese.
   c. taking high amounts of calcium in supplements.
   d. taking high amounts of vitamin D in supplements.

7. In addition to dietary sources, vitamin K is produced in our
   a. skin.
   b. stomach.
   c. small intestine.
   d. large intestine.

8. Give two reasons why adults over the age of 65 years may be more at risk for vitamin D deficiency than younger adults.

9. Explain the differences between osteoporosis and osteomalacia.

10. Explain how a person with breast cancer or prostate cancer may develop osteoporosis.

11. Explain why people with diseases that cause a malabsorption of fat may suffer from deficiency of vitamins D and K.

12. Most people reach their peak height by the end of adolescence, maintain that height for several decades, and then start to lose height in their later years. Describe the two processes behind this phenomenon.

13. Your best friend has fair skin and lives in Montreal. How much time does your friend need to spend out of doors with exposed skin on summer days to avoid the need for vitamin D from supplements? Should your friend take vitamin D supplements anyways?

14. Sinead's children are trying to convince her to have a DXA test to check her bone density. She is a 68-year-old woman living by herself, and she is refusing to go and see her doctor. She tells her children that she is much too young to have osteoporosis, and that she has always watched her weight and goes for walks at least three times a week. Her children argue that she's always had a penchant for diet pop and rarely drinks milk, so her bones must be in poor shape. What risk factors for osteoporosis apply to Sinead? What lifestyle factors are helping to reduce her risk for osteoporosis? Would you suggest that Sinead have the DXA test?

CASE STUDY

Chloe and Andrea are at the convenience store, looking for something to quench their thirst. Andrea reaches for a big carton of chocolate milk and Chloe comments that there are tons of calories and sugar in that. Instead, Chloe grabs a big bottle of diet pop. She explains that diet pop has fewer calories and no real sugar in it, making it the healthier choice. Andrea exchanges her milk for a diet pop and the two girls head back to school.

a. Was Chloe's diet pop really a healthier choice than Andrea's chocolate milk? Why or why not?

b. How do you think schools and parents could help persuade children to choose milk over soft drinks?

Test Yourself Answers

1. **False** By selecting foods that are good sources of calcium each day, most people can consume enough calcium in their diets to maintain bone health. People at risk for low calcium intakes include older adults, people who do not consume enough minerals in their diets, and people who do not consume enough food to maintain a healthful weight.

2. **False** Osteoporosis is more common among older women, but older men are also at risk for osteoporosis. Athletic young women who suffer from an eating disorder and menstrual cycle irregularity may also have osteoporosis, referred to as the female athlete triad.

3. **True** Our bodies can convert a cholesterol compound in our skin into vitamin D.

4. **True** Kale, broccoli, and turnip greens are good sources of calcium.

5. **True** Cigarette smoking has an unhealthy impact on the hormones that influence bone density. People who smoke have an increased risk for osteoporosis and fractures.

WEB LINKS

www.cda-adc.ca
Canadian Dental Association
Visit this site for more information about dental care, new techniques, and cosmetic procedures.

www.osteoporosis.ca
Osteoporosis Canada
This charitable organization provides information and advice for individuals with osteoporosis, the public, and health professionals. Try the Calcium Calculator to see if you are getting enough calcium in your diet.

www.nlm.nih.gov/medlineplus
MEDLINE Plus Health Information
Search for "rickets" or "osteomalacia" to learn more about these vitamin D–deficiency diseases.

www.iofbonehealth.org
International Osteoporosis Foundation
Find out more about this foundation and its mission to increase awareness and understanding of osteoporosis worldwide.

www.niams.nih.gov/Health_Info/Bone
National Institutes of Health
Osteoporosis and Related Bone Diseases—National Resource Center
Access this site for additional resources and information on metabolic bone diseases including osteoporosis and osteogenesis imperfecta.

Are the Amounts of Soft Drinks Consumed by Teens a Cause for Concern?

What is it about the latest soft drinks, like Fruitopia's Raspberry Kiwi Karma and carbonated beverages now available in everything—blue, vanilla, and carbohydrate reduced—that have so many teens choosing these drinks over milk? Why are dietitians and other health professionals keeping a watchful eye on the amount of soft drinks that teens are drinking?.

Dr. Susan Whiting is well-qualified to address these questions.

Dr. Susan Whiting, University of Saskatchewan

As a member of the American Society for Bone and Mineral Research, a consultant to the Scientific Advisory Board of the Osteoporosis Society of Canada, and chair of the Nutrition Subcommittee for the Osteoporosis Practice-Based Guidelines project, Dr. Whiting is one of Canada's leading researchers on bone health. And her findings suggest that the growing popularity of carbonated and uncarbonated soft drinks (the latter includes fruit drinks with less than 50% real fruit juice) is a threat to proper bone development among adolescents.

Adolescence is a critical time of growth when 30% to 40% of a person's bone accumulates (bone accrual). Calcium is an important constituent in bone mineralization, and dairy products are the most common sources of calcium in the Canadian diet. Insufficient amounts of calcium in teens' diets may compromise their bone development and put them at risk for osteoporosis in later life.

Dr. Whiting and her colleagues have examined the levels, sources, and seasonality of calcium intakes in Saskatchewan and found that fluid milk provides approximately 44% of the calcium in the diets of adolescents (Iuliano-Burns et al. 1999). However, adolescent girls appear to have low calcium intakes, with about 50% of their Calories from beverages coming from soft drinks rather than milk, and this puts teen girls at more risk for suboptimal bone development than boys (Vatanparast et al. 2006). Whiting and her colleagues have, in fact, shown that the high amounts of soft drinks, coupled with the inadequate calcium intakes, are resulting in less than optimum bone accrual for adolescent girls

(Whiting et al. 2001). Later, in Ireland, McGartland et al. (2003), using more than 10 times as many subjects, showed a similar impact on bone mineral density in adolescents. In both studies, girls had less bone accrual when intakes of soft drinks were high, while boys were spared an adverse effect on bone accrual (Whiting et al. 2001; McGartland et al. 2003). Whiting urges that, because females lose bone mineral mass faster than males later in life, it is especially important for females to achieve their maximal bone accrual and peak bone mass during adolescence (Whiting et al. 2004).

This work by these research teams strongly suggests that the direct substitution of soft drinks for milk beverages is the likely cause of the suboptimal bone health observed in teen girls, but this is difficult to prove conclusively. Other factors may cloud the picture, including smoking (perhaps the girls drinking soft drinks are also teen smokers?), overall poor diet quality (maybe less calcium-rich vegetables and legumes are consumed?), and low activity levels (a sedentary lifestyle may lead to less bone accrual). An earlier theory about the relationship between soft drink consumption and bone health was that the phosphorus in some cola beverages causes an imbalance between calcium and phosphorus in blood, which triggers the release of parathyroid hormone. Parathryoid hormone, in turn, stimulates osteoclasts to break down bone tissue, releasing calcium. However, it is more likely that the direct substitution of soft drinks for milk is related to suboptimal bone health.

Other Health Risks Associated with More Soft Drinks in the Diet

In addition to the impact on bone development, the shift away from milk in favour of soft drinks is thought to present other health risks to adolescents. More and more evidence supports the hypothesis that soft drinks may be an important contributor to the obesity epidemic, in part through the larger portion sizes of these beverages ("Would you like to supersize that?") and the high amounts of fructose (from high-fructose corn syrup) and sucrose they contain.

An often overlooked consequence of soft drink consumption is dental caries. Little attention has been given to the fact that sipping on acidic soft drinks loaded with simple carbohydrates can lead to tooth decay over time, spoiling a picture-perfect smile.

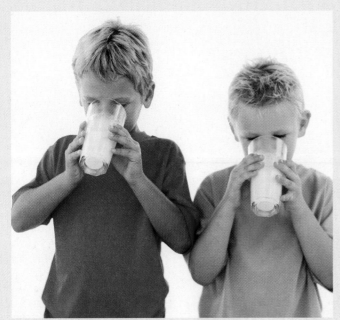

Encourage children to drink milk instead of soft drinks.

Why Are Soft Drinks the Beverage of Choice?

One of the factors driving the consumption of soft drinks is that many adolescents have complete freedom to consume whatever foods and beverages appeal to them. Food choices are influenced by peer groups, cost, and convenience. A large, ice-cold soft drink in a resealable container from a nearby vending machine may be more appealing and convenient than a small, overpriced carton of milk from the school cafeteria. In addition, the fast-food industry has made it hard to resist "supersizing" a soft drink for only pennies more. And any consumer who has tried to substitute milk or 100% fruit juice for a soft drink in a fast-food combo meal knows that it isn't easy to choose healthier options.

Who Is at Fault?

Adolescents are certainly capable of making informed decisions about the food and beverages they consume. And parents are obliged to provide growing children and teens with nutritious food options at home, and to set an appropriate example. But is it that straightforward?

If we consider for just a moment how much the food industry spends on child- and adolescent-specific marketing, shouldn't we point a finger in its direction, too? Soft drink team sponsorship, endorsements, advertising, and product placement in popular movies—is it possible for Canadian adolescents to avoid the message that soft drinks are the most convenient, affordable, and satisfying beverages out there?

Or is the marketplace to blame for providing cheap soft drinks and higher-priced milk? For the price of a 250 mL carton of milk at a fast-food restaurant, a cost-conscious teen could pick up a two-litre bottle of cola at a local convenience store. And what about schools that sign exclusive contracts with major soft drink manufacturers?

The concerns of researchers like Dr. Susan Whiting, the Dietitians of Canada, and parent lobbying groups have recently made a difference. The Coca-Cola Company and PepsiCo have pledged to stop selling carbonated soft drinks in cafeterias and vending machines in elementary and high schools in Canada, and they will replace them with water, fruit juices, and uncarbonated soft drinks. Even so, fruit drinks, flavoured waters, and other uncarbonated soft drinks are often high in sugar, so it is important to educate students on the most nutritious choices in the vending machines and cafeterias.

Is the ban on pop taking away students' freedom of choice? Where do you stand in this debate? Do you think the soft drinks you consume might be putting your bones at risk? What will it take for you to decide to put down the bottled soft drink and pick up a carton of milk now and then?

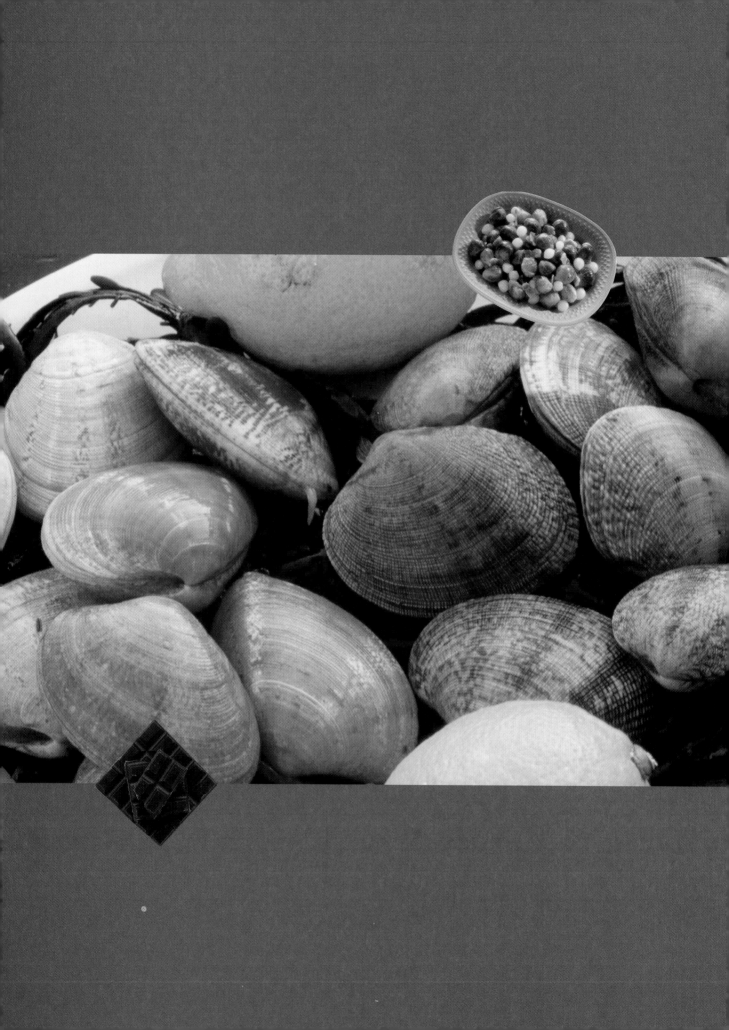

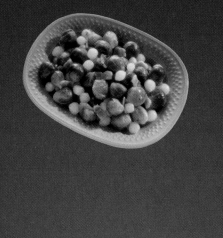

CHAPTER 10

Nutrients Involved in Energy Metabolism and Blood Health

CHAPTER OBJECTIVES

After reading this chapter you will be able to:

1. Describe how coenzymes enhance the activities of enzymes, pp. 350–352.

2. Identify the eight B vitamins and describe how they are involved in energy metabolism, pp. 352–358.

3. Identify the deficiency disorders of three B vitamins, pp. 352–358.

4. Identify at least two minerals that function as coenzymes in energy metabolism, pp. 359–361.

5. Describe the four components of blood, p. 362.

6. Discuss the role that iron plays in oxygen transport, pp. 364–365.

7. Distinguish among iron-deficiency anemia, pernicious anemia, and macrocytic anemia, pp. 373–379.

8. Describe the association among folate, vitamin B_{12}, and vascular disease, p. 373.

Test Yourself True or False

1. The B vitamins are an important source of energy for our bodies. **T or F**

2. Blood is a tissue. **T or F**

3. Excess amounts of the B vitamins are excreted, and therefore there are no Tolerable Upper Intake Levels (ULs) for these vitamins. **T or F**

4. Iron deficiency is the most common nutrient deficiency in the world. **T or F**

5. Taking a daily multivitamin-mineral supplement is a waste of money. **T or F**

Test Yourself answers can be found at the end of the chapter.

Dr. Leslie Bernstein looked in astonishment at the 80-year-old man in his office. A leading gastroenterologist and professor of medicine at Albert Einstein College of Medicine in New York City, he had admired Pop Katz for years as one of his healthiest patients, a strict vegetarian and athlete who just weeks before had been going on five-kilometre runs as if he were 40 years younger. Now he could barely stand. He was confused, cried easily, was wandering away from home partially clothed, and had lost control of his bladder. Tests showed that he was not suffering from Alzheimer's disease, had not had a stroke, did not have a tumour or an infection, and had no evidence of exposure to pesticides, metals, drugs, or other toxins. Blood tests were normal except that his red blood cells were slightly enlarged. Bernstein consulted with a neurologist, who diagnosed "rapidly progressive dementia of unknown origin."

Bernstein was unconvinced: "In a matter of weeks, a man who hadn't been sick for 80 years suddenly became demented—*Holy smoke!* I thought, *I'm an idiot! The man's been a vegan for 38 years. No meat. No fish. No eggs. No milk. He hasn't had any animal protein for decades. He has to be B_{12} deficient!*" Bernstein immediately tested Katz's blood, then gave him an injection of B_{12}. The blood test confirmed Bernstein's hunch: the level of B_{12} in Katz's blood was too low to measure. The morning after his injection, Katz could sit up without help. Within a week of continuing treatment, he could read, play card games, and hold his own in conversations. Unfortunately, the delay in diagnosis left some permanent neurological damage, including alterations in his personality and an inability to concentrate. Bernstein notes, "A diet free of animal protein can be healthful and safe, but it should be supplemented periodically with B_{12} by mouth or by injection" (Bernstein 2000).

It was not until 1906, when the English biochemist F. G. Hopkins discovered what he called *accessory factors,* that scientists began to appreciate the many critical roles of micronutrients in maintaining human health. Vitamin B_{12}, for instance, was not even isolated until 1948! In Chapters 7 through 9, we explored several key roles of vitamins and minerals, including regulation of fluids and nerve-impulse transmission, protection against the damage caused by oxidation, and maintenance of healthy bones. In this chapter, we conclude our exploration of the micronutrients with a discussion of two final roles: their contribution to the metabolism of carbohydrates, fats, and proteins, and their role in the formation and maintenance of our blood.

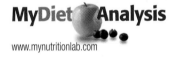

www.mynutritionlab.com

How Do Our Bodies Regulate Energy Metabolism?

We explored the digestion and metabolism of carbohydrates, fats, and proteins in Chapters 3 through 6 of this text. In those chapters, you learned that the regulation of energy metabolism is a complex process involving numerous biological substances and chemical pathways. Here, we describe how the micronutrients we consume in our diet assist us in generating energy from the carbohydrates, fats, and proteins we eat along with them.

Our Bodies Require Vitamins and Minerals to Produce Energy

Although vitamins and minerals do not directly provide energy, we are unable to generate energy from the macronutrients without them. The B vitamins are particularly important in assisting us with energy metabolism. Also referred to as the B-complex vitamins, this group includes thiamin, riboflavin, vitamin B_6, niacin, folate, vitamin B_{12}, pantothenic acid, and biotin.

The primary role of the B vitamins is to act as coenzymes. Remember from Chapter 6 that an *enzyme* is a protein that accelerates the rate of chemical reactions but is not used up or changed during the reaction. A coenzyme is a molecule that combines with an enzyme to activate it and help it do its job. Figure 10.1 illustrates how coenzymes work. Without coenzymes, we would be unable to produce the energy necessary for sustaining life and supporting daily activities.

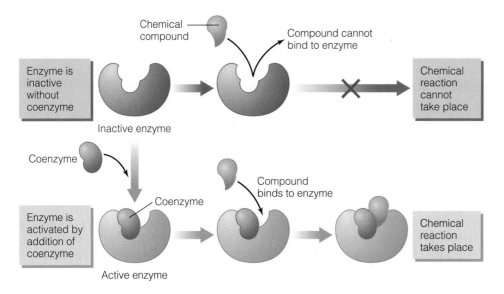

Figure 10.1 Coenzymes combine with enzymes to activate them, ensuring that the chemical reactions that depend upon these enzymes can occur.

Figure 10.2 provides an overview of how some of the B vitamins act as coenzymes to promote energy metabolism. For instance, thiamin is part of the coenzyme thiamin pyrophosphate, or TPP, which assists in the breakdown of glucose. Riboflavin is a part of two coenzymes, flavin mononucleotide (FMN) and flavin adenine dinucleotide (FAD), which help break down both glucose and fatty acids. The specific functions of each B vitamin are described in detail shortly.

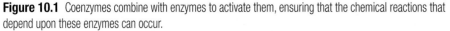

(a)

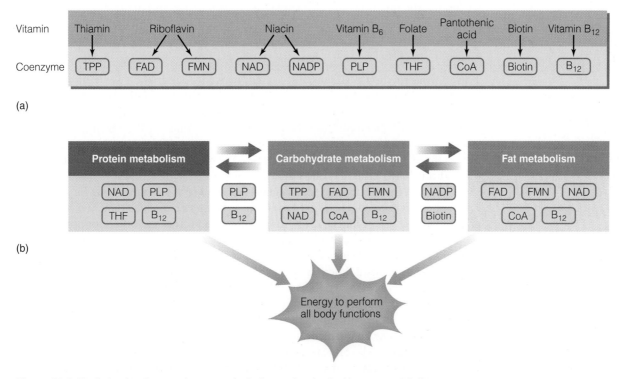

(b)

Figure 10.2 The B vitamins play many important roles in the reactions involved in energy metabolism. (a) B vitamins and the coenzymes they are a part of. (b) This chart illustrates many of the coenzymes essential for various metabolic functions; however, this is only a small sample of the thousands of roles that the B vitamins serve in our bodies.

Some Micronutrients Assist with Nutrient Transport and Hormone Production

Some micronutrients promote energy metabolism by facilitating the transport of nutrients into the cells. For instance, the mineral chromium helps improve glucose uptake into cells. Other micronutrients assist in the production of hormones that regulate metabolic processes; the mineral iodine, for example, is necessary for synthesis of thyroid hormones, which regulate our metabolic rate and promote growth and development. The details of these processes and their related nutrients are discussed in the following section.

> **Recap:** Vitamins and minerals are not direct sources of energy, but they help generate energy from carbohydrates, fats, and proteins. Acting as coenzymes, nutrients, such as the B vitamins, assist enzymes in metabolizing nutrients to produce energy. Minerals, such as chromium and iodine, assist with nutrient uptake into the cells and with regulating energy production and cell growth.

A Profile of Nutrients Involved in Energy Metabolism

In addition to the B vitamins, other nutrients involved in energy metabolism include a vitamin-like substance called choline and the minerals iodine, chromium, manganese, and sulphur. Let's take a closer look at these nutrients.

B Vitamins Act as Coenzymes in Energy Metabolism

Thiamin (vitamin B_1), riboflavin (vitamin B_2), niacin (nicotinamide and nicotinic acid), vitamin B_6 (pyridoxine), folate (folic acid), vitamin B_{12} (cobalamin), pantothenic acid, and biotin are the nutrients identified as the B vitamins. In this section we discuss the functions, recommended intakes, toxicity, and deficiency symptoms for these vitamins. For a summary of this discussion, see Table 10.1.

Thiamin (Vitamin B_1)

Thiamin was the first B vitamin discovered, hence its designation as vitamin B_1. Thiamin is part of the coenzyme thiamin pyrophosphate, or TPP. As a part of TPP, thiamin plays a critical role in the breakdown of glucose for energy and acts as a coenzyme in the metabolism of the branched-chain amino acids, which include leucine, isoleucine, and valine. TPP assists in producing DNA and RNA, and plays a role in the synthesis of neurotransmitters, or chemicals that transmit messages throughout our central nervous system.

The RDA for thiamin for adults aged 19 and older is 1.2 mg per day for men and 1.1 mg per day for women. Good food sources of thiamin include enriched cereals and grains, whole-grain products, ready-to-eat cereals, and ham and other pork products.

As the B vitamins are involved in most energy-generating processes, many of the deficiency symptoms include a combination of fatigue, apathy, muscle weakness, and detriments in cognitive function (see Table 10.1). Thiamin-deficiency disease is called **beriberi** and it comes in two forms: wet (the cardiovascular system is affected) and dry (the nervous system is affected) (Shils et al. 1999). In this disease, the body's inability to metabolize energy leads to muscle wasting and nerve damage; in later stages, patients may be unable to move at all. The heart muscle may also be affected, and the patient may die of heart failure.

Beriberi is seen in countries in which unenriched, processed grains are a primary food source; for instance, beriberi was widespread in China when rice was processed and refined, and it still occurs in refugee camps and other settlements dependent on poor-quality food supplies. Beriberi is also seen in industrialized countries in people with heavy alcohol consumption and limited food intake, where it is known as cerebral

beriberi A disease caused by thiamin deficiency.

Table 10.1   Functions, Recommended Intakes, and Toxicity and Deficiency Symptoms of B Vitamins and Choline

Nutrient	Primary Functions	Recommended Intake	Toxicity Symptoms/ Side Effects	Deficiency Symptoms/ Side Effects
Thiamin (vitamin B$_1$)	Part of the coenzyme thiamin pyrophosphate (TPP) involved in carbohydrate metabolism Coenzyme involved in branched-chain amino acid metabolism	RDA for 19 years and older: Men = 1.2 mg/day Women = 1.1 mg/day	None known at this time	Beriberi Anorexia and weight loss Apathy Decreased short-term memory Confusion and irritability Muscle weakness Enlarged heart
Riboflavin (vitamin B$_2$)	Coenzymes including flavin mononucleotide (FMN) and flavin adenine dinucleotide (FAD), involved in oxidation-reduction reactions for metabolism of carbohydrates and fats	RDA for 19 years and older: Men = 1.3 mg/day Women = 1.1 mg/day	None known at this time	Ariboflavinosis Sore throat Swelling of mouth and throat Cheilosis–dry, cracked lips Angular stomatitis–inflammation of the mucous membranes of the mouth Glossitis–magenta tongue Seborrheic dermatitis–inflammation of oil glands in the skin Anemia–lower than normal amount of red blood cells
Niacin (nicotinamide and nicotinic acid)	Coenzymes in carbohydrate and fatty acid metabolism, including nicotinamide adenine dinucleotide (NAD$^+$ and NADH) and nicotinamide adenine dinucleotide phosphate (NADP$^+$) Plays role in DNA replication and repair and cell differentiation	RDA for 19 years and older: Men = 16 mg/day Women = 14 mg/day	Excessive supplementation causes: Flushing Liver dysfunction and damage Glucose intolerance Blurred vision and edema of eyes	Pellagra Pigmented rash Vomiting Constipation or diarrhea Bright red tongue Depression Apathy Headache Fatigue Loss of memory
Vitamin B$_6$ (pyridoxine)	Part of coenzyme (pyridoxal phosphate, or PLP) involved in amino acid metabolism, synthesis of blood cells, and carbohydrate metabolism	RDA for 19 to 50 years of age: Men and women = 1.3 mg/day RDA for 51 years and older: Men = 1.7 mg/day Women = 1.5 mg/day	Excessive supplementation causes: Sensory neuropathy Lesions of the skin	Seborrheic dermatitis Microcytic anemia Convulsions Depression and confusion
Folate (folic acid)	Coenzyme tetrahydrofolate (THF), (or tetrahydrofolic acid, THFA) involved in DNA synthesis and amino acid metabolism Involved in the metabolism of homocysteine	RDA for 19 years and older: Men and women = 400 µg/day	Excessive supplementation causes: A masking of symptoms of vitamin B$_{12}$ deficiency Neurological damage	Macrocytic anemia Weakness and fatigue Difficulty concentrating Irritability Headache Palpitations Shortness of breath Elevated levels of homocysteine in the blood Neural tube defects in the developing fetus

(continued)

Table 10.1 Continued

Nutrient	Primary Functions	Recommended Intake	Toxicity Symptoms/ Side Effects	Deficiency Symptoms/ Side Effects
Vitamin B$_{12}$ (cobalamin)	Part of coenzymes that assist with formation of blood, nervous system function, and homocysteine metabolism	RDA for 19 years and older: Men and women = 2.4 µg/day	None known at this time	Pernicious anemia Pale skin Diminished energy and low exercise tolerance Fatigue Shortness of breath Palpitations Tingling and numbness in extremities Abnormal gait Memory loss Poor concentration Disorientation Dementia
Pantothenic acid	Component of coenzymes (coenzyme A, or CoA) that assist with fatty acid metabolism	AI for 19 years and older: Men and women = 5 mg/day	None known at this time	Rare; only seen in people who eat diets with virtually no pantothenic acid
Biotin	Component of coenzymes involved in carbohydrate, fat, and protein metabolism	AI for 19 years and older: Men and women = 30 µg/day	None known at this time	Red, scaly skin rash Depression Lethargy Hallucinations Burning, tingling, tickling Paresthesia of the extremities
Choline	Assists with homocysteine metabolism Accelerates the synthesis and release of the neurotransmitter acetylcholine Assists in synthesis of phospholipids and other components of cell membranes Assists in the transport and metabolism of fats and cholesterol	AI for 19 years and older: Men = 550 mg/day Women = 425 mg/day	Excessive supplementation causes: Fishy body odour Vomiting Excess salivation Sweating Diarrhea Low blood pressure	Increased fat accumulation in the liver, leading to liver damage

Wernicke-Korsakoff syndrome A form of thiamin deficiency seen in chronic alcoholics that results in mental confusion and a loss of memory.

beriberi or **Wernicke-Korsakoff syndrome**. Individuals with this condition show mental confusion, an inability to remember events in the past, and a lack of insight and ambition (Shils et al. 1999). Some individuals can improve when treated with thiamin supplements. There are no known adverse effects from consuming excess amounts of thiamin.

Riboflavin (Vitamin B$_2$)

Riboflavin is an important component of coenzymes that are involved in oxidation-reduction reactions occurring within the energy-producing metabolic pathways. These coenzymes, flavin mononucleotide (FMN) and flavin adenine dinucleotide (FAD), are involved in the metabolism of carbohydrates and fat. Riboflavin is also a part of the antioxidant enzyme glutathione peroxidase, thus assisting in the fight against oxidative damage.

The RDA for riboflavin for adults aged 19 and older is 1.3 mg per day for men and 1.1 mg per day for women. Note that milk is a good source of riboflavin; however, riboflavin is destroyed when it is exposed to light. Thus, milk is generally stored in opaque containers to prevent the destruction of riboflavin. Other good food sources include yogurt, enriched bread and grain products, ready-to-eat cereals, and organ meats.

There are no known adverse effects from consuming excess amounts of riboflavin. Riboflavin deficiency is referred to as **ariboflavinosis**. Symptoms of ariboflavinosis include inflamed, scaly, and greasy-looking skin, swelling of the mucus membranes in the mouth and throat, lips that are dry, cracked, and scaly (cheilosis), a purple-coloured tongue, and painful cracks at the corner of the mouth (angular stomatitis) (Shils et al. 1999). Severe riboflavin deficiency can impair the metabolism of vitamin B_6 (or pyridoxine).

Niacin

Niacin refers to the compounds nicotinamide and nicotinic acid. Interestingly, our bodies can make niacin from the amino acid tryptophan (60 mg tryptophan = 1 mg niacin). Niacin is a coenzyme that assists in the metabolism of carbohydrates and fatty acids, and it also plays an important role in DNA replication and repair and in the process of cell differentiation.

The RDA for niacin for adults aged 19 and older is 16 mg per day for men and 14 mg per day for women. The UL for niacin is 35 mg per day. Good food sources include meat, fish, poultry, enriched bread products, and ready-to-eat cereals.

Niacin can cause toxicity symptoms when taken in supplement form at high doses (such as 3 g/day). These symptoms include *flushing,* which is defined as burning, tingling, and itching sensations accompanied by a reddened flush primarily on the face, arms, and chest. Liver damage, glucose intolerance, blurred vision, and edema of the eyes can be seen with very large doses of niacin taken over long periods.

Pellagra results from severe niacin or tryptophan deficiency. Pellagra commonly occurred in the United States and parts of Europe in the early twentieth century in areas where corn or maize was the dietary staple. These foods are low in niacin and the amino acid tryptophan. Areas of the skin that are exposed to the sun become affected with a dermatitis that causes the skin to become rough, crusty, and dark coloured. It used to be known as the disease of the 4-Ds: dermatitis, diarrhea, dementia (although depression is more common than dementia), and, eventually, death (WHO 2000). At the present time, pellagra is rarely seen in industrialized countries, except in cases of chronic alcoholism. Pellagra is still found in such countries as India, China, and Africa. (For more information on pellagra, see the Highlight "Solving the Mystery of Pellagra" in Chapter 1.)

Vitamin B_6 (Pyridoxine)

Vitamin B_6 is actually a group of six related compounds: pyridoxine, pyridoxal, pyridoxamine, and the phosphate forms of these compounds, which include PNP, PLP, and PMP (respectively). Vitamin B_6 is part of a coenzyme for more than 100 enzymes involved in the metabolism of amino acids. It plays a critical role in transamination, which is the key process in making non-essential amino acids; without adequate vitamin B_6, all amino acids become essential, as our bodies cannot make them in sufficient quantities. Vitamin B_6 also assists in the metabolism of carbohydrate and the amino acid homocysteine and plays a role in the synthesis of hemoglobin and in oxygen transport.

The RDA for vitamin B_6 for adult men and women aged 19 to 50 years is 1.3 mg per day. For adults 51 years of age and older, the RDA increases to 1.7 mg per day for men and 1.5 mg per day for women. The UL for vitamin

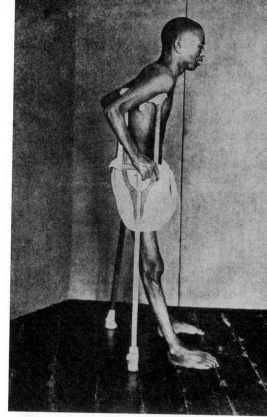

Dry beriberi, with wasting and nerve damage.

ariboflavinosis A condition caused by riboflavin deficiency.

pellagra A disease that results from severe niacin deficiency, characterized by dermatitis, diarrhea, depression, and in later stages, dementia and sometimes death.

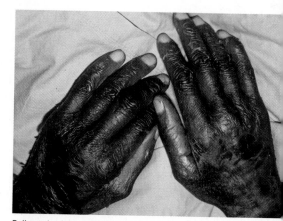

Pellagra is characterized by dermatitis in areas of the skin exposed to sunlight.

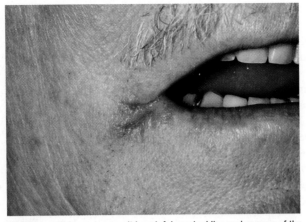

Riboflavin deficiency can result in painful cracked lips and corners of the mouth, and a magenta-coloured tongue.

B$_6$ is 100 mg per day. Good food sources include enriched ready-to-eat cereals, meat, fish, poultry, white potatoes and other starchy vegetables, organ meats, and fortified soy-based meat substitutes.

Vitamin B$_6$ supplements have been used to treat such conditions as premenstrual syndrome and carpal tunnel syndrome. You need to use caution, however, when using such supplements. Whereas consuming excess vitamin B$_6$ from food sources does not cause toxicity, supplementing in megadoses can result in nerve damage and lesions of the skin. Vitamin B$_6$ deficiency is uncommon, and the symptoms include depression and confusion. Severe cases of deficiency show symptoms of anemia, convulsions, and inflamed, irritated patches on the skin (Shils et al. 1999).

Folate

Folate is involved in DNA synthesis and amino acid metabolism. Its role in assisting with cell division makes it a critical nutrient during the first few weeks of pregnancy, when the combined sperm–egg cell multiplies rapidly to form the primitive tissues and structures of the human body. Folate, vitamin B$_{12}$, and vitamin B$_6$ are closely interrelated in some metabolic functions, including homocysteine metabolism.

The RDA for folate for adult men and women aged 19 years and older is 400 µg per day. The UL for folate is 1000 µg per day. Because of its critical role during the first few weeks of pregnancy and the fact that many women of childbearing age do not consume adequate folate, this nutrient has been added to wheat flour in Canada. Good food sources include breads, orange juice, leafy green vegetables, such as spinach and romaine lettuce, lentils, oatmeal, and asparagus.

Toxicity can occur when taking supplemental folate (in the form of folic acid). One especially frustrating problem with folate toxicity is that it can mask a simultaneous vitamin B$_{12}$ deficiency. This often results in failure to detect the B$_{12}$ deficiency and, as you saw in the chapter-opening case, a delay in diagnosis of B$_{12}$ deficiency can contribute to severe damage to the nervous system. There do not appear to be any clear symptoms of folate toxicity independent from its interaction with vitamin B$_{12}$ deficiency.

A folate deficiency can cause many adverse health effects, including *macrocytic (large cell) anemia*. Folate and vitamin B$_{12}$ deficiencies can cause elevated levels of homocysteine in the blood, a condition that is associated with heart disease. When folate intake is inadequate in pregnant women, *neural tube defects* (major malformations of the central nervous system that occur during the growth and development of the fetus) can occur. All of these conditions are discussed in more detail in the disorders section at the end of this chapter.

Vitamin B$_{12}$ (Cobalamin)

Vitamin B$_{12}$ is part of coenzymes that assist with formation of our blood. Also, as you saw in the chapter-opening scenario, B$_{12}$ is essential for healthy functioning of the nervous system because it helps maintain the sheath that coats nerve fibres. When this sheath is damaged or absent, the conduction of nervous signals is altered, causing numerous neurological problems.

Adequate levels of folate and vitamin B$_{12}$ are also necessary to break down the amino acid **homocysteine**. This amino acid is produced as a byproduct during the metabolism of another amino acid: methionine. When folate and vitamin B$_{12}$ consumption is inadequate, homocysteine levels rise. A high level of homocysteine in the blood is related to an increased risk of heart disease. We discuss the relationship between homocysteine and heart disease in more detail on page 373.

The RDA for vitamin B$_{12}$ for adult men and women aged 19 and older is 2.4 μg per day. Vitamin B$_{12}$ is found in only dairy products, meats, fish, eggs, and poultry; as discussed in Chapter 6, individuals consuming a vegan diet need to eat vegetable-based foods that are fortified with vitamin B$_{12}$ or take vitamin B$_{12}$ supplements or injections to ensure that they maintain adequate blood levels of this nutrient.

As we age, our sources of vitamin B$_{12}$ may need to change. Individuals younger than 51 years are generally able to meet the RDA for vitamin B$_{12}$ by consuming it in foods. However, it is estimated that about 10% to 30% of adults older than 50 years have a condition referred to as **atrophic gastritis** (Institute of Medicine 1998) that results in low stomach-acid secretion. Since stomach acid separates food-bound vitamin B$_{12}$ from dietary proteins, if the acid content of the stomach is inadequate, then we cannot free up enough vitamin B$_{12}$ from food sources alone. Because atrophic gastritis can affect almost one third of the older adult population, it is recommended that people older than 50 years of age consume foods fortified with vitamin B$_{12}$, take a vitamin B$_{12}$–containing supplement, or have periodic B$_{12}$ injections.

It is believed that vitamin B$_{12}$ insufficiency and deficiency are relatively common but often undiagnosed, particularly in older adults. Vitamin B$_{12}$ deficiency causes general symptoms of anemia, including pale skin, diminished energy and exercise tolerance, fatigue, and shortness of breath. Neurological symptoms include tingling and numbness of extremities, abnormal gait, memory loss, dementia, disorientation, visual disturbances, insomnia, and impaired bladder and bowel control. One of the primary causes of vitamin B$_{12}$ deficiency is a condition called *pernicious anemia*. People with pernicious anemia lack adequate amounts of a specialized protein secreted by the stomach, called intrinsic factor, that binds with vitamin B$_{12}$ and allows for its absorption into the bloodstream. Pernicious anemia is discussed in more detail with other micronutrient-related disorders on page 374.

There are no known adverse effects from consuming excess amounts of vitamin B$_{12}$.

Pantothenic Acid

Pantothenic acid is a component of coenzymes that assist with the metabolism of fatty acids. It is also critical for building new fatty acids. The AI for pantothenic acid for adult men and women aged 19 years and older is 5 mg per day. Food sources include chicken, beef, egg yolk, potatoes, oat cereals, tomato products, whole grains, and organ meats. There are no known adverse effects from consuming excess amounts of pantothenic acid. Deficiencies of pantothenic acid are very rare.

Biotin

Biotin is a component of coenzymes involved in the various steps of carbohydrate, fat, and protein metabolism. It also plays an important role in gluconeogenesis.

The AI for biotin for adult men and women aged 19 and older is 30 μg per day. The biotin content has been determined for very few foods, and these values are not reported in food composition tables or dietary analysis programs. Biotin appears to be

- Vitamin B$_{12}$ Absorption

homocysteine An amino acid that requires adequate levels of folate, vitamin B$_6$, and vitamin B$_{12}$ for its metabolism. High levels of homocysteine in the blood are associated with an increased risk for vascular diseases, such as cardiovascular disease.

atrophic gastritis A condition that results in low stomach-acid secretion; is estimated to occur in about 10% to 30% of adults older than 50 years of age.

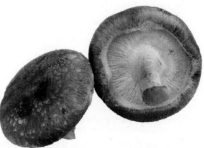

Shiitake mushrooms contain pantothenic acid.

Table 10.2 Common Foods That Contain at Least 50% of the RDA or AI for Select B Vitamins

Food Group	Thiamin	Riboflavin	Niacin	Vitamin B₆	Folate	Vitamin B₁₂	Pantothenic Acid
Meat, Poultry, Fish, Legumes	Pork loin, fried, 90 g (3 oz.) Pork ham, canned, 90 g (3 oz.)	Beef liver, fried, 90 g (3 oz.) Shrimp, breaded and fried, 6–8 shrimp	Beef liver, fried, 90 g (3 oz.) Chicken breast, breaded and fried, 1/2 breast Halibut, baked, 1/2 fillet Tuna fish, canned in oil, drained, 90 g (3 oz.)	Beef liver, fried, 90 g (3 oz.) Halibut, baked, 1/2 fillet Chickpeas, canned, 250 mL (1 cup)	Turkey giblets, simmered, 250 mL (1 cup) Lentils, boiled, 250 mL (1 cup) Pinto beans, boiled, 250 mL (1 cup)	Clams, canned, 90 g (3 oz.) Beef liver, fried, 90 g (3 oz.) New England clam chowder soup, 250 mL (1 cup) Salmon, baked, 1/2 fillet Tuna fish, canned in water, drained 90 g (3 oz.)	Beef liver, fried, 90 g (3 oz.)
Dairy	No dairy source	Chocolate milk-shake, 500 mL (16 fl. oz.)	No dairy source	No dairy source	No dairy source	New England clam chowder soup (a milk- or cream-based soup), 250 mL (1 cup)	Yogurt, plain, skim milk, 250 mL (1 cup)
Grains	Trail mix, with chocolate chips, salted nuts, and seeds, 250 mL (1 cup)	No grain source	No grain source	Long-grain white rice, dry, 250 mL (1 cup)	Long-grain white rice, dry, 250 mL (1 cup)	No grain source	Sunflower seeds, dry roasted, 60 mL (1/4 cup) Long-grain white rice, dry, 250 mL (1 cup)
Vegetables and Fruits	Sweet potato, baked with skin— 1 potato	No vegetable or fruit source	Tomato paste, 250 mL (1 cup)	Hash brown potatoes, 250 mL (1 cup)	No vegetable or fruit source	No vegetable or fruit source	Shiitake mush-rooms, cooked, 250 mL (1 cup)

Source: Data from U.S. Department of Agriculture, Agricultural Research Service, USDA Nutrient Database for Standard Reference, Release 16, 2003, Nutrient Data Laboratory homepage, www.ars.usda.gov/main/site_main.htm?modecode=12354500 (accessed January 2004).

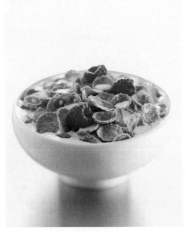

Ready-to-eat cereals are a good source of B vitamins.

widespread in foods. There are no known adverse effects from consuming excess amounts of biotin. Biotin deficiencies are typically seen only in people who consume a large number of raw egg whites over long periods. This is because raw egg whites contain a protein that binds with biotin and prevents its absorption. Biotin deficiencies are also seen in people fed total parenteral nutrition (nutrients are administered by a route other than the GI tract) that is not supplemented with biotin. Symptoms include thinning of hair; loss of hair colour; development of red, scaly rash around the eyes, nose, and mouth; depression; lethargy; and hallucinations.

Consuming Adequate B Vitamins Is Easy for Most People

In general, such foods as whole grains, enriched breads and ready-to-eat cereals, meat, poultry, fish, milk and dairy products, and some fruits and vegetables are good sources of the B vitamins. Although there are other food sources that contain more of these vitamins, ready-to-eat enriched cereals are regularly eaten by many adults and children in Canada and are consequently a consistently good source of the B vitamins. Table 10.2 summarizes other good sources of B vitamins.

Because most of the B vitamins are so widespread in foods, consuming adequate quantities from food sources is relatively easy for people who consume a varied diet and are able to adequately absorb these vitamins. Notice that, as shown in Table 10.1 on page 353, most of the B vitamins have an RDA value. At the present time, Tolerable Upper Intake Levels (UL) can only be set for niacin, vitamin B₆, and folate (Institute of Medicine 1998).

Recap: The B vitamins include thiamin, riboflavin, niacin, vitamin B_6 (pyridoxine), folate, vitamin B_{12} (cobalamin), pantothenic acid, and biotin. These vitamins primarily act as coenzymes in the metabolism of carbohydrates, fats, and protein. They are commonly found in whole grains, enriched breads, enriched ready-to-eat cereals, meats, dairy products, and some fruits and vegetables. B-vitamin toxicity is rare unless a person consumes large doses as supplements. Thiamin deficiency causes beriberi, niacin deficiency causes pellagra, folate deficiency causes macrocytic (large cell) anemia and can lead to neural tube defects in a fetus, and vitamin B_{12} deficiency leads to pernicious anemia and nervous system damage.

Choline

Choline is an essential vitamin-like substance found in many foods. It is typically grouped with the B vitamins because of its role in assisting homocysteine metabolism (see Table 10.1). Choline also accelerates the synthesis and release of **acetylcholine**, a neurotransmitter that is involved in many functions, including muscle movement and memory storage. Choline is also necessary for the synthesis of phospholipids and other components of cell membranes; thus, choline plays a critical role in the structural integrity of cell membranes. It appears to be especially critical during pregnancy, when it aids in the production of stem cells. There is some evidence that, like folate, choline may play a role in neural tube defects (Sanders and Zeisel 2007). Finally, choline can be metabolized to form phosphatidylcholine (lecithin), a key component of very low density lipoproteins (VLDL), which transport triglycerides out of the liver. Thus choline plays an important role in the transport and metabolism of fats and cholesterol, and one of the first clinical signs of a choline deficiency is a fatty liver, caused by the inability to move VLDL out of the liver (Sanders and Zeisel 2007).

Choline has an AI of 550 mg per day for men aged 19 and older and an AI of 425 mg per day for women aged 19 and older. The choline content of foods is not typically reported in nutrient databases. However, we do know that choline is widespread in foods, especially milk, liver, eggs, legumes, and peanuts. Inadequate intakes of choline can lead to increased fat accumulation in the liver, which eventually leads to liver damage. Excessive intake of supplemental choline results in various toxicity symptoms, including a fishy body odour, vomiting, excess salivation, sweating, diarrhea, and low blood pressure. The UL for choline for adults 19 years of age and older is 3.5 grams per day.

Iodine

Iodine is a trace mineral needed to support energy regulation. In our foods, iodine is mostly found in the form of iodide. Iodine is critical for the synthesis of thyroid hormones. Our bodies require thyroid hormones to regulate body temperature, maintain resting metabolic rate, and support reproduction and growth.

Although our bodies need relatively little iodine, adequate amounts are necessary to maintain health. The RDA for adults 19 years of age and older is 150 µg per day. The UL for iodine is 1100 µg per day.

Very few foods naturally contain iodine. Saltwater foods tend to have higher amounts of iodine because marine animals concentrate iodine from seawater. Good food sources include saltwater fish, shrimp, iodized salt, white and whole wheat breads made with iodized salt and bread conditioners, and milk and other dairy products. Interestingly, iodine is added to dairy cattle feed and used in sanitizing solutions in the dairy industry, making dairy foods an important source of iodine. Iodine has been added to salt in North America since the twentieth century to combat iodine deficiency resulting from poor iodine content of soils. For many people, iodized salt is their only source of iodine, and approximately 2 mL (1/2 tsp) of iodized salt meets the entire adult RDA for iodine.

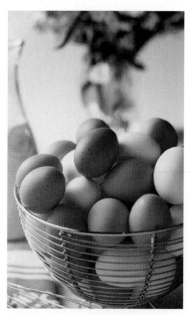

Choline is widespread in foods and can be found in eggs and milk.

acetylcholine A neurotransmitter that is involved in many functions, including muscle movement and memory storage.

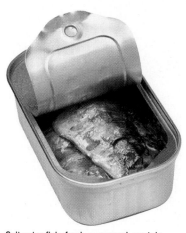

Saltwater fish, fresh or canned, contain iodine.

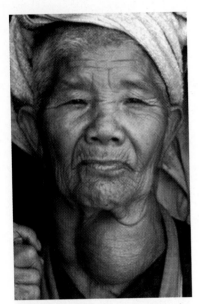

Goiter, or enlargement of the thyroid gland, occurs with both iodine toxicity and deficiency.

goiter Enlargement of the thyroid gland; can be caused by either iodine toxicity or deficiency.

cretinism A special form of mental retardation that occurs in infants when the mother experiences iodine deficiency during pregnancy.

Too much iodine blocks the synthesis of thyroid hormones. As the thyroid attempts to produce more hormones, it may enlarge, a condition known as **goiter**. (Goiter refers only to the enlarged thyroid gland, regardless of its cause.) Iodine toxicity generally occurs due to excessive supplementation.

Paradoxically, goiter is also the primary symptom of iodine deficiency. Iodine deficiency suppresses the production of thyroid hormones, leading to *hypothyroidism* (low levels of thyroid hormones) and goiter. Other symptoms of hypothyroidism are decreased body temperature, inability to tolerate cold environmental temperatures, weight gain, fatigue, and sluggishness. If a woman experiences iodine deficiency during pregnancy, her infant has a high risk of being born with a developmental disorder that results in a lower than normal IQ, referred to as **cretinism**. In addition to this mental disability, these infants may suffer from stunted growth, deafness, and muteness. Iodine deficiency during early pregnancy has also been associated with stillbirths, spontaneous abortions, and neonatal deaths (Shils et al. 1999).

Chromium

Chromium is a trace mineral that plays an important role in carbohydrate metabolism. You may be interested to learn that the chromium in our bodies is the same metal used in the chrome plating for cars.

Chromium enhances the ability of insulin to transport glucose from the bloodstream into cells. Chromium also plays important roles in the metabolism of RNA and DNA, in immune function, and in growth. Chromium supplements are marketed to reduce body fat and enhance muscle mass and have become popular with bodybuilders and other athletes interested in improving their body composition. (For more on this topic, see Chapter 12.) We have only very small amounts of chromium in our bodies. Whether our diets provide adequate chromium is controversial; our bodies appear to store less chromium as we age.

The AI for chromium for adults aged 19 to 50 years is 35 µg per day for men and 25 µg per day for women. For adults 51 years of age and older, the AI decreases to 30 µg per day and 20 µg per day for men and women, respectively.

Foods that have been identified as good sources of chromium include mushrooms, prunes, dark chocolate, nuts, whole grains, cereals, asparagus, brewer's yeast, some beers, and red wine. Dairy products are typically poor sources of chromium.

There appears to be no toxicity related to consuming chromium in the diet or in supplement form. Chromium deficiency appears to be uncommon in North America. When induced in a research setting, chromium deficiency inhibits the uptake of glucose by the cells, causing a rise in blood glucose and insulin levels. Chromium deficiency can also result in elevated blood lipid levels and in damage to the brain and nervous system.

Manganese

A trace mineral, manganese is a coenzyme involved in energy metabolism and in the formation of urea, the primary component of our urine. It also assists in the synthesis of the protein matrix found in bone tissue and in building cartilage, a tissue supporting our joints. As reviewed in Chapter 8, manganese is also an integral component of superoxide dismutase, an antioxidant enzyme. Thus, manganese assists in the conversion of free radicals to less damaging substances, protecting our bodies from oxidative damage.

The AI for manganese for adults 19 years of age and older is 2.3 mg per day for men and 1.8 mg per day for women. The UL for manganese is 11 mg per day for adults 19 years of age and older. Manganese requirements are easily met, as this mineral is widespread in foods and is readily available in a varied diet. Whole-grain foods, such as oat bran, wheat flour, whole wheat spaghetti, and brown rice are good sources of manganese (see Figure 10.3). Other foods that are good sources of manganese include pineapple, pine nuts, okra, spinach, and raspberries.

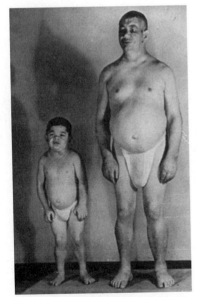

If a pregnant woman suffers from iodine deficiency, her child may have a mental disability called cretinism.

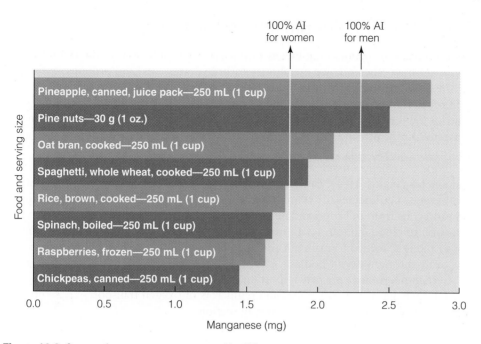

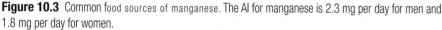

Figure 10.3 Common food sources of manganese. The AI for manganese is 2.3 mg per day for men and 1.8 mg per day for women.

(Data from U.S. Department of Agriculture, Agricultural Research Service, USDA Nutrient Database for Standard Reference, Release 16, 2003, Nutrient Data Laboratory homepage, www.ars.usda.gov/main/site_main.htm?modecode=12354500, accessed January 2004.)

Manganese toxicity can occur in occupational environments in which people inhale manganese dust and can also result from drinking water high in manganese. Toxicity results in impairment of the neuromuscular system, causing symptoms similar to those seen in Parkinson's disease, such as muscle spasms and tremors. Manganese deficiency is rare in humans. Symptoms of manganese deficiency include impaired growth and reproductive function, reduced bone density and impaired skeletal growth, impaired glucose and lipid metabolism, and skin rash.

Sulphur

Sulphur is a major mineral and a component of the B vitamins thiamin and biotin. In addition, as part of the amino acids methionine and cysteine, sulphur helps stabilize the three-dimensional shapes of proteins in our bodies. Our liver requires sulphur to assist in the detoxification of alcohol and various drugs, and sulphur assists us in maintaining acid–base balance.

We are able to synthesize ample sulphur from the protein-containing foods we eat; as a result, we do not need to consume sulphur in the diet, and there is no DRI for sulphur. There are no known toxicity or deficiency symptoms associated with sulphur.

Recap: Choline is a vitamin-like substance that assists in homocysteine metabolism and the production of acetylcholine. Iodine is necessary for the synthesis of thyroid hormones, which regulate metabolic rate and body temperature. Chromium enhances the transport of glucose into the cell, is important in the metabolism of RNA and DNA, and plays a role in immune function and growth. Manganese is involved in energy metabolism, the formation of urea, the synthesis of bone protein matrix and cartilage, and protection against free radicals. Sulphur is part of the B vitamins thiamin and biotin and also part of the amino acids methionine and cysteine.

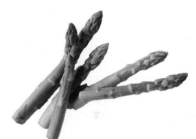

Our bodies contain very little chromium. Asparagus is a good dietary source of this trace mineral.

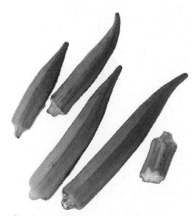

Okra is one of the many foods that contain manganese.

What Is the Role of Blood in Maintaining Health?

Blood is critical to maintaining life, as it transports virtually everything in our bodies. No matter how efficiently we metabolize carbohydrates, fats, and proteins, without healthy blood to transport those nutrients to our cells, we could not survive. In addition to transporting nutrients and oxygen to our cells to support life, blood removes the waste products generated from metabolism so that they can be properly excreted. Our health and our ability to perform daily activities are compromised if the quantity and quality of our blood is diminished.

Blood is actually a tissue, the only fluid tissue in our bodies. Blood comprises four components (Figure 10.4). **Erythrocytes**, or red blood cells, are the cells that transport oxygen. **Leukocytes**, or white blood cells, are the key to our immune function and protect us from infection and illness. **Platelets** are cell fragments that assist in the formation of blood clots and help stop bleeding. **Plasma** is the fluid portion of the blood, and it is needed to maintain adequate blood volume so that the blood can flow easily throughout our bodies.

Certain micronutrients play important roles in the maintenance of blood health through their actions as coenzymes and regulators of oxygen transport. These nutrients are discussed in detail in the following section.

A Profile of Nutrients That Maintain Healthy Blood

The nutrients recognized as playing a critical role in maintaining blood health include vitamin K, iron, zinc, and copper. A summary of the functions, requirements, and toxicity and deficiency symptoms of these nutrients is provided in Table 10.3.

Vitamin K

Vitamin K is a fat-soluble vitamin important for both bone and blood health. The role of vitamin K in the synthesis of proteins involved in maintaining bone density was discussed in detail in Chapter 9. In this section we focus primarily on its role in blood health.

erythrocytes The red blood cells, which are the cells that transport oxygen in our blood.
leukocytes The white blood cells, which protect us from infection and illness.
platelets Cell fragments that assist in the formation of blood clots and help stop bleeding.
plasma The fluid portion of the blood; needed to maintain adequate blood volume so that blood can flow easily throughout our bodies.

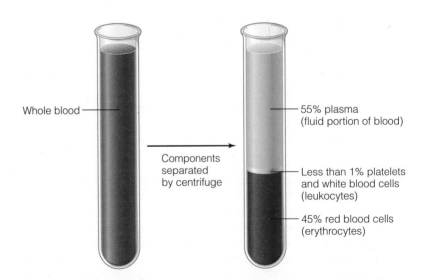

Whole blood

Components separated by centrifuge

55% plasma (fluid portion of blood)

Less than 1% platelets and white blood cells (leukocytes)

45% red blood cells (erythrocytes)

Figure 10.4 Blood has four components, which are visible when the blood is drawn into a test tube and spun in a centrifuge. The bottom layer is the erythrocytes, or red blood cells. The milky layer above the erythrocytes contains the leukocytes and platelets. The yellow fluid on top is the plasma.

Table 10.3   Nutrients Involved in Maintaining Blood Health

Nutrient	Primary Functions	Recommended Intake	Toxicity Symptoms/ Side Effects	Deficiency Symptoms/ Side Effects
Vitamin K (fat-soluble vitamin)	Coenzyme that assists in the synthesis of proteins involved in the coagulation of blood Coenzyme involved in the synthesis of proteins that assist in maintaining bone density	AI for 19 years and older: Men = 120 µg/day Women = 90 µg/day	None known at this time	Excessive bleeding or severe hemorrhaging caused by inability to form blood clots Effect on bone health is controversial
Iron (trace mineral)	As a component of hemoglobin, assists with oxygen transport in our blood As a component of myoglobin, assists in the transport of oxygen into muscle cells Coenzyme for enzymes involved in energy metabolism Part of the antioxidant enzyme system that combats free radicals	RDA for 19 to 50 years: Men = 8 mg/day Women = 18 mg/day RDA for 51 years and older: Men = 8 mg/day Women = 8 mg/day RDA for pregnant females = 27 mg/day	Nausea Vomiting Diarrhea Dizziness, confusion Rapid heartbeat Damage to heart, central nervous system, liver, kidneys Death	First stage of iron deficiency is marked by a decrease in iron stores with no physical symptoms Second stage of iron deficiency is marked by a decrease in iron transport, causing reduced work capacity Third stage of iron deficiency is marked by anemia, causing impaired work performance, general fatigue, pale skin, depressed immune function, impaired cognitive and nerve function, and impaired memory
Zinc (trace mineral)	Coenzyme that assists with hemoglobin production Part of superoxide dismutase antioxidant enzyme system that combats free radicals Assists enzymes in metabolizing carbohydrates, fats, and proteins and in activating vitamin A to facilitate vision Facilitates folding of proteins, which assists in gene regulation Plays role in cell replication and normal growth and sexual maturation Plays a role in proper development and function of immune system	RDA for 19 years and older: Men = 11 mg/day Women = 8 mg/day	Intestinal pain and cramps Nausea Vomiting Loss of appetite Diarrhea Headaches Depressed immune function Decreased concentration of high-density lipoprotein Reduced absorption of copper	Growth retardation Diarrhea Delayed sexual maturation and impotence Eye and skin lesions Hair loss Impaired appetite Increased incidence of illness and infections
Copper (trace mineral)	Coenzyme in metabolic pathways that produce energy Coenzyme that assists in production of collagen and elastin Part of superoxide dismutase antioxidant enzyme system that combats free radicals Component of ceruloplasmin, which facilitates the proper transport of iron	RDA for 19 years of age and older: Men and women = 900 µg/day	Abdominal pain and cramps Nausea Diarrhea Vomiting Liver damage occurs in extreme cases that result from Wilson's disease and other rare disorders	Anemia Reduced levels of white blood cells Osteoporosis in infants and growing children

Functions of Vitamin K

Vitamin K acts as a coenzyme that assists in the synthesis of a number of proteins that are involved in the coagulation of blood, including *prothrombin* and the *procoagulants*, and *factors VII, IX,* and *X.* Without adequate vitamin K, our blood does not clot properly: clotting time can be delayed, or clotting may even fail to occur. The failure of our blood to clot can lead to increased bleeding from even minor wounds, as well as internal hemorrhaging.

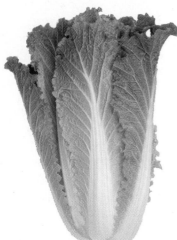

Green, leafy vegetables are a good source of vitamin K.

How Much Vitamin K Should We Consume?

Our needs for vitamin K are relatively small, but intakes of this nutrient are highly variable because vitamin K is found in few foods (Booth and Suttie 1998). Healthful intestinal bacteria produce vitamin K in our large intestine, providing us with an important non-dietary source of vitamin K.

The AI for vitamin K for adults 19 years of age and older is 120 µg per day and 90 µg per day for men and women, respectively. There is no UL established for vitamin K at this time (Institute of Medicine 2001).

Green, leafy vegetables are good sources of vitamin K. Examples include collard greens, spinach, broccoli, Brussels sprouts, and cabbage. Soybean and canola oils are also good sources. Refer to Figure 9.7 for a description of the vitamin K content of these foods.

What Happens If We Consume Too Much Vitamin K?

There are no known side effects associated with consuming large amounts of vitamin K from supplements or from food (Institute of Medicine 2001). In the past, a synthetic form of vitamin K was used for therapeutic purposes and was shown to cause liver damage; this form is no longer used.

What Happens If We Don't Consume Enough Vitamin K?

Vitamin K deficiency inhibits our ability to form blood clots, resulting in excessive bleeding and even severe hemorrhaging in some cases. Vitamin K deficiency is rare in humans. People with diseases that cause malabsorption of fat, such as celiac disease, Crohn's disease, and cystic fibrosis, can suffer secondarily from a deficiency of vitamin K. Newborns are typically given an injection of vitamin K at birth, as they lack the intestinal bacteria necessary to produce this nutrient.

As discussed in Chapter 9, the impact of vitamin K deficiency on bone health is controversial. Although a study found that low intakes of vitamin K were associated with a higher risk of bone fractures in women (Feskanich et al. 1999), there is not enough scientific evidence to strongly illustrate that vitamin K deficiency causes osteoporosis (Institute of Medicine 2001).

hemoglobin The oxygen-carrying protein found in our red blood cells; almost two thirds of all the iron in our bodies is found in hemoglobin.

heme The iron-containing molecule found in hemoglobin.

> **Recap:** Vitamin K is a fat-soluble vitamin and coenzyme that is important for blood clotting and bone metabolism. Bacteria manufacture vitamin K in our large intestine. The AIs for adult men and adult women are 120 µg per day and 90 µg per day, respectively.

Iron

Iron is a trace mineral that is needed in small amounts in our diets. Despite the small amount needed, iron deficiency is the most common nutrient deficiency in the world.

Functions of Iron

Iron is a component of many proteins in our bodies, including various enzymes and **hemoglobin**, which is the oxygen-carrying protein found in our red blood cells. In fact, almost two thirds of all the iron in our bodies is found in hemoglobin. As shown in Figure 10.5, the hemoglobin molecule consists of four polypeptide chains studded with four iron-containing **heme** groups. You know that we cannot survive for more than a few minutes without oxygen. Thus, hemoglobin's ability to transport oxygen throughout the body is absolutely critical to life. To carry oxygen, hemoglobin depends on the iron in its heme groups. Iron is able to bind with and release atoms, such as oxygen, nitrogen, and sulphur, very easily. It does this by transferring electrons to and from the other atoms as it

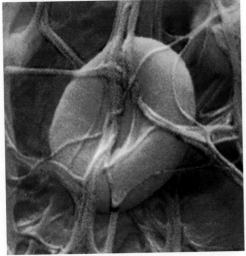

Blood clotting. Without enough vitamin K, our blood will not clot properly.

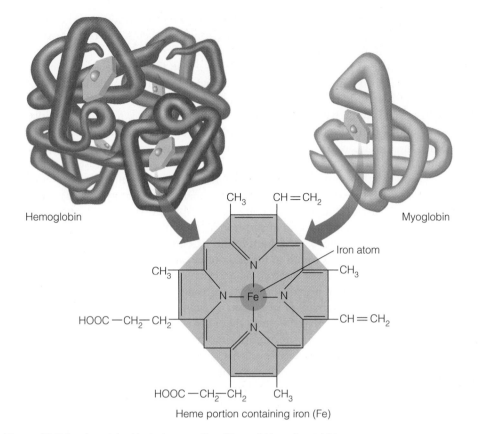

Hemoglobin

Myoglobin

Heme portion containing iron (Fe)

Figure 10.5 Iron is contained in the heme portion of hemoglobin and myoglobin.

moves between various oxidation states. In the bloodstream, iron acts as a shuttle, picking up oxygen from the environment, binding it during its transport in the bloodstream, and then dropping it off again in our tissues.

In addition to being a part of hemoglobin, iron is a component of **myoglobin**, a protein similar to hemoglobin but found in muscle cells. As a part of myoglobin, iron assists in the transport of oxygen into muscle cells.

Finally, iron is found in the body in certain enzymes. As a component of *cytochromes,* iron is a coenzyme involved in energy production. Cytochromes are electron carriers within the metabolic pathways that result in the production of energy from carbohydrates, fats, and protein. Also, as you learned in Chapter 8, iron is a part of the antioxidant enzyme system that assists in fighting free radicals. Interestingly, excess iron can also act as a pro-oxidant and promote the production of free radicals.

myoglobin An iron-containing protein similar to hemoglobin except that it is found in muscle cells.

How Much Iron Should We Consume?

Our bodies contain relatively little iron; men have less than 4 grams of iron in their bodies, while women have just more than 2 grams. Our bodies are capable of storing excess iron in two storage forms, **ferritin** and **hemosiderin**. The most common areas of iron storage in our bodies are the liver, bone marrow, intestinal mucosa, and spleen.

Our ability to absorb iron from the diet is influenced by a number of factors, including iron status, stomach acid content, the amount and type of iron in foods, and the presence of dietary factors that can either enhance or inhibit the absorption of iron. Absorption of iron is highest when our iron stores are low. Thus, people who have poor iron status, such as those with iron deficiency, pregnant women, or people who have recently experienced blood loss (including menstruation), have the highest iron absorption rates. In addition, adequate amounts of stomach acid are necessary for iron absorption. People with low levels of stomach acid, including many older adults, have a decreased ability to absorb iron.

ferritin A storage form of iron in our bodies found primarily in the intestinal mucosa, spleen, bone marrow, and liver.

hemosiderin A storage form of iron in our bodies found primarily in the intestinal mucosa, spleen, bone marrow, and liver.

heme iron Iron that is a part of hemoglobin and myoglobin; found only in animal-based foods such as meat, fish, and poultry.

non-heme iron The form of iron that is not a part of hemoglobin or myoglobin; found in animal- and plant-based foods.

MPF (meat protein factor) A special factor found in meat, fish, and poultry that enhances the absorption of non-heme iron.

The total amount of iron in your diet influences your absorption rate. People who consume low levels of dietary iron absorb more iron from their foods than those with higher dietary iron intakes. The type of iron in the foods you eat is a major factor influencing your iron absorption. There are two types of iron found in foods: heme iron and non-heme iron. **Heme iron** is a part of hemoglobin and myoglobin and is found only in animal-based foods, such as meat, fish, and poultry. **Non-heme iron** is the form of iron that is not a part of hemoglobin or myoglobin. It is found in both plant-based and animal-based foods. Heme iron is much more absorbable than non-heme iron. Since the iron in animal-based foods is about 40% heme iron and 60% non-heme iron, animal-based foods are good sources of absorbable iron. In contrast, all the iron found in plant-based foods is non-heme iron. Meat, fish, and poultry also contain a special factor, **MPF (meat protein factor)**, that enhances the absorption of non-heme iron. Vitamin C (or ascorbic acid) also enhances the absorption of non-heme iron.

Dietary factors that impair iron absorption include phytates, polyphenols, vegetable proteins, and calcium. Phytates are found in legumes, rice, and whole grains. Polyphenols include tannins found in tea and coffee, and polyphenols are also present in oregano and red wine. Soybean protein and calcium inhibit iron absorption. Because of the variability of iron absorption as a result of these dietary factors, it is estimated that the bioavailability of iron from a vegan diet is approximately 10%, while it averages 18% for a mixed Western diet (Institute of Medicine 2001).

To optimize our absorption of iron, it is important to consume either foods rich in heme iron or iron-rich foods with food that is high in vitamin C. For instance, eating meat with beans or vegetables enhances the absorption of the non-heme iron found in the beans and vegetables. Drinking a glass of orange juice with your breakfast cereal will increase the absorption of the non-heme iron in the cereal. Cooking foods in cast-iron pans will also significantly increase the iron content of foods, as the iron in the pan is absorbed into the food during the cooking process. It is best to avoid taking calcium supplements or drinking milk when eating iron-rich foods, as iron absorption will be impaired.

Recommended Dietary Intakes for Iron   The variability of iron availability from food sources was taken into consideration when estimating dietary recommendations for iron. The RDA for iron for men aged 19 years and older is 8 mg per day. The RDA for iron for women aged 19 to 50 years is 18 mg per day and decreases to 8 mg per day for women 51 years of age and older. The higher iron requirement for younger women is due to the excess iron and blood lost during menstruation. Pregnancy is a time of very high iron needs, and the RDA for pregnant women is 27 mg per day. The UL for iron for adults aged 19 and older is 45 mg per day.

There are a number of special circumstances that significantly affect iron requirements. These are identified in Table 10.4.

Shopper's Guide: Good Food Sources of Iron   Good food sources of heme iron include meats, poultry, and fish (Figure 10.6). Clams, oysters, and beef liver are particularly good sources of iron. Many breakfast cereals and breads are enriched with iron; although this iron is the non-heme type and less absorbable, it is still significant because these foods are a major part of the Canadian diet. Some vegetables and legumes are also good sources of iron, and the absorption of their non-heme iron can be enhanced by eating them with foods that contain MPF and heme iron or with vitamin C–rich foods.

What Happens If We Consume Too Much Iron?

Accidental iron overdose is the most common cause of poisoning deaths in children younger than six years of age in the United States (U.S. FDA 1997). (No comparable data for Canada could be found.) It is important for parents to take the same precautions with dietary supplements as they would with other drugs, keeping them in a locked cabinet or well out of reach of children. Symptoms of iron toxicity include nausea, vomiting, diarrhea, dizziness, confusion, and rapid heart beat. If iron toxicity is not treated quickly, significant damage to the heart, central nervous system, liver, and kidneys can result in death.

Cooking foods in cast-iron pans significantly increases their iron content.

Table 10.4 Special Circumstances Affecting Iron Status

Circumstances That Improve Iron Status	Circumstances That Diminish Iron Status
Use of oral contraceptives—use of oral contraceptives reduces menstrual blood loss in women. Breastfeeding—breastfeeding delays resumption of menstruation in new mothers and so reduces menstrual blood loss. It is therefore an important health measure, especially in developing nations. Consumption of iron-containing foods and supplements.	Use of hormone replacement therapy—use of hormone replacement therapy in postmenopausal women can cause uterine bleeding, increasing iron requirements. Eating a vegan diet—vegan diets contain no sources of heme iron or MPF. Because of the low absorbability of non-heme iron, vegans have iron requirements that are 1.8 times higher than non-vegetarians. Intestinal parasitic infection—approximately one billion people suffer from intestinal parasite infection. Many of these parasites cause intestinal bleeding and occur in countries in which iron intakes are inadequate. Iron-deficiency anemia is common in people with intestinal parasitic infection. Blood donation—blood donors have lower iron stores than non-donors; people who donate frequently, particularly premenopausal women, may require iron supplementation to counter the iron losses that occur with blood donation. Intense endurance exercise training—people engaging in intense endurance exercise appear to be at risk for poor iron status because of many factors, including suboptimal iron intake and increased iron loss caused by rupture of red blood cells and increased fecal losses.

Source: Data from Institute of Medicine, Food and Nutrition Board, *Dietary Reference Intakes for Vitamin A, Vitamin K, Arsenic, Boron, Chromium, Copper, Iodine, Iron, Manganese, Molybdenum, Nickel, Silicon, Vanadium, and Zinc.* © 2000 by the National Academy of Sciences, Washington, DC: National Academies Press, 2000.

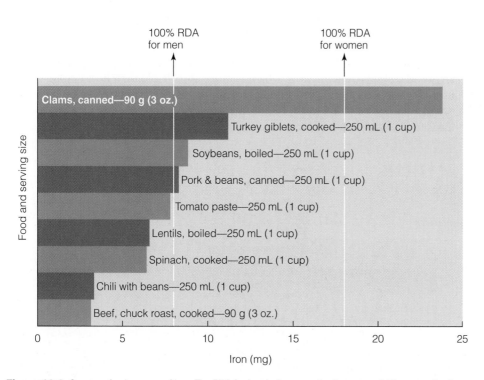

Figure 10.6 Common food sources of iron. The RDA for iron is 8 mg per day for men and 18 mg per day for women aged 19 to 50 years.
(Data from U.S. Department of Agriculture, Agricultural Research Service, USDA Nutrient Database for Standard Reference, Release 16, 2003, Nutrient Data Laboratory homepage, www.ars.usda.gov/main/site_main.htm?modecode=12354500, accessed January 2004.)

Adults who take iron supplements even at prescribed doses commonly experience constipation. Taking vitamin C with the iron supplement not only enhances absorption but also can help reduce constipation. Other gastrointestinal symptoms include nausea, vomiting, and diarrhea.

As introduced in Chapter 8, some individuals suffer from a hereditary disorder called hemochromatosis. This disorder affects between 1 in 200 and 1 in 400 individuals of northern European descent (Bacon et al. 1999). Hemochromatosis is characterized by excessive absorption of dietary iron and altered iron storage. The accumulation of iron in these individuals over many years causes cirrhosis of the liver, liver cancer, heart attack and heart failure, diabetes, and arthritis. Men are more at risk for this disease than women because of the higher losses of iron in women through menstruation. Treatment includes reducing dietary intake of iron, avoiding high intakes of vitamin C, and withdrawing blood occasionally.

What Happens If We Don't Consume Enough Iron?

Iron deficiency is the most common nutrient deficiency in the world. People at particularly high risk for iron deficiency include infants and young children, adolescent girls, premenopausal women, and pregnant women. Refer to the Highlight box on page 369 to learn more about the impact of iron deficiency on people around the world.

Iron deficiency progresses through three stages (Figure 10.7). The first stage of iron deficiency causes a decrease in iron *stores*, resulting in reduced levels of ferritin. During this first stage, there are generally no physical symptoms because hemoglobin levels are not yet affected. The second stage of iron deficiency causes a decrease in the *transport* of iron. This manifests as a reduction in the transport protein for iron, called **transferrin**. The production of heme also starts to decline during this stage, leading to symptoms of reduced work capacity. During the third and final stage of iron deficiency, **iron-deficiency anemia** results. In iron-deficiency anemia, the production of normal, healthy red blood cells decreases and hemoglobin levels are inadequate. Iron-deficiency anemia is discussed in detail on page 373.

transferrin The transport protein for iron.
iron-deficiency anemia A form of anemia that results from severe iron deficiency.

> **Recap:** Iron is a trace mineral that, as part of the hemoglobin protein, plays a major role in the transportation of oxygen in our blood. Iron is also a coenzyme in many metabolic pathways involved in energy production. The RDA for adult men aged 19 years and older is 8 mg per day. The RDA for adult women aged 19 to 50 years is 18 mg per day. Meat, fish, and poultry are good sources of heme iron, which is more absorbable than non-heme iron. Toxicity symptoms for iron range from nausea and vomiting to organ damage and potentially death. If left untreated, iron deficiency eventually leads to iron-deficiency anemia.

Stage 3 iron deficiency

- Iron-deficiency anemia
- Decreased production of normal red blood cells
- Reduced production of heme
- Inadequate hemoglobin to transport oxygen
- Symptoms include pale skin, fatigue, reduced work performance, impaired immune and cognitive functions

Stage 2 iron deficiency

- Decreased iron transport
- Reduced transferrin
- Reduced production of heme
- Physical symptoms include reduced work capacity

Stage 1 iron deficiency

- Decreased iron stores
- Reduced ferritin level
- No physical symptoms

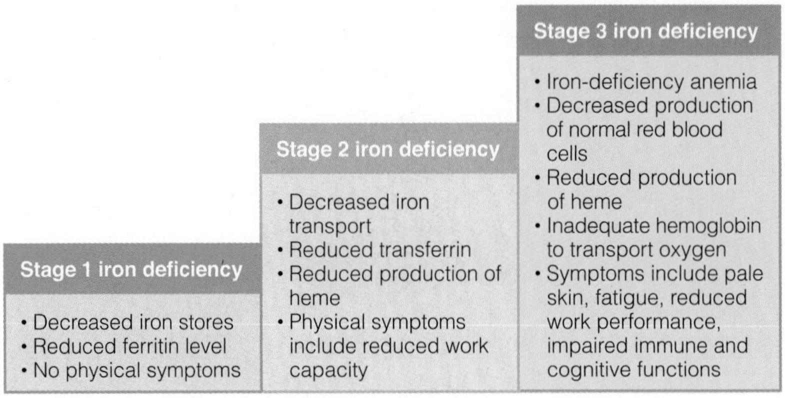

Figure 10.7 Iron deficiency passes through three stages. The first stage is identified by decreased iron stores, or reduced ferritin levels. The second stage is identified by decreased iron transport, or a reduction in transferrin. The final stage of iron deficiency is iron-deficiency anemia, which is identified by decreased production of normal, healthy red blood cells and inadequate hemoglobin levels.

▶ **HIGHLIGHT**

Global Nutrition: Iron Deficiency Around the World

Iron deficiency is the most common nutritional deficiency in the world. According to the World Health Organization (2003), approximately four billion to five billion people, or 66% to 80% of the world's population, are iron deficient. Because of its high prevalence worldwide, iron deficiency is considered an epidemic.

As you have learned in this chapter, severe iron deficiency results in anemia. Iron deficiency appears to be the main cause of anemia around the world. Other factors that can cause anemia include deficiencies of folate, vitamin B_{12}, and vitamin A, and infections, such as hookworm and malarial parasites. In fact, it is estimated that two billion people suffer from worm infections, while 300 million to 500 million people suffer from malaria.

Those who are particularly susceptible to iron deficiency include people living in developing countries, pregnant women, and young children. But iron deficiency does not hurt only individuals. Because it results in increased health care needs, premature death and resultant family breakdown, and lost work productivity, it also damages communities and entire nations.

Among children, the health consequences of iron-deficiency anemia are particularly devastating:

- premature birth
- low birth weight
- increased risk of infections
- increased risk of premature death
- impaired cognitive and physical development
- behavioural problems and poor school performance

To date, it is still unclear if iron supplementation in children already suffering from iron-deficiency anemia can effectively and consistently reverse the cognitive and behavioural damage that has occurred (Grantham-McGregor and Ani 2001).

The World Health Organization (2003) has developed a comprehensive plan to address all aspects of iron deficiency and anemia. This plan is being implemented in developing countries that suffer high rates of iron deficiency and anemia. This plan involves the following:

1. Increasing iron intake with iron supplements (see the work of Dr. Zlotkin in Chapter 9), iron-rich foods, and foods that enhance iron absorption
2. Controlling infections that cause anemia, including hookworm infections and malaria
3. Improving overall nutritional status by controlling major nutrient deficiencies and improving the quality and diversity of people's diets

By implementing this plan around the world, it is hoped that the devastating effects of iron deficiency can be reduced and potentially even eliminated.

Zinc

Zinc is a trace mineral that acts as a coenzyme for approximately 100 different enzymes. It thereby plays an important role in many physiologic processes in nearly every body system.

Functions of Zinc

As a coenzyme, zinc assists in the production of hemoglobin, indirectly supporting the adequate transport of oxygen to our cells. Zinc is also part of the superoxide dismutase antioxidant enzyme system and thus helps fight the oxidative damage caused by free radicals. It assists enzymes in generating energy from carbohydrates, fats, and protein and in activating vitamin A in the retina of the eye.

Zinc also plays a role in facilitating the folding of proteins into biologically active molecules used in gene regulation. Zinc is critical for cell replication and normal growth. In fact, zinc deficiency was discovered in the early 1960s when researchers were trying to determine the cause of severe growth retardation, anemia, and poorly developed testicles in a group of Middle Eastern men. These symptoms of zinc deficiency illustrate its critical role in normal growth and sexual maturation.

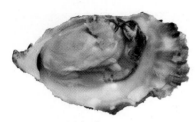

Oysters are high in zinc.

Zinc is vital for the proper development and functioning of the immune system. In fact, zinc has received so much attention for its contribution to immune system health that zinc lozenges have been formulated to fight the common cold. The Nutrition Debate at the end of this chapter explores the question of whether or not these lozenges are effective in combating the common cold.

How Much Zinc Should We Consume?

As with iron, our need for zinc is relatively small, but our intakes are variable and absorption is influenced by a number of factors. Overall, zinc absorption is similar to that of iron, ranging from 10% to 35% of dietary zinc. People with poor zinc status absorb more zinc than individuals with optimal zinc status, and zinc absorption increases during times of growth, sexual development, and pregnancy.

Several dietary factors influence zinc absorption. High non-heme iron intakes can inhibit zinc absorption, which is a primary concern with iron supplements (which are non-heme), particularly during pregnancy and lactation. High intakes of heme iron appear to have no effect on zinc absorption. Although calcium is known to inhibit zinc absorption in animals, this has not been demonstrated to occur in humans. The phytates and fibre found in whole grains and beans strongly inhibit iron absorption. In contrast, dietary protein enhances zinc absorption, with animal-based proteins increasing the absorption of zinc to a much greater extent than plant-based proteins.

It's not surprising, then, that the primary cause of the zinc deficiency in the Middle Eastern men just mentioned was their low consumption of meat and high consumption of beans and unleavened breads (also called *flat breads*). In leavening bread, the baker adds yeast to the dough. This not only makes the bread rise but also helps reduce the phytate content of the bread.

The RDA values for zinc for adult men and women aged 19 and older are 11 mg per day and 8 mg per day, respectively. The UL for zinc for adults aged 19 and older is 40 mg per day. Good food sources of zinc include red meats, some seafood, whole grains, and enriched grains and cereals. The dark meat of poultry has a higher content of zinc than white meat. As zinc is significantly more absorbable from animal-based foods, zinc deficiency is a concern for people eating a vegan diet. Figure 10.8 shows various foods that are relatively high in zinc.

What Happens If We Consume Too Much Zinc?

Eating high amounts of dietary zinc does not appear to lead to toxicity. Zinc toxicity can occur from consuming zinc in supplement form and in fortified foods. Toxicity symptoms include intestinal pain and cramps, nausea, vomiting, loss of appetite, diarrhea, and headaches. Excessive zinc supplementation has also been shown to depress immune function and decrease high-density lipoprotein concentrations. High intakes of zinc can also reduce copper status, as zinc absorption interferes with the absorption of copper.

What Happens If We Don't Consume Enough Zinc?

Zinc deficiency is uncommon in North America but occurs more often in countries in which people consume predominantly grain-based foods. Symptoms of zinc deficiency include growth retardation, diarrhea, delayed sexual maturation and impotence, eye and skin lesions, hair loss, and impaired appetite. As zinc is critical to a healthy immune system, zinc deficiency also results in increased incidence of infections and illnesses.

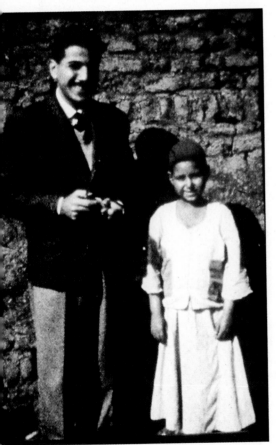

Growth retardation due to zinc deficiency. The boy on the right is 17 years old but is only four feet tall; his genitalia are like those of a six year old.

Copper

Copper is a trace mineral that functions as a coenzyme in many physiologic reactions. Copper is widely distributed in foods, and copper deficiency is rare.

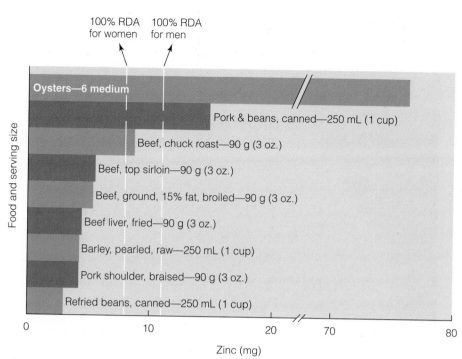

Figure 10.8 Common food sources of zinc. The RDA for zinc is 11 mg per day for men and 8 mg per day for women.

(Data from U.S. Department of Agriculture, Agricultural Research Service, USDA Nutrient Database for Standard Reference, Release 16, 2003, Nutrient Data Laboratory homepage, www.ars.usda.gov/main/site_main.htm?modecode=12354500, accessed January 2004.)

Copper functions as a coenzyme in the metabolic pathways that produce energy, in the production of the connective tissues collagen and elastin, and as part of the superoxide dismutase enzyme system that fights the damage caused by free radicals. Copper is a component of *ceruloplasmin*, a protein that is critical for the proper transport of iron. If ceruloplasmin levels are inadequate, iron accumulation results, causing symptoms similar to those described with the genetic disorder hemochromatosis (Chapter 8). Copper is also necessary for the regulation of certain neurotransmitters important to brain function.

Copper needs are very small, and people who eat a varied diet can easily meet their requirements. As we saw with iron and zinc, people with low dietary copper intakes absorb more copper than people with high dietary intakes. Also recall that high zinc intakes can reduce copper absorption, and, subsequently, copper status. In fact, zinc supplementation is used as a treatment for a rare disorder called Wilson's disease, in which copper toxicity occurs. High iron intakes can also interfere with copper absorption in infants.

The RDA for copper for men and women aged 19 years and older is 900 μg per day. The UL for adults ages 19 years and older is 10 mg per day.

Good food sources of copper include organ meats, seafood, nuts, and seeds. Whole-grain foods are also relatively good sources. Figure 10.9 reviews some foods relatively high in copper.

The long-term effects of copper toxicity are not well studied in humans. Toxicity symptoms include abdominal pain and cramps, nausea, diarrhea, and vomiting. Liver damage occurs in the extreme cases of copper toxicity that occur with Wilson's disease and other health conditions associated with excessive copper levels.

Copper deficiency is rare but can occur in premature infants fed milk-based formulas and in adults who eat prolonged formulated diets that are deficient in copper. Deficiency symptoms include anemia, reduced levels of white blood cells, and osteoporosis in infants and growing children.

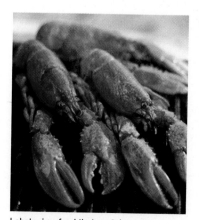

Lobster is a food that contains copper.

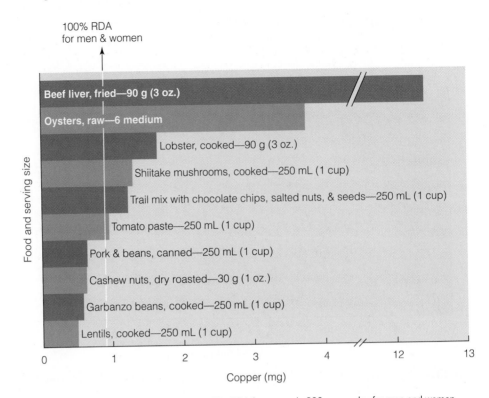

Figure 10.9 Common food sources of copper. The RDA for copper is 900 μg per day for men and women. (Data from U.S. Department of Agriculture, Agricultural Research Service, USDA Nutrient Database for Standard Reference, Release 16, 2003, Nutrient Data Laboratory homepage, www.ars.usda.gov/main/site_main.htm?modecode=12354500, accessed January 2004.)

Recap: Zinc is a trace mineral that is a part of almost 100 enzymes that affect virtually every body system. Zinc plays a critical role in hemoglobin synthesis, physical growth and sexual maturation, and immune function and assists in fighting the oxidative damage caused by free radicals. Copper is a trace mineral that is a coenzyme in the metabolic pathways that produce energy, in the production of the connective tissues collagen and elastin, and as part of the superoxide dismutase enzyme system that fights the damage caused by free radicals. Copper is also a component of ceruloplasmin, a protein that is critical for the proper transport of iron.

What Disorders Can Result from Inadequate Intakes of Nutrients Involved in Energy Metabolism and Blood Health?

A number of illnesses and disorders can occur if our intake of the nutrients related to energy metabolism and blood health is inadequate. Following is a brief review of some of these disorders.

Neural Tube Defects

A woman's requirement for folate substantially increases during pregnancy. This is because of the high rates of cell development needed for enlargement of the uterus, development of the placenta, expansion of the mother's red blood cells, and growth of the fetus. Inadequate folate intake during pregnancy can not only cause macrocytic (large cell) anemia but is also associated with major malformations in the fetus that are classified as neural tube defects.

Neural tube defects are the most common malformations of the central nervous system that occur during fetal development. The neural tube is formed by the fourth week of pregnancy, and it eventually develops into the brain and the spinal cord of the fetus. In folate deficiency, the tube will fail to fold and close properly. The resultant defect in the newborn depends on the degree of failure and can range from protrusion of the spinal cord outside of the spinal column to an absence of some brain tissue. Some forms of neural tube defects are minor and can be surgically repaired, while other forms are fatal. Neural tube defects are described in more detail in Chapter 15.

The challenging aspect of neural tube defects is that they occur very early in a woman's pregnancy, almost always before a woman knows she is pregnant. Thus, adequate folate intake is extremely important for all sexually active women of childbearing age, whether or not they intend to become pregnant. To prevent neural tube defects, it is recommended that all women capable of becoming pregnant consume 400 μg of folate daily from supplements, fortified foods, or both in addition to the folate they consume in their standard diet (Institute of Medicine 1998). The importance of folate in early pregnancy is also discussed in more detail on page 544.

neural tube defects The most common malformations of the central nervous system that occur during fetal development. A folate deficiency can cause neural tube defects.

Vascular Disease and Homocysteine

Folate and vitamin B_{12} are necessary for the metabolism of the amino acid homocysteine. When intakes of these two nutrients are insufficient, homocysteine cannot be properly metabolized, and it becomes more concentrated in our blood. A thorough review of recent studies on this topic showed that elevated levels of homocysteine are associated with a 1.5 to 2 times greater risk for cardiovascular, cerebrovascular, and peripheral vascular diseases (Beresford and Boushey 1997). These diseases substantially increase a person's risk for a heart attack or stroke.

The exact mechanism by which elevated homocysteine levels increase the risk for vascular diseases is currently unknown. It has been speculated (Mayer, Jacobsen, and Robinson 1996) that homocysteine may damage the lining of our blood vessels and stimulate the accumulation of plaque, which can lead to hardening of the arteries. Homocysteine also increases the clotting of our blood, which could lead to an increased risk of blocked arteries.

Although there is growing research evidence to suggest that low intakes of folate and vitamin B_{12} are associated with elevated homocysteine levels, the Institute of Medicine (1998) states that the DRI values for these two nutrients cannot be established based on this evidence at the present time. However, the importance of consuming adequate amounts of folate and vitamin B_{12} cannot be minimized. By eating foods that contain ample amounts of these nutrients, we not only reduce our risk for macrocytic and pernicious anemias, but we may also decrease our risk for a heart attack or stroke.

Anemia

The term *anemia* literally means "without blood"; it is used to refer to any condition in which hemoglobin levels are low. Some anemias are caused by genetic problems. For instance, you've probably heard of *sickle cell anemia,* a genetic disorder in which the red blood cells have a sickle shape. Another inherited anemia is *thalassemia,* a condition characterized by red blood cells that are small and short-lived. Other anemias are due to micronutrient deficiencies. Earlier in this chapter, we introduced three common deficiency-related anemias: iron-deficiency anemia, pernicious anemia, and macrocytic anemia. We discuss these in more detail here.

Iron-Deficiency Anemia

Red blood cells that are produced in an iron-deficient environment are smaller than normal and do not contain enough hemoglobin to transport adequate oxygen or to allow the proper transfer of electrons to produce energy. As normal cellular death occurs over time, more and more healthy red blood cells are replaced by these deficient cells, and the classic symptoms of oxygen and energy deprivation develop.

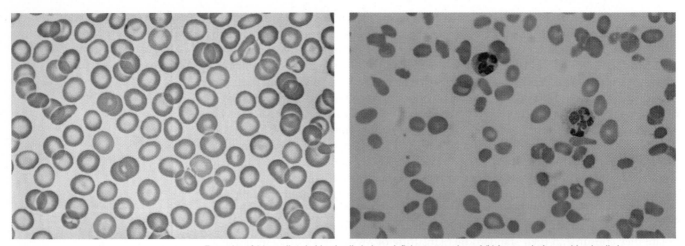

Examples of (a) small, pale blood cells in iron-deficiency anemia and (b) large, misshapen blood cells in macrocytic anemia.

These symptoms include impaired work performance, general fatigue, pale skin, depressed immune function, impaired cognitive and nerve function, and impaired memory. Pregnant women with severe anemia are at higher risk for low-birth-weight infants, premature delivery, and increased infant mortality.

Pernicious Anemia

As mentioned earlier in this chapter, **pernicious anemia** is a special form of anemia that is the primary cause of a vitamin B_{12} deficiency. Pernicious anemia occurs at the end stage of an autoimmune disorder that causes the loss of various cells in the stomach. The most common cause of the vitamin B_{12} deficiency seen with pernicious anemia is lack of a protein called **intrinsic factor**, which is normally secreted by these particular cells in the stomach. Intrinsic factor binds to vitamin B_{12} and aids its absorption in the small intestine. Pernicious anemia results in a reduction or complete cessation of intrinsic factor production. Without intrinsic factor, vitamin B_{12} cannot cross the intestinal lining. Inadequate production of intrinsic factor occurs more commonly in older people, making them at higher risk for vitamin B_{12} deficiency and pernicious anemia. Pernicious anemia can also occur in people who consume little or no vitamin B_{12} in their diets, such as people following a vegan diet. It is also commonly seen in people with malabsorption disorders, as well as in people with tapeworm infestation of the gut, as the worms take up the vitamin B_{12} before it can be absorbed by the intestines.

Symptoms of pernicious anemia include pale skin, reduced energy and exercise tolerance, fatigue, and shortness of breath. In addition, because nerve cells are destroyed, patients with pernicious anemia lose the ability to perform coordinated movements and maintain their body's positioning. Central nervous system (CNS) involvement can lead to irritability, confusion, depression, and even paranoia. As we saw in the case of Mr. Katz in the chapter opener, even with prompt administration of vitamin B_{12} after onset of CNS-involved symptoms, such symptoms are only partially reversible.

Macrocytic Anemia

A severe folate deficiency results in a condition called **macrocytic anemia**. Folate deficiency impairs DNA synthesis, which impairs the normal production of red blood cells. Macrocytic anemia is manifested as the production of larger-than-normal red blood cells containing insufficient hemoglobin, thus inhibiting adequate transport of oxygen. Because larger-than-normal red blood cells are produced in this situation, another term for macrocytic anemia is *megaloblastic anemia*. Symptoms of macrocytic anemia are similar to the symptoms that occur with other types of anemia,

pernicious anemia A special form of anemia that is the primary cause of a vitamin B_{12} deficiency; occurs at the end stage of an autoimmune disorder that causes the loss of various cells in the stomach.

intrinsic factor A protein secreted by cells of the stomach that binds to vitamin B_{12} and aids its absorption in the small intestine.

macrocytic anemia A form of anemia manifested as the production of larger-than-normal red blood cells containing insufficient hemoglobin, which inhibits adequate transport of oxygen; also called megaloblastic anemia. Macrocytic anemia can be caused by a severe folate deficiency.

including weakness, fatigue, difficulty concentrating, irritability, headache, shortness of breath, and reduced exercise tolerance.

Recap: Neural tube defects are potentially serious and even fatal malformations of the central nervous system in a developing fetus that can result from folate deficiency in the first few weeks of pregnancy. Low intakes of folate and vitamin B_{12} are associated with elevated blood homocysteine levels, which increase the risk of cardiovascular, cerebrovasular, and peripheral vascular disease. Anemia refers to any condition in which hemoglobin levels are low. Inadequate intake of iron causes iron-deficiency anemia, an autoimmune disorder causes pernicious anemia, and an inadequate intake of folate causes macrocytic anemia.

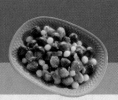

CHAPTER SUMMARY

- The B vitamins include thiamin, riboflavin, vitamin B_6, niacin, folate, vitamin B_{12}, pantothenic acid, and biotin.

- The primary role of the B vitamins is to act as coenzymes. In this role, they activate enzymes and assist them in the metabolism of carbohydrates, fats, and amino acids; the repair and replication of DNA; cell differentiation; the formation and maintenance of the central nervous system; and the formation of blood.

- Deficiencies of the B-complex vitamins can cause beriberi (thiamin), pellagra (niacin), neural tube defects (folate), and elevated homocysteine levels (folate and vitamin B_{12}).

- Choline is a vitamin-like substance that assists with homocysteine metabolism. Choline also accelerates the synthesis and release of acetylcholine, a neurotransmitter that is involved in a variety of functions, such as muscle function and memory storage.

- Iodine is a trace mineral needed for the synthesis of thyroid hormones. Thyroid hormones are integral to the regulation of body temperature, maintenance of resting metabolic rate, and healthy reproduction and growth.

- Chromium is a trace mineral that enhances the ability of insulin to transport glucose from the bloodstream into the cell. Chromium is also necessary for the metabolism of RNA and DNA, and supports normal growth and immune function.

- Manganese is a trace mineral that acts as a coenzyme in energy metabolism and in the formation of urea. Manganese also assists in the synthesis of the protein matrix found in bone, assists in building cartilage, and is a component of the superoxide dismutase antioxidant enzyme system.

- Sulphur is a major mineral that is a component of the B-complex vitamins thiamin and biotin. It is also a part of the amino acids methionine and cysteine. Sulphur helps stabilize the three-dimensional shapes of proteins and helps the liver detoxify alcohol and various drugs.

- Blood is the only fluid tissue in our bodies. It has four components: erythrocytes, or red blood cells; leukocytes, or white blood cells; platelets; and plasma, or the fluid portion of our blood.

- Blood is critical for transporting oxygen and nutrients to our cells and for removing waste products from our cells so they can be properly excreted.

- Vitamin K is a fat-soluble vitamin that acts as a coenzyme assisting in the coagulation of blood. Vitamin K is also a coenzyme in the synthesis of proteins that assist in maintaining bone density.

- Iron is a trace mineral. Almost two thirds of the iron in our bodies is found in hemoglobin, the oxygen-carrying protein in our blood. One of the primary functions of iron is to assist with the transportation of oxygen in our blood. Iron is a coenzyme for many of the enzymes involved in the metabolism of carbohydrates, fats, and protein. It is also a part of the superoxide dismutase antioxidant enzyme system that fights free radicals.

- Zinc is a trace mineral that acts as a coenzyme in the production of hemoglobin, in the superoxide dismutase antioxidant enzyme system, in the metabolism of carbohydrates, fats, and proteins, and in activating vitamin A in the retina. Zinc is also critical for cell reproduction and growth and for proper development and functioning of the immune system.

- Copper is a trace mineral that functions as a coenzyme in the metabolic pathways that produce energy, in the production of collagen and elastin, and as part of the superoxide dismutase antioxidant enzyme system. Copper is also a component of ceruloplasmin, a protein needed for the proper transport of iron.

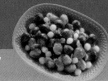

CHAPTER SUMMARY

- Neural tube defects, which can result from inadequate folate intake during the first four weeks of pregnancy, are the most common malformations of the fetal central nervous system. Some neural tube defects are minor and can be treated with surgery; other neural tube defects are fatal.

- Inadequate intakes of folate and vitamin B_{12} are associated with elevated homocysteine levels. Elevated homocysteine levels are associated with a greater risk of suffering from cardiovascular, cerebrovascular, and peripheral vascular diseases. These diseases significantly increase the risk for a heart attack or stroke.

- *Anemia* is a term that means "without blood." Severe iron deficiency results in iron-deficiency anemia, in which the production of normal, healthy red blood cells decreases and hemoglobin levels are inadequate. Iron deficiency is the most common nutrient deficiency in the world.

- Pernicious anemia is caused by a lack of intrinsic factor, which in turn results in vitamin B_{12} deficiency. Pernicious anemia causes reduced energy and exercise tolerance, as well as signs of nervous system damage, including impaired movement and cognitive and personality changes.

- Macrocytic anemia results from folate deficiency and causes the formation of excessively large red blood cells that have reduced hemoglobin. Symptoms are similar to those of iron-deficiency anemia.

mynutritionlab Go to MyNutritionLab at www.pearsoned.ca/mynutritionlab and enrich your understanding of nutrition! You'll find key animations, interactive exercises, access to My DietAnalysis, and much more.

REVIEW QUESTIONS

Quizzes

1. The B vitamins include
   a. niacin, folate, and iodine.
   b. cobalamin, iodine, and chromium.
   c. manganese, riboflavin, and pyridoxine.
   d. thiamin, pantothenic acid, and biotin.

2. The micronutrient most closely associated with blood clotting is
   a. iron.
   b. vitamin K.
   c. zinc.
   d. vitamin B_{12}.

3. Which of the following statements about iron is true?
   a. Iron is stored primarily in the liver, the blood vessel walls, and the heart muscle.
   b. Iron is a component of hemoglobin, myoglobin, and certain enzymes.
   c. Iron is a component of red blood cells, platelets, and plasma.
   d. Excess iron is stored primarily in the form of ferritin, cytochromes, and intrinsic factor.

4. Homocysteine is
   a. a byproduct of glycolysis.
   b. a trace mineral.
   c. an amino acid.
   d. a B vitamin.

5. Which of the following statements about choline is true?
   a. Choline is found exclusively in foods of animal origin.
   b. Choline is a B vitamin that assists in the metabolism of fatty acids.
   c. Choline is a neurotransmitter that is involved in muscle movement and memory storage.
   d. Choline is necessary for the synthesis of phospholipids and other components of cell membranes.

6. Which of the following is not a component of blood?
   a. Erythrocyte
   b. Leukocytes
   c. Biotin
   d. Plasma

7. Which trace mineral has no DRI, UL, or RDA?
   a. Sulphur
   b. Manganese
   c. Iodine
   d. Choline

8. Pernicious anemia is the primary cause of
   a. an iron deficiency.
   b. a zinc deficiency.
   c. a folate deficiency.
   d. a B_{12} deficiency.

9. Jackie was thrilled about her first pregnancy and was eager to share the news to her friends. As they chattered excitedly, they told her about seeing advice about folate supplements. Unfortunately, none of them were familiar with the details so Jackie consulted her health care provider about it. What foods are good sources of folate? When should Jackie start taking folate supplements? Why is folate recommended for young women?

10. Copper toxicity may lead to
    a. beriberi.
    b. Wilson's disease.
    c. pellagra.
    d. cheilosis.

11. In the chapter-opening story, Mr. Katz was given an injection of vitamin B_{12}. Why didn't his physician simply give him the vitamin in pill form?

12. Cassandra is 11 years old and has just begun menstruating. She and her family members are vegans (that is, they consume only plant-based foods). Explain why Cassandra's parents should be careful that their daughter consumes not only adequate iron but also adequate vitamin C.

13. Create a simple flow chart showing how loss of intrinsic factor in an older adult can lead to symptoms of dementia.

14. Avery is a lacto-ovo-vegetarian. His typical daily diet includes milk, yogurt, cheese, eggs, nuts, seeds, legumes, whole grains, and a wide variety of fruits and vegetables. He does not take any supplements. What, if any, micronutrients are likely to be inadequate in his diet?

15. Janine is 23 years old and engaged to be married. She is 18.2 kg (40 lb.) overweight, has hypertension, and her mother suffered a mild stroke recently, at age 45. For all these reasons, Janine is highly motivated to lose weight and has put herself on a strict low-carbohydrate diet recommended by a friend. She now scrupulously avoids breads, pastries, pasta, rice, and "starchy" fruits and vegetables. Identify two reasons why Janine should consider taking a folate supplement.

16. It has been three months since Eli's wife, Monica, lost her job. As they live in a small town in New Brunswick, the job market is tight and Monica feels hopeless. Eli is growing more concerned every day because his wife doesn't get out of bed, seems disoriented and confused, and constantly cries. Once an avid hockey player, Monica no longer skates or even goes outside. She claims that she is too tired to even get up and have dinner. After hearing that B vitamins increase your energy, Eli immediately goes to the nearest health food store and grabs every B vitamin supplement he can get his hands on. Is this claim that B vitamins increase energy true? After learning about Monica's situation, do you think that taking a B vitamin supplement would help? Why or why not? Does her situation give rise to any other concerns? What additional advice might you give her?

CASE STUDY

During class, the topic of vitamin and mineral supplements comes up. Your teacher asks the students if anyone takes multivitamin and mineral supplements, and many volunteer to explain why they have chosen to take these supplements. Chantal swears by her vitamins to help her lose weight, and Jamal claims that his multivitamin and mineral supplement gives him more energy and focus. Li-Mei claims to take a supplement "just for insurance," and Muna simply says that for as long as she can remember, she's always taken a multivitamin and mineral capsule at breakfast, so she continues to do so because it's a habit.

All those who responded are healthy university students. Would you suggest that they all continue taking a supplement? Are the claims that the multivitamin and mineral supplements help reduce weight and enhance energy correct? Where do you think these students got their ideas, and what source of information would you suggest they turn to when seeking facts about multivitamin and mineral supplements?

WEB LINKS

www.nlm.nih.gov/medlineplus/vitamins.html
U.S. National Library of Medicine and National Institutes of Health
This great website has information on the latest research on health and vitamins and minerals.

http://fnic.nal.usda.gov
USDA Food and Nutrition Information Center: Dietary Supplements
Click "dietary supplements" for a wealth of information about macronutrients, phytonutrients, vitamins, and minerals. The individual fact sheets for dietary supplements are very informative.

www.cfsan.fda.gov/~dms/ds-warn.html
U.S. Food and Drug Administration and Center for Food Safety and Applied Nutrition. Dietary Supplements: Warnings and Safety Information
This site provides information about product recalls and consumer advisories for many different types of dietary supplements, including herbal remedies, products to enhance athletic performance, and over-the-counter weight loss substances.

www.unicef.org/nutrition
UNICEF—Nutrition
This site provides information about micronutrient deficiencies in developing countries and the efforts to combat them.

www.thearc.org
The Arc
Search this site for "neural tube defects" and find information on the development and prevention of these conditions.

Test Yourself Answers

1. **False** B vitamins do not directly provide energy for our bodies. However, they play critical roles in ensuring that our bodies are able to generate energy from carbohydrates, fats, and proteins.

2. **True** Blood is the only fluid tissue in the body.

3. **False** Niacin, vitamin B_6, and folate have Tolerable Upper Intake Levels.

4. **True** This deficiency is particularly common in infants, children, and women of childbearing age.

5. **True** and **False** For an individual who consumes a varied diet that provides adequate energy and nutrients, this statement is true. However, many people do not consume a varied diet that provides adequate levels of micronutrients, and others have health issues that increase their requirements or affect their ability to absorb micronutrients from food. For these individuals, a daily multivitamin-mineral supplement is not a waste of money and is important to optimize health.

Do Zinc Lozenges Help Fight the Common Cold?

The common cold has plagued human beings since the beginning of time. Children suffer from six to ten colds each year, and adults average two to four per year. Although colds are typically benign, they result in significant absenteeism from work and cause discomfort and stress. Finding a cure for the common cold has been at the forefront of modern medicine for many years.

The most frequent causes of the adult colds are viruses called coronaviruses; rhinovirus is another virus that causes about one third of all adult colds. It is estimated that there are more than 200 viruses that can cause a cold. Because a cold can be caused by so many different viruses, finding treatments or potential cures for a cold is extremely challenging.

The role of zinc in the health of our immune system is well known. Zinc has been shown to inhibit the replication of rhinovirus and other viruses that cause the common cold (Prasad 1996), thus leading to speculation that taking zinc supplements may reduce the length and severity of colds. Consequently, zinc lozenges were formulated as a means of providing potential relief from cold symptoms. These lozenges are readily found in most drugstores.

Does taking zinc in lozenge form actually reduce the length and severity of a cold? Over the past 20 years, numerous research studies have been conducted to try to answer this question. Unfortunately, the results of these studies are inconclusive because about half have found that zinc lozenges do reduce the length and severity of a cold, while about half find that zinc lozenges have no effect on cold symptoms or duration (Jackson, Lesho, and Peterson 2000). Some reasons that various studies report different effects of zinc on a cold include

- Inability to truly "blind" participants to the treatment—Because zinc lozenges have a unique taste, it may be difficult to keep the research participants uninformed as to whether they are getting zinc lozenges or a placebo. Knowing which lozenge they are taking could lead participants to report biased results.

- Self-reported symptoms are subject to inaccuracy—Many studies had the research participants self-report changes in symptoms, which may be inaccurate and be influenced by mood and other emotional factors.

- Wide variety of viruses that cause a cold—Because more than 200 viruses can cause a cold, it is

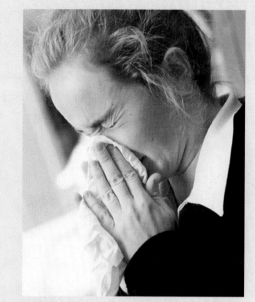

Zinc lozenges may help fight cold symptoms.

highly unlikely that zinc can combat them all. It is possible that people who do not respond favourably to zinc lozenges are suffering from a cold virus that cannot be treated with zinc.

- Differences in zinc formulations and dosages— The type of zinc formulation and the dosages of zinc consumed by study participants differed across studies. These differences most likely contributed to various responses across studies. It is estimated that for zinc to be effective, at least 80 mg of zinc should be consumed each day, and that people should begin using zinc lozenges within 48 hours of onset of cold symptoms. Also, sweeteners and flavourings found in many zinc lozenges, such as citric acid, sorbitol, and mannitol, may bind the zinc and inhibit its ability to be absorbed into the body, limiting its effectiveness.

Based on what you have learned here, do you think taking zinc lozenges can be effective in fighting the common cold? Have you ever tried zinc lozenges, and did you find them effective? Even if you only have about a 50% chance of reducing the length and severity of your cold by taking zinc lozenges, would you take these to combat your cold? Because there is no conclusive evidence supporting or refuting the effectiveness of zinc lozenges on the common cold, the debate on whether people should take them to treat their colds will most likely continue for many years.

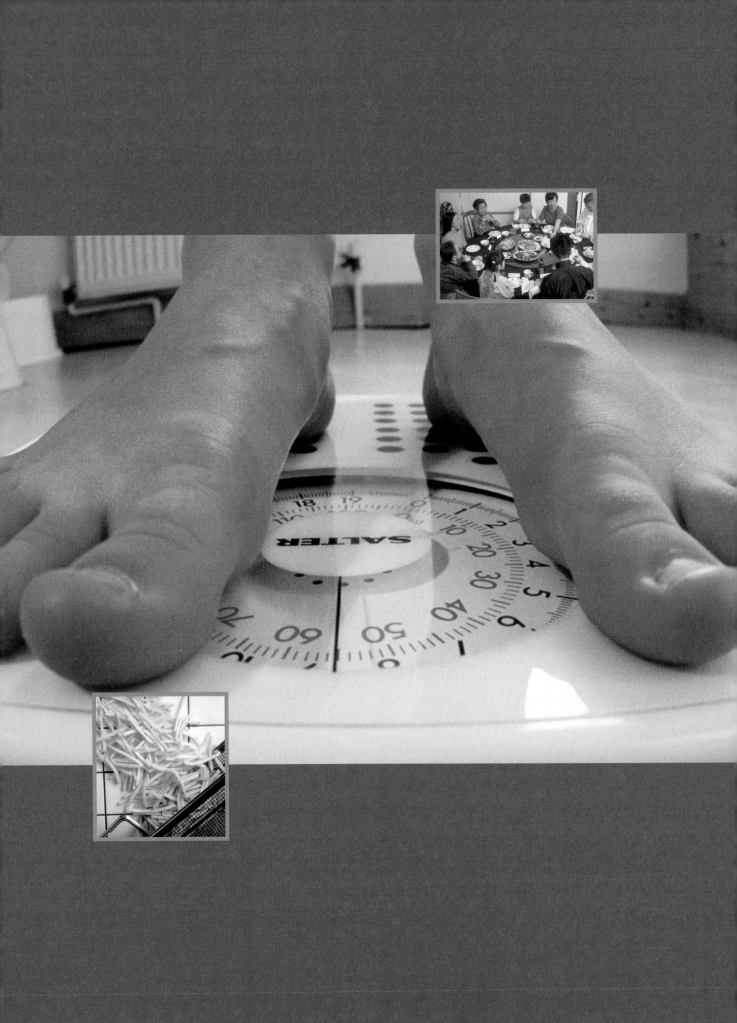

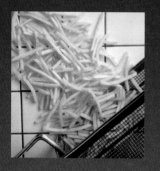

CHAPTER 11

Achieving and Maintaining a Healthy Body Weight

Test Yourself   True or False

1. Being underweight can be just as detrimental to our health as being obese. **T or F**

2. Obesity is a condition that is simply caused by people eating too much food and not getting enough exercise. **T or F**

3. Getting my body composition measured at the local fitness club will give me an accurate assessment of my body fat level. **T or F**

4. By staying physically active as we get older, we can prevent some of the decline in our muscle mass and our basal metabolic rate. **T or F**

5. People who are moderately overweight and physically active should not be considered healthy. **T or F**

Test Yourself answers can be found at the end of the chapter.

As a teenager, she won a full athletic scholarship to Syracuse University, where she was honoured for her "significant contribution to women's athletics and to the sport of rowing." After graduating, she became a television reporter and anchor for an NBC station in Flagstaff, Arizona. Then she went into modelling, and soon her face smiled out from the covers of fashion magazines, cosmetics ads, even a billboard in Times Square. Now considered a supermodel, she hosts her own television show, has her own website, her own clothing line, and even a collection of dolls. *People* magazine has twice selected her as one of the 50 Most Beautiful People and *Glamour* magazine named her Woman of the Year. So who is she? Her name is Emme Aronson . . . and by the way, her average weight is 86 kilos (190 pounds).

Emme describes herself as "very well-proportioned." She focuses not on maintaining a certain weight, but instead on keeping healthy and fit. So she eats when she's hungry and works out regularly. Observing that "we live in a society that is based on the attainment of unrealistic beauty," Emme works hard to get out the message that self-esteem should not be contingent on size. In fact, she says, "I don't know if I'll ever be perfect, but I'm happy with who I am" (Emme 2004; PBS 2004).

Are you happy with your weight, shape, body composition, and fitness? If not, what needs to change—your attitude, your diet, your level of physical activity? What role do diet and physical activity play in maintaining a healthy body weight? How much of your body size and shape is due to genetics? What influence does society—including food advertising—have on your weight? And if you decide that you do need to lose weight, what's the best way to do it? In this chapter, we will explore these questions and provide some answers.

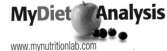

www.mynutritionlab.com

What Is a Healthy Body Weight?

As you begin to think about achieving and maintaining a healthy weight, it's important to make sure you understand what a healthy body weight actually means. We can define a healthy weight as all of the following (Manore and Thompson 2000):

- a weight that is appropriate for your age and physical development

- a weight that you can achieve and sustain without severely curtailing your food intake or constantly dieting

- a weight that is acceptable to you

- a weight that is based upon your genetic background and family history of body shape and weight

- a weight that promotes good eating habits and allows you to participate in regular physical activity

As you can see, a healthy body weight is not one in which a person must be extremely thin or overly muscular. In addition, there is no one particular body type that can be defined as healthy. Thus, achieving a healthy body weight should not be dictated by the latest fad or current societal expectations of what is acceptable.

Now that we know what a healthy body weight is, let's look at some terms applying to underweight and overweight. Physicians, nutritionists, and other scientists define **underweight** as having too little body fat to maintain health, causing a person to have a weight that is below an acceptably defined standard for a given height. **Overweight** is defined as having a moderate amount of excess body fat, resulting in a person having a weight that is greater than some accepted standard for a given height but is not considered obese. **Obesity** is defined as having excess body fat that adversely affects health, resulting in a person having a weight that is substantially greater than some accepted standard for a given height. In the next section we discuss how these terms are defined by using certain indicators of body weight and body fat.

underweight Having too little body fat to maintain health, causing a person to have a weight that is below an acceptably defined standard for a given height.

overweight Having a moderate amount of excess body fat, resulting in a person having a weight that is greater than some accepted standard for a given height but is not considered obese.

obesity Having excess body fat that adversely affects health, resulting in a person having a weight that is substantially greater than some accepted standard for a given height.

Recap: A healthy body weight is one that is appropriate for your age and physical development, can be achieved and sustained without constant dieting, is acceptable to you, is based upon your genetic background and family history of body shape and weight, promotes good eating habits, and allows for regular physical activity. Underweight is having too little body fat to maintain optimum health. Overweight occurs when someone has a moderate amount of excess body fat, while obesity occurs when someone has excess body fat that adversely affects health.

How Can You Evaluate Your Body Weight?

Various methods are available to help you determine whether or not you are currently maintaining a healthy body weight. Let's review a few of these methods.

Determine Your Body Mass Index (BMI)

Body mass index (BMI, or *Quetelet's index*) is a commonly used index representing the ratio of a person's body weight to the square of his or her height. Table 11.1 helps to interpret the resulting ratio. You can calculate your BMI by using the following equation:

$$BMI = weight\ (kg) \div height\ (m)^2$$

A less exact but often useful method is to use the graph in Figure 11.1, which shows approximate BMIs for your height and weight and whether your BMI is in a healthy range. You can also calculate your BMI on the internet by using the BMI calculator found at ww1.heartandstroke.ca/page.asp?PageID=1192.

Why Is BMI Important?

Your body mass index provides an important clue to your overall health. Research studies show that a person's risk for type 2 diabetes, high blood pressure, heart disease, and other diseases largely increases when their BMI is at or above a value of 30 kg/m². Having a very low BMI, defined as a value below 18.5 kg/m², is also associated with increased risk of health problems and death.

Figure 11.2 on page 385 shows how the *mortality rate,* or death rate, from all diseases increases significantly above a value of 30 kg/m². Having a BMI value within the normal weight range means that your risk of dying prematurely is within the

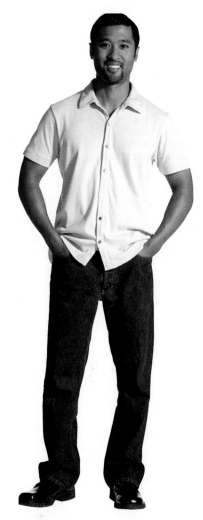

A healthy body weight varies from person to person.

body mass index (BMI) A measurement representing the ratio of a person's body weight to his or her height.

Table 11.1 BMI Classifications and Risk of Developing Health Problems

Classification	BMI Category (kg/m²)	Risk of Developing Health Problems
Underweight	< 18.5	Increased
Normal weight	18.5–24.9	Least
Overweight	25.0–29.9	Increased
Obese		
Class I	30.0–34.9	High
Class II	35.0–39.9	Very high
Class III	> 40.0	Extremely high

Source: Canadian Guidelines for Body Weight Classification in Adults. Health Canada, 2003 © Reproduced with the permission of the Minister of Public Works and Government Services Canada, 2008.

Note: For persons 65 years and older, the "normal" range may begin slightly above BMI 18.5 and extend into the "overweight" range.

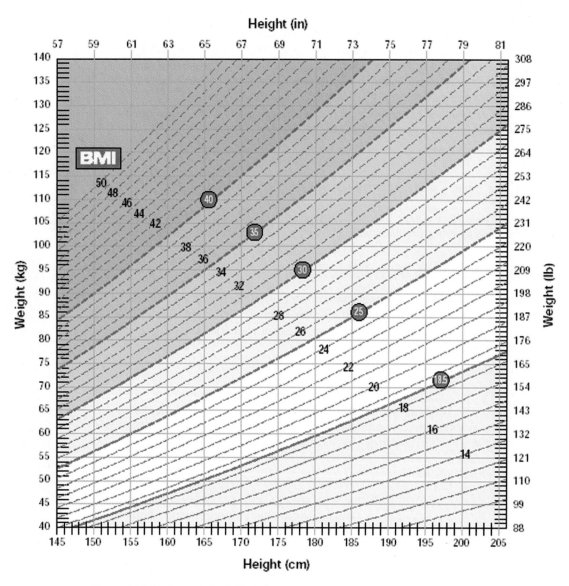

Figure 11.1 Body mass index (BMI) nomogram.

(*Source:* Canadian Guidelines for Body Weight Classification in Adults. Health Canada, 2003 © Reproduced with the permission of the Minister of Public Works and Government Services Canada, 2008.)

expected average. If your BMI value falls outside of this range, either higher or lower, your risk of dying prematurely becomes greater than the average risk. For example, men with a BMI equal to or greater than 35 kg/m^2 have a risk of dying prematurely that is more than twice that of men with a BMI value in the range of 22 to 25 kg/m^2.

Limitations of BMI

Although calculating your BMI can be very helpful in estimating your health risk, this method is limited when used with people who have a disproportionately higher muscle mass for a given height. For example, one of Matthew's friends, Randy, is a 23-year-old weightlifter who is 1.7 metres (5'7") tall and weighs 95.5 kg (210 lb.). According to our BMI calculations, Randy's BMI is 32.9 kg/m^2, placing him in the obese and high-risk category for many diseases. Is Randy really obese? In cases such as his, an assessment of body composition is necessary.

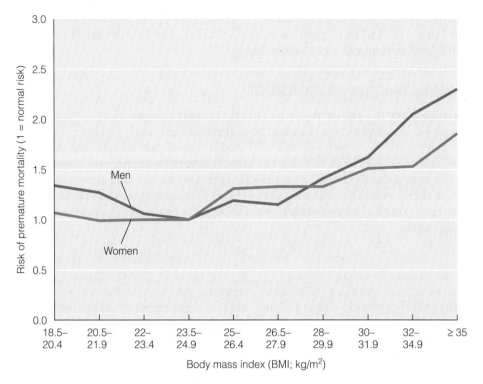

Figure 11.2 Increased body mass index is associated with an increased risk for premature mortality. These results pertain only to U.S. adults who have never smoked and have no history of disease. (Adapted from E. E. Calle, M. J. Thun, J. M. Petrelli, C. Rodriguez, and C. W. Heath, Jr., Body-mass index and mortality in a prospective cohort of U.S. adults, *N. Engl. J. Med.* 341 [1999]:1097–1105.)

It is important to know that this classification system was not designed for children or adolescents under the age of 18 years, or for pregnant or nursing women. It may under- or overestimate body fatness and thus health risks in teens who have not yet reached their full adult weight and height, and women who are carrying extra weight during pregnancy and lactation. The BMI is also not accurate with adults who naturally have a very lean body build, adults who have very muscular builds, adults over the age of 65 years, and certain ethnic and racial groups (Health Canada 2005). Recent research has suggested that the BMI categories for Asian populations should

▶ **YOU DO THE MATH**

Calculating Your Body Mass Index

Calculate your personal BMI value based on your height and weight. Let's use Matthew's values as an example:

$$BMI = weight\ (kg) \times height\ (m)^2$$

1. Matthew's weight is 200 pounds. To convert his weight to kg, divide his weight in pounds by 2.2 pounds per kg:

   200 pounds/2.2 pounds per kg = 90.91 kg

2. Matthew's height is 6 feet 8 inches, or 80 inches. To convert his height to metres, multiply his

   height in inches by 0.0254 metres per inch:

   80 inches × 0.0254 metres per inch = 2.03 metres

3. Find the square of his height in metres:

   $$2.03\ m \times 2.03\ m = 4.13\ m^2$$

4. Then, divide his weight in kg by his height in m^2 to get his BMI value:

   $$90.91\ kg \times 4.13\ m^2 = 22.01\ kg/m^2$$

Is Matthew underweight according to this BMI value? As you can see in Figure 11.1, this value shows that he is maintaining a normal, healthy weight.

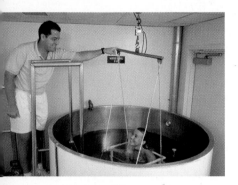

Underwater weighing

body composition The ratio of a person's body fat to lean body mass.

be different from the BMIs for Caucasians. For example, some researchers have proposed that a BMI of 23.0 kg/m² in Asian populations may be equivalent to a BMI of 25.0 kg/m² in Caucasians (Gallagher 2004).

Measure Your Body Composition

There are many methods available to assess your **body composition,** or the amount of body fat (or *adipose tissue*) and lean body mass (or *lean tissue*) you have. Table 11.2 lists some of the more common methods used to assess body composition. It is important to remember that measuring body composition provides only an estimate of your body fat and lean body mass, meaning that we cannot measure your exact level of these tissues. Because the range of error of these methods can be from 3% to more than 20%, body composition results should not be used as the only indicator of health status.

Underwater Weighing Method

In underwater weighing, a technician submerges a person underwater, the person exhales fully while underwater, and then the technician measures the person's weight. Although this method is available in most exercise physiology laboratories across North America, it is not readily available or affordable for many people. It is therefore used mostly for research purposes.

If you have access to a laboratory performing underwater weighing, it is worth having the procedure done, as this method of determining body composition is considered to be one of the most accurate. Under the best of circumstances, underwater weighing can estimate body fat within a 2% to 3% margin of error. This means that if your underwater weighing test shows you have 20% body fat, this value could be no lower than 17% nor higher than 23%. This test can only be done with people who are comfortable in water and does not work well with obese people. Before participating in this test, you must abstain from food for at least 8 hours, and you should not have exercised during the previous 12 hours.

Table 11.2   Overview of Various Body Composition Assessment Methods

Method	Strength	Limitations
Underwater weighing	Fairly accurate Inexpensive	Must be comfortable in water Requires trained technician and specialized equipment
Skinfolds	Fairly accurate if technician is well trained Inexpensive Easy for person being measured Can be done anywhere	Less accurate unless technician is well trained Proper prediction equation must be used to improve accuracy Person being measured may not want to be touched or may not want to expose their skin Cannot be used to measure obese people
Bioelectrical impedance analysis (BIA)	Inexpensive Easy for person being measured Can be done anywhere May be more accurate for obese people	Less accurate Body fluid levels must be normal Proper prediction equation must be used to improve accuracy
Near infrared reactance (NIR)	Inexpensive Easy for person being measured Can be done anywhere	Accuracy is very low Only one equation is used to compute body fat, which limits its use with a wide variety of people
Bod Pod	Easy for the person being measured Does not require a trained technician	Expensive Less accurate

Skinfold Measurements

Measuring skinfolds involves pinching a person's fold of skin (with its underlying layer of fat) at various locations of the body. The fold is measured by using a specially designed caliper. This method cannot be used with many obese people, as their skin folds are too large to be measured by the caliper. Himes (2001) found that almost 25% of women aged 50 years and older have skinfolds that are too large to measure. When we consider that the North American population is getting heavier each year, it is possible that this method will soon be useless for more than half of the population.

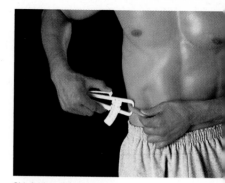

Skinfold measurement

Another major challenge of measuring body fat by using skinfolds is that this method relies on a technician predicting a person's body fat by using one of more than 400 equations developed in research studies, and it is accurate only if the correct prediction equation is applied. Many places that offer this measurement have untrained technicians performing the measurement, and they use only one equation for their entire client base, which severely limits the accuracy of this method.

When performed by a skilled technician, skinfold measurement can estimate your body fat with an error of 3% to 4%. This means that if your skinfold test shows you have 20% body fat, your actual value could be as low as 16% or as high as 24%.

Bioelectrical Impedance Analysis

Bioelectrical impedance analysis (BIA) is a method of determining body composition that involves sending a very low level of electrical current through a person's body. As water is a good conductor of electricity and lean body mass is made up of mostly water, the rate at which the electricity is conducted gives an indication of a person's lean body mass and body fat. This method can be done while lying down, with electrodes attached to the feet, the hands, and the BIA machine. There are also hand-held and standing models (that look like bathroom scales) now available, where only half of the body's impedance to electricity is measured, and total body fat is determined by estimating the impedance of the remainder of the body.

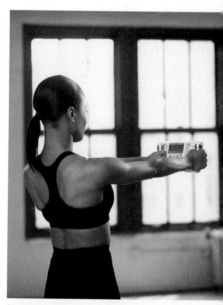

One of the challenges of the BIA method is that the person being measured must follow certain guidelines to improve accuracy of the test. This includes no eating for 4 hours and no exercise for 12 hours prior to the test and no alcohol consumption within 48 hours of the test. Females should not be measured if they are retaining water because of menstrual cycle changes. Another challenge is that, as with the skinfold method, most places that offer BIA only use one prediction equation for all clients; this limits the accuracy of the BIA method. When done under the best of circumstances, BIA can estimate your body fat with an error of 3% to 4%.

Bioelectrical impedance analysis

Near Infrared Reactance

The brand name of the machine most commonly used to estimate body fat using *near infrared reactance (NIR)* technology is the Futrex 5000. The technology is based on the principles of light absorption and reflection. A probe, or wand, is attached to the biceps (upper arm) by using a Velcro-type strip. An infrared beam then penetrates the arm and is reflected back into the probe.

Although this method is widely used at the present time, especially in health clubs, its accuracy has been shown to be very poor, and there is no way to know if the results you obtain from this test are of any real value. The few studies done with this method show that the margin of error for predicting a person's body fat ranges from 2% to as high as 10% (Panotopoulos et al. 2001; Heyward and Stolarczyk 1996). Most researchers consider this wide range of potential error unacceptable.

Bod Pod

The Bod Pod is the brand name of a machine that uses air displacement to measure body composition. This machine is a large, egg-shaped chamber made from fibreglass.

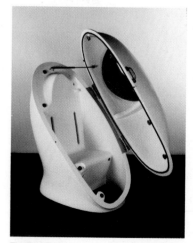

The Bod Pod

Table 11.3 Percent Body Fat Standards for Health

	Body Fat Levels (%)				
	Unhealthily Low	**Low**	**Mid**	**Upper**	**Obesity**
Men:					
Young adult	<8	8	13	22	>22
Middle adult	<10	10	18	25	>25
Elderly	<10	10	16	23	>23
Women:					
Young adult	<20	20	28	35	>35
Middle adult	<25	25	32	38	>38
Elderly	<25	25	30	35	>35

Source: Reprinted from T. G. Lohman, L. Houtkooper, and S. B. Going, Body fat measurement goes high-tech: Not all are created equal, 1997, *ACSM's Health Fitness Journal* 7:30–35. Used by permission.

The person being measured wears a swimsuit and sits in the machine, and the door to the machine is closed. The machine measures how much air is displaced once the person being measured enters the chamber, and this value is used to calculate body composition. The Bod Pod is expensive and is currently used mostly in research settings. Although this method appears to be fairly accurate in Caucasians, a recent study indicates that it overestimates body fat in some African-American men (Wagner, Heyward, and Gibson 2000). Despite these limitations, this technology appears promising as an easier and equally accurate alternative to underwater weighing in many populations.

Dual Energy X-Ray Absorptiometry

In Chapter 9 you learned about dual energy x-ray absorptiometry, also called DEXA or DXA, as a simple, non-invasive technique for measuring bone density. It is also a technology that is increasingly used to measure whole body composition. Very low dose x-rays can identify and quantify soft tissue (lean and fat tissue) and bone separately. See the Highlight Box on Dr. Linda McCargar on page 390 to learn more about the use of this technology in body composition research.

Let's return to Randy, whose BMI of 32.9 kg/m² places him in the obese category. Is he obese? Randy trains with weights four days per week, rides the exercise bike for about 30 minutes per session three times per week, and does not take drugs, smoke cigarettes, or drink alcohol. Through his local gym, Randy contacted a technician who assesses body composition. The results of his skinfold measurements show that his body fat is 9%. See Table 11.3 for a list of the percentage of body fat standards that are appropriate for health. According to this table, Randy's body fat values are within the healthy (low to mid) range. Randy is an example of a person whose BMI appears very high but who is not actually obese.

Assess Your Fat Distribution Patterns

To evaluate your body weight, it is also helpful to consider the way fat is distributed throughout your body. This is because your fat distribution pattern is known to affect your risk for various diseases. Figure 11.3 shows two types of fat patterning. *Apple-shaped fat patterning,* or upper-body obesity, is known to significantly increase a person's risk for many chronic diseases, such as type 2 diabetes, heart disease, and high blood pressure. It is thought that the apple-shaped patterning causes problems with the metabolism of fat and carbohydrate, leading to unhealthy changes in blood cholesterol, insulin, glucose, and blood pressure. In contrast, *pear-shaped fat patterning,* or lower-body obesity, does not seem to significantly

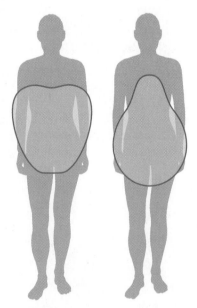

(a) Apple-shaped fat patterning (b) Pear-shaped fat patterning

Figure 11.3 Fat distribution patterns. (a) An apple-shaped fat distribution pattern increases an individual's risk for many chronic diseases. (b) A pear-shaped distribution pattern does not seem to be associated with an increased risk for chronic disease.

Table 11.4 Strengths and Limitations of Various Tools for Defining Overweight

	Strengths	Limitations
BMI	Gives ratio of weight to height Accurately predicts health risks related to obesity in large groups of people	Cannot indicate pattern of fat or amount of fat or lean body mass Does not account for differences in gender, frame size, or activity level
Body composition	If done properly, most accurate way to measure body fat	Can be expensive Equipment not always available
Fat patterning	Tells us about a person's body shape Can indicate if a person has a higher risk of certain chronic diseases	Does not directly measure body fat content

increase your risk for chronic diseases. Women tend to store fat in their lower body, and men in their abdominal region. In 2004, a study involving more than 10 000 people found that 64% of women are pear-shaped and 38% of men are apple-shaped (Zernike 2004).

Two methods, the waist-to-hip ratio and the waist circumference, can determine type of fat patterning. The *waist-to-hip ratio* is determined by measuring the waist circumference at the level of the natural waist (or the narrowest part of the torso as observed from the front). The hip circumference is measured at the maximal circumference (includes the maximal width of the buttocks as observed from the side). The waist value is divided by the hip value. If a man's waist-to-hip ratio is higher than 1.00 or a woman's is higher than 0.80, then they are considered to have a higher risk for chronic diseases.

For the waist circumference, a man's risk is increased above 102 cm (40 in.), and a woman's risk is increased above 88 cm (35 in.). Recent Canadian research suggests that waist circumference is more useful in predicting obesity-related health risk than BMI (Janssen, Katzmarzyk, and Ross 2004). It is a practical and easy way of identifying central obesity, in particular, visceral adipose tissue or the fat found around internal organs (as opposed to subcutaneous fat) (Kuk et al. 2005).

It is important to understand how BMI, body composition assessment, and fat distribution patterning differ in their ability to define a person's overweight status. Table 11.4 lists the strengths and limitations of these techniques in determining whether you are maintaining a healthy weight. There is no single best way to determine overweight or obesity; each technique has its own advantages and disadvantages.

Recap: Body mass index, body composition, and the waist-to-hip ratio and waist circumference are tools that can help you evaluate the health of your current body weight. None of these methods is completely accurate, but most may be used appropriately as general health indicators.

What Makes Us Gain and Lose Weight?

Have you ever wondered why some people are thin and others are overweight, even though they seem to eat about the same diet? If so, you're not alone. For hundreds of years, researchers have puzzled over what makes us gain and lose weight. In this section, we explore some information and current theories that may shed some light on this question.

We Gain or Lose Weight When Our Energy Intake and Expenditure Are Out of Balance

Fluctuations in body weight are a result of changes in our **energy intake** (the food we eat) and our **energy expenditure** (or the amount of energy we expend at rest and

energy intake The amount of food a person eats; in other words, it is the number of kilocalories consumed.

energy expenditure The energy the body expends to maintain its basic functions and to perform all levels of movement and activity.

Dr. Linda McCargar: Sarcopenic Obesity: An Emerging Health Problem

Can a person have too little muscle and be over-fat? Do you know an older person who has lost a lot of muscle mass, but has ample body fat?

Dr. Linda McCargar, a professor at the University of Alberta and the Director of the Human Nutrition Research Unit there, is a leading expert in body composition. Recently she's been interested in a condition called sarcopenic obesity. Literally, sarco means "muscle" and penia means "lack of"; sarcopenic obesity, therefore, refers to a condition of low muscle mass and high body fat (McCargar 2007). A person may not necessarily look obese, but they have too little lean body mass relative to their fat mass.

How can you tell if an individual has too little muscle and too much fat? The new imaging techniques available today can quantify the amount of fat and lean tissue fairly accurately. Dual energy x-ray absorptiometry is a simple, non-invasive technique that, according to Dr. McCargar (2007), "is rapidly becoming the method of choice for body composition research, because it is precise and overcomes some disadvantages of other commonly used methods." This technique has been widely used to measure bone density and mineral content, but it is also an excellent choice to measure whole body composition. It uses very low dose x-rays to identify and quantify soft tissue (lean and fat tissue) and bone separately.

As we learned already in this chapter, if you have a pear body shape and you carry much of your body fat in your hips and thighs, you don't have the same health risks as someone who has an apple body shape or a "spare tire" around their middle. In other words, the more fat deposited centrally (around your abdomen), the greater the health risks. Dr. McCargar's colleague and collaborator Dr. Geoff Ball, also from the University of Alberta, has shown that there can be significant differences in the amount of abdominal fat among 10-year-old children who have the same BMI values and are at the same stage of development. These findings may help health professionals to predict which children will be at greatest risk for possible future health problems, such as type 2 diabetes.

Who is most at risk of sarcopenic obesity? Most of the research to date has examined the muscle wasting commonly seen in older adults. However, sarcopenia has also been seen in breast cancer survivors and patients with other types of cancer. Dr. McCargar notes that "recent studies have confirmed a unique pattern of weight gain often observed in breast cancer patients: usually fat gain with a loss or no change in lean tissue" (McCargar 2007). This suggests that women recovering from breast cancer may benefit from following a healthy diet and an exercise regime that includes both aerobic and resistance training. A loss of lean body mass has also been observed in patients with colon cancer. An abnormal body composition may influence the distribution and efficacy of chemotherapy drugs in the body. In general, our population has become more obese and less active over the last two decades; thus an increased incidence of sarcopenic obesity may be seen in the future.

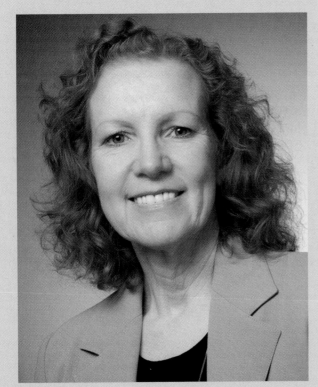

Dr. Linda McCargar is a leading expert in body composition.

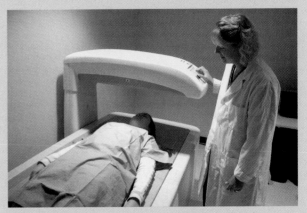

DEXA has been widely used to assess bone density, but it is also an excellent choice to measure whole body composition.

during physical activity). This relationship between what we eat and what we do is defined by the energy balance equation:

Energy balance occurs when energy intake = energy expenditure

This means that our energy is balanced when we consume the same amount of energy that we burn each day. Figure 11.4 shows how our weight changes when we change either side of this equation. From this figure, you can see that to lose body weight, we must expend more energy than we consume. In contrast, to gain weight, we must consume more energy than we expend. Finding the proper balance between energy intake and expenditure allows us to maintain a healthy body weight.

Energy Intake Is the Food We Eat Each Day

Energy intake is equal to the amount of energy in the food we eat each day. This value includes all foods and beverages. Daily energy intake is expressed as *kilocalories*

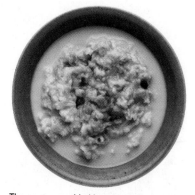

The energy provided by a bowl of oatmeal is derived from its protein, carbohydrate, and fat content.

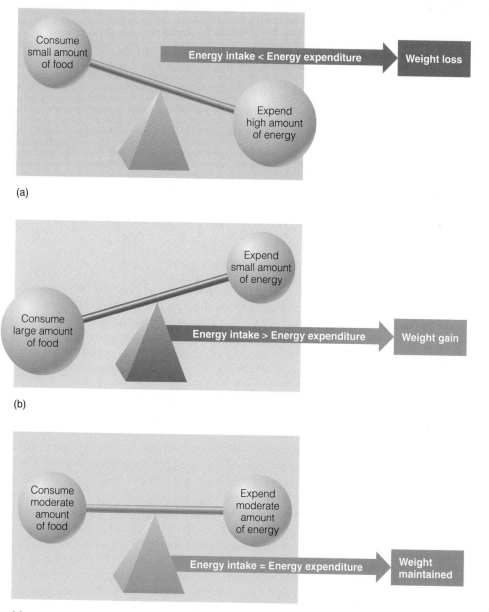

(a)

(b)

(c)

Figure 11.4 Energy balance describes the relationship between the food we eat and the energy we burn each day. (a) Weight loss occurs when food intake is less than energy output. (b) Weight gain occurs when food intake is greater than energy output. (c) We maintain our body weight when food intake equals energy output.

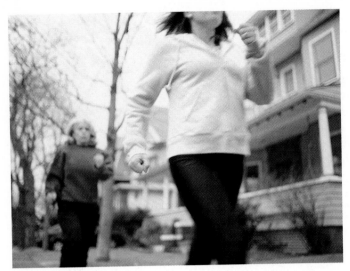

Brisk walking expends energy.

(kJ) per day (kcal/d or kJ/d). Energy intake can be estimated manually by using food composition tables or by using computerized dietary analysis programs. The energy content of each food is a function of the amount of carbohydrate, fat, protein, and alcohol that each food contains; vitamins and minerals have no energy value, so they contribute zero kcal (kJ) to our energy intake.

Remember that the energy value of carbohydrate and protein is 4 kcal (17 kJ) per gram and the energy value of fat is 9 kcal (37 kJ) per gram. The energy value of alcohol is 7 kcal (29 kJ) per gram. By multiplying the energy value (in kcal per gram) times the amount of the nutrient (in grams), you can calculate how much energy is in a particular food. For instance, 250 mL (1 cup) of quick oatmeal has an energy value of 142 kcal (600 kJ). How is this energy value derived? The 250 mL (1 cup) of oatmeal contains 6 grams of protein, 25 grams of carbohydrate, and 2 grams of fat. By using the energy values for each nutrient, you can calculate the total energy content of oatmeal:

6 grams protein × 4 kcal per gram = 24 kcal from protein

25 grams carbohydrate × 4 kcal per gram = 100 kcal from carbohydrate

2 grams fat × 9 kcal per gram = 18 kcal from fat

Total kcal for 250 mL (1 cup) oatmeal = 24 kcal (100kJ) + 100 kcal (420 kJ) + 18 kcal (80 kJ) = 142 kcal (600 kJ)

When someone's total daily energy intake exceeds the amount of energy expended, then weight gain results. An excess intake of approximately 3500 kcal or 14 640 kJ will result in a gain of 0.5 kg (1 lb.). Without exercise, this gain will likely be fat.

Energy Expenditure Includes More Than Just Physical Activity

Energy expenditure (also known as energy output) is the energy our body expends to maintain its basic functions and to perform all levels of movement and activity. Total 24-hour energy expenditure is calculated by estimating the energy used during rest and as a result of physical activity. There are three components of energy expenditure: basal metabolic rate (BMR), thermic effect of food (TEF), and energy cost of physical activity (Figure 11.5).

basal metabolic rate (BMR) The energy the body expends to maintain its fundamental physiologic functions.

Our Basal Metabolic Rate Is Our Energy Expenditure at Rest Our **basal metabolic rate,** or **BMR,** is the energy we expend just to maintain our body's basal, or resting, functions. These functions include respiration, circulation, maintenance of body temperature, synthesis of new cells and tissues, secretion of hormones, and nervous system activity. The majority of our energy output each day (about 60%–70%) is a result of our BMR. This means that 60% to 70% of our energy output goes to fuel the basic activities of staying alive, aside from any physical activity.

BMR varies widely among people. The primary determinant of our BMR is the amount of lean body mass that we have. People with a higher lean body mass have a higher BMR, as lean body mass is more metabolically active than body fat. Thus, it takes more energy to support this active tissue. One common assumption is that obese people have a depressed BMR. This is usually not the case. Most studies of obese people show that the amount of energy they expend for every kilogram of lean body mass is similar to that of a non-obese person. In general, people who weigh more also have more lean body mass and

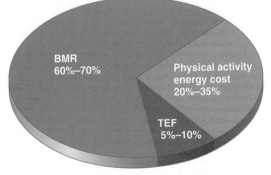

Components of energy expenditure

Figure 11.5 The components of energy expenditure include basal metabolic rate (BMR), the thermic effect of food (TEF), and the energy cost of physical activity. BMR accounts for 60% to 70% of our total energy output, whereas TEF and physical activity together account for 25% to 45%.

Key:
■ Lean body mass
■ % body fat

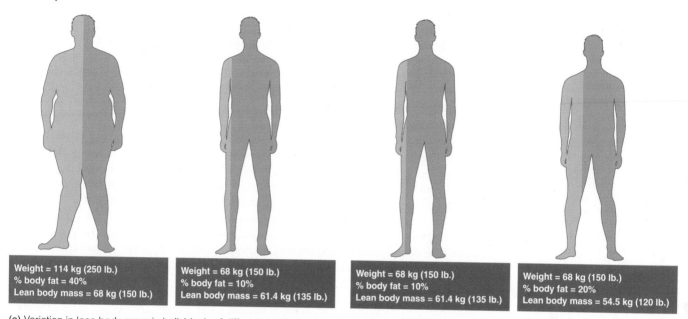

Weight = 114 kg (250 lb.)	Weight = 68 kg (150 lb.)	Weight = 68 kg (150 lb.)	Weight = 68 kg (150 lb.)
% body fat = 40%	% body fat = 10%	% body fat = 10%	% body fat = 20%
Lean body mass = 68 kg (150 lb.)	Lean body mass = 61.4 kg (135 lb.)	Lean body mass = 61.4 kg (135 lb.)	Lean body mass = 54.5 kg (120 lb.)

(a) Variation in lean body mass in individuals of different weights (b) Variation in lean body mass in individuals of same weight

Figure 11.6 Lean body mass varies in people with different body weights and body fat levels. (a) The person on the left has a higher body weight, body fat, and lean body mass than the person on the right, who is very lean. (b) Both people are the same weight but the person on the right has more body fat and less lean body mass than the person on the left.

consequently have a *higher* BMR. See Figure 11.6 for an example of how lean body mass can vary for people with different body weights and body fat levels.

BMR decreases with age, approximately 3% to 5% per decade after age 30. This age-related decrease results partly from hormonal changes, but much of this change is due to the loss of lean body mass resulting from physical inactivity. Thus, a large proportion of this decrease may be prevented with regular physical activity. There are other factors that can affect a person's BMR, and some of these are listed in Table 11.5.

How can you estimate the amount of energy you expend for your BMR? Of the many equations that can be used, one of the simplest ways to estimate your BMR is to multiply your body weight in kilograms (kg) by 1.0 kcal per kg of body weight per hour for men or by 0.9 kcal per kg of body weight per hour for women. A little later

Table 11.5 Factors Affecting Basal Metabolic Rate (BMR)

Factors That Increase BMR	Factors That Decrease BMR
Higher lean body mass	Lower lean body mass
Greater height (more surface area)	Lower height
Younger age	Older age
Elevated levels of thyroid hormone	Depressed levels of thyroid hormone
Stress	Starvation or fasting
Male gender	Female gender
Pregnancy and lactation	
Certain drugs, such as stimulants, caffeine, and tobacco	

in this chapter you will have an opportunity to calculate BMR and determine your total daily energy needs.

The Thermic Effect of Food Is the Energy Expended to Process Food   The **thermic effect of food (TEF)** is the energy we expend as a result of processing the food we eat. A certain amount of energy is needed to digest, absorb, transport, metabolize, and store the nutrients we eat. The TEF is equal to about 5% to 10% of the energy content of a meal, a relatively small amount. Thus, if a meal contains 500 kcal (2100 kJ), the thermic effect of processing that meal is about 25 to 50 kcal (105 to 210 kJ). These values apply to eating what is referred to as a mixed diet, or a diet containing a mixture of carbohydrate, fat, and protein. Most of us eat some combination of these nutrients throughout the day. Individually, the processing of each nutrient takes a different amount of energy. Although fat requires very little energy to digest, transport, and store in our cells, protein and carbohydrate require relatively more energy to process.

At one time, it was thought that obese people had a blunted (or reduced) TEF, which was identified as an important contributor to obesity. We now know that there are a lot of errors associated with measuring the TEF. These errors make our previous assumptions about the link between obesity and the thermic effect of food questionable. One of the most important contributors to obesity in industrialized countries is having an inactive lifestyle, which significantly reduces the energy output through physical activity, our next topic.

The Energy Cost of Physical Activity Is Highly Variable   The **energy cost of physical activity** represents about 20% to 35% of our total energy output each day. This is the energy that we expend for any movement or work above basal levels. This includes lower intensity activities, such as sitting, standing, and walking, and higher intensity activities, such as running, skiing, and bicycling. One of the most obvious ways to increase how much energy we expend as a result of physical activity is to do more activities for a longer time.

Table 11.6 lists the energy costs for certain activities. As you can see, the activities, such as running, swimming, and cross-country skiing, that involve moving our larger muscle groups (or more parts of the body) require more energy. The amount of energy we expend during activities is also affected by our body size, the intensity of the activity, and how long we perform the activity. This is why the values in Table 11.6 are expressed as kcal of energy per kg of body weight per minute.

By using the energy value for running at 6 miles (9.5 km) per hour (or a 10-minute per mile running pace) for 30 minutes, let's calculate how much energy Matthew would expend doing this activity:

- Matthew's body weight (in kg) = 200 pounds ÷ 2.2 pounds per kg = 90.91 kg
- Energy cost of running at 6 mph = 0.175 kcal/kg body weight/minute
- At Matthew's weight, the energy cost of running per minute = 0.175 kcal/kg body weight/min × 90.91 kg = 15.91 kcal/minute
- If Matthew runs this pace for 30 minutes, his total energy output = 15.91 kcal/minute × 30 minutes = 477 kcal

Recap: The energy balance equation relates food intake to energy expenditure. Eating more energy than you expend causes weight gain, while eating less energy than you expend causes weight loss. The three components of energy expenditure are basal metabolic rate, the thermic effect of food, and the energy cost of physical activity.

Genetic Factors Affect Body Weight

Our genetic background influences our height, weight, body shape, and metabolic rate. A classic study shows that the body weights of adults who were adopted as children are similar to the weights of their biological parents, not their adoptive parents

---

thermic effect of food (TEF) The energy expended as a result of processing food consumed.

energy cost of physical activity The energy that is expended on body movement and muscular work above basal levels.

Table 11.6 Energy Costs of Various Physical Activities

Activity	Intensity	Energy Cost (kcal/kg body weight/min)
Sitting, knitting or sewing	Light	0.026
Cooking or food preparation (standing or sitting)	Light	0.035
Walking, shopping	Light	0.04
Walking, 2 mph (slow pace)	Light	0.044
Cleaning (dusting, straightening up, vacuuming, changing linen, carrying out trash)	Moderate	0.044
Stretching—Hatha Yoga	Moderate	0.044
Weightlifting (free weights, Nautilus, or universal type)	Light or moderate	0.052
Bicycling < 10 mph	Leisure (work or pleasure)	0.07
Walking, 4 mph (brisk pace)	Moderate	0.088
Aerobics	Low impact	0.088
Weightlifting (free weights, Nautilus, or universal type)	Vigorous	0.105
Bicycling 12 to 13.9 mph	Moderate	0.14
Running, 5 mph (12 minutes per mile)	Moderate	0.14
Running, 6 mph (10 minutes per mile)	Moderate	0.175
Running, 8.6 mph (7 minutes per mile)	Vigorous	0.245

Source: B. E. Ainsworth, W. L. Haskell, M. C. Whitt, M. L. Irwin, A. M. Swartz, S. J. Strath, W. L. O'Brien, D. R. Bassett, Jr., K. H. Schmitz, P. O. Emplaincourt, D. R. Jacobs, Jr., and A. S. Leon, Compendium of physical activities: An update of activity codes and MET intensities, 2000, *Medicine and Science in Sports and Exercise* 32:S498–S516.

(Stunkard et al. 1986). Figure 11.7 shows that about 25% of our body fat is accounted for by genetic influences. Some proposed theories linking genetics with our body weight are the thrifty gene theory and the set-point theory.

The Thrifty Gene Theory

The **thrifty gene theory** suggests that some people possess a gene (or genes) that causes them to be energetically thrifty. This means that at rest and even during active times these individuals expend less energy than people who do not possess this gene. The proposed purpose of this gene is to protect a person from starving to death during times of extreme food shortages. This theory has been applied to some Aboriginal peoples, as these societies were exposed to centuries of feast and famine. Those with a thrifty metabolism survived when little food was available, and this trait was passed on to future generations. Although an actual thrifty gene (or genes) has not yet been identified, researchers continue to study this explanation as a potential cause of obesity.

If this theory is true, think about how people who possess this thrifty gene might respond to today's environment. Low levels of physical activity, inexpensive food sources that are high in fat and energy, and excessively large serving sizes are the norm in our society. A person with a thrifty metabolism will experience a great amount of weight gain, and their bodies are more resistant to weight loss. Theoretically,

thrifty gene theory A theory that suggests that some people possess a gene (or genes) that causes them to be energetically thrifty, resulting in their expending less energy at rest and during physical activity.

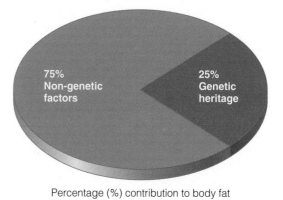

Percentage (%) contribution to body fat

Figure 11.7 Research indicates that about 25% of our body fat is accounted for by our genetic heritage. However, non-genetic factors, such as diet and exercise, play a much larger role.

having thrifty genetics appears advantageous during times of minimal food resources; however, this state could lead to very high levels of obesity in times of plenty.

The Set-Point Theory

set-point theory A theory that suggests that the body raises or lowers energy expenditure in response to increased and decreased food intake and physical activity. This action serves to maintain an individual's body weight within a narrow range.

The **set-point theory** suggests that our bodies are designed to maintain our weight within a narrow range, or at a set point. In many cases, our bodies appear to respond in such a way as to maintain our present weight. When we dramatically reduce energy intake (such as with fasting or strict diets), our body responds with physiologic changes that cause our BMR to drop. This causes a significant slowing of our energy output. In addition, being physically active while fasting or starving is difficult because we just don't have the energy for it. These two mechanisms of energy conservation may contribute to some of the rebound weight gain many dieters experience after they quit dieting.

Conversely, in some people overeating may cause an increase in BMR and is thought to be associated with an increased thermic effect of food as well as an increase in spontaneous movements, or fidgeting. This in turn increases energy output and prevents weight gain. These changes may explain how some people fail to gain all the weight expected from eating excess food. We don't eat the exact same amount of food each day; some days we overeat, other days we eat less. When you think about how much our daily energy intake fluctuates (about 20% above and below our average monthly intake), our ability to maintain a certain weight over long periods of time suggests that there is some evidence to support the set-point theory.

Can we change our weight set point? It appears that, when we maintain changes in our diet and activity level over a long time, weight change does occur. This is obvious in the case of obesity, since many people become obese during middle adulthood, and they are not able to maintain the lower body weight they had as a younger adult. Also, many people do successfully lose weight and maintain that weight loss over long periods. Thus, the set-point theory cannot entirely account for our body's resistance to weight loss. An interesting study on weight gain in twins demonstrates how genetics may affect our tendency to maintain a set point; this study is reviewed in the Highlight box on page 397.

Hormones Affect Body Weight

The Leptin Theory

leptin A hormone that is produced by body fat that acts to reduce food intake and to decrease body weight and body fat.

Leptin, first discovered in mice, is a hormone produced by fat cells (specifically, adipocytes in white adipose tissue). Thus, the amounts found circulating in the blood are proportional to the amount of body fat—that is, the higher the BMI (more body fat), the more leptin produced. Leptin acts to reduce food intake and to increase physical activity and energy expenditure, leading to a reduction in body fat and body weight.

Obese mice were found to have genetic mutations in the *obesity gene,* or *ob gene,* and these mutations caused overeating, reduced energy expenditure, and extreme obesity. When the ob gene is functioning normally, it produces leptin. When there is a genetic mutation of the ob gene, leptin is not secreted in sufficient amounts, food intake increases dramatically, and energy output is reduced. Researchers believe that leptin is the hormone that relays information about fat cell and fat tissue metabolism and body weight to the appetite centres in the hypothalamus (Kieffer and Habener 2000). They have found that mice bred to become obese (the ob/ob strain) are not only leptin deficient but also have type 2 diabetes. Several studies have demonstrated that these obese mice respond well to leptin injections, and not only do they lose weight, but their blood insulin levels also drop. The relationships among overweight, leptin, insulin, and type 2 diabetes are an exciting area of research (see the Highlight box on Dr. Timothy Kieffer in Chapter 4).

▶ **HIGHLIGHT**

Overfeeding Responses of Identical Twins

A classic study done by researchers at Laval University in Quebec shows how genetics plays a role in our responses to overeating (Bouchard et al. 1990). Twelve pairs of male identical twins volunteered to stay in a dormitory where they were supervised 24 hours a day for 120 consecutive days. Researchers measured how much energy each man needed to maintain his body weight at the beginning of the study. For 100 days, the subjects were fed 1000 kcal (4200 kJ) more per day than they needed to maintain body weight. Daily physical activity was limited, but each person was allowed to walk outdoors for 30 minutes each day, read, watch television and videos, and play cards and video games. The research staff stayed with these men to ensure that they did not stray from the study protocol.

The average weight gain experienced by this group of men was almost 8.2 kg (18 lb.). Although they were all overfed enough energy to gain about 11.8 kg (26 lb.), the average weight gain was 3.6 kg (8 lb.) less than expected. These men gained mostly fat but also gained about 2.7 kg (6 lb.) of lean body mass. Interestingly, there was a very wide range of weight gained. One man gained only 4.3 kg (9.5 lb.), while another man gained more than 13.2 kg (29 lb.)! Keep in mind that the food these men ate and the activities they performed were tightly controlled.

This study shows that when people overeat by the same amount of food, they can gain very different amounts of weight and body fat. Although each twin gained a similar amount of weight to his twin pair, there was a lot of difference in how each set of twins responded. It is suggested that those more resistant to weight gain when they overeat have the ability to increase BMR, store more excess energy as lean body mass instead of fat, and increase spontaneous movements, such as fidgeting. Thus, genetic differences may explain why some people have a better ability to maintain a certain weight set point than others.

Recap: There are many factors that affect our ability to gain and lose weight. Our genetic background influences our height, weight, body shape, and metabolic rate. The thrifty gene theory suggests that some people possess a thrifty gene, or set of genes, that causes them to expend less energy at rest and during physical activity than people who do not have this gene. The set-point theory suggests that our bodies are designed to maintain weight within a narrow range, also called a set point. Leptin is a hormone produced by body fat that reduces food intake and decreases body weight and fat. The role of leptin in weight regulation and obesity is still under investigation.

Childhood Weight Influences Adult Weight

In addition to genetic and hormonal factors, the environmental factors present in our childhood can influence our food choices, activity level, and other behaviours as adults and cause us to weigh more or less than others of similar body type. For example, children who are very physically active and eat nutritious diets that do not contain a lot of excess fat and sugar are less likely to be overweight or obese as children. In contrast, children who spend most of their time on the computer or watching television and who eat a lot of foods that contain excess fat and sugar are more likely to be overweight or obese as children. These patterns can very likely be carried into adulthood and result in adult overweight and obesity. We know that being overweight or obese as a child can be detrimental to our health as we age, as childhood overweight has been shown to significantly increase a person's risk of heart disease and premature death in adulthood (Gunnell et al. 1998).

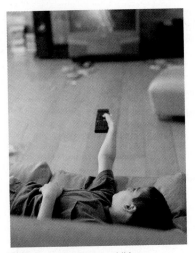

Behaviours learned as a child can affect adult weight and physical activity patterns.

Behavioural Factors Affect Food Choices and Body Weight

We know that there are a number of behavioural factors that can contribute to obesity. Behavioural factors include such things as how we select the carbohydrate, fat, and protein composition of our diet and which motivators drive us to eat, including hunger and appetite.

Composition of the Diet

As we have said, when we eat more energy than we expend, we gain weight. Most people eat what is referred to as a "mixed" diet, meaning it contains a mix of carbohydrate, fat, and protein. Scientists used to think that people would gain the same amount of weight if they ate too much food of any type, but now there is evidence to support the theory that when we overeat dietary fat, we store it much more easily as adipose tissue than we do either carbohydrate or protein (Hellerstein, Christiansen, and Kaempfer 1991). This may be due to the fact that eating fat doesn't cause much of an increase in metabolic rate, and the body stores fat in the form of adipose tissue quite easily. In contrast, when we overeat protein or carbohydrate, our body's initial response is to use this extra food for energy, storage, or the building of tissues, with a smaller amount of the excess stored as fat. This does not mean, however, that you can eat as many low-fat foods as you want and not gain weight! Consistently overeating protein or carbohydrate will also lead to weight gain. Instead, maintain a balanced diet combining fat, carbohydrate, and protein, and reduce your dietary fat to 20% to 35% of total energy. This strategy may help reduce your storage of fat energy as adipose tissue.

Hunger Versus Appetite

As introduced in Chapter 3, *hunger* is our innate, physiologic drive or need to eat. We can tell when we are hungry by paying attention to our body's signals, such as a growling stomach and light-headedness. This need for food is triggered by physiologic changes, such as low blood glucose, that affect the chemicals in our brain. The hypothalamus is the part of the brain that plays an important role in hunger regulation. Special cells referred to as *feeding cells* in the hypothalamus respond to conditions of low blood glucose, causing us to be hungry and to eat.

Once we have eaten and our bodies respond accordingly, other centres in the hypothalamus are triggered, and our desire to eat is reduced. The state we reach in which we no longer desire to eat is referred to as *satiety*. It may be that some people have an insufficient satiety mechanism, which prevents them from feeling full after a meal, allowing them to overeat. Some of the factors that increase satiety (or decrease food intake) include

- stomach expansion;
- nutrient absorption from the small intestine;
- increased blood glucose;
- hormones, such as leptin, serotonin, and cholecystokinin (CCK). Leptin is produced by adipose tissue; serotonin is made from the amino acid tryptophan; and CCK is produced by the intestinal cells and stimulates the gallbladder to secrete bile.

There are also many factors that can decrease satiety (or increase food intake):

- Hormones, such as beta-endorphins. Beta-endorphins increase a sense of pleasure while eating, which can increase food intake.
- Neuropeptide Y, which is an amino-acid-containing compound produced in the hypothalamus, stimulates appetite.
- Decreased blood glucose.

We explored in Chapter 3 the concept that *appetite* can be experienced in the absence of hunger. Appetite may therefore be considered a psychological drive to eat,

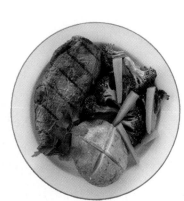

A balanced diet contains protein, carbohydrate, and fat.

being stimulated by learned preferences for food and particular situations that promote eating. For instance, some people learn as children to love or hate certain foods. This may explain why such foods as frogs' legs, cactus, and cultured yeast extract (Marmite) appeal to people in certain cultures who were raised on them but are almost never adopted into the diet as new foods by an adult. Others may follow learned behaviours related to timing and size of meals. In addition, the sight and fragrance of certain foods stimulate the pleasure centres of the brain, whether or not we happen to be hungry at the time. Mood can also affect appetite, as some people will eat more or less if they feel depressed or happy. As you can imagine, appetite leads many people to overeat.

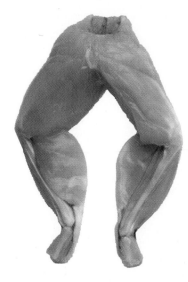

Food preferences often depend on culture. Some cultures enjoy foods such as frogs' legs, while others do not.

Social Factors Influence Behaviour and Body Weight

Social factors can encourage us to overeat or choose high-energy foods. For example, pressure from family and friends to eat the way they do and easy access to large servings of inexpensive and high-fat foods contribute to overeating. Think about how you might eat differently when you attend a birthday celebration with family or friends. You are offered hot dogs, pizza, birthday cake, ice cream, and many other dishes that taste great but are relatively high in fat and energy. The pressure to overeat during holidays is also high, with constant encouragement to eat extra servings of your favourite holiday foods and to finish a very large meal with dessert.

We also have numerous opportunities to overeat because of easy access to foods high in fat and energy throughout our normal daily routine. Vending machines selling junk foods are everywhere: at schools, in business offices, and even at laundromats. Shopping malls are filled with fast-food restaurants, where inexpensive, large serving sizes are the norm. Even foods we have traditionally considered nutritious, such as peanut butter, yogurt, and milk, can contain added sugars and other ingredients that are high in energy and fat. We don't even have to spend time or energy preparing our food anymore, as everything is either ready to serve or requires just a few minutes to cook in a microwave oven. This easy access to high-fat and high-energy foods leads many of us to overeat.

Similarly, social factors can cause people to be less physically active. Social factors restricting physical activity include watching a lot of television, maintaining a busy lifestyle that does not include a lot of physical activity, coping with family responsibilities, and living in an area with harsh weather conditions. Many overweight people identify such factors as major barriers to maintaining a healthy body weight, and research seems to confirm their influence. There is growing evidence that sedentary behaviours, such as television watching, are associated with obesity in both children and adults. A study of 11- to 13-year-old schoolchildren found that children who watched more than two hours of television per night were more likely to be overweight or obese than children who watched less than two hours of television per night. Interestingly, adults who reported an increase in television watching of 20 hours per week (approximately three hours per day) over a nine-year period had a significant increase in waist circumference (Koh-Banerjee et al. 2003), indicating significant weight gain in these adults.

Conversely, social pressures to maintain a lean body are great enough to encourage many of us to undereat or to avoid foods we perceive as "bad," especially fats. Our society ridicules and often ostracizes overweight people, many of whom even face job discrimination. Media images of waiflike fashion models and men in tight jeans with washboard abdomens and muscular chests encourage many people—especially adolescents and young adults—to skip meals, resort to crash diets, and exercise obsessively. Even some people of normal body weight push themselves to achieve an unrealistic and unattainable weight goal, in the process threatening their health and even their life (see Chapter 13 for consequences of disordered eating).

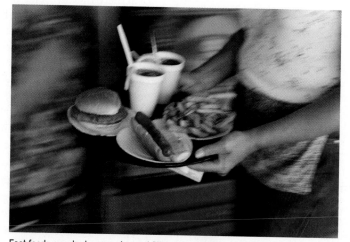

Fast foods may be inexpensive and filling but are often high in fat and sugar.

It should be clear that how we gain, lose, and maintain our body weight is a complex matter. Most people who are overweight have tried several weight loss programs but have been unsuccessful in maintaining long-term weight loss. A significant number of these people have consequently given up all weight loss attempts. Some even suffer from severe depression related to their body weight. Should we condemn these people as failures and continue to pressure them to lose weight? Should people who are overweight but otherwise healthy (e.g., low blood pressure, cholesterol, and glucose levels) feel compelled to lose weight? The Nutrition Debate at the end of this chapter addresses these issues and provides an opportunity to discuss how we should deal with the growing concerns and prejudices related to obesity in our society.

> **Recap:** Our diet and activity patterns as children influence our body weight as adults. Behavioural factors, such as the amount of dietary fat, carbohydrate, and protein, and alterations in satiety and appetite, also influence our body weight. Social factors influencing our weight include ready availability of high-energy foods, lack of physical activity, and too much television watching. There are prejudices and social pressures against those who are overweight and obese, and these pressures can even drive many normal-weight individuals to use unhealthy and even dangerous approaches in an attempt to achieve an unrealistic body weight.

How Many Calories Do You Need?

Given everything we've discussed so far, you're probably asking yourself, "How much should I eat?" This question is not always easy to answer, as our energy needs fluctuate from day to day according to our activity level, environmental conditions, and other factors, such as the amount and type of food we eat and our intake of caffeine. However, you can get a general estimate of how much energy your body needs to maintain your present weight.

One potential way to estimate how much energy you need each day is to record your total food and beverage intake for a defined time, such as three or seven days. You can then use a food composition table or computer dietary assessment program to estimate the amount of energy you eat each day. Assuming that your body weight is stable over this period, your average daily energy intake should represent how much energy you need to maintain your present weight.

Unfortunately, many studies of energy intake in humans have shown that dietary records estimating energy needs are not very accurate. Most studies show that people underestimate the amount of energy they eat by 10% to 30%. Overweight people tend to underestimate by an even higher margin, at the same time overestimating the amount of activity they do. This means that someone who really eats about 2000 kcal or 8370 kJ per day may only record eating 1400 to 1800 kcal or 5860 to 7530 kJ per day. So one reason that many people are confused about their ability to lose weight is that they are eating more than they realize.

A simpler and more accurate way to estimate your total daily energy needs is to calculate your BMR, and then add the amount of energy you expend as a result of your activity level. Refer to the You Do the Math box, "Calculating BMR and Total Daily Energy Needs," for an example of how to do this. As the energy cost for the thermic effect of food is small, you don't need to include it in your calculations.

> **Recap:** Accurately determining daily energy needs is difficult because of the limitations of currently available estimation methods. A less accurate way to estimate energy needs is to record food intake for three to seven days; if body weight is stable, average energy intake should be representative of daily energy needs. A simpler and more accurate way to estimate daily energy needs is to calculate your BMR and then add your estimated daily activity level to that value.

▶ **YOU DO THE MATH**

Calculating BMR and Total Daily Energy Needs

1. *Calculate your BMR:* If you are a man, you will need to multiply your body weight in kg by 1 kcal per kg body weight per hour. Assuming you weigh 175 pounds, your body weight in kg would be 175 pounds ÷ 2.2 pounds per kg = 79.5 kg. Next, multiply your weight in kg by 1 kcal per kg body weight per hour:

$$1 \text{ kcal per kg body weight per hour} \times 79.5 \text{ kg} = 79.5 \text{ kcal per hour}$$

Calculate your BMR for the total day (or 24 hours):

$$79.5 \text{ kcal per hour} \times 24 \text{ hours per day} = 1909 \text{ kcal (8020 kJ) per day}$$

(If you are a woman, multiply your body weight in kg by 0.9 kcal per kg body weight per hour.)

	Men	Women
Sedentary/inactive Involves mostly sitting, driving, or very low levels of activity.	25%–40%	25%–35%
Lightly Active Involves a lot of sitting; may also involve some walking, moving around, and light lifting.	50%–70%	40%–60%
Moderately Active Involves work plus intentional exercise, such as an hour of walking, four to five days per week; may have a job requiring some physical labour.	65%–80%	50%–70%
Heavily Active Involves a great deal of physical labour, such as roofing, carpentry work, or regular heavy lifting and digging.	90%–120%	80%–100%
Exceptionally Active Involves a lot of physical activities for work and intentional exercise; also applies to athletes who train for many hours each day, such as triathletes and marathon runners or other competitive athletes performing heavy, regular training.	130%–145%	110%–130%

2. *Estimate your activity level by selecting the description that most closely fits your general lifestyle.* The energy cost of activities is expressed as a percentage of your BMR. Refer to the values in the table below when estimating your own energy output.

3. *Multiply your BMR by the decimal equivalent of the lower and higher percentage values for your activity level.* Let's use the man referred to in Step 1 above. He is a college student who lives on campus. He walks to classes located throughout campus, carries his book bag, and spends most of his time reading and writing. He does not exercise on a regular basis.

His lifestyle would be defined as lightly active, meaning he expends 50% to 70% of his BMR each day in activities. You want to calculate how much energy he expends at both ends of this activity level. How many kilocalories does this equal?

$$1909 \text{ kcal per day} \times 0.50 \text{ (or 50\%)} = 955 \text{ kcal per day}$$

$$1909 \text{ kcal per day} \times 0.70 \text{ (or 70\%)} = 1336 \text{ kcal (5610 kJ) per day}$$

These calculations show that this man expends about 955 to 1336 kcal (4010 to 5610 kJ) per day doing daily activities.

4. *Calculate total daily energy output by adding together BMR and the energy needed to perform daily activities.* In this man's case, his total daily energy output is:

$$1909 \text{ kcal per day} + 955 \text{ kcal per day} = 2864 \text{ kcal (12 030 kJ) per day}$$

$$1909 \text{ kcal per day} + 1336 \text{ kcal per day} = 3245 \text{ kcal (13 630 kJ) per day}$$

Assuming this man is maintaining his present weight, he requires between 2864 and 3245 kcal (12 000 to 13 580 kJ) per day to stay in energy balance.

How Can You Achieve and Maintain a Healthy Body Weight?

Achieving and maintaining a healthy body weight involves many factors, including a good diet and participation in regular physical activity. In this section we discuss these factors and review the use of prescribed medications and dietary supplements in losing or gaining body weight.

Safe and Effective Weight Change Involves Moderation and Consistency

There are an unlimited number of weight loss and weight gain programs available. How can you know which plan or program is based on sound dietary principles and whether it will result in long-term weight change? There are three primary components of a sound weight change plan:

- gradual changes in energy intake

- incorporation of regular and appropriate physical activity

- application of behaviour modification techniques

Following a lifestyle plan that includes these components will help ensure a sound approach to weight change. Beware of fad diets! They are just what their name implies—fads that do not result in long-term, safe weight changes. Most of these programs will die only to be born again as a "new and improved" fad diet. See the Highlight box "The Anatomy of Fad Diets" on page 403 to learn more about this issue.

Safe and Effective Weight Loss

Setting realistic weight loss goals is an important part of a weight loss plan. Although making gradual changes in body weight is frustrating for most people, this slower change is much more effective in maintaining weight loss over the long term. Ask yourself the question, "How long did it take me to gain this extra weight?" A fair expectation for weight loss is that it should take about the same amount of time to lose the weight as it took to gain it. In general, a sound weight loss plan involves a modest reduction in energy intake, incorporating physical activity into each day, and practising changes in behaviour that can assist you in meeting your weight loss goals. The guidelines for a sound weight loss plan are outlined in the Highlight box on page 404.

Eat Smaller Portions of Lower-Fat Foods

What changes can you make to reduce your energy intake and stay healthy? Here are some helpful suggestions:

1. Follow the serving sizes recommended in *Eating Well with Canada's Food Guide*. Making this change involves understanding what constitutes a serving size and measuring foods to determine if they meet or exceed the recommended serving size. Remember that one pound of fat is equal to about 3500 kcal (14 640 kJ); to lose one pound of fat, you must eat less food and expend more energy to create an energy deficit of 3500 kcal.

2. Reduce the amount of foods that are high in fat and energy from your daily diet. Reduce dietary fat to 20% to 35% of total energy. This goal can be achieved by eliminating extra fats, such as butter, margarine, and mayonnaise, and snack foods, such as ice cream, doughnuts, and cakes. Save these foods as occasional special treats. Select lower-fat versions of the foods listed in *Eating Well with Canada's Food Guide*. This means selecting leaner cuts of meat (such as the white meat of poultry and extra-lean ground beef) and reduced-fat or skim dairy products, and selecting lower-fat preparation methods (baking and broiling instead of frying).

By following these suggestions, you can make simple changes that are effective in reducing energy intake and help contribute to a more nutritious diet overall.

Participate in Regular Physical Activity

Why is being physically active so important for achieving changes in body weight and for maintaining a healthy body weight? Of course, we expend extra energy during

▶ **HIGHLIGHT**

The Anatomy of Fad Diets

Fad diets are programs that enjoy short-term popularity and are sold based on a marketing gimmick that appeals to the public's desires and fears. There are hundreds of these types of diets on the market today, and the goal of the person or company designing and marketing these diets is to make money. How can you tell if the program you are interested in is a fad diet? Here are some pointers to help you:

- The promoters of the diet claim that the program is new, improved, or based on some new discovery; however, no scientific data are available to support these claims.
- The program is touted for its ability to result in rapid weight loss or body fat loss, usually more than 1 kg (2.2 lb.) per week, and may include the claim that weight loss can be achieved with little or no physical exercise.
- The diet includes special foods and supplements, many of which are expensive or difficult to find or can only be purchased from the diet promoter. Common recommendations for these diets include avoiding certain foods, only eating a special combination of certain foods, or including magic foods in the diet that "burn" fat and speed up metabolism.

- The diet may include a rigid menu that must be followed daily or may limit participants to eating a few select foods each day. Variety and balance are discouraged, and certain foods (such as fruits and vegetables) may be restricted.
- Many programs include supplemental foods or nutritional supplements that are identified as substances critical to the success of the diet and usually include claims that these supplements can cure or prevent a variety of health ailments or that the diet can stop the aging process.

The success of fad diets lies in their ability to appeal to the concerns of many people: being overweight or not being muscular enough; reducing the effects of aging, such as wrinkles, loose skin, and tissue damage; and eating anything you want or desire and still losing weight. It is estimated that Americans currently spend more than $33 billion on fad diets each year (American Dietetic Association 2001). In a world where many of us feel we have to meet a certain physical standard to be attractive and "good enough," these types of diets flourish. Unfortunately, the only people who usually benefit from them are their marketers, who can become very wealthy promoting programs that do not produce permanent results.

---

physical activity, but there's more to it than that, because exercise alone (without a reduction of energy intake) does not result in dramatic decreases in body weight. Instead, one of the most important reasons for being regularly active is that it helps us maintain or increase our lean body mass and our BMR. In contrast, energy restriction alone causes us to lose lean body mass. As you've learned, the more lean body mass we have, the more energy we expend over the long term.

The U.S. National Weight Control Registry (NWCR) is an ongoing project documenting the habits of people who have lost at least 13.6 kg (30 lb.) and kept their weight off for at least one year. Of the more than 5000 people registered thus far, average weight loss was 30 kg (66 lb.), and the group maintained the minimum weight loss criterion of 13.6 kg (30 lb.) for 5.5 years (NWCR n.d.). Virtually all the people (98%) reported changing their food intake to lose weight and maintain weight loss and 94% became more physically active. Walking was the most popular form of exercise, and 90% said they averaged one hour a day of physical activity.

They also tended to watch less television—62% reported watching fewer than 10 hours of TV weekly. Although very few weight loss studies have documented long-term maintenance of weight loss, those that have find that only people who are regularly active are able to maintain most of their weight loss.

In addition to expending energy and maintaining lean body mass and BMR, regular physical activity improves our mood, results in a higher quality of sleep, increases self-esteem, and gives us a sense of accomplishment (see Chapter 12 for more benefits

▶ **HIGHLIGHT**

Recommendations for a Sound Weight Loss Plan

Dietary Recommendations:

- Reasonable weight loss is defined as 0.25 to 1 kg (0.5 to 2 lb.) per week. To achieve this rate of weight loss, energy intake should be reduced by approximately 250 to no more than 1000 kcal per day of present intake. A weight loss plan should never provide fewer than a total of 1200 kcal (5020 kJ) per day.

- Total fat intake should be 20% to 35% of total energy intake.

- Saturated fat intake should be 5% to 10% of total energy intake.

- Monounsaturated fat intake should be 10% to 15% of total energy intake.

- Polyunsaturated fat intake should be no more than 10% of total energy intake.

- Protein intake should be approximately 10–39% of total energy intake.

- Carbohydrate intake should be around 45–65% of total energy intake, with less than 10% of energy intake coming from simple sugars.

- Fibre intake should be 25 to 35 grams per day.

- Calcium intake should be 1000 to 1500 mg per day.

Physical Activity Recommendations:

- A long-term goal for physical activity should be a minimum of 30 minutes of moderate physical activity most, or preferably all, days of the week. (See Canada's Physical Activity Guide)

- Doing 45 minutes or more of an activity, such as walking, at least five days per week is ideal.

Behaviour Modification Recommendations:

- Eliminate inappropriate behaviours by shopping when you are not hungry, eating only at set times in one location, refusing to buy problem foods, and avoiding vending machines, convenience stores, and fast-food restaurants.

- Suppress inappropriate behaviours by taking small food portions, eating foods on smaller serving dishes so they appear larger, and avoiding feelings of deprivation by eating regular meals throughout the day.

- Strengthen appropriate behaviours by sharing food with others, learning appropriate serving sizes, planning nutritious snacks, scheduling walks and other physical activities with friends, and keeping clothes and equipment for physical activity in convenient places.

- Repeat desired behaviours by slowing down eating, always using utensils, leaving food on your plate, moving more throughout the day, and joining groups who are physically active.

- Reward yourself for positive behaviours by getting a massage, buying new clothes or tickets to non-food amusements, taking a walk, or reading a book (for fun).

- Use the buddy system by exercising with a friend or relative or calling this support person when you need an extra boost to stay motivated.

- Don't punish yourself if you deviate from your plan (and you will—everyone does). Ask others to avoid responding to any slips you make.

Source: Adapted from National Heart, Lung, and Blood Institute Expert Panel, National Institutes of Health, *Clinical Guidelines on the Identification, Evaluation, and Treatment of Overweight and Obesity in Adults,* Washington, DC: Government Printing Office, 1998.

of regular physical activity). All these changes enhance our ability to engage in long-term healthful lifestyle behaviours.

Weight Loss Can Be Enhanced with Prescribed Medications

The biggest complaint about the recommendations for weight loss is that they are too difficult for most people to follow. Many people are looking for a "magic bullet" that will allow them to lose weight quickly and easily, requiring little sustained effort on their part to achieve their weight goals. Other people have tried to follow sound weight loss suggestions for years and have not been successful. In response to these challenges, prescription drugs have been developed to assist people with weight loss.

Table 11.7   Side Effects of Two Prescription Weight Loss Drugs

Sibutramine (brand name Meridia)	Orlistat (brand name Xenical)
Increased blood pressure	Abdominal pain
Dry mouth	Fatty and loose stools
Anorexia	Leaky stools
Constipation	Flatulence
Insomnia	Decreased absorption of fat-soluble nutrients, such as vitamins E and D
Dizziness	
Nausea	

Source: G. A. Bray, Drug treatment of obesity, 1999, *Baillière's Clinical Endocrinology and Metabolism* 13:131–148.

Two prescription weight loss drugs are available, and their long-term safety and efficacy are still being explored. Sibutramine (brand name Meridia) is an appetite suppressant that can cause increased blood pressure in some people. Orlistat (brand name Xenical) is a drug that acts to inhibit the absorption of dietary fat from the intestinal tract, which can result in weight loss in some people. A one-year study of orlistat found that it was effective in minimizing weight regain in obese people who lost weight by using a low-energy diet (Hill et al. 1999). Orlistat (Xenical) is now available in the United States without a prescription, in capsules with half the dosage of the prescription capsules. The side effects of these drugs are identified in Table 11.7.

Health Canada (2007) has received 65 reports of "adverse reactions to sibutramine, including rapid heart beats (tachycardia), irregular heart rhythm (arrhythmia), and unstable hypertension linked to sibutramine." The large increases in blood pressure associated with the drug are believed to be responsible for the heart problems.

Rimonabant is the first of a new class of weight loss drug approved for use in Europe in 2006. This drug acts on parts of the central and peripheral nervous systems that help to control food intake. To date, it has not been approved in Canada or the United States. In clinical trials, those people taking the drug have lost significantly more weight than people in control groups, but there have been reports of psychiatric side effects including depression and anxiety (Christensen et al. 2007).

Prescribed weight loss medications can be associated with serious side effects and a certain level of risk. The medications may be justified for people who are severely obese but should be used only while under a physician's supervision so that the progress and health risks can be closely monitored. They are most effective when combined with a program that supports energy restriction, regular exercise, and increasing physical activity throughout the day.

Over-the-Counter Substances Used and Abused for Weight Loss

Over-the-counter (OTC) dietary and herbal supplements and prescription medications are also marketed for weight loss. A growing number of these products increase metabolic rate and suppress appetite through one or several combined ingredients, including caffeine, ephedrine, and phenylpropanolamine (PPA), a substance commonly found in many cold medications. Use of these substances is being closely monitored by Health Canada, as it is thought that abnormal increases in heart rate and blood pressure can occur and the substances may be dangerous if used improperly.

Ephedrine, also known as ephedra, Chinese ephedra, or ma huang, is commonly found in products that claim to suppress appetite, promote weight loss, aid bodybuilding, and speed up metabolism. In addition to increasing stamina, ephedrine is claimed to aid in the reduction of body weight and body fat in sedentary women, which has piqued the interest of a growing number of Canadians. Those looking to find ephedrine as their answer for weight loss can find hundreds of aggressively marketed American fitness and weight loss ads on the internet, promoting ephedrine-containing products as "fat burners" and "rapid fat loss catalysts." (Stricter regulation of labels in Canada prevents the same American-made brands sold here from making such claims.)

However, side effects of ephedrine include headaches, nausea, nervousness, anxiety, irregular heart rate, and high blood pressure. At least one death in Canada has been linked to the use of a product that combined large doses of ephedrine with caffeine, and at least 60 adverse events had been reported in Canada related to the use of ephedrine. Most such reactions involved the use or overuse of combination products, which combine ephedrine with caffeine (Health Canada 2003).

In January 2002, Health Canada issued a warning for Canadians not to use certain products containing ephedrine—especially those containing caffeine and other stimulants with labelled or implied claims, such as weight loss, bodybuilding, or increased energy (Health Canada 2003). At the time, all products combined with caffeine or stimulants and over the maximum dosage of ephedrine were recalled. Currently, the maximum allowable dosages for ephedrine in products is 8 mg per single dose, or 32 mg per day. Products containing ephedrine that are marketed for traditional uses, such as in cold remedies and allergy medications, remain available in Canadian stores so long as they do not exceed the maximum allowable dosages. Despite the warnings, many Canadians continue to buy ephedrine-containing products for use as a weight loss supplement.

Phenylpropanolamine (PPA) is another ingredient used in many OTC and prescription cough and cold medications as a decongestant and in OTC weight loss products. In 2000, both Canada and the United States banned PPA from the market when several women died of hemorrhagic stroke, or bleeding into the brain, after taking the prescribed dose. The increased risk of hemorrhagic stroke was detected among women using the drug for weight control in the three days after starting to use the medication (USFDA 2000).

Fenfluramine, dexfenfluramine, and a combination of phentermine and fenfluramine (called phen-fen) are appetite-suppressing drugs commonly promoted for the management of obesity. In 1996, the drugs made shocking headlines when drug manufacturers around the world pulled diet drugs containing fenfluramine and dexfenfluramine after studies revealed a link between the drugs and serious heart valve disease. Further studies also concluded that people taking the drugs for more than three months have a 23 times greater chance of developing primary pulmonary hypertension (PPH), a rare and deadly lung condition.

As you can see, Canada has had a history of identifying and advising against weight loss aids. Clearly, using weight loss supplements can have dangerous consequences. Even the use of prescribed weight loss medications is associated with side effects and a certain level of risk. Recently, several Canadian provinces have seen a rise in the incidence of abuse of an illegal drug known as methamphetamine, more commonly known by its street name, crystal meth. Young adolescent females are vulnerable to use of the drug as a weight control measure. Sadly, many teenage girls begin taking this stimulant in an attempt to lose weight but end up highly addicted and faced with severe long-term effects. Side effects can include irritability, heart palpitations, confusion, severe anxiety, paranoia, violence, or psychosis. Long-term use may cause structural changes to the brain, memory loss, difficulty completing complex tasks, and permanent psychotic symptoms.

Recap: Maintaining a healthy body weight involves sound dietary approaches and participation in regular physical activity. Weight loss can be accomplished by eating smaller portion sizes, eating less dietary fat, incorporating regular physical activity, and applying appropriate behavioural modification techniques. Maintenance of weight loss is enhanced by healthful eating habits and regular physical activity. When necessary, drugs can be used to reduce obesity with a doctor's prescription and supervision. Using dietary supplements to lose weight is controversial and can be dangerous in some instances.

Safe and Effective Weight Gain

With so much emphasis in North America on obesity and weight loss, some find it surprising that many people are trying to gain weight. People looking to gain weight include those who are underweight to the extent that it is compromising their health, and many athletes who are attempting to increase strength and power for competition.

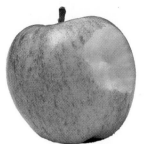

Eat More Energy Than Is Expended

To gain weight, people must eat more energy than they expend. Although overeating large amounts of high-saturated-fat foods (such as bacon, sausage, and cheese) can cause weight gain, doing this without exercising is not wise because most of the weight gained is fat, and high-fat diets increase our risks for cardiovascular and other diseases. Unless there are medical reasons to eat a high-fat diet, it is recommended that people trying to gain weight eat a diet that is relatively low in dietary fat (less than 30% of total energy) and relatively high in complex carbohydrates (55% of total energy). Recommendations for weight gain include these:

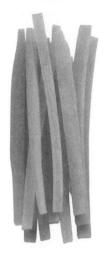

- Eat a diet that includes about 500 to 1000 kcal (2100 to 4200 kJ) per day more than is needed to maintain present body weight. Although we don't know exactly how much extra energy is needed to gain 0.5 kg (1 lb.), estimates range from 3000 to 3500 kcal (12 600 to 14 700 kJ). Thus, eating 500 to 1000 kcal (2100 to 4200 kJ) per day in excess should result in a gain of 0.5 to 1.0 kg (1 to 2 lb.) of weight each week.

- Eat a diet that contains about 55% of total energy from carbohydrate, 25% to 30% of total energy from fat, and 15% to 20% of total energy from protein.

- Eat frequently, including meals and numerous snacks throughout the day. Many underweight people do not take the time to eat often enough.

- Avoid the use of tobacco products, as they depress appetite and increase metabolic rate, which prevent weight gain. They also cause lung, mouth, and esophageal cancers.

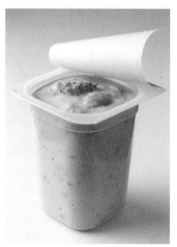

- Exercise regularly and incorporate weightlifting or some other form of resistance training into your exercise routine. This form of exercise is most effective in increasing muscle mass. Performing aerobic exercise (such as walking, running, bicycling, or swimming) at least 30 minutes for three days per week will help maintain a strong cardiovascular system.

The key to gaining weight is to eat frequent meals throughout the day and to select energy-dense foods. When selecting foods that are higher in fat, make sure you select foods higher in polyunsaturated and monounsaturated fats (such as peanut butter, olive and canola oils, and avocados). For instance, smoothies and milkshakes made with low-fat milk or yogurt are a great way to take in a lot of energy. Eating peanut butter with fruit or celery and including salad dressings on your salad are other ways to increase the energy density of foods. The biggest challenge to weight gain is setting aside time to eat; by packing a lot of foods to take with you throughout the day, you can enhance your opportunities to eat more.

Protein Supplements Do Not Increase Muscle Growth or Strength

As with weight loss, there are many products marketed for weight gain. One of the most common claims is that these products are *anabolic;* that is, that they increase muscle mass.

These products include protein and amino acid supplements, which are legal in Canada and the United States. Do these substances really work? A growing body of evidence exists to show that protein and amino acid supplements do not enhance muscle gain or result in improvements in strength (Kreider, Miriel, and Bertun 1993). The health consequences of using protein supplements are unknown.

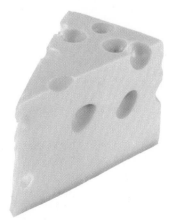

Eating frequent nutrient-dense snacks can help promote weight gain.

A substance called androstenedione, or "Andro," became popular after baseball player Mark McGwire claimed he was using it during the season he hit 70 home runs. Androstenedione is technically an "androgenic steroid precursor," because it gets converted in the body to the male sex hormone testosterone (an androgen). Testosterone is also an anabolic steroid, because it enhances muscle development and athletic performance. Although the case of Mark McGwire may seem to suggest that androstenedione is an extremely effective product for building muscle mass, gaining strength, and improving performance, some studies have found that it did not have any benefits (Joyner 2000; Broeder et al. 2000; Brown et al. 2000).

In Canada, androstenedione is a controlled substance, which means that it is available only with a doctor's prescription. In the United States, it is legal, but the FDA recently issued warning letters to 23 companies that manufacture products containing androstenedione, warning them that the safety of the substance has not been established and they should not be marketing products containing androstenedione as dietary supplements. Many health and sports organizations have warned against using androgenic and anabolic steroids and their precursors, such as androstenedione, because these substances increase the risk of serious health problems (Center for Food Safety and Applied Nutrition 2004). See Chapter 12 for more discussion of anabolic steroid use.

> **Recap:** Weight gain can be achieved by eating more and performing weightlifting and aerobic exercise. Protein and amino acid supplements do not increase muscle growth or strength, and their potential side effects are unknown. Anabolic steroids and their precursors, such as androstenedione, can increase body weight and muscle mass but are known to cause major health problems.

What Disorders Are Related to Energy Intake?

At the beginning of this chapter, we provided some definitions of underweight, overweight, and obesity. Let's take a closer look at these disorders.

Underweight

As defined earlier in this chapter, underweight occurs when a person has too little body fat to maintain health. People with a BMI of less than 18.5 kg/m^2 are typically considered underweight. Many people are underweight because of heavy smoking; an underlying disease, such as cancer or HIV infection; or an eating disorder, such as anorexia nervosa (see Chapter 13). Being underweight increases the risk for infections and illness, and it can even be fatal.

Although childhood overweight and obesity are major health concerns in most developed countries, wasting (or starvation) is still a critical health crisis for children in many developing countries. Refer to the Highlight box on global nutrition to learn more about overweight and wasting in preschool children around the world.

Overweight

Overweight is defined as having a moderate amount of excess body fat, resulting in a person having a weight for a given height that is greater than some accepted standard but is not considered obese. People with a BMI between 25 and 29.9 kg/m^2 are considered to be overweight. Being overweight does not appear to be as detrimental to our health as being obese, but some of the health risks of overweight include an increased risk for high blood pressure, heart disease, type 2 diabetes, sleep disorders, osteoarthritis, gallstones, and gynecological abnormalities (National

Institutes of Health 1998). It is possible that some people who are overweight will become obese, which can lead to an even higher risk for these diseases and for premature death. Because of these concerns, health professionals recommend that overweight individuals adopt a lifestyle that incorporates nutritious eating and regular physical activity in an attempt to prevent additional weight gain, to reduce body weight to the normal level, and to support long-term health even if body weight is not significantly reduced.

Obesity

Obesity is defined as having an excess body fat that adversely affects health, resulting in a person having a weight for a given height that is substantially greater than some accepted standard. People with a BMI between 30 and 34.9 kg/m^2 are in the Class I obese category; a BMI of 35.0 to 39.9 kg/m^2 is Class II obese; and a BMI greater than 40.0 kg/m^2 is Class III.

Both overweight and obesity are now considered an epidemic in North America. In 2004, an estimated 5.5 million adult Canadians were obese and an additional 8.6 million were overweight (Tjepkema 2005). The prevalence of obesity is a major health concern because it is linked to many chronic diseases, including heart disease, high blood pressure, type 2 diabetes, some cancers, and osteoarthritis. At least six of the ten leading causes of death in Canada are associated with obesity (see Table 11.8).

It has been estimated that the financial costs associated with obesity total more than $99 billion. These costs affect not just the person with obesity but all of society, as they increase the costs of health care and medications, reduce productivity because of days of lost work, and reduce future earnings because of premature death.

Ironically, up to 40% of women and 25% of men are dieting at any given time. How can obesity rates be so high when there are so many people dieting? Certainly some people dieting at any given time are actually at a normal or even below-normal weight, and these people account for a small percentage of this total; however, many

Table 11.8 Top 10 Causes of Death, 1997

Cause of Death	No. of Deaths: Males	No. of Deaths: Females
Cancer	31 555	27 148
Heart diseases	30 149	27 268
Cerebrovascular disease	6 675	9 376
Pulmonary diseases	5 607	4 011
Unintentional injuries	5 305	3 321
Pneumonia/influenza	3 749	4 283
Suicide	2 914	*
Diabetes	2 767	2 932
Diseases of arteries	2 505	2 262
Diseases of central nervous system (e.g., Alzheimer's)	2 104	2 945
Psychoses	**	3 084

Source: "Deaths due to top 10 causes, 1997," from the Statistics Canada publication "Health Reports", 2000, Catalogue 82-003, Vol. 12, No. 3, April 26, 2001, page 45, available at: http://www.statcan.ca/english/freepub/82-003-XIE/0030082-003-XIE.pdf

Note: Six of the top 10 causes of death for men and for women are associated with obesity.

* Did not rank in top 10 causes for females.

** Did not rank in top 10 causes for males.

▶ **HIGHLIGHT**

Global Nutrition: Overweight and Wasting Among Preschool Children

We know that wealthy, developed countries are experiencing significant upward trends of obesity in adults and children. In contrast, in developing countries, wasting (or starvation) has generally been considered one of the most significant health concerns. Recently, however, poverty and low socioeconomic status have been linked with higher rates of obesity worldwide. In fact, the United Nations now estimates that more than one billion people are overweight or obese worldwide, including 22 million children under age 5 (Arnst 2004). So is childhood obesity on the rise in developing countries, too?

A recent study documents the prevalence and trends of overweight among children aged 0 to 6 years in developed and developing countries (de Onis and Blössner 2000). Figure 11.8 shows a graph of some of the countries studied.

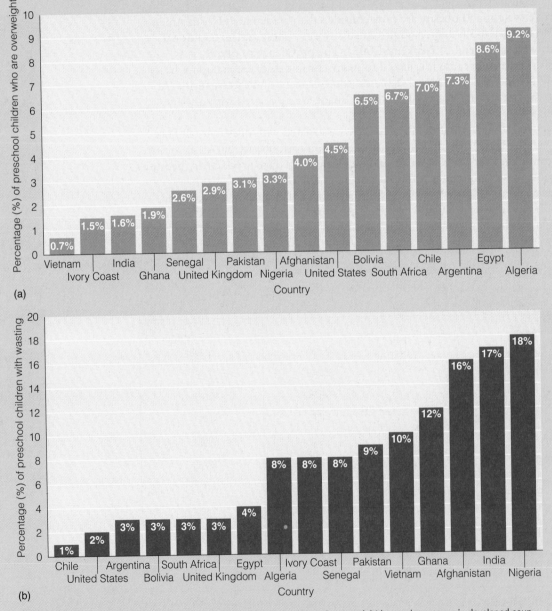

Figure 11.8 Rates of overweight (a) versus wasting (b) worldwide. Although overweight is a major concern in developed countries, wasting is still a major concern in developing countries.

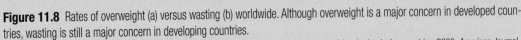
(Adapted from M. de Onis and M. Blössner, Prevalence and trends of overweight among preschool children in developing countries, 2000, *American Journal of Clinical Nutrition* 72:1032–1039.)

Of the 94 countries surveyed, 76% reported less than 5% of their young children to be overweight. In contrast, 21% of these countries reported that 5% to 10% of their children were overweight, and 2% reported more than 10% of their children as overweight. As you might suspect, the countries with the fewest overweight children were developing countries, such as those in Africa and Asia. The countries with the highest rates of overweight were developed countries, such as the United States.

Although overweight appears to be on the rise in some developing countries, it is important to note that wasting rates are much higher in these countries than are rates of overweight. Forty-five of the countries studied reported greater than 5% of their children as malnourished. These findings show that although the overall global rate of obesity may be increasing, we must not focus on reducing overweight in young children at the expense of solving problems with wasting.

obese people who are dieting are somehow failing to lose weight or to maintain long-term weight loss.

What Causes Obesity?

Obesity is known as a **multifactorial disease**, meaning that there are many things that cause it. This makes obesity extremely difficult to treat. Although it is certainly true that obesity, like overweight, is caused by eating more energy than is expended, it is also true that some people are more susceptible to becoming obese than others.

In addition, as we saw with the twin study, some people are more resistant to weight loss and maintaining weight loss than others. Research on the causes and best treatments of obesity is ongoing, but let's explore some current theories.

multifactorial disease Any disease that may be attributable to one or more of a variety of causes.

Genetic Factors Because our genetic background influences our height, weight, body shape, and metabolic rate, it also affects our risk for obesity. The thrifty gene theory (page 395) suggests that some people possess a thrifty gene (or genes), which causes them to expend less energy at rest and during physical activity. This theory has been used to try to explain the high rates of obesity among Aboriginal North Americans and other indigenous peoples. The set-point theory (page 396) suggests that our bodies work to maintain our weight at a set point, which could partially explain why most obese people are very resistant to weight loss. As we learn more about genetics, we will gain a greater understanding of the role that our genetic background plays in the development and treatment of obesity.

Childhood Overweight and Obesity Are Linked to Adult Obesity The prevalence of overweight in children and adolescents is increasing at an alarming rate in North America. There was a time when having extra "baby fat" was considered good for the child. We assumed that childhood overweight and obesity were temporary and that the child would grow out of it. Although it is important for children to have a certain minimum level of body fat to maintain health and to grow properly, researchers are now concerned that overweight and obesity are harmful to children's health and increase their risk of overweight and obesity in adulthood.

Health data demonstrate that obese children are already showing signs of disease while they are young, including elevated blood pressure, high cholesterol levels, and changes in insulin and glucose metabolism that may increase the risk for type 2 diabetes. In some communities, children as young as 6 years of age have been diagnosed with type 2 diabetes. Unfortunately, many of these children are maintaining these disease risk factors into adulthood.

Does being an obese child guarantee that obesity will be maintained during adulthood? Not all obese adults were obese as children, and some children who are obese grow up to have a normal body weight. However, it has been estimated that about 50% of children who are obese will maintain their higher weight as adults. This has important consequences for their health.

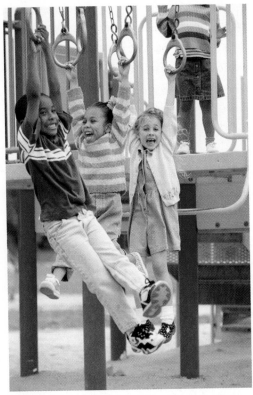
Adequate physical activity is instrumental in preventing childhood obesity.

What factors contribute to obesity in children? For young people, it has been suggested that there are three critical periods during which weight gain can increase the risk of obesity and related diseases in adulthood:

- gestation and early infancy
- the period of weight gain (called *adiposity rebound*) that occurs between five and seven years of age
- adolescence (or puberty)

Substantial weight gain during these periods can increase the risk for adult obesity and related diseases. Having either one or two overweight parents increases the risk of obesity two to four times (Dietz 1994).

An additional important contributor to childhood obesity includes low physical activity levels. There was a time when children played outdoors regularly and when physical education was offered daily in school. In today's society, many children cannot play outdoors because of safety concerns and lack of recreational facilities, and few schools have the resources to regularly offer physical education to children. In addition, many popular activities for children today are sedentary in nature, including playing video games, watching television, using the computer, and playing with hand-held toys. As childhood and adolescence are critical times for forming activity habits, many young people today are not getting an opportunity to be physically active, which will likely have a significant impact on their physical activity levels and potential for obesity as adults.

How Is Obesity Treated?

The first line of defence in treating obesity is a low-energy diet and regular physical activity. Overweight and obese individuals should work with their health care practitioner to design and maintain a low-fat diet (less than 30% of total energy from fat) that has a deficit of 500 to 1000 kcal per day (about 2100 to 4200 kJ) (National Institutes of Health 1998). Physical activity should be increased gradually so that the person can build a program in which they are exercising at least 30 minutes per day, five times per week; see Canada's Activity Guide.

As discussed earlier in this chapter, prescription medications are used to treat some cases of obesity. Again, these medications should be used only while under a physician's supervision, and they appear to be most effective when combined with energy restriction and regular physical activity.

Surgery may be recommended for people with a BMI greater than or equal to 35 kg/m^2 who have not been able to lose weight with energy restriction and exercise. The three most common types of weight loss surgery performed are gastroplasty, gastric bypass, and gastric banding (Figure 11.9).

- *Gastroplasty* involves partitioning or stapling a small section of the stomach to reduce total food intake.
- *Gastric bypass surgery* involves attaching the lower part of the small intestine to the stomach, so that most of the food bypasses the stomach and small intestine. This results in significantly less absorption of food in the intestine and is the most frequently performed type of surgery for weight loss.
- *Gastric banding* is a relatively new procedure in which stomach size is reduced by using a constricting band, thus restricting food intake.

The risks of surgery in people with obesity are extremely high and include increased infections, higher formation of blood clots, and more adverse reactions to anaesthesia. After the surgery, these people may face a lifetime of problems with

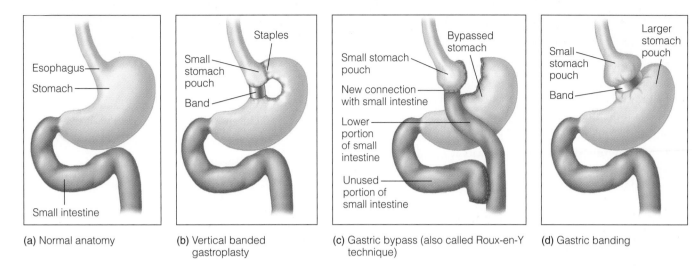

(a) Normal anatomy

(b) Vertical banded gastroplasty

(c) Gastric bypass (also called Roux-en-Y technique)

(d) Gastric banding

Figure 11.9 Various forms of surgery alter the normal anatomy of the gastrointestinal tract (a) to result in weight loss. Vertical banded gastroplasty (b), gastric bypass (c), and gastric banding (d) are three surgical procedures used to reduce obesity.

chronic diarrhea, vomiting, intolerance to dairy products and other foods, dehydration, and nutritional deficiencies resulting from alterations in nutrient digestion and absorption. Thus, the potential benefits of the procedure must outweigh the risks. It is critical that each surgery candidate be carefully screened by a trained medical professional. If the immediate threat of serious disease and death is more dangerous than the risks associated with surgery, then the procedure is justified.

Are these surgical procedures successful in reducing obesity? About one third to one half of people who received obesity surgery lose significant amounts of weight and keep this weight off for at least five years. The reasons that one half to two thirds do not experience long-term success include that some are unable to eat less over

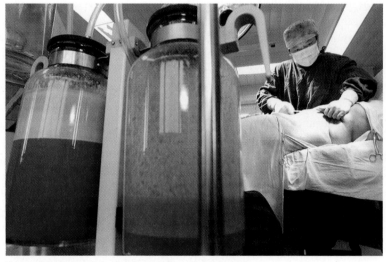

Liposuction removes fat cells from specific areas of the body.

time, even with a smaller stomach. For others, staples and gastric bands loosen and stomach pouches enlarge. Some individuals do not survive the surgery. Although these surgical procedures may seem extremely risky, those who lose weight, keep it off, and improve their health feel that the eventual benefits are worth the risks.

Liposuction is a cosmetic surgical procedure that removes fat cells from localized areas in the body. It is not recommended or typically used to treat obesity. This procedure is not without risks; blood clots, skin and nerve damage, adverse drug reactions, and perforation injuries can and do occur as a result of liposuction. It can also result in deformations in the area where the fat is removed. This procedure is not the solution to long-term weight loss, as the millions of fat cells that remain in the body after liposuction enlarge if the person continues to overeat.

Recap: Obesity is caused by many factors. Genetic theories about obesity include the thrifty gene theory, set-point theory, and leptin theory. In addition, childhood obesity is strongly associated with adult obesity. Treatments for overweight and obesity include low-energy, low-fat diets in combination with regular physical activity, weight loss prescription medications, and weight loss surgery.

CHAPTER SUMMARY

- Definitions of a healthy body weight include one that is appropriate for someone's age and level of development, that can be achieved and sustained without constant dieting, and that promotes good eating habits and allows for regular physical activity.

- Underweight is defined as having too little body fat to maintain health, causing a person to have a weight for a given height that is below an acceptably defined standard.

- Obesity is defined as having excess body fat that adversely affects health, resulting in a person having a weight for a given height that is substantially greater than some accepted standard.

- Body mass index (BMI) is an index of weight/height^2. It is useful to indicate health risks associated with overweight and obesity in groups of people; however, it has some important limitations.

- Body composition assessment involves estimating the proportions of a person's body fat (or adipose tissue) and lean body mass. Methods include underwater weighing, skinfold measures, bioelectrical impedance analysis, near infrared reactance, and the Bod Pod.

- The waist-to-hip ratio and waist circumference are used to determine patterns of fat storage. People with large waists (as compared with hips) have an apple-shaped fat pattern. People with large hips (as compared to the waist) have a pear-shaped fat pattern. Having an apple-shaped pattern increases your risk for heart disease, type 2 diabetes, and other chronic diseases.

- We lose or gain weight based on changes in our energy intake, the food we eat, and our energy expenditure (both at rest and when physically active).

- Basal metabolic rate (BMR) is the energy needed to maintain our body's resting functions. BMR accounts for 60% to 70% of our total daily energy needs.

- The thermic effect of food is the energy we expend to process the food we eat. It accounts for 5% to 10% of the energy content of a meal and is higher for processing proteins and carbohydrates than for processing fats.

- The energy cost of physical activity represents energy that we expend for physical movement or work we do above basal levels. It accounts for 20% to 35% of our total daily energy output.

- Our genetic heritage influences our risk for obesity, and such factors as possessing a thrifty gene (or genes)

- or maintaining a weight set point may affect a person's risk for obesity.

- Being overweight or obese as a child can lead to adult obesity, and childhood obesity is linked with the risk for heart disease and premature death later in adulthood.

- Behavioural factors contributing to obesity include eating a high-energy diet and alterations in the cues for hunger, appetite, and satiety. Social factors that may contribute to obesity include pressure to eat from family and peers, easy access to inexpensive and high-fat foods, watching too much television, and not taking time to exercise. Mood and emotional state also affect appetite.

- A sound weight change plan involves a modest change in energy intake, incorporating physical activity into each day, and practising changes in behaviour that can assist in meeting realistic weight change goals.

- Prescription drugs can be used to assist with weight loss when the risks of obesity override the risks associated with the medications.

- Various dietary supplements are marketed as weight loss products. Many of these products cause dangerous changes in heart rate and blood pressure.

- Most of the products marketed for weight gain have been shown to be ineffective. The risks associated with these products are not well documented; many of these may have no effect on a person's weight and are simply a waste of money. Safe weight gain involves consuming more energy than is expended by selecting ample servings of nutritious, high-energy foods and exercising regularly by including resistance training and aerobic exercise.

- Being underweight can be dangerous to our health, and wasting (or starvation) among children is still a health crisis in many developing countries.

- Overweight is not as detrimental to health as obesity, but it is associated with an increased risk for high blood pressure, heart disease, type 2 diabetes, sleep disorders, osteoarthritis, gallstones, and gynecological abnormalities.

- Obesity is associated with significantly increased risks for many diseases and for premature death. Obesity can be treated with low-energy diets and regular physical activity, prescription medications, and surgery when necessary.

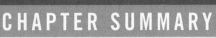 **mynutritionlab** Go to MyNutritionLab at www.pearsoned.ca/mynutritionlab and enrich your understanding of nutrition! You'll find key animations, interactive exercises, access to My DietAnalysis, and much more.

REVIEW QUESTIONS

1. The ratio of a person's body weight to height is represented as his or her
   a. body composition.
   b. basal metabolic rate.
   c. bioelectrical impedance.
   d. body mass index.

2. The body's total daily energy expenditure includes
   a. basal metabolic rate, thermal effect of food, and effect of physical activity.
   b. basal metabolic rate, movement, standing, and sleeping.
   c. effect of physical activity, standing, and sleeping.
   d. body mass index, thermal effect of food, and effect of physical activity.

3. All people gain weight when they
   a. eat a high-fat diet (> 30% fat).
   b. take in more energy than they expend.
   c. fail to exercise.
   d. take in less energy than they expend.

4. The set-point theory proposes that
   a. obese people have a gene not found in slender people that regulates their weight so that it always hovers near a given set point.
   b. obese people have a gene that causes them to be energetically thrifty.
   c. all people have a genetic set point for their body weight.
   d. all people have a hormone that regulates their weight so that it always hovers near a given set point.

5. Our innate, physiologic drive to eat is called
   a. hunger.
   b. appetite.
   c. satiety.
   d. our basal metabolic rate.

6. To lose one pound (0.5 kg) of weight, you need to create a deficit of approximately
   a. 1000 kcal.
   b. 3500 kcal.
   c. 7000 kcal.
   d. 14 700 kcal.

7. What percentage of adult Canadians are estimated to be overweight or obese?
   a. 10%
   b. 25%
   c. 40%
   d. More than 50%

8. Which one of the following is *not* a component of a sound weight change plan?
   a. Make gradual changes in energy intake
   b. Incorporate regular physical activity
   c. Aim to lose more than 1 kg (approx. 2.2 lbs.) per week
   d. Choose a variety of foods

9. As part of recovery from surgery, Sydney has been trying to put on some weight and muscle. However, he has not been listening to the dietitian. He hates going to the gym and has been eating high-caloric foods to gain instead. His doctor has been worried about Sydney since he has an apple-shaped pattern of body fat. What are the risks associated with apple-shaped fat patterning? What do you think the dietitian suggested Sydney to do to gain weight?

10. Vincent loves his mother-in-law's cooking. As a matter of fact, he has put on 13.6 kg (30 lb.) since getting married last year. At a recent visit to the doctor, he found out that his BMI is 32 kg/m^2. Since then, he has joined a gym and has been working hard toward weight loss. During a fitness class, he overheard a fellow classmate talk about weight loss surgery. Is Vincent a good candidate for weight loss surgery? Why or why not?

11. Identify at least four characteristics of a healthy weight.

12. Describe a sound weight loss program, including recommendations for diet, physical activity, and behavioural modifications.

13. Can you increase your basal metabolic rate? Is it wise to try? Defend your answer.

14. Identify at least four societal factors that may have influenced the rise in obesity rates in North America. Think especially of the effect of advances in technology that have occurred in the last 40 years.

15. Your friend Misty joins you for lunch and confesses that she is discouraged about her weight. She says that she has been trying "really hard" for three months to lose weight, but that no matter what she does, she cannot drop below 67.2 kg (148 lb.). Based on her height, you know Misty is not overweight, and she exercises regularly. What questions would you suggest she think about? How would you advise her?

16. Simon has always had a lean build, but recently he's finding it even harder to keep his weight up. Constantly playing hockey, soccer, and badminton for his high school teams, Simon is always on the go. His mom always makes him a big breakfast of bacon and eggs, and Simon makes sure to eat a couple of ham sandwiches at lunchtime. Dinner is usually a couple

of hamburgers after soccer practice, and sometimes he'll have his favourite protein bar before bed. He's never hungry between meals, so he rarely snacks during the day. Simon would really like to beef up so he can be a little more intimidating on the field, but he feels this is impossible.

Given what you've learned about energy balance and weight management, do you think there are any problems with Simon's food intake? What might you advise him to change about his food choices that could help stimulate his appetite? Are there any other suggestions you might give Simon to help him gain weight?

CASE STUDY

While babysitting, you notice that Haruki, the youngest child, isn't playing in the wading pool. His older siblings and their friends are all having a great time escaping the heat, so you ask Haruki why he isn't joining them. You discover that he is constantly picked on in school, and he is always called names like "elephant" and "fatty." He tries not to show that it bothers him, but he confides to you that he often goes home and cries by himself. Haruki states that he will never put on his bathing suit, no matter how hot it gets. Instead of playing in the wading pool, he asks if he can go get an ice cream cone and sit on the bench.

a. Think back to your own childhood. Were you ever teased for some aspect of yourself that you felt unable to change?

b. Can Haruki change his weight? What kinds of obstacles does he face?

c. As overweight children are often made to feel ashamed and worthless by their peers, how would you propose that adults increase their awareness of social stigmatization and reduce incidents of teasing and insensitivity?

Test Yourself Answers

1. **True** Being underweight increases our risk for illness and premature death and in many cases can be just as unhealthful as being obese.

2. **False** Obesity is a multifactorial disease with many contributing factors. Although eating too much food and not getting enough exercise can lead to being overweight and obese, the disease of obesity is complex and is not simply caused by overeating.

3. **False** Body composition assessments can help give us a general idea of our body fat levels, but most methods are not extremely accurate.

4. **True** Staying physically active helps us maintain our muscle mass, which in turn assists us in preventing a dramatic drop in our basal metabolic rate. These changes can help reduce our risk for becoming obese as we get older.

5. **False** Health can be defined in many ways. An individual who is overweight but who exercises regularly and has no additional risk factors for various diseases, such as heart disease and type 2 diabetes, is considered a healthy person.

WEB LINKS

http://women.webmd.com/fad-diets
WebMD—Spotting Fad Diets
Visit this site to learn about the dangers of fad diets and how to identify them.

www.hc-sc.gc.ca/fn-an/food-guide-aliment/index_e.html
Health Canada—*Eating Well with Canada's Food Guide*
See this site for information about *Canada's Food Guide*.

www.hc-sc.gc.ca/fn-an/nutrition/weights-poids/vitalit/index_e.html
Health Canada—Vitality
Visit this site to learn about healthy eating, your own fat patterning, and self esteem.

www.eatrightontario.ca
Eat Right Ontario
Learn more about a Canadian service designed to help you improve your health through nutritious eating.

www.eatracker.ca
Eat Tracker
This online tool by the Dietitians of Canada allows you to track your day's food intake and activity expenditure and compares them with Health Canada guidelines.

www.cdc.gov/nccdphp/dnpa/healthyweight
Centers for Disease Control and Prevention. Healthy Weight—It's Not a Diet, It's a Lifestyle!
This is a new interactive site from the CDC for consumers who want to change their lifestyle to achieve and maintain a healthy weight.

www.nhlbisupport.com/bmi
National Heart, Lung, and Blood Institute BMI calculator
Calculate your body mass index (BMI) on the internet.

www.ftc.gov
Federal Trade Commission
Click on For Consumers and then Diet Health and Fitness to find how to avoid false weight loss claims.

www.consumer.gov/weightloss
Partnership for Healthy Weight Management
Visit this site to learn about successful strategies for achieving and maintaining a healthy weight.

www.eatright.org
American Dietetic Association
Go to this site to learn more about fad diets.

www.niddk.nih.gov/health/nutrit/nutrit.htm
National Institute of Diabetes and Digestive and Kidney Diseases
Find out more about healthy weight loss.

www.sne.org
Society for Nutrition Education
Click on Resources and Relationships and then Weight Realities Division for additional resources related to positive attitudes about body image and healthful alternatives to dieting.

The Criminalization of Fat: Have We Gone Too Far?

Although prejudice of all kinds still exists, our society espouses values of tolerance and compassion toward all people, despite their disease state, religious beliefs, sexual orientation, or racial and ethnic background. However, there seems to be one group of people against whom prejudice is still acceptable, and that is obese people. They remain the punch line of many jokes, are socially ostracized, and experience widespread harassment and embarrassment at work and in many avenues of life.

Most people do not understand that obesity is a disease, just as heart disease and diabetes are diseases. Contrary to this fact, society generally views obesity as a condition that results from being lazy and having no willpower. As you have learned in this chapter, obesity is a complex, multifactorial disease that is not caused solely by overeating or doing too little exercise. As we continue to struggle with how best to prevent and treat obesity, our society must take measures to reduce the social stigma of living with this disease. Such measures might include using more overweight men and women in print and television advertisements and increasing public awareness of regulations prohibiting job and housing discrimination based on weight.

Recently, some compelling arguments have been put forth that we should stop our obsession with weight. Although more than US$30 billion is spent every year in the United States on weight loss efforts, the average weight loss is only about 10% of body weight. Even more discouraging is that most of the weight lost is regained within five years. As most diets are not effective over the long term, many nutrition and exercise professionals are proposing that we encourage a healthy lifestyle defined by eating a balanced diet and staying physically active on a regular basis and stop defining a person's health by his or her body weight.

Dr. Glen Gaesser (1999) and others have challenged long-held assumptions that increased body weight is associated with increased mortality. According to these researchers, there is no clear-cut evidence to define the "best" body weight to increase our lifespan. In contrast, evidence does support the contention that regular physical activity leads to significant improvements in health without weight loss. For instance, increasing aerobic fitness helps reduce mortality rates, whether or not the person performing the aerobic activity also loses weight. Thus, experts question whether it makes sense to spend limited health care resources encouraging individuals who are moderately overweight, particularly those with no significant disease risk factors, to meet a predefined ideal weight.

This topic will most likely remain controversial for many years. However, some professional organizations are beginning to embrace a new way of thinking about the definition of ideal body weight and the negative effects of dieting. The Society for Nutrition Education has a division called Weight Realities to assist dietitians, nutrition educators, and the general public in coping with unrealistic body image expectations and an unhealthy pursuit of thinness. Refer to the website at www.sne.org/weightrealitiesdivision.htm to gain access to weblinks and other resources related to positive attitudes about body image and healthful alternatives to dieting. For instance, About Face (www.about-face.org) is a media literacy organization focused on the impact that mass media has on the mental, emotional, and physical well-being of girls. Bullying (www.bullying.org) is a website written by students on the topic of bullying and weight prejudice among youth. The Body Positive (www.thebodypositive.org) is an organization whose goal "is to empower people of all ages, especially our youth, to celebrate their natural size and shape instead of what society promotes as the ideal body." There are award-winning videos with accompanying curricula that teachers and health educators can use with young children and adolescents, to help them with age-specific self-esteem and body image issues.

Earlier, we identified a few measures for reducing the social stigma of obesity. What other measures can you think of? How can we deal with practical concerns, such as small seats in food courts and movie theatres and narrow department store aisles? Can you think of ways we can be more compassionate toward obese family members, friends, and acquaintances, and support them in their quest for health? As the obesity epidemic continues to grow, our need to answer these questions becomes more critical.

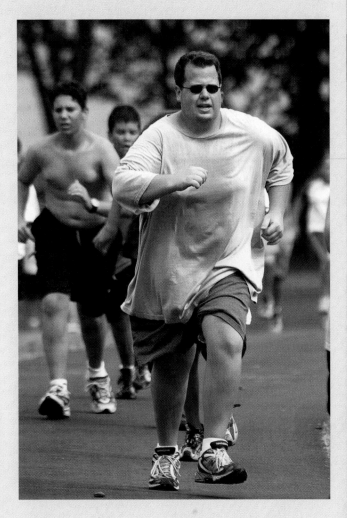

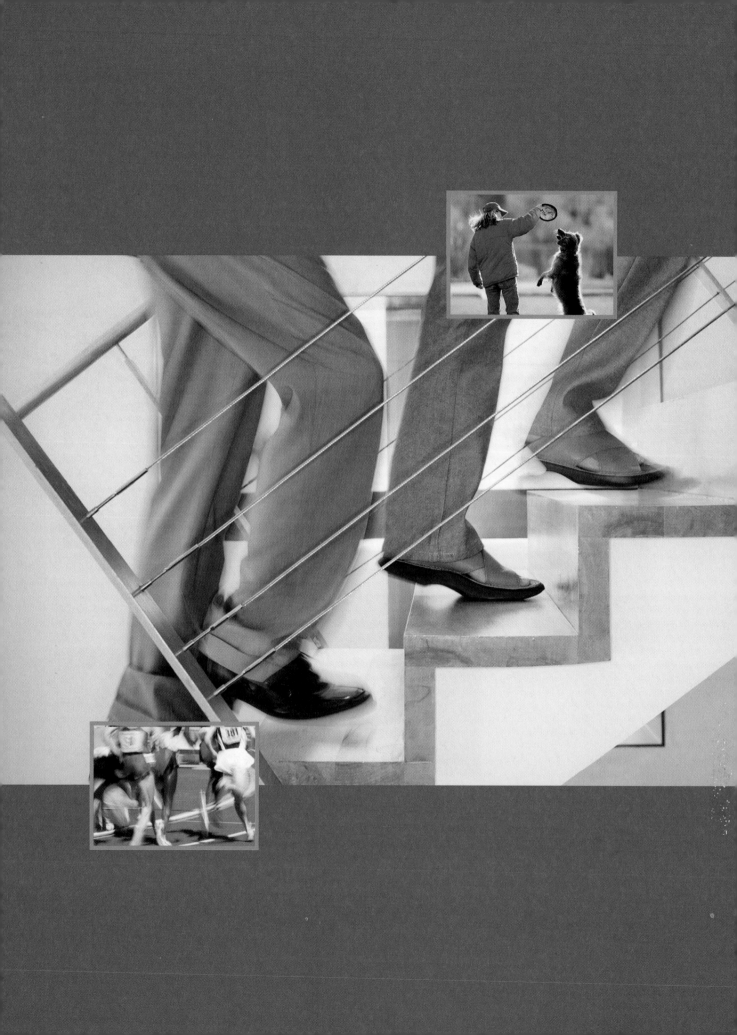

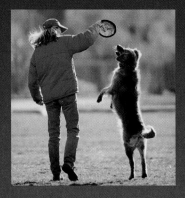

CHAPTER 12

Nutrition and Physical Activity: Keys to Good Health

Test Yourself True or False

1. *Physical activity* and *exercise* mean basically the same thing and are terms that can be used interchangeably. **T or F**

2. Despite the multitude of health benefits of participating in regular physical activity, half of Canadian adults report being inactive. **T or F**

3. To achieve fitness, a person needs to exercise at least one hour each day. **T or F**

4. Lactic acid is not a major contributor to muscle soreness. **T or F**

5. Most ergogenic aids are not effective, and many can be dangerous or cause serious health consequences. **T or F**

Test Yourself answers can be found at the end of the chapter.

In June 2003, Harold Hoffman of North Carolina won several gold medals in track and field at the National Senior Olympics. He clocked 38.36 seconds in the 100-metre dash to beat the listed American record of 38.66. He also won the 200-metre dash (in 1:37.46), the 5K (in 38.3 minutes), and the long jump. If Hoffman's performance times don't amaze you, perhaps they will when you consider his age: at the time he gave these winning performances, he was 95 years old!

There's no doubt about it: regular physical activity dramatically improves our strength, stamina, health, and longevity. But what qualifies as "regular physical activity"? In other words, how much do we need to do to reap the benefits? And if we do become more active, does our diet have to change, too?

Healthy eating practices and regular physical activity are like two sides of the same coin, interacting in a variety of ways to improve our strength and stamina and to increase our resistance to many chronic diseases and acute illnesses. In fact, the nutrition and physical activity recommendations for reducing your risk of heart disease also reduce your risk of high blood pressure, type 2 diabetes, obesity, and some forms of cancer! In this chapter, we define physical activity, identify its many benefits, and discuss the nutrients needed to maintain an active life.

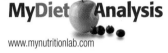

www.mynutritionlab.com

physical activity Any movement produced by muscles that increases energy expenditure; includes occupational, household, leisure-time, and transportation activities.

leisure-time physical activity Any activity not related to a person's occupation; includes competitive sports, recreational activities, and planned exercise training.

exercise A subcategory of leisure-time physical activity; any activity that is purposeful, planned, and structured.

physical fitness The ability to carry out daily tasks with vigour and alertness, without undue fatigue, and with ample energy to enjoy leisure-time pursuits and meet unforeseen emergencies.

cardiorespiratory fitness Fitness of the heart, lungs, and circulatory system; achieved through regular participation in aerobic-type activities.

musculoskeletal fitness Fitness of the muscles and bones.

muscular strength A subcomponent of musculoskeletal fitness defined as the maximal force or tension level that can be produced by a muscle group.

muscular endurance A subcomponent of musculoskeletal fitness defined as the ability of a muscle to maintain submaximal force levels for extended periods of time.

Physical Activity, Exercise, and Physical Fitness: What's the Difference?

Do the terms *physical activity, exercise,* and *physical fitness* mean the same thing? They are used interchangeably in many situations, but they actually represent quite different concepts. **Physical activity** describes any movement produced by muscles that increases energy expenditure. Different categories of physical activity include occupational, household, leisure-time, and transportation (U.S. Department of Health and Human Services 1996). **Leisure-time physical activity** is any activity not related to a person's occupation and includes competitive sports, planned exercise training, and recreational activities, such as hiking, walking, and bicycling. **Exercise** is therefore considered a subcategory of leisure-time physical activity and refers to activity that is purposeful, planned, and structured (Caspersen, Powell, and Christensen 1985).

Physical fitness is a state of being that arises largely from the interaction between nutrition and physical activity. It is defined as the ability to carry out daily tasks with vigour and alertness, without undue fatigue, and with ample energy to enjoy leisure-time pursuits and meet unforeseen emergencies (U.S. Department of Health and Human Services 1996). Physical fitness has many components (Table 12.1) (Heyward 1998). These include **cardiorespiratory fitness**, which is defined as the ability of the heart, lungs, and circulatory system to efficiently supply oxygen and nutrients to working muscles. **Musculoskeletal fitness** involves fitness of both the muscles and the bones and includes *muscular strength* and *muscular endurance*. **Muscular strength** is the maximal force or tension level that can be produced by a muscle group, and **muscular endurance** is the ability of a muscle to maintain submaximal

Table 12.1 The Components of Fitness

Fitness Component	Examples of Activities People Can Do to Achieve Fitness in Each Component
Cardiorespiratory	Aerobic-type activities, such as walking, running, swimming, cross-country skiing
Musculoskeletal fitness:	Resistance training, weightlifting, calisthenics, sit-ups, push-ups
Muscular strength	Weightlifting or related activities using heavier weights with few repetitions
Muscular endurance	Weightlifting or related activities using lighter weights with greater number of repetitions
Flexibility	Stretching exercises, yoga
Body composition	Aerobic exercise and resistance training can help optimize body composition

force levels for extended periods. **Flexibility** is the ability to move a joint fluidly through the complete range of motion, and **body composition** is the amount of bone, muscle, and fat tissue in the body. Although many people are interested in improving their physical fitness, some are more interested in maintaining general fitness, while others are interested in achieving higher levels of fitness to optimize their athletic performance.

flexibility The ability to move a joint fluidly through its full range of motion.

body composition The amount of bone, muscle, and fat tissue in the body.

> **Recap:** Physical activity is any movement produced by muscles that increases energy expenditure. Leisure-time physical activity is any activity not related to a person's occupation. Exercise is a subcategory of leisure-time physical activity and is purposeful, planned, and structured. Physical fitness is the ability to carry out daily tasks with vigour and alertness, without undue fatigue, and with ample energy to enjoy leisure-time pursuits and meet unforeseen emergencies. The components of physical fitness include cardiorespiratory fitness, musculoskeletal fitness, flexibility, and body composition.

Why Engage in Physical Activity?

Many people are looking for a "magic pill" that will help them maintain weight loss, reduce their risk of diseases, make them feel better, and improve their quality of sleep. Although many people are not aware of it, regular physical activity is this magic pill. Regular physical activity has many benefits:

- *Reduces our risks for, and complications of, heart disease, stroke, and high blood pressure:* Regular physical activity increases high-density lipoprotein cholesterol (HDL, the "good" cholesterol) and lowers triglycerides in the blood; improves the strength of the heart; helps maintain healthy blood pressure; and limits the progression of atherosclerosis (or hardening of the arteries).

- *Reduces our risk for obesity:* Regular physical activity maintains lean body mass and promotes more healthful levels of body fat; may help in appetite control; and increases energy expenditure and the use of fat as an energy source.

- *Reduces our risk for type 2 diabetes:* Regular physical activity enhances the action of insulin, which improves the cells' uptake of glucose from the blood and can improve blood glucose control in people with diabetes, which in turn reduces the risk for, or delays the onset of, diabetes-related complications.

- *Potential reduction in our risk for colon cancer:* Although the exact role that physical activity may play in reducing colon cancer risk is still unknown, we do know that regular physical activity enhances gastric motility, which reduces the transit time of potential cancer-causing agents through the gut.

- *Potential reduction in our risk for breast cancer and endometrial cancer.*

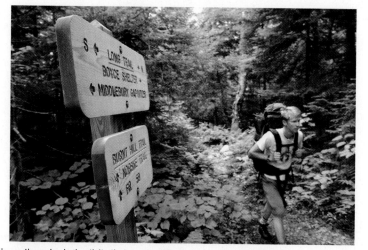

Hiking is a leisure-time physical activity that can contribute to your physical fitness.

• *Reduces our risk for osteoporosis:* Regular physical activity strengthens bones and enhances muscular strength and flexibility, thereby reducing the likelihood of falls and the incidence of fractures and other injuries when falls occur.

Regular physical activity is also known to improve our sleep patterns, reduce our risk for upper respiratory infections by improving immune function, and reduce anxiety and mental stress. It also can be effective in treating mild and moderate depression. In women receiving chemotherapy treatment for breast cancer, regular physical activity may reduce fatigue (Schwartz et al. 2001). During pregnancy, regular physical activity helps maintain the mother's fitness and muscle tone and helps control weight gain. It is also associated with lower fetal distress during labour, shorter labour, lower risk of cesarean birth, and improved recovery for the mother after the birth (Olds et al. 2003).

Despite the plethora of benefits derived from regular physical activity, most people find that this magic pill is not easy to swallow. In fact, most people in Canada are physically inactive. Results from the 2004–05 Canadian Community Health Survey (CCHS v.2) (Health Canada 2007) showed that 51% of adults surveyed were not physically active. This is lower than the estimate of 59% from the 2000–01 Canadian Community Health Survey (CCHS v.1) (Statistics Canada 2002) and 63% from the 1994–95 National Population Health Survey (NPHS) data (Statistics Canada 2002), suggesting that Canadian adults may be getting more physically active. The CCHS v.2 rates of inactivity were slightly higher among women (52%) than men (48%). Approximately one-quarter (25%) of adults were moderately active, and 24% were active. Although it is encouraging that more adults may be becoming physically active, more than half of the adult population have sedentary or inactive lifestyles.

Inadequate physical activity is also a problem in young people. Although 54% of schools claimed to have a policy requiring daily physical education classes, only 16% of schools were actually offering these classes in 2001 (CIHI 2004). On average, time allotted for physical activity ranged from 44 minutes (junior elementary school) to 60 minutes (senior secondary students) per week (Canadian Fitness and Lifestyle Research Institute 2005). For the Canadian Fitness and Lifestyle Research Institute's *Canadian Physical Activity Levels Among Youth* (CANPLAY) *Study,* children and youth were given pedometers to wear. On average, children and youth between the ages of 5 and 19 took 11 356 steps a day. As Figure 12.1 shows, children 5 to 10 years

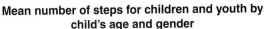
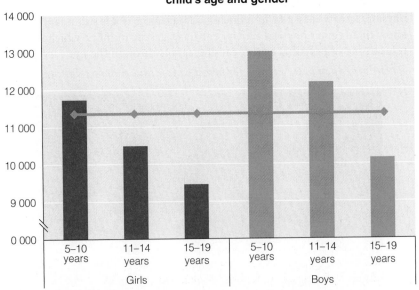

Figure 12.1 Mean number of steps for children and youth by child's age and gender.
(Canadian Fitness and Lifestyle Research Institute, 2005, *Physical activity among Canadians: The current situation.* www.cflri.ca/eng/statistics/surveys/documents/pam2005_sec1.pdf.) Reprinted with permission of the Canadian Fitness and Lifestyle Institute. www.cflri.ca

of age recorded the highest number of steps, and teens aged 15 to 19 recorded the fewest, with boys taking more steps than girls across all age categories (Canadian Fitness and Lifestyle Research Institute 2005). Since our habits related to eating and physical activity are formed early in life, it is imperative that we provide opportunities for children and adolescents to engage in regular, enjoyable physical activity. An active lifestyle during childhood increases the likelihood of a healthier life as an adult.

> **Recap:** Physical activity provides a multitude of health benefits, including reducing our risks for obesity and many chronic diseases and relieving anxiety and stress. Despite the many health benefits of physical activity, approximately half of Canadians, including many children, are inactive.

What Is a Sound Fitness Program?

There are several widely recognized qualities of a sound fitness program, as well as guidelines to help you design one that is right for you. These are explored here.

A Sound Fitness Program Meets Your Personal Goals

A fitness program that is ideal for someone else isn't necessarily right for you. Before you design or evaluate any program, you need to know what you intend to get from it; in other words, you need to define your personal fitness goals. Do you want to prevent osteoporosis, diabetes, or another chronic disease that runs in your family? Do you simply want to increase your energy and stamina? Or do you intend to compete in athletic events? Each of these scenarios requires a very different fitness program.

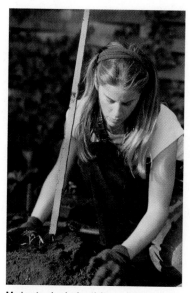

Moderate physical activity, such as gardening, helps maintain overall health.

For example, if you want to train for athletic competitions, a traditional approach that includes planned, purposive exercise sessions under the guidance of a trainer or coach would probably be most beneficial. Similarly, if you want to achieve cardiorespiratory fitness, you would likely be advised to participate in an aerobics class at least three times per week, or jog for at least 20 minutes three times per week.

In contrast, if your goal is to maintain your overall health, you might do better to follow *Canada's Physical Activity Guide to Healthy Active Living,* produced by Health Canada and the Canadian Society for Exercise Physiology. This guide emphasizes ways to build physical activity into everyday routines at home, school, or work to accumulate 60 minutes each day. The benefits of regular physical activity include

- better health;
- improved fitness;
- better posture and balance;
- higher self-esteem;
- easier weight control;
- stronger muscles and bones;
- increased energy;
- more relaxation and reduced stress;
- continued independent living in later life.

These health benefits occur even when the time spent performing the physical activities is cumulative (for example, brisk walking for 10 minutes three times per day). Although these guidelines are appropriate for achieving health benefits, they are not necessarily of sufficient intensity and duration to improve physical fitness.

Recently, the Institute of Medicine published guidelines that state that the minimum amount of physical activity that should be done each day to maintain health and fitness is 60 minutes, consistent with *Canada's Physical Activity Guide to Healthy*

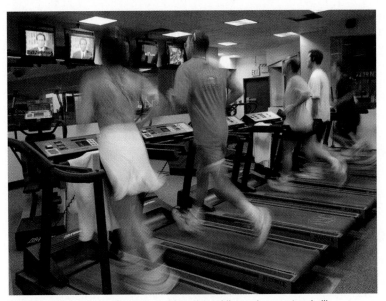

Watching television or reading can provide variety while running on a treadmill.

Active Living (Institute of Medicine 2002; Health Canada 2003). Refer to the Nutrition Debate at the end of this chapter to learn more about initiatives to increase physical activity.

A Sound Fitness Program Is Fun

One of the most important goals for everyone is fun; unless you enjoy being active, you will find it very difficult to maintain your physical fitness. What activities do you consider fun? If you enjoy the outdoors, hiking, camping, fishing, and rock climbing are potential activities for you. If you would rather exercise with friends on your lunch break, walking, climbing stairs, and bicycle riding may be more appropriate. Or you may find it more enjoyable to stay indoors and use the programs and equipment at your local fitness club . . . or purchase your own treadmill and free weights.

A Sound Fitness Program Includes Variety and Consistency

Variety is critical to maintaining your fitness. Although some people enjoy doing similar activities day after day, most of us get bored with the same fitness routine. Incorporating a variety of activities into your fitness program will help maintain your interest and increase your enjoyment while you are active. Variety can be achieved by combining indoor and outdoor activities throughout the week; taking a different route when you walk each day; watching a movie or reading a book while you ride a stationary bicycle or walk on a treadmill; or participating in different activities each week, such as walking, bicycling, swimming, taking the stairs, hiking, and gardening. This smorgasbord of activities can increase your activity level without leading to monotony and boredom.

Fortunately, a fun and useful tool has been developed to help you increase the variety of your physical activity choices (Figure 12.2). Like *Eating Well with Canada's Food Guide*, *Canada's Physical Activity Guide to Healthy Active Living* is shaped like a rainbow with the activities recommended most often in the outer yellow arc and the least desirable behaviour, sitting for long periods, in the inner red arc. The *Physical Activity Guide* recommends a variety of activities every week from three groups:

1. *Endurance:* Four to seven days a week. Continuous activities, such as walking, cycling, and skiing are good for your heart, lungs, and circulatory system.

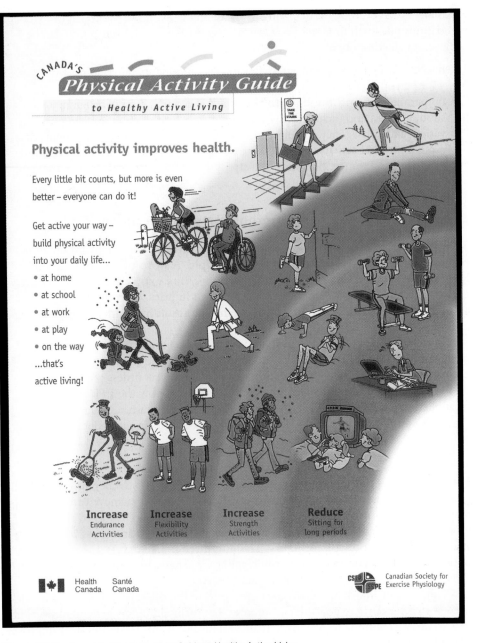

Figure 12.2 *Canada's Physical Activity Guide to Healthy Active Living.*
(Public Health Agency of Canada, 1999 © Reproduced with the permission of the Minister of Public Works and Government Services Canada, 2008.)

2. *Flexibility:* Four to seven days a week. Gentle reaching, bending, and stretching activities, especially before playing sports or running, will keep your muscles relaxed and your joints mobile.

3. *Strength:* Two to four days a week. Activities against resistance, such as lifting weights or doing sit-ups, will strengthen muscles and bones and improve posture.

It is important to understand you cannot do just one activity to achieve overall fitness. Refer back to Table 12.1, and notice that different activities are listed as examples to achieve the various components of fitness. For instance, participating in aerobic-type activities will improve our cardiorespiratory fitness but will do little to improve muscular strength. To achieve that goal, we must participate in some form of **resistance training,** or exercises in which our muscles work against resistance.

resistance training Exercises in which our muscles act against resistance.

Flexibility is achieved by participating in stretching activities. By following the recommendations put forth in *Canada's Physical Activity Guide*, physical fitness can be achieved in all components.

> **Recap:** A sound fitness program has many components. First, it must meet your personal fitness goals, such as reducing your risks for disease or preparing for competition in athletic events. Second, a fitness program should be fun and include activities you enjoy. Third, it should include variety and consistency to help you maintain interest and reap the benefits of regular physical activity. Physical fitness is specific to each of the components of fitness: endurance, flexibility and strength.

A Sound Fitness Program Appropriately Overloads the Body

overload principle Placing an extra physical demand on your body to improve your fitness level.

To improve your fitness level, you must place an extra physical demand on your body. This is referred to as the **overload principle**. A word of caution is in order here: *the overload principle does not advocate subjecting your body to inappropriately high stress* because this can lead to exhaustion and injuries. In contrast, an appropriate overload on various body systems will result in healthy improvements in fitness.

FIT principle The principle used to achieve an appropriate overload for physical training. Stands for frequency, intensity, and time of activity.

To achieve an appropriate overload, you should consider three factors, collectively known as the **FIT principle**: frequency, intensity, and time of activity. You can use the FIT principle to design either a general physical fitness program or a performance-based exercise program. Table 12.2 shows how the FIT principle can be applied to a cardiorespiratory and muscular fitness program.

Let's consider each of the FIT principle's three factors in more detail.

Frequency

frequency Refers to the number of activity sessions per week you perform.

Frequency refers to the number of activity sessions per week. Depending upon your goals for fitness, the frequency of your activities will vary. To achieve cardiorespiratory fitness, training should be more than two days per week; however, training more than five days per week does not cause significant gains in fitness but can substantially increase your risk for injury. Training three to five days per week appears optimal to achieve and maintain cardiorespiratory fitness. In contrast, only two to three days are needed to achieve muscular fitness.

Think about Matthew's goals for fitness during the off-season and the frequency needed to achieve these goals. He is interested in maintaining his general physical fitness so he can continue to play basketball, and he also wants to significantly improve muscular strength and size. By using *Canada's Physical Activity Guide* as a guide, Matthew should do the activities as suggested for every day and those prescribed three to five times a week. To further improve muscular strength and size, he should perform weightlifting at least two to three days each week. With this type of program,

Table 12.2 Using the FIT Principle to Achieve Cardiorespiratory and Muscular Fitness

	Cardiorespiratory Fitness	Muscular Fitness
Frequency	3–5 days per week	2–3 days per week
Intensity	55% to 90% of maximal heart rate	70% to 85% of maximal weight you can lift
Time	At least 20 consecutive minutes	1–3 sets of 8–12 lifts[1] for each set

Source: Adapted from American College of Sports Medicine Position Stand, The recommended quantity and quality of exercise for developing and maintaining cardiorespiratory and muscular fitness, and flexibility in healthy adults, 1998, *Medicine and Science in Sports and Exercises* 30:975–991. Used with permission.

[1] A minimum of 8 to 10 exercises involving the major muscle groups, such as arms, shoulders, chest, abdomen, back, hips, and legs, is recommended.

Matthew will be able to reach his goals. He should also regularly participate in flexibility activities to enhance his quality of training and to prevent potential injuries.

Intensity

Intensity refers to the amount of effort expended or, to put it another way, how difficult the activity is to perform. In general, **low-intensity activities** are those that cause very mild increases in breathing, sweating, and heart rate, while **moderate-intensity activities** cause moderate increases in these responses. **Vigorous-intensity activities** produce significant increases in breathing, sweating, and heart rate so that talking is difficult when exercising at a vigorous intensity.

Traditionally, heart rate has been used to indicate level of intensity during aerobic activities. Figure 12.3 shows an example of a heart rate training chart. You can calculate the appropriate range of exercise intensity for you by estimating your **maximal heart rate**, which is the rate at which your heart beats during maximal-intensity exercise (see the You Do the Math box on p. 430). Maximal heart rate is estimated by subtracting your age from 220 and is described in more detail below. For achieving and maintaining physical fitness, the intensity range typically recommended is 50% to 80% of your estimated maximal heart rate. People who are older or who have been inactive for a long time may want to exercise at the lower end of the range. Those who are more physically fit or are striving for a more rapid improvement in fitness may want to exercise at the higher end of the range. Competitive athletes generally train at a higher intensity, around 80% to 95% of their maximum heart rate.

Although the calculation *220 – age* has been used extensively for years to predict maximal heart rate, it was never intended to accurately represent everyone's true maximal heart rate or to be used as the standard of aerobic training intensity. There are limitations to using the calculation, and it has been challenged (Tanaka, Monahan, and Seals 2001). The most accurate way to determine your own maximal heart rate is to complete a maximal exercise test in a fitness laboratory; however, this test is not commonly conducted with the general public and can be very expensive. Although not completely accurate, the estimated maximal heart rate method can still be used to give you a general idea of your aerobic training range.

intensity Refers to the amount of effort expended during the activity, or how difficult the activity is to perform.
low-intensity activities Activities that cause very mild increases in breathing, sweating, and heart rate.
moderate-intensity activities Activities that cause moderate increases in breathing, sweating, and heart rate.
vigorous-intensity activities Activities that produce significant increases in breathing, sweating, and heart rate; talking is difficult when exercising at a vigorous intensity.
maximal heart rate The rate at which your heart beats during maximal intensity exercise.

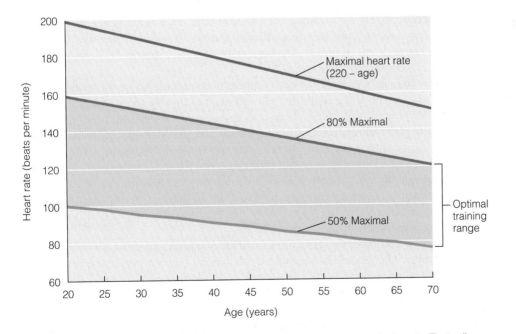

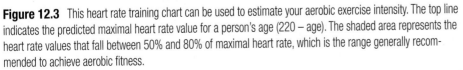

Figure 12.3 This heart rate training chart can be used to estimate your aerobic exercise intensity. The top line indicates the predicted maximal heart rate value for a person's age (220 – age). The shaded area represents the heart rate values that fall between 50% and 80% of maximal heart rate, which is the range generally recommended to achieve aerobic fitness.

▶ YOU DO THE MATH

Calculating Your Maximal and Training Heart Rate Range

Nadia's brother has type 1 diabetes, her mother has recently been diagnosed with type 2 diabetes, and Nadia is like the rest of her family, always struggling with being moderately overweight. She is interested in participating in a regular exercise program that will improve her cardiorespiratory fitness and help her maintain a healthier weight. As she enjoys walking and bike riding, Nadia plans to begin by either riding the stationary bicycle or walking on the treadmill at the gym three times per week for 30 minutes each time. She now needs to determine the aerobic exercise training intensity that will help her improve her cardiorespiratory fitness. Nadia is 28 years of age and healthy, and she does a lot of light walking and lifting in her work in the retail business. Based on this information, Nadia should set her training heart rate range between 50% and 80% of her maximal heart rate.

Let's work with Nadia while she calculates these values:

Maximal heart rate: 220 − age =
220 − 28 = 192 beats per minute (bpm)

Lower end of intensity range: 50% of
192 bpm = 0.50 × 192 bpm = 96 bpm

Higher end of intensity range: 80% of
192 bpm = 0.80 × 192 bpm = 154 bpm

When Nadia rides the bicycle or walks on the treadmill, her heart rate (when counted for an entire minute) should be between 96 and 154 bpm; this puts her in her aerobic training zone and will allow her to achieve cardiorespiratory fitness. Although Nadia does some walking at work, she is not accustomed to exercising for 30 minutes without stopping, and it is very likely that she will be unable to complete the entire 30 minutes of exercise when she first begins her program. It is important that she start at a level that she can achieve (for example, an intensity that allows her to exercise for 15 to 20 minutes) and that she slowly increase her exercise time and intensity until she meets her fitness goal.

Time of Activity

time of activity How long each exercise session lasts.

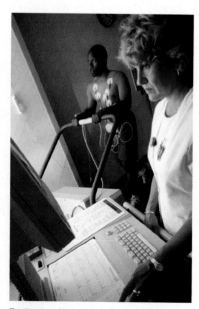

Testing in a fitness lab is the most accurate way to determine maximal heart rate.

Time of activity refers to how long each session lasts. To achieve general health, you can do multiple short bouts of activity that add up to 30 minutes each day. However, to achieve higher levels of fitness, it is important that the activities be done for at least 20 to 30 consecutive minutes.

For example, let's say you want to compete in triathlons. To be successful during the running segment of the triathlon, you will need to be able to run quickly for at least eight kilometres (five miles). Thus, it is appropriate for you to train so that you can complete eight kilometres during one session and still have enough energy to swim and bicycle during the race. Running for two or three 10-minute sessions each day would not be a sufficient overload to prepare you for this competition. You will need to consistently train at a distance of eight kilometres; you will also benefit from running longer distances. In contrast, bicycling for 10 minutes two or three times each day would be appropriate for someone like Nadia to achieve her health-related cardiorespiratory fitness goal.

Table 12.3 compares the guidelines for achieving health to those for achieving physical fitness. The guidelines you follow will depend on your personal goals. These recommendations apply to people of all ages, and following either set will allow you to improve and maintain your health. For people with established disease, these guidelines may help postpone complications and reduce their reliance on medications. People with heart disease, high blood pressure, diabetes, osteoporosis, or arthritis should get approval to exercise from their health care practitioner prior to starting a fitness program. In addition, a medical evaluation should be conducted before starting an exercise program for an apparently healthy but currently inactive man 40 years or older or woman 50 years or older.

Table 12.3   Physical Activity Guidelines for Achieving Health versus Physical Fitness

	Health	Physical Fitness
Frequency	Daily	2–5 days per week (3–5 days for cardiorespiratory fitness, 2–3 days for muscular fitness and flexibility)
Intensity	Any level	50%–80% of maximal heart rate
Time	Accumulation of a minimum of 30 minutes each day	20–60 minutes of continuous or intermittent activity
Type	Any activity	Aerobic-type activities, resistance exercises to enhance muscular strength and endurance, and flexibility exercises

Source: Adapted from American College of Sports Medicine Position Stand, The recommended quantity and quality of exercise for developing and maintaining cardiorespiratory and muscular fitness, and flexibility in healthy adults, 1998, *Medicine and Science in Sports and Exercise* 30:975–991; U.S. Department of Health and Human Services, *Physical Activity and Health: A Report of the Surgeon General,* Atlanta, GA: U.S. Department of Health and Human Services, Centers for Disease Control and Prevention, National Center for Chronic Disease Prevention and Health Promotion, 1996.

Recap: To improve fitness, you must place an extra physical demand, or an overload, on your body. To achieve appropriate overload, the FIT principle should be followed; FIT stands for frequency, intensity, and time of activity. Frequency refers to the number of activity sessions per week. Intensity refers to how difficult the activity is to perform. Time refers to how long each activity session lasts.

A Sound Fitness Plan Includes a Warm-Up and a Cool-Down Period

To properly prepare for and recover from an exercise session, warm-up and cool-down activities should be performed. **Warm-up**, also called preliminary exercise, includes general activities (such as stretching and calisthenics) and specific activities that prepare you for the actual activity (such as jogging or swinging a golf club). Your warm-up should be brief (5 to 10 minutes), gradual, and sufficient to increase muscle and body temperature but should not cause fatigue or deplete energy stores.

Warming up prior to exercise is important, as it properly prepares the muscles for exertion by increasing blood flow and temperature. It may also help to prepare a person psychologically for the exercise session or athletic event.

Cool-down activities are done after the exercise session is completed. Similar to the warm-up, the cool-down should be gradual and allow your body to slowly recover. Your cool-down should include some of the same activities you performed during the exercise session but done at a low intensity, and you should allow ample time for stretching. Cooling down after exercise assists in the prevention of injury and may help reduce muscle soreness.

warm-up Also called preliminary exercise; includes activities that prepare you for an exercise bout, including stretching, calisthenics, and movements specific to the exercise bout.

cool-down Activities done after an exercise session is completed. Should be gradual and allow your body to slowly recover from exercise.

adenosine triphosphate (ATP) The common currency of energy for virtually all cells of the body.

Recap: Warm-up, or preliminary exercise, is important to get prepared for exercise. Warm-up exercises prepare the muscles for exertion by increasing blood flow and temperature. Cool-down activities are done after an exercise session is complete. Cool-down activities should be done at a low intensity, and cooling down after activity assists in the prevention of injury and may help reduce muscle soreness.

What Fuels Our Activities?

To perform exercise, or muscular work, we must be able to generate energy. The common currency of energy for virtually all cells in the body is **ATP**, or **adenosine triphosphate.** As you might guess from its

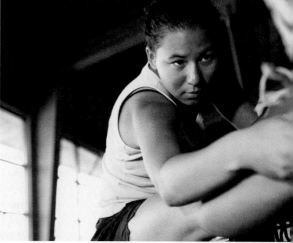

Stretching should be included in the warm-up and the cool-down for exercise.

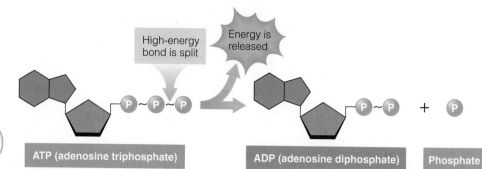

High-energy bond is split

Energy is released

ATP (adenosine triphosphate)

ADP (adenosine diphosphate)

Phosphate

Animations

• Energy Currency

Figure 12.4 Structure of adenosine triphosphate (ATP). Energy is produced when ATP is split into adenosine diphosphate (ADP) and inorganic phosphate (P$_i$).

name, a molecule of ATP includes an organic compound called adenosine and three phosphate groups (Figure 12.4). When one of the phosphates is cleaved, or broken away, from ATP, energy is released. The products remaining after this reaction are adenosine diphosphate (ADP) and an independent inorganic phosphate group (P1). In a mirror image of this reaction, the body regenerates ATP by adding a phosphate group back to ADP. In this way, we continually provide energy to our cells.

The amount of ATP stored in a muscle cell is very limited; it can keep the muscle active for about one to three seconds. Thus, we need to generate ATP from other sources to fuel activities for longer periods. Fortunately, we are able to generate ATP from the breakdown of carbohydrate, fat, and protein, providing our cells with a variety of sources from which to receive energy. The primary energy systems we rely upon to provide energy for physical activities are the adenosine triphosphate–creatine phosphate (ATP-CP) energy system and the anaerobic and aerobic breakdown of carbohydrates. Our bodies also generate energy from the breakdown of fats. As you will see, the type, intensity, and duration of the activities we perform determine the amount of ATP we need and therefore the energy system we use.

The ATP-CP Energy System Uses Creatine Phosphate to Regenerate ATP

As we said, muscle cells store only enough ATP to maintain activity for one to three seconds. When more energy is needed, a high-energy compound called **creatine phosphate (CP)** (also called **phosphocreatine**, or **PCr**) can be broken down to support the regeneration of ATP (Figure 12.5). Because this reaction can occur in the absence of oxygen, it is referred to as an **anaerobic** reaction (meaning "without oxygen").

Muscle tissue contains about four to six times as much CP as ATP, but there is still not enough CP available to fuel activities longer than two minutes. We tend to use CP the most during very intense, short bouts of activity, such as lifting, jumping, and sprinting (Figure 12.6). Together, our stores of ATP and CP can only support a *maximal* physical effort for about 3 to 15 seconds. We must rely on other energy sources, such as carbohydrate and fat, to support activities of longer duration.

creatine phosphate (CP) or **phosphocreatine (PCr)** A high-energy compound that can be broken down for energy and used to regenerate ATP.

anaerobic Means "without oxygen." Term used to refer to metabolic reactions that occur in the absence of oxygen.

Recap: Adenosine triphosphate, or ATP, is the common energy source for all cells of the body. When one of the phosphate groups is cleaved from the ATP molecule, energy is released. The amount of ATP stored in a muscle cell is limited and can keep a muscle active for about one to three seconds. For maximal-physical-effort activities lasting about 3 to 15 seconds, creatine phosphate can be broken down in an anaerobic reaction to provide energy and support the regeneration of ATP. To support activities that last longer than two minutes, we must derive energy from the breakdown of carbohydrates, fats, and protein.

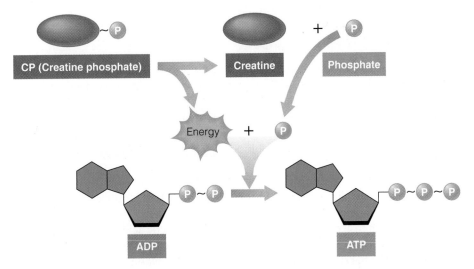

Figure 12.5 When the compound creatine phosphate (CP) is broken down into a molecule of creatine and an independent phosphate molecule, energy is released. This energy, along with the independent phosphate molecule, can then be used to regenerate ATP.

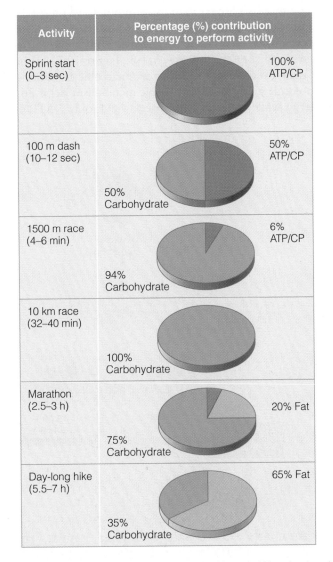

Figure 12.6 The relative contribution of ATP-CP, carbohydrate, and fat to activities of various durations and intensities.

glycolysis The breakdown of glucose; yields two ATP molecules and two pyruvic acid molecules for each molecule of glucose.

pyruvic acid The primary end product of glycolysis.

lactic acid A compound that results when pyruvic acid is metabolized in the presence of insufficient oxygen.

The Breakdown of Carbohydrates Provides Energy for Brief and Long-Term Exercise

During activities lasting about 30 seconds to 2 minutes, we cannot generate enough ATP from the breakdown of CP to fully support our efforts. Thus, we need an energy source that we can use quickly to produce ATP. The breakdown of carbohydrates, specifically glucose, provides this quick energy in a process called **glycolysis.** The most common source of glucose during exercise comes from glycogen stored in the muscles and glucose found in the blood. As shown in Figure 12.7, for every glucose molecule that goes through glycolysis, two ATP molecules are produced. The primary end product of glycolysis is **pyruvic acid.**

When oxygen availability is limited in the cell, pyruvic acid is converted to **lactic acid**. For years it was assumed that lactic acid was a useless, even potentially toxic, byproduct of high-intensity exercise. We now know that lactic acid is an important intermediate of glucose breakdown and that it plays a critical role in supplying fuel for working muscles, the heart, and resting tissues (see the Nutrition Myth or Fact, "Lactic Acid Causes Muscle Fatigue and Soreness," page 436).

The major advantage of glycolysis is that it is the fastest way that we can regenerate ATP for exercise, other than the ATP-CP system. However, this high rate of ATP production can be sustained only for a brief time, generally less than three minutes. To perform exercise that lasts longer than three minutes, we must rely on the aerobic energy system to provide adequate ATP.

To generate even more ATP molecules, pyruvic acid can go through additional metabolic pathways in the presence of oxygen (see Figure 12.7). Although this process is slower than glycolysis occurring under anaerobic conditions, the breakdown of one glucose molecule going through aerobic metabolism yields 36 to 38 ATP molecules for energy, while the anaerobic process yields only 2 ATP molecules.

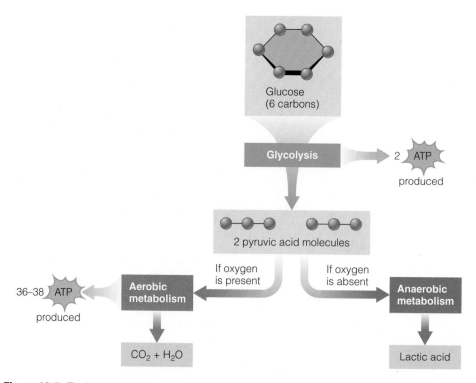

Figure 12.7 The breakdown of one molecule of glucose, or the process of glycolysis, yields two molecules of pyruvic acid and two ATP molecules. The further metabolism of pyruvic acid in the presence of insufficient oxygen (anaerobic process) results in the production of lactic acid. The metabolism of pyruvic acid in the presence of adequate oxygen (aerobic process) yields 36 to 38 molecules of ATP.

Thus, this aerobic process supplies 18 times more energy! Another advantage of the aerobic process is that it does not result in the significant production of acids and other compounds that contribute to muscle fatigue, which means that a low-intensity activity can be performed for hours. Aerobic metabolism of glucose is the primary source of fuel for our muscles during activities lasting from three minutes to four hours (see Figure 12.6).

As you learned in Chapter 4, we can store only a limited amount of glycogen in our bodies. An average, well-nourished man who weighs about 70 kg (154 lb.) can store about 200 to 500 grams of muscle glycogen, which is equal to 800 to 2000 kcal (3360 to 8400 kJ) of energy. Although trained athletes can store more muscle glycogen than the average person, there is still not enough glycogen stored in our bodies to provide an unlimited energy supply for long-term activities. Thus, we also need a fuel source that is very abundant and can be broken down under aerobic conditions so that it can support activities of lower intensity and longer duration. This fuel source is fat.

> **Recap:**   To support activities that last from 30 seconds to three minutes, energy is produced from the breakdown of glucose, in a process called glycolysis. Two ATP molecules are produced for every glucose molecule broken down, and pyruvic acid is the primary end product of this reaction. Lactic acid is formed when pyruvic acid is metabolized under anaerobic conditions. To support activities that last from three minutes to four hours, energy is produced from the aerobic metabolism of pyruvic acid. During this process, pyruvic acid is broken down in the presence of oxygen, and each molecule can yield 36 to 38 ATP molecules.

Aerobic Breakdown of Fats Supports Exercise of Low Intensity and Long Duration

When we refer to fat as a fuel source, we mean the triglyceride molecule, which is the primary storage form of fat in our cells. As you learned in Chapter 5, a triglyceride molecule comprises a glycerol backbone attached to three fatty acid molecules (see Figure 5.1). It is these fatty acid molecules that provide much of the energy we need to support long-term activity. Fatty acids are classified by their length; that is, by the number of carbons they contain. The longer the fatty acid, the more ATP that can be generated from its breakdown. For instance, palmitic acid is a fatty acid with 16 carbons. If palmitic acid is broken down completely, it yields 129 ATP molecules! Obviously, far more energy is produced from this one fatty acid molecule than from the aerobic breakdown of a glucose molecule.

There are two major advantages of using fat as a fuel. First, fat is a very abundant energy source, even in lean people. For example, a man who weighs 70 kg (154 lb.) who has 10% body fat has approximately 7 kg (15 lb.) of body fat, which is equivalent to more than 50 000 kcal (209 200 kJ) of energy! This is significantly more energy than can be provided by his stored muscle glycogen (800 to 2000 kcal or 3350 to 8370 kJ). Second, fat provides 9 kcal (37 kJ) of energy per gram, while carbohydrate provides only 4 kcal (17 kJ), which means that fat supplies more than twice as much energy per gram as carbohydrate. The primary disadvantage of using fat as a fuel is that the breakdown process is relatively slow; thus fat is used predominantly as a fuel source during activities of lower intensity and longer duration. Fat is also our primary energy source during rest, sitting, and standing in place.

What specific activities are primarily fuelled by fat? Walking long distances uses fat stores, as do other low- to moderate-intensity forms of exercise. Fat is also an important fuel source during endurance events, such as marathons (42 km, or 26.2 miles) and ultra-marathon races (80 km, or 49.9 miles). Endurance exercise training improves our ability to use fat for energy, which may be one reason that people who exercise regularly tend to have lower body fat levels than people who do not exercise.

> ▶ **NUTRITION MYTH OR FACT**

Lactic Acid Causes Muscle Fatigue and Soreness

Lactic acid is a byproduct of glycolysis. For many years it was believed that lactic acid caused both muscle fatigue and soreness. Does recent scientific evidence support this belief?

The exact causes of muscle fatigue are not known, and there appear to be many contributing factors. Recent evidence suggests that fatigue may be due not only to the accumulation of acids and other metabolic byproducts but also to the depletion of creatine phosphate and changes in calcium in the cells that affect muscle contraction. Depletion of muscle glycogen, liver glycogen, and blood glucose, as well as psychological factors, can all contribute to fatigue (Brooks et al. 2000). Thus, lactic acid contributes to fatigue but does not appear to cause fatigue independently.

So what factors cause muscle soreness? As with fatigue, there are probably many contributors. It is hypothesized that soreness usually results from microscopic tears in the muscle fibres as a result of strenuous exercise. This damage triggers an inflammatory reaction that causes an influx of fluid and various chemicals to the damaged area. These substances work to remove damaged tissue and initiate tissue repair, but they may also stimulate pain (Brooks et al. 2000). However, it appears highly unlikely that lactic acid is an independent cause of muscle soreness.

Recent studies indicate that lactic acid is produced even under aerobic conditions! This means it is produced at rest as well as during any intensity of exercise. The reasons for this constant production of lactic acid are still being studied. What we do know is that lactic acid is an important fuel for resting tissues and for working cardiac and skeletal muscles. That's right—skeletal muscles not only produce lactic acid but also use it for energy, both directly and after it is converted into glucose and glycogen in the liver (Brooks 2000; Gladden 2000). We also know that endurance training improves the muscle's ability to use lactic acid for energy. Thus, contrary to being a waste product of glucose metabolism, lactic acid is actually an important energy source for muscle cells during rest and exercise.

It is important to remember that we are almost always using some combination of carbohydrate and fat for energy. At rest, we use very little carbohydrate, relying mostly on fat. During maximal exercise (at 100% effort), we are using mostly carbohydrate and very little fat. However, most activities we do each day involve some use of both fuels (Figure 12.8).

When it comes to eating properly to support regular physical activity or exercise training, the nutrient to focus on is carbohydrate. This is because most people store more than enough fat to support exercise, whereas our storage of carbohydrate is limited. It is especially important that we maintain adequate stores of glycogen for moderate to intense exercise. Dietary recommendations for fat, carbohydrate, and protein are reviewed later in this chapter (pages 439–449).

Recap: Fat can be broken down aerobically to support activities of low intensity and long duration. Each fatty acid from a triglyceride molecule is broken down for energy, and the amount of energy derived depends upon the length of the fatty acid chain. The two major advantages of using fat as a fuel is that it is an abundant energy source and it provides more than twice the energy per gram as compared with carbohydrate. The primary disadvantage of using fat as a fuel is that the breakdown process is relatively slow so it cannot support quick, high-intensity activities.

Amino Acids Are Not Major Sources of Fuel During Exercise

Proteins, or more specifically amino acids, are not major energy sources during exercise. As discussed in Chapter 6, amino acids can be used directly for energy if necessary, but they are more often used to make glucose to maintain our blood glucose

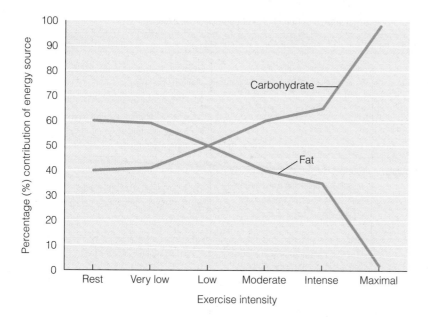

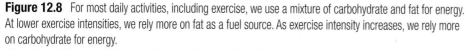

Figure 12.8 For most daily activities, including exercise, we use a mixture of carbohydrate and fat for energy. At lower exercise intensities, we rely more on fat as a fuel source. As exercise intensity increases, we rely more on carbohydrate for energy.
(Adapted from M. Manore and J. Thompson, *Sports Nutrition for Health and Performance,* Champaign, IL: Human Kinetics, 2000.)

levels during exercise. Amino acids also help build and repair tissues after exercise. Depending upon the intensity and duration of the activity, amino acids may contribute about 3% to 6% of the energy needed (Tarnolpolsky 2000).

Given this, why is it that so many people are concerned about their protein intakes? As you learned in Chapter 6, our muscles are not stimulated to grow when we eat extra dietary protein. Only appropriate physical training can stimulate our muscles to grow and strengthen. Thus, although we need enough dietary protein to support activity and recovery, consuming very high amounts does not provide an added benefit. The protein needs of athletes are only slightly higher than the needs of non-athletes, and most of us eat more than enough protein to support even the highest requirements for competitive athletes! Thus, there is generally no need for recreationally active people or even competitive athletes to consume protein or amino acid supplements.

> **Recap:** Amino acids may contribute from 3% to 6% of the energy needed during exercise, depending upon the intensity and duration of the activity. Amino acids help build and repair tissues after exercise. We generally consume more than enough protein in our diets to support regular exercise, and there is typically no need for protein or amino acid supplementation, even for competitive athletes.

What Kind of Diet Supports Physical Activity?

Many people wonder, "Do my nutrient needs change if I become more physically active?" The answer to this question depends upon the type, intensity, and duration of activity in which you participate. It is not necessarily true that our requirement for every nutrient is greater if we are physically active.

People who are performing moderate-intensity daily activities for health can follow the general guidelines put forth in *Eating Well with Canada's Food Guide.* For smaller or less active people, the lower end of the range of recommendations for each food group may be appropriate. For larger or more active people, the higher end of

Table 12.4   Suggested Intakes of Nutrients to Support Vigorous Exercise

Nutrient	Functions	Suggested Intake
Energy	Supports exercise, activities of daily living, and basic body functions	Depends upon body size and the type, intensity, and duration of activity. For many female athletes: 1800–3500 kcal (7530–14 650 kJ) per day For many male athletes: 2500–7500 kcal (10 460–31 380 kJ) per day
Carbohydrate	Provides energy, maintains adequate muscle glycogen and blood glucose; high-complex-carbohydrate foods provide vitamins and minerals	At least 60% of total energy intake Depending upon sport and gender, should consume 6–10 grams of carbohydrate per kg body weight per day
Fat	Provides energy, fat-soluble vitamins, and essential fatty acids; supports production of hormones and transport of nutrients	15%–25% of total energy intake
Protein	Helps build and maintain muscle; provides building material for glucose; energy source during endurance exercise; aids recovery from exercise	Endurance athletes: 1.2–1.4 grams per kg body weight Strength athletes: 1.6–1.7 grams per kg body weight
Water	Maintains temperature regulation (adequate cooling); maintains blood volume and blood pressure; supports all cell functions	Consume fluid before, during, and after exercise Consume enough to maintain body weight Consume at least 2 litres (or 64 fl. oz.) of water daily to maintain regular health and activity Athletes may need up to 10 litres (or 170 fl. oz.) every day; more is required if exercising in a hot environment
B vitamins	Critical for energy production from carbohydrate, fat, and protein	May need slightly more (1–2 times the RDA) for thiamin, riboflavin, and vitamin B6
Calcium	Builds and maintains bone mass; assists with nervous system function, muscle contraction, hormone function, and transport of nutrients across cell membrane	Meet the current AI: 14–18 yrs: 1300 mg per day 19–50 yrs: 1000 mg per day 51 and older: 1200 mg per day
Iron	Primarily responsible for the transport of oxygen in blood to cells; assists with energy production	Consume at least the RDA: Males: 14–18 yrs: 11 mg per day 19 and older: 8 mg per day Females: 14–18 yrs: 15 mg per day 19–50 yrs: 18 mg per day 51 and older: 8 mg per day

the range is suggested. Modifications may need to be made for people who exercise vigorously every day, and particularly for athletes training for competition. Table 12.4 provides an overview of the nutrients that can be affected by regular, vigorous exercise training. Each of these nutrients is described in more detail below (American College of Sports Medicine et al. 2000).

Vigorous Exercise Increases Energy Needs

Athletes generally have higher energy needs than moderately physically active or sedentary people. The amount of extra energy needed to support regular training is determined by the type, intensity, and duration of the activity. In addition, the energy needs of male athletes are higher than those of female athletes because male athletes weigh more, have more muscle mass, and will expend more energy during activity than women. This is relative, of course: a large woman who trains three to five hours each day will probably need more energy than a small man who trains one hour each day. The energy needs of athletes can range from only 2000 kcal (8400 kJ) per day for a small female gymnast to more than 7500 kcal (31 380 kJ) per day for a male cyclist competing in the Tour de France cross-country cycling race! Figure 12.9 shows a sample of meals that total 2000 kcal (8400 kJ) per day and 4000 kcal (16 800 kJ) per day, with the carbohydrate content of these meals meeting more than 60% of total energy intake. As you can see, athletes who need more than 4000 kcal (16 800 kJ) per day need to consume very large quantities of food. However, the heavy demands of daily physical training, work, school,

Small snacks can be helpful to meet daily energy demands.

2000 kcal (8400 kJ) per Day Diet	4000 kcal (16 800 kJ) per Day Diet
375 mL (1 1/2 cups) Cheerios	750 mL (3 cups) Cheerios
125 mL (4 fl. oz.) skim milk	250 mL (8 fl. oz.) skim milk
1 medium banana	1 medium banana
1 slice whole wheat toast	2 slices whole wheat toast
7 mL (1 1/2 tsp) butter	15 mL (1 Tbsp) butter
250 mL (8 fl. oz.) orange juice	250 mL (8 fl. oz.) orange juice
One turkey sandwich with:	Two turkey sandwiches with:
2 slices whole wheat bread	4 slices whole wheat bread
90 g (3 oz.) turkey lunch meat	180 g (6 oz.) turkey lunch meat
30 g (1 oz.) Swiss cheese slice	60 g (2 oz.) Swiss cheese slices
1 leaf iceberg lettuce	2 leaves iceberg lettuce
2 slices tomato	4 slices tomato
250 mL (8 fl. oz.) tomato soup made with water	500 mL (16 fl. oz.) tomato soup made with water
1 container (250 mL/1 cup) low-fat fruit yogurt	2 containers (each 250 mL/1 cup) low-fat fruit yogurt
375 mL (12 fl. oz.) Gatorade	750 mL (24 fl. oz.) Gatorade
90 g (3 oz.) grilled skinless chicken breast	180 g (6 oz.) grilled skinless chicken breast
375 mL (1 1/2 cups) mixed salad greens	750 mL (3 cups) mixed salad greens
25 mL (1 1/2 Tbsp) French salad dressing	45 mL (3 Tbsp) French salad dressing
250 mL (1 cup) steamed broccoli	500 mL (2 cups) cooked spaghetti noodles
125 mL (1/2 cup) cooked brown rice	250 mL (1 cup) spaghetti sauce with meat
250 L (8 fl. oz.) skim milk	500 mL (16 fl. oz.) skim milk

Figure 12.9 High-carbohydrate (approximately 60% of total energy) meals that contain approximately 2000 kcal (8400 kJ) per day (on left) and 4000 kcal (16 800 kJ) per day (on right). Athletes must plan their meals carefully to meet energy demands, particularly athletes with very high energy needs.

grazing Consistently eating small meals throughout the day; done by many athletes to meet their high energy demands.

and family responsibilities often leaves these athletes with little time to eat adequately. Thus, many athletes meet their energy demands by planning regular meals and snacks and **grazing** (eating small meals throughout the day) consistently. They may also take advantage of the energy-dense snack foods and meal replacements specifically designed for athletes participating in vigorous training. These steps help athletes to maintain their blood glucose and energy stores.

If an athlete is losing body weight, then his or her energy intake is inadequate. Conversely, weight gain may indicate that energy intake is too high. Weight maintenance is generally recommended to maximize performance. If weight loss is warranted, food intake should be lowered no more than 200 to 500 kcal (840 to 2100 kJ) per day, and athletes should try to lose weight prior to the competitive season if at all possible. Weight gain may be necessary for some athletes and can usually be accomplished by consuming 500 to 700 kcal (2100 to 2940 kJ) per day more than needed for weight maintenance. The extra energy should come from a healthy balance of carbohydrate (55% to 60% of total energy intake), fat (25% to 30% of total energy intake), and protein (10% to 20% of total energy intake).

Many athletes are concerned about their weight for reasons of performance or physical appearance. Jockeys, boxers, wrestlers, judo athletes, and others are required to "make weight," or meet a predefined weight category. Others, such as distance runners, gymnasts, figure skaters, and dancers, are required to maintain a very lean figure for performance and aesthetic reasons. These athletes tend to eat less energy than they need to support vigorous training, which puts them at risk for inadequate intakes of all nutrients. These athletes are at a higher risk of suffering from health consequences resulting from poor energy and nutrient intake, including eating disorders, osteoporosis, menstrual disturbances, dehydration, heat and physical injuries, and even death. Refer to the Highlight box "When Sports Nutrition Becomes a Matter of Life or Death" to learn more about the consequences of risky nutritional practices among athletes.

> **Recap:** The type, intensity, and duration of activities you participate in will determine your nutrient needs. Vigorous-intensity exercise requires extra energy, and male athletes typically need more energy than female athletes because of their higher muscle mass and larger body weight. Weight maintenance is recommended to maximize athletic performance. Some athletes who are concerned with making a competitive weight or with the aesthetic demands of their sport may be at risk for poor energy and nutrient intakes.

Carbohydrate Needs Increase for Many Active People

As you know, carbohydrate (in the form of glucose) is one of the primary sources of energy needed to support exercise. Both endurance athletes and strength athletes require adequate carbohydrate to maintain their glycogen stores and provide quick energy.

How Much of an Athlete's Diet Should Be Carbohydrates?

You may recall from Chapter 4 that the AMDR for carbohydrates is 45% to 65% of total energy intake. Athletes should consume at least 60% of their total energy intake as carbohydrates, which falls within this recommended range. Athletes who are participating in strength-type activities, sprinting, or other explosive-type events, or are not training for more than one hour each day, may find that consuming 55% of their total energy intake as carbohydrate is sufficient.

To illustrate how inadequate carbohydrate affects glycogen stores, let's see what happens to Matthew when he participates in a study designed to determine how carbohydrate intake affects glycogen stores during a period of heavy training. He was asked to come to the exercise laboratory at the university and ride a stationary bicycle for two hours a day for three consecutive days at 75% of his maximal heart rate. Before and after each ride, samples of muscle tissue were taken from his thighs to determine

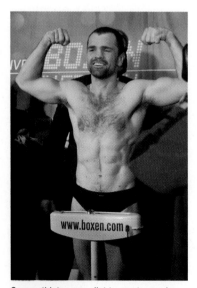

Some athletes may diet to meet a predefined weight category.

▶ **HIGHLIGHT**

When Sports Nutrition Becomes a Matter of Life or Death

Athletes are generally strong and very physically fit. However, some athletes push their bodies to the extreme, placing themselves in danger of illness and even death. The example described below illustrates how poor decisions about nutrition, specifically on inappropriate ways to achieve weight loss, can lead to serious, life-threatening consequences.

In 2003, at the age of 23, Baltimore Orioles baseball player Steve Bechler died of heatstroke and multiple organ failure after collapsing during spring training. At the beginning of training camp, Bechler's weight was approximately 114 kg (249 lb.), reportedly 4.5 kg (10 lb.) heavier than he had been the year before. With a height of approximately 1.9 metres (6'2"), the player's body mass index was about 32 (classified as obese Class I according to Canadian standards).

Bechler had been taking an over-the-counter sport supplement containing the stimulant ephedra to try to lose weight. The coroner noted that the concentration of ephedrine found in the blood sample taken before Bechler's death was consistent with reports from teammates that he had taken three capsules of the weight loss aid and energy stimulant. The ephedra- and caffeine-containing supplement, a history of borderline high blood pressure, liver abnormalities, warm and humid weather during the workout, and a weight loss diet restricting solid food intake were all critical factors converging together and resulting in a fatal heatstroke.

Likely faced with intense pressure to perform well at his sport, Bechler's use of a weight loss supplement, dieting, and training with multiple layers of clothing to increase sweat losses illustrates the risks that he and many other professional athletes are willing to take to remain competitive.

the amount of glycogen stored in the working muscles. Matthew performed these rides on two different occasions—once when he had eaten a high-carbohydrate diet (80% of total energy intake) and again when he had eaten a moderate-carbohydrate diet (40% of total energy intake). As you can see in Figure 12.10, Matthew's muscle glycogen levels decreased dramatically after each training session. More importantly, his muscle glycogen levels did not recover to baseline levels over the three days when Matthew ate the lower-carbohydrate diet. He was able to maintain his muscle glycogen levels only when he was eating the higher-carbohydrate diet. Matthew also told the researchers that completing the two-hour rides was much more difficult when he had eaten the moderate-carbohydrate diet as compared with when he ate the diet that was higher in carbohydrate.

When Should Carbohydrates Be Consumed?

It is important for athletes not only to consume enough carbohydrate to maintain glycogen stores but also to time their intake optimally. Our bodies store glycogen very rapidly during the first 24 hours of recovery from exercise, with the highest storage rates occurring during the first few hours (Burke 2000). If an athlete has to perform or participate in training bouts that are scheduled less than eight hours apart, then he or she should try to consume enough carbohydrate in the few hours following training to allow for ample glycogen storage. However, with a longer recovery time (generally 12 hours or more) the athlete can eat when he or she chooses, and glycogen levels should be restored as long as the total carbohydrate eaten is sufficient.

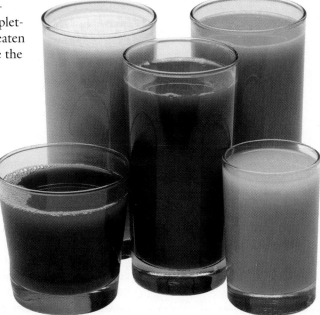

Fruit and vegetable juices can be a good source of carbohydrates.

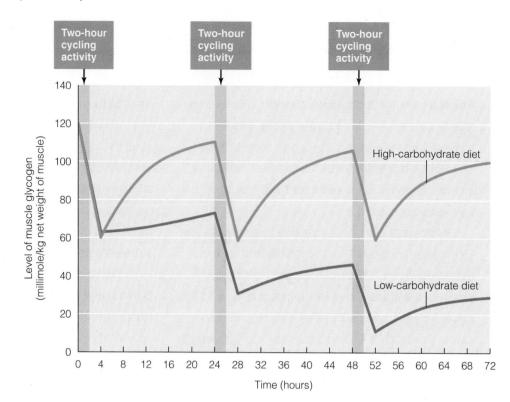

Figure 12.10 The effects of a low-carbohydrate diet on muscle glycogen stores. When a low-carbohydrate diet is consumed, glycogen stores cannot be restored during a period of regular vigorous training.
(Adapted from D. L. Costill and J. M. Miller, Nutrition for endurance sport: CHO and fluid balance, 1980, *International Journal of Sports Medicine* 1:2–14. Copyright © 1980 Georg Thieme Verlag. Used with permission.)

What Food Sources of Carbohydrates Are Good for Athletes?

What are good carbohydrate sources to support vigorous training? In general, complex, less-processed carbohydrate foods, such as whole grains and cereals, fruits, vegetables, and juices, are excellent sources that also supply fibre, vitamins, and minerals. Guidelines suggest intake of simple sugars be less than 10% of total energy intake, but some athletes who need very large energy intakes to support training may need to consume more. There are also many beverages and snack bars designed to assist athletes with increasing carbohydrate intake. Simple, inexpensive foods that contain 50 to 100 grams of carbohydrate are listed in Table 12.5, as are some snack bars designed for athletes.

When Does Carbohydrate Loading Make Sense?

carbohydrate loading Also known as glycogen loading. A process that involves altering training and carbohydrate intake so that muscle glycogen storage is maximized.

As you know, carbohydrate is a critical energy source to support exercise, particularly endurance-type activities. Because of the importance of carbohydrates as an exercise fuel and our limited capacity to store them, discovering ways to maximize our storage of carbohydrates has been at the forefront of sports nutrition research for many years. The practice of **carbohydrate loading**, also called *glycogen loading*, involves altering both exercise duration and carbohydrate intake such that it maximizes the amount of muscle glycogen. Table 12.6 reviews a schedule for carbohydrate loading for an endurance athlete. Athletes who may benefit from maximizing muscle glycogen stores are those competing in marathons, ultra-marathons, long-distance swimming, cross-country skiing, and triathlons. Athletes who compete in baseball, football, 10-kilometre runs, walking, hiking, weightlifting, and most swimming events will not gain any performance benefits from this practice, nor will people who regularly participate in moderately intense physical activities to maintain fitness.

Table 12.5   Nutrient Composition of Various Foods and Sport Bars

Food	Amount	Carbohydrate (grams)	Energy from Carbohydrate (%)	Protein (grams)	Fat (grams)	Energy (kcal)
Sweetened applesauce	250 mL (1 cup)	50	97	0.5	0.5	207
Large apple	1 each	50	82	3	4	248
Saltine crackers	8 each					
Whole wheat bread	30 g (1 oz.) slice	50	71	16	2	282
Jelly	20 mL (4 tsp)					
Skim milk	375 mL (12 fl. oz.)					
Spaghetti noodles (cooked)	250 mL (1 cup)	50	75	8	4	268
Tomato sauce	65 mL (1/4 cup)					
Brown rice (cooked)	250 mL (1 cup)	100	88	8	2	450
Mixed vegetables	125 mL (1/2 cup)					
Apple juice	375 mL (12 fl. oz.)					
Large bagel	1 (100 g/3.5 oz.)	100	81	19	2	494
Jelly	40 mL (8 tsp)					
Skim milk	250 mL (8 fl. oz.)					
Grape Nuts cereal	125 mL (1/2 cup)	100	84	16	1	473
Raisins	35 mL (1/8 cup)					
Skim milk	250 mL (8 fl. oz.)					
Balance food bar	50 g (1.76 oz.)	22	44	14	6	200
Clif Bar (chocolate chip)	69 g (2.4 oz.)	45	72	10	4	250
Kellogg's Nutri-grain Bar (raspberry)	37 g (1.3 oz.)	27	77	2	3	140
Nature Valley Granola Bar	43 g (1.5 oz.)	29	64	5	6	180
Power Bar (chocolate)	64 g (2.25 oz.)	42	75	10	2	225

Source: Adapted from M. Manore and J. Thompson, *Sport Nutrition for Health and Performance,* Champaign, IL: Human Kinetics, 2000, pp. 42, 49.

Table 12.6   Recommended Carbohydrate Loading Procedure for Endurance Athletes

Days Prior to Event	Exercise Duration (minutes)	Carbohydrate Content of Diet (grams per kg of body weight)
6	90	5
5	40	5
4	40	5
3	20	10
2	20	10
1	None (rest day)	10
Day of race	Competition	Precompetition food and fluid

Source: E. Coleman, Carbohydrate and exercise, in C. A. Rosenbloom, editor, *Sports Nutrition* (3d ed.), Chicago, IL: The American Dietetic Association 2000. Used with permission.

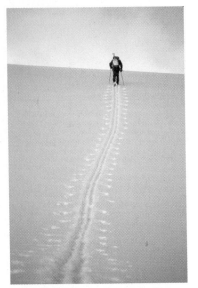

Carbohydrate loading may benefit endurance athletes, such as cross-country skiers.

It is important to emphasize that carbohydrate loading does not always improve performance. There are many adverse side effects of this practice, including extreme gastrointestinal distress, particularly diarrhea. We store water along with the extra glycogen in our muscles, which leaves many athletes feeling heavy and sluggish. Athletes who want to try carbohydrate loading should experiment prior to competition to determine if it is an acceptable and beneficial approach for them (Manore and Thompson 2000).

Recap: Carbohydrate needs increase for active people. In general, athletes should consume 55% to 60% of their total energy as carbohydrate. Consuming carbohydrate sources within the first few hours of recovery can maximize carbohydrate storage rates. Good food sources of carbohydrates for active people include whole grains and cereals, fruits, vegetables, and juices. Carbohydrate loading involves altering physical training and the diet such that the storage of muscle glycogen is maximized in an attempt to enhance endurance performance.

Moderate Fat Consumption Is Enough to Support Most Activities

As you have learned, fat is an important energy source for both moderate physical activity and vigorous endurance training. When athletes reach a physically trained state, they are able to use more fat for energy; in other words, they become better "fat burners." This can also occur in people who are not athletes but who regularly participate in aerobic-type fitness activities. This training effect occurs for a number of reasons, including an increase in the number and activity of various enzymes involved in fat metabolism, improved ability of the muscle to store fat, and improved ability to extract fat from the blood for use during exercise. By using fat as a fuel, athletes can spare carbohydrate so they can use it during prolonged, intense training or competition.

Many athletes concerned with body weight and physical appearance believe they should eat less than 15% of their total energy intake as fat, but this is inadequate for vigorous activity. Instead, a fat intake of 15% to 25% of total energy intake is generally recommended for most athletes, with less than 10% of total energy intake as saturated fat. These same recommendations can also be followed by people who are not competitive athletes. Recall from Chapter 5 that fat provides not only energy but also fat-soluble vitamins and essential fatty acids that are critical to maintaining general health. If fat consumption is too low, inadequate levels of these vitamins and essential fatty acids can eventually prove detrimental to training and performance. Athletes who have chronic disease risk factors, such as high blood lipids, high blood pressure, or unhealthful blood glucose levels, should work with their physician to adjust their intake of fat and carbohydrate according to their health risks.

Recap: Athletes and physically active people use more fat than carbohydrates for energy because they experience an increase in the number and activity of the enzymes involved in fat metabolism, and they have an improved ability to store fat and extract it from the blood for use during exercise. A dietary fat intake of 15% to 25% is generally recommended for athletes, with less than 10% of total energy intake as saturated fat.

Active People Need More Protein Than Do Inactive People, but Many Already Eat Enough

The protein intakes suggested for competitive athletes and moderately active people are in Table 12.7. Competitive male and female endurance athletes are those individuals who train five to seven days per week for more than an hour each day; many of these individuals may train for three to six hours per day. These athletes need protein in amounts similar to strength athletes, while the needs of moderate-intensity endurance athletes are slightly higher than the current RDA of 0.8 grams of protein

Table 12.7   Estimated Protein Requirements for Athletes

Group	Protein Requirements (grams per kg body weight)
Competitive male and female athletes	1.4–1.6
Moderate-intensity endurance athletes	1.2
Recreational endurance athletes	0.8–1.0
Football, power sports	1.4–1.7
Resistance athletes, weightlifters (early training)	1.5–1.7
Resistance athletes, weightlifters (steady-state training)	1.0–1.2

Source: Adapted from M. Tarnopolsky, Protein and amino acid needs for training and bulking up, in L. Burke and V. Deakin, editors, *Clinical Sports Nutrition*, Sydney, AUS: McGraw-Hill, 2000, p. 109.

per kg body weight. Moderate-intensity endurance athletes are people exercising four to five times per week for 45 to 60 minutes each time; these individuals may compete in community races and other activities. Recreational endurance athletes are people who exercise four to five times per week for 30 minutes at less than 60% of their maximal effort. These individuals have a protein need that is equal to or slightly higher than the needs of sedentary people. Strength athletes who are already trained need less protein than those who are initiating training. Studies do not support the contention that consuming more than 2 grams of protein per kg body weight improves protein synthesis, muscle strength, or performance (Tarnopolsky 2000).

As we mentioned earlier, most inactive people and many athletes in North America consume more than enough protein to support their needs (Manore and Thompson 2000). However, some athletes do not consume enough protein; these typically include individuals with very low energy intakes, vegetarians or vegans who do not consume high-protein food sources, and young athletes who are growing and are not aware of their higher protein needs.

As we discussed in Chapter 6, low-carbohydrate, high-protein diets have become quite popular, especially among people who want to lose weight (see Nutrition Debate in Chapter 6). Unlike many of these diets, the Zone Diet was developed and marketed specifically for competitive athletes. It recommends that athletes eat a 40–30–30 diet, or one comprising 40% carbohydrate, 30% fat, and 30% protein. Dr. Sears claims that high-carbohydrate diets impair athletic performance because of unhealthy effects of insulin. These claims have never been supported by research—in fact, many of Dr. Sears's claims are not consistent with human physiology. The primary problems with the Zone Diet for athletes are these:

- A low-carbohydrate diet is recommended. Years of research have shown that the only way to store sufficient glycogen for athletic performance is to consume a diet relatively high in carbohydrate. For most serious athletes, the Zone Diet is too low in carbohydrate to support training and performance.

- A high-protein diet is recommended, in levels much higher than can ever be used by the body. Some athletes have reported feeling better when eating the Zone Diet. It may be that their protein intake prior to trying the Zone Diet was inadequate, so their overall nutrient intake may have improved by following this diet.

- The Zone Diet, if followed as recommended, is a low-energy diet. This diet only provides 1200 to 1300 kcal (5020 to 5440 kJ) per day, which is not enough energy for any athlete or even for a recreationally active person.

- It is difficult for the average person to really know if they are eating a 40–30–30 diet. Estimating diet composition involves meticulous counting and recording of Calories and grams of fat, carbohydrate, and protein. Many people do not have the time, energy, desire, or expertise to make this determination.

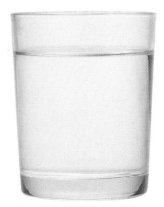

Water is essential for maintaining fluid balance and preventing dehydration.

As described in Chapter 6, high-quality protein sources include lean meats, poultry, fish, eggs and egg whites, low-fat dairy products, legumes, and soy products. By following *Eating Well with Canada's Food Guide* and meeting energy needs, people of all fitness levels can consume more than enough protein without the use of supplements or specially formulated foods.

Recap: Protein needs can be higher for athletes and active people. However, most people in North America already consume more than their daily needs for protein. Athletes at risk for low protein intakes include those with low-energy intakes, vegetarians or vegans who do not consume high-protein food sources, and young athletes who are growing and not aware of their higher protein needs. Although low-carbohydrate, high-protein diets have been marketed to athletes, these diets are generally too low in carbohydrate and energy to support regular training and competition.

Regular Exercise Increases Our Need for Fluids

A detailed discussion of fluid and electrolyte balance is provided in Chapter 7. In this chapter, we will briefly review some of the basic functions of water and its role during exercise.

Functions of Water

Water serves many important functions in the body:

- as a lubricant that bathes the tissues and cells
- as a transport medium for nutrients, hormones, and waste products
- as an important component of many chemical reactions, particularly those related to energy production
- as a structural part of body tissues, such as proteins and glycogen
- as a vital component in temperature regulation; without adequate water, we cannot cool our bodies properly through sweating and thereby can cause severe heat illness and even death

evaporative cooling Another term for sweating, which is the primary way in which we dissipate heat.

heat syncope Dizziness that occurs when people stand for too long in the heat or when they stop suddenly after a race or stand suddenly from a lying position; results from blood pooling in the lower extremities.

Cooling Mechanisms

When you exercise, your body generates heat. In fact, heat production can increase 15 to 20 times during heavy exercise! The primary way in which we dissipate this heat is through sweating, which is also called **evaporative cooling**. When body temperature rises, more blood (which contains water) flows to the surface of the skin. Heat is carried in this way from the core of our bodies to the surface of our skin. By sweating, the water (and body heat) leaves our bodies and the air around us picks up the evaporating water from our skin, cooling our bodies.

Dehydration and Heat-Related Illnesses

Exercising in extreme heat and humidity is very dangerous for two reasons: the extreme heat dramatically raises body temperature, and the high humidity prohibits evaporative cooling. During periods of high humidity, the environmental air is so saturated with water that it is unable to pull the water from the surface of our skin. Under these conditions, we are unable to cool ourselves adequately, and heat illnesses are likely to occur. It is important to remember that dehydration significantly increases our risk for heat illnesses. General signs of dehydration for adults and children were introduced in Chapter 3, and are listed in Table 3.1.

Heat illnesses include heat syncope, heat cramps, heat exhaustion, and heatstroke. **Heat syncope** is dizziness that occurs when people stand for too long in the heat, and the blood pools in their lower extremities rather than fully supplying their brains. It can also occur when people stop suddenly after a race or stand suddenly from a lying position. **Heat cramps** are muscle spasms that occur several hours after strenuous exercise. They occur during times when sweat losses and fluid intakes are high, urine volume is low, and sodium intake was inadequate to replace losses. These cramps generally are felt in the legs, arms, or abdomen after a person cools down from exercise.

Heat exhaustion and heatstroke occur on a continuum, with unchecked heat exhaustion leading to heatstroke. Early signs of heat exhaustion include excessive sweating, weakness, nausea, dizziness, headache, and difficulty concentrating. As this condition progresses, consciousness becomes impaired. Signs that a person is progressing to heatstroke are hot, dry skin, rapid heart rate, vomiting, diarrhea, a body temperature greater than or equal to 40°C or 104°F, hallucinations, and coma. It is critical that a person get proper medical care or death can result. These illnesses occur because during exercise in the heat, our muscles and skin are constantly competing for blood flow. When there is no longer enough blood flow to simultaneously provide adequate blood to our muscles and to our skin, muscle blood flow takes priority over the skin, which prevents us from cooling ourselves. Body temperature during these conditions becomes dangerously high, and the dehydration that occurs during this situation worsens this overheating condition. Heat cramps and heat exhaustion are highly likely to occur, and heatstroke is possible with prolonged exposure or exercise in environmental temperatures between 32°C and 54°C or 90°F and 130°F; heatstroke is highly likely in temperatures of at least 54°C or 130°F (National Weather Service 2003).

Guidelines for Proper Fluid Replacement

How can we prevent dehydration and heat illnesses? Obviously, adequate fluid intake is critical before, during, and after exercise. Unfortunately, our thirst mechanism cannot be relied upon to signal when we need to drink. If we rely only on our feelings of thirst, we will not consume enough fluid to support exercise.

General fluid replacement recommendations are based on maintaining body weight. As introduced in Chapter 7, athletes who are training and competing in hot environments should weigh themselves before and after the training session or event and should regain the weight lost over the subsequent 24-hour period. They should avoid losing more than 2% to 3% of body weight during exercise, as performance can be impaired with fluid losses as small as 1% of body weight.

Table 12.8 reviews guidelines for proper fluid replacement. For activities lasting less than one hour, plain water is generally adequate to replace fluid losses. However, for training and competition lasting longer than one hour in any weather, sport beverages containing carbohydrates and electrolytes are recommended. These beverages are also recommended for people who will not drink enough water because they don't like the taste. If drinking these beverages will guarantee adequate hydration, they are appropriate to use. For more specific information about sport beverages, refer to pages 241–242.

> **Recap:** Regular exercise increases our fluid needs. Fluid is critical to cool our internal body temperature and prevent heat illnesses. Dehydration is a serious threat during exercise in extreme heat and high humidity. Heat illnesses include heat syncope, heat cramps, heat exhaustion, and heatstroke. Adequate fluid intake before, during, and after exercise is critical to prevent heat illnesses.

Inadequate Intakes of Some Vitamins and Minerals Can Diminish Health and Performance

When individuals train vigorously for athletic events, their requirements for certain vitamins and minerals may be altered. Many highly active people do not eat enough food or a variety of foods that allows them to consume enough of these nutrients, yet it is imperative that active people do their very best to eat an adequate, varied, and balanced diet to try and meet the increased needs associated with vigorous training.

heat cramps Muscle spasms that occur several hours after strenuous exercise; most often occur when sweat losses and fluid intakes are high, urine volume is low, and sodium intake is inadequate.

heat exhaustion A heat illness that is characterized by excessive sweating, weakness, nausea, dizziness, headache, and difficulty concentrating. Unchecked heat exhaustion can lead to heatstroke.

Table 12.8 Guidelines for Fluid Replacement

Activity Level	Environment	Fluid Requirements (litres per day)
Sedentary	Cool	2–3
Active	Cool	3–6
Sedentary	Warm	3–5
Active	Warm	5–10 +

Before Exercise or Competition:
- Drink adequate fluids during 24 hours before event; should be able to maintain body weight.
- Drink about 500–750 mL (16–24 fl. oz.) of water or a sports drink 2–3 hours prior to exercise or event to allow time for excretion of excess fluid prior to event.
- Drink 250–375 mL (8–12 fl. oz.) of water or a sports drink 10–20 minutes prior to event.

During Exercise or Competition:
- Drink early and regularly throughout event to sufficiently replace all water lost through sweating, or consume the maximal amount of fluid that can be tolerated; generally 250–375 mL (8–12 fl. oz.) every 10 to 20 minutes is adequate.
- Fluids should be cooler than the environmental temperature and flavoured to enhance taste and promote fluid replacement.

During Exercise or Competition That Lasts More Than One Hour:
- Fluid replacement beverage should contain 4%–8% carbohydrate to maintain blood glucose levels; sodium and other electrolytes should be included in the beverage in amounts of 0.5–0.7 grams of sodium per litre of water to replace the sodium lost by sweating.

Following Exercise or Competition:
- Consume at least 500 mL (16 fl. oz.) of fluid for each 0.5 kg (1 lb.) of body weight lost.
- Fluids after exercise should contain water to restore hydration status, carbohydrates to replenish glycogen stores, and electrolytes (for example, sodium and potassium) to speed rehydration.
- Consume enough fluid to permit regular urination and to ensure the urine colour is very light or light yellow in colour; drinking about 125% to 150% of fluid loss is usually sufficient to ensure complete rehydration.

In General:
- Products that contain fructose should be limited, as these may cause gastrointestinal distress.
- Caffeine and alcohol should be avoided, as these products increase urine output and reduce fluid retention.
- Carbonated beverages should be avoided as they reduce the desire for fluid intake because of stomach fullness.

Sources: Adapted from R. Murray, Drink more! Advice from a world-class expert, 1997, *ACSM's Health and Fitness Journal* 1:9–23; American College of Sports Medicine Position Stand, Exercise and fluid replacement, 1996, *Medicine and Science in Sports and Exercise* 28:i–vii; D. J. Casa, L. E. Armstrong, S. K. Hillman, S. J. Montain, R. V. Reiff, B. S. E. Rich, W. O. Roberts, and J. A. Stone, National Athletic Trainers' Association position statement: Fluid replacement for athletes, 2000, *Journal of Athletic Training* 35:212–224.

B Vitamins

The B vitamins are directly involved in energy metabolism (see pages 350–359). There is reliable evidence that the requirements of active people for thiamin, riboflavin, and vitamin B_6 may be slightly higher than the current RDA (Manore and Thompson 2000). However, these increased needs are easily met by consuming adequate energy and a lot of complex carbohydrates, fruits, and vegetables. Athletes and physically active people at risk for poor B vitamin status are those who consume inadequate energy or who consume mostly refined carbohydrate foods, such as pop and sugary snacks. Vegan athletes and active individuals may be at risk for inadequate intake of vitamin B_{12}; food sources enriched with this nutrient include some soy and cereal products.

Calcium and the Female Athlete Triad

Calcium supports proper muscle contraction and ensures bone health (see pages 315–322). Calcium intakes are inadequate for most women in North America, including both sedentary and active women. This is most likely due to the failure to consume foods that are high in calcium, particularly dairy products. Although vigorous training does not appear to increase our need for calcium, we need to consume enough calcium to support bone health. If we do not, stress fractures and severe loss of bone can result.

Some female athletes suffer from what is referred to as the female athlete triad (see page 340 for more details). The triad includes three syndromes: eating disorders, osteoporosis, and **amenorrhea** (lack of menstruation for at least three consecutive months in the absence of pregnancy). In this triad, nutritional inadequacies from inadequate food and energy intake cause irregularities in the menstrual cycle; these in turn cause hormonal disturbances that lead to a significant loss of bone mass. Reduction in bone mass may cause poor bone strength and eventually lead to *osteoporosis,* a disease in which the bones become porous (less dense) and break easily (see page 337). Consuming the recommended amounts of calcium can help prevent osteoporosis. For female athletes who are physically small and consume lower energy intakes, supplementation may be needed to meet current recommendations.

amenorrhea Lack of menstruation for at least three consecutive months in the absence of pregnancy.

Iron

Iron is a part of the hemoglobin molecule and is critical for the transport of oxygen in our blood to our cells and working muscles. Iron also is involved in energy production. Research has shown that active individuals lose more iron in the sweat, feces, and urine than do inactive individuals and that endurance runners lose iron when their red blood cells break down in their feet because of the high impact of running (Weaver and Rajaram 1992). Female athletes and non-athletes lose more iron than male athletes because of menstrual blood losses, and females in general tend to eat less iron in their diet. Vegetarian athletes and active people may also consume less iron. Thus, many athletes and active people are at higher risk of iron deficiency. Depending upon its severity, poor iron status can impair athletic performance and our ability to maintain regular physical activity.

Not all athletes suffer from iron deficiency. A phenomenon known as *sports anemia* was identified in the 1960s. Sports anemia is not true anemia, but a transient decrease in iron stores that occurs at the start of an exercise program for some people, and it is also seen in athletes who increase their training intensity. Exercise training increases the amount of water in our blood (called *plasma volume*); however, the amount of hemoglobin does not increase until later into the training period. Thus, the iron content in the blood appears to be low but instead is falsely depressed because of increases in plasma volume. Sports anemia, since it is not true anemia, does not affect performance.

The stages of iron deficiency are described in pages 364–369. In general, it appears that physically active females are at relatively high risk of suffering from the first stage of iron depletion, in which iron stores are low (Haymes 1998; Haymes and Clarkson 1998). Because of this it is suggested that blood tests of iron stores and monitoring dietary iron intakes be routinely done for active females (Manore and Thompson 2000). In some cases, iron needs cannot be met through the diet, and supplementation is necessary. Iron supplementation should be done with a physician's approval and proper medical supervision.

Recap: Some athletes may have a greater need for certain vitamins and minerals. Active people may need more thiamin, riboflavin, and vitamin B$_6$ than inactive people. Exercise itself does not increase our calcium needs, but most women, including active women, do not consume enough calcium. Some female athletes suffer from the female athlete triad, a condition that involves the interaction of inadequate energy intake, poor bone strength, and amenorrhea. Many active individuals require more iron, particularly female athletes and vegetarian athletes.

Are Ergogenic Aids Necessary for Active People?

ergogenic aids Substances used to improve exercise and athletic performance.

Many competitive athletes and even some recreationally active people continually search for that something extra that will enhance their performance. **Ergogenic aids** are substances used to improve exercise and athletic performance. For example, nutrition supplements can be classified as ergogenic aids, as can anabolic steroids and other pharmaceuticals. Interestingly, people report using ergogenic aids not only to enhance athletic performance but also to improve their physical appearance, prevent or treat injuries, treat diseases, and help them cope with stress. Some people even report using them because of peer pressure.

As you have learned in this chapter, adequate nutrition is critical to athletic performance and to regular physical activity, and such products as sport bars and beverages can assist athletes with maintaining their competitive edge. However, as we will explore shortly, many of these products are not effective, some are dangerous, and most are very expensive. For the average consumer, it is virtually impossible to track the latest research findings for these products. In addition, many have not been adequately studied, and unsubstantiated false claims surrounding them are rampant. How can you become a more educated consumer about ergogenic aids?

It is important that independent laboratories conduct some of the research, as they are more likely to be unbiased. Many companies claim that research is being conducted but state that the findings cannot be shared with the public. This is a warning sign, as there is no need to hide research findings. The use of a celebrity spokesperson is also very common, as celebrity testimonials help to sell products. However, many times this spokesperson is simply being paid to endorse the product and does not actually use it. Finally, it is critical that consumers realize that a patent on a product does not guarantee the effectiveness or safety of that product. Patents are granted solely to distinguish differences among products; indeed, they can be granted on a product that has never been scientifically tested for effectiveness or safety.

New ergogenic aids are available virtually every month, and keeping track of these substances is a daunting task. It is therefore not possible to discuss every available product in this chapter. However, a brief review of a number of currently popular ergogenic aids is provided.

> **Recap:** Ergogenic aids are substances used to improve exercise and athletic performance. Some people also use these substances to improve physical appearance, prevent or treat injuries, treat diseases, or help them cope with stress. Many ergogenic aids are not effective, some are dangerous, and most are expensive.

Anabolic Products Are Touted as Muscle and Strength Enhancers

anabolic Refers to a substance that builds muscle and increases strength.

Many ergogenic aids are said to be **anabolic,** meaning that they build muscle and increase strength. Most anabolic substances promise to increase testosterone, which is the hormone associated with male sex characteristics and increased muscle size and strength. Although some anabolic substances are effective, they are generally associated with harmful side effects.

Anabolic Steroids

Anabolic steroids are testosterone-based drugs that have been used extensively by strength and power athletes. Anabolic steroids are known to be effective in increasing muscle size, strength, power, and speed. These products are illegal in North America, and their use is banned by all major college, university, and professional sports organizations, in addition to the International Olympic Committees. They cause dangerous side effects, including premature closure of growth plates in bones, which can stunt the growth of young athletes who use them. Other side effects include liver cysts, liver dysfunction, increased risk of heart disease, high blood pressure, and reproductive dysfunction. Some of the irreversible side effects experienced by women include increased growth of body and facial hair and an enlarged clitoris. Men may grow breast tissue that must be surgically removed. Anabolic steroids also cause mood disturbances, increased aggressiveness, and sleep disturbances.

Androstenedione and Dehydroepiandrosterone

Androstenedione and dehydroepiandrosterone (DHEA) are precursors of testosterone. Manufacturers of these products claim that taking them will increase testosterone levels and muscle strength. Recent studies have found that these products do not increase testosterone levels, and androstenedione has been shown to increase the risk of heart disease in men aged 35 to 65 years (Broeder et al. 2000). There are no studies that support the products' claims of improving strength or increasing muscle mass.

Gamma-Hydroxybutyric Acid

Gamma-hydroxybutyric acid, or GHB, has been promoted as an alternative to anabolic steroids for building muscle. The production and sale of GHB has never been approved in Canada or the United States; however, it was illegally produced and sold on the black market. For many users, GHB caused only dizziness, tremors, or vomiting, but others experienced severe side effects, including seizures. Many people were hospitalized and some died.

After GHB was banned, a similar product (gamma-butyrolactone, or GBL) was marketed in its place. This product was also found to be dangerous and was removed from the market. Recently, another replacement product called BD, or 1,4-butanediol, was banned because it has caused at least 71 deaths, with 40 more under investigation. BD is an industrial solvent and is listed on ingredient labels as tetramethylene glycol, butylene glycol, or sucol-B. Side effects include wild, aggressive behaviour, nausea, incontinence, and sudden loss of consciousness.

Creatine

Creatine is a supplement that has become very popular with strength and power athletes. Creatine, or creatine phosphate, is found in meat and fish and stored in our muscles. As described earlier in this chapter, we use creatine phosphate (or CP) to regenerate ATP. By taking creatine supplements, it is hypothesized that more CP is available to replenish ATP, which will prolong a person's ability to train and perform in short-term, explosive activities, such as swimming, cycling, weight-lifting, and sprinting (American College of Sports Medicine 2000). Between 1994 and 2004, more than 700 research articles related to creatine and exercise in humans were published. Creatine does not seem to enhance performance in aerobic-type events, and studies examining increases in the work performed and the amount of strength gained during resistance exercise are inconclusive (American College of Sports Medicine 2000). More research is needed on the use of creatine supplements over long periods, especially on the potential for kidney and liver damage.

> **Recap:** Anabolic products are marketed to build muscle and increase strength. Anabolic steroids are effective in increasing muscle size, power, and strength, but they are illegal and can cause serious health consequences. Androstenedione and dehydroepiandrosterone are precursors of testosterone; neither of these products has been shown to effectively increase testosterone levels or to increase strength or muscle mass. Gamma-hydroxybutyric acid was marketed as an alternative to steroids but was banned because of severe and sometimes fatal side effects. Creatine supplements are popular and can enhance sprint performance in swimming, running, and cycling. Little is known about the long-term use of creatine.

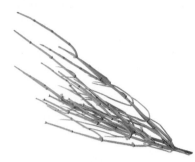

Ephedrine is made from the herb *Ephedra sinica* (Chinese ephedra).

Some Products Are Said to Optimize Fuel Use During Exercise

Certain ergogenic aids are touted as increasing energy levels and improving athletic performance by optimizing our use of fat, carbohydrate, and protein. The products reviewed here include caffeine, ephedrine, carnitine, chromium, and ribose.

Caffeine

Caffeine is a stimulant that makes us feel more alert and energetic, decreasing feelings of fatigue during exercise. Caffeine has been shown to increase the use of fat as a fuel during endurance exercise, which spares muscle glycogen and improves performance (Anderson et al. 2000; Spriet and Howlett 2000). Side effects of caffeine use include increased blood pressure, increased heart rate, dizziness, insomnia, headache, and gastrointestinal distress.

Ephedrine

Ephedrine, also known as ephedra, Chinese ephedra, or ma huang, is a strong stimulant marketed as a weight loss supplement and energy enhancer. In reality, many products sold as Chinese ephedra (or herbal ephedra) contain ephedrine from the laboratory and other stimulants, such as caffeine. The use of ephedra supplements does not appear to enhance performance, but supplements containing both caffeine and ephedra have been shown to prolong the amount of exercise that can be done until exhaustion is reached (Bucci 2000). Ephedra is known to reduce body weight and body fat in sedentary women, but its impact on weight loss and body fat levels in athletes is not well studied. Side effects of ephedra use include headaches, dizziness, nausea, reduced appetite, nervousness, anxiety, irregular or fast heart rate, high blood pressure, strokes, seizures, and death (Health Canada 2008). Ephedra has been banned by the International Olympic Committee for many years, and Health Canada advises Canadians that the only approved use of ephedra is in nasal decongestants (Health Canada 2008). Products containing ephedra for body building, weight loss, or increased physical energy are not approved for sale in Canada (Health Canada 2008).

Carnitine

Carnitine (also known as L-carnitine and levocarnitine) is a compound made from amino acids (lysine and methionine) in our liver and kidneys and found in nearly all cells in our body. Healthy children and adults make enough carnitine in their bodies, so carnitine is not an essential nutrient (National Institutes of Health 2006). Carnitine helps shuttle long chain fatty acids into the mitochondria so they can be used for energy. In theory, it has been proposed that exercise training depletes our cells of carnitine and that supplementation should increase the amount of carnitine in our cell membranes. By increasing cellular levels of carnitine, we should be able to improve the use of fat as a fuel source. Thus, carnitine is marketed not only as a performance-enhancing substance but also as a fat burner. The U.S. National Institutes of Health (2006) states that 20 years of research suggest that "carnitine supplements do not appear to increase the body's use of oxygen or improve metabolic status when exercising, nor do they necessarily increase the amount of carnitine in muscle."

Chromium

Chromium is a trace mineral that enhances insulin's action of increasing the transport of amino acids into the cell (see Chapter 10). It is found in whole-grain foods, cheese, nuts, mushrooms, and asparagus. Promoters of chromium supplements suggest that many people are chromium deficient and that supplementation will enhance the uptake of amino acids into muscle cells, which will increase muscle growth and strength. Like carnitine, chromium is marketed as a fat burner, as it is speculated that its effect on insulin stimulates the brain to decrease food intake.

However, a review of 24 studies found that chromium supplements had no significant effects on body composition (National Institutes of Health 2005). Another review of controlled clinical trials found that supplements were associated with weight loss but the differences were very small. The inconsistent findings are likely due to differences in the number of participants in studies, the length of the studies, and the chromium in participants' diets (National Institutes of Health 2005). Chromium supplements are available as chromium picolinate and chromium nicotinate. Early studies of chromium supplementation showed promise, but more recent, better-designed studies do not support any benefit of chromium supplementation on muscle mass, muscle strength, body fat, or exercise performance.

Ribose

Ribose is a five-carbon sugar that is critical to the production of ATP. Ribose supplementation is claimed to improve athletic performance by increasing work output and by promoting a faster recovery time from vigorous training. Although ribose has been shown to improve exercise tolerance in patients with heart disease (Pliml et al. 1992), no published studies have examined its impact on athletic performance (Coleman 2000).

From this review of ergogenic aids, you can see that most of these products are not effective in enhancing athletic performance or in optimizing muscle strength or body composition. It is important to be a savvy consumer when examining these products to make sure you are not wasting your money or putting your health at risk by using them.

> **Recap:** Caffeine is a stimulant that increases the use of fat during exercise. Ephedrine is a stimulant that has been recalled by Health Canada because of its potentially fatal side effects. Carnitine helps shuttle fatty acids into our mitochondria so they can be used for energy. Carnitine supplements do not enhance fat utilization during exercise or improve athletic performance. Chromium is a trace mineral that is marketed as a fat burner, but chromium supplements do not appear to enhance body composition or athletic performance. Ribose supplementation is claimed to increase work output and promote faster recovery time from training, but no studies have yet been done in athletes to support these claims.

CHAPTER SUMMARY

- Physical activity is any movement produced by muscles that increases energy expenditure and can be categorized as occupational, household, leisure-time, and transportation.

- Physical activity provides a multitude of health benefits, including reducing our risks for heart disease, stroke, high blood pressure, obesity, type 2 diabetes, some cancers, and osteoporosis. Despite these benefits, 51% of Canadian adults are sedentary.

- Leisure-time physical activity is any activity not related to a person's occupation and includes competitive sports and recreational activities. Exercise is a

subcategory of leisure-time physical activity and is purposeful, planned, and structured.

- Physical fitness has many components and is defined as the ability to carry out daily tasks with vigour and alertness, without undue fatigue, and with ample energy to enjoy leisure-time pursuits and meet unforeseen emergencies.

- The components of fitness include cardiorespiratory fitness, musculoskeletal fitness (which includes muscular strength and endurance), flexibility, and body composition.

CHAPTER SUMMARY

- To achieve the appropriate overload for fitness, the FIT principle (frequency, intensity, and time of activity) should be followed. Frequency refers to the number of activity sessions per week. Intensity refers to how difficult the activity is to perform. Time refers to how long each activity session lasts.

- Warm-up, or preliminary exercise, is important to get prepared for exercise. Warm-up exercises prepare the muscles for exertion by increasing blood flow and temperature.

- Cool-down activities are done after an exercise session is complete. Cool-down activities assist in the prevention of injury and may help reduce muscle soreness.

- Adenosine triphosphate, or ATP, is the common energy source for all cells of the body. The amount of ATP stored in a muscle cell is limited and can only keep a muscle active for about one to three seconds.

- For maximal activities lasting about 3 to 15 seconds, creatine phosphate can be broken down in an anaerobic reaction to provide energy and support the regeneration of ATP.

- To support activities that last from 30 seconds to 2 minutes, energy is produced from glycolysis. Glycolysis produces two ATP molecules for every glucose molecule broken down. Pyruvic acid is the final end product of glycolysis.

- The further metabolism of pyruvic acid in the presence of adequate oxygen provides energy for activities that last from three minutes to four hours. During this aerobic process, each molecule of glucose can yield 36 to 38 ATP molecules.

- Lactic acid is formed when pyruvic acid is metabolized under anaerobic conditions. Recent research suggests it is also produced under aerobic conditions, and may be an important energy source for muscle cells during rest and exercise.

- Fat can be broken down aerobically to support activities of low intensity and long duration. Fat is an abundant energy source and it provides more than twice the energy per gram as compared with carbohydrate, but its breakdown process is relatively slow, and it cannot support quick, high-intensity activities.

- Amino acids can be used to make glucose to maintain our blood glucose levels during exercise and can contribute from 3% to 6% of the energy needed during exercise. Amino acids also help build and repair tissues after exercise.

- Vigorous-intensity exercise requires extra energy, and male athletes typically need more energy than female athletes because of their higher muscle mass and larger body weight. Athletes who are concerned with making a competitive weight or with the aesthetic demands of their sport may be at risk for poor energy and nutrient intakes.

- It is generally recommended that athletes should consume 55% to 60% of their total energy as carbohydrate.

- Carbohydrate loading involves altering physical training and the diet such that the storage of muscle glycogen is maximized in an attempt to enhance endurance performance.

- A dietary fat intake of 15% to 25% of total energy is generally recommended for athletes, with less than 10% of total energy intake as saturated fat.

- Protein needs can be higher for athletes and regularly active people, but most people in Canada consume more than their daily needs for protein.

- Athletes at risk for low protein intake include those with low energy intakes, vegetarians or vegans who do not consume high-protein food sources, and young athletes who are growing and not aware of their higher protein needs.

- Regular exercise increases our fluid needs to help cool our internal body temperature and prevent heat illnesses. Heat illnesses include heat syncope, heat cramps, heat exhaustion, and heatstroke. Adequate fluid intake before, during, and after exercise will help prevent heat illnesses.

- Active people may need more thiamin, riboflavin, and vitamin B_6 than inactive people. Most women, including active women, do not consume enough calcium. Many active individuals also require more iron, particularly female athletes and vegetarian athletes.

- Ergogenic aids are substances used to improve exercise and athletic performance, to improve physical appearance, to prevent or treat injuries, to treat diseases, or to cope with stress. Many ergogenic aids are not effective, some are dangerous, and most are expensive.

mynutritionlab Go to MyNutritionLab at www.pearsoned.ca/mynutritionlab and enrich your understanding of nutrition! You'll find key animations, interactive exercises, access to My DietAnalysis, and much more.

REVIEW QUESTIONS

Quizzes

1. Using the FIT principle for achieving and maintaining cardiorespiratory fitness, the intensity range typically recommended is
   a. 25% to 50% of your estimated maximal heart rate.
   b. 35% to 75% of your estimated maximal heart rate.
   c. 55% to 90% of your estimated maximal heart rate.
   d. 75% to 95% of your estimated maximal heart rate.

2. The amount of ATP stored in a muscle cell can keep a muscle active for about
   a. 1 to 3 seconds.
   b. 10 to 30 seconds.
   c. 1 to 3 minutes.
   d. 1 to 3 hours.

3. To support a long afternoon of gardening, the body predominantly uses which nutrient for energy?
   a. Carbohydrate
   b. Fat
   c. Amino acids
   d. Lactic acid

4. Creatine
   a. seems to enhance performance in aerobic-type events.
   b. appears to increase an individual's risk for bladder cancer.
   c. seems to increase strength gained in resistance exercise.
   d. is stored in our muscles.

5. What percents of dietary fat and carbohydrate are recommended for athletes?
   a. 15% to 25% fat and 55% to 60% carbohydrate
   b. 55% to 60% fat and 15% to 25% carbohydrate
   c. 25% to 35% fat and 45% to 50% carbohydrate
   d. 45% to 50% fat and 25% to 35% carbohydrate

6. What practice do long distance athletes sometimes follow to maximize their race performance?
   a. Glycolysis loading
   b. Glucose loading
   c. Carbohydrate loading
   d. Mineral loading

7. What does FIT stand for?
   a. Frequency, interval, time
   b. Frequency, intensity, time
   c. Fast, interval, target heart rate
   d. Fitness, intensity, target heart rate

8. Catherine is an ultra-distance runner who has just started training for a 100-kilometre race. Being new to the event, Catherine has found the more intense training challenging. Although she is a vegetarian, Catherine makes sure she eats plenty of nuts and legumes to maintain her iron stores. However, during a routine blood test, one week into her training, the laboratory report indicated that Catherine's blood iron content was low. What do you think happened? List and explain the factors that put Catherine at risk for iron deficiency. Should Catherine begin iron supplementation?

9. Write a plan for a weekly activity/exercise routine that does the following:
   - meets your personal fitness goals
   - is fun for you to do
   - includes variety and consistency
   - uses all components of the FIT principle
   - includes a warm-up and cool-down period

10. Determine how many grams of carbohydrate, protein, and fat you need to consume daily to support the activity/exercise routine you described in the previous question.

11. You decide to start training for your school's annual marathon. After studying this chapter, which of the following preparation strategies would you pursue, and why?
    - use of B vitamin supplements
    - use of creatine supplements
    - use of sports beverages
    - carbohydrate loading

12. Your father is a slightly overweight couch potato. Would you advise him to begin a planned exercise program of low to moderate intensity? Why or why not? If so, what steps should he take before starting an exercise program?

13. Marisa and Conrad are students at the same city college. Marisa walks to and from school each morning from her home seven blocks away. Conrad lives in a suburb 19 kilometres (12 miles) away and drives to school. Marisa, an early childhood education major, covers the lunch shift, two hours a day, at the college's daycare centre, cleaning up the lunchroom and supervising the children in the playground. Conrad, an accounting major, works in his department office two hours a day, entering data into computer spreadsheets. On weekends, Marisa and her sister walk downtown and go shopping. Conrad goes to the movies with his friends. Neither Marisa nor Conrad participates in sports or scheduled exercise sessions. Marisa has maintained a normal, healthy weight throughout the school year, but in the same period, Conrad has gained several kilograms. Identify at least two factors that might play a role in Marisa's and Conrad's current weight.

14. While exercising at the gym, you notice a middle-aged woman on the treadmill next to you. Her shirt is soaked with sweat and she has no water bottle. Looking shaky, she breathlessly but proudly tells you that she's been running for 40 minutes straight on the second-highest level. Then she goes on to tell you that this is the first time she's exercised in 10 years! Five minutes later, she abruptly stops running and heads to the change room. How would you critique this woman's exercise routine? What is positive about her story? Is there anything about it that alarms you? What suggestions might you give this woman, keeping in mind that you don't want to discourage her?

CASE STUDY

Dylan is preparing for the upcoming soccer season by hitting the gym every day. His coach advises him to see a dietitian to make sure that he's eating properly. After keeping a food record, he calculates that he eats an average of about 500 grams of carbohydrates and 150 grams of protein each day. Dylan is 1.83 metres (6') tall and about 82 kg (180 lbs.) during practice season. Working out, he's been feeling sluggish, sometimes dragging himself through practice. A trainer at the gym overhears Dylan commenting on his concern about consuming too little protein and suggests trying one of the protein powders sold by the gym.

a. Given what you know about the role of energy nutrients in vigorous physical activity, what do you think might be causing Dylan to feel exhausted?
b. Would you recommend that he try the protein powder offered by the gym?
c. What other strategies might Dylan consider?

Test Yourself Answers

1. **False** *Physical activity* refers to any movement produced by muscles that increases energy expenditure, while *exercise* is a subcategory of leisure-time physical activity and refers to activity that is planned, purposeful, and structured.

2. **True** An estimated 51% of Canadian adults are physically inactive, and only 49% are moderately active or more.

3. **False** Each person has to design a fitness program based on his or her own interests and needs. Depending upon a person's fitness goals, being active 20 to 30 minutes each day could be enough for a given individual.

4. **True** Although lactic acid is one of many contributors to muscle fatigue, recent research has shown that it is not a primary cause of muscle soreness.

5. **True** Most ergogenic aids are ineffective or do not produce the results that are advertised. Many ergogenic aids, such as anabolic steroids and ephedrine, can actually cause serious health consequences and can even cause death in some instances.

WEB LINKS

www.phac-aspc.gc.ca/pau-uap/fitness/index.html
**Physical Activity Unit, Public Health Agency
of Canada**
This site has all the physical activity guides (for adults, older
adults, children, and youth) and good ideas about how to
incorporate physical activity into your daily work and leisure
activities.

www.caaws.ca
**Canadian Association for the Advancement of Women
and Sport and Physical Activity**
Visit this site to learn more about the opportunities for girls
and women to become active in sports and physical activity
through such programs as Mothers in Motion and On the
Move.

www.cahperd.ca/eng/index.cfm
**Canadian Association for Health, Physical Education,
Recreation and Dance**
CAHPERD describes itself on its website as "a national,
charitable, voluntary-sector organization whose primary
concern is to influence the healthy development of children
and youth by advocating for quality, school-based physical
and health education." Visit the site to learn more about its
unique initiatives.

www.cflri.ca
Canadian Fitness and Lifestyle Research Institute
This research institute monitors the physical activity
levels of Canadian adults and children on an
annual basis.

www.csep.ca
Canadian Society for Exercise Physiology (CSEP)
Interested in becoming a certified fitness consultant or a
professional fitness and lifestyle consultant? Visit this website
to learn about the certification programs available.

www.acsm.org
American College of Sports Medicine
Look under Health and Fitness Information for guidelines
on healthy aerobic activity, calculating your exercise heart
rate range, and the ACSM's *Fit Society Page* newsletter.

www.webmd.com
WebMD Health
Visit this site to learn about a variety of lifestyle topics,
including fitness and exercise.

www.hhs.gov
U.S. Department of Health and Human Services
Review this site for multiple statistics on health, exercise,
and weight, as well as information on supplements, wellness,
and more.

http://dietary-supplements.info.nih.gov
NIH Office of Dietary Supplements
Look on this National Institutes of Health site to learn more
about the health effects of specific nutritional supplements.

www.nal.usda.gov/fnic/etext/ds_ergogenic.html
Food and Nutrition Information Center
Visit this site for links to detailed information about
ergogenic aids and sports nutrition.

How Much Physical Activity Is Enough?

Your aerobics instructor tells you to work out at your target heart rate for 20 minutes a day, whereas your doctor tells you to walk for half an hour three or four times a week. A magazine article exhorts you to work out to the point of exhaustion, while a new weight loss book claims that you can be perfectly healthy without ever breaking a sweat. And as if these mixed messages about what constitutes "regular physical activity" weren't enough, a recent report from the Institute of Medicine (2002) has inadvertently added to the confusion. In this report, it is recommended that North Americans should be active 60 minutes per day to optimize health. This message is similar to *Canada's Physical Activity Guide to Healthy Active Living*, which suggests that 60 minutes a day of light activity is needed to stay healthy. Light activity or light effort includes regular walking, volleyball, stretching, and gardening. However, as the activity becomes more strenuous, the amount of time needed to stay healthy decreases. Activities requiring moderate effort, such as biking, brisk walking, and swimming laps, should be done for 30 to 60 minutes on most days of the week. The recommendation for vigorous or strenuous activities, such as aerobics, hockey, jogging,

and fast swimming, is 20 to 30 minutes a day on four days a week.

The publication of the report by the Institute of Medicine resulted in an immediate firestorm of responses from various health organizations condemning the recommendations. The primary concern of these organizations was that consumers would be confused about how much physical activity was enough and that this confusion would result in frustration and lead to people giving up on participating in any physical activity. Another concern was that 60 minutes of physical activity each day is too much to ask of a population in which more than half are already insufficiently active.

So how much activity is really enough? To try to answer this question, let's take a closer look at what we have learned from exercise training studies and from population-based epidemiological studies. *Exercise training studies* involve taking individuals, putting them through a clearly defined training program, and assessing fitness and health outcomes. These studies consistently show that less fit and older individuals can significantly improve their cardiorespiratory fitness and reduce their risk for chronic diseases by participating in

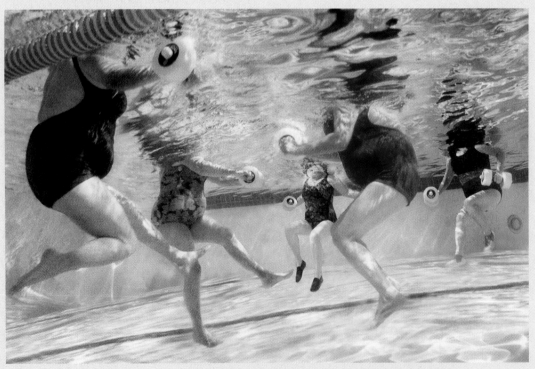

Older and less fit individuals can improve their health and physical fitness with moderate daily activity.

moderate levels of physical activity (King et al. 1991; Kohrt et al. 1991). In contrast, *population-based* epidemiological studies compare self-reports of physical activity or fitness to rates of illness and mortality (LaCroix et al. 1996; Blair et al. 1995). In other words, the direct effect of exercise training is not being assessed in these studies; instead, they assess only the relationship between level of physical activity/fitness and rates of disease and premature death. These studies show that unfit, sedentary people suffer from the highest rates of disease and premature mortality and that increased physical activity significantly correlates to decreased risks for chronic diseases and premature mortality.

Some studies indicate that expending an average of 150 Calories (630 kJ) per day, which is equivalent to about 30 minutes of moderate physical activity per day, is associated with significant reductions in disease risk and premature mortality (Paffenbarger et al. 1986; Leon et al. 1987; Slattery, Jacobs, and Nichaman 1989; Helmrich et al. 1991). It is important to emphasize that this recommendation is intended for individuals who are currently inactive. It is not intended to apply to individuals who are already physically active and doing more activity that results in moderate to high fitness levels. Additional health and fitness benefits will result by adding in more time doing moderate-intensity physical activity or by substituting vigorous physical activities for those that are moderate in intensity.

In contrast, the Institute of Medicine based their physical activity recommendations on the assumption of a healthful energy balance, in which energy intake should be equal to the energy expenditure associated with maintaining a healthy body weight. Thus, this group of experts examined studies that measured the amount of energy people expend to maintain a BMI of 18.5 to 25 kg/m^2. After reviewing a large number of studies that assessed energy expenditure and BMI, the Institute of Medicine concluded that participating in about 60 minutes of moderately intense physical activity per day will move people from a very sedentary to an active lifestyle and will allow them to maintain a healthy body weight.

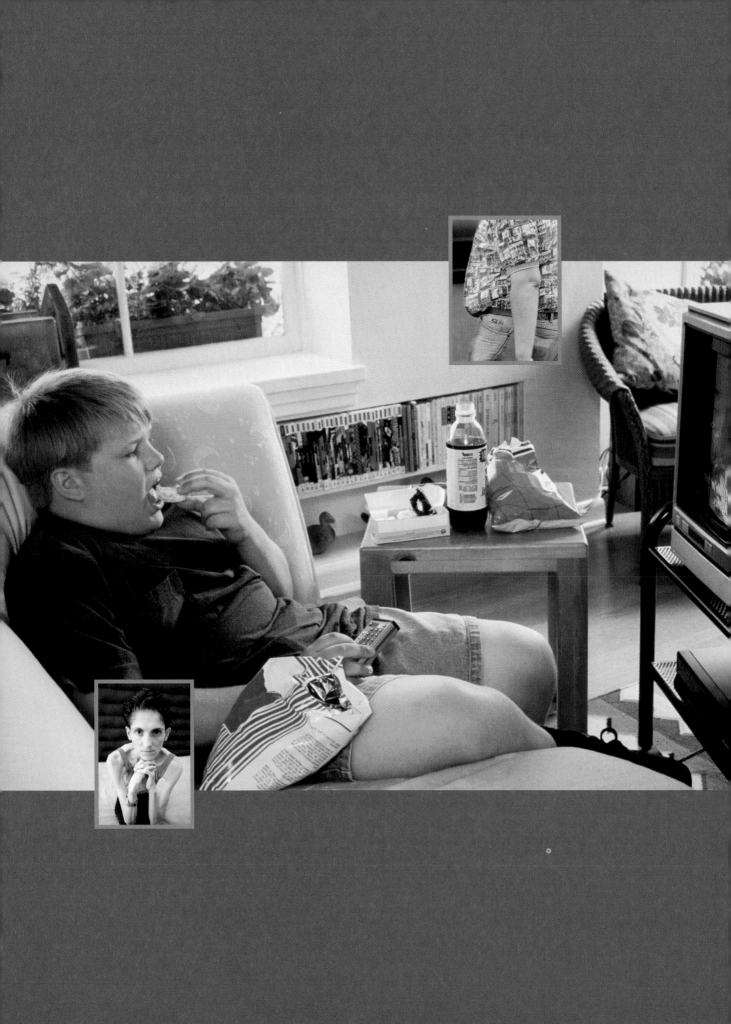

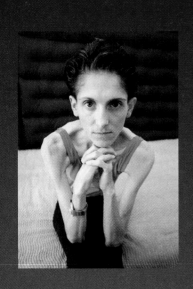

CHAPTER 13

Disordered Eating

CHAPTER OBJECTIVES

After reading this chapter you will be able to:

1. Explain what is meant by the statement that eating behaviours occur along a continuum, pp. 462–463.

2. Compare and contrast disordered eating behaviours and true clinical eating disorders, pp. 463–464.

3. Identify at least four factors that may contribute to the development of an eating disorder, pp. 464–471.

4. Create a table listing the symptoms and health risks of anorexia nervosa, bulimia nervosa, binge-eating disorder, and chronic dieting, pp. 471–482.

5. Discuss the steps you can use when discussing an eating disorder with a friend or family member, p. 475.

6. Explain the three components of the female athlete triad and explain how they are interconnected, pp. 483–484.

7. Discuss ways of preventing the development of eating disorders and disordered eating, pp. 487–488.

Test Yourself True or False

1. Only females get eating disorders. **T or F**

2. No one ever recovers from an eating disorder. **T or F**

3. Anorexia nervosa has one primary cause. **T or F**

4. Disordered eating behaviours may lead to the development of a true eating disorder. **T or F**

5. Obesity can be associated with an eating disorder. **T or F**

Test Yourself answers can be found at the end of the chapter.

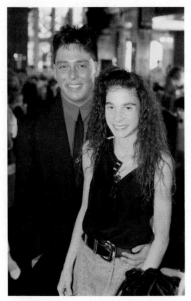

Former gymnast Christy Henrich and her fiancé, a year before she died.

In 1988, at age 16, gymnast Christy Henrich bragged to her coach that she could exist on three apples a day. In 1994, she died. A national champion, Henrich failed to make the 1988 Olympic team. During a critique session, a United States judge told her that, at 1.5 metres (4'11") tall and 44.5 kg or 98 pounds, she was too fat. Following that remark, she began restricting her food intake and exercising obsessively. Laxative abuse and forced vomiting soon followed. Her weight fell so dramatically that, a year later, her coach insisted she begin counselling with a psychotherapist and nutritionist. When she stopped attending the sessions, he removed her from the team. Her weight then plummeted to a low of 21.3 kg or 47 pounds, despite repeated hospital stays of several months and the loving concern of her fiancé, parents, coaches, and friends. In July of 1994, she suffered multiple organ failure, slipped into a coma, and died. When she heard of Henrich's death, Olympic gymnast Cathy Rigby, who twice suffered heart attacks during her own 12-year battle with eating disorders, burst into tears. Rigby called gymnastics "fertile ground" for eating disorders, which the American College of Sports Medicine confirms afflict a majority of young women in the sport.

Everybody knows that food is essential for life, so why would anyone stop eating? When does normal dieting cross the line into disordered eating? Are there any early warning signs that would tip you off that a friend was crossing that line? If you noticed the signs in one of your friends or teammates, would you confront him or her? If so, what would you say?

This chapter will discuss the continuum of eating behaviours and the negative consequences of moving from normal to disordered to abnormal eating behaviours. First, we describe eating behaviours and body image as a continuum. We then discuss specific eating disorders and disordered eating behaviours that commonly occur in adolescents and adults, including the female athlete triad. We will also discuss the various treatment options available to those with an eating disorder. Finally, we will look at ways to prevent eating disorders and disordered eating.

Eating Behaviours Occur on a Continuum

Over the past 20 years, food availability and lifestyle choices have changed dramatically, making it more difficult to describe "normal eating behaviours." The days of a nuclear family sitting down to a home-cooked meal together every evening at 6:00 p.m. seem part of our culture's distant past. Nowadays, our schedules are crammed with classes, jobs, and activities, and our meals are often packaged or eaten out. Skipping meals, eating at odd times, and trying a variety of fad diets are all behaviours commonly accepted as normal. So when does normal eating in a disorderly life cross over into disordered eating or a medically diagnosed eating disorder?

This question is tricky to answer because eating behaviours occur on a *continuum,* a spectrum that can't be divided neatly into parts. An example is a rainbow—where exactly does the red end and the orange begin? Thinking about eating behaviours as a continuum makes it easier to understand how a person could progress from relatively normal eating behaviours to a pattern that is disordered. For instance, let's say that for several years you've skipped breakfast in favour of a midmorning snack, but now you find yourself avoiding the cafeteria until early afternoon. Is this normal? To answer that question, you'd need to consider your feelings about food and your **body image**—the way you perceive your body.

Take a moment to study the Eating Issues and Body Image Continuum in Figure 13.1. Which of the five columns best describes your feelings about food and your body? If you find yourself identifying with the statements on the left side of the continuum, you probably have few issues with food or body image. Most likely you accept your body size and view food as a normal part of maintaining your health and fuelling your daily physical activity. As you progress to the right side of the continuum, food and body image become bigger issues, with food restriction becoming the norm. If you identify with the statements on the far right, you are probably afraid of

body image A person's perception of his or her body's appearance and functioning.

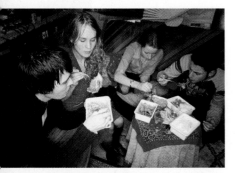

Hectic schedules often force us to grab a quick meal on the go.

• I am not concerned about what others think regarding what and how much I eat. • When I am upset or depressed I eat whatever I am hungry for without any guilt or shame. • I feel no guilt or shame no matter how much I eat or what I eat. • Food is an important part of my life but only occupies a small part of my time. • I trust my body to tell me what and how much to eat.	• I pay attention to what I eat in order to maintain a healthy body. • I may weigh more than what I like, but I enjoy eating and balance my pleasure with eating with my concern for a healthy body. • I am moderate and flexible in goals for eating well. • I try to follow guidelines for healthy eating.	• I think about food a lot. • I feel I don't eat well most of the time. • It's hard for me to enjoy eating with others. • I feel ashamed when I eat more than others or more than what I feel I should be eating. • I am afraid of getting fat. • I wish I could change how much I want to eat and what I am hungry for.	• I have tried diet pills, laxatives, vomiting, or extra time exercising in order to lose or maintain my weight. • I have fasted or avoided eating for long periods of time in order to lose or maintain my weight. • I feel strong when I can restrict how much I eat. • Eating more than I wanted to makes me feel out of control.	• I regularly stuff myself and then exercise, vomit, and use diet pills or laxatives to get rid of the food or calories. • My friends/family tell me I am too thin. • I am terrified of eating high-fat foods. • When I let myself eat, I have a hard time controlling the amount of food I eat. • I am afraid to eat in front of others.
FOOD IS NOT AN ISSUE	**CONCERNED WELL**	**FOOD PREOCCUPIED/ OBSESSED**	**DISRUPTIVE EATING PATTERNS**	**EATING DISORDERED**
BODY OWNERSHIP	**BODY ACCEPTANCE**	**BODY PREOCCUPIED/ OBSESSED**	**DISTORTED BODY IMAGE**	**BODY HATE/ DISASSOCIATION**
• Body image is not an issue for me. • My body is beautiful to me. • My feelings about my body are not influenced by society's concept of an ideal body shape. • I know that the significant others in my life will always find me attractive. • I trust my body to find the weight it needs to be at so I can move and feel confident of my physical body.	• I base my body image equally on social norms and my own self-concept. • I pay attention to my body and my appearance because it is important to me, but it only occupies a small part of my day. • I nourish my body so it has the strength and energy to achieve my physical goals. • I am able to assert myself and maintain a healthy body without losing my self-esteem.	• I spend a significant time viewing my body in the mirror. • I spend a significant time comparing my body to others. • I have days when I feel fat. • I am preoccupied with my body. • I accept society's ideal body shape and size as the best body shape and size. • I'd be more attractive if I was thinner, more muscular, etc...	• I spend a significant amount of time exercising and dieting to change my body. • My body shape and size keeps me from dating or finding someone who will treat me the way I want to be treated. • I have considered changing or have changed my body shape and size through surgical means so I can accept myself. • I wish I could change the way I look in the mirror.	• I often feel separated and distant from my body—as if it belongs to someone else. • I hate my body and I often isolate myself from others. • I don't see anything positive or even neutral about my body shape and size. • I don't believe others when they tell me I look OK. • I hate the way I look in the mirror.

Figure 13.1 The Eating Issues and Body Image Continuum. The progression from normal eating to eating disorders occurs on a continuum. People whose responses fall to the far left of the continuum have normal eating patterns and do not suffer from an eating disorder. People whose responses fall to the far right of the continuum most likely suffer from an eating disorder, such as anorexia nervosa or bulimia nervosa.
(Smiley/King/Avoy: Campus Health Service. Original Continuum, C. Shlaalak: Preventive Medicine and Public Health. Copyright © 1997 Arizona Board of Regents. Used with permission.)

eating and dislike your body. If so, what can you do to begin to move toward the left side of the continuum? How can you begin to develop a more healthful approach to food selection and to view your body in a more positive light? Before you can begin to find solutions, you need to understand the many complex factors that contribute to eating disorders and disordered eating and the differences between these terms.

What Is the Difference Between an Eating Disorder and Disordered Eating?

The media, consumers, and health professionals frequently use the terms *eating disorder* and *disordered eating* interchangeably. Do they mean the same thing? The answer is no! An **eating disorder** is a psychiatric condition that must be diagnosed

eating disorder A psychiatric disorder that must be clinically diagnosed by a physician and is characterized by severe disturbances in body image and eating behaviours. Anorexia nervosa and bulimia nervosa are two examples of eating disorders for which specific diagnostic criteria must be present for diagnosis.

by a physician and involves extreme body dissatisfaction and long-term eating patterns that negatively affect body functioning. The behaviours of someone with an eating disorder typically include severe food restriction, obsessive exercising, self-induced vomiting, and/or laxative abuse. Before a physician can diagnose an eating disorder, the patient's condition and behaviour must meet specific diagnostic criteria outlined by the American Psychiatric Association's (APA) *Diagnostic and Statistical Manual of Mental Disorders* (*DSM-IV-TR*) (APA 2000a).

It is estimated that approximately 3% of Canadian women will develop an eating disorder at some point in their lives (Health Canada 2002). The three most commonly diagnosed clinical eating disorders are anorexia nervosa, bulimia nervosa, and eating disorders—not otherwise specified.

- *Anorexia nervosa* is a potentially life-threatening eating disorder that is characterized by self-starvation, which eventually leads to severe nutrient deficiencies.

- *Bulimia nervosa* is characterized by recurrent episodes of extreme overeating and compensatory behaviours to prevent weight gain, such as self-induced vomiting, misusing of laxatives, fasting, or exercising excessively.

- *ED-NOS* is an acronym for "eating disorders—not otherwise specified." This cluster of symptoms and behaviours is diagnosed in an estimated 30% to 50% of all people seeking treatment for eating disorders. Although sometimes called *subclinical eating disorders,* ED-NOS can significantly impair an individual's health and daily functioning. *Binge-eating disorder* is a type of ED-NOS that shares some characteristics with bulimia nervosa but also has important differences.

A recent study conducted in Ontario estimated that 0.3% of men and 2.1% of women between the ages of 15 and 64 years had either anorexia nervosa or bulimia nervosa (Health Canada 2002). People admitted to hospitals for eating disorders stay an average of 27.5 days, or almost one month, and the hospitalization rates are highest among adolescents aged 10 to 19 with eating disorders. Both disorders will be discussed in detail later in the chapter.

disordered eating A general term used to describe a variety of abnormal or atypical eating behaviours that are used to keep or maintain a lower body weight. Individuals with disordered eating behaviours do not have severe enough eating disturbances to be medically diagnosed with an eating disorder, such as anorexia nervosa or bulimia nervosa. The designation of "eating disorders not otherwise specified" is the medical term used to describe these individuals.

In contrast, **disordered eating** is a general term used to describe a variety of abnormal or atypical eating behaviours that people use to meet their body size or image goals, regardless of whether or not these goals are realistic or achievable. People with disordered eating spend an inordinate amount of time thinking about food—what they are or are not going to eat—and engaging in behaviours to change their weight, shape, or size. These behaviours may be as simple as going on and off diets or as extreme as refusing to eat any high-fat foods. Such behaviours don't usually continue for long enough to make the person seriously ill, and they do not significantly disrupt the person's normal routine. In fact, most people who engage in disordered eating behaviours periodically don't consider what they're doing as abnormal. However, sometimes such behaviours disturb people enough to cause them to seek medical care.

> **Recap:** Eating behaviours occur along a continuum from normal to somewhat abnormal to disordered. Our feelings about food and our body images influence our eating behaviours. True eating disorders are psychiatric conditions characterized by long-term behaviour patterns that negatively affect body functioning, whereas disordered eating is a more general term applicable to any of a variety of abnormal or atypical eating behaviours that may not seriously impair health or functioning.

What Factors Contribute to the Development of Eating Disorders?

The factors that result in the development of an eating disorder are very complex, but research indicates that they can be grouped into two main categories: (1) genetic and biological factors, including personality and psychological traits, and

Table 13.1 Risk Factors That May Contribute to the Development of an Eating Disorder

Psychological Factors	Interpersonal Factors	Genetic and Social Factors	Biological Factors*
Low self-esteem Feelings of inadequacy or lack of control over life Depression, anxiety, anger, or loneliness	Troubled family and personal relationships Difficulty expressing emotions and feelings History of being teased or ridiculed based on size or weight History of physical or sexual abuse	Cultural pressures to be thin and the high value placed on a "perfect body" Narrow definitions of beauty that include only women and men of a certain body size Cultural norms that value people on the basis of physical appearances and not inner qualities and strengths	Chemical imbalances that control hunger, appetite, and digestion Possible gene or set of genes that predisposes an individual

* These factors are still under investigation.

Source: Adapted from National Eating Disorders Association (NEDA), *Causes of Eating Disorders,* © 2002. Used with permission. Available at www.nationaleatingdisorders.org/p.asp?WebPage_ID5322&Profile_ID541144 (accessed April 2004).

(2) environmental factors, such as family environment, interpersonal relationships and interactions, and social factors. Table 13.1 outlines examples of risk factors and characteristics in each of these categories.

Genetic and Biological Factors

If eating disorders are to be prevented, researchers must understand their causes. A variety of research efforts are currently focusing on the roles of genetics, biological factors, and personality traits.

Genetic Factors

Overall, the diagnosis of anorexia nervosa and bulimia nervosa is several times more common in biological relatives who also have the diagnosis than in the general population (Strober and Bulik 2002). This observation would imply that existence of some mechanism of transmission of the disease occurs within families; however, it is difficult to separate the impact of genetic and environmental components in many studies.

One way to address this issue is to look at the incidence of eating disorders in identical twins who were raised in different families. If genetics plays a significant role in this disease, then if one twin has an eating disorder, it would be highly likely that the other twin would have an eating disorder as well. In this way, the influence of genetics can be separated out from the influence of the environment. Research from the twin studies suggests that genetics is a factor but not the only determining cause of anorexia nervosa. Specifically, researchers found that genetics explained about 50% to 75% of the variability for anorexia nervosa in identical twins (Klump et al. 2002). This means that if one twin develops anorexia nervosa, there is a 50% to 75% chance that the other twin will also develop an eating disorder, even if they are raised in different households.

The same approach has been used to look at bulimia nervosa. Researchers found that if one twin has bulimia nervosa, there is a strong possibility that the other twin will also have bulimia nervosa, but the genetic link is not as strong as it is for anorexia nervosa. With bulimia nervosa, the environment in which an individual lives also plays a significant role in the development of the disorder (Klump et al. 2002).

Researchers now have strong evidence suggesting that a specific gene or sets of genes may influence the development of eating disorders, but more research is needed to confirm the theory and identify the genes involved. See the Highlight box "Biology May Cause Most Anorexia" to learn more about this research.

Biological Factors

Biological factors may play a role in the development of eating disorders, although this hypothesis is also under investigation. Currently, researchers are looking at imbalances in the chemicals that control hunger, appetite, and digestion. Among these are hormones produced in the central nervous system, such as serotonin, dopamine, and cholecystokinin, and ghrelin, a polypeptide released from the stomach and small intestine (Bailor and Kaye 2003; Tanaka et al. 2003).

One area of ongoing research examines the role that serotonin plays in explaining the biological mechanisms underlying the eating behaviours of individuals with either anorexia or bulimia nervosa (Attia 2003). Serotonin is a neurotransmitter that helps regulate appetite, with high levels of serotonin enhancing satiety and reducing food consumption (Kaye et al. 2003). The amino acid tryptophan is a precursor used in the synthesis of serotonin. It has been hypothesized that individuals with eating disorders may have altered production of serotonin compared with people without eating disorders (Bulik and Tozzi 2004). In these individuals, serotonin production may be higher because the excessive amounts of tryptophan may cross the blood-brain barrier after the person has eaten. It is also thought that this increased serotonin production may contribute to the changes in mood common in individuals with anorexia nervosa, such as anxiety. When food is restricted, less tryptophan is available for serotonin production, and these mood changes are less noticeable (Kaye et al. 2003). Whether or not serotonin plays a role in the development and persistence of anorexia nervosa is still not clear (Attia 2003).

Personality Traits

Researchers have long been interested in the question of whether certain personalities predispose people to the development of an eating disorder. In this context, personality is usually thought of as an inherited trait that runs in families. The reverse question has also been asked: Does an eating disorder modify personality traits, making changes in personality a consequence of the disorder instead of a cause?

Research suggests that people with anorexia nervosa have high rates of obsessive-compulsive disorder (OCD), which is an inherited illness characterized by intrusive thoughts or compulsions to repeat certain behaviours in a certain way (Lilenfeld et al. 2005). The higher incidence of OCD occurs not only in individuals with eating disorders but also in their families. For example, one child may have anorexia nervosa while another child has OCD.

Other personality traits associated with anorexia nervosa are perfectionism, drive for thinness, difficulty with social interactions, compliance, and emotional restraint (Lilenfeld et al. 2005, Wonderlich 2002). Unfortunately, many studies observe these behaviours only in individuals who are very ill and in a state of starvation, which may affect personality. Thus, it is difficult to determine if personality is the cause or effect of the disorder. For example, research shows that perfectionism is high in malnourished individuals and takes a long time to change after recovery (Wonderlich 2002). In contrast to individuals with anorexia nervosa, individuals with bulimia nervosa tend to be more impulsive, have low self-esteem, and demonstrate an extroverted, erratic personality style that seeks attention and admiration. For example, a comparison of diaries kept by individuals with bulimia nervosa and healthy controls indicated that those with bulimia nervosa showed greater self-criticism and deterioration in mood following a stressful interpersonal interaction (Steiger, Lehoux, and Gauvin 1999). In individuals with bulimia nervosa, negative moods are more likely to cause overeating than food restriction (Wonderlich 2002). Finally, individuals with bulimia nervosa are more likely to practise substance abuse and suffer from anxiety disorders.

Environmental Factors

Researchers have long suspected that an individual may have a genetic predisposition for an eating disorder that is not manifested until the environment triggers or activates

▶ **HIGHLIGHT**

Biology May Cause Most Anorexia: Scientists Now Believe Genes Account for up to 70 Percent of Risk of Developing the Disease

The insidious voice of anorexia nervosa is the most deadly of psychiatric disorders.

Yet contrary to dominant thinking about the condition for the past two decades, this slow slide into starvation is not about aspiring to a cultural ideal and becoming supermodel skinny. Other eating disorders, including bulimia nervosa, may be largely influenced by our culture's obsession with thinness. But scientists now say anorexia, which kills up to 15 per cent of those it afflicts, is likely rooted in a person's genes. And though environment does play a role, researchers believe a genetic predisposition for anorexia outweighs any psychological or cultural factors, and can account for up to 70 per cent of the risk for developing the disorder.

But perhaps the biggest clue that biology trumps culture is the fact that the incidence of anorexia has not changed dramatically in the past 30 years. Rates of bulimia, on the other hand, have risen sharply over the same period, along with societal pressure to be thin.

Cynthia Bulik, a professor of nutrition and director of the eating disorders program at the University of North Carolina at Chapel Hill, says a core of researchers have long believed anorexia has genetic origins—even before scientific studies bore out their theory. "These patients are not choosing this behaviour," says Bulik, who's considered an international expert on the disorder. "You could go to any eating disorder clinic around the world and the core clinical picture would be identical. There may be different cultural presentations or variations on the packaging, but the core signs of low body weight, an extreme drive for thinness, amenorrhea (absence of menstruation) and often hyperactivity and anxiety just jump out at you as saying this is biological in origin."

Right now there is no effective drug protocol, and doctors mainly try to help patients gain—and maintain—weight, says Dr. Allan Kaplan, head of the eating disorders program at Toronto General Hospital, part of the University Health Network. Developing new therapies based on genetic research will likely take years, but Kaplan says understanding the role of genes will help ease the guilt and stigma that afflict patients and their families. Sometimes parents feel responsible for their child's eating disorder or are accused of bad parenting.

Patients, meanwhile, may blame themselves for their condition. There is the long-held idea that anorexia is a self-imposed affliction, Kaplan observes—that people just need to "pull up their socks," to get better. Many people—even some medical professionals—get angry over a child or young adult's refusal to eat, seeing the patient as "a manipulative, kind of spoiled brat kid who is just acting out. When somebody says, 'I'm not eating' and they're 80 pounds and it's obvious that if they don't eat, they are going to die, this gets people very angry. They think, 'How hard is it to take food and put it on your fork and put it in your mouth.'"

Scientists first started to investigate whether biology was a factor in anorexia in the 1980s, after observing that identical twins, who share 100 per cent of their genes, were more likely to both get the disorder than non-identical, or fraternal, twins, who share only a portion of DNA. That led to family studies in the 1990s, in which investigators found that a person is more likely to have anorexia if she has a close relative who's affected. But it was unclear whether the increased risk was due to genetic predisposition or environmental factors, such as a child watching a mother obsessively diet, says Bulik.

To tease out that critical difference, researchers turned back to studying identical twins in very large groups, and found the chance of both twins having anorexia if one is afflicted was close to 60 per cent. In fraternal twins, that chance dropped to 10 per cent.

In the mid-1990s, a private foundation in Europe financed research to locate the specific region on the human genome that gives rise to anorexia. That effort, from data collected across Canada, Germany, Italy and the U.S., pinpointed the hotspot on chromosome 1.

Another genetic-linkage study, this one funded by the U.S. National Institute of Mental Health (NIMH), is wrapping up this spring. The five-year, $10-million study brings together 11 research groups, including Kaplan's at Toronto General, to analyze DNA samples from families with two or more members with anorexia.

So far, two genes have been identified, one associated with serotonin (a neurotransmitter that controls mood and appetite) and the other with opioid receptors (which modulate pain), says Bulik, who was involved with the NIMH study.

(Continued)

Bulik attributes the lack of attention to "the plausibility [of] the socio-cultural explanation" for anorexia. "It's so easy to believe, because we're so surrounded by these cultural pressures for thinness, that these (people with anorexia) are just vain people who are trying to diet down to reach some societal ideal. That plausibility hits you in the face when you're in the checkout line in your supermarket."

Experts stress anorexia is a complex disorder that can't be entirely explained by genetics, and not by just one or two genes. Unlike cystic fibrosis, for example, which is caused by a mutation on a single gene, anorexia is likely due to the interaction of a number of genes with a number of environmental factors.

Someone with a genetic predisposition for anorexia may be at higher risk for developing the disorder, much like someone with a family history of breast cancer. But that genetic risk does not guarantee a person will get anorexia, says Walter Kaye, the scientist who co-helmed both genetic studies of anorexia and who holds a joint professorship of psychiatry at the University of California at San Diego and the University of Pittsburgh. Environmental factors, including pressure to be thin, can trigger the underlying risk, he believes.

Kaplan suggests parents who have a strong history of anorexia in their families take some preventive measures: they should avoid talking about people's weight or shape, having diet products in the house or labelling foods as either good or bad. Self-esteem, he adds, has to be kept separate from weight and appearance, and even from successes at school or in sports.

Kaplan even suggests that a young girl who, for example, has a mother with anorexia or a father with some of the temperamental traits of compulsivity or perfectionism should not participate in activities that focus on shape, including competitive gymnastics or ballet.

Source: M. Ogilvie, Biology May Cause Most Anorexia. *Toronto Star.* Available from - http://healthzone.ca/health/article/413989 (accessed April 13, 2008). Reprinted with permission. Torstar Syndication Services.

the behaviour. One question that has puzzled scientists who study eating disorders is "Why does one sibling develop an eating disorder while a twin or other siblings in the home do not develop an eating disorder?" If individuals share the same genetic background and environment, wouldn't the incidence of an eating disorder be similar between siblings and twins?

One explanation is that the environment within families can be divided into shared and unshared experiences. This means that siblings within the same home may actually have very different experiences. Parents may treat children differently, siblings may treat each other differently, and how children respond to experiences within the home may be different. For example, one child may find a disruptive, chaotic family environment stressful, whereas that child's sibling may not be bothered by it. In addition, one child may have different environmental experiences outside the home than his or her sibling does.

Research now shows that the unshared environment, either within or outside the family, may play a role in the development of the disease in 20% to 40% of the individuals diagnosed with either anorexia nervosa or bulimia nervosa. In addition, it appears that for individuals diagnosed with anorexia nervosa, genetics and unshared environmental experiences are the best predictors of who develops the disease (Klump et al. 2002). Thus, identical twins who share genetic and family environments do not always both develop anorexia nervosa because unshared experiences may be very different.

Family Environment

Most of us recognize that family conditioning influences our eating behaviours. During childhood, our parents and other family members provided most of the food we ate, limiting our choices and influencing our developing concept of how much food to eat, when, how often, and so forth. As we grew, our

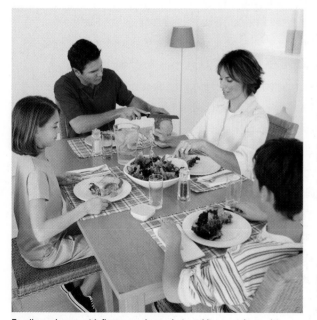

Family environment influences when, what, and how much we eat.

families developed unique mealtime rituals. For example, perhaps your family never sat down together at a meal, and you were responsible for getting your own meals. Or perhaps your family insisted on a shared mealtime, and one family member was responsible for preparing the meal for the whole family. We also had experiences that caused us to associate food with particular family members or shared activities. Maybe you really like hot oatmeal with brown sugar and raisins on winter days because your grandmother prepared this for you when you visited for the holidays. Because of such family patterns, rituals, and associations, our response to food and our eating behaviours are to some extent conditioned. Thus, it is not difficult to believe that the family eating environment might contribute to the development of an eating disorder.

Researchers have examined a number of family-related factors to determine whether or not they contribute to the development of eating disorders. Currently, there are no data to suggest that family size or birth order is influential. Research on siblings, however, does show a greater likelihood of developing an eating disorder if a sibling also has an eating disorder. The precise reason for this is unclear. Family structure and patterns of interaction have also been implicated. Based on observational studies, compared with families without an anorexic member, families with an anorexic member show more rigidity in their family structure, less clear interpersonal boundaries, and a tendency to avoid open discussions on topics of disagreement. In contrast, families with a member diagnosed with bulimia nervosa have a less stable family organization, are less nurturing, and more angry and disruptive than other families (Vandereycken 2002). In addition, childhood physical or sexual abuse can increase the risk of an eating disorder developing in a child (Patrick 2002). In short, family conditioning, structure, and patterns of interaction, including abuse, can influence the development of an eating disorder.

Unrealistic Media Images

Every day we are confronted with advertisements in which computer-enhanced images of lean, beautiful women promote everything from beer to cars. Most adult men and women understand that these images are unrealistic, but adolescents, who are still developing a sense of their identity and body image, lack the same ability to distance themselves from what they see (Steinberg 2002). Adolescent girls are likely to compare themselves unfavourably with these "perfect" female bodies and to develop a negative body image as a result. In examining the impact of media on how women and girls view their bodies, researchers carefully studied the research literature over the past 22 years (Groesz, Levine, and Murnen 2002). They found that females had more negative feelings about their bodies after they viewed images of thin models than they did after viewing average-size or plus-size models. This effect was stronger in women under age 20 than in older women. Because body image influences eating behaviours, the barrage of media models may be contributing to an increase in dieting behaviours, which may lead to an eating disorder. Unfortunately, scientific evidence demonstrating whether the media is *causing* increased eating disorders is difficult to obtain.

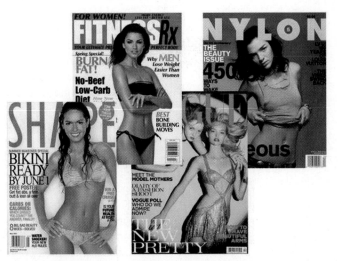

Sociocultural Values

Evidence suggesting that Western sociocultural values contribute to eating disorders is also hard to deny. For instance, consider the fact that eating disorders are significantly more common in white females in Western societies than in other women worldwide. This may be due in part to our culture's valuing of slenderness, not only for aesthetic reasons but also because Westerners tend to consider it as an indication that the person is self-disciplined,

Photos of celebrities or models are often airbrushed or altered to enhance their physical appearance. Unfortunately, many people believe that these are accurate images and strive to reach this unrealistic image of physical beauty.

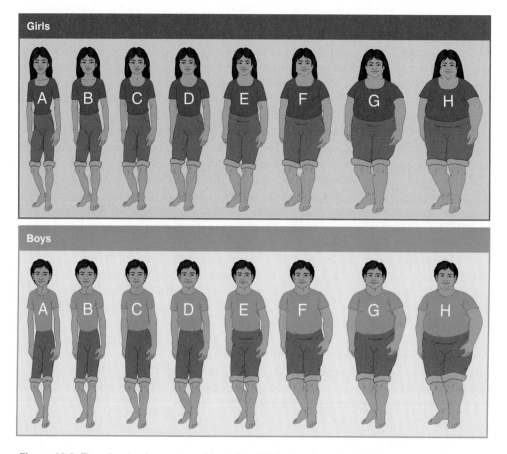

Figure 13.2 These line drawings were used in studies of Native American schoolchildren to assess levels of body dissatisfaction in this population.
(J. Stevens, M. Story, A. Becenti, S. A. French, J. Gittelsohn, S. B. Going, Juhaeri, S. Levin, and D. M. Murray, Weight-related attitudes and behaviors in fourth grade American Indian children, 1999, *Obesity Research* 7:34–42.)

a generally valued characteristic. Westerners also associate slenderness with health and often with wealth. In contrast, until quite recently the prevailing view in developing societies has been that excess body fat is desirable as a sign of wealth.

Recent research among Native American children illustrates that body dissatisfaction and desire for thinness are more common in this population than previously assumed. Rural (Davis and Lambert 2000; Stevens et al. 1999) and urban (Rinderknecht and Smith 2002) Native American children were asked to rate their own satisfaction with their bodies by using the images shown in Figure 13.2. In all of these studies, girls reported higher rates of body dissatisfaction than boys, and overweight children more often chose a thinner body size as more desirable. Surprisingly, 38% to 61% of children in grade 4 and grade 5 reported already trying to lose weight at this young age.

Only limited research has examined the prevalence of eating disorders in non-white populations and in non-Western cultures; thus, we have a lot to learn about how culture affects the development of eating disorders. However, as cross-cultural interactions increase, some researchers hypothesize that non-Western cultures will adapt Western norms for beauty, and this may increase the development of eating disorders in those cultures.

The members of society with whom we most often interact—our family members, friends, teachers, and co-workers—also influence the way we see ourselves. Their comments related to our body weight or shape can be particularly hurtful—enough so to cause some people to start down the path of disordered eating. For example, individuals with bulimia nervosa report that they perceived greater pressure from their peers to be thin than controls, while research shows that peer teasing about weight increases body dissatisfaction and eating disturbances (Stice 2002). Thus, our comments to others regarding their weight do count.

Recap: A number of factors are thought to influence the development of eating disorders. These include genetic and biological factors as well as environment—our family environment, the media, society, and culture. However, the combination of factors triggering the development of an eating disorder in any individual is probably unique.

What Does an Eating Disorder Look Like?

An eating disorder can be defined as a "persistent disturbance of eating behaviour which significantly impairs physical health or psychosocial functioning" (Fairburn and Walsh 2002). This section discusses anorexia nervosa, bulimia nervosa, and ED-NOS.

Anorexia Nervosa Is a Potentially Deadly Eating Disorder

Anorexia nervosa is a medical disorder in which an individual uses a number of unhealthful practices to maintain a body weight less than 85% of expected, as based on height and weight. Canadian data suggest that between 0.5% and 4% of women will be diagnosed with anorexia nervosa sometime during their lives (Health Canada 2002). According to the American Psychiatric Association (APA 1994), 90% to 95% of individuals with anorexia nervosa are young girls or women. Approximately 0.5% to 1% of U.S. females develop anorexia, and between 5% and 20% of these will die from complications of the disorder within 10 years of initial diagnosis (Patrick 2002). These statistics make anorexia nervosa the most common and deadly psychiatric disorder diagnosed in women and the leading cause of death in females between the ages of 15 and 24 years (Patrick 2002). Anorexia nervosa also occurs in males, but the prevalence is much lower than in females (Robb and Dadson 2002).

Characteristics of Anorexia Nervosa

For people who develop anorexia nervosa, the trigger factors that initiated the disorder may differ widely, but the results are the same: extremely restrictive eating practices that lead to self-starvation. These individuals have such an intense drive for thinness and need for weight loss that they may fast completely, restrict energy intake to only a few Calories per day, or eliminate all but one or two food groups from their diet. They also have an intense fear of weight gain or becoming fat, even though they are underweight. In anorexic individuals, small amounts of weight gain (e.g., one kilogram or two pounds) trigger high stress and anxiety. Finally, **amenorrhea** (no menstrual periods for at least three months) is a feature of anorexia nervosa in females. *Primary amenorrhea* occurs when a girl has not yet begun to menstruate by age 16, even though she has secondary sex characteristics; *secondary amenorrhea* is the absence of a menstrual period for three or more months after menarche. It occurs when a young woman consumes insufficient energy to maintain normal body functions.

The *DSM-IV-TR* (APA 2000a) identifies the following diagnostic criteria for anorexia nervosa:

- Refusal to eat adequate amounts of energy to maintain body weight at or above a minimally normal weight for age and height

- Intense fear of gaining weight or becoming fat, even though considered underweight by all medical criteria

- Disturbance in the way in which one's body weight or shape is experienced, undue influence of body weight or shape on self-evaluation, or denial of the seriousness of the current low body weight

- Amenorrhea in females who are past puberty. Amenorrhea is defined as the absence of at least three consecutive menstrual cycles. A woman is considered to have amenorrhea if her periods occur only when given hormones, such as estrogen or oral contraceptives.

anorexia nervosa A serious, potentially life-threatening eating disorder that is characterized by self-starvation, which eventually leads to a deficiency in energy and essential nutrients that are required by the body to function normally. For an individual to be considered to have anorexia nervosa, he or she must be medically diagnosed by a physician and meet specific diagnostic criteria.

amenorrhea The absence of a menstrual period. Primary amenorrhea is the absence of menstruation by the age of 16 years in a girl who has secondary sex characteristics, while secondary amenorrhea is the absence of the menstrual period for three or more months after menarche. The presence of amenorrhea is a criterion for the diagnosis of anorexia nervosa in females.

Table 13.2   Behavioural, Emotional, Mental, and Physical Signs of Anorexia Nervosa

Behavioural Signs	Emotional and Mental Signs	Physical Signs
Difficulty eating with others, lying about eating	Depression and social isolation (e.g., withdrawal from usual friends and avoiding any social situations where food is being served)	Low body weight (15% or more below what is expected for age, height, activity level)
Frequently weighing self; measuring food portions, calculating energy intake or fat grams	Strong need to be in control; rigid and inflexible	Lack of energy, fatigue, muscle weakness because of low energy intakes and malnutrition
Development of food rituals, such as eating foods in a certain order, excessive chewing, or rearranging food on the plate	Decreased interest in sex or fears around sex	Decreased balance and unsteady gait due to loss of muscle tissue and bone density
Refusal to eat certain foods, such as carbohydrates, fats, or foods of a particular colour	Low sense of self-worth—uses weight as a measure of worth	Lowered body temperature, blood pressure, and pulse rate and irregular heartbeat caused by malnutrition, poor maintenance of blood electrolytes, and loss of body fat and lean tissue
Avoidance of mealtimes or other situations involving food	Difficulty expressing feelings; afraid to discuss their food and body issues with others	
Excessive, rigid exercise regimen	Perfectionistic—strives to be the neatest, thinnest, or smartest person in the group	Tingling in hands and feet because of poor circulation
Frequent comments revealing disgust with body size or shape and focusing on parts of the body that are not perfect (e.g., buttocks, thighs, stomach)	Difficulty thinking clearly or concentrating because of malnutrition and poor energy intake	Thinning hair or hair loss, lanugo (downy growth of body hair) because of poor nutrition
Distortion of body size (e.g., feels fat even though others tell them they are too thin)	Irritability, denial—believes others are overreacting to their low weight or energy restriction	
Denial of hunger	Insomnia	

Do you know anyone who might have anorexia nervosa? How can you determine if they have this eating disorder? Table 13.2 lists behavioural, emotional, mental, and physical signs of anorexia nervosa that you might look for in someone you suspect may have this disorder. Remember, one person may not display all these characteristics, but you may observe one or two characteristics in each category.

Health Risks of Anorexia Nervosa

Left untreated, anorexia nervosa eventually leads to a deficiency in energy and other nutrients that are required by the body to function normally. During this period of self-imposed starvation, the body will use stored fat and lean tissue (e.g., organ and muscle tissue) as energy sources to maintain brain tissue and vital body functions. The body will also shut down or reduce non-vital body functions to conserve energy. For example, the menstrual cycle will stop, thus conserving the energy required for normal periods and eliminating the chance of pregnancy during a period when there are inadequate nutrients to support a growing fetus. In children and adolescents, growth slows or stops because the body does not have enough energy to support the formation of new tissue.

In addition, people with anorexia nervosa may have many of the following health problems (Figure 13.3). The severity of these problems will depend on the length of time they have had the disorder and the degree of weight loss that has occurred:

- Electrolyte imbalances—Imbalances in sodium, potassium, calcium, magnesium, and other electrolytes can lead to irregular heartbeats, heart failure, and death. The role of electrolytes in our health is discussed in detail in Chapter 7.

- Cardiovascular problems—Slowed heart rate, low blood pressure, dizziness, and fainting can all occur as a result of starvation.

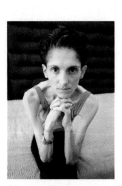
People with anorexia nervosa experience an extreme drive for thinness, resulting in potentially fatal weight loss.

- Gastrointestinal problems—The gastrointestinal tract can become weak and lose its ability to function. These changes result in irritable bowel syndrome, constipation, loss of peristalsis (the wavelike movements of the gastrointestinal tract that push food through the tract), and delayed emptying of food from the intestines. People with anorexia nervosa frequently complain of stomach pain.

- Bone problems—The malnutrition that accompanies starvation can deprive the body of bone-building nutrients such as calcium, magnesium, vitamins D and K, and protein. The amenorrhea that occurs is associated with a decrease in estrogen production, which causes poor bone health and can lead to osteoporosis (see Chapter 9).

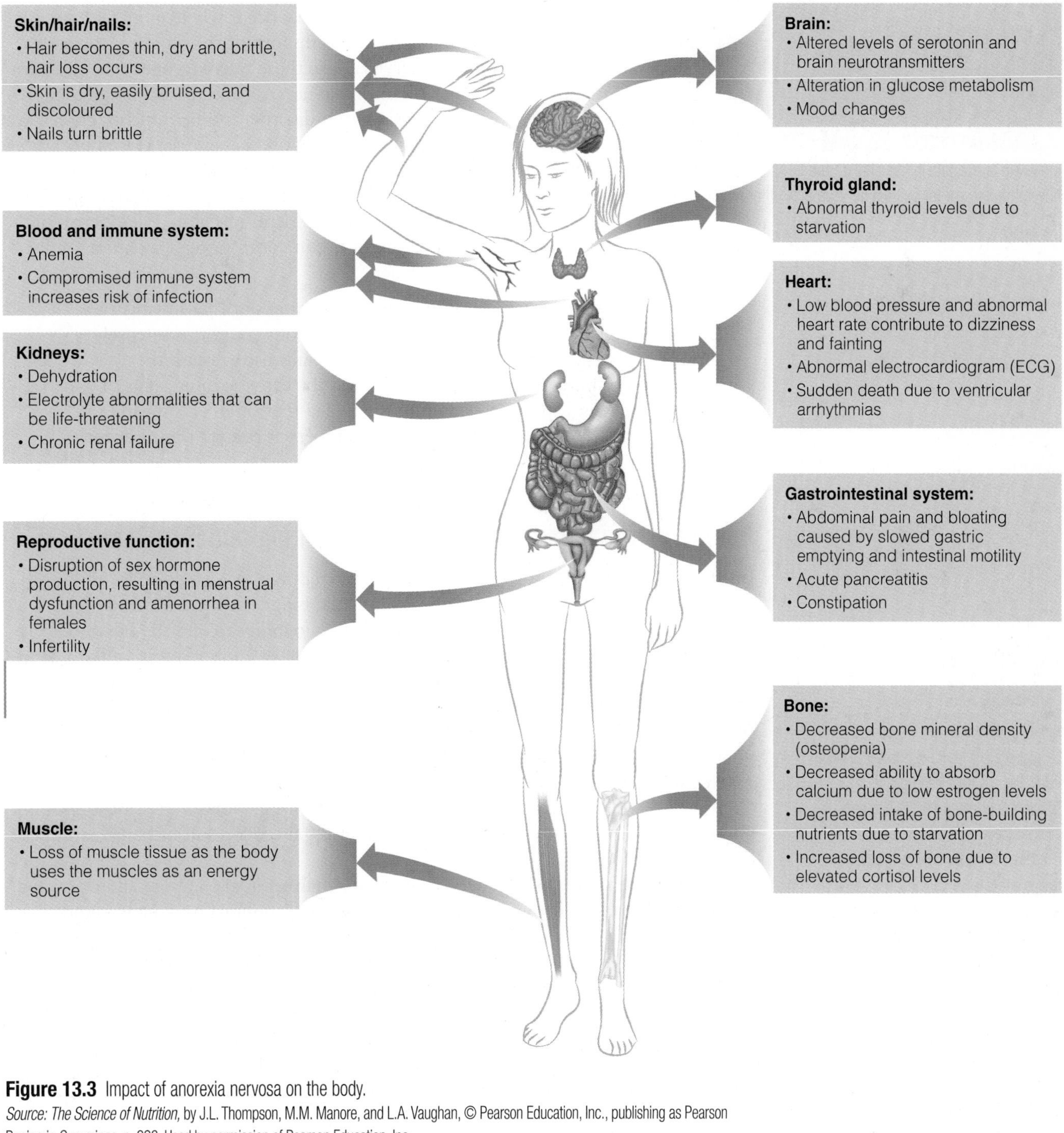

Figure 13.3 Impact of anorexia nervosa on the body.

Source: The Science of Nutrition, by J.L. Thompson, M.M. Manore, and L.A. Vaughan, © Pearson Education, Inc., publishing as Pearson Benjamin Cummings, p. 628. Used by permission of Pearson Education, Inc.

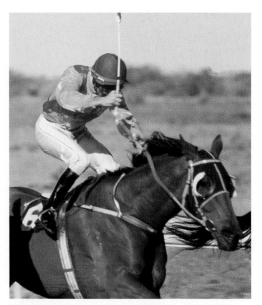

Men who participate in "thin build" sports, such as jockeys, have a higher risk for bulimia nervosa than other men.

- Muscle and organ wasting—The chronic undernutrition that accompanies anorexia nervosa reduces the body's ability to build, maintain, and repair its protein tissues, especially the muscles and organs. Eventually, the body begins to use these tissues as an energy source, which causes organ and muscle wasting, which in turn can lead to organ failure and death.

- Reproduction—Undernutrition causes the body to stop producing reproductive hormones so that pregnancy does not occur.

- Skin, hair, and nails—Deficiencies of protein, lipids, and micronutrients cause the skin to become dry and fragile, hair thins, and nails become brittle.

Because the best chances for recovery occur when an individual receives intensive treatment early, it is important to recognize the early warning signs of anorexia nervosa. Use these warning signs as a guide to help identify those at risk for anorexia nervosa and to encourage them to seek help. Discussing a friend's eating disorder can be difficult, especially if your friend is in denial about having anorexia nervosa. It is important to choose an appropriate time and place to raise your concerns, and to listen closely and with great sensitivity to their feelings. The Highlight box, "Discussing an Eating Disorder with a Friend or Family Member: What Do You Say?" outlines an approach you might use in confronting a friend or family member who might have an eating disorder.

Recap: Anorexia nervosa is a severe, life-threatening disorder in which the person refuses to maintain a minimally normal body weight, is intensely afraid of gaining weight, and exhibits a significant distortion in the perception of body size and shape. Knowing the early warning signs of anorexia nervosa, and understanding the denial that often accompanies it, can help you identify friends and family members at risk for this disorder.

Bulimia Nervosa Is Characterized by Binging and Purging

Bulimia nervosa is an eating disorder characterized by repeated episodes of **binge eating**, followed by some form of **purging**. While binge eating, the person feels a loss of self-control (Garfinkel 2002), including an inability to end the binge once it has started. At the same time, the person feels a sense of euphoria not unlike a drug-induced high. For practical purposes, a binge is usually determined on an individual basis, but generally it is a quantity of food that would be large for the individual, compared with what other people eat, and for the time period and social occasion (Garfinkel 2002). For example, a person may eat a dozen brownies with two litres of ice cream in 30 minutes. Binge episodes occur an average of twice a week or more (APA 1994). An individual with bulimia nervosa typically purges after most episodes, but not necessarily on every occasion, and weight gain as a result of binge eating can be significant.

The prevalence of bulimia nervosa is higher than anorexia nervosa and estimated to affect 0.5% to 4% of women. Like anorexia nervosa, bulimia nervosa is found predominantly in women, with the male–female prevalence ratio ranging from 1:6 to 1:10 (APA 2000b). This means that for every one male diagnosed with bulimia nervosa, six to ten females are diagnosed with this disorder. The mortality rate is much lower than for anorexia nervosa, with 1% of patients dying within 10 years of diagnosis (Patrick 2002). Statistics on bulimia nervosa are somewhat misleading, because about half of anorexic individuals will also be diagnosed with bulimia at some point. Thus, many of the women who die of anorexia nervosa may also have bulimia.

bulimia nervosa A serious eating disorder characterized by recurrent episodes of binge eating and recurrent inappropriate compensatory behaviours (such as self-induced vomiting; misuse of laxatives, diuretics, enemas, or other medications; fasting or excessive exercise) to prevent weight gain.

binge eating Consumption of a large amount of food in a short period, usually accompanied by a feeling of loss of self-control.

purging An attempt to rid the body of unwanted food by vomiting or other compensatory means, such as excessive exercise, fasting, or laxative abuse.

▶ **HIGHLIGHT**

Discussing an Eating Disorder with a Friend or Family Member: What Do You Say?

Background: Before approaching a friend or family member you suspect of having an eating disorder, learn as much as possible about the eating disorder. Make sure you know the difference between the facts and myths about eating disorders. Locate a health professional specializing in eating disorders to whom you can refer your friend, and be ready to go with your friend if he or she does not want to go alone. If you are at a university or college, check with your local health centre to see if it has an eating disorder team or can recommend someone to you. Set the stage for your discussion by finding a relaxed and private setting.

Steps to use in your discussion:

- Schedule a time to talk. Set aside a time and place for a private discussion where you can share your concerns openly and honestly in a caring and supportive way. Make sure the setting is quiet and away from other distractions.

- Communicate your concerns. Share your memories and knowledge of specific times when you felt concerned about your friend's eating or exercise behaviours. Explain that you think these things may indicate that there could be a problem that needs professional attention.

- Ask your friend to explore these concerns with a counsellor, doctor, dietitian, or other health professional who is knowledgeable about eating issues.

- Avoid conflicts or a "battle of the wills" with your friend. If your friend refuses to acknowledge that there is a problem, restate your feelings and the reasons for them and leave yourself open and available as a supportive listener.

- Avoid placing shame, blame, or guilt on your friend regarding his or her actions or attitudes. Do not use accusatory "you" statements, such as, "You just need to eat" or "You are acting irresponsibly." Instead use "I" statements, such as, "I am concerned about you because you refuse to eat breakfast and lunch" or "It makes me afraid when I hear you vomit."

- Avoid giving simple solutions. For example, "If you would just stop, everything would be fine."

- Express your continued support. Remind your friend that you care and want your friend to be healthy and happy.

Source: Adapted from National Eating Disorders Association, Communication: What Should I Say? 2002, www.nationaleatingdisorders.org/p.asp? WebPage_ID5322&Profile_ID541174 (accessed April 2004). Used with permission.

Although the prevalence of bulimia nervosa is much higher in women than men (Robb and Dadson 2002), rates for men are higher in some predominantly thin-build male sports in which participants are encouraged to maintain a low body weight (e.g., horse racing, wrestling, crew, and gymnastics). Individuals in these sports typically do not have all the characteristics of bulimia nervosa, however, and the purging behaviours they practise typically stop once the sport is discontinued.

The binge-purge pattern of disordered eating may begin as an infrequent occurrence in which a person attempts to deal with unwanted food in a social situation. For example, friends are having a pizza party and the person wants to join in but feels guilty about eating so much food. So upon returning home, the person induces vomiting, takes laxatives, or stays up late exercising to burn off the extra energy. What may begin as an isolated incident can develop into a daily event, with purging occurring even after the person has eaten only a small amount of food. Binging and purging behaviours can also be triggered by periods of dieting: depriving ourselves of adequate food and energy for a long period requires tremendous self-control, and when the control fails, such as if the person "cheats" even once, he or she can quickly lose any ability to deal with food rationally and will binge.

Many people with bulimia engage in vomiting as a way of purging unwanted foods. Other methods of purging are laxative or diuretic abuse, enemas, or excessive exercise. For example, after a binge a runner may increase her daily distance to equal the "calculated" energy content of the binge. Some people with bulimia fast for a day

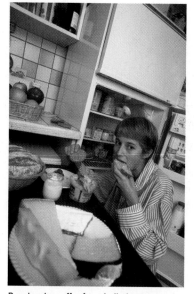

People who suffer from bulimia nervosa can consume relatively large amounts of food in brief periods.

or two until they feel they have compensated for the extra energy from the binge (Garfinkel 2002).

Characteristics of Bulimia Nervosa

As with anorexia nervosa, the *DSM-IV-TR* (APA 2000a) lists diagnostic criteria for bulimia nervosa. These are listed below. Unlike anorexia nervosa, individuals with bulimia nervosa are usually normal weight or overweight, which makes their eating disorder less visible and, thus, easier to hide.

- Recurrent episodes of binge eating (e.g., eating a large amount of food in a short period, such as within two hours)
- Recurrent inappropriate compensatory behaviour to prevent weight gain, such as self-induced vomiting, misuse of laxatives, diuretics, enemas, or other medications, fasting, or excessive exercise
- Binge eating occurs on average at least twice a week for three months
- Body shape and weight unduly influence self-evaluation
- The disturbance does not occur exclusively during episodes of anorexia nervosa. Some individuals will have periods of binge eating and then periods of starvation, which makes classification of their disorder difficult.

How can you tell if a family member or friend has bulimia nervosa? The National Eating Disorders Association (2008), identifies the following early warning signs:

- disappearance of large amounts of food in a short time, or the existence of wrappers or containers indicating the consumption of large amounts of food
- frequent trips to the bathroom after a meal, signs or smells of vomiting, presence of wrappers or packages of laxatives or diuretics
- excessive exercising
- visual signs, such as unusual swelling of the cheeks or jaw area, which is due to the swelling of the salivary glands as they increase saliva production to coat the mouth and esophagus and protect them from stomach acid, calluses on the back of the hands and knuckles from trauma during self-induced vomiting, or discolouration of the teeth from contact with stomach acids
- withdrawal from usual friends and family
- statements and behaviours indicating that weight loss, dieting, and control of food are becoming primary concerns

To learn more about the realities of having bulimia nervosa, refer to the Highlight box "A Day in the Life of a Bulimic."

Health Risks of Bulimia Nervosa

The destructive behaviours of bulimia nervosa can lead to illness and even death. The most common health consequences associated with bulimia nervosa are

- electrolyte imbalance—This can lead to an irregular heartbeat and even heart failure and death. The electrolyte imbalance seen in bulimia nervosa is caused by dehydration and the loss of potassium and sodium from the body with frequent vomiting;
- gastrointestinal problems—Inflammation, ulceration, and possible rupture of the esophagus and stomach from frequent binging and vomiting. Chronic irregular bowel movements and constipation may result in people with bulimia who regularly abuse laxatives;
- dental problems—Tooth decay and staining and mouth sores from stomach acids released during frequent vomiting;

- calluses on the back of the hands and knuckles from self-induced vomiting;
- swelling of the cheeks or jaw area from irritation of the salivary glands and other mouth tissues during recurrent vomiting.

As with anorexia nervosa, the chance of recovery from bulimia nervosa increases, and the negative effects on health decrease, if the disorder is detected at an early stage. Familiarity with the warning signs of bulimia nervosa can help you identify friends and family members who might be at risk.

> **Recap:** Bulimia nervosa is a severe eating disorder characterized by recurrent episodes of binge eating followed by self-induced vomiting or another method of purging (e.g., laxatives, diuretics, excessive exercise, fasting for days after a binge) in an attempt to avoid weight gain. Knowing the early warning signs of bulimia nervosa can help you identify friends and family members who may be at risk.

The precise disordered eating behaviours that can be classified as ED-NOS are not as well defined or well characterized as those involved with anorexia nervosa or bulimia nervosa. Typically, physicians and health professionals diagnose ED-NOS in someone whose disordered eating behaviours are serious but don't meet the diagnostic criteria for anorexia nervosa or bulimia nervosa. Such behaviours might include severe chronic dieting, extremely rigid eating behaviours, and binge-eating disorder.

In this section, we first discuss the characteristics, psychological profile, and health risks of ED-NOS. We then explore how chronic dieting, a common type of disordered eating, might lead to ED-NOS. We conclude the section with a detailed discussion of binge-eating disorder, which is a subtype of ED-NOS.

Characteristics of ED-NOS

The *DSM-IV-TR* (APA 2000a) criteria for ED-NOS are listed below. After reading through these criteria, you will recognize that the individual with ED-NOS does have a serious eating disorder, but the condition does not meet the specific criteria for classification as either anorexia nervosa or bulimia nervosa.

- For females, all the criteria for anorexia nervosa, except the individual has regular menses.
- All the criteria for anorexia nervosa, except that weight is still within the normal range although weight loss may have occurred.
- All the criteria for bulimia nervosa, except that the binge eating and the use of inappropriate compensatory behaviours are less than twice a week or the duration is less than 3 months.
- The regular use of inappropriate compensatory behaviours occurs in an individual with normal body weight after eating small amounts of food (for example, the person induces vomiting after eating only two small cookies).
- Repeated chewing and spitting out of food, without swallowing food.
- Binge eating not associated with the inappropriate compensatory behaviours that occur in either anorexia nervosa or bulimia nervosa.

Because ED-NOS includes many different types of disordered eating patterns, researchers have not clearly defined the characteristics of a person with ED-NOS. However, they believe that individuals diagnosed with ED-NOS have some of the same psychological issues as individuals with anorexia nervosa or bulimia nervosa. In moving along the eating issues continuum (see Figure 13.1) toward more disruptive and disordered eating behaviours, these individuals become increasingly preoccupied with their body faults, critical of their body shape and size, and concerned with comparing themselves with others. They also become increasingly preoccupied with what they eat, how much they eat, and whether the foods are "good" or "bad." Finally,

A Day in the Life of a Bulimic

Hi, my name is Katie.* Through high school and my first two years of college, I suffered from bulimia nervosa and used exercise as a method of purging. Initially, I was able to keep it a secret because people saw me eat meals, and I looked normal because I had learned to purge my Calories through exercise. After a few years, I knew I had a problem and so did people around me. My excessive exercise is what clued in my friends and family. Below, I give you an example of what a typical day was like for me during my first two years of college.

5:30 a.m.

Alarm goes off. I ate too much yesterday. I was the only one to finish my plate of food at dinner. I must get up and go running. If I can run this morning and eat only a small bowl of cereal at breakfast, then everything that happened last night won't matter.

6:10 a.m.

Two miles in 15:45 minutes. That's horrible. What is my problem? OK, if I won't run fast enough, I'll just have to increase my miles. Instead of running three miles, I'm going to run five. Why are my legs so heavy? I've got to run faster than this.

8:30 a.m.

The run was pathetic. It wasn't even worth going out. If I just skip going to the cafeteria, then I won't eat breakfast. That's what I should do. No breakfast today. Just get to class and then you'll be OK until lunch.

9:00 a.m.

Oh no, there's Julie. I know she's going to ask me to go into the cafeteria with her. I can't. Katie, do not let yourself go in to the cafeteria, no matter what Julie says or does. Just wait three more hours until lunch. Don't go.

9:25 a.m.

I can't believe I went to the cafeteria with Julie. Of course, they were serving my favourite scones and I ate two! They are huge—there must be 400 Calories in each of them. I'm so utterly disgusting. Julie does not even understand how hard that is for me. I'm so mad at myself. After class, I'll go to the gym. Katie, do not worry about the scones. You can get rid of them by taking the kickboxing class after your workout.

1:00 p.m.

If I can walk straight past the cafeteria and not eat lunch, I can get home faster, and get to the gym sooner.

1:15 p.m.

I did it—I walked past the cafeteria. Not eating lunch is going to make my workout feel so much better. I'll drink a Diet Coke first and then I'll go.

2:30 p.m.

Three hundred Calories burned on the treadmill and 400 burned on the elliptical machine. That's 700 Calories! If I go to the kickboxing class, then I can stop thinking about the scones I ate for breakfast and I'll be able to eat a normal dinner with my roommates.

4:00 p.m.

I'm exhausted. I've got to lie down.

4:15 p.m.

I can't lie down. You don't burn Calories while you're sleeping. Get up!

5:00 p.m.

I'm so dizzy. I hate that feeling, but I love it at the same time. It's good to know that I was strong enough to deny myself food long enough to feel dizzy. I get such a sense of strength from feeling so weak, it's strange. I'm safe to go to dinner now as long as I don't eat any dessert afterwards.

7:00 p.m.

It's amazing how normal I can act when I eat dinner. Even my roommates don't have any idea how hard it is for me to just enjoy a meal with them. I ate my complete dinner and took seconds—I couldn't believe I kept eating. I will add a couple of miles to my run in the morning to make up for the extra 300 Calories. I'm too tired to think about it now.

8:30 p.m.

I've got to go to bed. I can't move my body. I can't concentrate on my homework. I don't know when I'm ever going to get caught up in my classes. I'll have to read some after I run in the morning. I have to do better tomorrow—more exercise and less food.

*Not her real name. This true story was submitted by a student of one of the authors.

individuals diagnosed with ED-NOS can be depressed, be anxious, and experience loss of concentration and mood swings. These symptoms are similar to those of people diagnosed with other eating disorders.

Health Risks of ED-NOS

For most of us, going on a diet for a short time presents few nutritional or long-term health problems. However, if dieting or rigid eating behaviours progress to the point that an individual can be diagnosed with ED-NOS, a number of health problems can result. Listed below are some of the health risks associated with ED-NOS.

- Poor nutrient and energy intakes—If you restrict energy intake to fewer than 1500 kcal (6280 kJ) per day it becomes almost impossible to get adequate nutrients (protein, carbohydrates, vitamins, and minerals), even if you are not active. In general, most sedentary adults need at least 1600 to 1800 kcal (6700 to 7530 kJ) to maintain weight, and active adults need significantly more (see Chapter 11). Both inactive and active individuals who restrict their energy intake to lose weight frequently have poor vitamin and mineral intakes, especially calcium, magnesium, iron, zinc, B-complex vitamins, and antioxidants.

- Decreased total daily energy expenditure—It is well documented that as you severely restrict energy intake, your resting or basal metabolic rate (BMR) decreases at a greater rate than your change in body size. As you know, your BMR represents about 60% to 75% of the energy you need each day. Thus, when your BMR slows and your body uses less energy, you need to cut back on your energy intake even more to lose weight.

- Decreased ability to exercise—Remember that to maintain body weight, we must consume enough energy (kilocalories) to cover the energy costs of basic metabolism, the building and repair of muscle tissue, activities of daily living, and exercise. Females of reproductive age must also cover the energy costs of menstruation, while children and adolescents must cover the energy costs of growth. If, in addition, you are trying to maintain an exercise or training program or are competing regularly in sports or dance, the energy costs are much greater. Therefore, among athletes and dancers, chronic dieting not only reduces the level of nutrients available to cover these energy costs but also dramatically increases risk of injury and the time it takes to recover from injury, decreases the ability to concentrate, and reduces exercise performance (Beals and Manore 1998).

- Psychological stresses—A number of psychological stresses are reported with severe dieting and frequent energy restriction, especially in those who use exercise as a way of expending energy and maintaining a lean body shape. Some of these stressors include increased depression, obsession with food and body weight, and stress from constantly trying to maintain an unrealistic body weight (Beals and Manore 1998; Manore 2002).

- Increased risk of developing anorexia nervosa or bulimia nervosa—One fact that eating-disorder specialists agree on is that constant dieting can lead to an eating disorder, such as ED-NOS, anorexia nervosa, or bulimia nervosa. As individuals become more and more restrictive in their dieting behaviours, they move farther to the right on the eating continuum and their perception of what constitutes normal eating behaviours becomes more distorted.

Chronic Dieting May Lead to an Eating Disorder Such as ED-NOS

Do you find yourself dieting every January to make up for holiday eating or dieting every spring in preparation for beach season? If so, you're not alone. Many people diet occasionally to lose those two or three extra kilos (five pounds), and their behaviour certainly doesn't qualify as disordered eating. But at some point for some people, those occasional weight loss diets become habitual. Two common patterns of habitual energy restriction are weight cycling and chronic dieting.

Weight cycling or "yo-yo" dieting occurs when a person who is normal weight or overweight successfully diets to lose weight, then regains the lost weight, and then repeats the cycle all over again (Manore 1996). One reason why weight cyclers are thought to be unsuccessful at maintaining long-term weight loss is their failure to make permanent lifestyle changes in their eating and exercise behaviours.

Although energy restriction during the dieting phase can be severe, weight cycling is unlikely to cause serious illness unless the diet is long and not monitored by a physician. This is because the person overeats during the non-dieting phase, restoring the body's nutritional status. The long-term health consequences associated with this type of dieting, such as increased risk of heart disease, remain controversial. However, everyone agrees that there is a great deal of physiologic and psychological stress associated with losing and then regaining weight.

In contrast with weight cycling, **chronic dieting** is usually defined as consistently and successfully restricting energy intake to maintain an average or a below average body weight (Manore 1996). For most people, going on a diet for a short time presents few health risks. However, health problems may result for chronic dieters who are expending high amounts of energy in exercise. One example is the female athlete triad (discussed on page 482), which develops from chronic dieting in active females.

Chronic dieters experience a lot of stress related to eating. Notice that as you move from column 3 to column 4 of the eating continuum (see Figure 13.1), the comments related to dieting and body image become more extreme. That means that people who chronically diet are very aware of what they are eating and may constantly have negative thoughts related to food. If they allow themselves to eat foods they feel are "bad," they become upset with themselves for having so little self-control. Understandably, chronic dieters experience a lot of stress related to eating, and research has shown that their production of the stress hormone cortisol is higher. Some of the symptoms you may observe in a friend or family member who is chronically dieting are related to this increased stress.

weight cycling The condition of successfully dieting to lose weight, regaining the weight, and repeating the cycle again.

chronic dieting Consistently and successfully restricting energy intake to maintain an average or a below average body weight.

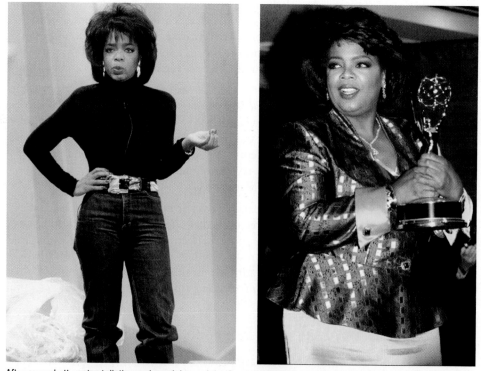

After several attempts at dieting and regaining weight, Oprah Winfrey has stated that she is now comfortable with her weight. Here are two extreme examples of her weight cycling. At left, Oprah in 1988, after losing 30.5 kg (67 lb.) At right, in 1992, having regained the weight.

As chronic dieting becomes more severe, the dieters become more preoccupied with food, the energy in food, and their weight. They may eliminate particular foods or food groups from their diet and consider some foods "off-limits." Activity patterns may also change as they increasingly use exercise to expend energy to keep their weight low. Chronic dieters may become compulsive about exercise, insisting that they need to exercise even when they are injured, fatigued, or sick. If you see these signs in an individual, recognize that their behaviours may be compromising their health and that they may have moved from disordered eating to ED-NOS.

> **Recap:** Weight cycling or "yo-yo" dieting occurs when a person who is normal weight or overweight successfully diets to lose weight, then regains the lost weight, and then repeats the cycle all over again A chronic dieter is an individual who consistently and successfully restricts energy intake to maintain an average or a below average body weight. Because this type of behaviour can last for years, the long-term health consequences may be poor nutrient status, loss of lean tissue, poor bone health, fatigue, and decreased ability to exercise. Chronic dieters are also at risk for developing a more severe eating disorder, such as anorexia nervosa or bulimia nervosa.

Binge-Eating Disorder Can Cause Significant Weight Gain

When was the last time a friend or relative confessed to you about "going on an eating binge"? Most likely, they explained that the behaviour followed some sort of stressful event, such as a problem at work, the breakup of a relationship, or a poor grade on an exam. As we noted earlier, binge eating is defined as the consumption of a large amount of food *in a short time*. This time factor distinguishes binge eating from "continual snacking" or "grazing." Many people have one or two binge episodes every year or so, in response to stress. But when the behaviour occurs an average of twice a week or more, the person is categorized in the *DSM-IV* as having a **binge-eating disorder** (APA 1994). Specifically, binge-eating disorder is a type of ED-NOS characterized by the consumption of a large amount of food within a short time without compensatory behaviours, such as vomiting or excessive exercise.

In Canada, an estimated 2% of the adult population is thought to have binge-eating disorder. U.S. statistics suggest that binge-eating disorder affects 2% to 3% of the adult population and 8% of the obese population; however, some obesity treatment programs report that 20% to 40% of their patients suffer from this disorder (Grilo 2002). In contrast to anorexia nervosa and bulimia nervosa, binge-eating disorder is also common in men (an approximate ratio of 1.5 female to 1 male) and minority groups.

binge-eating disorder A disorder characterized by binge eating an average of twice a week or more without compensatory behaviours, such as vomiting or excessive exercise.

Characteristics of Binge-Eating Disorder

Not surprisingly, people with binge-eating disorder are often overweight. This is not only because of the amount of food they eat, but also because they do not end the binge by purging themselves of the food. In the absence of purging, the increased energy intake that occurs with each binge can significantly increase the person's overall energy intake and contribute to weight gain. Some evidence suggests that a large proportion of people who suffer from binge-eating disorder (35% to 55%) experienced their first binge-eating episode prior to beginning a diet (Grilo 2002). As in bulimia nervosa, an individual suffering from binge-eating disorder has a sense of a lack of control during the binge episode and cannot stop eating. The *DSM-IV* (APA 1994) associates the binge-eating episode with three or more of the following experiences: eating much more rapidly than normal; eating until feeling uncomfortably full; eating large amounts of food when you are not feeling hungry; eating alone because you are embarrassed by how much you are eating; or feeling disgusted with yourself, depressed, or guilty about overeating.

In addition, individuals who suffer from binge-eating disorder generally have chaotic eating behaviours, low levels of dietary restraint (e.g., when food is available they cannot resist), and may suffer from more chronic overeating behaviours (e.g., regularly overeating but without losing control). As you would expect, our current food environment, which offers an abundance of good-tasting, cheap food any time of the day, makes it difficult for people with binge-eating disorder to avoid food triggers.

People with binge-eating disorder frequently suffer from low self-esteem, are distressed over their eating behaviours and body size, and have dysfunctional attitudes about their weight and shape (Grilo 2002). Depression is reported in 50% to 60% of people with binge-eating disorder. Substance abuse and anxiety disorders are also common.

Health Risks of Binge-Eating Disorder

As you would expect, the destructive overeating behaviours of people suffering from binge-eating disorder can have long-term health consequences. First, the increased energy intake associated with each binge significantly increases a person's risk of being overweight or obese. As discussed in detail in Chapter 11, obesity significantly increases the risk of other health problems, such as heart disease, high blood pressure, stroke, type 2 diabetes, cancer, depression, and arthritis. Second, the types of foods individuals typically consume during a binge episode are high in fat and sugar, which can increase blood lipids. Third, the stress associated with binge eating can have psychological consequences, such as low self-esteem, avoidance of social contact, depression, and negative thoughts related to body size. Constantly battling the negative thought processes that occur following each binge can be overwhelming and increase stress levels. In general, there is a high level of psychological distress associated with this disorder.

> **Recap:** Binge-eating disorder is a severe, life-threatening disorder characterized by recurrent episodes of compulsive overeating or binge eating. The binge occurs on average two times a week but is not associated with the regular use of inappropriate compensatory behaviours (including vomiting, fasting, excessive exercise) seen in bulimia nervosa. Many people suffering from binge-eating disorder are overweight and depressed.

What Is the Female Athlete Triad?

The female athlete triad is a term used to describe a serious syndrome that consists of three medical disorders frequently seen in female athletes: disordered eating, menstrual dysfunction, and osteoporosis (Figure 13.4). To emphasize the seriousness of this syndrome, the American College of Sports Medicine issued a position stand on the female athlete triad in 1997 (Otis et al. 1997), which outlined the seriousness of this syndrome in active women and girls and delineated its three components. These components are described in more detail on the following pages.

Sports That Emphasize Leanness Increase the Risk for the Female Athlete Triad

Sports that emphasize leanness or a thin body build may put a young girl or a woman at risk for the female athlete triad. The American College of Sports Medicine has identified these sports and activities as follows (Otis et al. 1997):

- sports that have subjective performance scoring, such as dance, skating, diving, and gymnastics

- endurance sports that emphasize a lean build or a low body weight, such as long-distance running, cycling, and cross-country skiing

- sports that require the athlete to wear body-contouring or body-revealing clothing, such as gymnastics, swimming, volleyball, aerobics, track, and dance

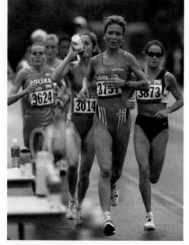

Sports that emphasize leanness or require the athlete to wear body-contouring clothing increase the risk for the female athlete triad.

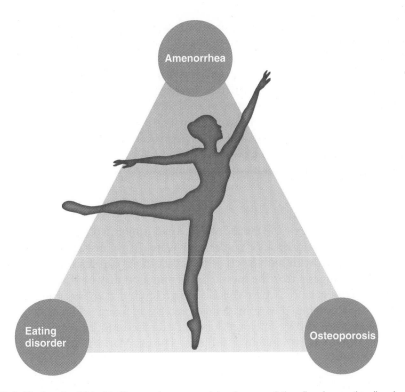

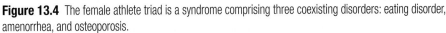

Figure 13.4 The female athlete triad is a syndrome comprising three coexisting disorders: eating disorder, amenorrhea, and osteoporosis.

- sports that require athletes to weigh in or that use weight-specific categories for participation, such as horse racing, martial arts, and rowing
- sports that emphasize a preadolescent body build for success, such as gymnastics, figure skating, and diving

Three Interrelated Disorders Characterize the Female Athlete Triad

Active females, like many women in our society, are often preoccupied with their body weight and shape. They feel pressure to conform to certain ideal body shapes and sizes; however, their source of pressure is twofold. These women experience the general social and cultural demands placed on women to be thin and also experience pressure from their coach, teammates, judges, or spectators to meet weight standards or body-size expectations for their sport. Failure to meet these standards can result in severe consequences, such as being cut from the team, losing an athletic scholarship, participating less with the team, or being eliminated from competition.

As the pressure to be thin mounts, active women may restrict their energy intake so much that they don't consume sufficient energy to support normal physiologic functioning. This undernutrition in turn disrupts the menstrual cycle and can result in amenorrhea. Without a normal menstrual cycle and adequate reproductive hormones, which play an important role in bone health, osteoporosis can result. Thus, for many female athletes, inadequate energy intake is the event that leads to absence of menstruation (amenorrhea) and premature bone loss (osteoporosis). In the following sections we describe each of the components of the female athlete triad.

Inadequate Energy Intake

The first component of the female athlete triad, inadequate energy intake to cover energy expenditure, frequently happens as part of an eating disorder (such as anorexia nervosa) or disordered eating. If a female athlete is required to lose weight to make the team or to please a coach or parent, she will often turn to harmful dieting practices to achieve her goal.

A number of factors may predispose active women to disordered eating, including a prolonged period of dieting, an increase in exercise, a stressful event, or the pressure to maintain a low body weight (Peterson et al. 1995; Sundgot-Borgen 1994). In addition, active women frequently avoid animal products and strictly limit their fat intake (Beals and Manore 1998), and these factors can increase their risk even further. Table 13.2 (page 472) lists some of the signs and symptoms that an active individual, either male or female, may not be eating enough.

Menstrual Dysfunction

The second component of the female athlete triad is menstrual dysfunction, such as irregular periods, amenorrhea, or failure to ovulate. As we discussed earlier, energy restriction combined with high levels of physical activity can disrupt the menstrual cycle. Research suggests that the menstrual dysfunction may be due in part to times of negative energy balance, where there is a high level of exercise and psychological or physical stress combined with inadequate intakes of energy (Dueck, Manore, and Matt 1996; Manore 2002). The prevalence of exercise-induced menstrual dysfunction may be as high as 50% in female athletes (Dueck, Manore, and Matt 1996; Beals and Manore 1998).

Poor Bone Strength

The final component of the female athlete triad is poor bone strength, which begins with osteopenia (low mineral density) and in its most severe form progresses to osteoporosis, a condition in which bones are weaker and more likely to fracture. (See Chapter 9 for more on osteoporosis and bone health.) Female athletes with menstrual dysfunction typically display reduced levels of the reproductive hormones estrogen and progesterone. When estrogen levels in the body are low, it is difficult for bone to retain calcium, and gradual loss of bone mass occurs. Research shows that in the lumbar region of the spine, bone mineral density is reduced by about 14% in amenorrheic athletes compared with athletes with regular menstrual cycles and by as much as 27% compared with normally menstruating sedentary women (Dueck, Manore, and Matt 1996). Loss of bone mineral density also increases the risk of muscle and bone injuries, such as stress fractures. Thus, despite the positive stimulus of exercise on bone, the hormonal changes associated with menstrual dysfunction compromise bone mineral density and increase the risk for fracture.

Recognizing and Treating the Female Athlete Triad Can Be Challenging

Recognition of an athlete with one or more of the components of the female athlete triad can be difficult, especially if the athlete is reluctant to be honest when questioned about the symptoms. For this reason, familiarity with the early warning signs is critical. These include excessive dieting or weight loss, excessive exercise, stress fractures, and self-esteem that appears to be dictated by body weight and shape. You may not know whether a female friend or teammate is experiencing irregular periods, but you might overhear her commenting negatively on her body or see her head off to the gym after eating only a lettuce salad for lunch.

Treating an athlete requires a multidisciplinary approach. This means that the sports medicine team, dietitian, exercise physiologist, psychologist, coach, trainer, parents, friends of the athlete, and the athlete all must work together. As with any health problem, prevention is the best treatment. Thus, recognition of the risk factors by the sports medicine team and education of athletes, coaches, and parents is imperative. If the athlete is having trouble with weight and body shape issues, care should be taken to deal with these issues before they develop into something more serious.

> **Recap:** The female athlete triad is a syndrome consisting of three distinct components: inadequate energy intake, menstrual dysfunction, and poor bone strength resulting in low mineral density or osteoporosis. This can increase the athlete's risk of fractures. Early warning signs include excessive dieting or weight loss, excessive exercise, stress fractures, and self-esteem that appears to be dictated by body weight and shape

What Therapies Work for People with an Eating Disorder?

Recognition and treatment of someone with an eating disorder can be difficult, especially if the person is reluctant to answer questions about the symptoms and does not want treatment. Since eating disorders can be triggered by any number of factors (discussed earlier), multiple issues may need to be addressed in treatment.

Most treatment programs use a multidisciplinary team-management approach that incorporates medical and nutritional management, psychological treatment, and a number of other therapies, depending on the individual problems and issues that need to be addressed.

A team-management approach to treating an individual suffering from an eating disorder will begin with a physical examination, diagnosis, and identification of underlying causes or trigger factors. The team will meet and decide on the approach each will use in working with the patient (Joy et al. 1997). At this time the team may choose to develop a contract for treatment that is then signed by the patient. Team members meet individually with the patient and on a regular basis as a team to determine the progress being made and the next steps in the treatment process. Team members may also meet with family and friends of the patient and involve them in the treatment plan; this is especially true if the patient is still living at home. Discussed below are the various steps and options for the treatment of eating disorders.

Choosing a Treatment Approach for an Eating Disorder

There are a variety of services available to treat eating disorders, ranging from intensive hospitalization to varied levels of outpatient care.

Conversely, patients who are underweight but are still medically stable may enter an outpatient program designed to meet their specific needs. For example, some outpatient programs are extremely intensive, requiring patients to come in each day for treatment, while others are less rigorous, requiring only weekly visits for meetings with a psychiatrist or eating-disorder specialist. The type of program an individual selects will be determined by his or her medical condition, options available, personal preference of the individual and family members involved, and affordability.

Treatment Options for Individuals with Anorexia Nervosa

The goals of treatment for individuals with anorexia nervosa are to achieve a healthy weight, treat any physical complications that may be present, motivate the person to restore healthy eating habits and lifestyle patterns, correct any dysfunctional feelings related to their eating disorder, treat associated psychiatric conditions, enlist the aid of family and friends to support the patient's healing, and prevent relapse. Nutritional rehabilitation, psychosocial interventions, and medications are the therapies most commonly used to reach these goals.

Nutritional Therapies Are Critical in Treating Anorexia Nervosa

The goals of nutritional therapies are to restore the individual to a healthy body weight and resolve the nutrition-related eating issues. For hospitalized patients, the expected weight gain per week ranges from 0.45 to 1.4 kg (1 to 3 lb.). For outpatient settings, the expected weight gain is much lower: 0.2 to 0.45 kg (0.5 to 1 lb.) per week. During the weight-gain phase of a treatment program, energy intake goals may be set at 1000 to 1600 Calories (4200 to 6700 kJ) per day, depending on body size, severity of the disease, and achievable levels of intake. Patients frequently try a variety of methods to avoid consuming the food presented to them. They may discard the food, vomit, exercise excessively, or engage in a high level of non-exercise motor activity to eliminate the calories they just consumed. In addition to increasing amounts of food, patients may be given vitamin and mineral supplements to ensure adequate micronutrients are consumed.

Nutrition counselling is an important aspect of the treatment to deal with the body image issues that occur as weight is regained. Once the individual reaches an acceptable body weight, nutrition counselling will address such issues as acceptability of certain foods, dealing with food situations, such as family gatherings and eating out, and learning to put together a nutritious food plan for weight maintenance.

Psychosocial Interventions Are Important

Most treatment programs for anorexia nervosa incorporate a variety of treatments aimed at addressing the underlying psychological issues related to the disorder. Individual psychotherapy along with both family therapy and group counselling sessions are usually recommended. Family therapy is useful in identifying and alleviating family dynamics or relationships that may be contributing to the maintenance of the disorder. Group counselling helps individuals realize that they are not alone in their struggles with the disorder and that others have similar issues.

Psychotropic Medications May Be Helpful

Psychotropic medications may be used in the treatment of anorexia nervosa. These medications are aimed primarily at preventing relapse in patients who have undergone treatment and in treating associated psychiatric disorders, such as depression or obsessive-compulsive disorder.

Treatment Options for Individuals with Bulimia Nervosa

The primary goals of treatment for individuals with bulimia nervosa are the identification and modification of events, behaviours, or environments that trigger binging and purging behaviours. As with anorexia nervosa, a variety of approaches are used to reach these goals. The most common include nutritional rehabilitation, psychosocial interventions, and medications.

Nutrition Counselling Is Important in Treating Bulimia Nervosa

Most individuals with bulimia nervosa are of normal weight or overweight, so restoring body weight is generally not the focus of treatment as it is with anorexia nervosa. Instead, nutrition counselling generally focuses on identifying and dealing with events and feelings that trigger binging, reducing purging, and establishing eating behaviours that can maintain a healthy body weight. In addition, nutrition counselling will address negative feelings about foods and the fear associated with uncontrolled binge eating.

Psychosocial Interventions Are Important

Cognitive therapy that helps patients monitor and alter their thought patterns related to eating issues and body image has been shown to be the most effective form of treatment for bulimia nervosa. Behaviour modification can help patients stop a binge episode from occurring or interrupt one in progress. As with anorexia nervosa, both group and family therapy are important. These approaches help identify food issues, body image concerns, interpersonal conflicts, difficulties with anger and aggression management, family dysfunctions, and coping styles that contribute to the disorder.

Antidepressant Medications May Be Helpful

The treatment of bulimia nervosa frequently involves the use of antidepressant medications in conjunction with nutritional and psychotherapy. Antidepressants are prescribed to alleviate the symptoms of depression, anxiety, obsessions, and overriding impulses that trigger a binge-and-purge event.

Treatment Options for Individuals with ED-NOS

The treatment of an individual with ED-NOS is similar to that discussed above for people with anorexia nervosa or bulimia nervosa, except that the interventions may not be as intense. Some individuals may need psychological and nutritional counselling as well as medications if coexisting psychiatric disorders are present. Early interventions and treatment may help prevent the eating disorder from becoming more severe.

> **Recap:** Treatments for individuals with an eating disorder may combine a variety of therapies, including nutrition counselling, individual psychotherapy, family counselling, support groups, and medications. Individuals may progress through various levels of treatment (e.g., hospitalization to weekly outpatient counselling) over months or years. Some individuals need ongoing counselling and medications to help prevent a recurrence of their eating disorder.

How Can We Prevent Eating Disorders and Disordered Eating?

We have suggested throughout this book to that, rather than trying to achieve an unrealistic body weight, you try to achieve a weight that is appropriate for you and one that can be maintained for life. This process requires you to think about your genetics, current body size and shape, environment, social life, exercise habits, and psychological factors. A healthy weight is one that can be realistically maintained, allows for involvement in physical activity, and reduces risk factors for chronic disease. It is not realistic to pick a body weight that you cannot maintain except by constant dieting or by resorting to disordered eating behaviours. At the end of this chapter is a list of Web Links to additional resources related to dieting and eating disorders.

As we noted earlier, it is difficult to delineate precisely what factors precipitate the development of eating disorders. Nevertheless, research does suggest that the following techniques may be useful in prevention (Piran 2002):

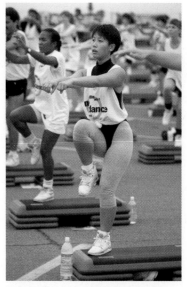

Maintaining a body weight that is appropriate for your body type allows you to be involved in physical activity, and that reduces risk factors for chronic disease.

- reducing peer and family weight-related criticism and teasing; educating parents and teachers about the destructiveness of such behaviour.

- teaching children and adolescents that changes of body shape and size are a natural part of human development.

- improving media literacy skills and helping children and adolescents identify unrealistic body images and subliminal messages.

- establishing public policies related to media messages about body weight and size aimed at children and adolescents.

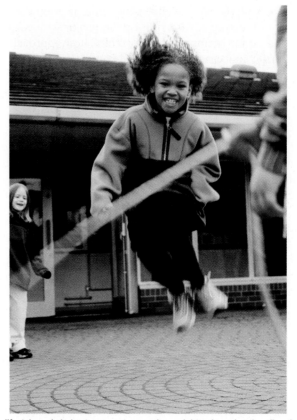

Encouraging an active lifestyle early helps to prevent excessive weight gain and eating disorders.

- identifying body weight and image concerns among children and adolescents early in the developmental years.

- encouraging participation in physical activity and sports early in life to help prevent excessive weight gain.

- establishing healthy eating behaviours within the home, school, and social environments, both for adults and for children. Making positive changes in the food environment to reduce unlimited access to high-fat, high-sugar foods in large portions. Finding alternative rewards for successful behaviours to replace the use of food (e.g., snacks, candy, sweets, fast food) and sedentary behaviour (e.g., more time at the computer or in front of the television) as rewards.

- establishing opportunities for activity throughout the day, at work, at school, and during periods of leisure time. Encouraging the development of walking programs that allow children and adolescents to walk safely to school and within their neighbourhoods.

- modelling of healthy diet and exercise habits by parents.

- commenting positively on attributes of children's and adolescents' bodies that are not related to appearance, such as strength, flexibility, endurance, and gross and fine motor skills.

Recap: The prevention of eating disorders is a relatively young field in which researchers are still developing models for prevention. The current goals of eating disorder prevention programs are to identify precipitating factors in the home, school, and social environment, and to implement strategies to reduce or eliminate these factors.

CHAPTER SUMMARY

- Eating behaviours occur along a continuum from normal to somewhat abnormal to disordered. Our feelings about food and our body images influence our eating behaviours.

- An eating disorder is a psychiatric disorder characterized by extreme body dissatisfaction and long-term eating patterns that negatively affect body functioning.

- *Disordered eating* is a general term used to describe a variety of abnormal or atypical eating behaviours that are used to achieve or maintain a lower body weight.

- The two most common clinically diagnosed eating disorders in Canada are anorexia nervosa and bulimia nervosa.

- A number of factors are thought to contribute to the development of eating disorders, including family environment, the media, social and cultural factors, personality traits, and genetics.

- Anorexia nervosa is a medical disorder in which an individual uses severe food restriction and other practices to maintain a body weight that is less than 85% of expected.

- Health risks associated with anorexia nervosa include electrolyte imbalance, cardiovascular and gastrointestinal problems, malnutrition, and poor bone health. Between 5% and 20% of people with anorexia will die from complications of the disorder within 10 years of initial diagnosis.

- Bulimia nervosa is an eating disorder characterized by recurrent episodes of binge eating, followed by some form of purging.

- The health consequences associated with bulimia nervosa include electrolyte imbalance, dental decay and mouth sores, gastrointestinal ulcerations from binging and vomiting, and constipation. Bulimia nervosa results in death in 1% of patients within 10 years of diagnosis.

- Eating disorders—not otherwise specified (ED-NOS) are serious eating disorders that do not meet the specific criteria for anorexia nervosa and bulimia nervosa. Binge-eating disorder is an example of an ED-NOS.

- Binge-eating disorder is the consumption of a large amount of food in a short time (such as within two hours) without compensatory behaviours (e.g., vomiting, excessive exercise, using laxatives). Increased rates of obesity, cardiovascular disease, diabetes, hypertension, cancer, arthritis, and depression are associated with binge-eating disorder.

- Chronic dieting is defined as consistently and successfully restricting energy intake to maintain an average or a below average body weight. Some of the health consequences of chronic dieting may include poor energy and nutrient intakes, poor nutritional status, decreased metabolic rate and total daily energy expenditure, increased psychological stress, increased risk of developing a clinical eating disorder (such as anorexia nervosa or ED-NOS), and increased risk of exercise-induced menstrual dysfunction.

- The female athlete triad is a syndrome characterized by the presence of three coexisting disorders: inadequate energy intake, amenorrhea, and poor bone strength and reduced bone mineralization, sometimes leading to osteoporosis.

- Treatment of a clinical eating disorder typically involves a team approach that includes nutritional management, psychological treatment, medications, and other treatment options as necessary.

- Individuals with life-threatening symptoms are hospitalized until their vital signs become stable. They may then be transferred to an inpatient facility specializing in the treatment of patients with eating disorders. Individuals with less severe symptoms typically receive outpatient care that may range from intensive daily appointments to weekly sessions.

- Strategies for preventing eating disorders include strategies to promote children's and adolescents' self-esteem and to help them develop and maintain healthy eating behaviours and exercise habits throughout life.

REVIEW QUESTIONS

1. Damage to the esophagus, dental decay, and electrolyte imbalances are health risks of what disorder?
   a. Binge-eating disorder
   b. Bulimia nervosa
   c. Chronic dieting
   d. Anorexia nervosa

2. Chronic dieting
   a. increases your risk of developing a psychiatric eating disorder.
   b. increases your basal metabolic rate.
   c. is a psychiatric eating disorder.
   d. is a characteristic of bulimia nervosa.

3. The components of the female athlete triad are
   a. disordered eating, amenorrhea, and osteoarthritis.
   b. anorexia nervosa, menstrual dysfunction, and increased injuries.
   c. binge-eating disorder, irregular periods, and osteoporosis.
   d. disordered eating, menstrual dysfunction, and osteoporosis.

4. One recommended strategy for maintaining a healthy body image is to
   a. exercise regularly.
   b. read sports magazines.
   c. reduce your fat intake to no more than 10% of your daily energy consumption.
   d. reduce your intake of sweets to no more than one "treat" a day.

5. Which of the following statements reflects a distorted body image?
   a. I am afraid that if I eat whenever I am hungry, I will get fat
   b. I wish I could change the way I look in the mirror
   c. I felt devastated yesterday when my best friend told me I was getting fat
   d. I think about food a lot

6. Which of the following is not used to characterize bulimia nervosa?
   a. Excessive exercising
   b. Binge eating at least twice a week
   c. Teeth discolouration
   d. Amenorrhea

7. Generally, the body slows its basal metabolic rate when energy intake is ____ and when energy expenditure is ____, in order to conserve energy.
   a. High, low
   b. Low, high

   c. Unchanged, high
   d. Low, low

8. Which of the following conditions is *not* typically associated with binge-eating disorder?
   a. Being overweight or obese
   b. Psychological disorders, such as depression
   c. Increased blood lipids
   d. Poor bone health

9. Explain why there is some truth to the saying that the more you diet, the harder it is to lose weight.

10. Create a flow chart showing how restricted energy intake in female athletes can eventually lead to loss of bone mineral density.

11. Compare and contrast anorexia nervosa and bulimia nervosa. In what ways are they similar? In what ways are they different?

12. You start a new aerobics class and make friends with another student named Kashi. Although Kashi wears oversized clothes in class, you notice right away that she is extremely thin. After class, you go out for coffee and are surprised when Kashi eats two large pastries with her skim-milk latte. Propose at least two theories as to what might be going on with Kashi.

13. You've noticed that your friend Carlo, who is on your crew team, has been losing a lot of weight over the last few months. Today you sit next to him in class and notice that his cheeks look swollen and the knuckles on the back of his right hand are scabbed. After class, you ask him if he is feeling okay and he frowns. "Never felt better!" he says—and abruptly walks away. What might you do next?

14. Your younger cousin, Ashley, complains to you that her mother won't let her eat anything but grapefruit for breakfast. Your aunt is notorious for following every fad diet and is always trying some crazy eating plan to try to lose weight—but it seems as if every time she diets, she ends up heavier than she was before! Ashley says she's so hungry by lunchtime, she eats anything and everything she can get her hands on. If you were to approach your aunt about her eating behaviours, what would you say? Specifically, what information might persuade her to change her pattern of disordered eating? What weight loss strategies might you suggest instead of chronic dieting? Most importantly, why would it be especially crucial to convince her to not involve Ashley in her fad diets?

15. Sharma has been a gymnast for as long as she can remember. Looking to become more competitive, she recently switched coaches and increased her training time. At 13 years old, she stands 1.58 metres

(5'2") tall and weighs about 45.5 kg (100 lbs). Sharma had never thought about her weight before, but her coach told her that if she doesn't lose at least 2.3 kg (5 lbs), she will never be able to compete at a high level. Immediately, Sharma stops eating breakfast and lunch, and only eats dinner because her parents insist. Her mother asks her if she is still menstruating, but Sharma lies and says yes. Constantly tired and sad, Sharma weighs herself religiously three times a day. She is now down to 41.4 kg (91 lbs).

Her coach is encouraging and congratulates her on her dedication and drive. What factors increase Sharma's risk for the female triad? If you were to explain osteoporosis, stress fractures and increased injury to her, do you think this might change her disordered eating behaviours? Why or why not? What role does Sharma's gymnastics coach play in this situation? What, if anything, do you think Sharma's parents should do? Do you think intervention is necessary, even though her coach says she is doing so well?

CASE STUDY

After your first four months of being away at college, you are returning home for winter break and you are very excited to see your family and friends. You and your best friend Carrie ventured off to different post-secondary schools but have kept in contact through email.

In high school, Carrie was captain of a figure skating team, a straight A student and always had a very active social life. Over the past several months, you have noticed a change in Carrie's emails—she does not sound like her usual happy and carefree self. You have also noticed her frequently commenting on her weight and the stress she is feeling with both the increased school workload and an upcoming skating competition.

The first time you see Carrie you are shocked! She has noticeably lost weight and appears very thin. When you question Carrie about her weight loss she comments that she "hates her body" and has been "too busy to eat."

a. After spending several days with Carrie, you determine that she falls within the "disruptive eating patterns" and "disordered body image" categories on the eating disorder continuum. Being an active female, what factors in Carrie's life do you suppose have influenced a change in both her eating patterns and her body image?

b. Being knowledgeable about eating disorders, you suspect that Carrie may be at risk of developing anorexia nervosa. List several signs and symptoms of this medical disorder that you could look for to help you in determining if Carrie is at risk.

Test Yourself Answers

1. **False** Males also are diagnosed with eating disorders, but the incidence is much lower than for females.

2. **False** People can and do recover from medically diagnosed eating disorders, with the best outcomes occurring in those who seek and get treatment early in their illness.

3. **False** There are a number of factors that may play a role in the development of anorexia nervosa in any one individual.

4. **True** As eating behaviours become increasingly atypical, there is an increased risk of a clinical eating disorder developing.

5. **True** Individuals who suffer from bulimia nervosa and binge-eating disorder may be obese. This is especially true of individuals who suffer from binge-eating disorder because they do not purge the extra energy consumed during the binge-eating episode. Overall, 8% of obese people have a problem with binge eating, and some clinics report the incidence to be as high as 20% to 40% of their obese clients.

WEB LINKS

www.nedic.ca
The National Eating Disorder Information Centre
This is a Toronto-based, nonprofit organization that provides information, referral, prevention resources, and support to persons with eating disorders.

www.harriscentermgh.org
Harris Center at Massachusetts General Hospital
This center, formerly called the Harvard Eating Disorders Center, provides information about current eating disorder research, as well as sections on understanding eating disorders and resources for those with eating disorders.

www.nimh.nih.gov
National Institute of Mental Health (NIMH)
Click on Health & Outreach and then "eating disorders" to find numerous articles on the subject.

www.anad.org
National Association of Anorexia Nervosa and Associated Disorders
Visit this site for information and resources about eating disorders offered to the public and to professional eating-disorder specialists.

www.nationaleatingdisorders.org
National Eating Disorders Association
This site is dedicated to expanding public understanding of eating disorders and promoting access to treatment for those affected and support for their families.

www.menstuff.org
Menstuff Eating Disorders
Search for "eating disorders" and find information about male anorexia and eating disorders in general, self-assessments, disordered eating statistics, and prevention information.

www.somethingfishy.org
Something Fishy Website on Eating Disorders
A comprehensive website about the dangers of eating disorders, eating disorder treatment, and signs of symptoms of disorders. This site includes first-hand survivors' stories and online chats.

Eating Disorders in Men: Are They Different?

David was tired of being called "fat boy." But the real motivation behind his weight loss was his coach's end-of-season threat: if he didn't lose at least 9 kg (20 lb.), he wouldn't make the soccer team again next year. David couldn't imagine his life without soccer, so he started cutting back on his snacks and running a couple of mornings a week at the gym. He lost 1 kg (2 lb.), but it took him four weeks. Discouraged by the slow pace, he eliminated all snacking, put less on his plate at mealtimes, and ran every day, first three kilometres (two miles), then five (three miles), then eight (five miles). His weight started dropping more dramatically, and he loved the high he got from "running on empty." Four months into his program, he'd lost the 9 kg (20 lb.), and he kept on going. By the time the soccer season started, he'd lost 14.5 kg (32 lb.), and his coach rewarded him with more time on the field. He knew he should slack off on the dieting and running now that he was in practice every day, but something made him keep at it. Every time he got on the scale and saw he weighed another bit less, he felt better, stronger, more in control.

Like many people, you might find it hard to believe that "real men" like David develop eating disorders . . . or if they do, their disorders must be somehow different, right? To explore this question, let's take a look at what research has revealed about similarities and differences between men and women with eating disorders.

Comparing Men and Women with Eating Disorders

Until about a decade ago, little research was conducted on eating disorders in males (Beals 2003, 2004). Recently, however, eating-disorder experts have begun to examine the gender-differences debate in detail and have discovered that "men with eating disorders are very similar to women with eating disorders on most variables" (Woodside et al. 2001). Or, to put it more simply, no current evidence suggests that eating disorders in males are atypical or somehow different from the eating disorders experienced by females (Anorexia Nervosa and Related Eating Disorders, Inc. 2002).

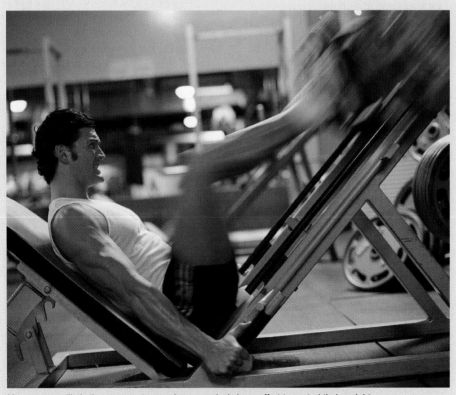

Men are more likely than women to exercise excessively in an effort to control their weight.

Following is a list of what *is* currently known regarding the similarities and differences between males and females with eating disorders.

Predisposing Factors, Personality Traits, and Dieting History Are Similar

Many of the factors that appear to predispose an individual to an eating disorder are similar for males and females. For example, both have a high probability of coming from families with mental health problems or have a personal history of mental health problems (Carlat, Camargo, and Herzog 1997; Andersen 1992; Beals 2003, 2004). Both males and females are also frequently connected with some type of social group, such as a family, peer group, or sports team, where leanness is encouraged (Andersen et al. 1995). In addition, media studies suggest that males are increasingly becoming the target of articles and ads promoting dieting and an ideal of lean muscularity that is difficult to achieve (Nemeroff et al. 1994).

Both males and females with eating disorders, especially anorexia nervosa, tend to be perfectionists, goal oriented, and introverted (Wonderlich 2002; Beals 2004). However, as with women, the extent to which these personality traits are effects of the illness rather than risk factors is not clear (Woodside et al. 2001).

Finally, dieting is one of the most powerful eating disorder triggers for both males and females (Anorexia Nervosa and Related Eating Disorders, Inc. 2002). Eating disorders in both males and females typically develop after a period of dieting that becomes increasingly stringent (in anorexia nervosa) or increasingly erratic (in bulimia nervosa).

History of Overweight, Triggers for Dieting, and Methods of Weight Loss Are Different

We discussed in this chapter the fact that females with eating disorders say they *feel* fat even though they typically are normal weight or even underweight before they develop the disorder. In contrast, males who develop eating disorders are more likely to have actually *been* overweight or even obese (Robb and Dadson 2002; Beals 2004). Thus, the male's fear of "getting fat again" is based on reality. In addition, males with disordered eating are less concerned with actual body weight (scale weight) than females are but are more concerned with body composition (percentage of muscle mass compared with fat mass). For example, Mangweth and colleagues (2001) found that male bodybuilders obsessed with eating and exercising focused on gaining muscle mass, as opposed to losing fat or weight, and were preoccupied with body image.

Whereas dieting itself is a common trigger for eating disorders in both males and females, research suggests that the factors *initiating* the dieting behaviour are different (Anderson 1992). There appear to be four reasons why males diet: to improve athletic performance, to avoid being teased for being fat, to avoid obesity-related illnesses observed in male family members, and to improve a homosexual relationship (Andersen 2001). Similar factors are rarely reported by women.

The methods that men and women use to achieve weight loss also appear to differ. Males are more likely to use excessive exercise as a means of weight control, while females use more passive methods, such as severe energy restriction, vomiting, and laxative abuse. These weight control differences may stem from the societal biases surrounding dieting and male behaviour; that is, dieting is considered to be more acceptable for women, whereas the overwhelming sociocultural belief is that "real men don't diet" (Beals 2004).

Reverse Anorexia Nervosa: The New Male Eating Disorder?

Is there an eating disorder unique to men? Recently, some eating disorder experts who work with men have suggested that there is. Observing men who are distressed by the idea that they are not sufficiently lean and muscular, who spend long hours lifting weights, and who follow an extremely restrictive diet, they have defined a disorder called *reverse anorexia nervosa*. (The disorder is also called *muscle dysphoria* or *muscle dysmorphia*.) Men with reverse anorexia nervosa perceive themselves as small and frail even though they are actually quite large and muscular. Thus, like men with true anorexia nervosa, they suffer from a body image distortion, but it is reversed. No matter how "buff" or "chiselled" he becomes, his biology cannot match his idealized body size and shape (Andersen 2001).

There are other reversals in these men compared with men with anorexia and other eating disorders. For instance, men with reverse anorexia nervosa frequently abuse performance-enhancing drugs: in one study, approximately half the participants reported using anabolic steroids (Pope, Phillips, and Olivardia 2000). Additionally, whereas people with anorexia eat little of anything, men with reverse anorexia tend to consume excessive high-protein foods and dietary supplements, especially products like protein powders that promise increased muscle mass and weight gain (Pope and Katz 1994).

Men with reverse anorexia do share some characteristics with men and women with other eating disorders. For instance, they too report "feeling fat" and engage in the same behaviours that indicate an obsession with appearance (such as looking in the mirror). They also express significant discomfort with the idea of having to expose their body to others (e.g., taking off their clothes in the locker room) and have increased rates of mental health problems (Pope, Phillips, and Olivardia 2000).

Do you know anyone who might have reverse anorexia nervosa? If you do, maybe you're wondering how you can tell whether your friend's concern about his body size is extreme or a simple enthusiasm for weightlifting. The warning signs listed in the accompanying box may help. If you think they apply to your friend, talk to him about it. Although reverse anorexia nervosa isn't typically life-threatening, it can certainly cause distress and despair; therapy—especially participation in an all-male support group—can help.

Warning Signs of Reverse Anorexia Nervosa

These are some of the outward indications that someone may be struggling with reverse anorexia nervosa. Not all of them apply to all men with the disorder. If you notice any of these behaviours in a friend or relative, talk about it with him and let him know that help is available:

- rigid and excessive schedule of weight training

- strict adherence to a high-protein, muscle-enhancing diet

- use of anabolic steroids, protein powders, or other muscle-enhancing drugs or supplements

- poor attendance at work, school, or sports activities because of interference with rigid weight-training schedule

- avoidance of social engagements where the person will not be able to follow his strict diet

- avoidance of situations in which the person would have to expose his body to others

- frequent and critical self-evaluation of body composition

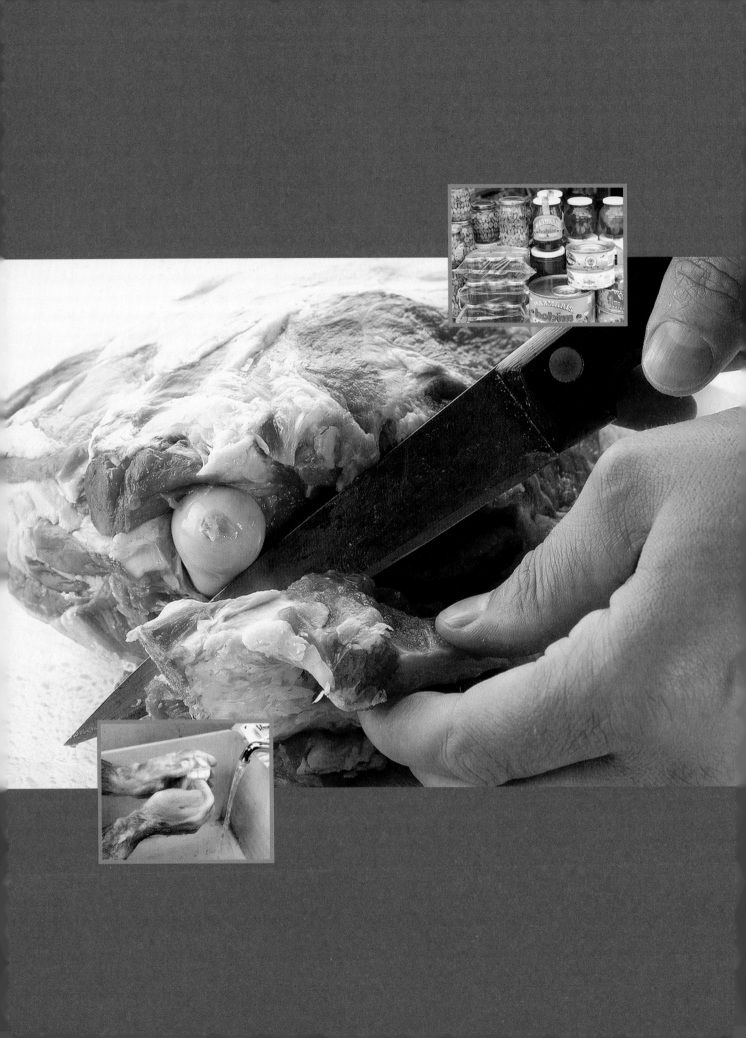

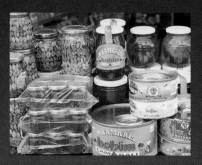

Food Safety and Technology: Impact on Consumers

CHAPTER OBJECTIVES

After reading this chapter you will be able to:

1. Discuss three reasons why food safety is an important concern, pp. 498–500.

2. Identify the types of microorganisms involved in food-borne illness, pp. 501–506.

3. Describe strategies for preventing food-borne illness at home and while eating out, pp. 508–516.

4. Explain the advantages and disadvantages of canning, pasteurizing, using preservatives, using aseptic packaging, and irradiating to preserve foods, pp. 516–521.

5. Identify at least five categories of food additives and explain why they are used, pp. 521–523.

6. Define the acronym FATTOM and describe the factors that promote microbial growth, pp. 507–508.

Test Yourself True or False

1. Freezing destroys any microorganisms that might be lurking in your food. **T** *or* **F**

2. The colour of hamburger is a good indicator of whether the food is sufficiently cooked. **T** *or* **F**

3. Mould is the most common cause of food poisoning. **T** *or* **F**

4. Bacteria grow best in slightly acidic environments with a pH of 4.6 to 7.0. **T** *or* **F**

5. In Canada, food additives are strictly regulated under the Food and Drugs Act. **T** *or* **F**

Test Yourself answers can be found at the end of the chapter.

Pre-washed and bagged baby spinach was the source of a 2006 outbreak of *E. coli* O157:H7 that sickened 205 people and caused three deaths in the United States.

Spinach—a good food source of iron, vitamins A and C, and . . . *E. coli*? In September 2006, U.S. consumers were shocked to learn of an outbreak of *E. coli* O157:H7 linked to the consumption of Dole Pre-Packaged Baby Spinach. How can fresh produce that has been sorted, washed, and bagged make people violently ill? The investigation centred on the 13 bags that were collected from ill consumers and used the product codes and a technique called "DNA fingerprinting" on the bacteria from the bags to identify the specific farmers' fields with contaminated spinach. The U.S. Food and Drug Administration identified three possible environmental risk factors: wild pigs nearby, irrigation wells used for the field crops, and waterways that potentially carried feces from cattle and wildlife. The FDA ultimately concluded that the exact cause of this outbreak, which killed 3 people and sickened at least 205 others, may never be known (USFDA 2007).

What is food poisoning? How common is it, and what causes it? Would spinach grown in Canada have caused the same outbreak? If consumers thoroughly washed the spinach at home, would it have prevented them from being infected with *E. coli*? Are there any guarantees that our food is safe? In this outbreak it appears that the spinach was irrigated with contaminated water, and washing the spinach would not have prevented consumers from getting this food-borne illness.

In this chapter, you'll discover how contaminants enter our food supply and learn some simple ways to protect yourself from getting sick. You will also learn about techniques for food preservation, food additives and residues, and the difference between organic and non-organic farming. But whether your food comes from South America, a corporate farm, an organic grower, or your own backyard, you'll see that safeguards must be in place at every step from field to table to ensure food safety.

Food Safety and Food Quality

Unsafe food is food that has been contaminated with a harmful substance that causes injury or illness when eaten. The harmful substances include chemicals (such as methylmercury), microorganisms (such as bacteria, fungi, or viruses), and substances that cause physical injury (such as a piece of glass or bone). **Food safety** refers to practices, guidelines, or legislation designed to protect our food supply from harmful substances. Food containing microorganisms and pathogens that cause illness may

food safety Practices, guidelines, or legislation designed to protect our food supply from harmful substances.

look and smell the same as safe food. You can't tell by looking at or smelling a cantaloupe, for example, whether or not the rind is harbouring salmonella bacteria. **Food quality** refers to food characteristics, such as taste, odour, colour, and texture. The breakdown or deterioration of food is due both to enzymes naturally found in the food and to microorganisms that colonize the food.

Spoilage affects food quality in several ways. Slice an apple and leave it exposed to air for a few minutes and you'll notice how it changes in appearance. At this point, it may have lost its appeal, but it is still safe to eat. As food proceeds along the path to spoilage, both fruits and meats turn brown, vegetables wilt, and milk starts to curdle and sometimes takes on a yellow tinge. The texture of foods also changes as components that give food their fibrous structure begin to break down. Think of the difference between a perfectly ripe tomato and one that has turned to mush. Taste and smell also change as a food spoils. The taste and smell of soured milk or an apple that is mealy are very distinct to anyone who has the misfortune of consuming them.

Most importantly, some of the microorganisms that cause food to decompose may make you sick, while others spoil the food but don't cause illness. You can't tell from smelling or looking at food that has spoiled whether or not it contains harmful pathogens. To avoid a food-borne illness, it is best to discard food that is spoiled.

food quality Food characteristics, such as taste, odour, colour, and texture.

Food-Borne Illness Affects an Estimated 11 Million to 13 Million Canadians Each Year

Food-borne illness is a term used to encompass any symptom or illness that arises from ingesting food or water that contains an infectious agent (such as bacteria, viruses, and parasites), a poisonous substance, or a protein that causes an immune reaction. Food-borne illness is commonly called *food poisoning*. Some researchers also consider *food allergy*, a topic we introduced in Chapter 3, a type of food-borne illness. In this chapter, we are focusing on microbial food safety, pathogens, and toxic chemicals in the environment.

An estimated 11 million to 13 million Canadians get food-borne illnesses each year (Canadian Food Inspection Agency 2007a). The symptoms can include stomach cramps, nausea, vomiting, diarrhea, and fever, and many people mistakenly think they have the flu. Infants and young children, older adults, pregnant women, and people with weak immune systems are most at risk of becoming seriously ill and even dying from a food-borne illness.

food-borne illness An illness transmitted through food or water; either by an infectious agent, by a poisonous substance, or by a protein that causes an immune reaction.

Technologic Manipulation of Food Raises Safety Concerns

Technologic manipulation of food also raises concerns related to food safety. Food producers manipulate their products by adding chemicals and other substances that can remain in food as residues, and by using techniques, such as irradiation and genetic modification, that cause some consumers concern.

Food additives are not foods in themselves but are chemicals added to foods to enhance them in some way. For instance, low-calorie margarines may include guar gum to make the product more spreadable, beta-carotene may be added to cheddar cheese as a colouring agent, and calcium increases the nutrient value of orange juice. One category of food additives are **food preservatives**, chemicals added to foods to help maintain their freshness and appearance.

Pesticides are a family of chemicals used in both the field and storage areas to destroy plant, fungal, and animal pests. Other residues, such as organic and industrial pollutants or growth hormones used in livestock, can also remain in foods. High levels of some residues can be harmful to human health. The use of food additives, pesticides, and other chemicals and processes for food production and preservation are discussed in more detail later in this chapter.

food additives A substance or mixture of substances intentionally put into food to enhance its appearance, palatability, and quality.

food preservatives Chemicals that help prevent microbial growth and enzymatic deterioration.

pesticides Chemicals used either in the field or in storage to destroy plant, fungal, and animal pests.

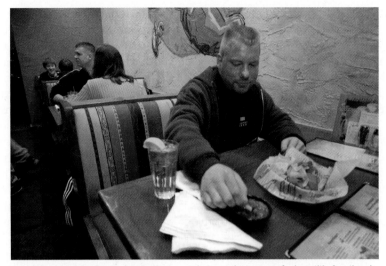

A customer samples salsa at the Pennsylvania restaurant that was the source of a hepatitis A outbreak. The restaurant no longer uses scallions, the cause of the deadly outbreak, in its salsa or other dishes.

Genetic Modification

genetic modification Changing an organism by manipulating its genetic material.

In **genetic modification**, the DNA of an organism is altered to bring about specific changes in its seeds or offspring, for instance making tomatoes plumper, juicier, and more pest-resistant or making beef cattle that produce a higher quality of meat. The relative benefits and harm of genetic modification have been debated worldwide. For instance, some environmentalists have raised the concern that seeds from genetically modified crops disrupt other crops through cross-pollination, even those many kilometres from where the altered ones are growing. Another concern is the long-term effect of genetically modified crops on the plants, insects, and animals that consume them or use them for their habitat.

Government Regulations Control Food Safety

The Canadian Food Inspection Agency (CFIA) is part of Agriculture and Agri-Food Canada, and reports to Health Canada. The agency is responsible for enforcing 14 federal acts related to food, plants, and animals and ensures that the food safety, animal health, and plant protection standards set out in those acts are followed. The CFIA inspects foods, plants, animals, restaurants, and food service establishments; checks that food-labelling regulations are followed; and issues allergy alerts and food recalls.

At the municipal level, Public Health Inspectors visit all eating and drinking establishments to ensure that the minimum standards for food temperatures, food handling, sanitation, dishwashing, and personal hygiene practices are being followed.

> **Recap:** Concerns about food safety centre on three areas: food-borne illness, food spoilage, and technologic manipulation of food. Food-borne illness arises from consuming food or water that causes illness or injury. Food spoilage affects a food's appearance, texture, taste, and smell, and may or may not affect its safety, depending upon the type of microbes involved. The food industry uses additives and other chemicals and techniques in food production and preservation that concern some people. The Canadian Food Inspection Agency monitors and regulates food production and preservation and helps to set standards to ensure food safety.

What Causes Food-Borne Illness?

Microbes or their toxic byproducts cause most cases of food-borne illness. However, as we will discuss later in the chapter, chemical residues in foods can also cause illness.

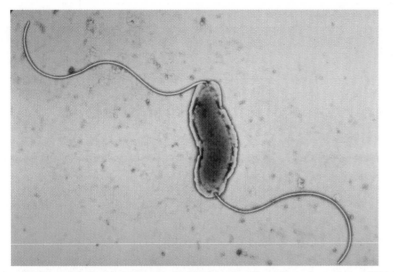

The bacteria called *Campylobacter jejuni* is found in the intestines of poultry, cattle, swine, rodents, wild birds, and household pets, like cats and dogs (CFIA 2007a).

Food-Borne Illness Is Caused by Microorganisms and Their Toxins

Two types of food-borne illness are common: *food infections* result from the consumption of food containing living microorganisms, whereas *food intoxications* result from consuming food in which microbes have secreted poisonous substances called *toxins* (Bauman 2004).

Several Types of Microbes Poison Foods

The microbes that most commonly cause food infections are bacteria and viruses; however, helminths, fungi, and prions also poison foods.

According to the CDC (2003), the majority of food infections are caused by **bacteria** (Table 14.1). Bacteria are microorganisms that lack a true nucleus and have a chemical called peptidoglycan in their cell walls. Of the several species involved, *Campylobacter jejuni* is thought to be the most common culprit. Most cases result from eating foods or drinking milk or water contaminated with infected animal feces. The bacteria cause fever, pain, and bloody and frequent diarrhea (Bauman 2004).

Salmonella is the second most common bacterial culprit in food infections. As with *Campylobacter*, most *Salmonella* infections result from eating food contaminated with animal feces. Poultry and eggs are commonly implicated but all foods, including fruits and vegetables, can become contaminated with *Salmonella*. Salmonellosis causes diarrhea, nausea, and vomiting, and cells of some strains of the bacteria can perforate the intestines and infect the blood. Approximately 6000 to 12 000 Canadians are diagnosed with Salmonellosis each year (Health Canada 2006c). It's thought that a much larger number of people are affected but attribute their symptoms to the "stomach flu." *Salmonella* bacteria can be difficult to eradicate, as some strains have developed a resistance to commonly prescribed antibiotics (Health Canada 2006c).

Escherichia coli, more commonly known as *E. coli*, are bacteria that are found in the intestines of cattle, poultry, and other animals. Although some strains are relatively harmless, other strains, such as *E. coli* O157:H7, can cause serious illness. One complication of an *E. coli* O157:H7 infection is hemolytic uremic syndrome (HUS). An infected person will experience bloody diarrhea, vomiting, abdominal cramping, and fever, usually commencing between two and four days after exposure to this bacterium. Interestingly, it takes only 10 to 100 colony-forming units (bacteria cells or parts of cells) for *E. coli* O157:H7 to become infectious, which is quite few compared with the 1 million to 100 million *E. coli* colony-forming units required for a person to become infected with traveller's diarrhea (University of Florida 2002). Although the

bacteria Microorganisms that lack a true nucleus and have a chemical called peptidoglycan in their cell walls.

Table 14.1   Common Bacterial Causes of Food-Borne Illness

Bacteria	Incubation Period	Duration	Symptoms	Foods Most Commonly Affected	Usual Sources of Contamination	Steps for Prevention
Campylobacter jejuni	1–7 days	7–10 days	Fever Headache and muscle pain followed by diarrhea (sometimes bloody) Nausea Abdominal cramps	Raw and undercooked meat, poultry, or shellfish Raw eggs Cake icing Untreated water Unpasteurized milk	Intestinal tracts of animals and birds Raw milk Untreated water and sewage sludge	Only drink pasteurized milk Cook foods properly Avoid cross contamination
Salmonella (more than 2300 types)	12–24 hours	4–7 days	Diarrhea Abdominal pain Chills Fever Vomiting Dehydration	Raw or undercooked eggs Undercooked poultry and meat Raw milk and dairy products Seafood Fruits and vegetables	Intestinal tract and feces of poultry *Salmonella enteritidis* in raw shell eggs	Cook thoroughly Avoid cross contamination Use sanitary practices
Escherichia coli (0157:H7 and other strains that can cause human illness)	2–4 days	5–10 days	Diarrhea (may be bloody) Abdominal cramps Nausea Can lead to kidney and blood complications	Contaminated water Raw milk Raw or rare ground beef, sausages Unpasteurized apple juice or cider Uncooked fruits and vegetables	Intestinal tracts of cattle Raw milk Unchlorinated water	Thoroughly cook meat Avoid cross contamination
Clostridium botulinum	12–36 hours	1–8 days	Nausea Vomiting Diarrhea Fatigue Headache Dry mouth Double vision Muscle paralysis (droopy eyelids) Difficulty speaking and swallowing Difficulty breathing	Improperly canned or vacuum-packed food Meats Sausage Fish Garlic in oil Honey	Widely distributed in nature Soil, water, on plants and in intestinal tracts of animals and fish Grows only in little or no oxygen	Properly can foods following recommended procedures Cook foods properly Children under 16 months should not consume raw honey
Staphylococcus	1–6 hours	2–3 days	Severe nausea and vomiting Abdominal cramps Diarrhea	Custard- or cream-filled baked goods Ham Poultry Dressing Gravy Eggs Mayonnaise-based salads and sandwiches Cream sauces	Human skin Infected cuts Pimples Noses and throats	Refrigerate foods Use sanitary practices

(continued)

Bacteria	Incubation Period	Duration	Symptoms	Foods Most Commonly Affected	Usual Sources of Contamination	Steps for Prevention
Shigella (more than 30 types)	12–50 hours	2 days–2 weeks	Bloody and mucus-containing diarrhea Fever Abdominal cramps Chills Vomiting	Contaminated water Salads Milk and dairy products	Human intestinal tract Rarely found in other animals	Use sanitary practices
Listeria monocytogenes	2 days–3 weeks	None reported	Fever Muscle aches Nausea Diarrhea Headache, stiff neck, confusion, loss of balance, or convulsions can occur if infection spreads to nervous system Infections during pregnancy can lead to miscarriage or stillbirth, premature delivery, or infection of newborn	Uncooked meats and vegetables Soft cheeses Lunch meats and hot dogs Unpasteurized milk	Intestinal tract and feces of animals Soil and manure used as fertilizer Raw milk	Thoroughly cook all meats Wash raw vegetables before eating Keep uncooked meats separate from vegetables and cooked foods Avoid unpasteurized milk or foods made from unpasteurized milk People at high risk should: not eat hot dogs or lunch meats unless they are reheated until steaming hot; avoid getting fluid from hot dog packages on foods, utensils, and surfaces; wash hands after handling hot dogs or lunch meats; avoid eating soft cheeses, such as feta, Brie, and Camembert; avoid eating refrigerated smoked seafood unless it is cooked.

Sources: Iowa State University Extension, Food safety and quality project 2000, Safe Food: It's Your Job Too! www.extension.iastate.edu/foodsafety/Lesson/L1.html (accessed July 2003); U.S. Food and Drug Administration, How can I prevent foodborne illness? www.cfsan.fda.gov/~dms/qa-fdb1.html (accessed June 2003); Centers for Disease Control and Prevention, Division of Bacterial and Mycotic Diseases, Disease information, foodborne illness www.cdc.gov/ncidod/dbmd/diseaseinfo/foodborneinfections_g.htm (accessed April 2004).

symptoms may resemble the flu, HUS is not to be taken lightly, as it can lead to permanent kidney damage, particularly in children younger than 5 years of age and adults over the age of 50 years. Of the children who become ill with this condition, upward of 80% will need blood transfusions and about 50% will require kidney dialysis (Kidney Foundation of Canada 2002); some will need kidney transplants.

How does a person become infected by *E. coli* O157:H7? This bacterium can be transferred several ways: food to person, food to food, person to person, or person to food. Coming into contact with fecal matter from an infected person or animal can lead to infection. Hamburger meat may become contaminated through the slaughtering and grinding processes, and contamination is estimated to cost meat producers $5 billion annually (Canadian Institutes of Health Research 2003). In fact,

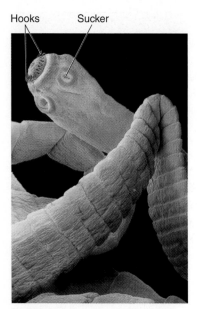

Hooks   Sucker

Tapeworms have long, wormlike bodies, hooks, and suckers, which help them to attach to human tissues.

viruses A group of infectious agents that are much smaller than bacteria, lack independent metabolism, and need a live host to reproduce.

helminth Multicellular microscopic worm.

giardiasis A diarrheal illness caused by the intestinal parasite *Giardia intestinalis* (or *Giardia lamblia*).

undercooked hamburger meat was responsible for two of the five biggest *E. coli* O157:H7 outbreaks on record (University of Florida 2002), and HUS is often referred to as *hamburger disease.*

But vegetarians beware—this illness is not limited to meat. In fact, the largest outbreak, which made 5727 people sick, was caused by improperly washed radish sprouts in Sakai, Japan (University of Florida 2002). Lettuce, sprouts, salami, and unpasteurized milk, cider, and juice are other sources of infection. A shocking 50 000 North Americans become infected each year, and, of those, 500 cases are fatal (Canadian Institutes of Health Research 2003).

Although there is no vaccine for humans, scientists at the University of British Columbia and the University of Saskatchewan have developed a vaccine for cattle. This exciting new research may prove to be invaluable in the fight against *E. coli* O157:H7. Avoiding unpasteurized milk and juices and following the food safety guidelines on pages 508 through 516 will reduce your chances of becoming infected with *E. coli* O157:H7.

Listeria monocytogenes is a bacterium that is commonly found in soil, plants, water, sewage, and manure. Humans and animals may carry it and not show any symptoms of ill health. When it is present in large amounts, pregnant women, the elderly, and people with poor immune systems are at high risk of a serious and sometimes fatal illness called listeriosis. Pregnant women may be 20 times more susceptible than women who are not pregnant, and their babies may be born early or seriously ill, or they may be stillborn.

Listeria is an unusual bacterium because it can live and grow slowly on refrigerated foods, and contaminated foods may appear safe and taste normal. In August 2008, an outbreak of listeriosis at an Ontario Maple Leaf meat processing plant resulted in the recall of approximately 200 ready-to-eat products, 53 confirmed cases of listeriosis, and 20 deaths (Canadian Public Health Agency 2008).

Although bacteria are the primary cause of food infections, some food-borne **viruses** also cause disease. Viruses are infectious agents that are much smaller than bacteria, lack independent metabolism, and need a live host to reproduce. The hepatitis A virus can contaminate raw produce and cause liver damage. Hepatitis E also damages the liver and is fatal in about 20% of infected pregnant women. In terms of sheer numbers, the rotaviruses are the most serious cause of acute diarrheal illness in the world, and in developing nations they are responsible for about one million childhood deaths. The Norwalk virus and Norwalk-like viruses (now called noroviruses), can live on door handles, sinks, railings, and glassware (PHAC 2005). They live year round but are most common in winter and affect all age groups, causing severe diarrhea, nausea, and vomiting. They are not affected by chlorine and can persist on hard surfaces despite cleaning with disinfectants.

Helminths are commonly called worms, and include tapeworms, flukes, and roundworms. These microbes release their eggs into the environment, such as in vegetation or water. Animals, most commonly cattle, pigs, or fish, then consume the contaminated matter. The eggs hatch inside their host, and larvae develop in the host's tissue. The larvae can survive in the flesh long after the host is killed for food. Thoroughly cooking beef, pork, or fish destroys the larvae. In contrast, if you eat the contaminated meat or fish either raw or undercooked, you consume living larvae, which then mature into adult worms in your small intestine. Some worms cause mild symptoms, such as nausea and diarrhea, but others can grow large enough to cause intestinal obstruction. Some spread beyond the gastrointestinal tract to damage other organs, such as the liver, bladder, or lungs. Some can cause death.

A parasite known as *Giardia intestinalis* (or *Giardia lamblia*) causes a diarrheal illness called **giardiasis**. *Giardia* lives in the intestines of animals and humans, and it is passed in the stool of infected people and animals. It is one of the most common causes of waterborne disease in humans in North America. You can consume *Giardia* by putting something in your mouth or by swallowing something that has come into contact with the stool of an infected person or animal, by drinking contaminated water (this includes water in lakes, streams, rivers, swimming pools, hot tubs, or fountains), or by eating uncooked food contaminated with *Giardia*. Symptoms include diarrhea,

▶ HIGHLIGHT

Bird Flu: The Next Pandemic Influenza?

Historical patterns suggest that pandemics can be expected to occur at least three to four times each century, and in this new century, the question is, when and what will be the next outbreak? Experts stress that a pandemic is unavoidable, and many believe that it is the H5N1 strain of the avian flu that will inevitably intensify to pandemic proportions.

Also known as bird flu, avian influenza (AI) is a viral infection carried mainly by birds, but it can also be transmitted to mammals. AI viruses can be classified into two categories: low pathogenic (LPAI) and high pathogenic (HPAI) forms based on the severity of the illness caused in poultry, with HPAI causing the greatest number of deaths. Domestic poultry are most at risk, but all types of birds can carry this virus. First identified in Italy more than 100 years ago, there are now 15 known subgroups of this virus, and they are classified by numbering their surface proteins: H for hemagglutinin, N for neuraminidase. The H5 and H7 subgroups are considered the most dangerous because they can quickly mutate and pick up genes from other viruses. In Hong Kong, the location of the first recorded case of human infection, 18 people were hospitalized, 6 people died, and more than 1.5 million birds were destroyed following the outbreak (World Health Organization 2005a). Avian influenza is most prevalent in Vietnam and Thailand, where 52 cases were confirmed and 39 people died of the H5N1 strain between January 2004 and January 2005 (World Health Organization 2005b).

In Canada, poultry farmers in British Columbia suffered a tremendous blow when 17 million birds were destroyed after a highly pathogenic avian flu H7 ravaged the Fraser Valley in March of 2004 (Canadian Food Inspection Agency 2008a). In total, 42 commercial flocks and 11 backyard flocks were exterminated by the CFIA, devastating farmers and their families. In September 2007, H7N3 avian influenza, another highly pathogenic strain, was discovered during a routine inspection at a commercial poultry operation in Saskatchewan. This strain is different from the one that has been associated with human illness in Asia, Africa, and Europe (CFIA 2008a).

At present, there is no vaccine for H5N1; however, a virus seed bank is being developed from a genetically modified strain of H5N1 for future production of vaccine. Consumers are advised that it is safe to eat cooked poultry and poultry products, as the virus is killed at temperatures above 70°C (158°F) (WHO 2005b). Still, the destruction and devastation in the wake of the avian flu crisis in British Columbia and the climbing death toll in Vietnam and Thailand may be a glimpse of what's in store for the future.

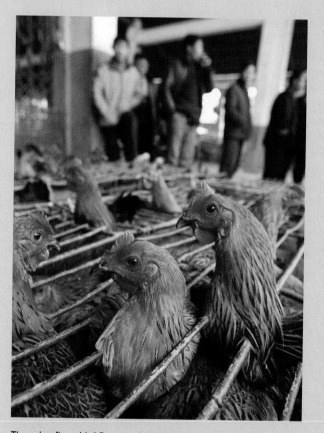

The avian flu or bird flu caused 39 deaths in Vietnam and Thailand between January 2004 and January 2005.

loose or watery stools, stomach cramps, and upset stomach, but some people show no symptoms. The symptoms usually begin within one to two weeks of being infected, and generally last two to six weeks. Symptoms last longer in some people.

Fungi are plant-like, spore-forming organisms that can grow either as single cells or as multicellular colonies. Two types of fungi are yeasts, which are globular, and moulds, which are long and thin. Growths of these microbes on foods rarely cause food infection. This is due in part to the fact that very few species of fungi cause

fungi Plant-like, spore-forming organisms that can grow either as single cells or as multicellular colonies. Yeasts and moulds are two types of fungi.

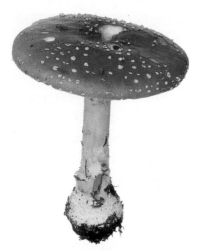

Some mushrooms, such as this fly agaric, contain toxins that can cause illness or even death.

mad cow disease A fatal brain disorder prompted by consumption of food containing prions, which are an abnormal form of protein found in the brains and other organs of infected sheep, cows, and other livestock.

prion A protein that is closely related to a virus but is self-replicating.

toxin Any harmful substance; specifically, a chemical produced by a microorganism that harms tissues or causes harmful immune responses.

neurotoxins A type of toxin that targets the nervous system cells.

enterotoxins A type of toxin that targets the gastrointestinal tract cells.

serious disease in people with healthy immune systems (Bauman 2004). In addition, unlike bacterial growth, which is invisible and often tasteless, fungal growth typically makes food look and taste so unappealing that we quickly discard it.

A food-borne illness that has had front-page exposure in recent years is **mad cow disease**, or *bovine spongiform encephalopathy* (*BSE*). Cattle contract this disease from eating feed contaminated with tissue and blood from other infected animals. First discovered in the early 1980s in Britain, this neurological disorder is caused by a **prion**, a proteinaceous infectious particle that is closely related to a virus but is self-replicating (Tortora, Funke, and Case 2003). Prions are not destroyed with cooking and are only found in the tissue of the central nervous system, retina, and lower intestines—not in the milk or muscle meats. BSE can be passed to humans who consume contaminated meat or tissue that has been ground into such items as sausages or ground beef.

Some Microbes Release Toxins

The microbes just discussed cause illness by directly infecting and destroying body cells. In contrast, other bacteria and fungi secrete chemicals called **toxins** that are responsible for serious and even life-threatening illnesses. These toxins bind to body cells and can cause a variety of symptoms, such as diarrhea, vomiting, organ damage, convulsions, and paralysis.

Toxins can be categorized depending on the type of cell they bind to; the two primary types of toxins associated with food-borne illness are **neurotoxins** and **enterotoxins**. Neurotoxins damage the nervous system, usually causing paralysis, while enterotoxins target the gastrointestinal system and generally cause severe diarrhea and vomiting.

One of the most common and deadly neurotoxins is produced by the bacteria *Clostridium botulinum*. The botulism toxin blocks nerve transmission to muscle cells and causes paralysis, including of the muscles required for breathing. Health Canada warns parents not to put honey in infant food or on infant soothers because there is a chance that it can carry *Clostridium botulinum* spores. Infants under the age of 1 year don't have protective bacterial flora in their gastrointestinal tracts or bile acids to prevent the spores from germinating and producing neurotoxins (Health Canada 2006b).

Some fungi produce poisonous chemicals called *mycotoxins*. (The prefix *myco* means "fungus.") These toxins are typically found in grains stored in moist environments. In some instances, moist conditions in the field encourage fungi to reproduce and release their toxins on the surface of growing crops. Long-term consumption of mycotoxins can cause organ damage or cancer, and they can be fatal if consumed in large doses. A mycotoxin called *aflatoxin* is produced by the mould *Aspergillus flavus*. Aflatoxin has been associated with peanuts, peanut butter, and other crops and, if ingested, can cause illness in livestock and humans.

A highly visible fungus that causes food intoxication is the poisonous mushroom. Most mushrooms are not toxic, but a few, such as the deathcap mushroom (*Amanita phalloides*), can be fatal. Some poisonous mushrooms are quite colourful, a fact that helps to explain why the victims of mushroom poisoning are often children (Bauman 2004).

Our Bodies Respond to Food-Borne Microbes and Toxins with Acute Illness

Many food-borne microbes are killed in the mouth by antimicrobial enzymes in saliva or in the stomach by hydrochloric acid. Any microbe that survives these chemical assaults will usually trigger vomiting or diarrhea as the gastrointestinal tract attempts to expel the offender. Simultaneously, the white blood cells of the immune system will be activated, and a generalized inflammatory response will cause the person to experience nausea, fatigue, fever, and muscle cramps. Refer back to Table 14.1 (page 502) to identify many possible symptoms resulting from food infection with various bacteria.

People most affected by food-borne illnesses are those with compromised immune systems, such as people with HIV or undergoing chemotherapy, older adults, infants and young children, and pregnant women. However, food-borne illness can

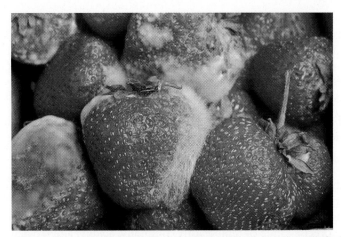

Moulds rarely cause human illness, in part because they look so unappealing that we throw the food away.

affect anyone. Depending on our state of health, the precise microbe involved, and the number of microbes ingested, the symptoms can range from mild to severe, including double vision, loss of muscle control, and excessive or bloody diarrhea. As noted earlier, some cases, if left untreated, can result in death.

To diagnose a food-borne illness, a specimen must be obtained and cultured. This means the specimen is analyzed in a laboratory setting in which the offending microorganisms are grown in a specific chemical medium. Stool (fecal) cultures are usually analyzed, especially if diarrhea is a symptom. Blood is cultured if the patient has a high fever. A physician who suspects that a patient is suffering from a food-borne illness will take a detailed history including a 24-hour dietary recall. Treatment usually involves keeping the person hydrated and comfortable, as most food-borne illness tends to be self-limiting; the person's vomiting and diarrhea, though unpleasant, serve to rid the body of the offending microbe. In severe illnesses, such as botulism, the patient's intestinal tract will be repeatedly treated to remove the microbe, and antibodies will be injected to neutralize its deadly toxin.

Certain Environmental Conditions Help Microbes Multiply in Foods

Given the correct conditions, microbes can thrive and multiply in many types of food. These growth-favouring conditions can be remembered with the acronym FATTOM. FATTOM stands for

- food—bacteria like high-protein and high-carbohydrate foods;

- acid—a mildly acidic environment with a pH of 4.6 to 7.0;

- time—when conditions are ideal, bacteria can double their numbers every 15 to 30 minutes. In general, bacteria grow to sufficient numbers to cause illness in about four hours;

- temperature—bacteria grow best between 5°C (41°F) and 60°C (140°F);

- oxygen—some bacteria are aerobic and need oxygen, while others are anaerobic and can't survive in the presence of oxygen;

- moisture—many microbes require a high level of moisture, and thus foods like boxed dried pasta and rice do not make suitable microbial homes, although cooked pasta and cooked rice left at room temperature might prove hospitable.

As just noted, many microbes cannot tolerate acidic foods. For example, *Clostridium botulinum* cannot grow or produce its toxin in an acidic environment, so the risk of botulism is lower in citrus fruits, sauerkraut, and pickles. In contrast, more alkaline foods, such as eggs and canned mushrooms are a magnet for *C. botulinum*.

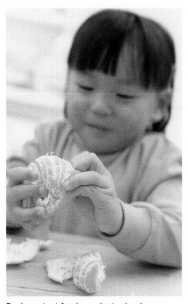

Peels protect foods against microbes.

In addition, microbes need an entryway into a food. Just as our skin protects our bodies from microbial invasion, the peels, rinds, and shells of many foods seal off access to microbes. Eggshells are a good example of a barrier that keeps bacteria, such as *Salmonella,* from entering the nutrient-rich environment within. Once such a barrier is removed, however, the food loses its primary defence against contamination.

> **Recap:** Food infections result from the consumption of food containing living microorganisms, such as bacteria, whereas food intoxications result from consuming food in which microbes have secreted toxins. Food infections can be caused by bacteria, viruses, fungi, helminths, and prions. The body has several defence mechanisms, such as saliva, stomach acid, vomiting, diarrhea, and the inflammatory response, which help rid us of offending microorganisms or their toxins. To reproduce in foods, microbes require a precise range of temperature, humidity, acidity, and oxygen content. Most bacteria prefer protein-rich or carbohydrate-rich foods and need about four hours to grow to numbers that cause illness.

How Can You Reduce Your Risk of Food-Borne Illness?

Most people associate foods of animal origin with food-borne illness. These include not only raw meat, poultry, and fish but also eggs, shellfish, and unpasteurized milk. Foods that may be the product of several animals (such as ground beef) can be especially hazardous. In addition, a bacteria or virus present in one animal has the potential to contaminate the entire herd.

However, recent outbreaks of food-borne illness have been in fruits and vegetables—spinach, lettuce, alfalfa sprouts, carrot juice, and cantaloupes in particular. Washing decreases, but cannot eliminate, all contaminants, and the quality of the water used in washing may be an important factor. If produce has been grown by using unsafe water, there is virtually nothing consumers can do to avoid food-borne illness (Dietitians of Canada 2007). Unpasteurized fruit or vegetable juices may also be contaminated if the produce used to make these juices contained pathogens (CDC 2003).

When Preparing Foods at Home

When you prepare foods at home, you can reduce your risk of food-borne illness by following these tips (Figure 14.1):

cross contamination Contamination of one food by another via the unintended transfer of microbes through physical contact.

1. Wash your hands and sanitize kitchen surfaces often. Wash raw fruits and vegetables thoroughly before you prepare and eat them.

2. Separate foods to prevent **cross contamination,** that is, the spread of bacteria or other microbes from one food to another. This commonly occurs when raw, unwashed foods are cut on the same cutting board or served together on the same plate.

3. Cook foods to their proper temperatures (discussed on page 512) by using a food thermometer.

4. Chill foods to prevent microbes from growing.

Wash Your Hands

One of the easiest and most effective ways to prevent food-borne illness is to wash your hands before, during, and after preparing food. Pay special attention to the areas underneath your fingernails and between your fingers. Also, it's a good idea to remove your rings while cooking, as they can harbour bacteria. See the Highlight box "Dude, Wash Your Hands."

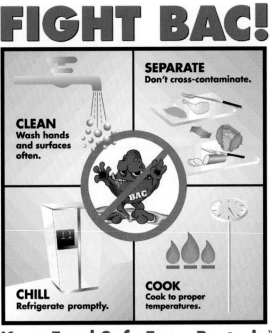

Figure 14.1 The Fight BAC! logo is the food safety logo of the Canadian Partnership for Consumer Food Safety Education and the United States Department of Agriculture. (See www.canfightbac.org.)

▶ **HIGHLIGHT**

Dude, Wash Your Hands

Proper handwashing with the proper tools—soap, water, and paper towels—can significantly reduce the chance of getting some foodborne and other illnesses, according to Kansas State University's Doug Powell, Associate Professor of Diagnostic Medicine and Pathobiology and scientific director of the International Food Safety Network. Powell says people should always wash their hands before handling or preparing food and

- after using the toilet;
- before handling ready-to-eat food;
- after handling raw food;
- after changing diapers;
- after playing with or cleaning up after pets;
- after handling garbage.

People are continuously exposed to various bacteria and viruses because of improper handwashing or lack of handwashing, Powell said. The steps in proper handwashing, based on the available evidence, are to

- wet hands with water;
- use enough soap to build a good lather;

- scrub hands vigorously, creating friction and reaching all areas of the fingers and hands for at least 10 seconds to loosen pathogens on the fingers and hands;
- rinse hands with thorough amounts of water while continuing to rub hands;
- then dry hands with a paper towel because the friction from rubbing hands with paper towels helps remove additional bacteria and viruses.

Powell said water temperature is not a critical factor when washing hands. Water hot enough to kill dangerous bacteria and viruses would scald hands, so use a temperature that is comfortable.

Powell also said that the next time you visit a bathroom that is missing soap, water, or paper towels, to let someone in charge know.

Source: Used with permission of Dr. Douglas Powell, Kansas State University, International Food Safety Network, http://foodsafety.ksu.edu/en/

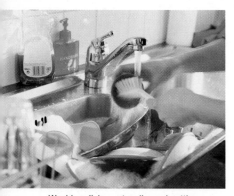

Washing dishes, utensils, and cutting boards with hot soapy water reduces the chances for food contamination.

Wash Kitchen Utensils and Sanitize Surfaces

A clean area and tools are also essential in reducing cross contamination. Wash utensils, containers, and cutting boards in the dishwasher or with hot soapy water before and after contact with food; this is especially critical with raw and cooked meat, poultry, and seafood (Food Marketing Institute 2003). It's also important to sanitize counter tops and wash utensils with hot soapy water after preparing each food type to reduce the chance of cross contamination. Use a non-porous, smooth plastic or stone cutting board because porous wood and scratched plastic can hold juices and harbour bacteria.

Dishtowels, cloths, and aprons should be washed in hot water often. It's a good idea to wash sponges in the dishwasher each time you run it and to replace them regularly. If you don't have a dishwasher, put sponges in boiling water for three minutes on a routine basis to sterilize them.

Wash Fruits and Vegetables

Wash raw fruits and vegetables well with clean, safe running water before you prepare and eat them. Use a brush to scrub produce with firm or rough surfaces, such as oranges, cantaloupes, potatoes, and carrots, before you peel or cut them, as their outer surfaces may carry microbes (Canadian Food Inspection Agency 2008b).

Isolate Raw Foods

Raw meat, poultry, and seafood harbour an array of microbes and can easily contaminate other foods through direct contact, as well as by the juices they leave behind on surfaces (including hands) that are not cleaned after each food's preparation. Contact between foods that won't be cooked, like salad ingredients, and these foods or their juices can result in food-borne illness. Also be careful not to place cooked food on a plate that previously held raw meat, seafood, or poultry. When preparing meals with a marinade, make sure you reserve some of the marinade in a clean container before adding raw ingredients if you will need some uncontaminated marinade to use later in the cooking process. Remember to always marinate raw food in the refrigerator.

Store Foods in the Refrigerator or Freezer

Different microbes thrive in different environmental temperatures. The majority of bacteria that cause food-borne illness prefer temperatures between 15°C and 50°C (60°F and 130°F), with the majority growing best in temperatures between 25°C and 40°C (80°F and 100°F) (Tortora, Funke, and Case 2003). Because of this, refrigeration (storage between 1°C and 4°C or 34°F and 40°F) and freezing (storage at or below 0°C or 32°F) are two of the most reliable methods of diminishing bacteria's ability to cause illness. Not all bacteria in cool environments are killed, but the rate at which they reproduce is drastically reduced. Also, naturally occurring enzymes that cause food decomposition are stopped at freezing temperatures.

Shopping Tips　When shopping for food, purchase refrigerated and frozen foods last. Many grocery stores are actually designed so that these foods are in the last aisles. When you are buying meats, poultry, seafood, and dairy products, look for the durable life information on their labels or on a poster near the food. The durable life of a food is the number of days that an unopened product will keep its freshness, taste, and nutritional value when stored properly (CFIA 2002). The best before (*meilleur avant*) date is another way of giving this information and is required on products that have a durable life of 90 days or less. It indicates the last day an unopened product will maintain its quality; proper storage instructions (e.g., "keep refrigerated") must also be provided. It is best to avoid buying foods past the best before date, even though they are generally still safe to eat. For foods that are packaged in the store, such as meat, fish, or poultry, the label must have a packaged-on date and durable life information (on the label or an accompanying poster); alternatively, the foods can carry a best before date and storage instructions (CFIA 2002). For less perishable foods, such as cereal and baking mixes, the "best if used by [or before]" dates indicate the shelf life of the product or the date at which the product is no longer at peak flavour, texture, and appearance. These foods can be safely eaten past the listed date if they have been stored properly, but they may not taste as good or be as nutritious as they were before this date. Proper storage for non-perishable items includes storage in a dry, clean, cool (less than 29°C or 85°F) cabinet or pantry.

After you purchase perishable foods, get them home and into the refrigerator or freezer within one hour. If your trip home will be longer than an hour, bring along a cooler in which to transport them.

Refrigerating Foods Once you get home, meat, poultry, and seafood should be put in the coldest part of the refrigerator. They should also be properly wrapped so their juices do not drip onto any other foods. If you are not going to use meat, poultry, or seafood within 48 hours of purchase, store them in the freezer (Food Marketing Institute 2003). Remember that eggs are also perishable and should be kept refrigerated. Avoid overstocking your refrigerator or freezer, as air needs to circulate around food to cool it quickly and discourage microbial growth.

After a meal, leftovers should be promptly refrigerated—even if still hot—to discourage microbial growth. The standard rule for storing leftovers is: *2 hours/2 inches/ 4 days*. Food should be refrigerated *within 2 hours* of serving. If the temperature is 32°C (90°F) or higher, such as at a picnic, then foods should be refrigerated within one hour (USDA 2003). Because a larger quantity of food takes longer to cool and will allow more microbes to thrive, food should be stored at a depth of no greater than *2 inches* (5 centimetres). The interior of deeper containers of foods can remain warm long enough to allow bacteria to multiply rapidly even when the surface of the food has cooled. Leftovers should only be refrigerated for *up to 4 days*. If you don't plan to use the food within four days, freeze it. A guide for storing foods in your refrigerator is provided in Figure 14.2.

Freezing and Thawing Foods The temperature in your freezer should not rise above 0°C (32°F). Use a freezer thermometer to check it periodically to make sure this temperature is being maintained. If your electricity goes out, avoid opening the freezer until the power is restored. When the power does come back on, check to make sure the temperature is at least −5°C (23°F) on the top shelf. If it is warmer, you should inspect your freezer's contents and discard any items that are not firmly frozen, thus lessening chances of an overgrowth of bacteria.

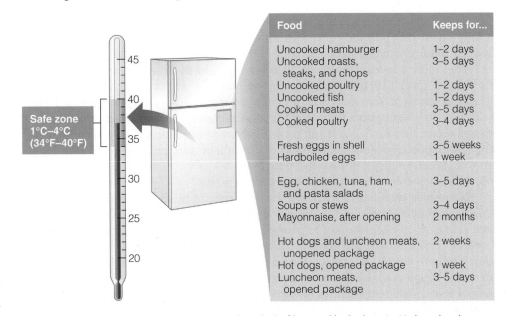

Food	Keeps for...
Uncooked hamburger	1–2 days
Uncooked roasts, steaks, and chops	3–5 days
Uncooked poultry	1–2 days
Uncooked fish	1–2 days
Cooked meats	3–5 days
Cooked poultry	3–4 days
Fresh eggs in shell	3–5 weeks
Hardboiled eggs	1 week
Egg, chicken, tuna, ham, and pasta salads	3–5 days
Soups or stews	3–4 days
Mayonnaise, after opening	2 months
Hot dogs and luncheon meats, unopened package	2 weeks
Hot dogs, opened package	1 week
Luncheon meats, opened package	3–5 days

Safe zone 1°C–4°C (34°F–40°F)

Figure 14.2 Although it's important to keep a well-stocked refrigerator, it's also important to know how long foods will keep.
(U.S. Department of Agriculture, Food Safety and Inspection Service, Consumer Education and Information, Refrigeration and Food Safety, January 1999, www.fsis.usda.gov/OA/pubs/focus_ref.htm, accessed April 2004.)

When freezing items, remember that smaller packages will freeze more quickly. So rather than attempting to freeze an entire casserole or a whole batch of homemade spaghetti sauce, divide the food into multiple portions in freezer-safe containers, and then freeze.

Sufficient thawing will ensure adequate cooking throughout, which is essential to preventing food-borne illness. Raw poultry is a good example of a food item that needs to be carefully contained as it thaws, so its juices don't contaminate other foods. Most references suggest that the perfect place to thaw poultry is on the bottom shelf of the refrigerator and in a large bowl to catch any of its juices. However, more research is needed to establish the safety of other methods, such as thawing in the microwave or in basins of cold water (Lacroix, Li, and Powell 2003). Perhaps more important is the need to use a meat thermometer to confirm that the internal temperatures are high enough to ensure that the poultry is fully cooked (Lacroix, Li, and Powell 2003).

Moulds in Refrigerated Foods Have you ever taken cheese out of the refrigerator and noticed that it had a fuzzy blue growth on it? This is mould, one of the two types of fungi. Interestingly, cool temperatures do not slow the growth of some moulds; in fact, some prefer refrigeration. For instance, when acidic foods, such as applesauce, leftover coffee, and spaghetti sauce, are refrigerated, they readily support the growth of mould. So how did the mould get into the sealed, refrigerated package? Mould spores are common in the atmosphere, and they randomly land on food either in the processing plant or in open containers at your home. If the temperature and acidity of the food is hospitable, they will grow.

Most people throw away mouldy foods because they are so unappealing, but as we noted earlier, food-borne illnesses aren't commonly caused by fungi. If a small portion of a solid food, such as cheese, becomes mouldy, it is generally safe to cut off that section and eat the unspoiled portion.

Some fungi are actually used in the food industry to create popular foods and beverages. The distinct flavour of Roquefort and blue cheeses can be attributed to the moulds used in their ripening process. Yeast, the globular form of fungi, gives a distinct flavour to fermented foods, such as sourdough bread, miso, soy sauce, beer, wine, and distilled spirits. Even the production of chocolate requires the help of yeasts, which ferment the cacao seeds, causing them to lose their bitter taste.

Cook Foods Thoroughly

Remember those intestinal worms we discussed earlier? Thoroughly cooking food is a sure way to kill these and other microbes. The appropriate temperatures for cooking raw meat, poultry, seafood, and eggs vary, as shown in Figure 14.3.

The colour of cooked meat can be deceiving. Grilled meat and poultry often brown very quickly on the outside but may not be thoroughly cooked on the inside. The only way to be sure meat is thoroughly cooked is with a food thermometer. Test your food in several places to be sure it's cooked evenly, and remember to wash the thermometer after each use. If you cook hamburger, use a meat thermometer rather than relying on colour—some hamburger may still be pink even when it is thoroughly cooked. Some poultry will also have pink-coloured juices when adequately cooked, so use a thermometer to be sure the poultry is safe to eat.

Microwave cooking is convenient, but you need to be sure your food is thoroughly cooked and there are no cold spots in the food where bacteria can thrive. For best results when microwaving, remember to cover food, stir often, rotate for even cooking (CFIA 2007b) and allow "standing time" if it is recommended. "Standing time" helps to ensure the temperature inside the product is uniform. If you are microwaving meat or poultry, use a thermometer to check internal temperatures in several spots, since temperatures vary in different parts of food more in microwave cooking than in conventional ovens (CFIA 2007b).

Raw fish delicacies, such as sushi, are tempting, but their safety cannot be guaranteed. Always cook fish thoroughly. When done, fish should be opaque and flake easily with a fork.

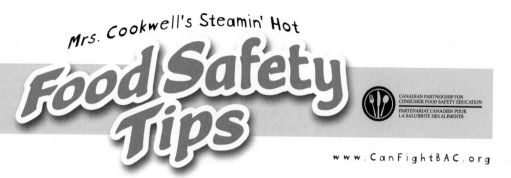

An Industry Standard Chart

Ground Meat	Recommended internal cooking temperature
Beef, pork, veal	71°C (160°F)
Chicken, turkey	80°C (176°F)

Fresh Beef	
Rare	60°C (140°F)
Medium	71°C (160°F)
Well done	77°C (170°F)
Rolled beef roasts or steaks	71°C (160°F)
Beef minute steak	71°C (160°F)

Fresh Pork	
Pork chops	71°C (160°F)
Roasts	71°C (160°F)
Fresh cured ham	71°C (160°F)
Cooked ham (to reheat)	60°C (140°F)

Poultry	Recommended internal cooking temperature
Chicken, turkey–whole, stuffed	82°C (180°F)
Chicken–whole, unstuffed	82°C (180°F)
Turkey–whole, unstuffed	77°C (170°F)
Chicken, turkey–pieces	77°C (170°F)

Stuffing	
Cooked alone	74°C (165°F)

Eggs & Egg Dishes	
Egg casseroles, sauces, custards	71°C (160°F)
Leftovers–reheated	74°C (165°F)

Thanks to the following industry groups for their input to the cooking chart:

  Beef Information Centre
  Canadian Egg Marketing Agency
  Canadian Pork Council
  Chicken Farmers of Canada
  Canadian Turkey Marketing Agency

Figure 14.3 Food Safety Tips.
(Canadian Partnership for Food Safety Education, www.canfightbac.org/en/_pdf/cooking_chart-eng.pdf.)

You may have memories of licking the cake batter off a spoon when you were a kid, but such practices are no longer considered safe. That's because cake batter contains raw eggs, which may be contaminated with *Salmonella*. For this reason, eggs should be cooked until the yolk and whites are firm. Scrambled eggs should not be runny. If you are using eggs in a casserole or custard, make sure that the internal temperature reaches at least 71°C (160°F) (Center for Science in the Public Interest [CSPI] 2004b).

Killing microorganisms with heat is an important step in keeping food safe, but it won't protect you against their toxins. That's because toxins may be unaffected by heat and are capable of causing severe illness even when the microbes that produced them have been destroyed. For example, let's say you prepare a casserole for a team picnic. Too bad you forget to wash your hands before serving it to your teammates, because you contaminate the casserole with the bacteria *Staphylococcus aureus*. You and your friends go off and play soccer, leaving the food in the sun, and a few hours later, you take the rest of the casserole home. At supper, you heat the leftovers thoroughly, thinking as you do so that this will kill any bacteria that might have multiplied while it was left out. That night you wake up with nausea, vomiting, diarrhea, and abdominal pain. What happened? While your food was left out, the bacteria from your hands multiplied and produced their toxin (Figure 14.4). When you reheated the food, you killed the microorganisms, but their toxin was unaffected by the heat.

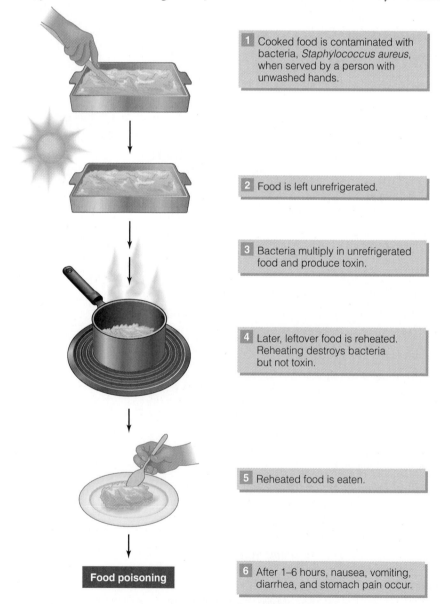

1 Cooked food is contaminated with bacteria, *Staphylococcus aureus*, when served by a person with unwashed hands.

2 Food is left unrefrigerated.

3 Bacteria multiply in unrefrigerated food and produce toxin.

4 Later, leftover food is reheated. Reheating destroys bacteria but not toxin.

5 Reheated food is eaten.

Food poisoning

6 After 1–6 hours, nausea, vomiting, diarrhea, and stomach pain occur.

Figure 14.4 Food intoxication can occur long after the microbe itself has been destroyed.

When you then ate the food, the toxin made you sick. Fortunately, in the case of *S. aureus,* symptoms typically resolve on their own in about 24 hours.

When Eating Out

When choosing a place to eat out, avoid restaurants that don't look clean. Grimy tabletops and dirty restrooms indicate indifference to hygiene. On the other hand, cleanliness of areas used by the public doesn't guarantee that the kitchen is clean and free of pathogens.

That is why health inspections are important. Public health inspectors randomly visit and inspect the food preparation areas of all businesses that serve food, whether eaten in or taken out. You can usually find the results of these inspections in the local newspaper or by contacting your local health department. In some Canadian cities, these establishments are required to post the report of the inspection for consumers to see (see an example in Figure 14.5).

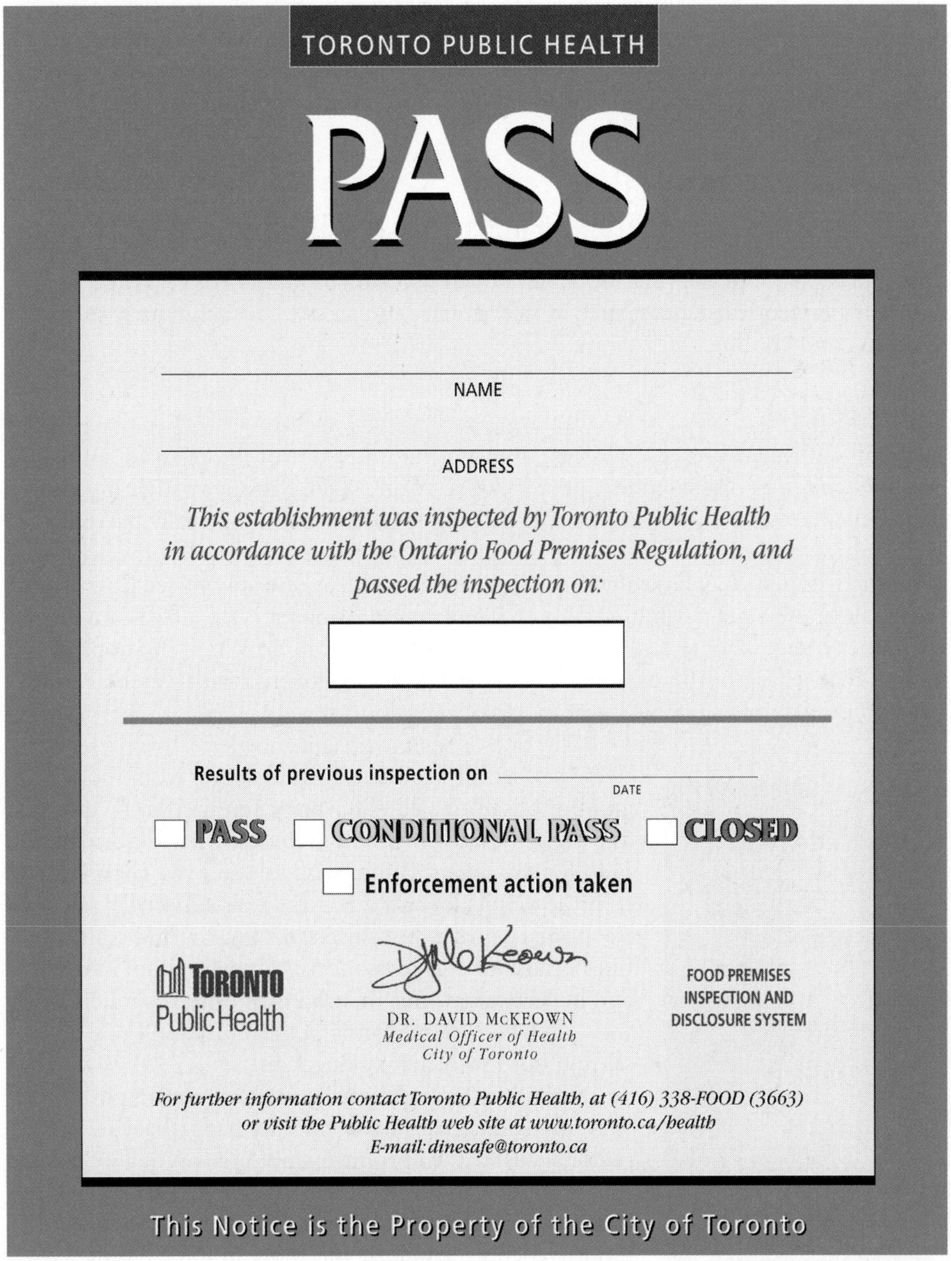

TORONTO PUBLIC HEALTH

PASS

_____
NAME

_____
ADDRESS

This establishment was inspected by Toronto Public Health in accordance with the Ontario Food Premises Regulation, and passed the inspection on:

Results of previous inspection on _____
DATE

☐ **PASS**   ☐ **CONDITIONAL PASS**   ☐ **CLOSED**

☐ **Enforcement action taken**

TORONTO
Public Health

DR. DAVID McKEOWN
Medical Officer of Health
City of Toronto

FOOD PREMISES
INSPECTION AND
DISCLOSURE SYSTEM

For further information contact Toronto Public Health, at (416) 338-FOOD (3663)
or visit the Public Health web site at www.toronto.ca/health
E-mail: dinesafe@toronto.ca

This Notice is the Property of the City of Toronto

Figure 14.5 An example of the Food Premises Inspection and Disclosure form used by Toronto Public Health. (Toronto Public Health, Food Premises Inspection and Disclosure Overview, www.toronto.ca/fooddisclosure/overview.htm, accessed March 2008.)

Another way to protect yourself when dining out is by asking for foods to be cooked thoroughly. If you order a hamburger that looks undercooked in the middle, send it back and ask for it to be cooked longer. If you order scrambled eggs that arrive runny, send them back or order something else.

> **Recap:** You can prevent food-borne illness at home by following these tips: wash your hands and kitchen surfaces often; separate raw foods from cooked foods to prevent cross contamination; cook foods to their proper temperatures; store foods in the refrigerator or freezer; thaw frozen foods in the refrigerator; and heat foods long enough and at proper temperatures to ensure proper cooking.

How Is Food Spoilage Prevented?

Any food that has been harvested and that people aren't ready to eat must be preserved in some way or, before long, it will degrade chemically and become home to a variety of microorganisms. Here, we look at some techniques that people have used for centuries to preserve food, as well as more modern techniques used in the food industry.

Tried and True—Preserving Foods Through Traditional Techniques

Some methods of preserving foods have been used for thousands of years and use naturally derived substances, such as salt, sugars, and smoke, or techniques, such as drying and cooling.

Salting and Sugaring

Both salt and sugar preserve food by drawing the water out of the plant or animal cells by *osmosis,* as discussed in Chapter 7 (see Figure 7.4). Salting or sugaring essentially dehydrates the food, making it inhospitable to microbes, especially bacteria. Dehydration also dramatically slows the action of enzymes that would otherwise continue to ripen or chemically break down the food. A good way to see how effectively salt draws water from food, and to understand osmosis, is to rub salt on cucumber or eggplant slices, and then let them sit for an hour. When the hour has passed, the surface of the cucumber or eggplant will be covered with water that has sweated out of the vegetable.

Salt, one of the oldest and most effective preservatives, is especially good at drawing water from food. The amount of salt or salt-water brine required to be effective as a preservative is much higher than what is normally used for seasoning. Brines with salt and vinegar are used to preserve pickles and sauerkraut. Traditionally, salt was the primary preservative used in all meats and seafood, but because of current concerns about sodium intake and hypertension, this method is not used as much as it was in the past. Some kinds of meat jerky still rely on salting, but few other products do.

Salt has been traditionally used for curing pork products. Many countries have specialty hams that rely on regional customs to produce a unique and quality meat.

A good example is the Parma ham from Italy, which is dry-salted with sea salt during the winter for about a month, then wiped clean and hung in huge curing rooms in long rows where plenty of fresh air can circulate around them. The curers must constantly adjust

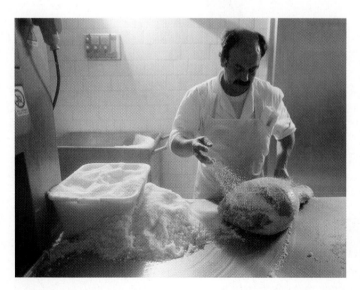
A worker salting a Parma ham

windows to accommodate changing winds. It takes almost nine months for a Parma ham to mature (Shephard 2000).

Sugar has a remarkable ability to preserve foods while retaining much of their shape, colour, and texture because some of the sugar is absorbed into the cells, replacing the water drawn out. The downside to using sugar is that fungi tend to flourish in sweet, acidic environments, such as jams. Sugar also adds Calories and can contribute to dental caries (cavities).

Honey, a natural sweetener, is also an effective preserver. Thousands of years ago, long before the processing of white or cane sugar, honey was used to preserve meats and fruits (Shephard 2000). Hams are often covered in honey to create an antibacterial coating to protect them during storage.

Drying

Drying is an ancient method of preserving food, used by many cultures in a variety of climates. There is evidence that the Egyptians dried fish and poultry in the hot desert sun as early as 12 000 B.C.E. (Shephard 2000). Beans, peas, and fruits are also commonly preserved by drying.

Drying works by the same principle as osmosis: by removing water, it makes a food inhospitable to bacteria, fungi, and other microorganisms and slows its chemical deterioration. However, depending on the method used, the food's colour, texture, and flavour may change, and the vitamin content can be decreased.

Another method of drying food is called *freeze-drying;* this is a rapid and complete drying of food. The food is first flash-frozen: any water is rapidly converted to fine ice crystals, which are evaporated in a vacuum. The product is then immediately packaged and sealed to ensure no penetration of moisture occurs. Freeze-drying preserves flavour, colour, and texture, and allows a shelf life of several years as long as the seal is not broken. Food manufacturers use freeze-drying for such products as coffee, tea, dried milk, gravy, and soup powders. This method is also used to make freeze-dried food products for camping and backpacking trips.

Smoking

Smoking has been used for centuries for preserving meats, poultry, and fish. If food was not drying well, it would be hung near the campfire or chimney so the smoke of the fire would permeate the food, further drying it.

For short-term preservation, food can be *cold-smoked* at a temperature no higher than 29°C (85°F). The smoke will give a mild, smoky flavour to the food as it dries but will not actually cook the food. This method is good for meat or fish but will only preserve them for a limited time before they start to spoil. Cold-smoking is commonly used for foods that are eaten raw, such as beef fillets or smoked salmon.

Hot-smoking uses temperatures above 55°C (130°F). It not only dries but also partially cooks the food. This process is used for such foods as venison, poultry, smoked trout, pork, lamb, and beef. Originally, heavy salting was used in conjunction with hot-smoking, but modern hot-smoked food uses much less salt.

The type of wood used to smoke foods contributes to the food's flavour. Birch, hickory, apple, juniper, mesquite, and willow are woods that have distinctive flavours. Smoked foods still need to be covered and stored in areas where air, heat, and insects cannot have easy access to them.

Cooling

As mentioned earlier, bacterial metabolism works best at temperatures at or above 15.5°C (60°F). As the temperature of a food is lowered, the bacteria's metabolism is slowed, and it becomes less able to reproduce or give off toxic byproducts. So what did people use to cool and store foods before they had electric refrigerators?

For thousands of years, people have stored foods in underground cellars, caves, running streams, and even cold pantries—rooms of the house that were kept dark and unheated and often were stocked with ice. The use of icehouses to store food is

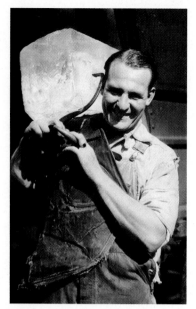

Before the modern refrigerator, an iceman would deliver ice to homes and businesses.

discussed in records from second-century China. Thirteenth- and fourteenth-century Egyptian royalty were also storing food in icehouses, stocked with ice brought from the mountains of Lebanon (Shephard 2000). The transport of freshly caught fish by using ice is also first attributed to the Chinese, and European merchants fascinated with the idea soon perfected the use of cold to design and build refrigerated vessels to transport all types of foods. Ice therefore became an important commodity. A Massachusetts company developed the forerunner of our refrigerator, the miniature icehouse, in the early 1800s, and in cities and towns, the local iceman would make rounds delivering ice to homes.

> **Recap:** Natural food preservation techniques include salting, sugaring, drying, and smoking, all of which draw water out of foods, making them inhospitable to microbes. Storage in icehouses, cold pantries, cellars, running streams, and other cold areas has been used for centuries to preserve food.

Industrial Techniques to Preserve Food and Improve Food Safety

To be successful, food producers have had to find ways to preserve the integrity of their products during the days, weeks, or months between harvesting and consumption. Until the latter part of the twentieth century, industrial techniques for food preservation were limited to drying, canning, pasteurization, and the addition of certain preservative chemicals. However, in the last few decades, the modern techniques of aseptic packaging, irradiation, and genetic modification have greatly expanded our food choices.

Industrial Canning

The French inventor Nicolas François Appert first developed the canning process in the late 1700s, and modern techniques have contributed to the retention of flavour, texture, and nutrients in canned foods.

Producers of canned foods are required by law to ensure that all endospores of *Clostridium botulinum* be eliminated from their goods. As you recall, if the spores of this bacteria were to germinate inside a can of food, the food would soon become saturated with the deadly botulism toxin. The same process that destroys *C. botulinum* endospores also kills other microorganisms that have food-poisoning potential. This process involves several steps:

pasteurization A form of sterilization using high temperatures for short periods.

1. The food to be canned is sorted, and any spoiled food is removed.
2. The food is washed.
3. The food is blanched. Blanching involves the use of hot water or steam to parboil or scald the food, thereby stopping enzymatic processes and killing microorganisms on the food's surface. It can also be used to help remove skins from certain fruits and vegetables.
4. Cans are filled and heated, air is siphoned out, and they are sealed.
5. The sealed cans are heated to a very high temperature by steam under pressure and then cooled in a water bath.

The U.S. Army has found canned meats, vegetables, and jam that have been in "excellent states of preservation" after 46 years. However, long storage of canned foods is not recommended. Canned food has an average shelf life of two years from the date of purchase. It is recommended that all canned food be stored in moderate temperatures (24°C or 75°F and below). When buying canned foods, look for cans that have no dents, cracks, or bulging lids or sides.

Pasteurization

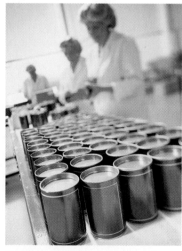

Canning food involves several steps to ensure all microorganisms in the food are killed.

Pasteurization was developed in 1864 by Louis Pasteur to destroy microorganisms that spoiled wine. Its quick use of heat to eliminate pathogens without altering the taste or quality of the food product makes it a particularly useful and important process in the dairy and juice industry. Heating to 72°C (162°F) for 15 seconds pasteurizes milk, while ice cream, which is higher in fat, requires pasteurization at 82°C (180°F) for 20 seconds. Pasteurization does not eliminate all microbes but significantly decreases the numbers of heat-sensitive microorganisms, which tend to be the most harmful. Some people claim that pasteurization robs food of vitamins and enzymes. For more information, see the Nutrition Debate "Is Unpasteurized Milk Healthier Than Pasteurized Milk?"

A newer technique called *flash pasteurization* uses higher temperatures and shorter times to destroy pathogens. It's commonly used with fruit juices, cider, and milk because it helps to maintain the nutrients and the flavour of the product. Beverages in tetra boxes or pouches have likely used flash pasteurization so that they can sit at room temperature on grocery shelves.

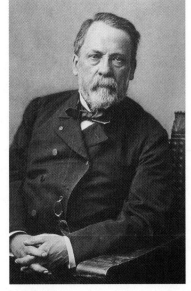

Louis Pasteur

Addition of Preservatives

Food preservatives are substances added to a variety of foods to prevent or slow food spoilage. There are many natural and synthetically derived preservatives used in our food supply and regulated by the Food and Drugs Act of Canada. One of the most commonly used natural preservatives is vitamin C. This nutrient is a powerful antioxidant and helps protect foods from damage caused by oxygen exposure. Sugar and salt can also be considered natural food preservatives, as discussed above. EDTA (ethylenediaminetetraacetic acid) is a commonly used synthetic preservative. It is used to trap trace amounts of metal impurities that can get into foods from containers and processing machinery.

Preservatives help extend the shelf life of many foods, decreasing costs and allowing consumers to buy items in bulk. Some preservatives, such as vitamin C, also enhance the nutrient quality of foods. However, a small segment of the population is sensitive to certain preservatives. These people can experience asthma, headaches, or other symptoms after eating food containing preservatives.

Most processed foods contain preservatives, unless the package states that it is "preservative free." All preservatives must be listed in the ingredients, but you must know a wide array of chemical names to know and understand which ingredients are preservatives. Table 14.2 lists some common preservatives and the types of foods you might expect to find them in. We discuss a few of these in more detail here.

Table 14.2 Common Food Preservatives

Preservative	Foods Found In
Alpha-tocopheral (vitamin E)	Vegetable oils
Ascorbic acid (vitamin C)	Breakfast cereal, cured meat, fruit drinks
BHA	Breakfast cereal, chewing gum, oil, potato chips
BHT	Breakfast cereal, chewing gum, oil, potato chips
Calcium proprionate/sodium proprionate	Breads, cakes, pies, rolls
EDTA	Canned shellfish, margarine, mayonnaise, processed fruits and vegetables, salad dressings, sandwich spreads, soft drinks
Propyl gallate	Mayonnaise, chewing gum, chicken soup base, vegetable oil, meat products, potato sticks, mashed potato flakes, fruits, ice cream
Sodium benzoate	Carbonated drinks, fruit juice, pickles, preserves
Sodium chloride (salt)	Most processed foods
Sodium nitrate/sodium nitrite	Bacon, corned beef, ham, lunch meat, hot dogs, smoked fish
Sorbic acid/potassium sorbate	Cakes, cheese, dried fruit, jelly, syrup, wine
Sulphites (sodium bisulphite, sulphur dioxide)	Dried fruit, processed potatoes, wine

BHT (butylated hydroxytoluene) An antioxidant used primarily to stop rancidity in fats and oils.

BHA (butylated hydroxyanisole) An antioxidant used primarily to stop rancidity in fats and oils.

BHA/BHT   **BHT (butylated hydroxytoluene)** and **BHA (butylated hydroxyanisole)** are two commonly used antioxidants in foods. BHT and BHA are found in a wide variety of products and are used to keep oils and fats from going rancid. BHT is frequently added to many breakfast cereal packages to decrease spoilage. BHA is stable at high temperatures and is often used in such products as soup bases, ice cream, potato flakes, gelatin desserts, dry mixes for desserts, unsmoked dry sausage, and chewing gum.

Propyl gallate, another antioxidant, works synergistically with both BHA and BHT to enhance their effectiveness. Propyl gallate is used in such products as mayonnaise, mashed potato flakes, fruits, chewing gum, ice cream, baked goods, and gelatin desserts.

Propionic Acid   The bread you bought, left on the counter, and finally got around to eating a week later would start to mould if it hadn't been treated with mould inhibitors, such as propionic acid, calcium propionate, or sodium propionate. *Propionic acid* occurs naturally in apples, strawberries, and tea and is used to prevent mould growth in baked goods and processed cheese. *Sodium propionate* and *calcium propionate* are salts synthesized from propionic acid and are used as mould inhibitors in a variety of foods.

sulphites Agents that are effective as preservatives, as antioxidants, and to prevent browning. Sulphites also have antibacterial properties, are used to bleach flour, and inhibit mould growth in grapes, wine, and other foods.

Sulphites   **Sulphites,** such as sodium bisulphite and sulphur dioxide, are effective preservatives, antioxidants, and antibrowning agents. Sulphites have antibacterial properties and are used as a bleaching agent for flour. They are also used in the beer and wine industry to inhibit mould growth, as well as in dehydrated foods, maraschino cherries, and processed potatoes. Sulphites are not used in enriched grain products because of their capacity to bind with thiamin (vitamin B_1), making it unavailable for absorption.

Sulphur dioxide is used to control mould growth on fresh fruits and vegetables. For example, it has become standard commercial practice to fumigate stored grapes every 10 days with this chemical. Because of such procedures, it's important to remember to wash all fresh fruit and vegetables before eating.

nitrates Chemicals used in meat curing to develop and stabilize the pink colour associated with cured meat; also function as antibacterial agents.

nitrites Chemicals used in meat curing to develop and stabilize the pink colour associated with cured meat; also function as antibacterial agents.

Nitrates and Nitrites   **Nitrates** and **nitrites** have been used in the processed meat industry for many years as antibacterial agents and colour enhancers. They give ham, hot dogs, and bologna their familiar pink colour. They also inhibit microbial growth, particularly *Clostridium botulinum* growth, and rancidity. However, nitrites can easily be converted to *nitrosamines* during the cooking process. Nitrosamines have been found to be carcinogenic in animals, so Health Canada has limited the amount of nitrites and nitrates that can be added to food to 200 parts per million (Food Safety Network 2008).

aseptic packaging Sterile packaging that does not require refrigeration or preservatives while the seal is maintained.

Aseptic Packaging   Many different packaging techniques have arisen over the past several decades. The newest and most environmentally sound one is **aseptic packaging**. You probably know it best as "juice boxes." Food and beverages that are packaged in aseptic containers are first sterilized in a flash-heating and cooling process, and then placed in the sterile container. Nutrient quality, as well as overall food quality, remains high without the need for preservatives or refrigeration as long as the package seals are not broken. The process uses less energy than traditional canning.

Aseptic packaging material consists of six layers: several outer polyethylene layers make the package liquid-tight. An inner paper layer gives strength and shape, while an ultrathin inner aluminum layer eliminates the need for refrigeration and preservatives by forming a barrier against light and oxygen (Aseptic Packaging Council 2003).

Although the six layers sounds like a lot of packaging, there is actually less packaging material used than in any other comparable container. A typical single-serving aseptic package provides a product-to-package ratio that is 96% product to only 4% packaging by weight. Aseptic cartons also use less energy to manufacture, fill, ship, and store, and they are recyclable. By eliminating the need for refrigeration or preservatives, aseptic packaging reduces subsequent energy use and its potential environmental burden (Aseptic Packaging Council 2003).

Irradiation

Irradiation is an effective process for eliminating harmful bacteria often found in foods, such as *Trichinella spirialis* and *Salmonella* in meats and poultry, and inhibits spoilage by fungus. It involves the use of x-rays, beams of high-energy electrons produced by electron accelerators, or gamma rays from cobalt 60 or cesium 137. Most of this energy simply passes through the food, leaving no residue.

In contrast to the many foods authorized for irradiation in the United States, Canada has a limited selection of foods that can be irradiated. Although amendments have been proposed to add fresh and frozen ground beef, poultry, fish, mangoes, and dried shrimp, currently only onions, potatoes, wheat, flour, whole wheat flour, dehydrated seasonings, and whole or ground spices can be irradiated.

A product must display the international symbol for irradiated food, the radura, if it has been wholly irradiated, and any irradiated ingredient that makes up more than 10% of a product must be stated as irradiated on the list of ingredients (Figure 14.6). Irradiation has been approved for use by 50 countries and endorsed by the World Health Organization (WHO), the Food and Agriculture Organization of the United Nations (FAO), and the International Atomic Energy Agency (IAEA).

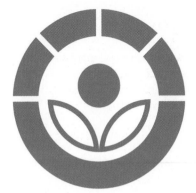

Figure 14.6 Radura—the international symbol of irradiated food—is found on products that have been wholly irradiated.

irradiation A sterilization process utilizing gamma rays or other forms of radiation, which does not impart any radiation to the food being treated.

> **Recap:** The canning process was developed in the late eighteenth century. Pasteurization has been in use for more than 100 years to destroy microbes, by using high heat for short durations on liquids, such as milk and juice. Natural and synthetic preservatives, such as salt, sugar, vitamin C, sulphites, and nitrates, are often added to keep foods fresher longer. Aseptic packaging is a relatively new form of packaging in which sterilized foods can be stored for long periods without refrigeration. Irradiation typically involves the use of gamma rays to destroy the microbes in foods.

What Are Food Additives, and Are They Safe?

Have you ever picked up a loaf of bread and started reading its ingredients? You'd expect to see flour, yeast, water, and some sugar, but what are all those other items? And why does it feel as if you have to have a degree in chemistry to understand what they are? They are collectively called food additives, and they are in almost every processed food. Without additives, that loaf of bread would go stale within a day or two.

Although their use is regulated by health authorities, food additives have been a source of controversy for the past 50 years. Nevertheless, their use has steadily increased, allowing food producers to offer consumers a greater variety of foods at lower costs.

Additives Can Enhance a Food's Taste, Appearance, Safety, or Nutrition

It's estimated that more than 3000 different additives are currently used in North America. By becoming familiar with some of the most common, you'll gain a better understanding of what's in your food.

Additives Can Be Natural or Synthetic

Many of the additives used by the food industry come from natural sources. Beet juice (a natural food colouring), salt, and citric acid are common, naturally derived food additives, but in cases when supply or cost would prohibit using naturally derived additives, additives are synthesized. For instance, vanillin, the main flavouring substance in vanilla beans, is synthesized at a cost considerably lower than the cost of extracting it from the natural beans. Even if the costs were comparable, it is doubtful that natural sources of vanillin could meet consumer demands.

Flavourings

flavouring agents Obtained from either natural or synthetic sources; allow manufacturers to maintain a consistent flavour from batch to batch.

Roughly half of all additives are flavourings used to replace the natural flavour lost during food processing (Winter 1994). **Flavouring agents** can be obtained from natural or synthetic sources. Essential oils, extracts, and spices supply most of the naturally derived flavourings. Flavourings are typically found in soft drinks, baked goods, and frozen confections.

Flavour enhancers are also widely used. These additives have little or no flavour of their own but accentuate the natural flavour of foods. They are often added when very little of a natural ingredient is used (CSPI 2004a). The most common flavour enhancers used are maltol and MSG (monosodium glutamate). MSG is the sodium salt of glutamic acid, one of the non-essential amino acids, which also serves as a neurotransmitter. Originally derived from sea kelp by the Japanese and introduced to Americans during World War II, MSG is found in many processed foods. However, in some people, MSG causes such symptoms as headaches, difficulty breathing, and heart palpitations. It has been demonstrated that the glutamate portion of MSG can cross the blood-brain barrier and cause overstimulation of neurons, especially in the young. Because of this research, the U.S. Congress mandated in the 1960s that MSG be removed from baby food (Blaylock 1996).

Colourings

coal tar A food additive made from thick or semisolid tar derived from bituminous coal, the byproducts of which have been found to cause cancer in animals.

Food colourings, derived from both natural and synthetic sources, are used extensively in processed foods. In the past, many food colourings were made from **coal tar**, a thick or semisolid tar derived from bituminous coal. Derivatives of coal tar have been found to cause cancer in animals, and most have been banned by health authorities from use in foods. Natural colourings, such as beet juice (which gives a red colour), beta-carotene (which gives a yellow colour), and caramel (which adds brown colour), are now used instead and do not need to be tested for safety. The colouring tartrazine (FD&C yellow #5) causes an allergic reaction in some people. Sudan I is a red dye that has caused cancer in lab animals and is not allowed in Canada (CFIA 2003).

Vitamins and Other Nutrients

texturizers A chemical used to improve the texture of various foods.
stabilizers Help maintain smooth texture and uniform colour and flavour in some foods.
thickening agents Natural or chemically modified carbohydrates that absorb some of the water present in food, making the food thicker while keeping food components balanced.
emulsifiers Chemicals that improve texture and smoothness in foods; stabilize oil-water mixtures.

Vitamin E is usually added to fat-based products to keep them from going rancid, and ascorbic acid is commonly added to such foods as frozen fruit, dry milk, apple juice, soft drinks, candy, and meat products containing sodium nitrates. Sodium ascorbate, a form of vitamin C with sodium added to produce a salt, is used as an antioxidant in such foods as concentrated milk products, cereals, and cured meats.

Iodine and vitamin D are purely nutritive additives. Their function in foods is to reduce the occurrence of a deficiency disease. Iodine was originally added to table salt to help decrease the incidence of goiter, a condition that causes the thyroid gland to enlarge. Vitamin D is added to milk and margarine because in northern latitudes it is not possible to produce adequate vitamin D from sun exposure during the late fall and winter. As you learned in Chapter 9, vitamin D is necessary for calcium metabolism and has been found to be important in preventing osteoporosis in adults and rickets in infants and children.

Texturizers, Stabilizers, and Emulsifiers

Texturizers, such as calcium chloride, are added to foods to improve their texture. For instance, they are added to canned tomatoes and potatoes so they don't fall apart. **Stabilizers** are added to products to give them body and help them maintain a desired texture or colour. **Thickening agents** are used to absorb water and keep the complex mixtures of oils, water, acids, and solids in foods balanced (CSPI 2004a). Natural thickeners include pectin, alginate, and carrageenan. **Emulsifiers**, like thickening agents and stabilizers, help to keep fats evenly dispersed within foods. Texturizers, stabilizers, thickening agents, and emulsifiers have no known adverse effect on humans when used according to regulations.

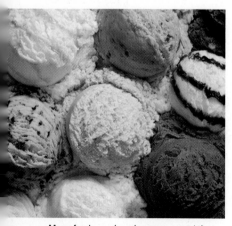
Many foods, such as ice cream, contain colourings.

Humectants and Desiccants

Moisture content is a critical component to food, and **humectants** and **desiccants** are added to maintain the correct moisture levels. Humectants keep such foods as marshmallows, chewing gum, and shredded coconut soft and stretchy. Common humectants are glycerin, sorbitol, and propylene glycol. Food-grade waxes used on produce also help maintain moisture content. The best way to remove wax from produce is to peel the outer layer off or scrub it with hot, soapy water and rinse well. Desiccants prevent moisture absorption from the air; for example, they are used to prevent table salt from forming clumps.

humectants Chemicals that help retain moisture in foods, keeping them soft and pliable.

desiccants Chemicals that prevent foods from absorbing moisture from the air.

Bleaching Agents

Bleaching agents are used primarily in baked goods. Fresh ground flour is pale yellow, and when stored it slowly becomes white. Processors have added bleaching agents to flour to speed this process and decrease the possibility of spoilage or insect infestation. Benzoyl peroxide is commonly used to bleach flour, as well as blue and Gorgonzola cheeses (Winter 1994).

bleaching agents Chemicals used to speed the natural process of ground flour changing from pale yellow to white.

Some Additives Get into Our Food Unintentionally

Trace amounts of substances (such as insects, fragments of packaging materials, pesticides, and hormones or antibiotics given to livestock) can get into our food during harvesting, processing, storage, or packaging. These are called *unintentional* or *incidental additives* and do not have to be included on the label. This small amount of incidental food additives present in food has not been shown to cause any problems with quality or safety.

Are Food Additives Safe?

Although there is often controversy over food additives, they have been tested and approved for use in the food industry, and they are strictly regulated according to Canada's Food and Drugs Act. These additives have allowed our food supply to increase and diversify, providing consumers more variety at lower costs. Without additives, such as flavourings, strawberry ice cream would only be available for a short time and only in limited quantities during the early summer. If you are interested in reducing the amount of food additives in your diet, you should start by comparing food labels of different brands of the same foods. Some brands use fewer additives than others, and some brands are additive-free.

> **Recap:** Food additives are chemicals intentionally added to foods to enhance their colour, flavour, texture, nutrient density, moisture level, or shelf life. Unintentional additives are trace amounts of substances that get into our food during harvesting, processing, storage, or packaging. Although there is sometimes controversy over food additives, they have been approved for use and are strictly regulated according to the Food and Drugs Act.

residues Chemicals that remain in the foods we eat despite cleaning and processing.

persistent organic pollutants (POPs) Chemicals released into the environment as a result of industry, agriculture, or improper waste disposal; automobile emissions also are considered POPs.

Do Residues Harm Our Food Supply?

Food **residues** are chemicals that remain in the foods we eat despite cleaning and processing. Two types of residues of global concern are pollutants and pesticides.

Persistent Organic Pollutants Can Cause Illness

Many different organic chemicals are released into the atmosphere as a result of industry, agriculture, automobile emissions, and improper waste disposal. These chemicals, collectively referred to as **persistent organic pollutants (POPs)**, eventually enter the food supply through the soil or water. If a pollutant gets into the soil, a

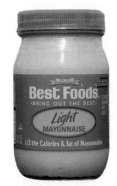

Mayonnaise contains emulsifiers to prevent separation of fats.

Acrylamide

What's not to love about a heaping order of fresh, crispy-brown french fries? As it turns out, a lot. Not only are these morsels full of fat (and sometimes trans fat) but new evidence also suggests that they may increase the risk of cancer. The formation of acrylamides in starch-based foods, which was first brought to the forefront in 2002 by scientists in Sweden, has been shown to cause cancer in laboratory animals. It is considered "probably carcinogenic to humans" by the International Agency for Research on Cancer and may also damage the nervous and reproductive systems.

Acrylamide is formed when asparagine, a natural amino acid, reacts with certain naturally occurring sugars during processing or cooking at temperatures above 120°C (250°F). Research shows that the process that browns food and increases flavour, known as the Maillard reaction, plays a key role in acrylamide formation. In the Maillard reaction, asparagine and glucose form the compound N-glycosylasparagine, which, when heated, produces large quantities of acrylamide. But french fries aren't the only culprits—acrylamide is found in many foods, most notably potato chips, bread, cereals, and coffee products.

Unfortunately, all the hype created by this new information about acrylamide's potential health risks often blurs the fact that a few simple steps can reduce the formation of this possible carcinogen. Health Canada recommends that when deep-frying, you should take care not to exceed temperatures of 170°C to 175°C (340°F to 350°F) and not to store potatoes below 8°C (46°F). Also, bread should be toasted to the lightest acceptable colour and crusts can be removed for further reduction of acrylamide consumption. All acrylamide found in ground coffee is transferred to the brew because of acrylamide's polar nature; however, because the roasting process virtually eliminates acrylamide, choosing a dark-roasted coffee will decrease the amount of acrylamide consumed.

Still have to have those french fries? Well, turn down the temperature and make them golden brown, not dark and crispy, and your body will thank you. If you take Health Canada's advice and choose a healthy diet full of a variety of foods, occasional consumption of fried or deep-fried food is not cause for alarm.

plant can absorb the chemical into its structure and can pass it on as part of the food chain. Animals can also absorb the pollutants into their tissues or can consume them when feeding on plants growing in the polluted soil. Fat-soluble pollutants are especially problematic, as they tend to accumulate in the animal's body tissues and are then absorbed by humans when the animal is used as a food source.

POP residues have been found in virtually all categories of foods, including baked goods, fruit, vegetables, fish, meat, poultry, and dairy products. The chemicals can travel long distance in trade winds and water currents, moving from tropical and temperate regions to concentrate in the northern latitudes. It is believed that all organisms on Earth carry a measurable level of POPs in their tissues (Schafer and Kegley 2002).

Mercury and Lead Are Nerve Toxins Found in the Environment

Mercury, a naturally occurring element, is found in soil and rocks, lakes, streams, and oceans. It is also released into the environment by pulp and paper processing and the burning of garbage and fossil fuels. As mercury is released into the environment, it falls from the air, eventually finding its way to streams, lakes, and the ocean, where it accumulates. Fish absorb mercury as they feed on aquatic organisms and convert it to methyl mercury. This methyl mercury is passed on to us when we consume the fish. As methyl mercury accumulates in the body, it has a toxic effect on the nervous system.

Predatory fish tend to accumulate higher levels of methyl mercury and therefore should be eaten less often by young children and women who are or may become pregnant or are breastfeeding. These fish species include fresh and frozen tuna, shark, swordfish, marlin, orange roughy, and escolar (sometimes called snake mackerel or oilfish). See Chapter 5 for the specific amounts recommended. Anchovy, capelin, char, hake, herring, Atlantic mackerel, mullet, pollock, salmon, smelt, rainbow trout, lake whitefish, shrimp, clam, mussel, oysters and canned light tuna are safe to consume (Health Canada 2007). Freshwater fish caught in local lakes and rivers have variable levels of methyl mercury; thus, provincial and territorial governments routinely monitor mercury levels and issue advisories when levels are too high.

Lead, another naturally occurring element, can be found in soil, water, and even air. It also occurs as industrial waste from leaded gasoline, lead-based paints, and lead-soldered cans, now outlawed but decomposing in landfills. Some ceramic mugs and other dishes are fired with lead-based glaze. Thus, residues can build up in foods. Excessive lead exposure can cause learning and behavioural impediments in children and cardiovascular and kidney disease in adults. It is impossible to avoid lead residues completely, but because of its health implications, everyone should try to limit their exposure.

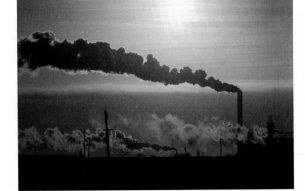

One of the ways mercury is released into the environment is by pulp mills.

Industrial Pollutants Also Create Residues

Polychlorinated biphenyls (PCBs) and **dioxins** are two industrial pollutants that have been found in food worldwide. Dioxins (byproducts of waste incineration) and PCBs (from discarded transformers) enter the soil and can persist in the environment for years, easily accumulating in fatty tissues. Many studies done in Belgium show that chicken, pork, and eggs have been found to have concentrations of these chemicals in excess of international standards (Larenbeke et al. 2002). PCBs and dioxins, along with other POPs, have been linked to cancer, learning disorders, impaired immune function, and infertility (Schafer and Kegley 2002).

polychlorinated biphenyls (PCBs) An industrial pollutant most commonly attributed to discarded transformers.
dioxins An industrial pollutant most commonly attributed to waste incineration.

Reducing POPs Is a Global Concern

International agreements sponsored by the United Nations seek to ban or restrict POPs. For example, the Stockholm Convention, originally drafted in May 2001, is intended to enable the international community to collaborate on an agreeable solution to reducing and eventually phasing out the use of POPs. Its mandate also includes the development of alternatives and the safe and environmentally sound disposal of POPs. If you're interested in reading the full text of the Stockholm Convention, go to www.pops.int.

> **Recap:** Persistent organic pollutants (POPs) have been found in virtually all categories of foods. Methyl mercury contaminates certain fish, and lead contaminates many foods. Both are toxic to the nervous system. Polychlorinated biphenyls (PCBs) and dioxins are two industrial pollutants that have been found in food worldwide. International agreements sponsored by the United States seek to ban or restrict POPs.

biopesticides Biopesticides include naturally occurring substances that control pests (biochemical pesticides), microorganisms that control pests (microbial pesticides), and pesticidal substances produced by plants containing added genetic material (plant-incorporated protectants) or PIPs.

Pesticides Protect Against Crop Losses

Pesticides are used to protect our food from damage by weeds, bacteria, fungi and other organisms, including birds and mammals.

Pesticides Can Be Natural or Synthetic

Many plants naturally produce pesticides to help protect themselves from predators and disease. Humans have found a way to use naturally derived or synthetic analogues of this protective mechanism for agricultural use. Despite the negative connotations associated with pesticides, many pesticides used today are naturally derived, or have a low impact on the environment. Gardeners and farmers are starting to use biopesticides. **Biopesticides** include naturally occurring substances that control pests (biochemical pesticides), microorganisms that control pests (microbial pesticides), and pesticidal substances produced by plants containing added genetic material (plant-incorporated protectants) or PIPs. Biopesticides are usually inherently less

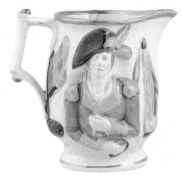

Antique porcelain is often coated with lead-based glaze.

toxic than conventional pesticides as they affect only the target pest and closely related organisms, in contrast to broad-spectrum conventional pesticides that may affect organisms as different as birds, insects, and mammals. Biopesticides are species-specific and work to suppress a pest's population, not eliminate it. Biopesticides do not leave residues on crops—most degrade rapidly and are easily washed away with water. As well, biopesticides may be effective in very small quantities, resulting in lower exposures. When used as a component of Integrated Pest Management (IPM) programs, biopesticides can greatly decrease the use of conventional pesticides, while maintaining a high crop yield.

Pheromones are a type of biochemical biopesticide. In nature, insects use pheromones to attract mates. Synthetic pheromones are used to disrupt insect mating by attracting males into traps. Microbial biopesticides are derived from naturally occurring or genetically altered microorganisms like bacteria, viruses, or fungi. A widely used microbial biopesticide is *Bacillus thuringiensis*, or *Bt*. This is a common soil bacterium that is genetically altered to be toxic to one group of insects—Lepidoptera.

Aside from biopesticides, many common products, such as boric acid or diatomaceous earth, are used as pesticides. Pesticides can also be synthetically derived. Many are made from petroleum-based products. Examples of commonly used synthetic pesticides include thiabendazole (a fungicide used on potatoes) and fungicides commonly used to prevent apple diseases (such as dithane, manzate, and polyram).

Some Pesticides Are Potential Toxins

Years of studies show that chemicals, whether natural or synthetic, can remain on food and affect immune system function in people whose systems are already compromised. The liver is responsible for detoxifying the chemicals that enter our bodies; but if diseases, such as cancer, or toxins, such as alcohol, already stress it, then the liver cannot effectively remove pesticide residues. When pesticide residues are not effectively removed, they can damage body tissues. Some are fat-soluble and can be deposited in adipose tissues, which may later be metabolized for energy—and the residues then may be released into the body and cause damage. Others target nervous system and endocrine system cells. Thus, although originally intended for other organisms, pesticides do have the potential to cause problems in humans.

Children may be more susceptible to pesticide residues, as they consume more food and water per unit of body weight than adults and may have a limited ability to detoxify these substances. Because of the potential risks from chemicals to a developing child, pregnant and breastfeeding women should peel fruit and vegetable rinds to decrease their exposure to residues. This is also a sensible precaution when preparing fruit or vegetables for small children.

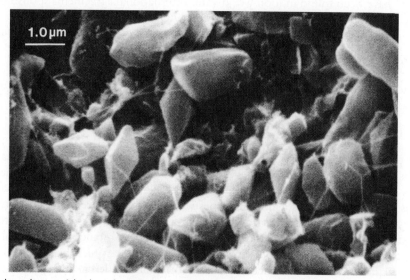

Bt bacteria produce crystals, shown here, that are a widely used microbial biopesticide.

To protect people from any possible harm arising from pesticide residues, Maximum Residue Limits (MRLs) have been set for each pesticide–crop combination. The Canadian Food Inspection Agency monitors all commercially available fruits and vegetables for pesticide residues and issues recalls of products that may not be safe. Special consideration is given to products like fruit juice that children may consume in higher than average amounts. No groups of the population are exposed to residues in food at levels that threaten their health.

Government Regulations Control the Use of Pesticides

Through the Pest Control Products Act, Health Canada's Pest Management Regulatory Agency is the government agency responsible for the registration of pesticides and assessment of the human health and safety aspects and environmental impacts of pesticides in Canada. Regulations concerning the transportation, sale, storage, use, and disposal of pesticides are at the provincial or territorial levels. Bylaws for the use of pesticides in residential and commercial areas are put in place and enforced at the municipal level.

> **Recap:** Pesticides are chemicals used to prevent or reduce food crop losses caused by weeds, insects, fungi, and other organisms, including birds and mammals. Biopesticides may be biochemical or microbial. Many synthetic pesticides are petroleum-based products. Some pesticides are potential toxins; therefore, it is essential to wash all produce carefully. Pregnant and breastfeeding women and young children should eat produce without the peel.

What Are Organic Foods?

Organic food is produced by farmers who emphasize the use of renewable resources and the conservation of soil and water to protect the environment for future generations. Organic meat, poultry, eggs, and dairy products come from animals that are given no antibiotics or growth hormones and that are treated humanely. Organic food is produced without using most conventional pesticides, fertilizers made with synthetic ingredients or sewage sludge, bioengineering, or ionizing radiation (Canadian General Standards Board 2006).

The General Principles and Management Standards set out by the Canadian General Standards Board (2006) for organic production state the following principles:

1. Protect the environment, minimize soil degradation and erosion, decrease pollution, optimize biological productivity, and promote a sound state of health.
2. Maintain long-term soil fertility by optimizing conditions for biological activity within the soil.
3. Maintain biological diversity within the system.
4. Recycle materials and resources to the greatest extent possible within the enterprise.
5. Provide attentive care that promotes the health and meets the behavioural needs of livestock.
6. Prepare organic products, emphasizing careful processing and handling methods in order to maintain the organic integrity and vital qualities of the products at all stages of production.
7. Rely on renewable resources in locally organized agricultural systems.

How Are Organic Foods in Canada Regulated?

In the 1990s, when organic foods first began appearing in major grocery chains, the organic food industry was small and there was no pressing reason for it to be regulated by government. Now Canada exports organic products, mostly grains, worth an estimated $63 million annually, with approximately one third of this going to Europe (Doering 2005). CODEX organic standards regulate international trade, and Canada complies with these standards.

In Canada, the Organic Products Regulations were passed by parliament in December 2006 and will be fully in place by mid 2009. These regulations are intended for all organic agricultural products, whether they are imported, exported, or traded among provinces and territories. Labels are allowed to carry the terms *organic, organically produced, organically grown,* and *organically raised* if 95% of the ingredients in the product are organic. If the product contains 70% to 95% organic ingredients, the label may specify the percentage of organic material—for example, "contains 75% Organic"—and must state which ingredients are organic in the ingredient list.

Recap: Pesticides are used to protect our food from damage by weeds, bacteria, fungi, and other organisms, including birds and mammals. Biopesticides are species-specific and less toxic to humans and to the environment. Organic food is produced without using most conventional pesticides, fertilizers made with synthetic ingredients or sewage sludge, bioengineering, or ionizing radiation. Organic products are strictly regulated by a new set of standards which will be in full effect by mid 2009.

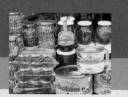

CHAPTER SUMMARY

- Concerns about food safety typically focus on food-borne illness, food spoilage, and technologic manipulation of food.

- Approximately 11 million to 13 million Canadians experience food-borne illness each year.

- Food infections result from the consumption of food containing living microorganisms, such as bacteria, whereas food intoxications result from consuming food in which microbes have secreted toxins.

- Food infections can be caused by bacteria, viruses, fungi, helminths, and prions.

- The body has several defence mechanisms, such as saliva, stomach acid, vomiting, diarrhea, and the inflammatory response, that help rid us of offending microorganisms and toxins.

- The conditions most favourable for bacterial growth are summarized by the acronym FATTOM: food, acidity, time, temperature, oxygen, and moisture. Most bacteria thrive in protein or carbohydrate foods at a mildly acidic pH, and can grow to harmful numbers in about four hours.

- You can reduce your risk for food-borne illness at home by following these tips: Wash your hands and kitchen surfaces often. Separate raw foods from cooked foods to prevent cross contamination. Cook foods to their proper temperatures. Store foods in the refrigerator or freezer. Thaw frozen foods in the refrigerator, and heat them long enough and at the required temperature to ensure proper cooking.

- Food spoilage affects a food's appearance, texture, taste, smell, and may or may not affect food safety.

- Both fresh and processed foods are vulnerable to spoilage.

- Some natural techniques for food preservation include salting and sugaring, drying, smoking, and cooling.

- Synthetic food preservation techniques include canning, pasteurization, flash pasteurization, addition of preservatives, aseptic packaging, irradiation, and genetic modification.

- Food additives are natural or synthetic ingredients added to foods during processing to enhance them in some way. They include flavourings, colourings, nutrients, texturizers, and other additives.

- Persistent organic pollutants (POPs) are chemicals released into the atmosphere as a result of industry, agriculture, automobile emissions, and improper waste disposal. Plants, animals, and fish absorb the chemicals from contaminated soil or water and pass them on as part of the food chain.

- Large predatory fish, such as swordfish, shark, and fresh and frozen tuna, tend to contain high levels of methyl mercury, which is especially toxic to the developing nervous system.

- All produce should be washed carefully before eating. Produce prepared for pregnant women, breastfeeding women, and young children should be peeled whenever possible.

- Organic foods must follow a strict set of standard practices in order to be certified in Canada. The legislation governing organic foods will be in full effect by mid 2009.

REVIEW QUESTIONS

1. The factors that promote bacterial growth can be summarized as
   a. food, acid, oxygen, heat, and light.
   b. food, acid, time, temperature, moisture, and light.
   c. food, acid, time, moisture, heat, and cold.
   d. food, acid, time, temperature, oxygen, and moisture.

2. Yeasts are
   a. a type of mould used to make bread rise.
   b. a type of bacteria that can cause food intoxication.
   c. a type of fungus used to ferment foods.
   d. a type of mould inhibitor used as a food preservative.

3. Monosodium glutamate (MSG) is
   a. a thickening agent used in baby foods.
   b. a flavour enhancer used in a variety of foods.
   c. a mould inhibitor used on grapes and other foods.
   d. an amino acid added as a nutrient to some foods.

4. You should store uncooked meat, poultry, and seafood in the refrigerator and use within
   a. 24 hours.
   b. 48 hours.
   c. three days.
   d. a week.

5. Beginning with the most ancient method, what is the correct chronological order for the following techniques for food preservation?
   a. Freezing, drying, pasteurization, aseptic packaging
   b. Freeze-drying, smoking, irradiation, pasteurization
   c. Freezing, pasteurization, canning, aseptic packaging
   d. Cooling, canning, pasteurization, irradiation

6. Hemolytic uremic syndrome (HUS) is a complication of
   a. *E. coli* O157:H7 poisoning.
   b. salmonellosis.
   c. *Clostridium botulinum* poisoning.
   d. avian influenza.

7. Which one of the following microbes secretes a toxin that causes food intoxication?
   a. *Campylobacter jejuni*
   b. *E. coli* O157:H7
   c. *Clostridium botulinum*
   d. Hepatitis A

8. Steven and Dante go to a convenience store after a tennis match looking for something to quench their thirst. Steven chooses a national brand of orange juice, and Dante chooses a bottle of locally produced, organic, unpasteurized apple juice. Steven points out to Dante that his juice is not pasteurized, but he shrugs and says, "I'm more afraid of the pesticides they used on the oranges in your juice than I am about microorganisms in mine!" Which juice would *you* choose, and why?

9. Pickling is a food-preservation technique that involves soaking such foods as cucumbers in a solution containing vinegar (acetic acid). Why would pickling be effective in preventing food spoilage?

10. In the 1950s and 1960s in Minamata, Japan, more than 100 cases of a similar illness were recorded: patients, many of whom were infants or young children, suffered irreversible damage to the nervous system. A total of 46 people died. Adults with the disease and mothers of afflicted young children had one thing in common: they had frequently eaten fish caught in Minamata Bay. What do you think might have been the cause of this disease? Using key words from this description, research the event on the internet and identify the culprit(s).

11. Your sister Joy, who attends a culinary arts school, is visiting you for dinner. You want to impress her, so you've decided to make chicken marsala. You begin that afternoon by removing two chicken breasts from the freezer and putting them in a bowl in the refrigerator to thaw. Then you go shopping for fresh salad ingredients. When you get home from the market, you wash your hands in cold water, then take the chicken breasts from the refrigerator and wash them thoroughly. You set them aside on a clean cutting board. You then take the lettuce, red pepper, and scallions you just bought, put them in a colander, and rinse them. Next, you slice them with a clean knife on your marble counter top and toss them together in a salad. You put the chicken breasts in a frying pan and cook them until they lose their pink colour. In a separate pan, you prepare the sauce, using a new carton of cream and the marsala. Finally, using a clean knife, you slice some freshly baked bread on the counter top. You then wash the knives and the cutting board you used for the chicken. Joy arrives and admires your skill in cooking. Later that night, you both wake up vomiting. Identify *at least two* aspects of your food preparation that might have contributed to your illness.

12. A couple of hours after a family potluck picnic where Vakeesh ate some turkey casserole and potato salad and drank a soft drink, he starts to feel terribly sick. He spends the whole evening in the bathroom and can barely move without feeling ill. The next morning he feels a bit better, but is still very weak and exhausted. When he calls his relatives to find out if

anybody else got sick, he is surprised to hear that nobody else fell ill—but he is still convinced that it was a dish at the picnic that made him sick. Do you think that the illness was food-borne? If so, what food(s) do you most suspect? What precautions might you advise Vakeesh to take in the future to prevent food-borne illness?

13. Louis's family owns a farm in Saskatchewan that has been passed from generation to generation since his family immigrated to Canada. Louis is refusing to take it over, however, because he feels very strongly that pesticides are ruining the environment and poisoning people. Louis's father argues that pesticides are necessary to prevent disease-causing microorganisms, but Louis will not agree. Who do you think is correct in this case: Louis, who says pesticides are dangerous, or his father, who argues that they prevent disease? How do you think this situation could be resolved?

CASE STUDY

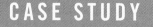

A local high school was having a barbeque to celebrate the end of the year on a Saturday around 11:30 a.m. They chose to serve hamburgers, hot dogs from Chuck's meat packaging plant, and potato salad and coleslaw catered from Sal's. The hamburgers were prepared by Chuck's employees on the Friday prior to the barbeque. Chuck went to the washroom and without washing his hands he removed the hamburger meat from the refrigerator and gave it to his employees.

They then began preparing the processor to make the hamburger patties, which took two hours to get running. After waiting for all the hamburgers to be processed, which took another half-hour, they wrapped them up and placed them back in the refrigerator in an open pan. Sal's potato salad and coleslaw contained fresh cabbage, onions, potatoes, celery, and carrots in addition to mayonnaise and seasonings. Sal thoroughly washed her hands before beginning to chop, dice, and slice the vegetables for the potato salad and coleslaw. She then took out the mayonnaise only as she needed it, mixed the salads, covered them, and quickly returned them to the refrigerator.

The hamburgers arrived at the school at 8 a.m. on Saturday, and the potato salad and coleslaw were delivered around 11:15 a.m. Ms. Crump began cooking the hamburgers and hot dogs at 9:30 a.m. and once they were finished, they were wrapped in tinfoil, which was around 10:30 a.m. The students and teachers arrived around 11:30 a.m. and there were complaints that the hamburgers and hot dogs were cold. On Monday at 8 a.m. a few of the teachers and several students were complaining of abdominal cramps, vomiting, diarrhea, dehydration, and listlessness.

a. As a CFIA inspector what would your first steps be to determine the cause of the illness?

b. Which bacteria do you suspect based on the incubation period, symptoms, and possible sources?

c. What types of things can you identify as possible causes of the illness?

Test Yourself Answers

1. **False** Freezing inhibits the ability of microbes to reproduce, but when the food is thawed, reproduction resumes.

2. **False** Some ground hamburger meat will still look slightly pink even when thoroughly cooked. It is important to use a meat thermometer to check doneness, even with hamburger patties.

3. **False** Bacteria cause the vast majority of cases of food-borne illness.

4. **True**

5. **True** The Canadian Food Inspection Agency (CFIA) is responsible for monitoring food safety and ensuring that manufacturers follow the Food and Drugs Act and its regulations and other legislation. Health Canada oversees the work of the CFIA.

WEB LINKS

www.phac-aspc.gc.ca/id-mi/index-eng.php
Public Health Agency of Canada—Infectious Diseases
This website provides information on infectious diseases—everything from avian flu, cholera, and *E. coli* to SARS, *salmonella*, and West Nile virus.

www.canfightbac.org
The Canadian Partnership for Consumer Food Safety Education
This is a national association of public and private organizations dedicated to helping consumers understand the importance of safe food handling practices at home. Click on Consumers for practical information and tips on keeping food safe to eat.

www.kidney.ca
The Kidney Foundation of Canada
A great site for anyone interested in learning more about hemolytic uremic syndrome (HUS), other kidney diseases, and research in progress.

www.foodsafety.gov
Foodsafety.gov
Use this website as a gateway to government food safety information; it contains news and safety alerts, an area to report illnesses and product complaints, information on food-borne pathogens, and much more.

www.fsis.usda.gov
The USDA Food Safety and Inspection Service
A comprehensive site providing information on all aspects of food safety. Click on Publications for links to the informative publications about food preparation, storage, handling, and other specific safety issues.

www.cspinet.org/foodsafety/index.html
Center for Science in the Public Interest: Food Safety
Visit this website for summaries of food additives and their safety, alerts and other information, and interactive quizzes.

www.inspection.gc.ca
Canadian Food Inspection Agency
This site contains information about food safety standards in Canada.

www.consumerreports.org/cro/food/food-safety/index.htm
Consumer Reports: Food Safety
On this site, you'll find information on such topics as benzene in soft drinks, mercury in fish, irradiated meat, produce washes, poultry safety, and mad cow disease.

www.cfsan.fda.gov
The USDA Center for Food Safety and Applied Nutrition
This site contains thorough information on such topics as national food safety programs, recent news, and food labelling. It also contains links to special program areas, such as regulation of mercury levels in fish, food colourings, and biotechnology.

www.extension.iastate.edu/foodsafety/
Food Safety From Farm to Table
This excellent University of Iowa website has lots of materials for consumers. View the cross-contamination or temperature monitoring videos; see the food-borne pathogen of the day, hot topics, and much more!

www.epa.gov/pesticides
The U.S. Environmental Protection Agency: Pesticides
This site provides information about agricultural and home-use pesticides, pesticide health and safety issues, environmental effects, and government regulation.

www.organicagcentre.ca
Organic Agriculture Centre of Canada
This partnership of federal and provincial governments, industry groups, commodity boards, and universities calls itself "Canada's national website for organic research and education." You can look at student job postings, take a virtual tour of a farm, and see consumer resources on a variety of topics.

www.ams.usda.gov
The USDA National Organic Program
Click on National Organic Program to find the website describing the NOP's standards and labelling program, consumer information, and publications.

Is Unpasteurized Milk Healthier Than Pasteurized Milk?

Although the sale of raw milk, or unpasteurized milk, has been banned for more than a decade, a growing number of consumers have been choosing to drink unpasteurized milk again (Jayarao et al. 2006). Advocates strongly believe that raw milk is healthier and more nutritious. In processing milk, they claim that important nutrients and enzymes are destroyed by the heat (Bren 2004). Moreover, they attribute growth problems, osteoporosis, arthritis, heart disease, and cancer to pasteurized milk (Campaign for Real Milk n.d.).

"Go for the real thing! Boycott counterfeits! Join a campaign for real milk!" states one popular raw milk advocate webpage. With slogans, such as "Pasture fed," "Unprocessed," and "Full-fat," splashed across their main page, it is confusing for consumers to sort out pro-raw-milk claims and government warnings. In a society where processed foods are considered unhealthy foods, where does pasteurized milk fit in? Is raw milk really healthier than pasteurized milk?

When you purchase milk in a Canadian supermarket, you can be sure that it has been pasteurized. Why is this? In its natural state, milk may contain microorganisms, such as *Listeria monocytogenes, Salmonella, Campylobacter,* and *Escherichia coli* (Perkin 2007). These pathogens can lead to illness, such as vomiting, diarrhea, fever, and even kidney failure (Health Canada 2006a). Before pasteurization became common, 25% of all food-borne diseases were milk-related (National Environmental Health Association 2008).

Young children, seniors, and other persons with compromised immune systems are most susceptible to illnesses from raw milk. Moreover, pregnant mothers who become ill from *L. monocytogenes* found in unpasteurized milk may risk fetal death or miscarriage (Bren 2004).

Cows with infections, such as mastitis, may pass on the pathogens into their milk. Moreover, unsanitary farm environments and poor equipment care can potentially introduce contaminants as well (Wier et al. 2007). Some dairy operators, on the other hand, maintain that practicing sound animal care and sanitary milk collection reduces the spread of pathogens, so that pathogens are not passed along to consumers who drink raw milk (Tauxe 2001).

Pasteurization is a process in which a food item is heated to a temperature at which a majority of bacteria is eliminated. However, this process cannot remove all pathogens from milk, and it is possible for pasteurized milk to cause illness. Nevertheless, since the introduction of pasteurization, milk-borne illnesses have been extremely rare (Gillespie et al. 2003).

There are vitamins in pasteurized milk that are not available in raw milk. In a northern country, such as Canada, the sun's rays are not strong enough for our skin to synthesize adequate amounts of vitamin D during the winter months. Therefore, milk in Canada is fortified with vitamin D. Vitamin D is involved in normal bone metabolism as well; it helps protect against childhood rickets, osteoporosis, and bone fractures (Bischoff et al. 2003).

Raw milk advocates claim that pasteurization denatures important enzymes and destroys vitamins. Although it is true that some vitamins are destroyed in the pasteurization process, the loss is, on average, less than 10% (Bren 2004). Furthermore, the enzymes present in cow's milk are bovine enzymes that are not needed for human use (Bren 2004). Some scientists argue that the bacteria found in raw milk have protective effects against allergic conditions (Perkin 2007). However, there is no strong evidence that this is truly the case. Pasteurization will slightly alter the composition of milk, but the losses are not great enough to compromise the consumer (Currier 1981). Scientific evidence still suggests that the benefits of pasteurized milk far outweigh any losses accounted in the treatment process.

Despite the benefits of heat-treating milk, many people are choosing raw over pasteurized milk. Why is this? Farming families are the largest consumers of raw milk for reasons of taste, convenience, and cost (Oliver et al. 2005). Moreover, many are not aware of the pathogens present in raw milk and thus are twice as likely to choose unpasteurized milk. There are growing numbers of urban people becoming raw milk consumers as well. Not only do they believe that the nutritional content of raw milk is far superior, but many also praise the creamy texture of raw milk. This texture is not found in processed milk's standardized fat contents (Bren 2004).

Hundreds of cases of illness caused by unpasteurized milk have been reported each year in the United States (Bren 2004). In response to this danger, Health Canada has prohibited the sale of raw milk since 1991 under Food and Drug Regulations (Health Canada 2006a). Regardless of this precaution, raw-milk supporters are able to purchase unpasteurized milk illegally from local farms. It is legal for farmers to consume the milk of their

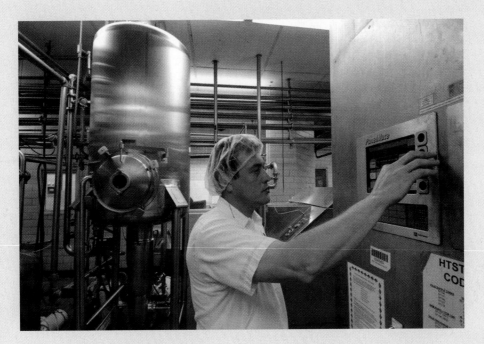

own animals; however, it is illegal to sell it to others. To bypass legal issues, milk co-operatives have sprung up across the country. Members of these co-op farms lease a cow and therefore own the animal. Furthermore, farm operators do not sell but rather distribute raw milk to their members (Eldeib 2007).

Raw milk is also consumed in the form of cheeses. In Europe, cheeses made from unpasteurized milk are popular. Since the cheesemaking process limits the growth of pathogens, they are not prohibited in Canada so long as they are stored according to regulations (Wier et al. 2007).

What do you think about this issue? Should consumers be able to consume raw milk if they like its taste and "all natural" state? Do you think it is wise to let young children drink raw milk?

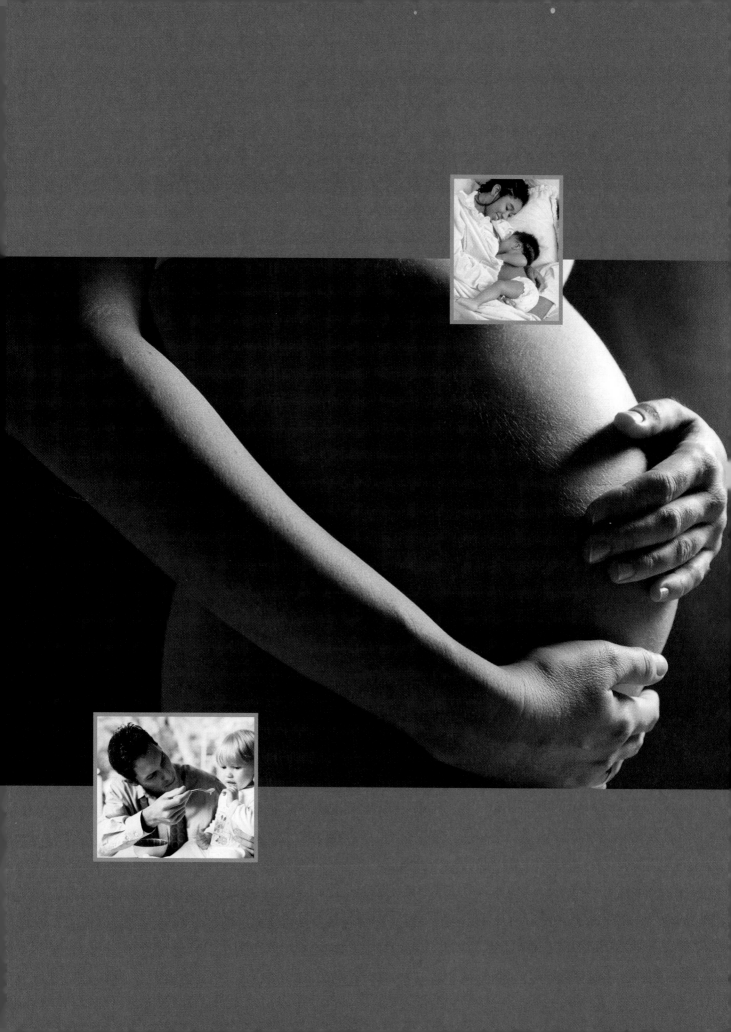

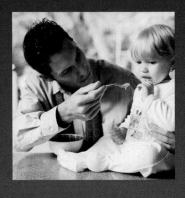

CHAPTER 15

Nutrition Through the Life Cycle: Pregnancy and the First Year of Life

CHAPTER OBJECTIVES

After reading this chapter you will be able to:

1. Explain why maintaining a nutritious diet is important for prospective parents even before conception, p. 536.

2. Explore the relationship among fetal development, changes in the mother, and increasing nutrient requirements during a pregnancy, pp. 537–540.

3. Identify the range of optimal weight gain for a pregnant woman in each trimester, pp. 540–542.

4. Describe the physiologic events that lead to lactation, pp. 556–557.

5. Compare and contrast the nutrient requirements of pregnant and lactating women, pp. 557–559.

6. Identify the advantages of breastfeeding, for both the baby and the mother, pp. 559–563.

7. Relate the growth and activity patterns of infants to their nutrient needs, pp. 563–570.

8. Discuss some common nutrition-related concerns for infants, pp. 568–570.

Test Yourself True or False

1. The amount of weight a woman gains during pregnancy has little influence on the outcome of the pregnancy. **T or F**

2. Despite popular belief, very few pregnant women actually experience morning sickness, food cravings, or food aversions. **T or F**

3. There have been fewer cases of neural tube defects, such as spina bifida, since Canada required folate to be added to wheat flour. **T or F**

4. Physical growth is the best way to assess whether an infant is adequately nourished. **T or F**

5. Most infants begin to require solid foods by about 3 months (12 weeks) of age. **T or F**

Test Yourself answers can be found at the end of the chapter.

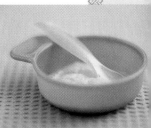

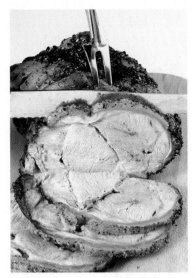

Meats, like pork roast, provide protein and heme iron that are important for maternal and fetal nutrition.

Pregnancy shouldn't be a death sentence . . . but for a malnourished woman, it often is. A report in the *Journal of the Indian Medical Association* found that maternal nutritional deficiency was one of the most important factors contributing to death during pregnancy or childbirth (Mitra and Chowdhury 2002). Statistics from the United Nations Children's Fund indicate that more than 100 000 women worldwide die each year during pregnancy or childbirth as a result of iron-deficiency anemia alone (UNICEF 2004). Deficiencies of iodine, folate, vitamin A, zinc, and protein also dramatically increase the risk of the mother or her newborn dying. Perhaps maternal malnutrition partly explains the traditional Filipino saying quoted in the UNICEF report: "A woman giving birth has one foot in the grave."

Is maternal malnutrition a problem only in developing nations? What role, if any, does nutrition play in maternal-newborn illness and death in the industrialized countries, such as Canada and the United States? Why is inadequate iron especially dangerous to a pregnant woman and her fetus? What role do protein, folate, iron, omega-3 fatty acids, and other nutrients play in maternal health and fetal development? In this chapter, we discuss how adequate nutrition supports fetal development, maintains the pregnant woman's health, and contributes to lactation. We then explore the nutrient needs of breastfeeding and formula-feeding infants.

Starting Out Right: Nutrition in Pregnancy

At no stage of life is nutrition more crucial than during fetal development and infancy. Especially from conception through the end of the first year of life, adequate nutrition is essential for tissue formation, neurological development, and bone growth, modelling, and remodelling. Your ability to reach your peak physical and intellectual potential in adult life is in part determined by the nutrition you received during the earliest years of your development.

Is Nutrition Important Before Conception?

conception (also called *fertilization*) The uniting of an ovum (egg) and sperm to create a fertilized egg, or zygote.

Several factors make adequate nutrition important even before **conception**, the point at which a woman's ovum (egg) is fertilized with a man's sperm. First, some deficiency-related problems develop extremely early in the pregnancy, typically before the mother even realizes she is pregnant. An adequate and varied preconception diet reduces the risk of such problems, providing insurance during those first few weeks of life. For example, failure of the spinal cord to close results in *neural tube defects*; these defects are closely related to inadequate levels of folate during the first few weeks following conception. For this reason, all sexually active women of childbearing age capable of becoming pregnant are encouraged to consume 400 µg of folic acid daily, whether or not they plan to become pregnant.

teratogen Any substance that can cause a birth defect.

Second, adopting a nutritious diet prior to conception includes the avoidance of alcohol, illegal drugs, and other known **teratogens** (substances that cause birth defects). Women should also consult their health care provider about their consumption of caffeine, medications, herbs, and supplements, and if they smoke, they should attempt to quit. Finally, maintaining a balanced and nourishing diet before conception reduces a woman's risk of developing a nutrition-related disorder during her pregnancy. These disorders, which we discuss later in the chapter, include gestational diabetes and pre-eclampsia, a form of hypertension specific to pregnant women. Although genetic and metabolic abnormalities are beyond the woman's control, following a nutritious diet prior to conception is something a woman can do to help her fetus develop into a healthy baby.

The man's nutrition prior to pregnancy is important as well, since malnutrition contributes to abnormalities in sperm (Olds et al. 2003). Both sperm number and motility (ability to move) are reduced by alcohol consumption, as well as the use of certain prescription and illegal drugs. Finally, infections accompanied by a high fever can destroy sperm; so, to the extent that adequate nutrition keeps the immune system strong, it also promotes a man's fertility.

Why Is Nutrition Important During Pregnancy?

A plentiful, nourishing diet is important throughout pregnancy to provide the nutrients needed to support fetal development without depriving the mother of nutrients she needs to maintain her own health.

The First Trimester

In clinical practice, the calculation of weeks in a pregnancy begins with the date of the first day of a woman's last menstrual period. A full-term pregnancy lasts 38 to 42 weeks and is divided into three **trimesters**, with each trimester lasting about 13 to 14 weeks. The first trimester begins when the ovum and sperm unite to form a single, fertilized cell called a **zygote**. As the zygote travels through the uterine (fallopian) tube, it further divides into a ball of 12 to 16 cells which, at about day four, arrives in the uterus (Figure 15.1). By day 10, the inner portion of the zygote, called the *blastocyst,* implants into the uterine lining. The outer portion becomes part of the placenta, which is discussed shortly.

Further cell growth and multiplication occurs, and the blastocyst differentiates into distinct layers of cells. At this stage, approximately day 15, the mass is called an **embryo**. Over the next six weeks, embryonic tissues differentiate and fold into a primitive tubelike structure with limb buds, organs, and facial features recognizable as human (Figure 15.2). It isn't surprising, then, that the embryo is most vulnerable to teratogens during this time. Not only alcohol and illegal drugs but also prescription and over-the-counter medications, megadoses of supplements, such as vitamin A, certain herbs, viruses, cigarette smoking, and radiation can interfere with embryonic development and cause birth defects (Olds et al. 2003). In some cases, the damage is so severe that the pregnancy is naturally terminated in a **spontaneous abortion** (*miscarriage*), most of which occur in the first trimester.

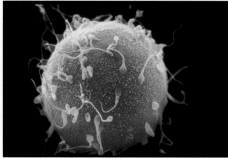

Adequate nutrition before conception is important for fetal development.

trimester Any one of three stages of pregnancy, each lasting 13 to 14 weeks.

zygote A fertilized egg (ovum) consisting of a single cell.

embryo Human growth and developmental stage lasting from the third week to the end of the eighth week after fertilization.

spontaneous abortion (also called miscarriage) Natural termination of a pregnancy and expulsion of pregnancy tissues because of a genetic, developmental, or physiologic abnormality that is so severe that the pregnancy cannot be maintained.

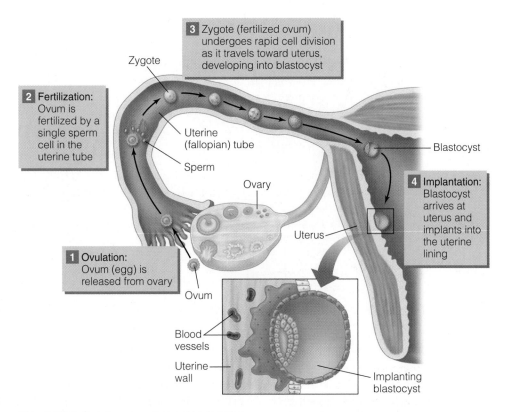

Figure 15.1 Ovulation, conception, and implantation.

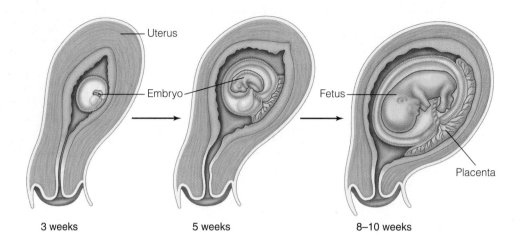

Uterus

Embryo

Fetus

Placenta

3 weeks   5 weeks   8–10 weeks

Figure 15.2 Human embryonic development during the first 10 weeks. Organ systems are most vulnerable to teratogens during this time, when cells are dividing and differentiating.

placenta A pregnancy-specific organ formed from both maternal and embryonic tissues. It is responsible for oxygen, nutrient, and waste exchange between mother and fetus.

During the first weeks of pregnancy, the embryo obtains its nutrients from cells lining the uterus. But by the fourth week, a primitive **placenta** has formed in the uterus from both embryonic and maternal tissue. Within a few more weeks, the placenta will be a fully functioning organ through which the mother will provide nutrients and remove fetal wastes (Figure 15.3).

By the end of the embryonic stage, about eight weeks postconception, the embryo's tissues and organs have differentiated dramatically: a primitive skeleton, including fingers and toes, has formed (Figure 15.4). Since muscles have begun to develop in the trunk, limbs, and head, some movement is now possible. A primitive

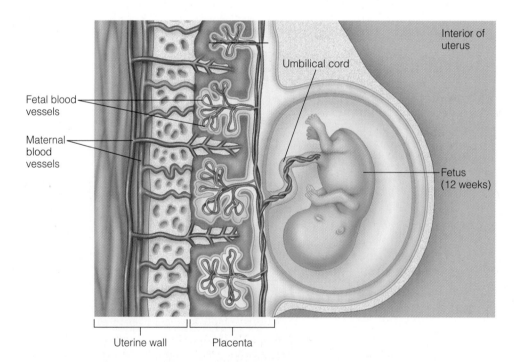

Interior of uterus

Umbilical cord

Fetal blood vessels

Maternal blood vessels

Fetus (12 weeks)

Uterine wall   Placenta

Figure 15.3 Placental development. The placenta is formed from both embryonic and maternal tissues. When the placenta is fully functional, fetal blood vessels and maternal blood vessels are intimately intertwined, allowing the exchange of nutrients and wastes between the two. The mother transfers nutrients and oxygen to the fetus, and the fetus transfers wastes to the mother for disposal.

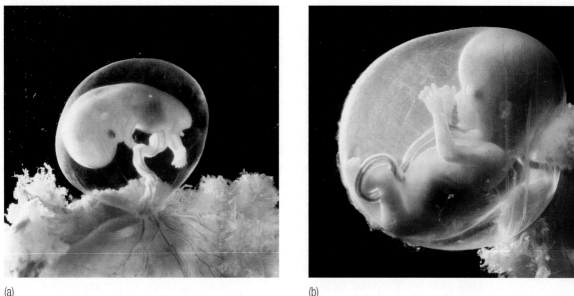

(a)   (b)

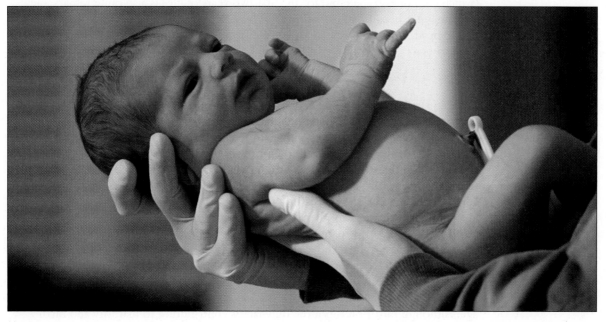

(c)

Figure 15.4 Stages of fetal development. (a) An embryo at 8 weeks. (b) A fetus at 16 weeks. (c) A full-term baby at birth.

heart has also formed and begun to beat, and the digestive system is differentiating into distinct organs (stomach, liver, etc.). The brain and cranial nerves have differentiated, and the head has a mouth, eyespots with eyelids, and primitive ears (Olds et al. 2003).

The third month of pregnancy marks the transition from embryo to **fetus**. The fetus requires abundant nutrients from the mother's body to support its dramatic growth during this period. The placenta is now a mature organ that can provide these nutrients. It is connected to the fetal circulatory system via the **umbilical cord**, an extension of fetal blood vessels emerging from the fetus's navel (called the *umbilicus*). Blood rich in oxygen and nutrients flows through the placenta and into the umbilical vein (see Figure 15.3). Once inside the fetus's body, the blood travels to the fetal liver and heart. Wastes are excreted in blood returning from the fetus to the placenta via the umbilical arteries.

fetus Human growth and developmental stage lasting from the beginning of the ninth week after conception to birth.

umbilical cord The cord containing arteries and veins that connects the baby (from the navel) to the mother via the placenta.

The Second Trimester

During the second trimester (weeks 14 to 27 of pregnancy), the fetus continues to grow and mature. The torso begins to elongate, bones are getting harder and stronger, and the arms and legs are moving. Organ systems also continue to develop and mature. During this period, the fetus can suck its thumb, its ears begin to hear and distinguish sounds, and its eyes can open and close and react to light. The placenta is now fully functional.

At the beginning of the second trimester, the fetus is about 7.5 cm (3 in.) long and weighs about 0.7 kg (1.5 lb.). By the end of the second trimester, the fetus is generally more than 30 cm (1 foot) long and weighs approximately 1 kg (2.2 lb.). Some babies born prematurely in the last weeks of the second trimester survive with intensive **neonatal** care.

neonatal A term referring to a newborn.

The Third Trimester

The third trimester (weeks 28 to 40) is a time of remarkable growth for the fetus. During three short months, the fetus gains nearly half its body length and three quarters of its body weight! At the time of birth, an average baby will be approximately 45 to 55 cm (18 to 22 in.) long and about 3.4 kg (7.5 lb.) in weight. Brain growth (which continues to be rapid for the first two years of life) is also quite remarkable, and the lungs become fully mature. The fetus acquires eyebrows, eyelashes, and hair on the head. Because of the intense growth and maturation of the fetus during the third trimester, it is critical that the mother eat an adequate and balanced diet.

Impact of Nutrition on Maturity and Birth Weight

An adequate, nourishing diet is one of the most important modifiable variables increasing the chances for birth of a mature newborn (at 38 to 42 weeks of **gestation**). If a baby is mature, sufficient fetal development, particularly of the lungs, will usually have occurred to ensure survival. Proper nutrition also increases the likelihood that the newborn's weight will be appropriate for his or her gestational age. Generally, a birth weight of at least 2500 grams, or 2.5 kg (5.5 lb.), is considered a marker of a successful pregnancy.

gestation The period of intrauterine development from conception to birth.

An undernourished mother is likely to give birth to a **low-birth-weight** baby (UNICEF 2004). Any infant weighing less than 2.5 kg (5.5 lb.) at birth is considered to be of low birth weight and is at increased risk of infection, learning disabilities, impaired physical development, and death in the first year of life (Figure 15.5). Many low-birth-weight babies are born **preterm**; that is, before 38 weeks of gestation. Others are born at term but weigh less than would be expected for their gestational age. Although nutrition is not the only factor contributing to maturity and birth weight, its role cannot be overstated.

low birth weight A weight of less than 2500 grams, or 2.5 kg (5.5 lb.) at birth.
preterm Birth of a baby prior to 38 weeks of gestation.

> **Recap:** A full-term pregnancy lasts from 38 to 42 weeks and is traditionally divided into trimesters lasting 13 to 14 weeks. During the first trimester, cells differentiate and divide rapidly to form the various tissues of the human body. The fetus is especially susceptible to teratogens during this time. The second trimester is characterized by continued growth and maturation of organ systems and body structures. The third trimester is a time of profound growth and maturation, especially of the fetal lungs and brain. Nutrition is important before and throughout pregnancy to support fetal development without depleting the mother's reserves. An adequate, nourishing diet increases the chance that a baby will be born after 37 weeks and weighing at least 2500 grams (2.5 kg or 5.5 lb.).

How Much Weight Should a Pregnant Woman Gain?

Recommendations for weight gain vary according to a woman's weight *before* she became pregnant (Table 15.1). As you can see in this table, the average recommended

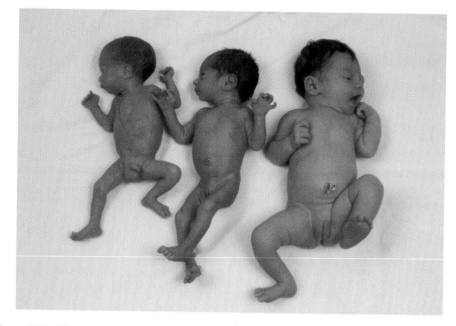

Figure 15.5 A healthy 2-day-old infant (right) compared with two low-birth-weight infants.

weight gain for women of normal pre-pregnancy weight is 11.5 to 16 kg (25 to 35 lb.); underweight women should gain a little more than this amount, and overweight and obese women should gain less.

As stated earlier, women who gain too little weight increase their risk of having a preterm or low-birth-weight baby and of dangerously depleting their own nutrient reserves, but gaining *too* much weight is also risky. Excessive weight gain increases the risk that the baby will be large for his or her gestational age, increasing the likelihood of trauma during vaginal delivery and of cesarean birth. In addition, the more weight gained during pregnancy, the more difficult it is to return to pre-pregnancy weight; therefore, women who gain excessive weight have an increased risk of permanent weight gain that can become especially problematic if the woman has two or more children.

In addition to amount of weight, the *pattern* of weight gain is important. During the first trimester, a woman of normal weight should gain no more than 1.4 to 2.3 kg (3 to 5 lb.). During the second and third trimester, about 0.5 kg (1 lb.) a week is considered appropriate. If weight gain is excessive in a single week, month, or trimester, the woman should not attempt to lose weight. Dieting during pregnancy jeopardizes the health of both mother and fetus by depriving both of critical nutrients and energy. Instead, the woman should merely attempt to slow the rate of weight gain. On the other hand, if a woman has not gained sufficient weight in the early months of her pregnancy, she should gradually increase her nutrient intake but not attempt to catch up all at once. In short, weight gain throughout pregnancy should be slow and steady.

Table 15.1   Recommended Weight Gain for Women during Pregnancy

Pre-Pregnancy Weight Status	Body Mass Index (kg/m²)	Recommended Weight Gain
Underweight	< 20	12.5–18.0 kg (28–40 lb.)
Normal	20–27	11.5–16.0 kg (25–35 lb.)
Overweight	> 27	7.0–11.5 kg (15–25 lb.)

Source: The Sensible Guide to a Healthy Pregnancy, Public Health Agency of Canada. 2008.) © Reproduced with the permission of the Minister of Public Works and Government Services Canada, 2008.

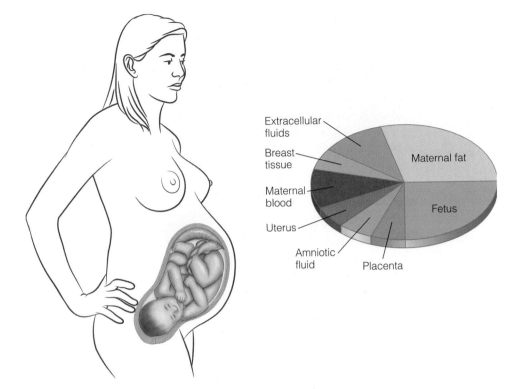

Figure 15.6 The weight gained during pregnancy is distributed between the mother's own tissues and the pregnancy-specific tissues.

In a society obsessed with thinness, it is easy for pregnant women to worry about weight gain. Focusing on the quality of food consumed, rather than the quantity, can help women feel more in control. In addition, following a physician-approved exercise program helps women maintain a positive body image and prevent excessive weight gain.

A pregnant woman may also feel less anxious about her weight gain if she understands how that weight is distributed. Of the total weight gained in pregnancy, 4.5 to 5.5 kg (10 to 12 lb.) are accounted for by the fetus itself, the amniotic fluid, and the placenta (Figure 15.6). Since these are delivered at birth, a woman can expect to be about 4.5 to 5.5 kg (10 to 12 lb.) lighter immediately afterward. In addition, within about two weeks, another 2.3 to 3.6 kg (5 to 8 lb.) of fluid (from increased blood volume and extracellular fluid) is lost. After that, losing the remainder of pregnancy weight depends on more energy being expended than is taken in. Since production of breast milk requires significant energy, breastfeeding helps many new mothers lose the remaining weight. We discuss breastfeeding on pages 559–563.

What Are a Pregnant Woman's Nutrient Needs?

The requirement for nearly all nutrients increases during pregnancy to accommodate the growth and development of the fetus without depriving the mother of the nutrients she needs to maintain her own health.

Macronutrient Needs of Pregnant Women

In pregnancy, macronutrients provide necessary energy for building tissue. They are also the building blocks for the physical form and structure of the fetus, as well as for other pregnancy-associated tissues.

Energy   Given what you've just learned about pregnancy weight gain, you've probably figured out that energy requirements increase only modestly during pregnancy. In

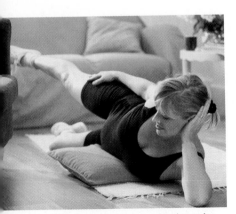

Following a physician-approved exercise program helps pregnant women maintain a positive body image and prevent excess weight gain.

fact, during the first trimester, a woman should consume approximately the same amount of energy daily as during her non-pregnant days. Instead of eating more, she should attempt to maximize the nutrient density of what she eats. For example, drinking low-fat milk is preferable to drinking soft drinks. Low-fat milk provides valuable protein, vitamins, and minerals to feed the fetus's rapidly dividing cells, while soft drinks provide nutritionally empty calories.

During the second and third trimesters, energy needs increase by about 340 kcal/day and 452 kcal/day respectively. For a woman normally consuming 2000 kcal or 8370 kJ per day, an extra 300 kcal represents only a 15% increase in energy intake, a goal that can be met more easily than many pregnant women realize. For example, 250 mL (1 cup) of non-fat yogurt and a graham cracker with jam is about 300 kcal (1260 kJ). At the same time, some vitamin and mineral needs increase by as much as 50%, so again, the key for getting adequate micronutrients while not consuming too much energy is choosing nutrient-dense foods.

Protein and Carbohydrate During pregnancy, protein needs increase to 1.1 grams/kg/day over the entire nine-month period. This is an increase of 25 grams of protein per day over the needs for non-pregnant, adult women. Keep in mind that many women already eat this much protein each day, especially in North America. Dairy products, meats, eggs, and soy products are all rich sources of protein, as are legumes, whole grains, nuts, and seeds.

Carbohydrate intake should be at least 130 grams per day to prevent ketosis (discussed on page 125). Additional carbohydrate is also needed to support daily physical activity. This recommendation is easily met by consuming a sensible diet but should be verified in each individual case. The majority of carbohydrate intake should come from whole foods, such as whole-grain breads and cereals, brown rice, fruits, vegetables, and legumes. Not only are these carbohydrates good sources of micronutrients, such as the B vitamins, but they also contain a lot of fibre, which can help prevent constipation. They are fairly filling and can be a boon to women who need to be careful not to gain too much weight. Refined carbohydrates in cakes, cookies, and so on, are both energy dense and nutrient poor. Although there's nothing wrong with an occasional treat, it is more healthful for a pregnant woman to satisfy her sweet tooth with fresh or dried fruits, which contain vitamins, fibre, and phytochemicals.

Fat The percentage of daily energy that comes from fat does not change during pregnancy. Pregnant women should be aware that, because new tissues and cells are being built, some fat in the diet is essential. In addition, during the third trimester the fetus stores fat that is a critical source of fuel in the newborn period. Without adequate fat stores, for example, newborns cannot effectively regulate their body temperature.

Moderation and eating the right kinds of fats is important. Like anyone else, pregnant women should limit saturated fat and avoid trans fats because of their negative impact on cardiovascular health (as discussed in Chapter 5). Polyunsaturated and monounsaturated fats should be chosen whenever possible. An omega-3 polyunsaturated fatty acid known as *docosahexaenoic acid (DHA)* has been found to be critical for both brain growth and eye development. Since the fetal brain grows dramatically during the third trimester, DHA is especially important in the maternal diet then and also after birth, for those who breastfeed, because of the rapid brain growth that occurs during the first three months of life outside the womb. Good sources of DHA are the oily fish: anchovies, mackerel, salmon, and sardines. It is also found in lesser amounts in tuna, shrimp, and lean fish, such as cod and haddock.

Pregnant women who eat fish should be aware of the potential for mercury contamination, as even a limited intake of mercury during pregnancy can impair a fetus's developing nervous system. For this reason, pregnant and breastfeeding women should limit their consumption of fresh and frozen tuna, shark, swordfish, marlin, orange roughy, and escolar (sometimes called snake mackerel or oilfish) to 150 grams per month. Canned tuna that is "light" (such as Skipjack or Yellowfin) is safe, but canned tuna from the large Albacore or Bluefin species (often labelled as "white") should be limited to 300 grams (4 *Canada's Food Guide* Servings) a month (Health Canada 2007). See Chapter 5 for more information about food sources of DHA.

Micronutrient Needs of Pregnant Women

During pregnancy, expansion of the mother's blood supply and growth of the uterus, placenta, breasts, body fat levels, and the fetus itself all contribute to an increased need for micronutrients. In addition, the increased need for energy during pregnancy correlates with an increased need for micronutrients involved in the metabolism of macronutrients and ATP production. Discussions of the micronutrients most critical during pregnancy follow. Refer to Table 15.2 for an overview of the changes in micronutrient needs with pregnancy.

Folate Folate is the form of the vitamin that occurs naturally in food; folic acid is the synthetic form used in fortified foods (such as wheat) and supplements (Health Canada 2008). Since folate, or folic acid, is necessary for cell division, it follows that during a time when both maternal and fetal cells are dividing rapidly, the requirement for this vitamin would be increased. Adequate folate is also needed for the proper development of the spine, skull, and brain (Health Canada 2008). For this reason it is especially critical during the first 28 days after conception, when it is required for the formation and closure of the **neural tube**, an embryonic structure that eventually becomes the brain and spinal cord. Folate deficiency is associated with neural tube defects, such as **anencephaly** and **spina bifida**. Anencephaly is a fatal defect in which there is partial absence of brain tissue most likely caused by failure of the neural tube to close (Institute of Medicine 1998). Spina bifida is associated with an incomplete development of the spinal cord. In the mildest form, occulta, there is a break between spinal vertebrae that is covered by skin but can be seen on x-rays. In meningocele, the spinal cord develops normally but the meninges (the protective covering) protrudes through an opening in the lower back. In myelomeningocele, which is the most severe form, both the spinal nerves and their protective covering protrude through the opening (see Figure 15.7). Sometimes surgery can help to repair the spinal opening; however, there is usually some permanent nerve damage and many children with spina bifida suffer some paralysis of their lower bodies and need braces, crutches, or wheelchairs.

Adequate folate intake does not guarantee normal neural tube development, as the precise cause of neural tube defects is unknown. However, in 2007, Dr. Philippe Gros, a biochemist at McGill University, and his team of researchers identified folate-responsive genes and non–folate-responsive genes associated with spina bifida,

neural tube Embryonic tissue that forms a tube, which eventually becomes the brain and spinal cord.

anencephaly A fatal neural tube defect in which there is partial absence of brain tissue most likely caused by failure of the neural tube to close.

spina bifida A neural tube defect in which vertebrae of the spine are not fully developed. In the most severe form, the spinal cord nerves and their protective sheath protrude through an opening in the skin causing permanent nerve damage.

Table 15.2 Changes in Nutrient Recommendations with Pregnancy for Adult Women

Micronutrient	Pre-Pregnancy	Pregnancy	% Increase
Folate	400 µg/day	600 µg/day	50
Vitamin B$_{12}$	2.4 µg/day	2.6 µg/day	8
Vitamin C	75 mg/day	85 mg/day	13
Vitamin A	700 µg/day	770 µg/day	10
Vitamin D	5 µg/day	5 µg/day	0
Calcium	1000 mg/day	1000 mg/day	0
Iron	18 mg/day	27 mg/day	50
Zinc	8 mg/day	11 mg/day	38
Sodium	1500 mg/day	1500 mg/day	0
Iodine	150 µg/day	220 µg/day	47

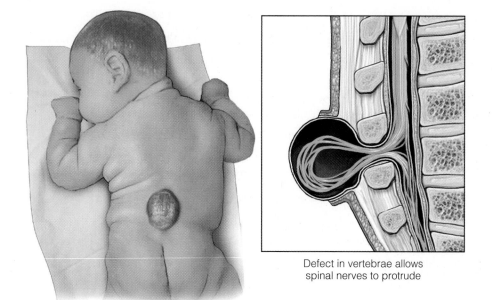

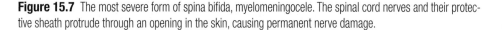

Defect in vertebrae allows
spinal nerves to protrude

Figure 15.7 The most severe form of spina bifida, myelomeningocele. The spinal cord nerves and their protective sheath protrude through an opening in the skin, causing permanent nerve damage.

moving scientists one step closer to one day eradicating this debilitating birth defect (Bourguignon 2007). Still, it is estimated that 70% of all neural tube defects could be prevented by simply consuming enough folate (CDC 2003).

To reduce the risk of a neural tube defect, all sexually active women of childbearing age who are capable of becoming pregnant are encouraged to take a multivitamin and mineral supplement that contains 400 µg (0.4 mg) of folic acid daily. If you are planning to become pregnant, the supplement should be taken at least three months before you get pregnant and you should take it daily through your pregnancy and for as long as you breastfeed (Health Canada 2008).

The RDA for folate for pregnant women is 600 µg per day, a full 50% increase over the RDA for non-pregnant females (Institute of Medicine 1998). A deficiency of folate during pregnancy can result in macrocytic anemia (a condition in which blood cells do not mature properly) and has been associated with low birth weight, preterm delivery, and failure of the fetus to grow properly. Types and sources of folate are discussed on pages 253–258 and include orange juice, fortified cereals and grains, spinach, and lentils.

An interesting fact about this vitamin is that the synthetic form, folic acid, is 1.7 times more bioavailable than the folate naturally found in food. All wheat flour in Canada is fortified with folic acid; 85% of the folic acid in a fortified product like bread is available for absorption, whereas only 50% of the folate naturally found in orange juice is available for absorption. Taking folic acid supplements on an empty stomach further increases the bioavailability (Health Canada 2008).

Vitamin B_{12}   Vitamin B_{12} (cobalamin) is vital during pregnancy because it regenerates the active form of folate. Not surprisingly, deficiencies of vitamin B_{12} can also result in macrocytic anemia. Yet the RDA for vitamin B_{12} for pregnant women is only 2.6 µg per day, a mere 8% increase over the RDA of 2.4 µg per day for non-pregnant women. How can this be? One reason is that during pregnancy, absorption of vitamin B_{12} is more efficient. However, recent Canadian research has suggested that 1 in 20 women may have inadequate vitamin B_{12} levels in their blood in early pregnancy, and, in fact, vitamin B_{12} deficiency could be another risk factor for neural tube defects (Ray et al. 2007, 2008).

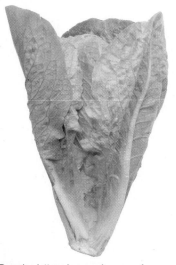

Romaine lettuce is a good source of folate.

Do Current Folate Recommendations Meet the Needs of Pregnant Women?

"Prior to folic acid fortification of the food supply in Canada, it was clear that most women did not consume the recommended intakes for folate. Unless their diet was meticulously planned, it was highly unlikely that women met their requirement for folate during pregnancy and lactation from dietary sources alone," explains Dr. Deborah O'Connor, director of Clinical Dietetics at the Hospital for Sick Children in Toronto. Dr. O'Connor's research career has been dedicated to increasing awareness of folate requirements before and during pregnancy and breastfeeding. She has been motivated by the growing body of evidence linking poor folate status during pregnancy and neural tube defects (NTD) in infants. Although she believes that Canada has made great improvements through the mandatory fortification of wheat flour with folic acid, her current research suggests that more needs to be done.

In her 2006 study published in the *Journal of Nutrition*, Dr. O'Connor demonstrates that almost one third of the pregnant and breastfeeding women participating in her research did not meet current folate recommendations from diet alone (Sherwood et al. 2006). She states that "this is of obvious concern as it looks like, at mandated fortification levels, even well-off women with higher education are at risk." Therefore she recommends that "women still consume a multivitamin containing 400 μg folic acid at least 3 months before and 3 months after conception to prevent neural tube defects, regardless of the quality of their diet."

What other strategies might help women increase their folate intakes? Dr. O'Connor believes that "education is the cornerstone of this issue," particularly education on *Eating Well with Canada's Food Guide* with a focus on healthy foods, such as leafy green vegetables. These foods are naturally high in folate, whereas foods "fortified with folic acid are mostly made with white flour and are low in fibre." We need to encourage healthy eating, rather than giving the impression that folic acid supplements are the answer to a healthy pregnancy.

Should Canada increase folic acid fortification in foods to improve the status of pregnant and lactating women? Dr. O'Connor's 2006 study also touches on the risk of folic acid supplementation masking vitamin B_{12} deficiencies (Sherwood et al. 2006). She explains that "B_{12} deficiency is becoming more common in pregnant and lactating women. It is a deficiency not just seen in the elderly and those who follow a vegan diet. And unlike most nutrients, B_{12} deficiency is often reflected in breast milk, which is why all prenatal multivitamins now have B_{12} in them." She notes that "more is not always better" and we need to be mindful that increasing the levels of supplemental folic acid could have negative health effects. So what does Dr. O'Connor see for the future of folate? She hopes that "more research is done on how much folate is actually in our food supply. We have to understand what we are eating now before we move ahead with changes in fortification policies."

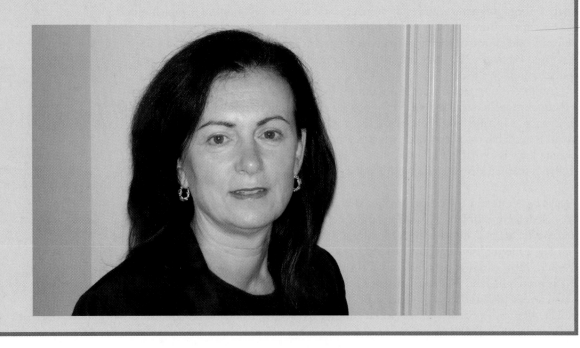

Vitamin C Vitamin C is necessary for the synthesis of collagen, a component of connective tissue (including skin, blood vessels, and tendons) and part of the organic matrix of bones. Because blood plasma volume increases during pregnancy, and because vitamin C is being transferred to the fetus, the concentration of vitamin C in maternal blood decreases. To make up the vitamin C deficit, the RDA for vitamin C during pregnancy is increased by a little more than 10% over the RDA for non-pregnant women (from 75 mg to 85 mg per day). A deficiency of vitamin C during pregnancy increases the risk for infections, preterm birth, and other problems. As described on pages 276–277, vitamin C is found abundantly in many food sources, such as citrus fruits, citrus juices, and numerous other fruits and vegetables.

Vitamin A Vitamin A needs increase during pregnancy by about 10%, to 770 µg per day. However, excess preformed vitamin A can cause fetal abnormalities, particularly in the kidneys and nervous system, even when it is not consumed in extremely high quantities. Since an adequate diet supplies sufficient vitamin A, supplementation is not recommended. Note that provitamin A, in the form of beta-carotene (which is converted to vitamin A in the body), has not been associated with birth defects.

Vitamin D Despite the role of vitamin D in calcium absorption, the AI for this nutrient does not increase during pregnancy. According to the Institute of Medicine (1997), the amount of vitamin D transferred from the mother to the fetus is relatively small and does not appear to affect overall vitamin D status. However, pregnant women with limited sun exposure who do not regularly drink milk will benefit from vitamin D supplementation. Most prenatal vitamin supplements contain 10 µg per day of vitamin D, which is considered safe and acceptable (Institute of Medicine 1997).

Calcium Growth of the fetal skeleton requires a significant amount of calcium. However, the AI for adult pregnant women is the same as that for non-pregnant adult women, 1000 mg per day, for two reasons. First, pregnant women absorb calcium from the diet more efficiently than do non-pregnant women. This increased absorption may be due to the fact that they have higher levels of the active form of vitamin D (Cross et al. 1995) and high levels of estrogen in their blood, both of which enhance calcium absorption. Second, the extra demand for calcium has not been found to cause de-mineralization of the mother's bones or to increase fracture risk (Institute of Medicine, 1997). Sources of calcium are discussed on pages 317–319.

Iron Recall from Chapter 10 the importance of iron in the formation of red blood cells, which transport oxygen throughout the body so that cells can produce ATP. During pregnancy, the demand for red blood cells increases to accommodate the needs of the growing uterus, placenta, and the fetus itself. Thus, more iron is needed. Fetal demand for iron increases even further during the last trimester, when the fetus stores iron in the liver for use during the first few months of life. This iron storage is protective because breast milk is low in iron.

Severely inadequate iron intake certainly has the potential to harm the fetus, resulting in an increased likelihood of low birth weight, preterm birth, stillbirth, and death of the newborn in the first weeks after birth. However, in most cases the fetus in a low-iron state builds adequate stores by taking maternal iron, prompting iron-deficiency anemia in the mother. During pregnancy, maternal iron deficiency causes pallor and exhaustion, but at birth, it endangers her life: anemic women are more likely to die during or shortly following childbirth because they are less able to tolerate blood loss and fight infection.

The RDA for iron for pregnant women is 27 mg per day, compared with 18 mg per day for non-pregnant women. This represents a 50% increase, despite the fact that iron loss is minimized during pregnancy because menstruation ceases. Typically, women of childbearing age have poor iron stores, and the demands of pregnancy are likely to produce deficiency. To ensure adequate iron stores during pregnancy, an iron supplement (as part of, or distinct from, a total prenatal supplement) is routinely prescribed during the last two trimesters. Vitamin C enhances iron absorption, as do dietary sources of heme iron, whereas substances in coffee, tea, milk, bran, and oxalates decrease absorption. Therefore, many health care providers recommend taking iron supplements with foods high in vitamin C or heme iron. Sources of iron are discussed on page 366.

Zinc   The RDA for zinc for adult pregnant women increases by about 38% over the RDA for non-pregnant adult women, from 8 mg per day to 11 mg per day. Since zinc has critical roles in DNA synthesis, RNA synthesis, and protein synthesis, it is imperative that adequate zinc status be maintained during pregnancy to facilitate proper growth and development of both maternal and fetal tissues. Inadequate zinc can lead to malformations in the fetus, premature delivery, and extended labour. It should be noted that the absorption of zinc is inhibited by iron when these two minerals are taken with water. However, when iron and zinc are consumed together in a meal, absorption of zinc is not affected (Whittaker 1998; Davidsson et al. 1995). In addition, the heme form of iron does not appear to inhibit zinc absorption. When iron supplements are prescribed during pregnancy, it is good practice to consume these supplements with food and with a good vitamin C source to enhance the absorption of both zinc and iron.

Sodium and Iodine   During pregnancy, the AI for sodium is the same as for a non-pregnant adult woman, or 1500 mg (1.5 g) per day (Institute of Medicine 2004). Although too much sodium is associated with fluid retention and bloating, as well as high blood pressure, increased fluids are a normal and necessary part of pregnancy, so some sodium is necessary to maintain fluid balance.

Iodine needs increase significantly during pregnancy, but the RDA of 220 µg per day is easy to achieve by using a modest amount of iodized salt (sodium chloride) during cooking. Sprinkling salt onto food at the table is unnecessary.

Do Pregnant Women Need Supplements?

Prenatal multivitamin and mineral supplements are not strictly necessary during pregnancy, but most health care providers recommend them. Meeting all the nutrient needs would otherwise take careful and somewhat complex dietary planning. Prenatal supplements are especially good insurance for special populations, such as vegans, adolescents, and others whose diet might normally be low in one or more micronutrients. It is important that pregnant women understand, however, that supplements are to be taken *in addition to,* not as a substitute for, a nutrient-rich diet. *Eating Well with Canada's Food Guide* recommends that pregnant women take a multivitamin containing folic acid and iron. Energy needs can be met by including an extra 2–3 *Food Guide* servings per day.

Fluid Needs of Pregnant Women

Fluid plays many vital roles during pregnancy. It allows for the necessary increase in the mother's blood volume, acts as a lubricant, aids in regulating body temperature, and is necessary for many metabolic reactions. Fluid that the mother consumes also helps maintain the **amniotic fluid** that surrounds, cushions, and protects the fetus in the uterus. The AI for total fluid intake, which includes drinking water, beverages, and food, is 3 litres per day (or about 12.7 cups). This recommendation includes approximately 2.3 litres (10 cups) of fluid as total beverages, including drinking water (Institute of Medicine 2004).

Drinking adequate fluid also helps combat fluid retention and constipation, two common discomforts of pregnancy. Drinking lots of fluids (and going to the bathroom as soon as the need is felt) will also help prevent **urinary tract infections**, which are very common in pregnancy. Urinary tract infections are bacterial infections of the urethra, which is the tube that leads from the bladder to the exterior of the body. Fluids also combat dehydration, which can develop if a woman with morning sickness has frequent bouts of vomiting. For these women, any non-diuretic fluid can help prevent dehydration, including soups, juices, and sport beverages.

amniotic fluid The watery fluid contained within the innermost membrane of the sac containing the fetus. It cushions and protects the growing fetus.

urinary tract infection A bacterial infection of the urethra, the tube leading from the bladder to the body exterior.

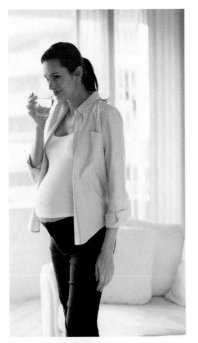

It is important that pregnant women drink about 2.3 litres (10 cups) of fluid a day.

Recap: Sufficient energy should be consumed so that a pregnant woman gains an appropriate amount of weight, typically 11.4 to 15.9 kg (25 to 35 lb.), to ensure adequate growth of the fetus. The food consumed during pregnancy should be nutrient dense so that both the mother and the fetus obtain the nutrients they need from food. Protein, carbohydrates, and fats provide the building blocks for fetal growth. Folate deficiency has been associated with neural tube defects. Most health care providers recommend prenatal supplements for pregnant women to ensure that sufficient micronutrients are consumed. Fluid provides for increased maternal blood volume and amniotic fluid.

Nutrition-Related Concerns for Pregnant Women

Pregnancy-related conditions involving a particular nutrient, such as iron-deficiency anemia, have already been discussed. The following sections describe some of the most common discomforts and disorders pregnant women experience that are related to their general nutrition.

Morning Sickness

Morning sickness, or *nausea and vomiting of pregnancy (NVP),* is increasingly gaining recognition as a legitimate and potentially serious medical condition worthy of study and treatment (von Dadelszen 2000). The symptoms vary in severity, from occasional mild queasiness to constant nausea with bouts of vomiting. In truth, "morning sickness" is not an appropriate name because the nausea and vomiting can begin at any time of the day, and about 80% of pregnant women who experience it report that it lasts all day. More than half of all pregnant women experience morning sickness, and some have it with one pregnancy but not with another. It usually begins shortly after the first missed period and abates by week 12 to 16, but a small number of women experience it throughout the pregnancy. Except in severe cases, the mother and fetus do not suffer lasting harm. However, some women experience such frequent vomiting that they are unable to nourish or hydrate themselves or their fetus adequately, and thus they require hospitalization.

Rising levels of two pregnancy-related hormones are thought to be at least partly responsible for morning sickness. Metabolic and emotional factors may also play some role.

There is no cure for morning sickness. However, here are some practical tips for reducing the severity:

- Eat lightly throughout the day. An empty stomach can actually trigger nausea, so eating small, frequent meals and snacks is usually helpful. Many women experiencing queasiness find that once they start eating, they begin to feel better. Protein and complex carbohydrates are especially useful in combating nausea.

- Some women find it helpful to keep snacks at their bedside to ease night-time queasiness. A small snack before rising in the morning helps some women, as does rising from bed slowly.

- Taking a prenatal supplement ensures that at least some vitamins and minerals are being absorbed. Obviously, the supplement should be taken at a time of day when vomiting is not likely.

- Women should also drink plenty of fluids to prevent dehydration from vomiting.

- Women should avoid sights, sounds, smells, and tastes that bring on or exacerbate queasiness.

- For some women, alternative therapies, such as acupuncture, acupressure wrist bands, biofeedback, meditation, and hypnosis, help. Raspberry tea soothes nausea in some women. Ginger tea may also be helpful but should be consumed in

morning sickness Varying degrees of nausea and vomiting associated with pregnancy, most commonly in the first trimester.

▶ **HIGHLIGHT**

Herbal Teas During Pregnancy and Breastfeeding

Although herbs seem to be healthy and all natural, there are some herbs that can have dangerous drug-like effects (Ernst 2002). Some may contain ingredients that can be toxic and harmful to both the mother and fetus (Health Canada 2005). Further, breastfeeding mothers may pass on harmful herbal ingredients to their baby through their breast milk.

In many cultures, the use of herbs is common and many benefits are cited. However the current research on herbs is still limited, thus the potential benefits of herbal products are difficult to evaluate and the safety of any specific herb can't be assured (Ernst 2002).

According to Health Canada, there are certain herbal teas that are generally considered to be safe if taken in moderation. Drinking tea in moderation refers to having two to three cups of weak tea infusions a day. These teas are ginger, linden flower, rose hip, lemon balm, orange peel, and citrus peel (Health Canada 2008). Drink a variety of these teas, rather than the same tea repeatedly, and make sure that tea is not replacing other nutrient-dense beverages, such as milk and juice.

Chamomile tea and teas with aloe, coltsfoot, juniper berry, pennyroyal, buckthorn bark, comfrey, sassafras, duck root, lobelia, and senna leaves are *not* recommended during pregnancy and breastfeeding (Health Canada 2008). Some herbal teas contain caffeine, which should be limited to a total of 300 mg from all sources (coffee, colas, etc.) a day. Overall, pregnant and breastfeeding mothers need to be cautious with herbal products and read ingredient lists on labels. When in doubt about a product's safety, consult a health care provider for advice.

---

moderation. Women should check with their health care provider regarding alternative therapies to ensure that the therapy they are using is safe and does not interact with other medications, supplements, or health considerations. See the Highlight on herbal teas.

- Decrease stress and get some rest and relaxation time, if possible.

Cravings and Aversions

It seems like nothing is more stereotypical about pregnancy than the image of a frazzled husband getting up in the middle of the night to run to the convenience store to get his pregnant wife some pickles and ice cream. This image, although humorous, is far from reality for most women. Although some women have specific cravings, most crave a particular type (such as "something sweet" or "something salty") rather than a particular food.

Why do pregnant women crave certain tastes? Does a desire for salty foods mean that the woman is experiencing a sodium deficit? Although there may be some truth to the assertion that we crave what we need, scientific evidence for this claim is lacking. It is thought more likely that cravings during pregnancy are due to hormonal fluctuations or physiologic changes or have familial or cultural roots. In some cases, when a woman improves her diet after learning she is pregnant, she simply misses the "forbidden" foods that she used to eat.

pica An abnormal craving to eat something not fit for food, such as clay, paint, and so on.

Most cravings are, of course, for edible substances. But a surprising number of pregnant women crave non-foods like freezer frost and clay. This craving, called **pica**, is the subject of the Highlight box.

Food aversions are also common during pregnancy but are by no means universal. Many women experience an aversion to coffee during the early months, for example. Does this mean a woman's body somehow "knows" she should avoid caffeine? Again, probably not, although this happens to be a fortuitous, convenient aversion if you're a habitual coffee drinker! It is also fairly common for deep-fried foods to elicit a gag response. Most likely food aversions have similar roots as food cravings.

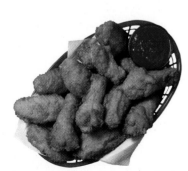

Deep-fried foods are often unappealing to pregnant women.

> ▶ **HIGHLIGHT**

The Danger of Non-Food Cravings

For most of her life, Darcy had thoroughly enjoyed good food. Her husband even bragged about her being a gourmet cook. But a few weeks after learning she was pregnant, her appetite seemed to disappear. She would wander through the aisles of the grocery store with an empty cart, knowing she should be choosing nutritious foods for her growing baby but feeling unable to find a single food that appealed to her. Eventually, she'd return home with a few things for her husband . . . and a large bag of ice. On weekends, she'd keep a cupful of ice with her almost constantly. She brought ice to work in a cold pack and ate it throughout the day, and she even kept a glass of ice by her bed at night. At her prenatal health care visits, her physician became concerned because she wasn't gaining weight. "I try to eat right," she confessed, "but nothing appeals to me." She was too embarrassed to admit to anyone, even her husband, that the only thing she really wanted to eat was ice.

Some people contend that a pregnant woman with unusual food cravings is intuitively seeking needed nutrients. Arguing against this claim is the phenomenon of pica—the craving and consumption of non-food material during pregnancy. A woman with pica may crave ice, freezer frost, clay, dirt, chalk, coffee grounds, baking soda, laundry starch, and many other substances. The cause of these non-food cravings is not known, though cultural factors, socioeconomic status, emotional support, and family tendencies seem to contribute to the incidence. No matter the cause, pica is dangerous. Consuming ice cubes or freezer frost can lead to inadequate weight gain if the substance substitutes for food. Ingestion of clay, starch, and other substances can cause deficiency of iron and other nutrients, as well as constipation, intestinal blockage, and even excessive weight gain.

Some women find it helpful to substitute food items for the craved non-food. For instance, frozen juice bars can be substituted for ice, and non-fat powdered milk can replace starch (Olds et al. 2003).

Heartburn

Heartburn (gastroesophageal reflux disease or GERD), along with indigestion, is common during pregnancy. Heartburn occurs when the sphincter between the esophagus and the stomach (the lower esophageal sphincter) relaxes, allowing acid and partially digested food from the stomach to well up and irritate the tissues of the lower esophagus. Because hormones released during pregnancy relax smooth muscle, heartburn incidence increases at this time. During the last two trimesters, enlargement of the uterus pushes up on the stomach, compounding the problem. Practical tips for minimizing the distress associated with heartburn and indigestion during pregnancy include the following:

- avoid excessive weight gain
- eat small, frequent meals and chew food slowly
- don't wear tight clothing
- avoid foods that seem to trigger the problem
- wait for at least one hour after eating before lying down
- sleep with your head elevated
- ask your doctor or midwife for an antacid that is safe for use during pregnancy

Constipation and Hemorrhoids

Hormone production during pregnancy causes the smooth muscles to relax, including the muscles of the large intestine. This causes movement of material through the colon to be sluggish. In addition, pressure exerted by the growing uterus on the colon can slow movement even further, making elimination difficult.

hemorrhoids Swollen varicose veins in the rectum.

Hemorrhoids—swollen varicose veins in the rectum—are caused by constipation or exacerbated by it. They are usually painful and may itch and bleed. Practical hints to avoid constipation include the following:

- Include 25 to 35 grams of fibre in the daily diet, concentrating on fresh fruits and vegetables, legumes, and whole grains. Dried fruits are fibre-rich and very portable snacks.

- Keep fluid intake high. Drink plenty of water, and eat water-rich fruits and vegetables to keep stools soft and moving, thus making them easier to eliminate.

- Exercise, as it helps increase motility of the large intestine.

- Don't hold bowel movements in. Go to the bathroom as soon as you feel the need.

Gestational Diabetes

gestational diabetes Insufficient insulin production or insulin resistance that results in consistently high blood glucose levels, specifically during pregnancy; condition typically resolves after birth occurs.

Gestational diabetes is generally a temporary condition in which a pregnant woman is unable to produce sufficient insulin or becomes insulin resistant. Either of these conditions results in elevated levels of blood glucose. Fortunately, gestational diabetes has no ill effects on either the mother or the fetus if blood glucose levels are strictly controlled through diet, exercise, or medication. Screening for gestational diabetes is routine for almost all health care practitioners and is necessary because the symptoms, which include frequent urination, fatigue, and an increase in thirst and appetite, among others, can be indistinguishable from normal pregnancy symptoms. If uncontrolled, gestational diabetes can result in *pre-eclampsia*, which is discussed in greater detail below. It can also result in a baby that is too large as a result of receiving too much glucose across the placenta during fetal life. Babies that are overly large are at risk for early delivery, trauma during birth, and other problems and may need to be born by cesarean section. There is also evidence that exposing a fetus to diabetes while in the womb significantly increases the risk for type 2 diabetes during adolescence and adulthood (Benyshek, Martin, and Johnston 2001; Dabelea et al. 1998). Women who are obese have a greater risk of developing gestational diabetes, and any woman who develops gestational diabetes remains at greater risk of developing type 2 diabetes later in life—particularly if she is obese to begin with or fails to maintain normal body weight after pregnancy. As with type 2 diabetes, attention to diet, weight control, and exercise reduce the risk of gestational diabetes.

Pre-eclampsia

pre-eclampsia High blood pressure that is pregnancy specific and accompanied by protein in the urine, edema, and unexpected weight gain.

Pre-eclampsia (also called *pregnancy-induced hypertension*) is characterized by sudden, high maternal blood pressure, swelling, excessive and rapid weight gain unrelated to food intake, and protein in the urine. If left untreated, it can result in death for both the mother and the fetus.

No one knows exactly what causes pre-eclampsia, but there appears to be a genetic link as well as a nutritional connection. Periconceptual use of a multivitamin with folic acid may lower the risk of pre-eclampsia, as may calcium supplements if calcium intake is low. High levels of blood triglycerides (associated with high-sugar diets) have been correlated with pre-eclampsia. Also at higher risk than the general population are women who are obese (BMI >35), women who already have chronic high blood pressure, women with diabetes (gestational or otherwise), women carrying multiple fetuses, and African-American women (Mostello et al. 2002).

Management of pre-eclampsia focuses mainly on blood pressure control. Typical treatment includes bed rest. Ultimately, the only thing that will cure the condition is childbirth. Depending on the severity of the symptoms and the gestational age of the fetus, delivery may be a viable treatment, either by inducing labour or by cesarean section. If the symptoms are mild and the onset is before the fetus would likely survive outside the womb, conservative treatment and bed rest are the usual course of action so that the fetus has the opportunity to mature further. Unfortunately,

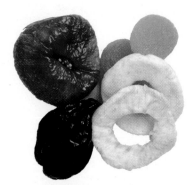

Foods high in fibre, such as dried fruits, reduce the chances of constipation.

sometimes severe pre-eclampsia occurs early in the pregnancy, and labour must be induced even though there is little chance of survival for the fetus. Today, with good prenatal care, pre-eclampsia is nearly always detected early and can be appropriately managed, and prospects for both mother and fetus are usually very good. In nearly all women without prior chronic high blood pressure, blood pressure returns to normal within about a day after the birth.

> **Recap:** About half of all pregnant women experience nausea or vomiting during pregnancy, called morning sickness, and many crave or feel aversions to specific types of foods. Pica is a craving for non-food items experienced by some pregnant women. Heartburn and constipation in pregnancy are related to the relaxation of smooth muscle caused by certain pregnancy-related hormones. Gestational diabetes and pre-eclampsia are nutrition-related disorders that can seriously affect maternal and fetal health.

Adolescent Pregnancy

Adolescents who become pregnant have greater nutritional risks than adult women. The adolescent body is still changing and growing. Peak bone mass has not yet been reached. Full physical stature may not have been attained, and teens are more likely to be underweight than are young adult women. This demand for tissue growth keeps nutrient needs during adolescence very high. In addition, many adolescents have not established healthy eating patterns; thus, the added burden of a pregnancy on an adolescent body creates a nutrient demand that can be very difficult to meet. Hence, adolescent mothers are more likely to have preterm births, low-birth-weight babies, and other complications related to nutritional deficiencies than are more mature women. With adequate and thorough prenatal care and close attention to proper nutrition and other healthy behaviours, the likelihood of a positive outcome for both the adolescent mother and the infant is greatly increased (Barnet, Duggan, and Devoe 2003).

Vegetarianism

Vegetarian women who consume dairy products and eggs (lacto-ovo-vegetarians) have no nutritional concerns beyond those encountered by every pregnant woman. In contrast, women who are totally vegetarian (vegan) need to be more vigilant than usual about their intake of nutrients that are derived primarily or wholly from animal products. These include vitamin D, vitamin B_6, vitamin B_{12}, calcium, iron, and zinc. Supplements containing these nutrients are usually necessary. A regular prenatal supplement will fully meet the vitamin and iron needs of a vegan woman but may not fulfill calcium needs, so a separate calcium supplement, or consumption of calcium-fortified soy milk or orange juice, might be required.

Dieting

Dieting to lose weight is not advisable during pregnancy. When energy is restricted, neither the woman nor the fetus obtains the nutrients necessary to grow and develop appropriately. Similarly, fad diets that are unbalanced in macronutrients (for example, high protein/low carbohydrate, or vice versa) are also unbalanced in micronutrients. Both total fasting and abstaining from carbohydrates are especially dangerous practices during pregnancy: recall from Chapter 4 that ketones are released when the body must rely on stored fats for fuel. These ketones are readily taken up and metabolized by the fetal brain, which could be detrimental to proper brain growth and development. Lack of glucose (carbohydrates) in the mother's diet also has been shown to result in reduced fetal growth (Harding 2001). The best strategy during pregnancy to ensure health of mother and baby is to consume a balance of all nutrients.

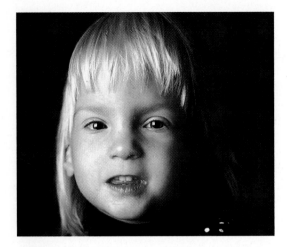

Figure 15.8 A child with fetal alcohol spectrum disorder (FASD). The facial features characteristic of children with FASD include a short nose with a low, wide bridge, drooping eyes with an extra skinfold, and a flat, thin upper lip. Behavioural problems and learning disorders are also characteristic. The effects of FASD are irreversible.

fetal alcohol spectrum disorder (FASD) A set of serious, irreversible alcohol-related birth defects characterized by certain physical and mental abnormalities.

Consumption of Caffeine

Caffeine is a stimulant found in several foods, including coffee, black tea, soft drinks, chocolate, and the herbs guarana and yerba mate. Caffeine crosses the placenta and reaches the fetus, but the fetus is unable to metabolize it. At what dose and to what extent caffeine causes harm is still a subject of controversy and study. Health Canada (2008) currently recommends that women should limit their consumption to 300 mg of caffeine per day from all sources. This is the equivalent of two 250 mL (two 8 fl. oz.) cups of coffee. Evidence suggests that consuming higher daily doses of caffeine (the higher the dose, the more compelling the evidence) may slightly increase the risk of miscarriage and low birth weight. In addition to its possible harm to the fetus, keep in mind that caffeine is a diuretic and will thus exacerbate maternal fluid loss and cause even more frequent trips to the bathroom.

Consumption of Alcohol

Alcohol is a known teratogen that readily crosses the placenta and accumulates in the fetal bloodstream. The immature fetal liver cannot readily metabolize alcohol, and its presence in the fetal tissues is associated with a variety of disabilities and birth defects called **fetal alcohol spectrum disorder (FASD)** (Health Canada 2006). The severity of these effects depends upon how much the mother drinks at one time, how often she drinks, and at what time during her pregnancy (Health Canada 2006).

Babies born with FASD have behavioural and learning problems, such as hyperactivity, attention deficit disorder, poor judgment, sleep disorders, and delayed learning. They may have characteristic malformations, particularly of the face, limbs, heart, and nervous system (see Figure 15.8). They have a high mortality rate, and those who survive typically have emotional, behavioural, social, learning, and developmental problems throughout life. Health Canada estimates that 3000 babies with FASD are born each year, and approximately 300 000 children and adults are living with FASD (Health Canada 2006).

Although some women do have the occasional alcoholic drink with no apparent ill effects, there is no amount of alcohol that is known to be safe. The best advice regarding alcohol during pregnancy is to abstain, if not from before conception, then as soon as pregnancy is suspected (Health Canada 2008).

Food-Borne Illnesses

Two food-borne illnesses are of particular concern during pregnancy because they can have serious outcomes and their symptoms are often mistaken for the flu (Health Canada 2005). Listeriosis is caused by the bacteria *Listeria monocytogenes,* which can survive at refrigerator temperatures and is found in dairy products, leafy vegetables, fish, and meats. A case of Listeriosis in the first trimester can cause miscarriage; in later pregnancy it may result in stillbirth. *Toxoplasma* is a parasite transmitted when a person eats contaminated raw meat or other raw foods, including fruits and vegetables. The illness, toxoplasmosis, can cause a severe infection in the fetus, especially if it occurs later in the pregnancy.

Pregnant women are advised to practise safe food handling techniques and to see a physician if they think they have the flu, to rule out a food-borne illness. It's worth remembering that food-borne pathogens don't always change the smell or look of foods, and "when in doubt, throw it out!" Other tips (Health Canada 2005) include these:

- Avoid eating raw or undercooked meats, fish, and poultry. Heat wieners until they are hot, and avoid unpasteurized dairy products.

- Don't eat runny eggs or foods that contain raw eggs (like Caesar salad dressings and some eggnogs).

- Avoid soft cheeses and pâtés as they may be sources of *Listeria monocytogenes.*
- Keep raw foods and cooked foods separated.
- Do not keep fresh or cooked meat and poultry products for more than two to three days in the refrigerator.
- Thoroughly clean and scrub all raw fruit and vegetables.

Exercise

Physical activity during pregnancy can be of tremendous benefit to a mother-to-be and is recommended for women experiencing normal pregnancies and who are otherwise in good health (Health Canada 2008). Exercise can help keep a woman physically fit during pregnancy, an important asset when enduring the physical stress of labour and delivery. In addition, exercise is a great mood booster, helping women feel more in control of their changing bodies. Expending additional energy through exercise will also allow intake of compensatory energy when a ravenous appetite kicks in. Moreover, regular moderate exercise will help keep blood pressure down and confer all the cardiovascular benefits that it does for non-pregnant women. Regular exercise can reduce the risks for pre-eclampsia (Yeo and Davidge 2001). Finally, a woman who keeps fit during pregnancy will have an easier time resuming a fitness routine and losing weight after pregnancy.

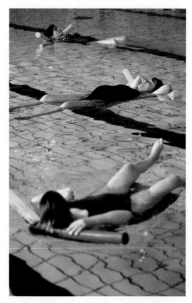

During pregnancy, women should adjust their physical activity to comfortable low-impact exercises.

If a woman was not active prior to pregnancy, then she should begin an exercise program slowly and progress gradually under the guidance of her health care provider. If a woman was physically active before pregnancy, she can continue to be physically active during pregnancy, within comfort and reason. The exercise should be comfortable for the woman. Low- or no-impact exercises are excellent choices for most women, although women who have been avid runners before pregnancy can often continue to run, as long as they feel comfortable. However, they should probably limit the distance and intensity of their runs.

All pregnant women should be careful not to unduly raise their heart rate or body temperature. They should avoid sports where there is potential for falling or jarring physical contact. Special care should also be taken when exercising in hot weather; careful attention should be given to fluid replenishment. Exercise while lying on your back should be avoided after the fourth month, since the growing weight of the uterus can compress important blood vessels. Generally, it is recommended that exercise gradually taper off during the last trimester, especially during the ninth month. Any exercise program should meet with the approval of the woman's health care provider, as some conditions encountered during pregnancy explicitly contraindicate exercise.

Recap: As adolescents' bodies are still growing and developing, their nutrient needs during pregnancy become so high that adequate nourishment for the mother and baby becomes difficult. Women who follow a vegan diet usually need to consume multivitamin and mineral supplements, plus supplemental calcium, during pregnancy. Dieting during pregnancy is not advised, as it leads to inadequate nutrition for mother and fetus. Caffeine intake should not exceed 300 mg (the equivalent of two 250 mL or two 8 fl. oz. cups of coffee) per day throughout pregnancy. Alcohol is a teratogen and should not be consumed in any amount during pregnancy. Exercise (provided the mother has no contraindications) can enhance the health of a pregnant woman.

Breastfeeding

Throughout most of human history, infants have thrived on only one food: breast milk. But during the first half of the twentieth century, commercially prepared infant formulas slowly began to replace breast milk as the mother's preferred feeding method. Aggressive marketing campaigns promoting formula as more nutritious than breast milk convinced many families, even in developing nations, to switch. Soon formula-feeding had become a status symbol, proof of the family's wealth and modern thinking. In the 1970s, this trend began to reverse with a renewed appreciation for the natural simplicity of breastfeeding and a distaste for corporate involvement in infant feeding. At the same time, several international organizations, including the World Health Organization, UNICEF, and La Leche League, began to promote the nutritional, immunologic, financial, and emotional advantages of breastfeeding and developed programs to encourage and support breastfeeding worldwide. These efforts have paid off: in Canada, 82% of new mothers begin breastfeeding in hospital. Worldwide, slightly more than half of all women breastfeed exclusively for at least six months (UNICEF 2003). However, Canadian women tend to breastfeed for shorter times. Of the 82% who start, only 63%, on average, choose or are able to continue breastfeeding past three months.

How, exactly, does breastfeeding occur? What nutrients are important for breastfeeding mothers? Is breastfeeding painful and difficult? And what exactly are the advantages that everyone is talking about? The answers to these questions are presented in the following sections.

How Does Lactation Occur?

lactation The production of breast milk.

Lactation, the production of breast milk, is a process that is set in motion during pregnancy in response to several hormones. Once established, lactation can be sustained as long as the mammary glands continue to receive the proper stimuli.

The Body Prepares During Pregnancy

Throughout pregnancy, the placenta produces estrogen and progesterone. In addition to performing various functions to maintain the pregnancy, these hormones prepare the breasts physically for lactation. The breasts increase in size, and milk-producing glands (alveoli) and milk ducts are formed (Figure 15.9). Toward the end of pregnancy, the hormone *prolactin* increases. Prolactin is released by the anterior pituitary gland and is responsible for milk synthesis. However, estrogen and progesterone suppress the effects of prolactin during pregnancy.

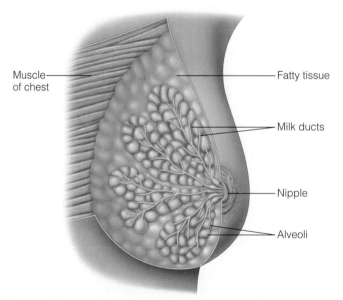

Figure 15.9 Anatomy of the breast. During pregnancy, estrogen and progesterone secreted by the placenta foster the preparation of breast tissue for lactation. This process includes breast enlargement and development of the milk-producing glands, or alveoli.

What Happens After Childbirth

By the time a pregnancy has come to full term, the level of prolactin is about 10 times as high as it was at the beginning of pregnancy. At birth, the suppressive effect of estrogen and progesterone ends, and prolactin is free to stimulate milk production. The first substance to be released from the breasts and to be ingested by a suckling infant is **colostrum**, sometimes called premilk or first milk. It is thick, yellowish, and rich in protein, and it includes antibodies that help protect the newborn from infection. It is also relatively high in vitamin and mineral content, compared with the mature milk that comes later. Colostrum also contains a factor that fosters the growth of a particular species of bacteria in the infant GI tract. These bacteria in turn prevent the growth of other bacteria that could potentially be harmful. Finally, colostrum has a laxative effect in infants, helping the infant to expel *meconium,* the sticky "first stool."

Within two to four days in most women, colostrum is fully replaced by mature milk. Mature breast milk contains protein, fat, and carbohydrate (in the form of the sugar lactose). Much of the protein and fat are synthesized in the breast, while the rest enter the milk from the mother's bloodstream.

colostrum The first fluid made and secreted by the breasts from late in pregnancy to about a week after birth. It is rich in immune factors and protein.

Mother-Infant Interaction Maintains Milk Production

Continued, sustained breast milk production depends entirely on infant suckling (or a similar stimulus like a mechanical pump). Infant suckling stimulates the continued production of prolactin, which in turn stimulates more milk production. The longer and more vigorous the feeding, the more milk will be produced. Thus, even twins can be successfully breastfed.

Prolactin allows for milk to be produced, but that milk has to move through the milk ducts to the nipple to reach the baby's mouth. The hormone responsible for this "let down" of milk is *oxytocin*. Like prolactin, oxytocin is produced by the pituitary gland and its production is dependent on the suckling stimulus at the beginning of a feeding (Figure 15.10). This response usually occurs within 10 to 30 seconds but can be significantly inhibited by stress, resulting in frustration on the part of both mother and baby. Finding a relaxed environment in which to breastfeed is therefore important. On the other hand, many women experience milk let down in response to other cues, such as breast fullness, hearing a baby cry, or even thinking about their infant.

What Are a Breastfeeding Woman's Nutrient Needs?

You might be surprised to learn that breastfeeding requires even more energy than pregnancy! This is because breast milk has to supply an adequate amount of all the nutrients an infant needs to grow and develop.

Nutrient Recommendations for Breastfeeding Women

It is estimated that milk production requires about 700 to 800 kcal (2930 to 3350 kJ) per day. It is generally recommended that lactating women consume 330 kcal/day for the first six months of lactation and 400 kcal/day for the second six months above their pre-pregnancy energy needs. This additional energy is sufficient to support adequate milk production. The resulting energy deficit of 200 to 300 kcal (840 to 1250 kJ) per day will assist in the gradual loss of excess fat and body weight gained during pregnancy. It is critical that lactating women avoid severe energy restriction, as this practice can result in decreased milk production.

The weight loss that occurs during breastfeeding should be gradual, approximately 0.5 to 2.0 kg (1 to 4 lb.) per month. Both breastfeeding and participating in regular physical activity can assist with weight loss. Interestingly, some active women may lose too much weight during breastfeeding and must either increase their energy intake or reduce their activity level to maintain health.

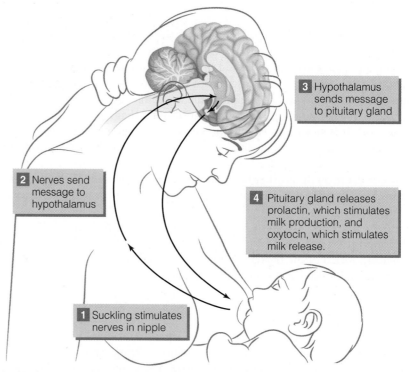

Figure 15.10 Sustained milk production depends on the mother-child interaction during breastfeeding, specifically the suckling of the infant. Suckling stimulates the continued production of prolactin, which is responsible for milk production, and also oxytocin, which is responsible for the milk let down response.

Of the macronutrients, only protein needs are different from pregnancy requirements. An increase of RDA 1.1 g per kilogram per day above pre-pregnancy requirements is recommended during lactation.

For the micronutrients, the need for several vitamins and minerals increases over the requirements of pregnancy. These include vitamins A, C, E, riboflavin, vitamin B_{12}, biotin, and choline, and the minerals copper, chromium, manganese, iodine, selenium, and zinc. The requirement for folate during lactation is 500 μg per day, which is decreased from the 600 μg per day required during pregnancy; but this requirement is higher than pre-pregnancy needs (400 μg per day).

Requirements for iron decrease significantly during lactation. For lactating women, iron needs are a mere 9 mg per day, compared with pregnant women at 27 mg per day and non-pregnant, non-lactating women at about 18 mg per day. This is because iron is not a significant component of breast milk, and, in addition, breastfeeding usually suppresses menstruation for at least a few months, reducing iron losses.

Calcium is a significant component of breast milk; but, as in pregnancy, calcium absorption is enhanced during lactation, and urinary loss of calcium is decreased.

In addition, some calcium appears to come from the demineralization of the mother's bones, and increased dietary calcium does not prevent this. Thus, the recommended intake for calcium for a lactating woman is unchanged from pregnancy; that is, 1000 mg per day. Because of their own continuing growth, however, teen mothers who are breastfeeding should continue to consume 1300 mg per day. Typically, a woman's bone density returns to normal after lactation ends.

Do Breastfeeding Women Need Supplements?

If a breastfeeding woman increases her energy intake by 330 kcal (1484 kJ) per day above pre-pregnancy levels, and does so with nutrient-dense foods, her nutrient needs can usually be met without supplements. However, there is nothing wrong with taking a basic multivitamin and mineral supplement for insurance, as long as it is not considered a substitute for proper nutrition. Lactating women should consume omega-3 fatty acids either in fish (with the same cautions as pregnant women with regard to mercury in fish) or supplements to support the infant's developing nervous system, and women who don't consume dairy products should monitor their calcium intake carefully. *Eating Well with Canada's Food Guide* recommends that women who are breastfeeding take a multivitamin containing folic acid. Energy needs are met by including an extra two to three *Food Guide* servings per day.

Fluid Recommendations for Breastfeeding Women

Since extra fluid is expended with every feeding, lactating women need to consume about an extra litre (about one quart) of fluid per day. This extra fluid facilitates milk production and staves off dehydration. Many women report that, within a minute or two of beginning to nurse their babies, they become intensely thirsty. To prevent this thirst and achieve the recommended fluid intake, women are encouraged to drink a nutritious beverage (water, juice, milk, etc.) each time they nurse their babies. However, it is not good practice to drink hot beverages while nursing because accidental spills could burn the infant.

> **Recap:** Lactation is the result of the coordinated effort of several hormones, including estrogen, progesterone, prolactin, and oxytocin. Breasts are prepared for lactation during pregnancy, and infant suckling provides the stimulus that sustains the production of prolactin and oxytocin needed to maintain the milk supply. Lactating women should consume an extra 500 kcal (2090 kJ) per day above pre-pregnancy energy intake, including increased protein, certain vitamins and minerals, and fluids. The requirements for folate and iron decrease from pregnancy levels, while the requirement for calcium remains the same.

Advantages of Breastfeeding

In 2004, Health Canada issued a statement that "exclusive breastfeeding is recommended for the first six months of life for healthy term infants, as it is the best possible food. Infants should be introduced to nutrient-rich, solid foods with particular attention to iron at six months, with continued breastfeeding for up to two years and beyond." The complete recommendation and supporting rationale can be accessed at www.hc-sc.gc.ca/fn-an/nutrition/child-enfant/infant-nourisson/excl_bf_dur-dur_am_excl_e.html.

As adept as formula manufacturers have been at simulating components of breast milk, an exact replica has never been produced. In addition, there are other benefits that mother and baby can access only through breastfeeding. However, illness, medication use, or other factors may make breastfeeding a difficult choice for some women. The decision to breastfeed or use formula must be made independently by each family after careful consideration of all the factors that apply to their particular situation.

Nutritional Quality of Breast Milk The main protein in breast milk, lactalbumin, is broken down easily in infants' immature GI tracts, and the whey-to-casein protein ratio in breast milk is more easily digested and absorbed than that of formula. Other proteins in breast milk bind iron and prevent the growth of harmful bacteria that require iron. Antibodies from the mother are additional proteins that help prevent infection while the infant's immune system is still immature. Cow's milk contains far too much protein. As we will discuss later, the infant's kidneys are not fully developed and are not able to process and excrete the excess amine groups from higher-protein milks.

The carbohydrate in milk is lactose, a disaccharide composed of glucose and galactose. The galactose component is important in nervous system development. Lactose provides energy and prevents ketosis in the infant, as well as promoting the growth of beneficial bacteria. It also aids in the absorption of calcium.

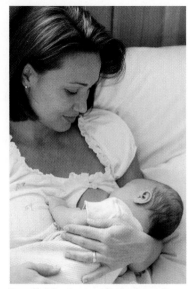

Breastfeeding has benefits for the mother and infant.

The fats in breast milk, especially DHA and arachidonic acid (ARA), have been shown to be essential for growth and development of the infant's nervous system and for development of the retina of the eyes. Interestingly, the concentration of DHA in breast milk varies considerably, is sensitive to maternal diet, and is highest in women who consume large quantities of fish. These fatty acids have now been added to commercial infant formulas in Canada and the United States. The fat content of breast milk changes according to the gestational age of the infant, providing a ratio of fatty acid types unique to the infant's needs. The fat content also changes during every feeding: the milk that is initially released is watery and low in fat, somewhat like skim milk. This milk is thought to satisfy the infant's initial thirst. As the feeding progresses, the milk acquires more fat and becomes more like whole milk. Finally, the very last 5% or so of the milk produced during a feeding (called the *hindmilk*) is very high in fat, similar to cream. This milk is thought to satiate the infant. It is important to let infants suckle for at least 20 minutes at each feeding so that they get this hindmilk.

Another important aspect of breastfeeding (or any type of feeding) is the fluid it provides the infant. Because of their small size, infants are at risk of dehydration, which is one reason why feedings must be consistent and frequent. This topic will be discussed at greater length in the section on infant nutrition.

In terms of micronutrients, breast milk is a good source of calcium and magnesium. It is low in iron, but the iron it does contain is easily absorbed (recall that infants store iron in preparation for the first few months of life). Health Canada (2007) recommends that breastfed infants receive 10 μg (micrograms) (400 IU) per day of a vitamin D supplement. It states: "**Supplementation should begin at birth and continue until the infant's diet includes at least 10 μg (400 IU) per day of vitamin D from other dietary sources or until the breastfed infant reaches one year of age.**" The complete recommendation and scientific rationale can be accessed at www.hc-sc.gc.ca/fn-an/nutrition/child-enfant/infant-nourisson/vita_d_supp_eng.php.

Breast milk composition continues to change as the infant grows and develops. Because of this ability to change as the baby changes, breast milk alone is entirely sufficient to sustain infant growth for the first six months of life. Throughout the next six months of infancy, as solid foods are gradually introduced, breast milk remains the baby's primary source of superior-quality nutrition.

Protection from Infections and Allergies   Immune factors from the mother, including antibodies and immune cells, are passed directly from the mother to the newborn through breast milk. These factors provide important disease protection for the infant while its immune system is still immature. Some studies have shown that breastfed infants have a lower incidence of respiratory tract, GI tract, and urinary tract infections than formula-fed infants. Even a few weeks of breastfeeding is beneficial, but the longer a child is breastfed, the greater the level of passive immunity from the mother. A report from the United Nations Children's Fund estimates that, in part because of this immunologic protection, if every baby were exclusively breastfed from birth for six months, 1.3 million lives would be saved (UNICEF 2003).

Breast milk is non-allergenic; however, there is conflicting evidence on the relationship between breastfeeding and the risk of allergies during childhood and adulthood. The duration of breastfeeding appears to be associated with the risk of overweight during adolescence and adulthood—the longer the infant is breastfed, the less likely the child will be overweight later in life (Harder et al. 2005; Arenz et al. 2004).

ovulation The release of an ovum (egg) from a woman's ovary.

Breastfeeding suppresses **ovulation** (the release of an ovum, or egg, from a woman's ovary), lengthening the time between pregnancies and giving a mother's body the chance to recover before she conceives again. This benefit can be lifesaving for malnourished women living in countries that discourage or outlaw the use of contraceptives. Ovulation may not cease completely, however, so it is still possible to become pregnant while breastfeeding. Health care providers typically recommend use of additional birth control methods while breastfeeding to avoid another conception occurring too soon to allow a mother's body to recover from the earlier pregnancy.

See the Highlight box to learn more about encouraging breastfeeding in developing nations.

Mother-Infant Bonding   Breastfeeding is among the most intimate of human interactions. Ideally, it is a quiet time away from distractions when mother and baby begin to develop an enduring bond of affection known as *attachment*. Breastfeeding enhances attachment by providing the opportunity for frequent, direct skin-to-skin contact, which stimulates the baby's sense of touch and is a primary means of communication (Olds et al. 2003). The cuddling and intense watching that occur during breastfeeding begin to teach the mother and baby about each other's behavioural cues. Breastfeeding also reassures the mother that she is providing the best possible nutrition for her baby.

Undoubtedly, bottle-feeding does not preclude parent-infant attachment! As long as attention is paid to closeness, cuddling, and skin contact, bottle-feeding can foster bonding as well.

Convenience and Cost   Breast milk is always ready, clean, at the right temperature, and available on demand, whenever and wherever it's needed. In the middle of the night, when the baby wakes up hungry, a breastfeeding mother can respond almost instantaneously, and both are soon back to sleep. In contrast, formula-feeding is a time-consuming process: parents have to continually wash and sterilize bottles, and each batch of formula must be mixed and heated to the proper temperature. Any leftover formula must be discarded.

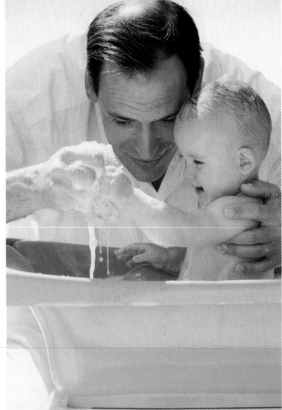

Fathers and siblings can bond with infants through such activities as bathing, changing diapers, and playing with and cuddling the infant.

In addition, breastfeeding costs nothing other than the price of a modest amount of additional food for the mother. In contrast, formula can be relatively expensive, and there are the additional costs of bottles and other supplies, as well as the cost of energy used for washing and sterilization.

A hidden cost of formula-feeding is its effect on the environment. Consider the energy used and waste produced during formula manufacturing, marketing, shipping and distribution, preparation, and disposal of used packaging. In contrast, breastfeeding is environmentally responsible, using no external energy and producing no external wastes.

Breastfeeding: Other Considerations

For some women and infants, breastfeeding is easy from the very first day. Others experience some initial difficulty because of mechanical factors, such as incorrect positioning or poor sucking technique, either of which can cause soreness or cracked nipples. With teaching from an experienced nurse, lactation consultant, or volunteer mother from La Leche League, these women are usually able to correct such problems, and the experience becomes mutually pleasurable. In contrast, some families encounter difficulties that make formula-feeding their best choice. This section discusses some social challenges for breastfeeding families.

Effects of Drugs and Other Substances on Breast Milk   Many substances make their way into breast milk. Among them are illegal and prescription drugs, over-the-counter drugs, and even substances from foods the mother eats. All illegal drugs should be assumed to pass into breast milk and should be avoided by breastfeeding mothers. Prescription drugs vary in the degree to which they pass into breast milk. Breastfeeding mothers should inform their physician that they are breastfeeding. Many drugs can be taken safely while lactating. If a safe and effective form of the necessary medication cannot be found, however, the mother will have to avoid breastfeeding while she is taking the drug. During this time, she can pump and discard her breast milk so that her milk

▶ **HIGHLIGHT**

Global Nutrition: Encouraging Breastfeeding in the Developing World

In Canada and other industrialized nations, the benefits of breast-feeding include its precise correspondence to the infant's nutritional needs, protection of the infant from infections and allergies, promotion of mother-infant bonding, low cost, and convenience. In developing countries, however, breastfeeding may also save the newborn's or mother's life. Here are some reasons why.

It is estimated that a quarter of the Earth's population may lack sanitary drinking water. Breastfeeding protects newborns from contaminated water supplies. The least expensive form of infant formula is a packaged powder that must be carefully measured and mixed with a precise quantity of sterilized water. If the water is not sterilized and is contaminated with disease-causing organisms, the baby will become ill. A baby who is fed formula instead of breast milk receives none of the mother's beneficial antibodies; this means that when formula-fed infants do contract an infection, whether from contaminated water or another source, they are not as well prepared to fight it off as breastfed infants would be. Many studies indicate that, for these reasons, a non-breastfed child living in disease-ridden and un-hygienic conditions is between 6 and 25 times as likely to die of diarrhea and 4 times as likely to die of pneumonia as breastfed infants living in the same region (UNICEF 2003).

In addition, in an attempt to make their supply of formula last longer, many impoverished parents add more water than the amount specified by the manufacturer. In this case, even when the water is sterilized, the child is at risk of malnutrition because the nutrients in the formula are being diluted (Elliot 2003; Reuters 2000).

These factors explain why breastfeeding is protective of the infant, but why does it help the mother? First, breastfeeding stimulates the uterus to contract vigorously after childbirth. This reduces the woman's risk of prolonged or excessive postpartum bleeding, a common cause of death in developing nations. Second, breastfeeding reduces a woman's risk of developing ovarian and breast cancer.

Third, as mentioned earlier, breastfeeding is a natural form of birth control. While her infant is exclusively breastfeeding, a mother is rarely fertile because frequent breastfeeding suppresses ovulation. In regions where access to contraceptives may be lacking, breastfeeding can help women to space births, giving their bodies a chance to fully recover from the physical and metabolic changes of pregnancy, and to nourish their baby adequately without also having to support the development of a growing fetus.

The human immunodeficiency virus (HIV), which causes AIDS, can be transmitted from mother to child via breast milk. For this reason, in areas with sanitary water supplies, women with HIV or AIDS may be counselled against breastfeeding. In contrast, in regions where the risk of infant death from infectious disease is high, mothers are counselled about the risks, benefits, and costs of all infant-feeding options. They are then encouraged to make an informed but independent feeding choice (Jackson et al. 2003; UNICEF 2003).

For these reasons, international organizations like the World Health Organization and UNICEF encourage all HIV-negative women to breastfeed exclusively until their baby is six months of age and to continue supplemented breastfeeding until at least the age of two.

supply will be adequate when she resumes breastfeeding. Similarly, a physician should be consulted before taking any over-the-counter medications. The Motherisk Program at the Hospital for Sick Children (www.motherisk.org) provides guidance about medications and drugs during breastfeeding.

Caffeine and alcohol do enter breast milk. Caffeine can make the baby agitated and fussy, whereas alcohol can make the baby sleepy, depress the central nervous system, and slow motor development, in addition to inhibiting the mother's milk supply. During the initial stages, when breastfeeding takes place nearly around the clock, caffeine is not recommended. When feedings become less frequent, an occasional cup of coffee is considered safe, as long as there is sufficient time before the next feeding to allow the caffeine to clear from the breast milk.

Nicotine also passes into breast milk; therefore, it is best for the woman to quit smoking altogether. Smoking can impair fetal growth and reduce the bioavailability of various nutrients (Berlanga et al. 2002).

Breast milk is absorbed more readily than formula, making more frequent feedings necessary. Newborns commonly require breastfeedings every one to three hours versus every two to four hours for formula feedings. After the first month, the infant's digestive system matures and the feedings become slightly less frequent. Nevertheless, mothers who are exclusively breastfeeding and return to work within the first six months after the baby's birth must leave several bottles of pumped breast milk for others to use in their absence each day. This means that, to keep up their milk supply, working women have to pump their breasts to express the breast milk during the workday. This can be a challenge in companies that do not provide the time, space, and privacy required. In addition, many in society do not feel it is appropriate for women to breastfeed in public places. Societal pressures against breastfeeding have led many community leaders and politicians who understand the importance of breastfeeding to introduce worksite policies and legislation that supports breastfeeding in public and to support working mothers who are breastfeeding. Refer to the Nutrition Debate at the end of this chapter to learn more about breastfeeding legislation.

> **Recap:** Breastfeeding provides many benefits to both mother and newborn, including superior nutrition, heightened immunity, mother-infant bonding, convenience, and cost. Breastfeeding mothers should avoid using illegal drugs and large amounts of alcohol and caffeine, as these substances enter the breast milk and can affect the infant. Workplaces and public spaces should be encouraged to accommodate the needs of breastfeeding mothers who need to express breast milk during the day.

Infant Nutrition: From Birth to One Year

Most first-time parents are amazed at how rapidly their infant grows. Optimal nutrition is extremely important during the first year, as the baby's organs and nervous system continue to develop and mature and as the baby grows physically and acquires new skills. In fact, health care providers use length and weight measurements as the main tools for assessing an infant's nutritional status. These measurements are plotted on growth charts (there are separate charts for boys and girls), which track an infant's growth over time (Figure 15.11). Although every infant is unique, in general, health care providers look for a correlation between length and weight. In other words, an infant who is in the 60th percentile for length is usually in about the 50th to 70th percentile for weight. An infant who is in the 90th percentile for weight but is in the 20th percentile for length might be overfed. Consistency over time is also a consideration: for example, an infant who suddenly drops well below her established profile for weight might be underfed or ill.

Typical Infant Growth and Activity Patterns

Babies' basal metabolic rates are high, in part because their body surface area is large compared with their body size. Still, their limited physical activity keeps total energy expenditure relatively low. For the first few months of life, an infant's activities consist mainly of eating and sleeping. As the first year progresses, the repertoire of activity gradually expands to include rolling over, sitting up, crawling, standing, and finally taking the first few wobbly steps. Nevertheless, relatively little energy is expended in movement, and the primary use of energy during the first year of life is to support growth.

In the first year of life, an infant generally grows about 25 cm (10 in.) in length and triples in weight—a growth rate more rapid than will ever occur again. Not surprisingly, energy needs per unit body weight are also the highest they will ever be to support this phenomenal growth and metabolism.

Part of the rapid growth of an infant involves the brain, the growth of which is more rapid during the first year than at any other time. To accommodate such a large

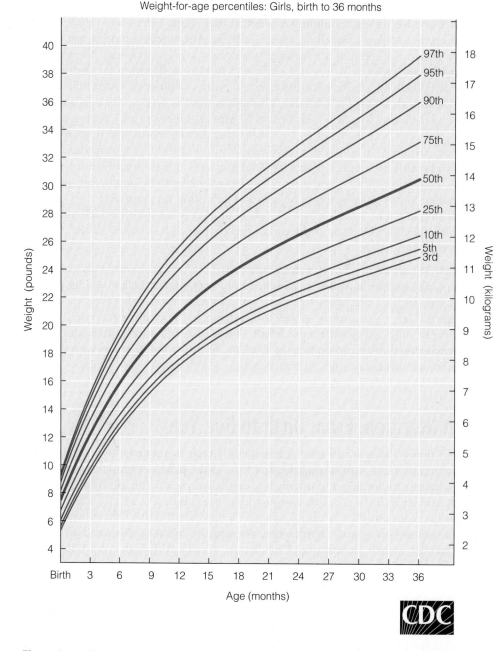

Weight-for-age percentiles: Girls, birth to 36 months

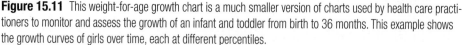

Figure 15.11 This weight-for-age growth chart is a much smaller version of charts used by health care practitioners to monitor and assess the growth of an infant and toddler from birth to 36 months. This example shows the growth curves of girls over time, each at different percentiles.
(Developed by the National Center for Health Statistics in collaboration with the National Center for Chronic Disease Prevention and Health Promotion 2000.)

increase in brain size, infants' heads are typically quite large in proportion to the rest of their bodies. Pediatricians use head circumference as an additional tool for the assessment of growth and nutritional status. After around 18 months of age, the rate of brain growth slows, and gradually the body catches up to head size.

Nutrient Needs for Infants

Three characteristics of infants combine to make their nutritional needs unique: (1) their high energy needs per unit body weight to support rapid growth; (2) their immature digestive tracts and kidneys; and (3) their small size.

Macronutrient Needs of Infants

An infant needs to consume about 110 kcal (460 kJ) per kilogram of body weight per day. This amounts to about 700 kcal (2930 kJ) per day at around 6 months of age. Given infants' immature digestive tracts and kidneys, as well as their high fluid needs, providing this much energy may seem difficult. Fortunately, breast milk and commercial formulas are energy dense, contributing about 690 kcal (2890 kJ) per litre. When solid foods are introduced after about 6 months of age, they provide even more energy in addition to the breast milk or formula.

Infants are not merely small versions of adults. The proportions of macronutrients they require differ from adult proportions, as do the types of food they can tolerate. It is generally agreed that about 40% to 50% of an infant's diet should come from fat during the first year of life and that fat intake below this level can be harmful before the age of 2. Given the high energy needs of infants just discussed, it makes sense to take advantage of the energy density of fat (9 kcal/g or 37 kJ/g) to help meet these requirements. Breast milk and commercial formulas are both high in fat (about 50% of total energy). In addition to being a dense source of energy, fats are essential for the rapid brain growth and nervous system development that happens in the first one to two years of life.

No more than 20% of an infant's daily energy requirement should come from protein. This is plenty to accommodate an infant's rapid growth. Immature infant kidneys are not able to process and excrete the excess amine groups from higher-protein diets. Breast milk and commercial formulas both provide adequate overall protein and appropriate essential amino acids to support growth and development.

Micronutrient Needs of Infants

An infant's micronutrient needs are also high to accommodate their rapid growth and development. Micronutrients of particular note include iron, vitamin D, zinc, and iodide. Fortunately, breast milk and commercial formulas provide most of the micronutrients needed for infant growth and development, with some special considerations discussed later in this chapter.

In addition, all infants are routinely given an dose of vitamin K shortly after birth. This provides vitamin K until the infant's intestine can develop its own healthful bacteria, which provide vitamin K thereafter.

Do Infants Need Supplements?

Breast milk and commercial formulas provide most of the vitamins and minerals infants need. However, there are several micronutrients that may warrant supplementation. For breastfed infants, a vitamin D supplement is recommended from birth. At around 6 months of age, the baby's iron stores become depleted, as breast milk is a poor source of iron. Iron is extremely important for cognitive development and prevention of iron-deficiency anemia. Starting solid foods (baby cereal) fortified with iron or meat and alternates at 6 months of age can serve as an additional iron source.

For formula-fed infants, supplementation depends on the formula composition and the water supply used to make the formula. Many formulas are already fortified with iron, for example, and some municipal water supplies contain fluoride. If the municipal water supply has fluoride at 0.3 parts per million or greater, then no fluoride supplements should be given for the first two years of life (Health Canada 2007). If the water supply has less than 0.3 ppm, babies between the ages of 6 months and 2 years may receive 0.25 mg/day of fluoride supplements. It should be noted that ready-to-serve infant formulas in Canada are not fortified with fluoride.

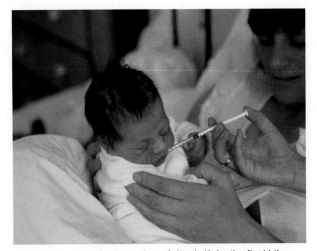

Newborns are routinely given a dose of vitamin K shortly after birth.

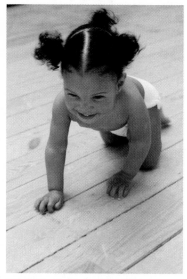

An infant's physical activity will progress beyond crawling before the first year of life is over.

Commercial infant formulas available in Canada come in two types: iron fortified and without added iron. Infants generally have enough iron stored in their bodies to meet their needs for the first 6 months; after that, formula-fed babies should receive iron-fortified formula. Because parents may forget to switch to an iron-fortified formula at 6 months, Health Canada (2007) recommends that infants not receiving breast milk be given iron-fortified formula from birth until 9 to 12 months at age. By 9 to 12 months of age, children should be receiving a variety of iron-rich table foods and can discontinue infant formula.

There are also special conditions in which additional supplements may be wise. For example, if a woman is a vegan, her breast milk may be low in vitamin B_{12}, and a supplement of this vitamin should be given to the baby.

If a supplement is given, careful consideration should be given to dosage. The supplement should be formulated specifically for infants, and the daily dose should not be exceeded. High doses of micronutrients can be dangerous. Too much iron can be fatal, and accidental iron poisoning is one of the leading causes of death in children under 6 years of age.

Fluid Recommendations for Infants

Fluid is critical for everyone, but for infants the balance is more delicate for two reasons. First, because infants are so small, they proportionally lose more water through evaporation than adults. Second, their kidneys are immature and unable to concentrate urine. Hence, they are at even greater risk of dehydration. An infant needs about 65 mL (2 fl. oz.) of fluid per 0.5 kg (1 lb.) of body weight, and either breast milk or formula is usually enough to provide this amount. However, there are certain conditions, such as diarrhea, vomiting, fever, or hot weather, that can exacerbate fluid loss. In these instances, supplemental fluid may be warranted. However, too much fluid can also be particularly dangerous for an infant. Thus, supplemental fluids (whether water or an infant electrolyte formula) should be given judiciously and under the advice of a physician. Generally, it is advised that supplemental fluids not exceed 125 mL (4 fl. oz.) per day. A guide for parents to determine whether fluid intake is appropriate is to look for six to eight wet diapers per day.

What Types of Formula Are Available?

We discussed the advantages of breastfeeding earlier in this chapter, and indeed both national and international health care organizations consider breastfeeding the best choice for infant nutrition, when possible. However, if breastfeeding is not feasible, several types of commercial formulas provide nutritious alternatives.

Most formulas are based on altered cow's milk proteins, casein and whey, which have been heated to denature them. The sugars lactose and sucrose, alone or in combination, provide carbohydrates, and vegetable oils or microbiologically-produced fatty acids provide the fat component (Usury and Mena 1999).

Soy-based formulas are a viable alternative for infants who cannot tolerate the proteins in cow's milk–based formulas, who have a genetic condition called galactosemia, or who need to avoid dairy products for reasons related to culture, religion, or a vegan lifestyle (Health Canada 2007). All soy-based formulas in Canada are iron fortified (Health Canada 2007). However, soy-based formulas are not without controversy. Because soy contains isoflavones, or plant forms of estrogens, there is some concern over the effects these compounds have on growing infants. Currently it is believed that soy formulas are safe, but they should be used only when breast milk or cow's milk–based formulas are contraindicated. Babies can also have allergic reactions to soy-based formulas (American Academy of Pediatrics 2000). Soy-based formulas are not the same as soy milk, which is not suitable for infant feeding.

Finally, there are specialized formula preparations for specific conditions. Some contain proteins that have been predigested, for example, or have compositions designed to accommodate certain medical conditions. Some have been specially formulated for older infants and toddlers. The final choice of formula depends on cost, infant tolerance, stage of infant development, and the advice of the infant's pediatrician.

When Do Infants Begin to Need Solid Foods?

Infants begin to need solid foods at around 6 months of age. Before this age, most infants are not physically able to consume solid food. The suckling response depends on a particular movement of the tongue that draws liquid out of breast or bottle. In response to solid foods introduced with a spoon, this tongue movement merely results in pushing most of the food back out of the mouth. Not only must the tongue's extrusion reflex begin to abate, but the infant must have gained muscular control of the head and neck and must be able to sit up (with or without support).

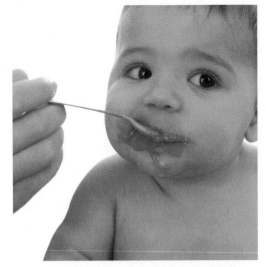

The suckling reflex will push solid food out of an infant's mouth.

Another part of being ready for solid foods is sufficient maturity of the digestive system, so that it can digest and absorb nutrients from solid food. If an infant is fed solid foods too soon, nutrient molecules (particularly proteins) can be absorbed intact and undigested, setting the stage for allergies. In addition, the kidneys must have matured so that they are better able to process proteins and concentrate urine.

Finally, the nutritional need for foods besides breast milk or formula becomes evident at about 6 months of age, when infant iron stores become depleted. Typically, the first foods introduced are iron-fortified infant cereals, starting with rice, which rarely provokes an allergic response and is easy to digest. Health Canada (2007) has recently updated its guidelines on the introduction of complementary foods (foods to accompany breast milk or formula). The new guidelines state: "In Canada, the most commonly used first food is iron-fortified infant cereal. Meat and alternatives are iron-containing foods that can also be introduced at this stage. The foods in this group include meats, fish, poultry, cooked egg yolks, and alternatives such as well-cooked legumes and tofu. Iron from meat sources is better absorbed than iron from non-meat sources." The complete recommendation can be accessed at www.hc-sc.gc.ca/fn-an/pubs/infant-nourrisson/nut_infant_nourrisson_term_6-eng.php.

Other grains, strained vegetables, and fruits can gradually be incorporated into the diet. Infant foods should be introduced one at a time, with no other new foods for a week, in order to watch for allergies. Gradually, a repertoire including a variety of foods should be built by the end of the first year. Throughout the first year, solid foods should only be a supplement to, not a substitute for, breast milk or formula. Infants still need the nutrient density and energy that breast milk and formula provide. Notice that it is not safe for infants to consume regular cow's milk.

What *Not* to Feed an Infant

The following foods should never be offered to an infant:

- *Foods that could cause choking.* Such foods as grapes, hot dogs, nuts, popcorn, raw carrots, raisins, and hard candies cannot be chewed adequately by infants and can cause choking.

- *Corn syrup and honey.* These may contain spores of the bacterium *Clostridium botulinum.* These spores can germinate and grow into viable bacteria in the immature digestive tracts of infants, whereupon they produce a potent toxin that can be fatal. Children older than one year can safely consume these substances because their digestive tracts are mature enough to kill any *C. botulinum* bacteria.

- *Goat's milk.* Goat's milk is notoriously low in many nutrients that infants need, such as folate, vitamin C, and iron. In Canada, goat's milk is fortified with vitamin D.

- *Cow's milk.* For children under 1 year, cow's milk is too concentrated in minerals and protein and contains too few carbohydrates to meet infant energy needs. Infants can begin to consume whole cow's milk after the age of 1 year. Infants and toddlers should not be given 1% or 2% partly-skimmed cow's milk before the age of 2, as it does not contain enough fat and is too high in mineral content for the kidneys to handle effectively. Infants should not be given evaporated milk or sweetened condensed milk.

- *Large quantities of fruit juices.* Fruit juices are poorly absorbed in the infant digestive tract, causing diarrhea if consumed in excess. Large quantities of fruit juice can make an infant feel full and reject breast milk or formula at feeding time, thus causing him or her to miss out on essential nutrients. It is considered safe for infants older than 6 months to consume 125 to 250 mL (4 to 8 fl. oz.) of pure fruit juice (no sweeteners added) per day, with no more than 65 to 125 mL (2 to 4 fl. oz.) given at a time; however, plain water will quench an infant's thirst. Diluting fruit juice with water is another option.

- *Too much salt and sugar.* Infant foods should not be seasoned with salt or other seasonings. Naturally occurring sugars, such as those found in fruits, can provide needed energy. Cookies, cakes, and other excessively sweet, processed foods should be avoided.

- *Too much breast milk or formula.* As nutritious as breast milk or formula are, once infants reach the age of 6 months, solid foods should be introduced gradually. Six months of age is a critical time, as it is when a baby's iron stores begin to be depleted and must be replenished with iron from enriched rice cereal. In addition, infants are physically and psychologically ready to incorporate solid foods at this time, and solid foods can help appease their increasing appetites. Between 6 months and the time of weaning (from breast or bottle), solid foods should gradually make up an increasing proportion of the infant's diet.

Nutrition-Related Concerns for Infants

Nutrition is one of the biggest concerns of new parents. Infants cannot speak, and their cries are sometimes indecipherable. Feeding time can be very frustrating for parents, especially if the child is not eating, not growing appropriately, or has problems like diarrhea, vomiting, or persistent skin rashes. Below are some nutrition-related concerns for infants.

Allergies

Many foods have the potential to stimulate an allergic reaction (see Chapter 3). Breastfeeding helps deter allergy development, as does delaying introduction of solid foods until the age of 6 months. One of the most common allergies in infants is to the proteins in cow's milk–based formulas. Some of these proteins are denatured with heat during the production process, but others remain intact. Symptoms include those of gastrointestinal distress, such as diarrhea, constipation, bloating, blood in the stool, and vomiting. In such cases, an alternative, such as a formula with predigested proteins, may be used.

As stated above, every food should be introduced in isolation, so that any allergic reaction can be spotted and attributed to a particular food, which can then be avoided.

Dehydration

Whether the cause is diarrhea, vomiting, or inadequate fluid intake, dehydration is extremely dangerous to infants, and if left untreated it can quickly result in death. The factors behind infants' increased risk of dehydration were discussed on page 566. Treatment includes providing fluids, a task that is difficult if vomiting is occurring. In some cases, the physician may recommend that a pediatric electrolyte solution be administered on a temporary basis. In more severe cases, hospitalization may be necessary. If possible, breastfeeding should continue throughout an illness.

Colic

Perhaps nothing is more frustrating to new parents than the relentless crying spells of some infants, typically referred to as **colic**. In this condition, newborns and young infants who appear happy, healthy, and well nourished suddenly begin to cry or even shriek, and continue no matter what their caregiver does to console them. The spells tend to occur at the same time of day, typically late in the afternoon or early in the evening, and often occur daily for several weeks. Crying lasts for hours at a time. Overstimulation of the nervous system, feeding too rapidly, swallowing of air, and intestinal gas pain are considered possible culprits, but the precise cause is unknown.

As with allergies, if a colicky infant is breastfed, breastfeeding should be continued, but the mother should try to determine whether eating certain foods seems to prompt crying and, if so, eliminate the offending food(s) from her diet. Avoidance of spicy or other strongly flavoured foods may also help. Formula-fed infants may benefit from a change in type of formula. In the worst cases of colic, a physician may prescribe medication. Fortunately, most cases disappear spontaneously, possibly because of maturity of the GI tract, around 3 months of age.

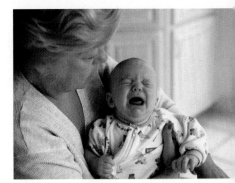

Colicky babies will begin crying for no apparent reason even if they otherwise appear well nourished and happy.

colic Inconsolable infant crying that lasts for hours at a time.

Anemia

As stated earlier, infants are born with sufficient iron stores to last for approximately the first six months of life. In older infants and toddlers, however, iron is the mineral most likely to be deficient. Iron-deficiency anemia causes pallor, lethargy, and impaired growth. Iron-fortified formula is a good source for formula-fed infants. Some pediatricians prescribe a supplement containing iron especially formulated for infants. Iron for older infants is typically supplied by iron-fortified rice cereal.

Nursing Bottle Syndrome

Infants should never be left alone with a bottle, whether lying down or sitting up. As infants manipulate the nipple of the bottle in their mouths, the high-carbohydrate fluid (whether breast milk, formula, or fruit juice) drips out, coming into prolonged contact with the developing teeth. This high-carbohydrate fluid provides an optimal food source for the bacteria that are the underlying cause of **dental caries** (cavities), which are defined as dental erosion and decay caused by acid-secreting bacteria in the mouth and on the teeth. Severe tooth decay can result. Encouraging the use of a cup around the age of 8 months helps prevent nursing bottle syndrome, along with weaning the baby from a bottle entirely by the age of 18 months.

dental caries Dental erosion and decay caused by acid-secreting bacteria in the mouth and on the teeth. The acid produced is a byproduct of bacterial metabolism of carbohydrates deposited on the teeth.

Lead Poisoning

Lead is especially toxic to infants and children because their brains and central nervous systems are still developing. Lead poisoning can result in decreased mental capacity, behavioural problems, impaired growth, impaired hearing, and other problems. Laws have been passed in recent decades to decrease lead exposure for everyone, including introducing unleaded gasoline, eliminating lead solder, and outlawing the use of lead-based paint. Unfortunately, lead in old pipes can still leach into a home's water supply, and lead paint can still be found in older homes and buildings. If the paint in an older home is flaking and peeling, infants or toddlers may easily pop these flakes into their mouths (as they do everything else). Measures to reduce lead exposure include

- allowing tap water to run for a minute or so before use, to clear the pipes of any lead-contaminated water that may have leached from solder

- using only cold tap water for drinking and cooking, as hot tap water is more likely to leach lead

- having lead-based paint professionally removed, painting it over with latex paint, or at least removing paint flakes and dust

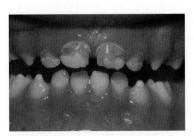

Leaving a baby alone with a bottle can result in the tooth decay of nursing bottle syndrome.

Recap: Infancy is characterized by the most rapid growth a human being will ever experience. Infants need large amounts of energy per unit of body weight to keep up with growth, but because they cannot consume large amounts of food, foods must be nutrient dense. Breast milk provides necessary nutrients for the first six months of life. Solid foods can gradually be introduced into an infant's diet thereafter. A supplement containing iron and fluoride may be prescribed after age 6 months. Infants must be monitored for allergies, dehydration, and other signs of distress. Growth is the most reliable longitudinal assessment of infant nutrition.

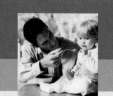

CHAPTER SUMMARY

- Nutrition is important before conception because critical stages of cell division, tissue differentiation, and organ development occur in the early weeks of pregnancy, often before a woman even knows she is pregnant.

- A plentiful, nourishing diet is important throughout pregnancy to provide the nutrients needed to support fetal development without depriving the mother of nutrients she needs to maintain her own health.

- A normal pregnancy progresses over the course of 38 to 42 weeks. This time is divided into three trimesters of 13 to 14 weeks. Each trimester is associated with particular developmental phases of the embryo or fetus.

- Pregnant women of normal weight should consume adequate energy to gain 11.5 to 16 kg (25 to 35 lb.) during pregnancy. Women who are underweight should gain slightly more, and women who are overweight or obese should gain less.

- Pregnant women need to be especially careful to consume adequate amounts of folate, vitamin B_{12}, vitamin C, vitamin D, calcium, iron, and zinc. A prenatal multi-vitamin and mineral supplement is often prescribed to ensure adequate intake of these nutrients.

- A majority of pregnant women experience nausea or vomiting during pregnancy, called morning sickness, and many crave or feel aversions to specific types of foods and non-food substances.

- Heartburn (or gastroesophageal reflux disease, GERD) and constipation in pregnancy are related to the relaxation of smooth muscle caused by certain pregnancy-related hormones.

- Gestational diabetes and pre-eclampsia are nutrition-related disorders that can seriously affect maternal and fetal health.

- Adolescents' bodies are still growing and developing; thus, their nutrient needs during pregnancy are higher than those of older pregnant women.

- Dieting during pregnancy leads to inadequate nutrition for mother and fetus.

- Alcohol is a teratogen and should be avoided during pregnancy.

- Successful breastfeeding requires the coordination of several hormones, including estrogen, progesterone, prolactin, and oxytocin. These hormones govern the preparation of the breasts, as well as actual milk production and the milk "let down" response.

- Breastfeeding women require more energy than during pregnancy. Protein needs increase, and an overall nutritious diet with plentiful fluids is important in maintaining milk quality and quantity, as well as in preserving the mother's health.

- The advantages of breastfeeding include the nutritional superiority of breast milk, protection from infections and allergies, the promotion of attachment, the convenience, and the lower cost.

- Breastfeeding exclusively for at least the first six months of a baby's life is recommended by both Health Canada and international health care organizations.

- Infants are characterized by their extremely rapid growth and brain development.

- Physicians use length and weight measurements as the main tools for assessing an infant's nutritional status.

- An infant needs to consume about 110 kcal per kg (460 kJ per kg) body weight per day.

- Since infant stores of iron become depleted after about six months, iron-rich foods, such as iron-fortified rice cereal and pureed meats, well-cooked legumes, and egg yolks, can be introduced.

- Table foods should be introduced one at a time, with a week between new foods in order to monitor for possible allergic reactions. Although the variety of foods gradually increases, breast milk or formula continues to be very important throughout the first year.

- Infants need to be monitored carefully for appropriate growth and six to eight wet diapers every day to assess adequate nutrient intake and hydration.

- Nutrition-related concerns for infants include the potential for allergies, dehydration, colic, nursing bottle syndrome, and ingestion of lead.

REVIEW QUESTIONS

Quizzes

1. Folate deficiency in the first weeks after conception has been linked with which of the following problems in the newborn?
   a. Anemia
   b. Neural tube defects
   c. Low birth weight
   d. Preterm delivery

2. Which of the following hormones is responsible for the milk let down response?
   a. Progesterone
   b. Estrogen
   c. Oxytocin
   d. Prolactin

3. Which of the following nutrients is not essential in a newborn's diet?
   a. Fibre
   b. Fat
   c. Iron
   d. Vitamin D

4. A pregnancy weight gain of 12.7 to 18 kg (28 to 40 lb.) is recommended for
   a. all women.
   b. women who begin their pregnancy underweight.
   c. women who begin their pregnancy overweight.
   d. women who begin their pregnancy at a normal weight.

5. The best solid food to introduce first to infants is
   a. Cream of Wheat cereal.
   b. applesauce.
   c. teething biscuits.
   d. iron-fortified rice cereal.

6. All women of childbearing age are encouraged to consume which of the following daily?
   a. 400 micrograms of folic acid
   b. 40 grams of folic acid
   c. 4 grams of folate
   d. 400 milligrams of folic acid

7. A woman weighs 78 kg (172 lbs.) and is 1.67 metres (5'7") tall. How much weight would you recommend she gain during pregnancy?
   a. 11.4–15.9 kg (25–35 lb.)
   b. 12.7–18.2 kg (28–40 lb.)
   c. 6.8–11.4 kg (15–25 lb.)
   d. no more than 6.8 kg (15 lb.)

8. If an infant weighs 5 kg, how many calories would it need to consume in a day?
   a. 550 kcal
   b. 100 kcal
   c. 110 kcal
   d. 5010 kcal

9. A family friend has just recently become pregnant; she comes to you and says, "Now I can start eating twice as much food, because I'm eating for two." What advice would you give her?

10. Explain the relationship between the increased need for iron and the increased need for fluid in a pregnant woman.

11. Your cousin, who is pregnant with her first child, tells you that her physician prescribed supplemental iron tablets for her but that she decided not to take them. "You know me," she says, "I'm a natural-food nut! I'm absolutely certain that my careful diet is providing all the nutrients my baby needs." Is it possible that your cousin is partly right and partly wrong? Explain.

12. You visit your neighbours one afternoon to congratulate them on the birth of their new daughter, Katie. While you are there, 2-week-old Katie suddenly starts crying as if she is in terrible pain. "Oh, no," Katie's dad says to his wife. "Here we go again!" He turns to you and explains, "She's been like this every afternoon for the past week, and it goes on until sunset. I just wish we could figure out what we're doing wrong." What would you say?

13. You are on a picnic at a park with your sister, who drapes a shawl over her shoulders and breastfeeds her

14-month-old son. A woman walking by stops and says, "Isn't that child getting too old for that?" What information could you share with her in response to her question?

14. Mary's doctor has just informed her that she has gestational diabetes. At this point, she does not need to give herself insulin shots as long as she watches what she eats. After hearing the list of foods she should avoid, Mary is worried that she will not be able to follow her doctor's orders. All the foods she is supposed to stay away from are the foods she has found she craves most during pregnancy. On top of this, Mary is also scared about the long-term effects of gestational diabetes. After learning about diabetes in Chapter 4, what foods do you think her doctor advised Mary to stay away from? What strategies might you suggest to help her control her cravings for carbohydrates? Besides diet, what other measures can Mary take to control her gestational diabetes? Assuming that her condition is under control, does she need to be afraid for her baby's health? Will she need to maintain her strict diet for the rest of her life?

15. Tera has a decision to make. She knows that breast milk is the best thing for her newborn but she is having trouble with the techniques involved. Her delivery was a smooth one and she was discharged early from the hospital before she could ask about how to breastfeed. Moreover, Tera wants to return to work within the next four months and is concerned with being able to continue breastfeeding her baby at that time. Explain to Tera the advantages of breastfeeding. Whom can Tera ask about correct breastfeeding techniques? What accommodations in Tera's workplace would help her to continue breastfeeding after she returns to work?

CASE STUDY

Daniel is 19 years old and his mother keeps hinting that he and his girlfriend, Samantha, should really settle down and start a family. In Nigeria, where Daniel's family is from, people marry young and usually have kids right away. Both Daniel and Samantha agree that they want to graduate from university before they consider marriage. This is a constant source of conflict between Daniel and his mother.

Considering what you've learned so far in this chapter, do you think there is any ideal age to have children? If so, what would that age be and why? What are the pros and cons of starting a family at a young age? What practical information could Daniel offer his mom to justify his decision to wait a few years before starting a family?

Test Yourself Answers

1. **False** Gaining too much weight might result in a large baby and difficult delivery, as well as difficulty in losing the weight after pregnancy. Gaining too little weight can result in a low-birth-weight baby, which increases the risk of various complications that can be life threatening.

2. **False** More than half of all pregnant women experience morning sickness, and food cravings or aversions are also common.

3. **True** The number of cases of neural tube defects in newborns has declined dramatically since Canada made folate fortification of wheat flour mandatory.

4. **True** Physical growth, including length, weight, and head circumference, is the best indicator for assessing an infant's nutrition status.

5. **False** Most infants do not have a physiologic need for solid food until about 6 months of age.

WEB LINKS

www.healthycanadians.gc.ca/hp-gs/index_e.html
Healthy Canadians: Healthy Pregnancy
This is a great site for anyone wanting easy-to-understand information about pregnancy. Click the link to *The Sensible Guide to a Healthy Pregnancy*.

www.womenshealthmatters.ca
Women's Health Matters: The New Women's College Hospital
This site is devoted to providing information on a range of current women's health topics.

www.caringforkids.cps.ca
Caring for Kids, Canadian Paediatric Association
This is a great site for parents who want credible and accurate information. It lists product recalls and has information about immunizations, pregnancy, healthy eating, and much more.

www.motherisk.org
The Motherisk Program at the Hospital for Sick Children
This is a clinical, research, and teaching program that provides information and guidance about the effects of drugs, chemicals, diseases, radiation, and environmental substances on the developing fetus.

www.aap.org
American Academy of Pediatrics
Visit this website for information on infants' and children's health. Searches can be performed on such topics as "neural tube defects" or "infant formulas."

www.nal.usda.gov/fnic
Food Nutrition Information Center
Click on Topics A–Z and then Child Nutrition and Health for a list of infant nutrition topics and a listing of child nutrition programs, links, and resources.

www.marchofdimes.com/pnhec/pnhec.asp
March of Dimes
Click on Pregnancy & Newborn to find links on nutrition during pregnancy, breastfeeding, and baby care.

www.diabetes.ca
Canadian Diabetes Association
Search for "gestational diabetes" to find information about diabetes that develops during pregnancy.

www.llli.org
La Leche League
Search this site to find multiple articles on the health effects of breastfeeding for mother and infant.

www.nofas.org
National Organization on Fetal Alcohol Syndrome
This site provides news and information relating to fetal alcohol syndrome.

Do Women Have a Right to Breastfeed in the Workplace and in Public?

Try to imagine the following scenarios. In the first, you have just finished grocery shopping and your 6-week-old infant decides it is time for his afternoon feeding. Without a second thought, you lift your shirt just enough to allow your son to feed while you wait in line at the checkout. Despite the stares and the disapproving looks from several customers, you continue to feed your newborn, reasoning that your baby has a right to eat when he's hungry. As you are leaving the store, you notice that some of the customers in line behind you are now talking with the manager and motioning in your direction. The manager approaches you awkwardly and informs you that the ladies' restroom has recently been remodelled to provide a "private" place for nursing mothers.

In the second scenario, you and your newborn are with a friend in a coffee house. Your infant daughter, sleeping quietly in your arms, wakes up from her nap and wants to be fed. You comfortably unbutton only the necessary number of buttons on your shirt and allow your daughter to nurse while your friend gets the lattes from the coffee counter. Within minutes, you are publicly humiliated by an insistent store manager who asks you to stop feeding because you are "disturbing other customers." Drawing even more attention to you, the manager then adds, "I will not tolerate nudity in my establishment!"

These scenarios, in fact, offer real-life examples of how mothers Sheryl Palmer and Elizabeth Ferencsik were treated by store managers and customers when trying to breastfeed in public. That this may be even more of a reality for some women than people choose to recognize is confirmed by recent Canadian newspaper headlines: "Nursing in public—a human right in BC," "Why, yes, she's sucking on me—get over it," "Mall management sorry nursing mother expelled," and "Into the mouths of babes—what exactly is repulsive about breastfeeding?" Each of these stories highlights women who have been expelled from a public establishment by security guards or store managers and who have been made to feel ashamed or embarrassed about the natural act of breastfeeding.

According to the human rights legislation under Canadian law, women have the right to breastfeed in the workplace and in public. However, only B.C. (www.ag.gov.bc.ca/human-rights-protection/pdfs/SexDiscrimination&Harassment.pdf) and Ontario (www.ohrc.on.ca/en/issues/pregnancy) have provincial human rights laws that specifically address breastfeeding. Despite this legal protection, many women find it extremely challenging to breastfeed in a public place or at work.

Not only are storeowners to blame, but employers have also been found guilty of making it less convenient for women to follow the Canadian recommendations for breastfeeding. In 1997, the British Columbia Human Rights Commission found that Michelle Poirier's employer discriminated against her by not permitting her to breastfeed her child in the workplace and at a public seminar sponsored by her employer. Poirier argued that not only was she inconvenienced by having to leave the office to breastfeed but that making other arrangements was also "stressful." As a nursing mother, she had experienced some physical discomfort at not being able to feed at regular times.

In a more recent case, an arbitrator ruled that an employer's refusal to allow employee Doris Degagne to breastfeed her child in the workplace constituted discrimination on the basis of gender. The arbitrator claimed "discrimination on the basis that a woman is breastfeeding is a form of sex discrimination." In this case, Degagne had requested permission to have her child brought into the workplace to breastfeed. When her request was denied, she asked for a six-month leave of absence to continue breastfeeding, which was also denied. Degagne's employer then terminated her employment when she did not return to work at the end of her maternity leave.

In Canada, the newest guidelines on infant feeding state that babies should be exclusively breastfed for six months, and then breastfeeding should continue with complementary foods up to the age of 2 years. When you consider the risk of humiliation, or the fear of being expelled from a local establishment, what type of message are women really receiving? How can women follow these guidelines when they feel shunned if they breastfeed in a public place or if there is nowhere—and no time—for breastfeeding at work? How can the work environment become more supportive of women's rights to breastfeed? When it is their responsibility to accommodate breastfeeding mothers, should employers also be offered incentives to provide lactation areas equipped with refrigerators and breastfeeding pumps?

In contrast to women's rights to breastfeed in Canada, only 13 states in the United States have

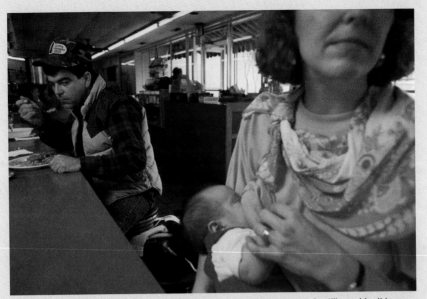

Although a much more common practice today than in the past, many people still consider it inappropriate to breastfeed in public.

legislation that specifically exempts breastfeeding from being classified as indecent exposure. It is important to emphasize that breastfeeding is not illegal, and legislation is not necessary to legalize this natural act. The primary purpose of legislation is to clarify that women have the right to breastfeed in public, and they should not be harassed or shunned if they do so. Porter (2003) reports that as of 2002, 32 states have enacted legislation that states breastfeeding is not illegal, and 17 states permit women to breastfeed in any public or private location where children and mothers are authorized to be. Five states exempt women from jury duty if they are breastfeeding, and Connecticut, Hawaii, Illinois, and Minnesota have laws that require employers to accommodate breastfeeding mothers who return to work (Weimer 2003).

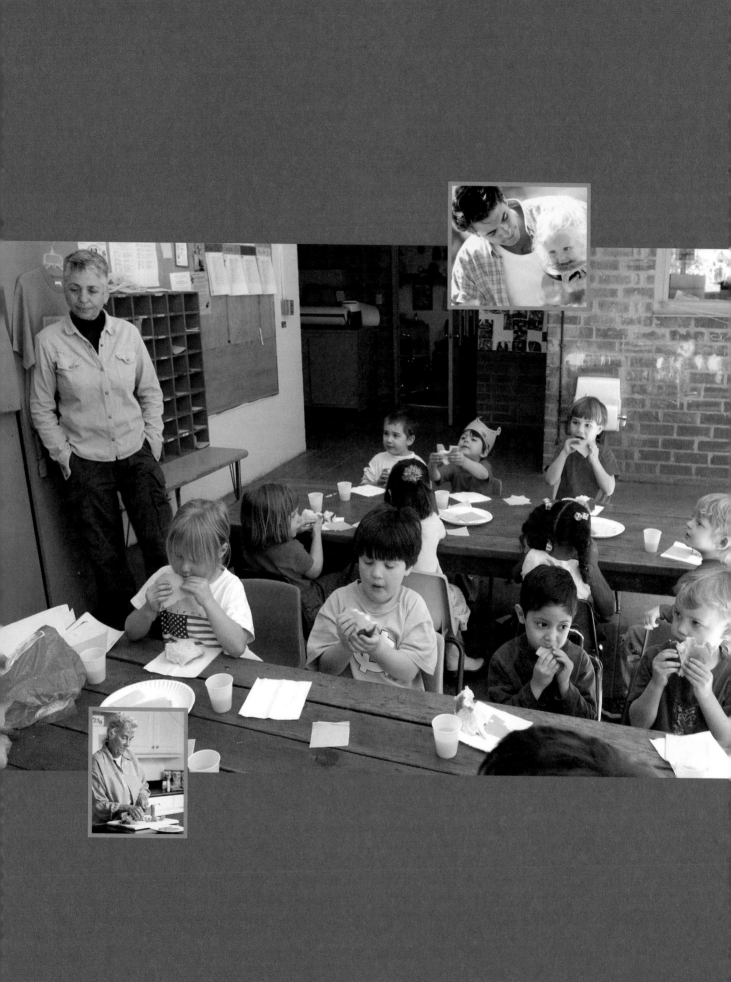

CHAPTER 16

Nutrition Through the Life Cycle: Childhood to Late Adulthood

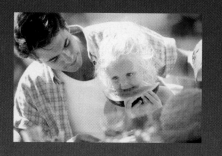

CHAPTER OBJECTIVES

After reading this chapter you will be able to:

1. Compare and contrast the growth and activity patterns of toddlers and preschoolers, pp. 578 and 585.

2. Identify at least three nutrients of concern when feeding a vegan diet to young children, pp. 583–584.

3. Describe how micronutrient needs change as a child matures from school-age years to adolescence, pp. 585–586 and 589.

4. Identify at least two factors that can result in obesity during childhood and adolescence, pp. 590–591 and 595.

5. Define puberty and describe how it influences changes in body composition, p. 592.

6. Identify at least three physiologic changes that occur with aging and describe how these changes affect nutrient needs of older adults, pp. 602–603.

7. Give two reasons why older adults may avoid drinking adequate amounts of fluid, p. 602.

8. Discuss how changes in oral health can affect nutrient intake in older adults, p. 603.

Test Yourself **True** or **False**

1. Toddlers should be fed non-fat milk products to reduce their risk for obesity. **T or F**

2. The average girl reaches almost full height by the onset of menstruation. **T or F**

3. The move toward consuming a heart-healthy diet should begin during the teen years. **T or F**

4. Participating in regular physical activity can delay or reduce some of the loss of muscle mass that occurs with aging. **T or F**

5. Older adults should take supplements whenever possible because they cannot consistently meet their nutritional needs by eating a nutritious diet. **T or F**

Test Yourself answers can be found at the end of the chapter.

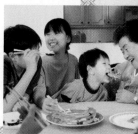

The second Canadian Community Health Survey was conducted in 2004, and for the first time in 25 years we have measured heights and weights of a sample of children and adolescents from across the country. The results have been disappointing, but not surprising. In 2004, 18% of children and youth aged 2 to 17 years were classified as being overweight and 8% were obese (Shields 2005). Among youth aged 12 to 17 years, the rate of obesity has tripled in the past 25 years. Since obesity is now so prevalent, chances are you know someone who struggles with this problem. Why have obesity rates skyrocketed in the past 10 years, and what can be done to promote weight management across the lifespan? How do our nutrient needs change as we grow and age, and what other nutrition-related concerns develop in each life stage? This chapter will help you answer these questions.

Nutrition for Toddlers, Age 1 to 3 Years

As babies begin to walk and explore, they transition out of infancy and into the active world of toddlers.

Toddler Growth and Activity Patterns

The rapid growth rate of infancy begins to slow during toddlerhood. During the second and third years of life, a toddler will grow a total of about 14 to 19 cm (5.5 to 7.5 in.) and gain an average of 4 to 5 kg (9 to 11 lb.). Toddlers expend more energy to fuel increasing levels of activity as they explore their ever-expanding world and develop new skills. They progress from taking a few wobbly steps to running, jumping, and climbing with confidence, and they begin to dress, feed, and toilet themselves. Thus, their diet should provide an appropriate quantity and quality of nutrients to fuel their growth and activity.

What Are a Toddler's Nutrient Needs?

Nutrient needs increase as a child progresses from infancy to toddlerhood. Refer to Table 16.1 for a review of specific nutrient recommendations.

Energy and Macronutrient Recommendations for Toddlers

Estimated Energy Requirements (EER)
The total amount of energy needed per day for any age group.

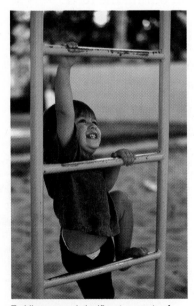

Toddlers expend significant amounts of energy actively exploring their world.

Although the energy requirement per kilogram of body weight for toddlers is just slightly less than for infants, *total* energy requirements are higher because toddlers are larger and much more active than infants. The **Estimated Energy Requirements (EER)**, or the total energy needed per day, varies according to the toddler's age, body weight, and level of activity. The equation to calculate EER for toddlers is as follows (Institute of Medicine 2002):

$$\text{kcal/day} = (89 \times \text{weight [kg]} - 100) + 20$$

Toddlers need more fat than adults. We know that fat provides a concentrated source of energy in a relatively small amount of food, and this is important for toddlers, especially those who are fussy eaters or have little appetite. Fat is also necessary during the toddler years to support the continuously developing nervous system. Although at the present time there is insufficient evidence available to set a DRI for fat for toddlers, it is recommended that toddlers consume 30% to 40% of their total daily energy intake as fat (Institute of Medicine 2002).

Toddlers' protein needs increase modestly because they weigh more than infants and are still growing rapidly. The RDA for protein for toddlers is 1.10 grams per kg body weight per day, or approximately 13 grams of protein daily (Institute of Medicine 2002).

The RDA for carbohydrate for toddlers is 130 grams per day, and carbohydrate intake should be about 45% to 65% of total energy intake (Institute of Medicine 2002). As is the case for older children and adults, most of the carbohydrates eaten should be complex, and refined carbohydrates from snack foods should be kept to a minimum. Fruits and fruit juices are nutritious sources of simple carbohydrates that can also be included. Keep in mind, however, that too much fruit juice can displace other foods and nutrients and can cause diarrhea.

Table 16.1 Nutrient Recommendations for Children and Adolescents

Nutrient	Toddlers (1–3 years)	Preschoolers (4–5 years)	School-Aged Children (6–8 years)	School-Aged Children (9–13 years)	Adolescents (14–18 years)
Total Fat	No RDA or AI	No RDA or AI	No RDA or AI	No RDA or AI	No RDA or AI
Protein	1.10 grams/kg body weight per day	0.95 grams/kg body weight per day	0.95 grams/kg body weight per day	0.95 grams/kg body weight per day	0.85 grams/kg body weight per day
Carbohydrate	130 g/day	130 g/day	130 g/day	130 g/day	130 g/day
Vitamin A	300 µg/day	400 µg/day	400 µg/day	600 µg/day	Boys = 900 µg/day Girls = 700 µg/day
Vitamin C	15 mg/day	25 mg/day	25 mg/day	45 mg/day	Boys = 75 mg/day Girls = 65 mg/day
Vitamin E	6 mg/day	7 mg/day	7 mg/day	11 mg/day	15 mg/day
Calcium	500 mg/day	800 mg/day	800 mg/day	1300 mg/day	1300 mg/day
Iron	7 mg/day	10 mg/day	10 mg/day	8 mg/day	Boys = 11 mg/day Girls = 15 mg/day
Zinc	3 mg/day	5 mg/day	5 mg/day	8 mg/day	Boys = 11 mg/day Girls = 9 mg/day
Fluid	1.3 litres/day	1.7 litres/day	1.7 litres/day	Boys = 2.4 litres/day Girls = 2.1 litres/day	Boys = 3.3 litres/day Girls = 2.3 litres/day
Vitamin D	5 µg	5 µg	5 µg	5 µg	5 µg

Adequate fibre is important for toddlers to maintain regularity and prevent constipation. The AI is 14 grams of fibre per 1000 kcal of energy, or 19 grams per day (Institute of Medicine 2002). Too much fibre can inhibit essential nutrient absorption, harm toddlers' small digestive tracts, and cause them to feel too full to consume adequate nutrients.

Determining the macronutrient requirements of toddlers can be challenging. See the You Do the Math box on p. 581 for analysis of the macronutrient levels in one toddler's daily diet.

Micronutrient Recommendations for Toddlers

As toddlers grow, their micronutrient needs increase. Of particular concern with toddlers are adequate intakes of the micronutrients associated with fruits and vegetables, such as vitamins A, C, and E, as well as the minerals calcium, iron, and zinc (Table 16.1).

Calcium is necessary for children to promote optimal bone mass, which continues to accumulate until early adulthood. For toddlers, the AI for calcium is 500 mg per day (Institute of Medicine 1997). Dairy products are excellent sources of calcium. When a child reaches the age of 1 year, whole cow's milk can be given; however, reduced-fat milk (2%) should *not* be given until age 2. If dairy products are not feasible, fortified orange juice or soy milk can supply calcium, or children's calcium supplements can be given. Toddlers generally cannot consume enough food to depend on alternative calcium sources, such as dark green vegetables.

Iron-deficiency anemia is the most common nutrient deficiency in young children around the world. Iron-deficiency anemia can affect a child's energy level, attention span, and mood. The RDA for iron for toddlers is 7 mg per day (Institute of Medicine 2001). Good sources of iron include lean meats, eggs, and fortified foods, such as breakfast cereals. If a toddler is willing to accept a non-heme source of iron, such as beans or greens, remember that consuming a source of vitamin C at the same meal will enhance the absorption of iron from these sources.

Fluid Recommendations for Toddlers

Toddlers lose less fluid from evaporation than infants do, and their more mature kidneys are able to concentrate urine, thereby sparing fluid. However, as toddlers become active, they start to lose significant fluid through sweat, especially in hot weather. Toddlers and young children sometimes become so busy playing that they ignore or fail to recognize the thirst sensation, so parents need to make sure an active toddler is drinking adequately. The recommended fluid intake for toddlers is 1.3 litres per day (or 5.5 cups per day), which includes about 0.9 litres (or 4 cups) as total beverages, including drinking water (Institute of Medicine 2004). Parents can also monitor the number and heaviness of wet diapers to make sure the child is urinating appropriately. Suggested beverages include plain water, milk and soy milk, diluted fruit juice, and foods high in water content, such as vegetables and fruits. Two cups of milk per day are recommended to meet vitamin D needs.

Do Toddlers Need Nutritional Supplements?

Toddlers can be well nourished by consuming a balanced, varied diet. But given their typically erratic eating habits, the child's physician may recommend a multivitamin and mineral supplement as a precaution against deficiencies. The toddler's physician or dentist may also prescribe a fluoride supplement, if the community water supply is not fluoridated. Supplements should always be considered for any child at risk for deficiency of one or more nutrients. These may include children in vegan families, children from families who are financially limited, children with certain medical conditions or dietary restrictions, or very picky or erratic eaters.

As always, if a supplement is given, it should be formulated especially for toddlers and the recommended dose should not be exceeded. A supplement should not contain more than 100% of the RDA or AI of any nutrient per dose.

> **Recap:** Growth during toddlerhood is slower than during infancy; however, toddlers are highly active and need to consume enough energy to fuel growth and activity. Energy, fat, and protein requirements are higher for toddlers than for infants. Many toddlers will not eat vegetables, so micronutrients of concern include vitamins A, C, and E. Until age 2, toddlers should drink whole milk rather than reduced-fat (2%) milk to meet calcium and vitamin D requirements. Iron deficiency is a concern in the toddler years and can be avoided by feeding toddlers lean meats, eggs, and iron-fortified foods.

Encouraging Nutritious Food Choices with Toddlers

Parents and pediatricians have long recognized that toddlers tend to be choosy about what they eat. Some avoid entire food groups, such as all meats or vegetables. Others will abruptly refuse all but one or two favourite foods (such as peanut butter on crackers) for several days or longer. Still others eat in extremely small amounts, seemingly satisfied by a single slice of apple or two bites of toast. These behaviours frustrate and worry many parents, but in fact, studies have consistently shown that, as long as food is abundant and choices varied, toddlers have an innate ability to match their intake with their needs. It is the whole nutrition profile over time that matters most, and the toddler will most likely make up for it later. Parents who offer only foods of high nutritional quality can feel confident that their children are

▶ YOU DO THE MATH

Is This Menu Good for a Toddler?

A dedicated mother and father want to provide the best nutrition for their young son, Ethan, who is now 1 1/2 years old and has just been completely weaned from breast milk. Ethan weighs about 11.8 kg (26 lb.). Below is a typical day's menu for Ethan. Grams of protein, fat, and carbohydrate, respectively, are given after each food in parentheses. The day's total energy intake is 1168 kcal (4900 kJ). Calculate the percentage of Ethan's energy intake from protein, fat, and carbohydrate (numbers may not add up to exactly 100% because of rounding). Where are Ethan's parents doing well, and where could they use some advice for improvement?

Note: This activity focuses on the macronutrients. It does not ask you to consider Ethan's intake of micronutrients or fluids.

Meal	Foods	Protein (grams)	Fat (grams)	Carbo-hydrate (grams)
Breakfast	Oatmeal, cooked (125 mL/½ cup)	2.5	1.5	13.5
	Brown sugar (5 mL/1 tsp)	0	0	4
	1% milk (125 mL/4 fl. oz.)	4	1.25	5.5
	Grape juice (125 mL/4 fl. oz.)	0	0	20
Mid-morning snack	1 small banana, sliced	0	0	16
	Yogurt, non-fat fruit-flavoured (90 mL/6 Tbsp)	5.5	0	15.5
	Orange juice (125 mL/ 4 fl. oz.)	1	0	13
Lunch	Whole wheat bread, 1 slice	1.5	0.5	10
	Peanut butter (15 mL/1 Tbsp)	4	8	3.5
	Strawberry jam (15 mL/1 Tbsp)	0	0	13
	Carrots, cooked (30 mL/2 Tbsp)	0	0	2
	Applesauce, sweetened (65 mL/¼ cup)	0	0	12
	1% milk (125 mL/4 fl. oz.)	4	1.25	5.5
Afternoon snack	Bagel, half	3	1	20
	Processed cheese, 1 slice	3	5	1
	Water	0	0	0
Dinner	Scrambled egg, 1	11	5	1
	Baby food spinach (90 mL/3 fl. oz.)	2	0.5	5.5
	Whole wheat toast, 1 slice	1.5	0.5	10
	Mandarin orange slices (65 mL/¼ cup)	0.5	0	10
	1% milk (125 mL/4 fl. oz.)	4	1.25	5.5

Calculations:

There is a total of 47.5 grams of protein in Ethan's menu.

$$47.5 \text{ grams} \times 4 \text{ kcal (17 kJ) per gram} =$$
$$190 \text{ kcal (800 kJ)}$$

$$190 \text{ kcal protein} \div 1168 \text{ total kcal} \times 100 =$$
$$16\% \text{ protein}$$

There is a total of 25.75 grams of fat in Ethan's menu.

$$27.75 \text{ grams} \times 9 \text{ kcal (37 kJ) per gram} =$$
$$232 \text{ kcal (970 kJ)}$$

$$232 \text{ kcal fat} \div 1168 \text{ total kcal} \times 100 = 20\% \text{ fat}$$

There is a total of 186.5 grams of carbohydrate in Ethan's menu.

$$186.5 \text{ grams} \times 4 \text{ kcal (17 kJ) per gram} =$$
$$746 \text{ kcal (3130 kJ)}$$

$$746 \text{ kcal protein} \div 1168 \text{ total kcal} \times 100 =$$
$$64\% \text{ carbohydrate}$$

Analysis: Ethan's parents are doing very well at offering a wide variety of foods from various food groups; they are especially doing well with fruits and vegetables. Also, according to his estimated energy requirement, Ethan requires about 970 kcal (4070 kJ) per day, and he is consuming 1168 kcal (4900 kJ), thus meeting his energy needs.

Ethan's total carbohydrate intake for the day is 186.5 grams, which is higher than the RDA of 130 grams per day; however, this value falls within the recommended 45% to 65% of total energy intake that should come from carbohydrates. Thus, high carbohydrate intake is adequate to meet his energy needs.

However, Ethan is being offered far more than enough protein. The DRI for protein for toddlers is about 13 grams per day, and Ethan is being offered more than three times as much!

It is also readily apparent that Ethan is being offered too little fat for his age. Toddlers need at least 30% to 40% of their total energy intake from fat, and Ethan is only consuming about 20% of his Calories from fat. He should be drinking whole milk, not 1% milk. He should occasionally be offered higher-fat foods like cheese for his snacks or macaroni and cheese for a meal. Yogurt is fine, but it shouldn't be non-fat at Ethan's age.

In conclusion, Ethan's parents should be commended for offering a variety of nutritious foods but should be counselled that a little more fat is critical for toddlers' growth and development. Some of the energy currently being consumed as protein and carbohydrate should be shifted to fat.

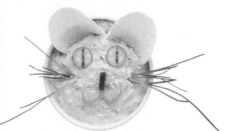

Most toddlers are delighted by food prepared in a fun way.

getting the nutrition they need even if their choices seem odd or erratic on any particular day. Food should never be forced on a child, as doing so sets the stage for eating and control issues later in life.

To encourage nutritious food choices in toddlers, it's important to recognize that their stomachs are still very small and they cannot consume all of the energy they need in three meals. They need small meals, interspersed with nutritious snacks, every two to three hours, and should not be forced to sit still until they finish every bite. A successful snack-time technique used by many experienced parents is to create a snack tray filled with small portions of nutritious food choices, such as one-third of a banana, two pieces of cheese, and three whole-grain pretzels, and leave it within reach of the child's play area. The child can then graze on these nutritious foods while he or she plays. A snack tray plus a spill-proof cup of milk or water is particularly useful on car trips.

Foods prepared for toddlers should be developmentally appropriate. Firm, raw foods, such as nuts, carrots, grapes, raisins, and cherry tomatoes, are difficult for a toddler to chew and pose a choking hazard. Foods should be soft and sliced into strips or wedges that are easy for children to grasp. As the child develops more teeth and becomes more coordinated, the food repertoire can become more varied.

Foods prepared for toddlers should also be fun. Parents can use cookie cutters to turn a peanut-butter sandwich into a pumpkin face, or arrange cooked peas or carrot slices to look like a smiling face on top of mashed potatoes. Juice and low-fat yogurt can be frozen onto sticks or blended like milkshakes.

A positive mealtime environment helps toddlers develop good mealtime habits as well. Parents should seat the toddler in the same place at the table consistently and make sure that the child is served first. Television and other distractions should be turned off, and pleasant conversation should include the toddler, even if the toddler is preverbal.

Even at mealtime, portion sizes should be small. One tablespoon (15 mL) of a food for each year of age constitutes a serving throughout the preschool years. Realistic portion sizes can give toddlers a sense of accomplishment when they "eat it all up" and allay parents' fears that their child is not eating enough.

Introduce new foods gradually. Most toddlers are leery of new foods, spicy foods, hot (temperature) foods, mixed foods, such as casseroles, and foods with strange textures. A helpful rule is to require the child to eat at least one bite of a new food: if the child does not want the rest, nothing negative should be said and the child should be praised just for the willingness to try. The food should be reintroduced a few weeks later. Eventually, the child might accept the food; however, some foods won't be accepted until well into adulthood as tastes expand and develop. One tactic that parents should not resort to is bribing; for example, promising dessert if the child finishes her squash. Bribing teaches children that food can be used to reward and manipulate. Instead, try to positively reinforce good behaviours; for example, "Wow! You ate every bite of your squash! That's going to help you grow big and strong!"

Role modelling is important when teaching toddlers how to make nutritious food choices. Toddlers emulate older children and adults: if they see their parents eating a variety of nutritious foods, they will be likely to do so as well.

Providing limited healthy alternatives early on will also help toddlers to make nutritious food choices. For example, parents might say, "It's snack time! Would you like apples and cheese or bananas and yogurt?" Toddlers can also help select from a limited range of nutritious foods at the grocery store. Finally, toddlers are more likely to eat food they help prepare: encourage them to assist in the preparation of simple foods, such as helping pour a bowl of cereal or helping to arrange the raw vegetables on a plate.

Nutrition-Related Concerns for Toddlers

Just as toddlers have their own specific nutrient needs, they also have toddler-specific nutrition concerns. Some continue from infancy, while others are new.

Continued Allergy Watch

As during infancy, new foods should be presented one at a time, and the toddler should be monitored for allergic reactions for a week before introducing additional

Portion sizes for preschoolers are much smaller than for older children. Use the following guideline: 15 mL (1 Tbsp) of the food for each year of age equals 1 serving. For example, the meal shown here—30 mL (2 Tbsp) of rice, 30 mL (2 Tbsp) of black beans, and 30 mL (2 Tbsp) of chopped tomatoes—is appropriate for a 2-year-old toddler.

new foods. To prevent the development of food allergies, even foods that are established in the diet should be rotated rather than served every day.

Obesity: A Concern Now?

Believe it or not, signs indicating a tendency toward overweight can occur as early as the toddler years. Toddlers should *not* be denied nutritious food; however, they should not be force fed, nor should they be encouraged to eat when they are full. In the toddler years, a child who is above the 80th percentile for weight (that is, who weighs more than 80% of children of the same age and height) should be monitored. These children should be encouraged and supported in increasing their physical activity, and, as for all children, foods with low nutrient density should be limited.

Vegetarian Families

For toddlers, a vegetarian diet in which eggs and dairy foods are included can be as wholesome as a diet including meats and fish. However, since red meat is an excellent source of heme iron, the most bioavailable form, families who do not serve red meat must be careful to include enough iron from other sources in their child's diet.

In contrast, a vegan diet, in which no foods of animal origin are consumed, poses several potential nutritional risks for toddlers:

- Protein—Vegan diets can be too low in protein for toddlers, who need protein for growth and increasing activity. Few toddlers can consume enough legumes and whole grains to provide sufficient protein.
- Iron, calcium, and zinc—Iron is a greater concern in vegan diets than in vegetarian diets that include eggs. Calcium is a concern because of the avoidance of milk, yogurt, and cheese. As with protein, few children can consume enough calcium from plant sources to meet their daily requirement, and supplementation is advised. Zinc is also commonly low in vegan diets.
- Vitamins D and B_{12}—Both vitamins are typically lower in strict vegan diets. Vitamin B_{12} is not available in any amount from plant foods and must be supplemented.
- Fibre—Vegan diets often contain a higher percentage of fibre than is recommended for toddlers.

If parents are very dedicated to planning a vegan diet for their toddler, such choices as fortified juices, soy milk, and other soy products, along with judicious supplement use, should be used to ensure adequate nutrition.

The practice of feeding a vegan diet to infants and young children is highly controversial. See the Nutrition Myth or Fact box for more information about this controversy.

> **Recap:** Toddlers require small, frequent, nutritious meals and snacks, and food should be cut in small pieces so it is easy to handle and swallow. Because toddlers are becoming more independent and can self-feed, parents need to be alert for choking and should watch for allergies and monitor weight gain. Role modelling by parents and access to ample nutritious foods can help toddlers make healthy choices for snacks and meals. Feeding vegan diets to toddlers is controversial and poses potential deficiencies for iron, calcium, zinc, vitamin D, and vitamin B_{12}.

Nutrition for Preschoolers, Age 4 to 5 Years

Distinct developmental markers, such as increased language fluency, decision-making skills, and physical coordination and dexterity, are characteristic of the preschool years. Here, we discuss preschooler growth and activity, nutrient requirements, and nutrition issues that reflect these changes.

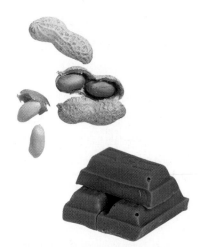

Foods that may cause allergies, such as peanuts and chocolate, should be introduced to toddlers one at a time.

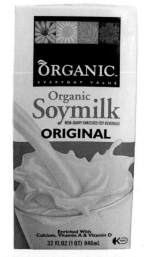

Soy milk can be a part of a healthy vegan diet for toddlers.

▶ **NUTRITION MYTH OR FACT**

Vegan Diets Are Not Appropriate for Young Children

It only takes a look at the headlines to realize that feeding a vegan diet to young children is a controversial issue. Strong proponents of veganism state that any consumption of animal products is wrong and that feeding animal products to children is forcing them into a life of obesity, clogged arteries, and chronic diet-related diseases. In addition, many people who consume a vegan diet feel that consumption of animal products wastes natural resources, contributes to environmental damage, and is therefore morally wrong. In contrast, strong antagonists of veganism emphasize that feeding a vegan diet to young children deprives them of essential nutrients that can only be found in animal products. Some people even suggest that veganism for young children is, in essence, a form of child abuse.

As with many controversies, there are truths on both sides. For example, there have been documented cases of children failing to thrive, and even dying, on extreme vegan diets (Bailey 2001; CDC 2001; Second Opinions 2002). Cases have been cited of vitamin B_{12} and probable calcium, zinc, and vitamin D deficiencies in vegan children. These nutrients are found primarily or almost exclusively in animal products, and deficiencies can have serious and lifelong consequences. For example, not all of the neurologic impairments caused by vitamin B_{12} deficiency can be reversed by timely B_{12} supplement intervention. In addition, inadequate zinc, calcium, and vitamin D can result in impaired bone growth and strength, failure to reach peak bone mass, and retarded growth in general.

However, close inspection of the cases of nutrition-related illness in children that cite veganism as the culprit reveals that lack of education, fanaticism, or extremism is usually at the root of the problem. Informed parents following responsible vegan diets are rarely involved. On the other hand, such cases do point out that veganism is not a lifestyle people can safely undertake without thorough education regarding the necessity of supplementation of those nutrients not available in plant products. Parents also need to understand that typical vegan diets are high in fibre and low in fat, a combination that can be dangerous for very young children (Mangels 2001). Moreover, certain staples of the vegan diet, such as wheat, soy, and nuts, commonly provoke allergic reactions in children;

when this happens, finding a plant-based substitute that contains adequate nutrients can be challenging.

On the other hand, the Dietitians of Canada, the American Dietetic Association, and the American Academy of Pediatrics have stated that a vegan diet can promote normal growth and development—provided that adequate supplements and fortified foods are consumed to account for the nutrients that are normally found in animal products. However, most health care organizations stop short of outright endorsement of a vegan diet for young children. Instead, many advocate a more moderate approach during the early childhood years. Reasons for this level of caution include acknowledgment of several factors:

- Some vegan parents are not adequately educated on the planning of meals, the balancing of foods, and the inclusion of supplements to ensure adequate levels of all nutrients.
- Most young children are picky eaters and are hesitant to eat certain food groups, particularly vegetables, a staple in the vegan diet.
- The high fibre content of vegan diets may not be appropriate for very young children.
- Young children have small stomachs, and they are not able to consume enough plant-based foods to ensure adequate intakes of all nutrients and energy.

Because of these concerns, most nutrition experts advise parents to take a more moderate dietary approach, one that emphasizes plant foods but also includes some animal based foods, such as fish, dairy, or eggs.

Once children reach school age, the low fat, abundant fibre, antioxidants, and many micronutrients in a vegan diet will promote their health as they progress into adulthood. However, those who consume animal products can also live a healthy life and reduce their risk for chronic diseases by choosing low-fat, nutrient-dense foods, such as lean meats, non-fat dairy products, whole grains, and fruits and vegetables. Since animal products are consumed, there are fewer worries about consuming adequate amounts of micronutrients such as vitamin B_{12}, calcium, vitamin D, iron, and zinc.

Preschooler Growth and Activity Patterns

During the preschool years, the growth rate continues to slow. Preschoolers experience an average growth of 7.5 to 10 cm (3 to 4 in.) per year, accompanied by an annual weight gain of 2.3 to 2.7 kg (5 to 6 lb.). Because of the slowed growth, the appetite of preschoolers is often noticeably diminished.

Activity levels in preschool children generally increase as they become more skillful and confident in running, jumping, and climbing. Most preschoolers can kick, throw, catch, and hit balls. Many ride their bikes, skate, swim, or perform other vigorous activities nearly every day. Sometimes it is hard to get preschoolers to stop for snacks and meals because they are so involved in their play and so intent on exerting their independence.

Preschool children have acquired all of their baby teeth, so they can chew most foods adequately enough to prevent choking. They can also use a cup, spoon, and fork with relative ease.

> **Recap:** Preschoolers have a slower growth rate than toddlers and may have a reduced appetite. Preschoolers are more physically active than toddlers, and playing can sometimes interfere with eating adequate food.

What Are a Preschooler's Nutrient Needs?

By age three, children exposed to a wide variety of foods typically have developed a varied diet. Nevertheless, since they are still small, they cannot be expected to consume the required amounts of nutrients in three main meals. Thus, nutrient-dense snacks continue to be important.

Energy and Macronutrient Recommendations for Preschoolers

Fat remains a key macronutrient in the preschool years. During this time, the total fat in a child's diet should gradually be reduced to a level closer to that of an adult, to around 25% to 35% of total energy (Institute of Medicine 2002). One easy way to start reducing dietary fat is to gradually introduce preschoolers to lower-fat dairy products, such as 2% milk.

Total needs for protein and energy increase for preschoolers because of their larger size, even though their growth rate has slowed. For preschoolers, the RDA for protein is 0.95 grams per kg body weight per day, or approximately 19 grams of protein per day (Institute of Medicine 2002).

The RDA for carbohydrate for preschoolers is 130 grams per day. By the end of the preschool years, carbohydrate intake should resemble the pattern of the recommended adult diet. That is, carbohydrates should make up about 45% to 65% of total daily energy intake, and carbohydrates should be mostly complex in nature. Simple sugars should come from fruits and fruit juices, with refined-sugar items, such as cakes, cookies, and candies, saved for occasional indulgences. The AI for fibre for children of preschool age is 14 grams of fibre per 1000 kcal (4200 kJ) of energy consumed, or 25 grams per day (Institute of Medicine 2002). As was the case with toddlers, too much fibre can be detrimental because it can make a child feel full and interfere with food intake and nutrient absorption.

Micronutrient Recommendations for Preschoolers

Children who fail to consume the recommended 5 servings of fruits and vegetables each day may become deficient in vitamins A, C, and E. Minerals of concern continue to be calcium, iron, and zinc, which come primarily from animal-based foods. For preschoolers, the AI for calcium is increased to 800 mg per day (Institute of Medicine 1997). The RDAs for iron and zinc increase slightly to 10 mg per day and 5 mg per day, respectively (Institute of Medicine 2001). Refer to Table 16.1 for a review of the nutrient needs of preschoolers.

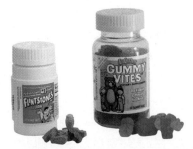

Children's multivitamins often appear in shapes or bright colours.

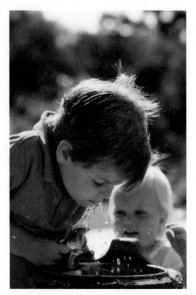

Fluid intake is important for preschoolers, who may become so involved in their play that they ignore the sensation of thirst.

A multivitamin and mineral supplement for preschoolers, though not strictly necessary, may help to make up for those times when the preschooler's appetite is low or when particular food groups are not being consumed with regularity. As is always the case with children, vitamin and mineral supplements for preschoolers should be specific for their age, and the recommended dose (not more than 100% RDA or AI) should not be exceeded.

Fluid Recommendations for Preschoolers

The fluid recommendation for preschoolers is 1.7 litres (or about 7 cups) of total water per day, which includes approximately 1.2 litres (or about 5 cups) as total beverages, including drinking water (Institute of Medicine 2004). The exact amount of fluid a preschooler needs varies according to level of physical activity and weather conditions. Preschoolers can use the bathroom on their own, but parents should keep an eye on the number of trips to the bathroom and occasionally check the child's urine to make sure it is pale. Preschoolers can easily become dehydrated because they get so involved in their play that they ignore or fail to recognize the sensation of thirst. Offer fluid breaks to preschoolers during prolonged periods of play, especially if the weather is hot. Two cups of milk a day are recommended to meet vitamin D needs.

> **Recap:** Preschoolers have teeth and can better chew their food, and they also can use dishes and eating utensils. Preschoolers need less fat than toddlers but slightly more than adults. Protein and energy needs are higher for preschoolers because of their larger size and higher activity levels. Calcium, iron, and zinc requirements are slightly higher for preschoolers than toddlers. Preschoolers can become easily dehydrated because they ignore or fail to recognize their thirst.

Encouraging Nutritious Food Choices with Preschoolers

Preschoolers can understand that some foods will "give them energy" and "help them grow up healthy and strong," and that other foods should be used only for treats. Thus, parents can now teach their children, by using age-appropriate language and concepts, what makes some foods better choices than others. Most preschoolers want to grow as quickly as possible, so parents can capitalize on this natural desire when they encourage foods high in protein, for example, and micronutrients.

Nutrition-Related Concerns for Preschoolers

In addition to potential nutrient deficiencies that have already been discussed, new concerns arise during the preschool years.

Obesity Watch: Encouraging an Active Lifestyle

The preschool years are an important time for parents to be watchful of potential overweight and obesity. This is the time when most children are becoming seriously active in their play. In addition, most preschoolers are prone to a decreased appetite. Combined, these two factors should work to combat obesity and overweight. If a preschooler is overweight, energy balance is disrupted at some level.

A child with a BMI at or above the 85th percentile is considered to be at risk of overweight; that is, the child's body mass is heavier than that of 85% children of the same age and height. (See BMI for age growth charts at www.cdc.gov/growthcharts.) A child is considered overweight if his or her BMI is at or above the 95th percentile (Roberts and Dallal 2001).

childhood overweight Having a body mass index (BMI) at or above the 95th percentile.

Overweight children are at higher risk of becoming overweight adults than are normal weight children, so preventing **childhood overweight** is important for the long-term health and happiness of the child. It is also important for the child's current health and happiness: even in early childhood, significant overweight can exacerbate asthma, cause sleep apnea, impair the child's mobility, and lead to intense teasing, low self-esteem, and social isolation.

The preschool years are formative; thus, establishing healthy eating and physical activity practices is very important during this time. One important guideline is to limit television watching to no more than two hours per day. Studies have linked higher rates of television watching to higher rates of obesity in children (Torgan 2002). Too much television can also interfere with the acquisition of physical skills and can hinder preschoolers' use of their own imagination, dampening creativity. Moreover, an abundance of television commercials during children's programs advertise less nutritious foods, such as sweetened breakfast cereals made with refined grains, high-sugar yogurt products, candies, pastries, and high-fat snacks. Even parents who limit television watching should sit with their children during several commercials and explain to them, in age-appropriate language, that these foods are made to look appealing to kids and are not nutritious choices.

Because of the high nutrient needs of preschoolers, restrictive diets are not advised even when the child is diagnosed as overweight. Rather, parents should strive to consistently provide more nutritious food choices, sitting down together to a shared family meal each evening. The television should be off throughout dinner to encourage slow eating and true enjoyment of the food. To encourage activity throughout the day, parents should limit their own and their children's television watching, computer games, and other sedentary activities and instead encourage increased physical activity, especially shared activities, such as ball games, hikes, and so on. When parents and children are active together, healthy activity patterns are established early. Over time, overweight children who are offered nutritious foods and encouraged to be active can "catch up" to their weight as they grow taller without restricting food (and thus nutrient) intake. Increased activity also helps young children acquire motor skills and muscle strength and develop self-esteem as they feel themselves becoming faster, stronger, and more skilled.

Active, healthy weight children are less likely to become overweight adults.

Dental Caries

As discussed in Chapter 4, *dental caries*, or cavities, occur when bacteria in the mouth feed on carbohydrates deposited on teeth. As a result of metabolizing the carbohydrates, the bacteria then secrete acid that begins to erode tooth enamel, leading to tooth decay. The occurrence of dental caries can be minimized by limiting sugary sweets, especially those that stick to teeth, like jelly beans. Frequent brushing helps to eliminate the sugars on teeth, as well as the bacteria that feed on them.

During the preschool years, children begin learning to brush their own teeth. Because preschoolers' fine-motor skills are not yet mature, parents should help, or at least supervise, to make sure that brushing is effective and thorough. Fluoride, either through a municipal water supply or through supplements, will also help deter the development of dental caries. Even though the teeth of a preschooler will be replaced by permanent teeth in several years, it is critical to keep them healthy and strong. This is because they make room for and guide the permanent teeth into position. Children should start having regular dental visits at the age of 3.

> **Recap:** Parents can communicate effectively with preschoolers to encourage healthy eating and can act as role models in regard to food choices, preparation, and level of physical activity. Overweight and obesity are potential concerns for preschoolers and can be prevented with a healthy diet and regular physical activity. An additional concern with preschoolers is dental caries, and they should be taught to brush their teeth regularly, limit sweets, and visit the dentist regularly beginning at age 3.

Nutrition for School-Age Children, Age 6 to 13 Years

The beginning of school marks the first time for many children to make some of their own food choices. The impact these decisions can make on the health of children can be profound and habit forming, so the education and training of school-age children to make nutritious food choices is critical.

School-Age Growth and Activity Patterns

School-age children can be expected to grow an average of 5 to 7.5 cm (2 to 3 in.) per year at a slow and steady pace. In fact, these years are sometimes referred to as the "calm before the storm" of adolescence, when growth rates again become very rapid. Activity levels among school-age children vary dramatically—some love sports and physical activity, while others prefer quieter activities like reading and drawing. All children can be encouraged to enjoy walking, to appreciate nature and exploration, and to have fun by using their minds and their muscles in various ways that suit their interests.

> **Recap:** School-age children are more independent and can make more of their own food choices. Their physical growth is slow and steady, and physical activity levels can vary dramatically between children.

What Are a School-Age Child's Nutrient Needs?

The beginning of sexual maturation is an important phenomenon that has a dramatic impact on the nutrient needs of children. Boys' and girls' bodies develop differently in response to gender-specific hormones. These changes in sexual maturation can begin subtly between the ages of 8 and 9 years; because of this, the DRI values for the macronutrients, fibre, and micronutrients are grouped together for children aged 1 to 3 years and 4 to 8 years, and are redefined for boys and girls between the ages of 9 and 13 years (Institute of Medicine 2002). Table 16.1 (page 579) identifies the nutrient needs of school-age children and adolescents.

Energy and Macronutrient Recommendations for School-Age Children

Children of school age should ideally consume a variety of foods from each major food group. Children should be guided to eat a diet that contains about 25% to 35% of total energy from fat. A diet lower in fat is not recommended for children of school age, as they are still growing, developing, and maturing. Such foods as meats and dairy products should not be withheld solely because of their fat content since they otherwise have important nutrient value. Indeed, too much emphasis should not be placed on fat at this age. Impressionable and peer-influenced school-age kids can easily be led to categorize foods as "good" or "bad"; this can lead to skewed views of food, eating, and body image, and, ultimately, can even lead to eating disorders.

As you can see in Table 16.1, the protein recommendation for school-age boys and girls is 0.95 grams per kg body weight per day. Although the recommended protein intake per kg body weight for children aged 4 to 13 years is lower than that of toddlers, the total protein intake of school-age children is higher because of their higher body weight.

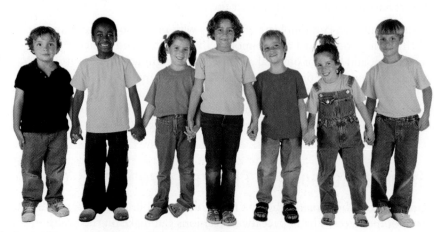

School-age children grow an average of 5 to 7.5 cm (2 to 3 in.) per year.

The RDA for carbohydrate for school-age children is the same as for toddlers through adults: 130 grams per day. Carbohydrate intake should be about 45% to 65% of total daily energy intake. As always, most carbohydrates eaten should be complex. The recommended fibre intake for school-age children is 14 grams per 1000 kcal (4200 kJ).

Micronutrient Recommendations for School-Age Children

The need for most micronutrients increases slightly for school-age children up to 8 years old because of their increasing size. A sharper increase in micronutrient needs occurs during the transition into full adolescence; this increase is due to the beginning of sexual maturation and in preparation for the impending adolescent growth spurt. Of continued interest during the school-age years are the minerals calcium and iron. The AI for calcium increases from 800 mg per day for children aged 4 to 8 years to 1300 mg per day for children aged 9 to 13 years (Institute of Medicine 1997). The RDA for iron for children aged 4 to 8 years is 10 mg per day, and this value drops to 8 mg per day for boys and girls aged 9 to 13 years. These recommendations are based on the assumption that most girls do not begin menstruation until after age 13 (Institute of Medicine 2001).

If there is any doubt that a child's nutrient needs are not being met for any reason (for instance, breakfasts are skipped, lunches are traded, parents lack money for nourishing food) a vitamin-mineral supplement that provides no more than 100% of the RDA or AI for the micronutrients may help to correct any existing deficit.

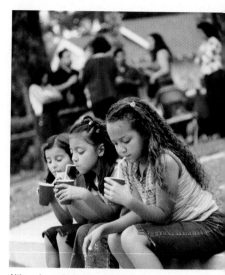

Although reminders to drink help keep school-age children hydrated, they mostly control their own fluid intake.

Fluid Recommendations for School-Age Children

The AI for school-age children aged 4 to 8 years is 1.7 litres per day (or about 7 cups) of total water, with about 1.2 litres (or 5 cups) as total beverages, including drinking water. The AI for fluid for school-age boys aged 9 to 13 years is 2.4 litres per day (or about 10 cups) of total water, with about 1.8 litres (or 8 cups) as total beverages, including drinking water. The AI for fluid for school-age girls aged 9 to 13 years is 2.1 litres per day (or about 9 cups) of total water, with about 1.6 litres (or 7 cups) as total beverages, including drinking water (Institute of Medicine 2004).

At this point in life, children are mostly in control of their own fluid intake. However, as they engage in physical activity classes at school and in extracurricular sporting activities and general play, reminders to drink when they are thirsty are important to assist them in staying properly hydrated.

> **Recap:** Sexual maturation begins during the school-age years. The DRI values reflect these changes by differentiating between nutrient needs for children 4 to 8 years and 9 to 13 years. School-age children should eat 25% to 35% of their total energy as fat and 45% to 65% of their total energy as carbohydrate. Micronutrient needs increase because of growth and maturation. Calcium needs increase as children mature, while iron needs decrease slightly.

Encouraging Nutritious Food Choices with School-Age Children

Peer pressure can be extremely difficult for both parents and their children to deal with during this life stage. Most children want to feel as if they belong, and they admire and like to emulate children they believe to be popular. If the popular children at school are eating chips and drinking regular soft drinks, it may be hard for a child to eat her tuna on whole wheat, apple, and milk without embarrassment.

Parents and children can work together to find compromises they can both live with by regularly communicating about nutrition. One strategy that parents might consider is to introduce to their kids "cool" role models, such as star athletes who follow nutritious diets. Emphasize that to perform at elite levels, athletes must pay close attention to their nutrition. Elite athletic performance cannot be sustained on chips and regular soft drinks! However, the common practice of athletes endorsing fast-food restaurants can be confusing for some children. One way to help deal with this confusion is to explain that even an occasional fast-food meal can be part of a healthy diet, but it is not the type of food that star athletes eat every day.

Continuing to involve children in food choices for the family and in meal preparation is also a good idea. If they have input into what is going into their bodies, they may be more likely to take an active role in their health. In addition, parents should continue to act as role models throughout this time to maintain consistent messages and images that children can rely upon when establishing their own eating and physical activity patterns.

What Is the Effect of School Attendance on Nutrition?

School attendance can affect a child's nutrition in several ways. First, in the hectic time between waking and getting out the door, many children minimize or skip breakfast completely. School children who don't eat breakfast may not get a chance to eat until lunch. If the entire morning is spent in a state of hunger, they are more likely to do poorly on schoolwork, have decreased attention spans, and have more behavioural problems than their peers who do eat breakfast (USDA Food and Nutrition Service 2003; USDA/ARS Children's Nutrition Research Center at Baylor College of Medicine 1999). For this reason, some schools now offer breakfast programs that are free to all children in the school. These breakfasts help children to optimize their nutrient intake and avoid the behavioural and learning problems associated with hunger in the classroom.

Another consequence of attending school is that, with no one monitoring what they eat, children do not always consume adequate amounts of food. They may spend their lunchtime conversing or playing with friends rather than eating. If a school lunch is purchased, they might not like the foods being served, or their peers might influence them to skip certain foods with comments such as, "This broccoli is yucky!" Even homemade lunches that contain nutritious foods may be left uneaten or traded for less nutritious fare.

Finally, many schools have become places where soft drink and snack food companies advertise and sell their products to children in exchange for providing important revenues to maintain necessary school programs (see the Nutrition Debate in Chapter 4 for more information on this topic). Many schools provide vending machines filled with snacks that are high in energy, sugar, and fat. Eating too many of these foods, either in place of or in addition to lunch, can lead to overweight and potential nutrient deficiencies.

The first years of school are an exciting time for learning, meeting new friends, and exerting a new degree of independence. However, it can also be a time of stress, the first real exposure to peer pressure, and the first real awareness of who and what are popular or acceptable to peers. Peer pressure and popularity influence food choices as much as they do friends, fashion, and other lifestyle choices.

> **Recap:** Peer pressure has a strong influence on nutritional choices in school-age children. Involving children in food purchasing, meal planning, and preparation can help them make more nutritious food choices. Attending school can interfere with eating breakfast, and children may not always choose nutritious foods during school lunch. Peer pressure and popularity are strong influences on food choices.

Nutrition-Related Concerns for School-Age Children

The nutrition-related concerns for school-age children revolve around weight concerns and body-image issues. These concerns are discussed below.

Obesity Watch: Keeping Active for Life

In the past decade, the skyrocketing rate of childhood obesity has become a concern for nutritionists, physicians, educators, policy makers, and parents across North

America. Experts agree that the main culprits are the same as those involved in adult obesity: eating too much and moving too little (Torgan 2002). Rather than placing school-age children on restrictive diets, however, experts advise encouraging physical activity.

In the past, children played freely outdoors and were relatively active indoors in times of bad weather and in the evening hours. In recent years, however, several factors have prompted childhood activities to become increasingly sedentary. One such factor is simply the availability of entertainment technologies, including television, video games, and computer games. Another factor is that the number of households in which no adult is at home after school has risen in recent decades, either because of single-parent families or because both parents have to work to support their families. Safety concerns cause working parents to forbid their children to venture

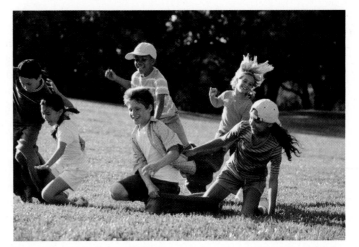

Encouraging physical play with friends is a good way to combat childhood obesity.

out of the house when they are at home alone after school. Given these circumstances and limited options for indoor physical activities at home, the television or the computer are quite logical choices. Children often eat snack foods while they watch television or play video games, and they don't have sufficient parental guidance to curb overeating or encourage physical play when they are at home alone.

What are some strategies for encouraging daily physical activity in children of working parents? Many communities and even public school districts offer after-school programs that include team sports, running, swimming, and other physical activities. If these are not available, working parents can form partnerships with classmates' families in which a parent is at home after school and agrees to encourage after-school physical activity. If children must return from school to an empty house, a phone call from a parent can encourage them to complete their homework and promise them an hour of quality time shooting hoops or bike riding as soon as the parent returns from work. Children can also be paid an allowance to complete a list of active chores, such as vacuuming, while they are waiting for their parents to come home.

Children should be very active for at least 90 minutes each day. For younger children, this can be divided into two or three shorter sessions, allowing them to regroup, recoup, and refocus in between activity sessions. Older children may be able to be active for an hour without stopping. Children should be exposed to a variety of activities so that they move different muscles, play at various intensities, avoid boredom, and find out what they like and don't like to do. In 2002, Health Canada, the Canadian Society for Exercise Physiology, the College of Family Physicians of Canada, and the Canadian Paediatric Society published *Canada's Physical Activity Guide for Children* (see Appendix C).

The ACTIVATE/Kidnetic.com Program is another approach aimed at encouraging children and their families to communicate and work together to be more physically active and to eat a more nutritious diet. This is done through an interactive computer-based program. This program was developed through a partnership of many organizations that are committed to improving the nutritional status and physical activity levels of children and families, including the International Food Information Council, the American Academy of Family Physicians, and the American College of Sports Medicine. The interactive computer-based program can be found at www.kidnetic.com.

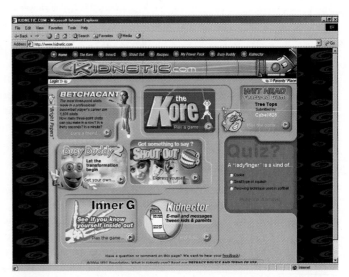

Kidnetic.com is an on-line program focused on increasing physical activity levels and promoting healthy eating among children and their families.

Body-Image Concerns

As children, particularly females, approach puberty, appearance and body image play increasingly important roles in food choice. Concerns about appearance and body image are not necessarily detrimental to health, particularly if they result in children making healthier food choices, such as eating more whole grains, fruits, and vegetables. However, it is important for children to understand that being thin does not guarantee health, popularity, or happiness and that a healthy body image includes accepting our own individual body type and recognizing that we can be physically fit and healthy at a variety of weights, shapes, and sizes. Excessive concern with thinness can lead children to experiment with fad diets, food restriction, and other behaviours that can result in undernutrition and perhaps even trigger a clinical eating disorder. (Refer to Chapter 13 to learn more about disordered eating and eating disorders and how they can be prevented and treated.)

Inadequate Calcium Intake

Another nutrition-related concern for school-age children is an inadequate intake of calcium. Adequate calcium is necessary to achieve peak bone mass, as well as for numerous other critical body and cell functions. As you learned in Chapter 9, we achieve peak bone mass in our late teens or early 20s, and childhood and adolescence are critical times to ensure adequate deposition of bone tissue. Inadequate calcium intake during childhood and adolescence leads to poor bone health and potential osteoporosis in our later years.

Dairy products are the most common source of calcium for children in North America (Institute of Medicine 1997). During the infant, toddler, and preschool years, milk consumption can largely be monitored by parents or caregivers. However, once children begin to attend school, they may choose to spend the money intended for milk on soft drinks, if available. This "milk displacement" is a recognized factor in low calcium intake and poor bone health (Heaney and Rafferty 2001). Diets that are low in calcium also tend to be low in other nutrients, so attention to calcium intake can help ensure a healthy overall diet for children. *Canada's Food Guide* recommends three to four servings of milk and alternates for children 9–13 years.

> **Recap:** Obesity is an important concern for school-age children. All children should be active at least 90 minutes every day. Appearance and body image play increasingly important roles in this age group, and disordered eating and eating disorders can result from these concerns. Consuming adequate calcium to support the development of peak bone mass is also a primary concern for school-age children.

Nutrition for Adolescents, Age 14 to 18 Years

puberty The period in life in which secondary sexual characteristics develop and people are biologically capable of reproducing.

The adolescent years begin with the onset of **puberty,** the period in life in which secondary sexual characteristics develop and we become capable of reproducing. This is a physically and emotionally tumultuous time for adolescents and their families. The nutritional needs of adolescents are influenced by their rapid growth in height, increased weight, changes in body composition, and their individual levels of physical activity.

Adolescent Growth and Activity Patterns

Growth during adolescence is primarily driven by hormonal changes, including increased levels of testosterone for boys and estrogen for girls. Both boys and girls experience *growth spurts,* or periods of accelerated growth, during later childhood and adolescence. Growth spurts for girls tend to begin around 10 to 11 years of age, while growth spurts for boys begin around 12 to 13 years of age. These growth periods last about two years.

Adolescents experience an average 20% to 25% increase in height during the pubertal years. On average, girls tend to grow 5 to 20 cm (2 to 8 in.) and boys tend to grow 10 to 30 cm (4 to 12 in.) (Polan and Taylor 2003). The average girl reaches almost full height by the onset of menstruation (called **menarche**). Boys typically experience continual growth throughout adolescence, and some may even grow slightly taller during early adulthood.

Skeletal growth ceases once closure of the *epiphyseal plates* occurs (Figure 16.1). The **epiphyseal plates** are plates of cartilage located toward the end of the long bones that provide for growth in length of the long bones. In some circumstances, the epiphyseal plates can close early in adolescents and result in a failure to reach full stature. The most common causes of this failure are malnourishment during childhood and adolescence or use of anabolic steroids during this critical growth period.

Weight and body composition also change dramatically during adolescence. Weight gain is extremely variable during this time and reflects the adolescent's energy intake, physical activity level, and genetics. The average weight gained by girls and boys during this time is 16 and 20 kg (35 and 45 lb.), respectively. The weight gained by girls and boys is dramatically different in terms of its composition. Girls tend to gain significantly more body fat than boys, with this fat accumulating around the buttocks, hips, breasts, thighs, and upper arms. Although many girls are uncomfortable or embarrassed by these changes, they are a natural result of maturation. Boys gain significantly more muscle mass than girls, and they experience an increase in muscle definition. Both girls and boys experience significant growth of their internal organs, including the liver, kidneys, heart, lungs, and sexual organs. Other changes that occur with sexual maturation include a deepening of the voice in boys and growth of pubic hair in both boys and girls.

The physical activity levels of adolescents are highly variable. Many are physically active in sports or other organized physical activities, whereas others become less interested in sports and more interested in intellectual or artistic pursuits. This variability in activity levels of adolescents results in highly individual energy needs. Although the rapid growth and sexual maturation that occur during puberty require a significant amount of energy, adolescence is often a time in which overweight begins. The following section discusses the unique nutrient needs of adolescents.

> **Recap:** Adolescence is predominated by puberty, or the period in life in which secondary sexual characteristics develop and the physical ability to reproduce begins. Adolescents experience rapid increases in height, weight, and lean body mass and fat mass. Physical activity levels of adolescents are highly variable, and overweight may begin during this period.

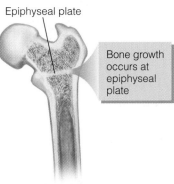

Figure 16.1 Skeletal growth ceases once closure of the epiphyseal plates occurs.

menarche The beginning of menstruation, or the menstrual period.

epiphyseal plates Plates of cartilage located toward the end of long bones that provide for growth in the length of long bones.

What Are an Adolescent's Nutrient Needs?

The nutrient needs of adolescents are influenced by rapid growth, weight gain, and sexual maturation, in addition to the demands of physical activity.

Energy and Macronutrient Recommendations for Adolescents

Adequate energy intake is necessary to maintain adolescents' health, support their dramatic growth and maturation, and fuel their physical activity. Because of these competing demands, the energy needs of adolescents can be quite high. The EER for adolescents can be calculated by using one of the equations presented in Table 16.2. To calculate the EER for this life stage, you must know the person's age, physical activity level, weight, and height.

As with the younger age groups, there is no DRI for fat for adolescents. However, adolescents are at risk for the same chronic diseases as adults, including type 2 diabetes, obesity, coronary heart disease, and various cancers. Thus, it is prudent for adolescents to consume 25% to 35% of total energy from fat and to keep saturated and trans fat as low as possible.

Table 16.2   Equations Used to Calculate the Estimated Energy Requirements (EER) of Children and Adolescents Ages 9 to 18 Years

Gender	EER Equation	Physical Activity (PA) Values
Males	EER (Cal/day) = 88.5 − (61.9 × Age [yrs]) + {Physical Activity × [(26.7 × Weight [kg]) + (903 × Height [m])]} + 25	PA = 1.00 if physical activity level is sedentary PA = 1.13 if physical activity level is low active PA = 1.26 if physical activity level is active PA = 1.42 if physical activity level is very active
Females	EER (Cal/day) = 135.3 − (30.8 × Age [yrs]) + {Physical Activity × [(10.0 × Weight [kg]) + (934 × Height [m])]} + 25	PA = 1.00 if physical activity level is sedentary PA = 1.16 if physical activity level is low active PA = 1.31 if physical activity level is active PA = 1.56 if physical activity level is very active

Source: Institute of Medicine, Food and Nutrition Board, *Dietary Reference Intakes for Energy, Carbohydrates, Fiber, Fat, Protein and Amino Acids (Macronutrients),* Washington, DC: National Academy of Sciences, 2002, pp. 5–55 and 5–56.

The RDA for carbohydrate for adolescents is 130 grams per day. As with adults, this amount of carbohydrate covers what is needed to supply adequate glucose to the brain, but it does not cover the amount of carbohydrate needed to support daily activities. Thus, it is recommended that adolescents consume more than the RDA, or about 45% to 65% of their total energy as carbohydrate, and most carbohydrate should come from complex carbohydrate sources. The AI for fibre for adolescents is 26 grams per day for females and at least 38 g per day for males, which is similar to adult values.

The RDA for protein for adolescents is similar to that of adults at 0.85 grams of protein per kg body weight per day. This value was selected because data are not available to determine protein maintenance requirements for this age group, and the amount of nitrogen needed to maintain protein balance in children is similar to that of adults (Institute of Medicine 2002). This amount is assumed to be sufficient to support health and to cover the additional needs of growth and development during the adolescent stage.

Micronutrient Recommendations for Adolescents

Micronutrients of particular concern for adolescents include calcium, iron, and vitamin A. Adequate calcium intake is critical to achieve peak bone density, and the AI for calcium for adolescents is 1300 mg per day. This amount of calcium can be difficult to consume for many adolescents because the quality of foods they select is often less than optimal to meet their nutrient needs. This level of calcium intake can be achieved by eating at least 3 servings of dairy foods or calcium-fortified products daily.

The iron needs of adolescents are relatively high; this is because iron is needed to replace the blood lost during menstruation in girls and to support the growth of muscle mass in boys. The RDA for iron for boys is 11 mg per day, while the RDA for girls is 15 mg per day. If energy intake is adequate and adolescents consume heme-iron food sources, such as animal products, each day, they should be able to meet the RDA for iron. However, many young people adopt a vegetarian lifestyle during this life stage, or they consume foods that have limited nutrient density. Both of these situations can prevent adolescents from meeting the RDA for iron.

Vitamin A is critical to support the rapid growth and development that occurs during adolescence. The RDA for vitamin A is 900 µg per day for boys and 700 µg per day for girls. These individuals can meet this RDA by consuming at least 7 servings of fruits and vegetables each day. As with iron and calcium, meeting the RDA for vitamin A can be a challenging goal in this age group because of their potential to make less nutritious food choices.

If an adolescent is unable or unwilling to eat adequate amounts of nutrient-dense foods, then a multivitamin and mineral supplement that provides no more than 100% of the RDA or AI for the micronutrients could be very beneficial as a safety net. As with younger children and adults, a supplement should not be considered a substitute for a balanced, nutritious diet.

Fluid Recommendations for Adolescents

The fluid needs of adolescents are higher than those for children because of their higher physical activity levels and the extensive growth and development that occurs during this phase of life. The AI for total fluid for adolescent boys is 3.3 litres per day (or 14 cups), which includes about 2.6 litres (or 11 cups) as total beverages, including drinking water. The AI for total fluid for adolescent girls is 2.3 litres per day (or 10 cups), which includes about 1.8 litres (or 8 cups) as total beverages, including drinking water. Boys are generally more active than girls and have more lean tissue, thus they require a higher fluid intake to maintain fluid balance. Highly active adolescents who are exercising in the heat may have higher fluid needs than the AI, and these individuals should be encouraged to drink often to quench their thirst and avoid dehydration.

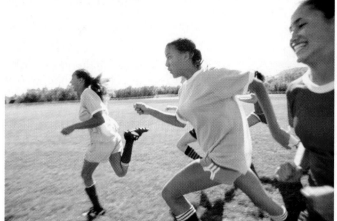

Regular physical activity is good for adolescents.

> **Recap:** Energy needs for adolescents can be very high, and adequate energy is needed to support growth, maturation, and physical activity. Fat intake should be 25% to 35% of total energy, and carbohydrate intake should be 45% to 65% of total energy intake. Because many adolescents fail to eat a variety of nutrient-dense foods, intakes of many nutrients, such as calcium, iron, and vitamin A, may be deficient. Calcium is needed to optimize bone growth and to achieve peak bone density, and iron needs are increased because of increased muscle mass in boys and menstruation in girls.

Encouraging Nutritious Food Choices with Adolescents

At this point in their lives, adolescents are making most of their own food choices, and many are also buying and preparing a significant amount of the foods they consume. Although parents can still be effective role models, adolescents are generally strongly influenced by their peers, their preferences, and their own developing sense of what foods compose a nutritious and adequate diet.

One particular area of concern in the adolescent diet is a lack of vegetables, fruits, and whole grains. Many teens eat on the run, skip meals, and select fast foods and convenience foods because they are inexpensive, are accessible, and taste good. Parents, caretakers, and school food service programs can capitalize on adolescents' preferences for pizza, burgers, spaghetti, and sandwiches by providing more nutritious meat and cheese alternatives, whole-grain breads, and plenty of appealing vegetable-based sides or additions to these foods. In addition, keeping nutritious snacks, such as fruits and vegetables that are already cleaned and prepared in easy-to-eat pieces, may encourage adolescents to consume more of these foods as between-meal snacks. Teens should also be encouraged to consume adequate milk and other calcium-enriched beverages (three to four servings per day of milk and alternatives).

Nutrition-Related Concerns for Adolescents

Nutrition-related concerns for adolescents continue to include weight concerns and body-image issues. Additional concerns include cigarette smoking and the use of alcohol and illegal drugs.

Obesity Watch: Balancing Food and Physical Activity to Encourage Healthful Weight Gain

Although expected and desirable, weight gain during adolescence can become excessive if increased energy intake is not balanced with adequate physical activity.

Many overweight and obese adolescents already have at least one risk factor for heart disease, such as high blood pressure, elevated blood cholesterol, or type 2 diabetes.

As with younger children, a reduction in regular physical activity is a significant factor in adolescent obesity. Nearly one quarter (24.4%) of youth aged 12 to 17 years spend 30 hours or more a week doing sedentary activities, such as watching television or playing computer games (Shields 2005). By offering daily physical education in school and by providing more opportunities and encouragement for adolescents to participate in regular physical activity outside of school, the prevalence of overweight and obesity among adolescents can be reduced.

Disordered Eating and Eating Disorders

An initially normal concern about body image and weight can turn into a dangerous obsession during this emotionally challenging life stage. Clinical eating disorders frequently begin during adolescence and can occur in boys as well as girls. Parents, teachers, and friends should be aware of the warning signs, which include rapid and excessive weight loss, a preoccupation with weight and body image, going to the bathroom regularly after meals, and signs of frequent vomiting or laxative use. Refer to Chapter 13 for a full discussion of eating disorders.

Other Nutrition-Related Concerns

Cigarette smoking and alcohol and illegal drug use are additional nutritional concerns that adolescents face. Adolescents are naturally curious, and most are open to experimenting with tobacco, illegal drugs, and alcohol. Cigarette smoking diminishes appetite and can interfere with nutrient absorption. Indeed, it is frequently used by adolescent girls to maintain a low body weight. The short-term effects of smoking include damage to the lungs and respiratory system, addiction to nicotine, and increased incidence of participation in other risky behaviours, such as alcohol and drug abuse, fighting, and engaging in unprotected sex. Most people who begin smoking during adolescence continue to smoke throughout adulthood, increasing their risks for lung cancer, heart disease, osteoporosis, and emphysema. Other consequences of cigarette smoking for adolescents include (CDC 2000)

- reduced physical fitness and poor exercise endurance;
- inhibition of normal lung growth and maximal lung function;
- increased incidence of respiratory illnesses;
- increased risk of addiction to nicotine;
- poor overall health.

Alcohol and drug use can start at early ages, even in school-age children. The primary cause of death among high-school-age youth is motor vehicle accidents; the risk of being involved in an accident is greatly increased by using alcohol and illegal drugs. Alcohol can also interfere with proper nutrient absorption and metabolism, and it can take the place of foods in an adolescent's diet; these adverse effects of alcohol put adolescents at risk for various nutrient deficiencies. Alcohol and marijuana use are also associated with getting "the munchies," a feeling of food craving that usually results in people eating large quantities of high-fat, high-sugar, nutrient-poor foods. This behaviour can result in overweight or obesity, and also increases the risk of nutrient deficiencies. Teens who use drugs and alcohol are typically in poor condition, are either underweight or overweight, have poor appetites, and perform poorly in school.

In addition, the number of homeless youth in Canada has been rising, and these young people face special nutritional challenges. With no food storage or cooking facilities, they may need to rely on charitable programs, such as soup kitchens and food banks. Read the Highlight box on the research being conducted by one University of Toronto nutrition researcher, Dr. Valerie Tarasuk, on this and other such issues.

Cigarette smoking may interfere with nutrient absorption.

▶ **HIGHLIGHT**

Dr. Valerie Tarasuk: Hunger in Canada

Hunger. The word conjures up images of emaciated third-world children with pathetically distended bellies and sad, hopeless eyes. Years of watching commercials to sponsor a child—to say nothing of news reports—have ingrained the knowledge of hunger elsewhere, but Canadians often see their own country as somehow immune. Many are shocked to discover that an estimated 2.3 million Canadians experience food insecurity (Statistics Canada 2005), defined as "the limited or uncertain availability of nutritionally adequate and safe foods or limited or uncertain ability to acquire acceptable foods in socially acceptable ways" (Tarasuk and Beaton 1999)

The subject is rarely addressed in Canada, but researchers like Dr. Valerie Tarasuk are helping to bring it to the forefront. Through research examining how hunger affects specific populations, Dr. Tarasuk, a Professor in the Department of Nutritional Sciences at the University of Toronto, is attempting to paint a clearer picture of who is affected by hunger in Canada..

Food Insecurity Takes Many Forms

The term *food insecurity* includes households with a chronic shortage of food and those with a constant worry that their food may run out. In 2004, an estimated 715 616 Canadians experienced severe food insecurity and did not have enough food to eat (Statistics Canada 2005). It is common for parents to short-change their own nutritional needs to feed their children better, leading to potentially inadequate intake of important nutrients. In 1999, Dr. Tarasuk and Dr. George Beaton examined 153 women in families receiving emergency food assistance in Toronto and found that women's intakes of energy, protein, vitamin A, iron, folate, magnesium, and zinc were lower when the food insecurity of their households was worse. Another study found that those who reported being food insecure were also more likely to report poor to fair overall health, depression, heart disease, type 2 diabetes, high blood pressure, and food allergies (Tarasuk and Vozoris 2003). In effect, food insecurity affects every member of the household.

Homeless Youth: A Growing Population At Risk

We've all heard the saying "I'm so hungry, I could eat a horse"—but what about "I'm so hungry I could eat out of a dumpster"?

Homeless youth are particularly vulnerable to food insecurity. Lacking economic and social support and unable to get jobs, these young adults are caught in a vicious cycle of hunger and poverty. According to a study of 261 homeless youths by Tarasuk, Naomi Dachner, and Jinguang Li (2005), on any one day 10% of male and 6% of female participants resorted to stealing food or taking it from the garbage in their struggles to get enough to eat. A true census of this population is nearly impossible, but it is estimated that a growing proportion of the homeless population are young adults. This raises questions about the nutritional vulnerability of young adults living on the street.

Using five trained interviewers with direct experience with homelessness, Tarasuk, Dachner, and Li (2005) were able to clarify how homeless youth obtain food, as well as their nutrient intake. Purchased food and charitable food programs were cited as the most common sources, but participants also relied on food given to them by acquaintances or strangers. In this study, more than 50% of participants had inadequate intakes of folate, vitamin A, vitamin C, magnesium, and zinc, illustrating that food received by homeless youth is insufficient in quality, quantity, or both. Furthermore, the intrinsic link among shelter, income, and food underlined the fact that it is impossible to study one of these challenges without examining the role of the others.

Measures to Alleviate Food Insecurity

Ultimately, the cause of food insecurity is poverty, and the most widely publicized method of easing hunger in the short term remains the food bank. In the 1980s, food banks were set up as a "temporary" measure to distribute donated goods to people devastated by the recession at the start of the decade. Contrary to expectation, use of food banks did not decline as the economy improved. In fact, it increased—and itself became part of the problem. Dr. Tarasuk has argued that "food banks give the illusion of effectively responding to hunger, [and] they unwittingly facilitate the further erosion of income supports to those at the bottom, leading to increased poverty and income inequality and a continued growing need for charitable assistance" (Eakin and Tarasuk 2003). In any event, it is by now apparent

(Continued)

that the need for food banks is unrelated to fluctuations in the Canadian economy, but instead is rooted in fundamental changes in Canadian social policy, such as major changes in how social assistance ("welfare") and employment insurance programs are delivered and the levels of support they provide. Programs and policies to provide affordable housing for low-income households are also required. Although food banks try to help people meet their immediate needs for food, they are powerless to solve the underlying issue of poverty (Tarusak 2001).

Many communities have initiated other programs to help ease hunger. These alternatives stress the importance of social support and community. For example, community kitchens try to foster a safe environment to learn skills that will allow individuals to purchase and prepare meals that are both cost efficient and nutritionally sound. Dr. Tarasuk (2001) describes community kitchens as "community-based cooking programs in which small groups of individuals regularly come together to prepare one or more meals, which may be taken home for later consumption or consumed together." This is a good start—but there is a limit to how much cooking skills can compensate for problems of poverty.

Canada is blessed with an abundance of rich and productive land, but many of its people go without food. Poverty thrusts families, and thus children and youth, into a perpetual cycle of food shortage and uncertainty. The statistics are cause for serious concern—especially since these figures exclude such high-risk populations as the homeless. Researchers like Dr. Valerie Tarasuk are giving us insight into Canada's food insecurity and drawing much-needed attention to this issue and the ineffective ways we have dealt it with so far. The way forward, though still far from clear, needs more of such signposts.

Recap: Adolescents' food choices are influenced by peer pressure, personal preferences, and their own developing sense of what foods are nutritious. Adolescents are at risk for skipping meals and selecting fast foods and snack foods in place of whole grains, fruits, and vegetables. Milk is commonly replaced with regular soft drinks. Obesity can occur during adolescence because of increased appetite and food intake and decreased physical activity. Disordered eating behaviours, eating disorders, cigarette smoking, and use of alcohol and illegal drugs are also concerns for this age group. Homeless youth have special nutritional challenges.

Nutrition for Young and Middle Adults, Age 19 to 64 Years

The majority of information in this text is directed toward nutrition for young and middle-aged adults. Thus, here we provide simply a brief summary for this age group.

Adult Growth and Activity Patterns

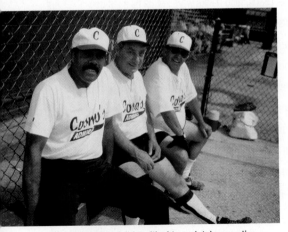

During adulthood, it is critical to maintain an active lifestyle; a sports team is one way to stay active.

The young adult and middle-aged years are primarily concerned with maintenance of health and our body tissues. Maximal height has been attained, and our goal is to maintain a healthy body weight. Peak bone mass is generally achieved by some time in our 20s, and bone mass starts to decline in our mid to late 30s. Thus, our goal in relation to bone is to build as much as we can during our childhood and adolescence and to maintain as much as we can during young and middle adulthood so we can decrease our risk for osteoporosis as we age. We can accomplish this by being physically active on a regular basis, getting enough sun or taking a supplement to maintain an optimum vitamin D status, and eating a balanced diet that contains adequate energy, calcium, phosphorus, and magnesium.

Young and middle adulthood is also a time when we become more concerned with our risk for chronic diseases, such as heart disease, type 2 diabetes, and various cancers. This is a critical time to establish and maintain a physically active lifestyle and to pay particularly close attention to consuming adequate amounts of fruits, vegetables, whole grains, and lower-fat foods.

What Are an Adult's Nutrient Needs?

The nutrient needs for young and middle-aged adults are covered in detail throughout this text. Refer to the appropriate chapter to review needs related to specific nutrients and illnesses. In addition, the DRIs for all life stages can be found in Appendix H.

Nutrition-Related Concerns for Adults

The primary nutrition-related concerns of young and middle-aged adults are maintaining a balanced, nutritious diet and a physically active lifestyle that can help reduce our risks for chronic diseases and the disabilities and premature death that can accompany them. This age group also needs to consume a diet that supports optimal functioning of the immune system and the maintenance and repair of body tissues.

> **Recap:** The majority of this text is directed toward the nutritional needs of young and middle-aged adults. The young adult and middle-aged years are primarily concerned with the maintenance of health and body tissues. Nutritional concerns include bone loss and increased risk for osteoporosis, obesity, and chronic diseases, such as heart disease, type 2 diabetes, and various cancers. Eating a balanced diet, maintaining a healthy body weight, and being physically active on a regular basis reduces the risks for these diseases.

Nutrition for Older Adults, Age 65 Years and Older

In Canada, the population is getting older each year. Census 2001 reported that 13% of the population was aged 65 or above, a 10.2% increase since 1996. Come 2011, when Canada's oldest baby boomers will enter the 65+ age bracket, this number will further increase. An expected 1.3 million Canadians will be 80 years and older by 2011, a projected 43% increase from 2001. A nutritious diet and regular physical activity can help prevent chronic disease and keep us happy and productive in our later years, so living a healthy lifestyle when we are older begins with a foundation built far before we reach age 65. Let's now explore the distinct nutritional needs of older adults.

Older Adult Growth and Activity Patterns

Older adulthood is a time in which growth is complete and our body systems begin to slow and degenerate. Although aging of our body tissues is inevitable, eating a nutritious diet and living a physically active lifestyle can help slow this process.

Some of the physiologic changes that occur with aging include

- decreased muscle mass and lean tissue;
- increased fat mass;
- decreased bone density;
- decreased immune function;
- impaired ability to absorb or metabolize various nutrients.

If these changes disturb you, remember that they are at least partly within your control. For instance, some of the decrease seen in muscle mass, bone mass, and muscle strength is due to low physical activity levels. Older adults who regularly participate in strengthening exercises and aerobic-type activities have reduced risks for low bone mass and muscle atrophy and weakness, which in turn reduces their risk for falls and the

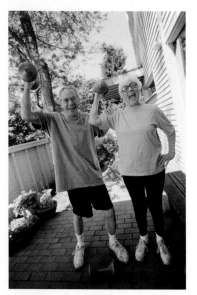

Older adults should participate in strengthening exercises to reduce the risks for low bone mass and muscle weakness.

fractures related to falls that commonly occur in this population. See *Canada's Physical Activity Guide to Healthy Active Living for Older Adults* in Appendix C.

> **Recap:** Older adults have the greatest risk for chronic diseases and related disabilities. Growth is complete, and body systems begin to degenerate with aging. The physiologic changes that occur with aging include loss of muscle mass and lean tissue, increased fat mass, decreased bone density, decreased immune function, and impaired ability to absorb and metabolize various nutrients. These changes influence the nutritional needs of older adults.

What Are an Older Adult's Nutrient Needs?

The requirements for many nutrients are the same for older adults as for young and middle-aged adults. A few nutrient requirements increase, and a few are actually lower. Table 16.3 identifies nutrient recommendations that do change, as well as the physiologic reason behind these changes.

Energy and Macronutrient Recommendations for Older Adults

The energy needs of older adults are lower than those of younger adults. This decrease is due to loss of muscle mass and lean tissue, a reduction in thyroid hormones, and a less physically active lifestyle. It is estimated that total daily energy expenditure decreases approximately 10 kcal each year for men and 7 kcal each year for women ages 19 and older (Institute of Medicine 2002). This means that a woman who needs 2000 kcal (8370 kJ) at age 20 needs just 1650 kcal (6900 kJ) at age 70. Some of this decrease in energy expenditure is an inevitable response to aging, but some of the decrease can be delayed or minimized by staying physically active. Because their total daily energy needs are lower, older adults need to pay particularly close attention to consuming a diet high in nutrient-dense foods but not too high in energy to avoid weight gain.

Because there is no evidence suggesting a minimal amount of dietary fat needed to maintain health, there is no DRI for total fat intake for older adults. However, to reduce the risk for heart disease and other chronic diseases, it is recommended that total fat intake remain within 20% to 35% of total daily energy intake, with saturated and trans fat as low as possible.

The RDA for carbohydrate for older adults is 130 grams per day. As with all other age groups, this level of carbohydrate is sufficient to support brain glucose utilization.

Table 16.3 Nutrient Recommendations That Change with Increased Age

Changes in Nutrient Recommendations	Rationale for Changes
Increased need for vitamin D from 5 µg/day for young adults to 10 µg/day for adults 51 to 70 years and to 15 µg/day for adults over age 70 years	• Decreased bone density • Decreased ability to convert vitamin D to its active form in our skin • Decreased absorption of dietary calcium
Increased need for calcium from 1000 mg/day for young adults to 1200 mg/day for adults 51 years of age and older	• Decreased bone density • Decreased absorption of dietary calcium
Decreased need for fibre from 38 grams/day for young men to 30 grams/day for men 51 years and older Decreases in fibre for women are from 25 grams/day for young women to 21 grams/day for women 51 years and older	• Decreased energy intake
Increased need for vitamins B_6 and B_{12}	• Lower levels of stomach acid • Decreased absorption from gastrointestinal tract • Increased need to reduce homocysteine levels and to optimize immune function

There is no evidence to indicate what percentage of carbohydrate should come from sugars or starches. However, it is recommended that older individuals consume a diet that contains no more than 30% of total energy intake as sugars (Institute of Medicine 2002). The fibre recommendations are slightly lower for older adults than for younger adults because older adults eat less energy. After age 50, 30 grams of fibre per day for men and 21 grams for women is assumed sufficient to reduce the risks for constipation and diverticular disease, maintain appropriate blood levels of glucose and lipids, and provide good sources of nutrient-dense, low-energy foods.

The recommendation for protein is the same for adults of all ages: 0.80 grams of protein per kg body weight per day. Protein is critically needed to help reduce the loss of muscle and lean tissue, and it is also critical to help prevent excessive loss of bone. Many protein foods are also important sources of vitamins and minerals that are typically low in the diets of older adults; thus, protein is an important nutrient for this age group.

Micronutrient Recommendations for Older Adults

The vitamins and minerals of particular concern for older adults are identified in Table 16.3 (page 600). Preventing or minimizing the consequences of osteoporosis is a top priority for older adults. The requirements for both calcium and vitamin D are higher because of a reduced absorption of calcium from the gut, along with reduced production of the active form of vitamin D in our skin as a result of aging. Many older adults are at risk for vitamin D deficiency because they are institutionalized and are not exposed to adequate amounts of sunlight. It is critical that older adults consume foods that are high in calcium and vitamin D, and in many cases supplements are necessary.

Iron needs decrease with aging. This decrease is primarily due to reduced muscle and lean tissue in both men and women and the cessation of menstruation in women. The decreased need for iron in older men is not significant enough to change the recommendations for iron intake in this group, thus the RDA for iron is the same for older men as for younger, 8 mg per day. However, the RDA for iron in older women is 8 mg per day, which is 10 mg per day lower than the RDA for younger women. Although zinc recommendations are the same for all adults, it is important to emphasize that zinc is a critical nutrient for optimizing immune function and wound healing in older adults. Intakes of both zinc and iron can be inadequate in older adults because they may eat less of the food sources that supply these nutrients, such as red meats, poultry, and fish. These foods are relatively expensive and many older adults on a limited income cannot afford to eat them regularly. Also, older adults may have a difficult time chewing meats because of the loss of teeth and the use of dentures.

Although it is speculated that older adults have increased oxidative stress, the recommendations for vitamin C and vitamin E are the same as for younger adults because there is insufficient evidence that consuming amounts higher than the current RDA for these nutrients has any additional health benefits (Institute of Medicine 2000).

Older adults need to pay close attention to consuming adequate amounts of the B vitamins, specifically vitamin B_{12}, vitamin B_6, and folate. As discussed in detail on pages 373–375, inadequate intake of these nutrients increases the levels of the amino acid homocysteine in the blood, and elevated homocysteine levels are associated with an increased risk for cardiovascular, cerebrovascular, and peripheral vascular diseases (Beresford and Boushey 1997). These diseases are common among older adults. The RDA for vitamin B_{12} is the same for younger and older adults, but up to 30% of older adults cannot absorb enough vitamin B_{12} from foods because of atrophic gastritis (see page 357). It is recommended that older adults consume foods that are fortified with vitamin B_{12} or supplements because the vitamin B_{12} in these sources is absorbed more readily. Vitamin B_6 recommendations are slightly higher for older adults, as these higher levels appear necessary to reduce homocysteine levels and optimize immune function in this population (Institute of Medicine 1998).

Vitamin A requirements are the same for adults of all ages; however, older adults should be careful not to consume more than the RDA, as absorption of vitamin A is actually greater in older adults. Thus, this group is at greater risk for vitamin A toxicity, which can cause liver damage and neurological problems. However, consuming foods high in beta-carotene or other carotenoids is safe and does not lead to vitamin A toxicity in this age group.

A variety of factors may limit an older adult's ability to eat a nutritious diet. These include limited financial resources that prevent some older people from buying nutrient-dense foods on a regular basis, reduced appetite, social isolation, inability to prepare foods, and illnesses and physiologic changes that limit the absorption and metabolism of many nutrients. Thus, some older adults may benefit from taking a multivitamin and mineral supplement that contains no more than the RDA for all nutrients contained in the supplement. Additional supplementation may be necessary for such nutrients as calcium, vitamin D, and vitamin B_{12}. However, supplementation with individual nutrients should be done only under the supervision of the individual's primary health care provider, as the risk of nutrient toxicity is high in this population.

Fluid Recommendations for Older Adults

The AI for fluid is the same for older and younger adults. Men should consume 3.7 litres (about 15.5 cups) of total water per day, which includes 3.0 litres (about 13 cups) as total beverages, including drinking water. Women should consume 2.7 litres (about 12 cups) of total water per day, which includes 2.2 litres (about 9 cups) as total beverages, including drinking water. It is important to emphasize that kidney function changes as we age, and the thirst mechanism of older people can be impaired. These changes can result in chronic dehydration and hypernatremia (elevated blood sodium levels) in this population. Some older adults will intentionally limit their beverage intake because they have urinary incontinence. This practice can endanger their health, so it is important for these individuals to seek treatment for the incontinence and continue to drink plenty of fluids.

> **Recap:** Older adults have lower energy needs because of their loss of lean tissue and lower physical activity levels. Older adults should consume 20% to 35% of total energy as fat and 45% to 65% of their energy as carbohydrate. Protein recommendations are the same as for younger adults. Micronutrients of concern for older adults include calcium, vitamin D, iron, zinc, vitamin B_{12}, vitamin B_6, and folate. Older adults need to carefully select nutrient-dense foods to meet their micronutrient needs, and supplementation of vitamin D is necessary. Older adults are at risk for chronic dehydration and hypernatremia, so ample fluid intake should be encouraged.

Nutrition-Related Concerns for Older Adults

Older adults have a number of unique nutritional concerns. In addition to body weight issues, they commonly experience changes in taste and appetite. They may also face dental problems, potential interactions between nutrients and medications, and diseases that affect their memory. Each of these concerns is discussed briefly in the following sections.

Overweight and Underweight: A Delicate Balancing Act

Not surprisingly, overweight and obesity are also a concern for older adults. This population has a high risk for heart disease, hypertension, type 2 diabetes, and cancer, and these diseases are more prevalent in people who are overweight or obese. In contrast, overweight can be protective against osteoporosis and fall-related fractures in older adults.

Underweight is also risky for older adults. Many older adults lose weight as a result of illness, disability, poor nutritional status, alcoholism, or smoking. Many lose the ability to smell and taste, and the loss of these senses is associated with lower appetite and reduced food and nutrient intakes (Kim et al. 2003). Limited income, mobility or transportation problems, or concerns about neighbourhood safety may make food shopping difficult. Other significant risk factors for underweight in older adults are depression and social isolation, which can develop following the death of family members and friends, or when adult children move out of the area. Depression and isolation can cause older adults to lose the desire to prepare nourishing meals for themselves. Any of these factors can result in underweight and frailty, significantly increasing the person's risk of serious illnesses and injuries. For homebound adults with disabilities and older adults, community programs, such as Meals on Wheels, provide nourishing, balanced meals, as well as vital social contact.

In summary, maintaining a healthy weight and a physically and socially active lifestyle helps older adults live stronger, healthier, and more satisfying lives.

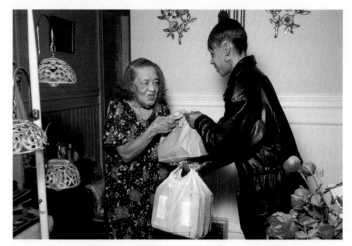

For homebound adults with disabilities and older adults, community programs, such as Meals on Wheels, provide nourishing, balanced meals and vital social contact.

Dental Health Issues

Many older adults have lost their teeth, suffer from gum disease, or have poorly fitting dentures. These conditions cause considerable mouth pain and make chewing difficult and sometimes embarrassing. Because of these dental health challenges, older adults may avoid eating such foods as meats and firm fruits and vegetables. Avoidance of these foods leads to nutrient deficiencies and an increased risk for illness and infection. Gum disease and other infections in the mouth can also increase the risk for heart disease. Maintaining good oral health and having regular dental checkups are thus critical to an older adult's nutrition and overall health.

Other Nutrition-Related Concerns

Many older adults take multiple medications daily. Some of these medications can alter nutrient absorption and metabolism, and many affect appetite. For example, people taking the blood-thinning drug Coumadin should avoid consuming excess vitamin E, as vitamin E magnifies the effects of this drug. Both ibuprofen (Motrin and Advil) and acetaminophen (Tylenol) are commonly prescribed for muscle, joint, and headache pain, but taking these drugs with alcohol increases the risk for liver damage and bleeding, so alcohol should not be consumed with these medications.

Older adults are also at higher risk for Alzheimer's disease and other forms of dementia. These illnesses affect memory and movement, interfering with and potentially preventing older adults from being able to choose, prepare, and consume a nutritious diet. Interestingly, recent studies show that eating a balanced, wholesome diet that includes ample folate, vitamin B_{12}, and macronutrients can improve memory and decrease the risk for Alzheimer's disease and other forms of dementia in older adults (Kaplan et al. 2001; Barberger-Gateau et al. 2002; Morris et al. 2003). These studies emphasize the critical importance to older adults of consuming a balanced diet and supplementing as needed.

Recap: Overweight and obesity are an important concern for older adults, as they increase the risk for chronic diseases. Underweight and frailty are also concerns, as these conditions can lead to increased illness and injury. Older adults may lose their sense of smell and taste, and dental problems can limit intake of meats, fruits, and vegetables; this can lead to nutrient deficiencies. Medications and certain nutrients can have adverse interactions. Alzheimer's disease and other forms of dementia affect memory and mobility and interfere with food preparation and consumption. Nutrient-rich diets have been shown to improve memory and reduce the risk of Alzheimer's disease and other forms of dementia in older adults.

CHAPTER SUMMARY

- Toddlers grow more slowly than infants but are far more active. They require small, frequent, nutritious snacks and meals, and food should be cut in small pieces so it is easy to handle and swallow.

- For toddlers and preschoolers, a serving of food equals 1 Tbsp (15 mL) for each year of age. For example, 4 Tbsp (60 mL) of yogurt is a full serving for a 4-year-old child.

- Energy, fat, and protein requirements are higher for toddlers than for infants. Many toddlers will not eat vegetables, so micronutrients of concern include vitamins A, C, and E.

- Until age 2, toddlers should drink whole milk rather than reduced-fat milk to meet calcium requirements. Iron deficiency is a concern in the toddler years and can be minimized by the consumption of foods naturally high in iron and iron-fortified foods.

- Toddlers are still at risk for choking. Parents should also watch for allergies and monitor weight gain.

- Feeding vegan diets to toddlers is controversial and poses potential deficiencies for protein, iron, calcium, zinc, vitamin D, and vitamin B_{12}.

- Preschoolers have a slower growth rate than toddlers and may have a reduced appetite. Preschoolers are more physically active than toddlers, and playing can sometimes interfere with eating adequate food.

- Preschoolers need less fat than toddlers but slightly more than adults. Protein and energy needs are higher for preschoolers because of their larger size and higher activity levels. Calcium, iron, and zinc requirements are slightly higher for preschoolers than for toddlers. Preschoolers can easily become dehydrated because they ignore or fail to recognize their thirst.

- Overweight and obesity are concerns for preschoolers and can be avoided by engaging in regular physical activity and eating a nutritious diet. Dental caries are also of concern, and preschoolers should brush their teeth regularly, limit sweets, and visit the dentist regularly beginning at age 3.

- School-age children are more independent and can make more of their own food choices. Physical activity levels can vary dramatically.

- School-age children should eat 25% to 35% of their total energy as fat and 45% to 65% of their total energy as carbohydrate. Calcium needs increase as children mature, while iron needs decrease slightly.

- Many school-age children skip breakfast and do not choose nutritious foods during school lunch. Peer pressure and popularity are strong influences on food choices. The foods that children choose to eat at school, both during and outside of the lunch break, can be high in fat, sugar, and energy and low in nutrients.

- Obesity is an increasing concern for school-age children. Children should be physically active at least one hour every day. Disordered eating behaviours and eating disorders can result from concerns about body image. Consuming adequate calcium to support the development of peak bone mass is a primary concern for school-age children.

- Puberty is the period in life in which secondary sexual characteristics develop and the physical capability to reproduce begins. Puberty results in rapid increases in height, weight, and lean body mass and fat mass.

- Energy needs for adolescents are variable and can be quite high; adequate energy is needed to support growth, maturation, and physical activity. Fat intake should be 25% to 35% of total energy, and carbohydrate intake should be 45% to 65% of total energy intake.

- Many adolescents replace whole grains, fruits, and vegetables with fast foods and snack foods, placing themselves at risk for deficiencies of calcium, iron, and vitamin A. Calcium is needed to optimize bone growth and to achieve peak bone density, and iron needs are increased because of increased muscle mass in boys and menstruation in girls.

- Obesity can occur during adolescence if food intake increases and physical activity decreases. Disordered eating, eating disorders, cigarette smoking, and use of alcohol and illegal drugs are also concerns for this age group.

- The young adult and middle-aged years are primarily concerned with the maintenance of health and body tissues. Nutritional concerns include bone loss and increased risk for osteoporosis, obesity, and chronic diseases, such as heart disease, type 2 diabetes, and various cancers.

- Growth is complete in older adults, and their body systems begin to degenerate as part of the normal aging process. Some of the physiologic changes that occur with aging include loss of muscle mass and lean tissue, increased fat mass, decreased bone density, decreased immune function, and impaired ability to absorb and metabolize various nutrients. A nutritious diet and regular physical activity can reduce the rate of some of these changes.

- Older adults have lower energy needs because of their loss of lean tissue and lower physical activity levels. Older adults should consume 20% to 35% of total energy as fat and 45% to 65% of their energy as carbohydrate. Protein recommendations are the same as for younger adults.

- Micronutrients of concern for older adults include calcium, vitamin D, iron, zinc, vitamin B_{12}, vitamin B_6, and folate. Older adults need to carefully select nutrient-dense foods to meet their micronutrient needs, and supplementation may be necessary. Older adults are at risk for chronic dehydration and hypernatremia, so ample fluid intake should be encouraged.

- Overweight and obesity are important concerns for older adults, as they increase the risk for chronic diseases. A variety of factors also increase the older adult's risk for underweight.

- Medications can interfere with nutrient absorption and metabolism, and nutrients can also interfere with the actions of medications.

- Alzheimer's disease and other forms of dementia affect memory and movement and interfere with food preparation and consumption. Varied, nutritious diets have been shown to improve memory and reduce the risk of Alzheimer's disease and other forms of dementia in older adults.

REVIEW QUESTIONS

Quizzes

1. Which of the following nutrients is needed in increased amounts in older adulthood?
   a. Fibre
   b. Vitamin D
   c. Protein
   d. Vitamin A

2. Carbohydrate should make up what percentage of total energy for school-age children?
   a. 25% to 40%
   b. 35% to 50%
   c. 45% to 65%
   d. 45% to 70%

3. Which of the following is a major nutrition-related concern for preschoolers?
   a. Choking
   b. Skipping breakfast
   c. Botulism
   d. Dental caries

4. Which of the following breakfasts would be most appropriate to serve a 20-month-old child?
   a. 125 mL (1/2 cup) of iron-fortified cooked oat cereal, 30 mL (2 Tbsp) mashed pineapple, and 250 mL (8 fl. oz.) whole milk
   b. 30 mL (2 Tbsp) of non-fat yogurt, 30 mL (2 Tbsp) applesauce, 1 slice of melba toast spread with strawberry jam, and 250 mL (8 fl. oz.) calcium-fortified orange juice
   c. 125 mL (1/2 cup) of iron-fortified cooked oat cereal, 65 mL (1/4 cup) pineapple tidbits, and 250 mL (8 fl. oz.) 1% milk
   d. 2 small link sausages, cut into small pieces, 30 mL (2 Tbsp) scrambled egg, 1 slice whole wheat toast,

4 cherry tomatoes, cut in pieces, 30 mL (2 Tbsp) applesauce, and 250 mL (8 fl. oz.) whole milk.

5. Which of the following statements about cigarette smoking is true?
   a. Cigarette smoking can interfere with the absorption of nutrients
   b. Cigarette smoking commonly causes food cravings, such as "getting the munchies"
   c. Cigarette smoking is the number-one cause of death in adolescents
   d. All of the above statements are true

6. Tom was raised by his parents to always finish all of his dinner; he was often told, "No dessert until you finish your plate." Since this is how he was raised, he feels it is the best strategy to use at meal time with his own 2-year-old son. Do you have any concerns about this approach?

7. Joe is a 65-year-old man who has a BMI of 28 and feels that he should lose some weight. He knows that you just recently took a nutrition course and asks for your advice. What would you recommend he do?

8. Identify some advantages and disadvantages of modern technology (such as television and computers) in terms of their impact on lifestyle and nutrition.

9. Explain why a toddler in a vegan family might be at risk for protein deficiency.

10. Imagine that you are taking care of four 5-year-old children for an afternoon. Design a menu for the children's lunch that is nutritious and that will be fun for them to eat.

11. Imagine that you manage a college cafeteria. Design a menu with three lunch choices that are nutritious and that are likely to be popular with 18- to 21-year-old students.

12. You and your parents live in Edmonton, where you attend university and your parents are employed as teachers. A year ago, your maternal grandmother, who lives in Halifax, stayed with you for several weeks following the death of your grandfather. She seemed fit at the time, going for walks with you and your dog, and cooking large meals for your family and special treats for you throughout her stay. Last night your mother received a phone call from a Halifax hospital saying that her mother had been admitted following a hip fracture suffered in a fall at home and was battling significant dehydration and moderate dementia as well. Identify several factors that might have contributed to your grandmother's condition.

13. Lillian is trying to no avail to convince her elderly parents to start taking vitamin-mineral supplements. Her mother has agreed, but her father refuses to even have them in his house. Even when her mother's doctor advised calcium and vitamin D supplements, her father decided it was just a hoax to make money. Lillian doesn't know what to do and is becoming increasingly worried about her parents' health. Do you agree with Lillian that her parents should be taking vitamin-mineral supplements? If you learned that her parents have never eaten dairy products regularly but enjoy a wide array of vegetables and whole grains, would this change your view? If you side with Lillian, which vitamin-mineral supplements would you recommend and why?

CASE STUDY

Elizabeth has always been a heavy-set child, but recently her weight has become a health concern. Elizabeth's mother is advised by their doctor to help her daughter lose weight, so they sit down and make a list of everything Elizabeth eats and all her physical activity. They realize that Elizabeth rarely eats a full breakfast and ends up eating hamburgers and french fries every day at lunch. Usually Elizabeth's mom is too tired to cook dinner, so they order in from the local Thai restaurant or the pizza place. Because Elizabeth is heavier than her classmates, she hates joining in their games at recess and won't even consider joining a sports team. She walks home from school every day and then watches her favourite television shows until dinnertime.

Given what you know about Elizabeth's lifestyle and the nutrients needed for school-age children, what would you say about the quality of her diet? What about her activity level? What could Elizabeth and her parents do to help her achieve a healthier body weight?

Test Yourself Answers

1. **False** Toddlers have a higher need for fat than do older children or adults, so they should consume foods that are higher in fat.

2. **True** Girls may grow only a few more centimetres after menstruation begins, while boys continue to grow throughout adolescence and even into early adulthood.

3. **True** Although growing children and teens need slightly more fat than adults, they should be encouraged to consume whole-grain foods, fruits, and vegetables.

4. **True** Although a reduction of muscle mass and lean tissue is inevitable with aging, some of this loss can be attenuated with regular physical activity.

5. **False** Older adults may need to supplement certain nutrients, such as vitamin D, calcium and vitamin B_{12}, but people in this age group are at increased risk for vitamin toxicity. In addition, certain nutrients and medications can interact to cause significant health problems, so supplementation with individual nutrients should occur only with the supervision of a trained health care professional.

WEB LINKS

www.dietitians.ca
Dietitians of Canada (DC)
Ask nutrition and diet questions or get the names of qualified dietitians in your community from this national professional organization.

www.hc-sc.gc.ca
Health Canada
Search this site for food and nutrition guidelines and policies, and for reports and statistics on the health of Canadians.

www.kidnetic.com
Kidnetic.com
This fun website developed to help children and families get active, providing instructions and ideas for physical games and challenges, recipes for kids to make, and information about nutrition and the body.

www.kidsnutrition.org
USDA/ARS Children's Nutrition Research Center at Baylor College of Medicine
This site provides information about current research projects, nutrition web links, and consumer and nutrition news.

www.mapmyrun.com
Map My Run
This fun site lets you plan your runs and calculates the distances for you. You can keep track of your training schedule or find new trails in your region.

www.keepkidshealthy.com
Keep Kids Healthy.com
This site has information about nutrition and health for toddlers, children, and adolescents.

www.cdc.gov
The Centers for Disease Control
Click on Life Stages & Populations, and then you can select topics, such as Older Adults & Seniors, Adolescents & Teens, and many others.

www.vrg.org
The Vegetarian Resource Group
Visit this website to learn more about vegetarianism for all ages. Included on the site are special sections for teens and kids, as well as recipes and guides for vegetarian and vegan eating in all kinds of situations.

www.fns.usda.gov/fns/
USDA Food & Nutrition Services
Read about U.S food assistance programs to provide food to all ages, including school meals programs; the Food Stamps Program, and the Women, Infants, and Children Program.

www.nlm.nih.gov/medlineplus/dentalhealth.html
MEDLINE Plus Dental Health
Contained on this site are links to articles about dental health for all ages.

www.healthandage.com
Health and Age
This site lists comprehensive information about nutrition, exercise, and preventative medicine with relation to aging. Features include a section for caregivers and a newsletter.

Should Governments Limit Food Advertising Directed to Children?

You can expect to find many things as you navigate the grocery store aisles. No doubt you'll see box upon box of sugary sweet cereals, row upon row of chocolaty cookies, can upon can of syrupy pop—and more than likely you'll also find a stubborn child, in mid-tantrum, demanding to stuff the shopping cart full of these tempting snacks.

Although this may seem a common occurrence, have you ever stopped to wonder why these children are so unrelenting in their quest for "junk" food? What motivates children to stop at nothing to convince their parents to purchase these foods? Is it that children are naturally attracted to novel sweet treats, or do advertisements program children to desire these products?

It's no secret that television commercials are intended to make a product more attractive and enticing to consumers. As adults, for the most part, we can take these incredible claims and advertising gimmicks with a grain of salt. But are children capable of separating opinion from fact? In a recent *Food and Drink Weekly*, Jeff McIntyre of the American Psychological Association claims that children younger than 8 years old "are easy targets for commercial persuasion because they lack the cognitive development to understand the persuasive intent of advertising" (2005). In other words, young children do not recognize that commercials are trying to influence their food choices; instead, they understand advertisements to be truthful representations of what a product has to offer. This makes them especially vulnerable to ads that feature their favourite cartoon character or athlete.

This wouldn't be such a problem if the products marketed to children were predominantly wholesome, nutrient-dense foods that promote a healthy lifestyle, but unfortunately this is hardly the case. In fact, according to the USDA's *Amber Waves: The Economics of Food, Farming, Natural Resources, and Rural America*, from 2000 to 2004, new food products directed at children in the United States were largely candies (46%), snacks (8%), cookies (6%), and breakfast cereals (5%) (Kuchler et al. 2005). And since Canadian children often view programs on networks that broadcast American commercials, these statistics are not relevant only to our neighbours to the south. On average, children view 40 000 television ads each year. More than half of these ads promote less healthy foods and account for about $1 billion of the $10 billion to $12 billion spent annually by the food and beverage industry on marketing aimed at children.

To address this advertising imbalance, the United States Congress enlisted the help of the National Academies' Institute of Medicine (IOM) to create an action plan that focuses on the prevention of obesity in children and youth, primarily by tackling broad environmental factors. The IOM released a report in September 2004 that has called for, among other things, "the food, beverage, and entertainment industries to voluntarily develop and implement guidelines for advertising and marketing directed at children and youth" and for schools to "implement new nutritional standards for all foods and beverages served or sold on their grounds." Advocacy groups, such as Campaign for a Commercial-Free Childhood (CCFC), are also fighting to prevent commercial exploitation of children. The CCFC points to product placement on hit TV shows and the creation of TV shows for the sole purpose of selling products as just a few examples of the many ways in which advertisers are able to get endorsements for their products outside a commercial, further masking their persuasive motives from young children.

This call for regulation is by no means a viewpoint shared by all—food and beverage industries are up in arms to protect the power of advertising to children. Some argue that freedom of speech is being infringed and that self-regulation is, in fact, effective. The Alliance for American Advertising claims that it is a "right" to advertise to children. Others completely deny the impact of advertisements on the obesity epidemic: the Center for Consumer Freedom, a non-profit organization, states that "there is simply no evidence proving food advertisement contributes to childhood obesity, but there is an abundance of research showing that lack of physical activity does, and this is where our efforts should be focused." Do companies truly have the right to advertise their products to children?

Another factor that must be considered is the loss of revenue schools will suffer if junk foods can no longer be advertised and sold in schools. Many schools have lucrative vending-machine deals that result not only in candy, chocolate bars, chips, and pop being within easy reach of children throughout the school day but also in more money to spend on school supplies and equipment. Will the health benefits to students outweigh the loss of funding that would result if vending-machine contracts were terminated?

In addition to limitations on advertising, the United States government is said to be considering a tax on junk food. This tax would be placed on items that

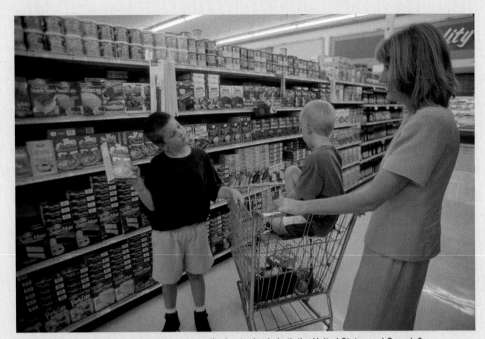

Is it really any wonder that obesity rates are continuing to rise in both the United States and Canada?

contain high numbers of Calories and added sugars, fats, and salt. In theory, this tax would deter consumers from purchasing unhealthy snack foods and encourage consumption of more nutritious products instead. Although the exact tax rate has yet to be decided, research has shown that the rate would have to be relatively high, approximately 30%, to have a significant impact on consumers. Would the taxation of junk food or the limitation of advertising be more effective in limiting the consumption of unhealthy snack products by children?

Although voluntary restrictions on advertising junk food to children are widely considered a failure, some companies are heeding the call to be more socially conscious. Kraft Foods has pulled ads promoting Oreos and Kool-Aid and instead shows commercials endorsing sugar-free Kool-Aid and white-meat chicken Lunchables during programs watched by children aged 6 to 11 years.

What is important to extract from all the information available is the lack of balance. According to the president of the American Dietetic Association, Susan H. Laramee, "Perhaps the most worrisome issue surrounding food marketing to children is that it's happening in a virtual absence of balanced and accurate nutrition education messages" (American Dietetic Association 2005). In Canada, organizations such as Concerned Children's Advertisers (www.cca-kids.ca) and policies such as the Canadian Broadcasting Code for Advertising to Children (www.adstandards.com/en/childrensinitiative) are attempting to ensure that appropriate messages are reaching Canadian children. Whether the government steps in and limits advertising to children or not, there should be more creative and effective programs in place to help shape the food choices of today's children.

If you were a member of the government, what would you do? Do you believe that advertising junk food to children is unfair and unbalanced, or would you fight for the freedom of industries to advertise their products?

References

Chapter 1

Institute of Medicine, Food and Nutrition Board. 2003. *Dietary Reference Intakes: Applications in Dietary Planning.* Washington, DC: National Academies Press.

Institute of Medicine, Food and Nutrition Board. 2002. *Dietary Reference Intakes for Energy, Carbohydrates, Fiber, Fat, Protein and Amino Acids (Macronutrients).* Washington, DC: National Academies Press.

Raine, K. 2004. *Overweight and Obesity in Canada: A Population Health Perspective.* Toronto: Canadian Institute for Health Information.

Shields, M. 2005. *Overweight Canadian Children and Adolescents.* Ottawa: Statistics Canada. www.statcan.ca/english/research/82-620-MIE/82-620-MIE2005001.htm. Accessed July 2005.

Tjepkema, M. 2005. *Adult Obesity in Canada: Measured Height and Weight.* Ottawa: Statistics Canada. www.statcan.ca/english/research/82-620-MIE/82-620-MIE2005001.htm. Accessed July 2005.

Chapter 2

Canadian Food Inspection Agency. 2003. Guide to Food Labelling and Advertising. Reference Standards, Tables 6.5 and 6.7. www.inspection.gc.ca/english/fssa/labeti/guide/ch6e.shtml#6.3.2. Accessed June 2008.

Canadian Food Inspection Agency. 2004. Information Letter: Carbohydrate Claims on Foods Sold in Canada. www.inspection.gc.ca/english/fssa/labeti/inform/choe.shtml. Accessed January 2006.

Fito, M., M. Guxens, D. Corella, G. Sáez, R. Estruch, R. de la Torre, F. Francés, C. Cabezas, M. Del Carmen López-Sabater, J. Marrugat, A. Garcia-Arellano, F. Arós, V. Ruiz-Gutierrez, E. Ros, J. Salas-Salvadó, M. Fiol, R. Solá, M-I. Covas, for the PREDIMED Study Investigators. 2007. *Arch. Intern. Med.* 167:1195–1203.

Friedman, J. M. 2003. A war on obesity, not the obese. *Science* 299:856–858.

Health Canada. 2003. Compendium of Templates for "Nutrition Facts" www.hc-sc.gc.ca/fn-an/label-etiquet/nutrition/reg/compend_nut_fact_tc-repertoire_etiquetage_nut_tm-eng.php. Accessed June 2008.

Health Canada. 2003. Frequently Asked Questions About Nutrition Labelling. http://hc-sc.gc.ca/fn-an/label-etiquet/nutrition/educat/te_quest-eng.php#18. Accessed September 2008.

Health Canada. 2008. Interactive Nutrition Label and Quiz. www.hc-sc.gc.ca/fn-an/label-etiquet/nutrition/cons/interactive-eng.php. Accessed June 2008.

Health Check. March 2008. Nutrient criteria. www.healthcheck.org/en/nutritional-information/nutrient-criteria-grocery.html. Accessed April 2008.

Hueter, J. S. 2002, August 30. Nutrition in schools. www.law.uh.edu/healthlawperspectives/Children/020830Nutrition.html. Accessed July 2003.

Jacobson, M. F., and K. D. Brownell. 2000. Small taxes on soft drinks and snack foods to promote health. *Am. J. Public Health* 90:854–857.

Nestle, M. 2002. *Food Politics. How the Food Industry Influences Nutrition and Health.* Berkeley, CA: University of California Press.

Oldways Preservation and Exchange Trust, The Food Issues Think Tank, Healthy Eating Pyramids & Other Tools, www.oldwayspt.org. Accessed September 2002.

Painter, J., R. Jee-Hyun, and L. Yeon-Kyung. 2002. Comparison of international food guide pictorial representations. *J. Am. Diet. Assoc.* 102:483–489.

Sacks, F. M., L. P. Svetkey, W. M. Vollmer, L. J. Appel, G. A. Bray, D. Harsha, E. Obarzanek, P. R. Conlin, E. R. Miller III, D. G. Simons-Morton, N. Karanja, and P.-H. Lin. 2001. Effects on blood pressure of reduced dietary sodium and the Dietary Approaches to Stop Hypertension (DASH) diet. *New Engl. J. Med.* 344:3–10.

Statistics Canada. February 2003. Food Expenditure in Canada. Catalogue no. 62-554. Ministry of Industry. www.statcan.ca/english/freepub/62-554-XIE/0010162-554-XIE.pdf. Accessed April 2008.

U.S. Department of Agriculture and U.S. Department of Health and Human Services (USDHHS). 2005. Dietary Guidelines for Americans, 2005. 6th ed. www.health.gov/dietaryguidelines/dga2005/recommendations.htm. Accessed April 2008.

Weschsler, H., G. W. Dowdall, A. Davenport, and E. B. Rimm. 1995. A gender-specific measure of binge drinking among college students. *Am. J. Public Health* 7:982–985.

Weschsler, H., J. E. Lee, M. Kuo, and H. Lee. 2000. College binge drinking in the 1990s: A continuing problem. *J. Am. Coll. Health* 48:199–210.

Wollin, S. D., and P. J. H. Jones. 2001. Alcohol, red wine and cardiovascular disease. *J. Nutr.* 131:1401–1404.

Chapter 3

American Physiological Society. June 30 2006. Celiac success: New enzyme efficiently degrades gluten in 'human stomach' environment. Press release.

Batterham, R. L., M. A. Cowley, C. J. Small, H. Herzog, M. A. Cohen, C. L. Dakin, A. M. Wren, A. E. Brynes, J. M. Low, M. A. Ghatei, R. D. Cone, and S. R. Bloom. 2002. Gut hormone PYY_{3-36} physiologically inhibits food intake. *Nature* 418:650–654.

Bell, E. A., and B. J. Rolls. 2001. Regulation of Energy Intake: Factors Contributing to Obesity. In *Present Knowledge in Nutrition*, 8th ed., edited by B. A. Bowman and R. M. Russell. Washington, DC: ILSI Press.

Blom, W. A. M., A. Stafleu, C. de Graaf, F. J. Kok, G. Schaafsma, G. Hendriks, and H. F. J. Hendriks. 2005. Ghrelin response to carbohydrate-enriched breakfast is related to insulin. *Am. J. Clin. Nutr.* 81:367–375.

Canadian Society for Intestinal Research. Celiac disease. www.badgut.com/index.php?contentFile=celiac& title=Celiac%20Disease. Accessed January 2006.

Chan, F. K. L., and W. K. Leung. 2002. Peptic-ulcer disease. *Lancet* 360:933–941.

Clancy, R. L. and G. Pang. 2007. Probiotics—Industry myth or practical reality? *J. Amer. Coll. Nutr.* 26(6):691S–694.

Crohn's and Colitis Foundation of Canada. 2008. What is Inflammatory Bowel Disease (IBD)? www.ccfc.ca/English/info/ibd.html. Accessed July 2008.

Davidson, N. O. 2003. Intestinal lipid absorption. In *Textbook of Gastroenterology*, Volume 1, 4th ed., edited by T. Yamada, D. H. Alpers, N. Kaplowitz, L. Laine, C. Owyang, and D. W. Powell. Philadelphia: Lippincott Williams & Wilkins.

Douglas, L. C. and M.E. Saunders. 2008. Probiotics and prebiotics in dietetic practice. *J. Amer. Diet. Assoc.*108:510–521.

Grajek, W., A. Olejnik, and A. Sip. 2005. Probiotics, prebiotics and antioxidants as functional foods. *Acta Biochimica Polonica*, 52(3), 665–671.

Guarner, F. and G.J. Schaafsma. 1998. Probiotics. *Inter. J. Food Micro.* 39:237–238.

Hauschildt, E. 2001. Prevalence of irritable bowel syndrome in Canada is approximately 6 percent. *Can. J. Gastroentero.* www.docguide.com/news/content.nsf/news. Accessed February 2005.

Health Canada. 2005. Food Allergens. www.hc-sc.gc.ca/ fn-an/securit/allerg/allergen_con_info_e.html. Accessed July 2005.

Huff, B. A. 2004. "Probiotics" might not be what they seem. *Can. Fam. Phys.* 50:583–587.

Kim, D-Y, M. Camilleri, J. A. Murray, D. A. Stephens, J. A. Levine, and D. D. Burton. 2001. Is there a role for gastric accommodation and satiety in asymptomatic obese people? *Obesity Res.* 9: 655–661.

Lenoir-Wijnkoop, I., M.E. Sanders, M. C. Cabana, E. Caglar, G. Corthier, N. Rayes, P.M. Sherman, H.M. Timmerman, M. Vaneechoutte, J. Van Loo, and D.A.W. Wolvers. 2007. Probiotic and prebiotic influence beyond the intestinal tract. *Nutr. Rev.* 65(11), 469–489.

Marsh, T. D. 1997. Nonprescription H_2-receptor antagonists. *J. Am. Pharm. Assoc.* NS37: 552–556.

Maton, P. N., and M. E. Burton. 1999. Antacids revisited. A review of their clinical pharmacology and recommended therapeutic use. *Drugs* 57:855–870.

Murray, J. A. 1999. The widening spectrum of celiac disease. *Am. J. Clin. Nutr.* 69:354–365.

National Digestive Diseases Information Clearinghouse (NDDIC). 2001, January. Diarrhea. NIH Publication No. 01-2749. http://digestive.niddk.nih.gov/ddiseases/pubs/diarrhea/index.htm. Accessed August 2003.

National Digestive Diseases Information Clearinghouse (NDDIC). 2002, December. H. pylori and Peptic Ulcer. NIH Publication No. 03–4225. http://digestive.niddk.nih.gov/ddiseases/pubs/hpylori/index.htm. Accessed August 2003.

National Digestive Diseases Information Clearinghouse (NDDIC). 2002, February. NSAIDs and Peptic Ulcers. NIH Publication No. 02–4644. http://digestive.niddk.nih.gov/ddiseases/pubs/ nsaids/index.htm. Accessed August 2003.

National Digestive Diseases Information Clearinghouse (NDDIC). 2003, April. Irritable Bowel Syndrome. NIH Publication No. 03–693. http://digestive.niddk.nih.gov/ddiseases/pubs/ibs/index.htm. Accessed August 2003.

National Digestive Diseases Information Clearinghouse (NDDIC). 2003, June. Heartburn, Hiatal Hernia, and Gastroesophageal Reflux Disease (GERD). NIH Publication No. 03–0882. http://digestive.niddk.nih.gov/ddiseases/pubs/gerd/index.htm. Accessed August 2003.

National Institute of Allergy and Infectious Diseases (NIAID). 2003, May. Food Allergy and Intolerances. NIAID Fact Sheet. www.niaid.nih.gov/factsheets/food.htm. Accessed August 2003.

Roberfroid, M. D. 2000. Prebiotics and probiotics: Are they functional foods? *Am. J. Clin. Nutr.* 71(suppl):1682S–1690S.

Sanders, M. E., D. C. Walker, K. M. Walker, K. Aoyama, and T. R. Klaenhammer. 1996.

Performance of commercial cultures in fluid milk applications. *J. Dairy Science* 79:943–955.

Saunders, M. E. 2003. Probiotics: considerations for human health. *Nutr. Rev.* 61(3):91–99.

Spiller, R. 2007. Clinical update: irritable bowel syndrome. *The Lancet* 369:1586–1588.

Stanley, S. L. 1999. Advice to travelers. In *Textbook of Gastroenterology*, Volume 1, 3rd ed., edited by T. Yamada. Philadelphia: Lippincott Williams & Wilkins.

Stepniak, D., L. Spaenij-Dekking, C. Mitea, M. Moester, A. de Ru, R. Baak-Pablo, P. van Veelen, L. Edens, and F. Koning. 2006. Highly efficient gluten degradation with a newly identified prolyl endoprotease: implications for celiac disease. *Am. J. Physiol. Gastrointest. Liver Physiol.* 291:G621–G629.

University of Guelph, Natural Hormone Has Potential to Aid Weight Loss, Researcher Finds. September 2007 News Release. http://www.uoguelph.ca/news/2007/09/natural_hormone.html

World Health Organization. 2001. *Health and nutritional properties of probiotics in food including powdered milk with live lactic acid bacteria.* Córdoba, Argentina.

Zorrilla, G. 1998. Hunger and satiety: Deceptively simple words for the complex mechanisms that tell us when to eat and when to stop. *J. Am. Dietetic Assoc.* 98:1111.

Chapter 4

American College of Sports Medicine (ACSM). 2000. Position stand: Exercise and type 2 diabetes. *Med. Sci. Sports Exerc.* 32:1345–1360.

American Dietetic Association. 2004. Position of the American Dietetic Association: Use of nutritive and nonnutritive sweeteners. *J. Am. Diet. Assoc.* 104:255–275.

Atkins, R. C. 1992. *Dr. Atkins' New Diet Revolution.* New York: M. Evans & Company, Inc.

Buyken, A. E., M. Toeller, G. Heitkamp, G. Karamanos, B. Rottiers, R. Muggeo, and M. Fuller. 2001. Glycemic index in the diet of European outpatients with type 1 diabetes: relations to glycated hemoglobin and serum lipids. *Am. J. Clin. Nutr.* 73:574–581.

Canadian Diabetes Association. 2003. Draft Blueprint for Action for the National Diabetes Strategy. www.diabetes.ca/Files/Blueprintv10.pdf. Accessed January 2006.

Canadian Diabetes Association. 2006b. The prevalence and costs of diabetes. www.diabetes.ca/Section_About/prevalence.asp. Accessed January 2006.

Canadian Food Inspection Agency. 2004. Guide to food labelling and advertising, Chapter 9.

www.inspection.gc.ca/english/fssa/labeti/guide/ch9ae.shtmL. Accessed February 2005.

Canadian Institute for Health Information, Canadian Population Health Initiative. February 2004. *Improving the Health of Canadians.* http://secure.cihi.ca/cihiweb/dispPage.jsp?cw_page=PG_39_E&cw_topic=39&cw_rel=AR_322_E.

Canadian Sugar Institute. 2006. Estimates of added sugars consumption in Canada. Nutrition Information Service. Toronto.

Centers for Disease Control. 2000. Non-polio enterovirus infections. www.cdc.gov/ncidod/dvrd/entrvirs.htm. Accessed February 2005.

Colditz, G. A., J. E. Manson, M. J. Stampfer, B. Rosner, W. C. Willett, and F. E. Speizer. 1992. Diet and risk of clinical diabetes in women. *Am. J. Clin. Nutr.* 55:1018–1023.

Dietitians of Canada. 2004. School food and nutrition recommendations for Ontario Ministry of Education regarding snacks and beverages dispensed by vending machines. www.dietitians.ca. Accessed February. 2005.

Dietitians of Canada. 2008. Current Issues: Understanding the glycemic index and glycemic load: Implications for health and prevention of disease. www.dietitians.ca. Accessed January 2008.

Garriguet, D. 2006. Canadians' Eating Habits 2004. Statistics Canada, 2006, Cat. No. 82–620-MIE. www.statcan.ca/bsolc/english/bsolc?catno=82–620-MIE2006002. Accessed January 2008.

Government of Canada. 2007. Regulations Amending the Food and Drug Regulations (1433 — Neotame). *Canada Gazette* 141, No. 17. canadagazette.gc.ca/partII/2007/20070822/html/sor176-e.html. Accessed May 2008.

Harnack, L., J. Stang, and M. Story. 1999. Soft drink consumption among U.S. children and adolescents: nutritional consequences. *J. Am. Diet. Assoc.* 99:436–441.

Health Canada. 2006. Health Canada comments on the recent study relating to the safety of aspartame. www.hc-sc.gc.ca/fn-an/securit/addit/sweeten-edulcor/aspartame_statement_e.html. Accessed May 2008.

Health Canada. 2007a. Canadian Community Health Survey, Cycle 2.2, Nutrition (2004) Nutrient Intakes from Food. Provincial, Regional and National Summary Data Tables, Volume 1. Cat.: H164-45/1-2007E-PDF. www.hc-sc.gc.ca/fn-an/pubs/cchs-nutri-escc/index_e.html. Accessed May 2008.

Health Canada. 2007b. What is saccharin? www.hc-sc.gc.ca/fn-an/securit/addit/sweeten-edulcor/saccharin_e.html. Accessed May 2008.

Health Canada: Canadian Community Health Survey, Cycle 2.2, Nutrition (2004)–Nutrient Intakes from Food Provincial, Regional and National Summary Data Tables, Volume 1. www.hc-sc.gc.ca/fn-an/pubs/cchs-nutri-escc/index_e.html. Accessed May 2008

Health Canada. Comments on the Recent Study Relating to the Safety of Aspartame, May 5, 2006. http://hc-sc.gc.ca/fn-an/securit/addit/sweeten-edulcor/aspartame_statement-eng.php

Heart and Stroke Foundation of Canada. 2007. Over 60? It's not too late to help your heart. ww1.heartandstroke.ca/Page.asp?PageID=1613&ContentID=24961&ContentTypeID=1. Accessed May 2008.

Howard, B. V., and J. Wylie-Rosett. 2002. Sugar and cardiovascular disease. A statement for healthcare professionals from the Committee on Nutrition of the Council on Nutrition, Physical Activity, and Metabolism of the American Heart Association. *Circulation* 106:523–527.

Institute of Medicine, Food and Nutritition Board. 2002. *Dietary Reference Intakes for Energy, Carbohydrates, Fibre, Fat, Protein and Amino Acids (Macronutrients)*. Washington, DC: The National Academy of Sciences.

Liu, S., J. E. Manson, M. J. Stampfer, M. D. Holmes, F. B. Hu, S. E. Hankinson, and W. C. Willett. 2001. Dietary glycemic load assessed by food-frequency questionnaire in relation to plasma high-density-lipoprotein cholesterol and fasting plasma triacylglycerols in postmenopausal women. *Am. J. Clin. Nutr.* 73:560–566.

Ludwig, D. S., K. E. Peterson, and S. L. Gortmaker. 2001. Relation between consumption of sugar-sweetened drinks and childhood obesity: A prospective, observational analysis. *Lancet* 357:505–508.

Meyer, K. A., L. H. Kushi, D. R. Jacobs, J. Slavin, T. A. Sellers, and A. R. Folsom. 2000. Carbohydrates, dietary fibre, and incident type 2 diabetes in older women. *Am. J. Clin. Nutr.* 71:921–930.

Nestle, M. 2002. *Food Politics: How the Food Industry Influences Nutrition and Health*. Berkeley, CA: University of California Press.

Ontario Ministry of Education. October 2004. Healthy foods and beverages in elementary school vending machines. Policy Memorandum No. 135. www.edu.gov.ca/extra/eng/ppm/ppm135.pdf. Accessed February 2005.

Pan, J. W., D. L. Rothman, K. L. Behar, D. T. Stein, and H. P. Hetherington. 2000. Human brain β-hydroxybutyrate and lactate increase in fasting-induced ketosis. *J. Cerebral Blood Flow Metabol.* 20:1502–1507.

Pan, X.-P., G.-W. Li, Y.-H. Hu, J. X. Wang, W. Y. Yang, Z. X. An, Z. X. Hu, J. Lin, J. Z. Xiao, H. B. Cao, P. A. Liu, X. G. Jiang, Y. Y. Jiang, J. P. Wang., H. Zheng, H. Zhang, P. H. Bennett, and B. V. Howard. 1997. Effects of diet and exercise in preventing NIDDM in people with impaired glucose tolerance. *Diabetes Care* 20:537–544.

Pi-Sunyer, X. 2005. Do gylcemic index, glycemic load, and fiber play a role in insulin sensitivity, disposition index, and type 2 diabetes? *Diabetes Care*. 28(12):2978–2979.

Public Health Agency of Canada. 2007. National diabetes fat sheet Canada 2007. www.phac-aspc.gc.ca/ccdpc-cpcmc/diabetes-diabete/english/pubs/ndfs-fnrd07-eng.html. Accessed May 2008.

Sears, B. 1995. *The Zone. A Dietary Road Map*. New York: HarperCollins Publishers.

Soffritti, M., F. Belpoggi, D. Degli Esposti, and L. Lambertini. 2005. Aspartame induces lymphomas and leukaemias in rats. *Eur. J. Oncol.* 10:107–116.

Statistics Canada. 2003. Food consumption in Canada 2003—Part II. www.statcan.ca/english/ads/23F0001XCB/1. Accessed February 2005.

Statistics Canada. 2005. Nutrition: Findings from the Canadian community health survey: Measured obesity. Ottawa: Statistics Canada Cat. No. 82–620-MWE.

Steward, H. L., M. C. Bethea, S. S. Andrews, and L. A. Balart. 1995. *Sugar Busters Cut Sugar to Trim Fat*. New York: Ballantine Books.

Suarez, F. L., J. Adshead, J. K. Furne, and M. D. Levitt. 1998. Lactose maldigestion is not an impediment to the intake of 1500 mg calcium daily as dairy products. *Am. J. Clin. Nutr.* 68:1118–1122.

Topping, D. L., and P. M. Clifton. 2001. Short-chain fatty acids and human colonic function: Roles of resistant starch and nonstarch polysaccharides. *Physiol. Rev.* 81:1031–1064.

Troiano, R. P., R. R. Briefel, M. D. Carroll, and K. Bialostosky. 2000. Energy and fat intakes of children and adolescents in the United States: Data from the National Health and Nutrition Examination Surveys. *Am. J. Clin. Nutr.* 72:1343S–1353S.

U.S. Food and Drug Administration, CFSAN/Office of Food Additive Safety. April 2007. FDA statement on European aspartame study. www.cfsan.fda.gov/~lrd/fpaspar2.html. Accessed May 2007.

Wannamethee SG, et al. Modifiable lifestyle factors and the metabolic syndrome in older men: effects of lifestyle changes. *Journal of the American Geriatrics Society*. 2006;54(12):1909-14.

Whiting, S. J., A. Healey, S. Psiak, R. Mirwald, K. Kowalski, and D. A. Bailey. 2001. Relationship between carbonated drinks and other low-nutrient-dense beverages and bone mineral content of adolescents. *Nutr. Res.* 21:1107–1115.

Wilkinson Enns, C., S. J. Mickle, and J. D. Goldman. 2002. Trends in food and nutrient intakes by children in the United States. *Family Econ. Nutr. Rev.* 14:56–68.

Chapter 5

Coyle, E.F. 1995. Substrate utilization during exercise in active people. *Am. J. Clin. Nutr.* 61: 968S–979S.

Hahn, R. A., and G. W. Heath. 1998. Cardiovascular disease risk factors and preventive practices among adults—United States, 1994: A behavioral risk factor atlas. *Morbid. Mortal. Wkly. Rep.* 47 (SS-5):35–69.

Harris, W. S. 1997. n-3 Fatty acids and serum lipoproteins: Human studies. *Am. J. Clin. Nutr.* 65 (Suppl.): 1645S–1654S.

Health Canada, Office of the Chief Scientist. 2005. Health Canada scientist leads trans fat research. www.hc-sc.gc.ca/ocs-besc/activ/consprod/trans_fat_e.htmL. Accessed August 2005.

Health Canada. 2007b. It's Your Health: Trans Fat. www.hc-sc.gc.ca/hl-vs/iyh-vsv/food-aliment/trans-eng.php. Accessed December 2007.

Health Canada. 2007c. Mercury in Fish. Consumption Advice: Making Informed Choices about Fish. www.hc-sc.gc.ca/fn-an/securit/chem-chim/mercur/cons-adv-etud_e.html. Accessed December 2007.

Health Canada. 2007a. Eating Well with Canada's Food Guide. www.hc-sc.gc.ca/fn-an/food-guide-aliment/index-eng.php. Accessed July 2008.

Health Canada. 2008. Trans fat monitoring program. Second set of trans fat monitoring data: July 2008. www.hc-sc.gc.ca/fn-an/nutrition/gras-trans-fats/tfa-age2-eng.php. Accessed August 2008.

Heart and Stroke Foundation of Canada. 2005, November 7. Cholesterol Article Updates.

Innis, S. 2004. Dietitians of Canada gives qualified support for replacing trans fat in the diet. www .dietitians.ca/members_only/resourceinventory. Accessed February 2005.

Institute of Medicine, Food and Nutrition Board. 2002. *Dietary Reference Intakes for Energy, Carbohydrate, Fiber, Fat, Fatty Acids, Cholesterol, Protein, and Amino Acids (Macronutrients)*. Washington, DC: National Academies Press.

International Food Information Council Foundation. April 2003. Functional foods fact sheet: Plant stanols and sterols. www.ific.org/publications/factsheets/sterolfs.cfm. Accessed September 2004.

Jebb, S. A, A. M. Prentice, G. R. Goldberg, P. R. Murgatroyd, A. E. Black, and W. A. Coward. 1996. Changes in macronutrient balance during over- and underfeeding assessed by 12-d continuous whole-body calorimetry. *Am. J. Clin. Nutr.* 64:259–266.

Kim, Y. I. 2001. Nutrition and cancer. In *Present Knowledge in Nutrition*, 8th ed., edited by B. A. Bowman and R. M. Russell. Washington, DC: International Life Sciences Institute Press.

Klingberg, S., L. Ellegard, I. Johansson, G. Hallmans, L. Weinehall, H. Andersson, and A. Winkvist. 2008. Inverse relation between dietary intake of naturally occurring plant sterols and serum cholesterol in northern Sweden. *Am. J. Clin. Nutr.* 87:993–1001.

Lau, V.W.Y., M. Journoud, and P.J.H. Jones. 2005. Plant sterols are efficacious in lowering plasma LDL and non-LDL cholesterol in hypercholesterolemic type 2 diabetic and nondiabetic persons. *Am. J. Clin. Nutr.* 81:1351–8.

Lichtenstein, A. H., and L. Van Horn. 1998. Very low fat diets. *Circulation* 98:935–939.

Manore, M. M., S. I. Barr, and G. E. Butterfield. 2000. Position of the American Dietetic Association, Dietitians of Canada, and the American College of Sports Medicine: Nutrition and athletic performance. *J. Am. Diet. Assoc.* 100:1543–1556.

Marangoni, A.G., S.H.J. Idziak, C. Vega, H. Batte, M. Ollivon, P.S. Jantzi, and J.W.E. Rush. 2007. Encapsulation-structuring of edible oil attenuates acute elevation of blood lipids and insulin in humans. *Soft Matter* 3:183–187.

National Institutes of Health (NIH). 2001. *Third Report of the National Cholesterol Education Program: Detection, Evaluation and Treatment of high blood cholesterol in adults (ATP:III)*. National Cholesterol Education Program, National Heart, Lung, and Blood Institute (NIH), May 2001. www.nhlbi.nih.gov/guidelines/cholesterol/atp3xsum.pdf.

Willett, W. C. 1999. Diet, nutrition and the prevention of cancer. In *Modern Nutrition in Health and Disease*, 9th ed., edited by M. E. Shils, J. A. Olsen, M. Shike, and A. C. Ross. Baltimore, MD: Williams & Wilkins, Publ.

Wootan, M. B. Lieberman, and W. Rosoesky. 1996. Trans: The phantom fat. *Nutrition Action Health Letter.* 23(7):10–13.

Chapter 6

Alekel, D. L., A. St. Germain, C. T. Peterson, K. B. Hanson, J. W. Stewart, and T. Toda. 2000. Isoflavone-rich soy protein isolate attenuates bone loss in the lumbar spine of perimenopausal women. *Am. J. Clin. Nutr.* 72:844–52.

Benson, J. E., K. A. Engelbert-Fenton, and P. A. Eisenman. 1996. Nutritional aspects of amenorrhea in the female athlete triad. *Int. J. Sport Nutr.* 6:124–145.

Bloch, A. S. 2005. Low-carbohydrate diets, pro: Time to rethink our current strategies. *Nutr. Clin. Prac.* 20:3–12.

Dietitians of Canada. 2003. Position of the American Dietetic Association and Dietitains of Canada: Vegetarian diets. *Can. J. Diet. Prac. Res.* 2003;64;62–81.

Fleming, R. M. 2000. The effect of high-protein diets on coronary blood flow. *Angiology* 51:817–26.

Fraser, G. E. 1999. Associations between diet and cancer, ischemic heart disease, and all-cause mortality in non-Hispanic white California Seventh Day Adventists. *Am. J. Clin. Nutr.* 70:532S–538S.

Health Canada. 2007. Canadian Community Health Survey, Cycle 2.2, Nutrition (2004) Nutrient Intakes from Food. Provincial, Regional and National Summary Data Tables, Volume 1. www.hc-sc.gc.ca/fn-an/pubs/cchs-nutri-escc/index-eng.php

Nutrient Intakes from Food. Provincial, Regional and National Summary Data Tables, Volume 1. Cat.: H164–45/1–2007E-PDF. www.hc-sc.gc.ca/fn-an/pubs/cchs-nutri-escc/index_e.html. Accessed April 2008.

Institute of Medicine, Food and Nutrition Board. 2002. *Dietary Reference Intakes for Energy, Carbohydrate, Fiber, Fat, Fatty Acids, Cholesterol, Protein, and Amino Acids (Macronutrients).* Washington, DC: National Academies Press.

Key, T. J., G. E. Fraser, M. Thorogood, P. N. Appleby, V. Beral, G. Reeves, M. L. Burr, J. Chang-Claude, R. Frentzel-Beyme, J. W. Kuzma, J. Mann, and K. McPherson. 1999. Mortality in vegetarians and nonvegetarians: Detailed findings from a collaborative analysis of five prospective studies. *Am. J. Clin. Nutr.* 70:516S–524S.

Kontessis, P., I. Bossinakou, L. Sarika, E. Iliopoulou, A. Papantoniou, R. Trevisan, D. Roussi, K. Stipsanelli, S. Grigorakis, and A. Souvatzoglou. 1995. Renal, metabolic, and hormonal responses to proteins of different origin in normotensive, non-proteinuric type 1 diabetic patients. *Diabetes Care* 18:1233–40.

Kushner, R. F. 2005. Low-carbohydrate diets, con: The mythical Phoenix or credible science? *Nutr. Clin. Prac.* 20:13–16.

Lemon, P. W. 2000. Beyond the Zone: Protein needs of active individuals. *J. Am. Coll. Nutr.* 19 (5 suppl.): 513S–521S.

Manore, M., and J. Thompson. 2000. *Sport Nutrition for Health and Performance.* Champaign, IL: Human Kinetics.

Merck Manuals. 2005. Protein Energy Malnutrition. www.merck.com/mrkshared/mmanual/section1/chapter2/2c.jsp. Accessed July 2005.

Messina, M. J. 1999. Legumes and soybeans: Overview of their nutritional profiles and health effects. *Am. J. Clin. Nutr.* 70 (suppl.): 439S–450S.

Messina, M., and V. Messina. 1996. *The Dietitian's Guide to Vegetarian Diets.* Gaithersburg, MD: Aspen Publishers.

Messina, V., V. Melina, and R. Mangels. 2003. A new food guide for North American vegetarians. *Can J. Diet. Prac. Res.* 64:82–86.

Munger, R. G., J. R. Cerhan, and B. C.-H. Chiu. 1999. Prospective study of dietary protein intake and risk of hip fracture in postmenopausal women. *Am. J. Clin. Nutr.* 69:147–52.

Musick, J. A., M. M. Harbin, S. A. Berkeley, G. H. Burgess, A. M. Eklund, L. Findley, R. G. Gilmore, J. T. Golden, D. S. Ha, G. R. Huntsman, J. C. McGovern, S. J. Parker, S. G. Poss, E. Sala, T. W. Schmidt, G. R. Sedberry, H. Weeks, and S. G. Wright. 2000. Marine, estuarine, and diadromous fish stocks at risk of extinction in North America (exclusive of Pacific Salmonids). *Fisheries* 25:6–30.

Phillips, R. L., and D. A. Snowdon. 1983. Association of meat and coffee use with cancers of the large bowel, breast, and prostate among Seventh-Day Adventists: preliminary results. *Cancer Res.* 43 (suppl.): 2403S–2408S.

Poortmans, J. R., and O. Dellalieux. 2000. Do regular high protein diets have potential health risks on kidney function in athletes? *Int. J. Sport Nutr.* 10:28–38.

Schaafsma, G. 2000. The protein digestibility–corrected amino acid score. *J Nutr* 130: 1865S–1867S.

Shai, I., D. Schwarzfuchs, Y. Henkin, D. R. Shahar, S. Witkow, I. Greenberg, R. Golan, D. Fraser, A. Bolotin, H. Vardi, O. Tangi-Rozental, R. Zuk-Ramot, B. Sarusi, D. Brickner, Z. Schwartz, E. Sheiner, R. Marko, E. Katorza, J. Thiery, G. M. Fielder, M. Bluher, M. Stumvoll, and M. J. Stampfer. 2008. Weight loss with a low-carbohydrate, Mediterranean, or low-fat diet. *NEJM* 359:229-241.

Statistics Canada. 2002. Endocrine, nutritional metabolic disease, by age, group and sex. www.statcan.ca/english/freepub/84–208-XIE/2002/tables/table4.htm. Accessed July 2005.

Taubes, G. 2002. What if fat doesn't make you fat? *The New York Times Magazine,* July 7, section 6.

Volek, J. S., M. J. Sharman, A. L. Gomez, C. DiPasquale, C. Roti, M. Pumerantz, A. Kraemer, and W. J. Kraemer. 2004. Comparison of a very low-carbohydrate and low-fat diet on fasting lipids, LDL subclasses, insulin resistance, and postprandial lipemic responses in overweight women. *J Am. Coll. Nutr.* 23(2):177–84.

Wegman, M. E. 2001. Infant mortality in the 20th century, dramatic but uneven progress. *J. Nutr.* 131 (suppl.):401S–408S.

World Bank (The). Health, Nutrition, and Population. 2005. *HNPFlash Newsletter* 54. www.worldbank.org/nutrition. Accessed August 2005.

World Health Organization. 2000. Protein energy malnutrition. www.emro.who.int/nutrition/PDF/Protein_Malnutrition.pdf. Accessed June 2006.

Yancy, W. S., M. K. Olsen, J. R. Gyton, R. P Bakst, and E. C. Westman. 2004. A low-carbohydrate, ketogenic diet versus a low-fat diet to treat obesity and hyperlipidemia: A randomized, controlled trial. *Ann. Intern. Med.* 140:769–777.

Chapter 7

American College of Sports Medicine (ACSM). 1996. Exercise and fluid replacement. *Med. Sci. Sports Exerc.* 28:i–vii.

American College of Sports Medicine (ACSM). 2000. Nutrition and athletic performance. *Med. Sci. Sports Exerc.* 32:2130–2145.

Appel, L. J., T. J. Moore, E. Obarzanek, W. M. Vollmer, L. P. Svetkey, F. M. Sacks, G. A. Bray, T. M. Vogt, J. A. Cutler, M. M. Windhauser, P.-H. Lin, and N. Karanja. 1997. A clinical trial of the effects of dietary patterns on blood pressure. *New Engl. J. Med.* 336:1117–1124.

Bilzon, J. L., A. J. Allsopp, and C. Williams. 2000. Short-term recovery from prolonged constant pace running in a warm environment: The effectiveness of a carbohydrate-electrolyte solution. *Eur. J. Appl. Physiol.* 82:305–312.

Canadian Hypertension Education Program. 2008. Hypertension: 2008 Public Recommendations. www.hypertension.ca/bpc/wp-content/uploads/2008/02/2008publicrecommendations.pdf. Accessed April 2008.

Cohen, A. J., and F. J. Roe. 2000. Review of risk factors for osteoporosis with particular reference to a possible aetiological role of dietary salt. *Food Chem. Toxicol.* 38:237–253.

Davis, D. P., J. S. Videen, A. Marino, G. M. Vilke, J. V. Dunford, S. P. Van Camp, and L. G. Maharam. 2001. Exercise-associated hyponatremia in marathon runners: A two-year experience. *J. Emerg. Med.* 21:47–57.

Galloway, S. D., and R. J. Maughan. 2000. The effects of substrate and fluid provision on thermoregulatory and metabolic responses to prolonged exercise in a hot environment. *J. Sports Sci.* 18:339–351.

Garriguet, D. 2007. Sodium consumption at all ages. Statistics Canada, Catalogue 83–003. *Health Reports* 18:47–52.

Health Canada. 2006. It's Your Health: Stroke. www.hc-sc.gc.ca/iyh-vsv/diseases-maladies/stroke-vasculaire_e.html. Accessed April 2008.

Health Canada. 2007. Water quality. www.hc-sc.gc.ca/fn-an/securit/facts-faits/faqs_bottle_water-eau_embouteillee_e.html. Accessed April 2008.

Heart and Stroke Foundation of Canada. 2008. High blood pressure. www.heartandstroke.com. Accessed April 2008.

Institute of Medicine. 2004. *Dietary Reference Intakes for Water, Potassium, Sodium, Chloride, and Sulfate.* Washington, DC: The National Academies Press.

International Council of Bottled Water Associations. n.d. Global bottled water statistics 2000–2003. www.icbwa.org/2000-2003_Zenith_and_Beverage_Marketing_Stats.pdf. Accessed August 2008.

International Food Information Council Foundation. 2005. Sodium in food and health. www.ific.org. Accessed March 2005.

Manore, M., and J. Thompson. 2000. *Sport Nutrition for Health and Performance.* Champaign, IL: Human Kinetics.

National Research Council. Food and Nutrition Board. 1989. *Recommended Dietary Allowances.* 10th ed. Washington, DC: National Academies Press.

Natural Resources Canada. 2004. The Atlas of Canada: Groundwater. atlas.nrcan.gc.ca/site/english/maps/freshwater/distribution/groundwater/1. Accessed August 2008.

Picard, A. Sports drinks even worse for your teeth than pop, study finds. *Globe and Mail,* Wednesday, March 23, 2005: A19.

Sacks, F. M., L. P. Svetkey, W. M. Vollmer, L. J. Appel, G. A. Bray, D. Harsha, E. Obarzanek, P. R. Conlin, E. R. Miller III, D. G. Simons-Morton,

N. Karanja, and P.-H. Lin. 2001. Effects on blood pressure of reduced dietary sodium and the Dietary Approaches to Stop Hypertension (DASH) diet. *New Engl. J. Med.* 344:3–10.

Speedy, D. B., T. D. Noakes, I. R. Rogers, J. M. Thompson, R. G. Campbell, J. A. Kuttner, D. R. Boswell, S. Wright, and M. Hamlin. 1999. Hyponatremia in ultradistance triathletes. *Med. Sci. Sports Exerc.* 31:809–815.

Statistics Canada, "Canadians' Eating Habits 2004," 2006, no. 2, Cat. No. 82-620-XIE, July 6, 2006, page 39, available at www.statcan.gc.ca/pub/ 82-620-m/82-620-m2006002-eng.pdf. Accessed Jan. 2008.

Touyz, R. M., N. Campbell, A. Logan, N. Gledhill, R. Petrella, and R. Padwal. 2004. The 2004 Canadian recommendations for the management of hypertension: Part III—Lifestyle modifications to prevent and control hypertension. *Can. J. Cardiol.* 20(1):55–59.

Chapter 8

Age-Related Eye Disease Study Research Group. 2001a. A randomized, placebo-controlled, clinical trial of high-dose supplementation with vitamins C and E, beta-carotene, and zinc for age-related macular degeneration and vision loss: AREDS Report No. 8. *Arch. Ophthalmol.* 119:1417–1436.

Age-Related Eye Disease Study Research Group. 2001b. A randomized, placebo-controlled, clinical trial of high-dose supplementation with vitamins C and E and beta-carotene for age-related cataract and vision loss: AREDS Report No. 9. *Arch. Ophthalmol.* 119:1439–1452.

Ahmed, F. 1999. Vitamin A deficiency in Bangladesh: A review and recommendations for improvement. *Public Health Nutr.* 2:1–14.

Albanes, D., O. P. Heinonen, J. K. Huttunen, P. R. Taylor, J. Virtamo, B. K. Edwards, J. Haapakoski, M. Rautalahti, A. M. Hartman, J. Palmgren, and P. Greenwald. 1995. Effects of a-tocopherol and b-carotene supplements on cancer incidence in the Alpha-Tocopherol Beta-Carotene Cancer Prevention Study. *Am. J. Clin. Nutr.* 62 (suppl.):1427S–1430S.

Alpha-Tocopherol, Beta-Carotene Cancer Prevention Study Group, The. (The ATBC Study Group). 1994. The effect of vitamin E and beta carotene on the incidence of lung cancer and other cancers in male smokers. *N. Engl. J. Med.* 330:1029–1035.

Bender, D. 2002. Daily doses of multivitamin tablets. *BMJ*, 325:173–174.

Blot, W. J., J.-Y. Li, P. R. Taylor, W. Guo, S. M. Dawsey, and B. Li. 1995. The Linxian trials: Mortality rates by vitamin-mineral intervention group. *Am. J. Clin. Nutr.* 62 (suppl.): 1424S–1426S.

Burri, B. J. 1997. Beta-carotene and human health: A review of current research. *Nutr. Res.* 17:547–580.

Canadian Cancer Society. 2008. General cancer statistics for 2008. www.cancer.ca/ccs/internet/ standard/0,2283,3172_14423__langId-en, 00.html. Accessed May 2008.

Chylack, L. T. Jr., N. P. Brown, A. Bron, M. Hurst, W. Kopcke, U. Thien, and W. Schalch. 2002. The Roche European American Cataract Trial (REACT): A randomized clinical trial to investigate the efficacy of an oral antioxidant micronutrient mixture to slow progression of age-related cataract. *Ophthalmic Epidemiol.* 9:49–80.

Clark, L. C., B. Dalkin, A. Krongrad, G. F. Combs Jr., B. W. Turnbull, E. H. Slate, R. Witherington, J. H. Herlong, E. Janosko, D. Carpenter, C. Borosso, S. Falk, and J. Rounder. 1998. Decreased incidence of prostate cancer with selenium supplementation: Results of a double-blind cancer prevention trial. *Br. J. Urol.* 81:730–734.

Dancho, C., and M. M. Manore. 2001. Dietary supplement information on the World Wide Web: Sorting fact from fiction. *ACSM's Health and Fitness J.* 5:7–12.

de Ferranti, S., and N. Rifai. 2002. C-reactive protein and cardiovascular disease: A review of risk prediction and interventions. *Clinica Chimica Acta* 317:1–15.

Delcourt, C., J. P. Cristol, F. Tessier, C. L. Léger, B. Descomps, and L. Papoz. 1999. Age-related macular degeneration and antioxidant status in the POLA study. POLA Study Group. Pathologies Oculaires Liées à l'Age. *Arch. Ophthalmol.* 117:1384–1390.

Fairfield, K., and R. H. Fletcher. 2002. Vitamins for chronic disease prevention in adults: Scientific review. *JAMA.*, 287:3116–3126.

Ford, E. S., and A. Sowell. 1999. Serum alpha-tocopherol status in the United States population: Findings from the Third National Health and Nutrition Examination Survey. *Am. J. Epidemiol.* 150(3): 290–300.

Gale, C. R., N. F. Hall, D. I. Phillips, and C. N. Martyn. 2001. Plasma antioxidant vitamins and carotenoids and age-related cataract. *Ophthalmology* 108:1992–1998.

Geleijnse, J. M., L. J. Launer, D. A. M. van der Kuip, A. Hofman, and J. C. M. Witteman. 2002. Inverse association of tea and flavonoid intakes with incident myocardial infarction: The

Rotterdam Study. *Am. J. Clin. Nutr.* 75:880–886.

Greenwald, P., C. K. Clifford, and J. A. Milner. 2001. Diet and cancer prevention. *Eur. J. Cancer* 37:948–965.

Gutteridge, J. M. C., and B. Halliwell. 1994. *Antioxidants in Nutrition, Health, and Disease.* Oxford, UK: Oxford University Press.

Haider, J., and T. Demissie. 1999. Malnutrition and xerophthalmia in rural communities of Ethiopia. *East Afr. Med. J.* 76:590–593.

Health Canada. 2003. Natural Health Products Regulations, Part II. *Canada Gazette,* vol. 137, no. 13.

Heart and Stroke Foundation of Canada. 2003. The Growing Burden of Heart Disease and Stroke in Canada 2003. www.cvdinfobase.ca/cvdbook/CVD_En03.pdf. Accessed July 2004.

Heart and Stroke Foundation of Canada. 2008. Statistics. www.heartandstroke.com/site/c.ikIQLcMWJtE/b.3483991/k.34A8/Statistics.htm#heartdisease. Accessed May 2008.

Heart Outcomes Prevention Evaluation Study Investigators, The (The HOPE Investigators). 2000. Vitamin E supplementation and cardiovascular events in high-risk patients. *N. Engl. J. Med.* 342:154–160.

Heinonen, O. P., D. Albanes, J. Virtamo, P. R. Taylor, J. K. Huttunen, A. M. Hartman, J. Haapakoski, N. Malila, M. Rautalahti, S. Ripatti, H. Maepaa, L. Teerenhovi, L. Koss, M. Virolainen, and B. K. Edwards. 1998. Prostate cancer and supplementation with a-tocopherol and b-carotene: Incidence and mortality in a controlled trial. *J. Natl. Cancer Inst.* 90:440–446.

Hemila, H. 1997. Vitamin C intake and susceptibility to the common cold. *Br. J. Nutr.* 77:59–72.

Institute of Medicine. 2000. *Dietary Reference Intakes for Vitamin C, Vitamin E, Selenium, and Carotenoids.* Washington, DC: The National Academies Press.

Josefson, D. 2002. Popping a multivitamin daily can keep disease at bay. *BMJ* 324:1544.

Joshipura, K. J., F. B. Hu, J. E. Manson, M. J. Stampfer, E. B. Rimm, F. E. Speizer, G. Colditz, A. Ascherio, B. Rosner, D. Spiegelman, and W. C. Willett. 2001. The effect of fruit and vegetable intake on risk for coronary heart disease. *Ann. Intern. Med.* 134:1106–1114.

Liu, S., I.-M. Lee, U. Ajani, S. R. Cole, J. E. Buring, and J. E. Manson. 2001. Intake of vegetables rich in carotenoids and risk of coronary heart disease in men: The Physicians' Health Study. *Intl. J. Epidemiol.* 30:130–135.

Livrea, M. A., L. Tesoriere, A. Bongiorno, A. M. Pintaudi, M. Ciaccio, and A. Riccio. 1995. Contribution of vitamin A to the oxidation resistance of human low-density lipoproteins. *Free Radic. Biol. Med.* 18:401–409.

Puuponen-Pimiä, R., S. T. Häkkinen, M. Aarni, T. Suortti, A-M. Lampi, M. Eurola, V. Piironen. A. M. Nuutila, K-M. Oksman-Caldentey. 2003. Blanching and long-term freezing affect various bioactive compounds of vegetables in different ways. *J. of Sc. and Ag.* 83 (14):1389–1402.

Thune I., and A. S. Furberg. 2001. Physical activity and cancer risk: Dose-response and cancer, all sites and site-specific. *Med. Sci. Sports Exerc.* (suppl.) 33:S530–S550.

U.S. Department of Agriculture (USDA), Agricultural Research Service. 1998. USDA–NCC Carotenoid Database for U.S. Foods. Nutrient Data Laboratory homepage, www.nal.usda.gov/fnic/foodcomp. Accessed August 2002.

U.S. Food and Drug Administration (FDA). 1998. An FDA guide to dietary supplements. *FDA Consumer Magazine.* September/October. www.fda.gov/fdac/features/1998/598_guid.html. Accessed August 2002.

West S., S. Vitale, J. Hallfrisch, B. Munoz, D. Muller, S. Bressler, and N. M. Bressler. 1994. Are antioxidants or supplements protective for age-related macular degeneration? *Arch. Ophthalmol.* 112:222–227.

Wooltorton, E. 2003. Too much of a good thing? Toxic effects of vitamin and mineral supplements. *Can. Med. Assoc. J.* 169:47–48.

World Cancer Research Fund/American Institute for Cancer Research. 2007. *Food, Nutrition, Physical Activity, and the Prevention of Cancer: A Global Perspective.* Washington, DC:AICR.

World Health Organization (WHO). 2002. Vitamin A. www.who.int/vaccines/en/vitaminamain.shtml. Accessed October 2002.

Zhang S., D. J. Hunter, M. R. Forman, B. A. Rosner, F. E. Speizer, G. A. Colditz, J. E. Manson, S. E. Hankinson, and W. C. Willett. 1999. Dietary carotenoids and vitamins A, C, and E and risk of breast cancer. *J. Natl. Cancer Inst.* 91:547–556.

Chapter 9

Arthur, P., and S. Zlotkin. 2002. Reply to NW Solomons and K Schumann. *Am. J. Clin. Nutr.* 76:693–694. www.ajcn.org. Accessed June 2005.

Ball, J. W., and R. C. Bindler. 2003. *Pediatric Nursing: Caring for Children.* Upper Saddle River, NJ: Pearson Education.

Barrett, S. 2004. Be wary of coral calcium and Robert Barefoot. *Quackwatch*, www.quackwatch.org/01QuackeryRelatedTopics/DSH/coral.html. Accessed April 2008.

Bell, J. 2004. Good things come in small packages. *Childview* (Spring) vol. 16, no. 4: 9–13.

Canadian Cancer Society. 2007. Canadian Cancer Society announces vitamin D recommendation. www.cancer.ca/ccs/internet/mediareleaselist. Accessed January 2008.

Canadian Multicentre Osteoporosis Study. 2004. *Camoscope* 8 (January). www.camos.org/Camoscope_Jan04_ENG.pdf. Accessed April 2005.

Dawson-Hughes, B., and S. S. Harris. 2002. Calcium intake influences the association of protein intake with rates of bone loss in elderly men and women. *Am. J. Clin. Nutr.* 75:773–779.

Felson, D. T., Y. Zhang, M. T. Hannan, W. B. Kannel, and D. P. Kiel. 1995. Alcohol intake and bone mineral density in elderly men and women: The Framingham Study. *Am. J. Epidemiol.* 142:485–492.

Feskanich, D., S. A. Korrick, S. L. Greenspan, H. N. Rosen, and G. A. Colditz. 1999. Moderate alcohol consumption and bone density among post-menopausal women. *J. Women's Health* 8:65–73.

Health Canada. 2008b. Fluoride and human health. www.hc-sc.gc.ca/hl-vs/iyh-vsv/environ/fluor-eng.php. Accessed August 2008.

Health Canada. 2008a. Findings and recommendations of the Fluoride Expert Panel (January 2007). www.hc-sc.gc.ca/ewh-semt/pubs/water-eau/2008-fluoride-fluorure/index-eng.php. Accessed August 2008.

Health Canada. 2004. Vitamin D Supplementation for Breastfed Infants - 2004 Health Canada Recommendation. www.hc-sc.gc.ca/fn-an/nutrition/child-enfant/infant-nourisson/vita_d_supp_e.html. Accessed April 2008.

Health Canada. 2007. Vitamin D and Health: Information Update. www.hc-sc.gc.ca/ahc-asc/media/advisories-avis/_2007/2007_130_e.html. Accessed April 2008.

Heaney, R. P., and K. Rafferty. 2006. The settling problem in calcium-fortified soybean drinks. *J. Am. Diet. Assoc.* 106:1753.

Holbrook, T. L., and E. Barrett-Connor. 1993. A prospective study of alcohol consumption and bone mineral density. *BMJ* 306:1506–1509.

Holick, M. F. 2004. Sunlight and vitamin D for bone health and prevention of autoimmune diseases, cancers, and cardiovascular disease. *Am. J. Clin. Nutr.* 80:1678S–1688S.

IFIC Foundation. 2007. Food Insight. Vitamin D in the spotlight: An expanded role emerges for promoting health. Washington, DC: International Food Information Council (IFIC) Foundation.

Institute of Medicine, Food and Nutrition Board. 1997. *Dietary Reference Intakes for Calcium, Phosphorus, Magnesium, Vitamin D, and Fluoride.* Washington, DC: National Academies Press.

Institute of Medicine, Food and Nutrition Board. 2002. *Dietary Reference Intakes for Vitamin A, Vitamin K, Arsenic, Boron, Chromium, Copper, Iodine, Iron, Manganese, Molybdenum, Nickel, Silicon, Vanadium, and Zinc.* Washington, DC: National Academies Press.

International Osteoporosis Foundation. 2003. The facts about osteoporosis and its impact. www.osteofound.org/press_centre/fact_sheet.html. Accessed December 2003.

Iuliano-Burns, S., S. J. Whiting, R. A. Faulkner, and D. A. Bailey. 1999. Levels, sources, and seasonality of dietary calcium intake in children and adolescents enrolled in the University of Saskatchewan Pediatric Bone Mineral Accrual Study. *Nutr. Res.* 19:1471–1483.

Jackson, R.D., A.Z. LaCroix, M. Gass, R.B. Wallace, J. Robbins, C.E. Lewis et al. 2006. Calcium plus vitamin D supplementation and the risk of fractures. *N. Engl. J. Med.* 354:669–683.

Keller, J. L., A. J. Lanou, and N. D. Barnard. 2002. The consumer cost of calcium from food and supplements. *J. Am. Diet. Assoc.* 102:1669–1671.

Laitinen, K., M. Valimaki, and P. Keto. 1991. Bone mineral density measured by dual-energy x-ray absorptiometry in healthy Finnish women. *Calcif. Tissue Int.* 48:224–231.

Lappe, J.M., D. Travers-Gustafson, K.M. Davies, R.R. Recker, and R.P. Heaney. 2007. Vitamin D and calcium supplementation reduces cancer risk: Results of a randomized trail. *Am. J. Clin. Nutr.* 85:1586–1591.

Massey, L. K. 2001. Is caffeine a risk factor for bone loss in the elderly? *Am. J. Clin. Nutr.* 74:569–570.

McGartland, C., P. J. Robson, G. Cran, M. J. Savage, D. Watkins, M. Rooney, and C. Boreham. 2003. Carbonated soft drink consumption and bone mineral density in adolescence: The Northern Ireland Young Hearts Project. *J. Bone Min. Res.* 18:1563–1569.

Osteoporosis Canada. 2007a. Osteoporosis Update: A Practical Guide for Physicians. www.osteoporosis.ca/

local/files/health_professionals/pdfs/Osteo1103Fal
l07_WebEdit.pdf. Accessed January 2008.

Osteoporosis Canada. 2007b. 25 Facts About
Osteoporosis. www.osteoporosis.ca/english/
Media%20Room/Background/2007_25facts/
default.asp?s=1. Accessed January 2008.

Osteoporosis Canada. 2007c. Zoledronic acid
(Aclasta) approved for osteoporosis.
www.osteoporosis.ca/english/news/aclasta-
short-nov1/default.asp?s=1. Accessed January
2008.

Osteoporosis Canada. 2007d. 10 top things you need
to know about osteoporosis. www.osteoporosis.ca/
english/Media%20Room/Background/
Top%2010/default.asp?s=1. Accessed January
2008.

Raiten, D. J., and M. F. Picciano. 2004. Vitamin D
and health in the 21st century: Bone and beyond.
Executive Summary. *Am. J. Clin. Nutr.* 80(suppl):
1673S–1677S.

Rapuri, P. B., J. C. Gallagher, H. K. Kinyamu, and
K. L. Ryschon. 2001. Caffeine intake increases the
rate of bone loss in elderly women and interacts
with vitamin D receptor genotypes. *Am. J. Clin.
Nutr.* 74:694–700.

Rapuri, P. B., J. C. Gallagher, K. E. Balhorn, and K. L.
Ryschon. 2000. Alcohol intake and bone
metabolism in elderly women. *Am. J. Clin. Nutr.*
72:1206–1213.

Ross, E. A., N. J. Szabo, and I. R. Tebbett. 2000.
Lead content of calcium supplements. *JAMA*
284:1425–1433.

Rucker, D., J. A. Allan, G. H. Fick, and D. A. Hanley.
2002. Vitamin D insufficiency in a population of
healthy Western Canadians. *Can. Med. Assoc. J.*
166: 1517–1524.

South-Pal, J. E. 2001. Osteoporosis: Part II.
Nonpharmacologic and Pharmacologic Treatment.
Am. Fam. Physician 63:1121–1128.

Statistics Canada. 2007. Canadian Community Health
Survey, Cycle 2.2, Nutrition (2004) – Share File
Volume 1, Table 12.13. Calcium (mg/d): Usual
intakes from food by DRI age-sex group,
household population, Canada excluding
territories, 2004. www.hc-sc.gc.ca/
fn-an/pubs/cchs-nutri-escc/tab12_calcium_e
.html#12_13. Accessed January 2008.

Tucker, K. L., H. Chen, M. T. Hannan, L. A.
Cupples, P. W. F. Wilson, D. Felson, and D. P. Kiel.
2002. Bone mineral density and dietary
patterns in older adults: The Framingham
Osteoporosis Study. *Am. J. Clin. Nutr.*
76:245–252.

Tucker, K. L., M. T. Hannan, H. Chen, L. A. Cupples,
P. W. F. Wilson, and D. P. Kiel. 1999. Potassium,
magnesium, and fruit and vegetable intakes are
associated with greater bone mineral density in
elderly men and women. *Am. J. Clin. Nutr.*
69:727–736.

Vatanparast, H., E. Lo, C. J. Henry, and S. J. Whiting.
2006. Trends of beverage intake from 1991–2003
in Grade 9 students living in Saskatoon show
substitution of milk by non-carbonated soft drinks.
Nutr. Rev. 26:325–329.

Whiting, S. J., A. Healey, S. Psiuk, R. Mirwald,
K. Kowalski, and D. A. Bailey. 2001.
Relationship between carbonated and other low
nutrient dense beverages and bone mineral
content of adolescents. *Nutr. Res.* 21:
1107–1115.

Whiting, S. J., H. Vatanparast, A. Baxter-Jones,
R. A. Faulkner, R. Mirwald, and D. A. Bailey.
2004. Factors that affect bone mineral accrual
in the adolescent growth spurt. *J. Nutr.* 134:
696S–700S.

Wyshak, G. 2000. Teenaged girls, carbonated beverage
consumption, and bone fractures. *Arch. Pediatr.
Adolesc. Med.* 154:610–613.

Wyshak, G., and R. E. Frisch. 1994. Carbonated
beverages, dietary calcium, the dietary calcium/
phosphorus ratio, and bone fractures in girls and
boys. *J. Adolesc. Health* 15:210–215.

Wyshak, G., R. E. Frisch, T. E. Albright, N. L.
Albright, I. Schiff, and J. Witschi. 1989.
Nonalcoholic carbonated beverage consumption
and bone fractures among women former college
athletes. *J. Orthop. Res.* 7:91–99.

Zlotkin, S., P. Arthur, K. A. Antwi, and G. Yeung.
2001. Treatment of anemia with microencapsulated
ferrous fumarate plus ascorbic acid supplied as
Sprinkles. *Am. J. Clin. Nutr.* 74:791–795.

Chapter 10

Bacon, B. R., J. K. Olynyk, E. M. Brunt, R. S. Britton,
and R. K. Wolff. 1999. HFE genotype in patients
with hemochromatosis and other liver diseases.
Ann. Intern. Med. 130:953–962.

Beresford, S. A., and C. J. Boushey. 1997.
Homocysteine, folic acid, and cardiovascular
disease risk. In *Preventive Nutrition: The
Comprehensive Guide for Health Professionals,*
edited by A. Bendich and R. J. Deckelbaum.
Totowa, NJ: Humana Press.

Bernstein, L. 2000, February. Dementia without a
cause: Lack of vitamin B$_{12}$ can cause dementia.

Discover. www.discover.com/issues/feb-00/ departments/featdementia. Accessed March 2004.

Booth, S. L., and J. W. Suttie. 1998. Dietary intake and adequacy of vitamin K. *J. Nutr.* 128: 785–788.

Feskanich, D., S. A. Korrick, S. L. Greenspan, H. N. Rosen, and G. A. Colditz. 1999. Moderate alcohol consumption and bone density among post-menopausal women. *J. Women's Health* 8:65–73.

Grantham-McGregor, S., and C. Ani. 2001. A review of studies on the effect of iron deficiency on cognitive development in children. *J. Nutr.* 131:649S–668S.

Institute of Medicine, Food and Nutrition Board. 1998. *Dietary Reference Intakes for Thiamin, Riboflavin, Niacin, Vitamin B$_6$, Folate, Vitamin B$_{12}$, Pantothenic Acid, Biotin, and Choline*. Washington, DC: National Academies Press.

Institute of Medicine, Food and Nutrition Board. 2001. *Dietary Reference Intakes for Vitamin A, Vitamin K, Arsenic, Boron, Chromium, Copper, Iodine, Iron, Manganese, Molybdenum, Nickel, Silicon, Vanadium, and Zinc*. Washington, DC: National Academies Press.

Jackson, J. L., E. Lesho, and C. Peterson. 2000. Zinc and the common cold: A meta-analysis revisited. *J. Nutr.* 130:1512S–1515S.

Mayer, E. L., D. W. Jacobsen, and K. Robinson. 1996. Homocysteine and coronary atherosclerosis. *J. Am. Coll. Cardiol.* 27:517–527.

Prasad, A. 1996. Zinc: The biology and therapeutics of an ion. *Ann. Intern. Med.* 125:142–143.

Sanders, L.M. and S.H. Zeisel. 2007. Choline: Dietary requirements and role in brain development. *Nutr. Today* 42:181–186.

Shils, M.E., J.A. Olson, M. Shike, and A.C. Ross. 1999. *Modern Nutrition in Health and Disease*, 9th ed. Philadelphia: Lippincott Williams & Wilkins.

U.S. Food and Drug Administration. 1997. Preventing Iron Poisoning in Children. FDA Backgrounder. www.fda.gov/opacom/ backgrounders/ironbg.html. Accessed January 2004.

World Health Organization. 2000. Pellagra: Its Prevention and Control in Major Emergencies. WHO/NHD 00.10. www.wpro.who.int/ internet/files/eha/toolkit/Technical%20Guidelin es/Nutrition/Pellagra%20in%20Emergencies.pdf. Accessed August 2008.

World Health Organization. 2003. Nutrition. Micronutrient Deficiencies. Battling iron deficiency anemia. www.who.int/nut/ida.htm. Accessed January 2004.

Chapter 11

American Dietetic Association. 2001. Send fad diets down the drain. www.eatright.org. Accessed February 2004.

Arnst, C. 2004. Let them eat cake—if they want to. *Business Week*. February 23, 110–111.

Bouchard, C., A. Tremblay, J. P. Després, A. Nadeau, P. J. Lupien, G. Thériault, J. Dussault, S. Moorjani, S. Pinault, and G. Fournier. 1990. The response to long-term overfeeding in identical twins. *N. Engl. J. Med.* 322: 1477–1482.

Broeder, C.E., J. Qundry, K. Brittingham, L. Panton, J. Thompson, S. Appakondu, K. Brel, R. Byrd, J. Douglas, C. Earnest, C. Mitchell, M. Olson, T. Roy, and C. Yarlagadda. 2000. The Andro Project: Physiological and hormonal influences of androstenedione supplementation in men 35 to 65 years old participating in a high-intensity resistance training program. *Arch. Int. Med.* 160: 3093–3104.

Brown, G. A., M. D. Vukovich, T. A. Reifenrath, N. L. Uhl, K. A. Parsons, R. L. Sharp, and D. S. King. 2000. Effects of anabolic precursors on serum testosterone concentrations and adaptations to resistance training in young men. *Intl. J. Sport Nutr. Ex. Metab.* 10:340–359.

Center for Food Safety and Applied Nutrition. U.S. Food and Drug Administration. 2004. Questions and Answers: Androstenedione. www.cfsan.fda.gov/~dms/androqa.html. Accessed August 2005.

Christensen, R., P.K. Kristensen, E.M. Bartels, H. Bliddal, and A. Astrup. 2007. Efficacy and safety of the weight-loss drug rimonabant: a meta-analysis of randomized trials. *The Lancet*, 370:1706–1713.

de Onis M., and M. Blössner. 2000. Prevalence and trends of overweight among preschool children in developing countries. *Am. J. Clin. Nutr.* 72:1032–1039.

Dietz, W. H. 1994. Critical periods in childhood for the development of obesity. *Am. J. Clin. Nutr.* 59:955–959.

Emme. 2004. Bio profile. www.safesearching .com/officialemme/allaboutemme/bio.shtml. Accessed February 2004.

Gaesser, G. A. 1999. Thinness and weight loss: beneficial or detrimental to longevity? *Med. Sci. Sports Exerc.* 31:1118–1128.

Gallagher, D. 2004. Overweight and obesity cut-offs and their relation to metabolic disorders in Koreans/Asians. *Obes. Res.* 12:440–441.

Gunnell, D. J., S. J. Frankel, K. Nanchahal, T. J. Peters, and G. Davey Smith. 1998. Childhood obesity and adult cardiovascular mortality: A 57-y follow-up study based on the Boyd Orr cohort. *Am. J. Clin. Nutr.* 67:1111–1118.

Health Canada. 2003. Health Canada Reminds Canadians of the Dangers of *Ephedra*/Ephedrine Products. www.hc-sc.gc.ca/ahc-asc/media/advisories-avis/2003/2003_43_e.html. Accessed July 2005.

Health Canada. 2005. Canadian Guidelines for Body Weight Classification in Adults. www.hc-sc.gc.ca/fn-an/nutrition/weights-poids/guide-ld-adult/qa-qr-pub-eng.php#5. Accessed August 2008.

Health Canada. 2007. Contraindicated Use of Sibutramine and Cardiovascular Adverse Reactions. www.docguide.com/news/content.nsf/news/852571020057CCF68525737500703C4A. Accessed May 2008.

Hellerstein, M., K. Christiansen, and S. Kaempfer. 1991. Measurement of de novo hepatic lipogenesis in humans using stable isotopes. *J. Clin. Invest.* 87:1841–1852.

Heyward, V. H., and L. M. Stolarczyk. 1996. *Applied Body Composition Assessment.* Champaign, IL: Human Kinetics.

Hill, J. O., J. Hauptman, J. W. Anderson, K. Fujioka, P. M. O'Neil, D. K. Smith, J. H. Zavoral, and L. J. Aronne. 1999. Orlistat, a lipase inhibitor, for weight maintenance after conventional dieting: a 1-y study. *Am. J. Clin. Nutr.* 69:1108–1116.

Himes, J. H. 2001. Prevalence of individuals with skinfolds too large to measure. *Am. J. Public Health* 91:154–155.

Janssen, I., P.T. Katzmarzyk, and R.Ross. 2004. Waist circumference and not body mass index explains obesity-related health risk. *Am. J. Clin. Nutr.* 79:379–384.

Joyner, M. J. 2000. Over-the-counter supplements and strength training. *Exerc. Sport Sci. Rev.* 28:2–3.

Kieffer, T. J., and J. F. Habener. 2000. The adipoinsular axis: Effects of leptin on pancreatic β-cells. *Am. J. Phys. Endo. Metab.* 278:E1–E14.

Koh-Banerjee, P., N. F. Chu, D. Spiegelman, B. Rosner, G. Colditz, W. Willett, and E. Rimm. 2003. Prospective study of the association of changes in dietary intake, physical activity, alcohol consumption, and smoking with 9-y gain in waist circumference among 16,587 U.S. men. *Am. J. Clin. Nutr.* 78:719–27.

Kreider, R. B., V. Miriel, and E. Bertun. 1993. Amino acid supplementation and exercise performance. *Sports Med.* 16:190–209.

Kuk, J.L., S. Lee, S.B. Heymsfield, and R. Ross. 2005. Waist circumference and abdominal adipose tissue distribution: influence of age and sex. *Am. J. Clin. Nutr.* 81:1330–1334.

Manore, M. M., and J. Thompson. 2000. *Sport Nutrition for Health and Performance.* Champaign, IL: Human Kinetics.

McCargar, L. 2007. New insights into body composition and health through imaging analysis. *Can. J. Diet. Prac. Res.* 68:160–165.

National Institutes of Health. National Heart, Lung, and Blood Institute. 1998. *Clinical Guidelines on the Identification, Evaluation, and Treatment of Overweight and Obesity in Adults.* Executive Summary. www.nhlbi.nih.gov/guidelines/obesity/ob_exsum.pdf. Accessed February 2004.

National Weight Control Registry. (n.d.) Research Facts. www.nwcr.ws/Research/default.htm. Accessed August 2008.

Panotopoulos, G., J. C. Ruiz, B. G. Grand, and A. Basdevant. 2001. Dual x-ray absorptiometry, bioelectrical impedance, and near infrared interactance in obese women. *Med. Sci. Sports Exerc.* 33:665–670.

PBS. 2004. Beyond the scale. *Healthweek.* www.pbs.org/healthweek/featurep3_428.htm. Accessed February 2004.

Stunkard, A. J., T. I. A. Sørensen, C. Hanis, T. W. Teasdale, R. Chakraborty, W. J. Schull, and F. Schulsinger. 1986. An adoption study of human obesity. *N. Engl. J. Med.* 314:193–198.

Tjepkema, M. 2005. *Nutrition: Findings from the Canadian Community Health Survey. Measured Obesity: Adult obesity in Canada,* issue no. 1. Cat. No. 82–620-MWE, Statistics Canada. www.statcan.ca/english/research/82–620-MIE/82–620-MIE2005001.htm. Accessed July 2005.

U.S. Food and Drug Administration (USFDA). FDA Talk Paper: FDA issues public health warning on phenylpropanolamine. November 6, 2000. www.fda.gov/bbs/topics/ANSWERS/ANS01051.html. Accessed July 2005.

Wagner, D. R., V. H. Heyward, and A. L. Gibson. 2000. Validation of air displacement plethysmography for assessing body composition. *Med. Sci. Sports Exerc.* 32:1339–1344.

Zernike, K. 2004. U.S. body survey, head to toe, finds signs of expansion. *The New York Times.* March 1, 1, 12.

Chapter 12

American College of Sports Medicine, American Dietetic Association, and Dietitians of Canada. 2000. Nutrition and athletic performance. Joint position statement. *Med. Sci. Sports Exerc.* 32:2130–2145.

American College of Sports Medicine. 2000. The physiological and health effects of oral creatine supplementation. *Med. Sci. Sports Exerc.,* 32:706–717.

Anderson, M. E., C. R. Bruce, S. F. Fraser, N. K. Stepto, R. Klein, W. G. Hopkins, and J. A. Hawley. 2000. Improved 2000-meter rowing performance in competitive oarswomen after caffeine ingestion. *Int. J. Sport Nutr. Exerc. Metab.* 10:464–475.

Blair, S. N., H. W. Kohl III, C. E. Barlow, R. S. Paffenbarger Jr., L. W. Gibbons, and C. A. Macera. 1995. Changes in physical fitness and all-cause mortality: A prospective study of healthy and unhealthy men. *JAMA* 273: 1093–1098.

Broeder, C. E., J. Quindry, K. Brittingham, L. Panton, J. Thomson, S. Appakondu, K. Breuel, R. Byrd, J. Douglas, C. Earnest, C. Mitchell, M. Olson, T. Roy, and C. Yarlagadda. 2000. The Andro Project: Physiological and hormonal influences of androstenedione supplementation in men 35 to 65 years old participating in a high-intensity resistance training program. *Arch. Intern. Med.* 160:3093–3104.

Brooks, G. A, T. D. Fahey, T. P. White, and K. M. Baldwin. 2000. *Exercise Physiology. Human Bioenergetics and Its Applications.* Mountain View, CA: Mayfield Publishing.

Brooks, G. A. 2000. Intra- and extra-cellular lactate shuttles. *Med. Sci. Sports Exerc.* 32: 790–799.

Bucci, L. 2000. Selected herbals and human exercise performance. *Am. J. Clin. Nutr.* 72: 624S–636S.

Burke, L. 2000. Nutrition for recovery after competition and training. In *Clinical Sports Nutrition,* 2nd ed., edited by L. Burke and V. Deakin, 396–427.

Canadian Fitness and Lifestyle Research Institute. 2005. Physical activity among Canadians: The current situation. www.cflri.ca/eng/statistics/ surveys/documents/pam2005_sec1.pdf. Accessed May 2008.

Canadian Institute for Health Information. 2004. *Improving the Health of Canadians.* Ottawa: CIHI.

Caspersen, C. J., K. E. Powell, and G. M. Christensen. 1985. Physical activity, exercise, and physical fitness: Definitions and distinctions for heath-related research. *Public Health Reports* 100: 126–131.

Coleman, E. 2000. Ribose—an ergogenic aid? *Sports Med. Digest* 22:54.

Costill, D. L., and J. M. Miller, Nutrition for endurance sport: CHO and fluid balance. *Int. J. Sports Med.* 1(1980): 2–14.

Gladden, L. B. 2000. Muscle as a consumer of lactate. *Med. Sci. Sports Exerc.* 32:764–771.

Haymes, E. M. 1998. Trace minerals and exercise. In *Nutrition and Exercise and Sport,* edited by I. Wolinsky. Boca Raton, FL: CRC Press, 1997–2218.

Haymes, E. M., and P. M. Clarkson. 1998. Minerals and trace minerals. In *Nutrition and Sport and Exercise,* edited by J. R. Berning and S. N. Steen. Gaithersburg, MD: Aspen Publishers, 77–107.

Health Canada. 2003. Why Physical Activity is Important for You. www.phac-aspc.gc.ca/pau-uap/ paguide/why.html. Accessed July 2005.

Health Canada. 2008. Health Canada reminds Canadians not to use ephedra/ephedrine products. www.hc-sc.gc.ca/ahc-asc/media/ advisories-avis/_2008/2008_41-eng.php. Accessed May 2008.

Helmrich, S. P., D. R. Ragland, R. W. Leung, and R. S. Paffenbarger Jr. 1991. Physical activity and reduced occurrence of non-insulin-dependent diabetes mellitus. *N. Engl. J. Med.* 325:147–152.

Heyward, V. H. 1998. *Advanced Fitness Assessment and Exercise Prescription,* 3d ed. Champaign, IL: Human Kinetics.

Institute of Medicine, Food and Nutrition Board. 2002. *Dietary Reference Intakes for Energy, Carbohydrates, Fiber, Fat, Protein and Amino Acids (Macronutrients).* Washington, DC: The National Academies of Sciences.

King, A. C., W. L. Haskell, C. B. Taylor, H. C. Kraemer, and R. F. DeBusk. 1991. Group- vs home-based exercise training in healthy older men and women: A community-based clinical trial. *JAMA* 266:1535–1542.

Kohrt, W. M., M. T. Malley, A. R. Coggan, R. J. Spina, T. Ogawa, A. A. Ehsani, R. E. Bourey, W. H. Martin 3rd, and J. O. Holloszy. 1991. Effects of gender, age, and fitness level on response of Vo_{2max} to training in 60–71 yr olds. *J. Appl. Physiol.* 71:2004–2011.

LaCroix, A. Z., S. G. Leveille, J. A. Hecht, L. C. Grothaus, and E. H. Wagner. 1996. Does walking decrease the risk of cardiovascular disease hospitalizations and death in older adults? *J. Am. Geriatr. Soc.* 44:113–120.

Leon, A. S., J. Connett, D. R. Jacobs Jr., and R. Rauramaa. 1987. Leisure-time physical activity levels and risk of coronary heart disease and death: The Multiple Risk Factor Intervention Trial. *JAMA* 258:2388–2395.

Manore, M., and J. Thompson. 2000. *Sports Nutrition for Health and Performance.* Champaign, IL: Human Kinetics.

National Institutes of Health, Office of Dietary Supplements. 2006. Carnitine. ods.od.nih.gov/factsheets/carnitine.asp. Accessed May 2008.

National Institutes of Health, Office of Dietary Supplements. 2005. Chromium. http://ods.od.nih.gov/factsheets/chromium.asp. Accessed May 2008.

National Weather Service. 2003. National Oceanic and Atmospheric Administration, Department of Commerce. December, 2003 Heat Index Chart. www.crh.noaa.gov/pub/heat.htm. Accessed April 2004.

Olds, S. B., M. L. London, P. W. Ladewig, and M. R. Davidson. 2003. *Maternal-Newborn Nursing and Women's Health Care,* 7th ed. Upper Saddle River, NJ: Prentice Hall Health, 373–374.

Paffenbarger, R. S. Jr., R. T. Hyde, A. L. Wing, and C.-C. Hsieh. 1986. Physical activity, all-cause mortality, and longevity of college alumni. *N. Engl. J. Med.* 314:605–613.

Pliml, W., T. von Arnim, A. Stablein, H. Hofmann, H. G. Zimmer, and E. Erdmann. 1992. Effects of ribose on exercise-induced ischaemia in stable coronary artery disease. *Lancet* 340(8818): 507–510.

Schwartz, A. L., M. Mori, R. Gao, L. M. Nail, and M. E. King. 2001. Exercise reduces daily fatigue in women with breast cancer receiving chemotherapy. *Med. Sci. Sports Exerc.* 33:718–723.

Slattery, M. L., D. R. Jacobs Jr., and M. Z. Nichaman. 1989. Leisure-time physical activity and coronary heart disease death: the U.S. Railroad Study. *Circulation* 79:304–311.

Spriet, L. L., and R. A. Howlett. 2000. Caffeine. In *Nutrition in Sport,* edited by R. J. Maughan. Oxford: Blackwell Science, 379–392.

Tanaka, H., K. D. Monahan, and D. R. Seals. 2001. Age-predicted maximal heart rate revisited. *J. Am. Coll. Cardiol.* 37:153–156.

Tarnopolsky, M. 2000. Protein and amino acid needs for training and bulking up. In *Clinical Sports Nutrition,* edited by L. Burke and V. Deakin, Sydney, Australia: McGraw-Hill.

U.S. Department of Health and Human Services. 1996. *Physical Activity and Health: A Report of the Surgeon General.* Atlanta, GA: U.S. Department of Health and Human Services, Centers for Disease Control and Prevention, National Centers for Chronic Disease Prevention and Health Promotion.

Weaver, C. M., and S. Rajaram. 1992. Exercise and iron status. *J. Nutr.* 122:782–787.

Chapter 13

Chapter 13 contains material from *The Science of Nutrition,* by J.L. Thompson, M.M. Manore, and L.A. Vaughan, © Pearson Education, Inc., publishing as Pearson Benjamin Cummings, pp. 620–645. Used by permission of Pearson Education, Inc.

American Psychiatric Association (APA). 1994. *Diagnostic and Statistical Manual of Mental Disorders (DSM-IV),* 4th ed. Washington, DC: American Psychiatric Association.

American Psychiatric Association. 2000. *Practice Guidelines for the Treatment of Patients with Eating Disorders.* Washington, DC: American Psychiatric Association.

Andersen, A. E. 1992. Eating disorders in male athletes: A special case? In *Eating, Body Weight and Performance in Athletes: Disorders of Modern Society,* edited by K. D. Brownell, J. Rodin, and J. H. Wilmore. Philadelphia, PA: Lea and Fegiger, 172–188.

Andersen, A. E. 2001, Spring. Eating disorders in males: Gender divergence management. *Currents.* Volume 2, Number 2. University of Iowa Health Care. www.uihealthcare.com/news/currents/vol2issue2/eatingdisordersinmen.html. Accessed February 2004.

Andersen, R. E., S. J. Bartlett, G. D. Morgan, and K. D. Brownell. 1995. Weight loss, psychological and nutritional patterns in competitive male body builders. *Int. J. Eating Disord.* 18:49–57.

Anorexia Nervosa and Related Eating Disorders, Inc. (ANRED). 2002. Males with eating disorders. www.anred.com/males.html. Accessed February 2004.

Attia, E. 2003. Serotonin in anorexia nervosa: A new study supports a familiar hypothesis. *Int. J. Eating Disord.* 33:268–270.

Bailor, U. F., and W. H. Kaye. 2003. A review of neuropeptide and neuroendocrine dysregulation in anorexia and bulimia nervosa. *Curr. Drug Target CNS Neurol. Disord.* 2:53–59.

Beals, K. A. 2003. Mirror, Mirror on the Wall, who is the most muscular one of all? Disordered eating and body image disturbances in male athletes. *ACSM Health and Fitness J.* 7(2):6–11.

Beals, K. A. 2004. *Disordered Eating in Athletes: A Comprehensive Guide for Health Professionals.* Champaign, IL: Human Kinetics.

Beals, K. A., and M. M. Manore. 1998. Nutritional status of female athletes with subclinical eating disorders. *J. Am. Diet. Assoc.* 98:419–425.

Bulik, C. M. and F. Tozzi. 2004. The genetics of bulimia nervosa. *Drugs Today.* 40(9):741–749.

Carlat, D. J., C. A. Camargo, and D. B. Herzog. 1997. Eating disorders in males: A report on 135 patients. *Am. J. Psychiatry* 154(8): 1127–1132.

Davis, S. M., and L. C. Lambert. 2000. Body image and weight concerns among Southwestern American Indian preadolescent schoolchildren. *Ethn. Dis.* 10:184–194.

Dueck, C. A., M. M. Manore, and K. S. Matt. 1996. Role of energy balance in athletic menstrual dysfunction. *Int. J. Sport Nutr.* 6:90–116.

Fairburn, C. G., and T. B. Walsh. 2002. Atypical eating disorders. In *Eating Disorders and Obesity: A Comprehensive Handbook,* 2nd ed., edited by D. G. Fairburn and K. D. Brownell. New York: Guilford Press, 171–177.

Garfinkel, P. E. 2002. Classification and diagnosis of eating disorders. In *Eating Disorders and Obesity: A Comprehensive Handbook,* 2nd ed., edited by D. G. Fairburn and K. D. Brownell. New York: Guilford Press, 155–161.

Grilo, C. M. 2002. Binge eating disorder. In *Eating Disorders and Obesity: A Comprehensive Handbook,* 2nd ed., edited by D. G. Fairburn and K. D. Brownell. New York: Guilford Press, 178–182.

Groesz, L. M., M. P. Levine, and S. K. Murnen. 2002. The effect of experimental presentation of thin media images on body satisfaction: A meta-analysis review. *Int. J. Eating Disord.* 31–1-16.

Health Canada. 2002. *A Report on Mental Illnesses in Canada.* Chapter 6: Eating Disorders. Health Canada: Ottawa. www.phac-aspc.gc.ca. Accessed April 2005.

Joy, E., N. Clark, M. L. Ireland, J. Martie, A. Nattiv, and S. Varechok. 1997. Team management of the female athlete triad. Part 2: Optimal treatment and prevention tactics. *Physician Sports Med.* 25(4):55–69.

Kaye, W. H., N. C. Barbarich, K. Putnam, K. A. Gendall, J. Fernstrom, M. Fernstrom, C. W. McConada, and A. Kishore. 2003. Anxiolytic effects of acute tryptophan depletion in anorexia nervosa. *Int. J. Eating Disord.* 33:257–267.

Klump, K. L., S. Wonderlich, P. Lehoux, L. R. R. Lilenfeld, and C. M. Bulik. 2002. Does environment matter? A review of nonshared environment and eating disorders. *Int. J. Eating Disord.* 31:118–135.

Lilenfeld, L. R. R., S. Wonderlich, L. P. Riso, R. Crosby, and J. Mitchell. 2005. Eating disorders and personality: A methodological and empirical review. *Clin. Psych. Rev.* 26(3):299–320.

Mangweth, B., H. G. Pope, G. Kemmler, C. Ebenbichler, A. Hausmann, C. DeCol, B. Kreutner, J. Kinzl, and W. Biebl. 2001. Body image and psychopathology in male bodybuilders. *Psychother. Psychosom.* 70:38–43.

Manore, M. M. 1996. Chronic dieting in active women: What are the health consequences? *Women's Health Issues* 6(6):332–341.

Manore, M. M. 2002. Dietary recommendations and athletic menstrual dysfunction. *Sports Med.* 32(14):887–901.

Nemeroff, C. J., R. I. Stein, N. S. Diehl, and K. M. Smilack. 1994. From the Cleavers to the Clintons: Role choices and body orientation as reflected in magazine article content. *Int. J. Eating Disord.* 16:167–176.

Ogilvie, M. 2008. Biology May Cause Most Anorexia. *Toronto Star.* healthzone.ca/health/article/413989. Accessed April 2008.

Otis, C. L., B. Drinkwater, M. Johnson, A. Loucks, and J. Wilmore. 1997. American College of Sports Medicine Position Stand: The female athlete triad. *Med. Sci. Sports Exerc.* 29:i–ix.

Patrick, L. 2002. Eating disorders: A review of the literature with emphasis on medical complication and clinical nutrition. *Altern. Med. Rev.* 7(3): 184–202.

Peterson, A. L., W. Talcott, W. J. Kelleher, and S. D. Smith. 1995. Bulimic weight-loss behaviors in military versus civilian weight-management programs. *Military Med.* 160:616–620.

Piran, N. 2002. Prevention of eating disorders. In *Eating Disorders and Obesity: A Comprehensive Handbook,* 2nd ed., edited by D. G. Fairburn and K. D. Brownell. New York: Guilford Press, 367–371.

Pope, H. G., and D. L. Katz. 1994. Psychiatric and medical effects of anabolic-androgenic steroid use:

A controlled study of 160 athletes. *Arch. Gen. Psychiatry* 51:375–382.

Pope, H. G., K. A. Phillips, and R. Olivardia. 2000. *The Adonis Complex: The Secret Crisis of Male Body Obsession.* New York: The Free Press.

Rinderknecht, K., and C. Smith. 2002. Body-image perceptions among urban Native American youth. *Obes. Res.* 10:315–327.

Robb, A. S., and M. J. Dadson. 2002. Eating disorders in males. *Child Adolesc. Psychiatr. Clin. N. Am.* 11:399–418.

Steiger, H., P. M. Lehoux, and L. Gauvin. 1999. Impulsivity, dietary control and the urge to binge in bulimic syndromes. *Inter. J. Eating Disord.* 26:261–274.

Steinberg, L. 2002. *Adolescence,* 6th ed. New York: McGraw-Hill.

Stevens, J., M. Story, A. Becenti, S. A. French, J. Gittelsohn, S. B. Going, Juhaeri, S. Levin, and D. M. Murray. 1999. Weight-related attitudes and behaviors in fourth grade American Indian children. *Obes. Res.* 7:34–42.

Stice, E. 2002. Sociocultural influences on body image and eating disturbances. In *Eating Disorders and Obesity: A Comprehensive Handbook,* 2nd ed., edited by D. G. Fairburn and K. D. Brownell. New York: Guilford Press, 103–107.

Strober, M., and C. M. Bulik. 2002. Genetic epidemiology of eating disorders. In *Eating Disorders and Obesity: A Comprehensive Handbook,* 2nd ed., edited by D. G. Fairburn and K. D. Brownell. New York: Guilford Press, 238–242.

Sundgot-Borgen, J. 1994. Risk and trigger factors for the development of eating disorders in female elite athletes. *Med. Sci. Sport Exerc.* 26: 414–419.

Tanaka, M., T. Naruo, N. Nagai, N. Kuroki, T. Shiiya, M. Nakazato, S. Matsukura, and S. Nozoe. 2003. Habitual binge/purge behavior influences circulating ghrelin levels in eating disorders. *J. Psychiat. Res.* 37:17–22.

Vandereycken, W. 2002. Families of patients with eating disorders. In *Eating Disorders and Obesity: A Comprehensive Handbook,* 2nd ed., edited by D. G. Fairburn and K. D. Brownell. New York: Guilford Press, 215–220.

Wonderlich, S. A. 2002. Personality and eating disorders. In *Eating Disorders and Obesity: A Comprehensive Handbook,* 2nd ed., edited by D. G. Fairburn and K. D. Brownell. New York: Guilford Press, 204–209.

Woodside, D. B., P. E. Garfinkel, E. Lin, P. Goering, A. S. Kaplan, D. S. Goldbloom, and S. H. Kennedy. 2001. Comparisons of men with full or partial eating disorders, men without eating disorders, and women with eating disorders in the community. *Am. J. Psychiatry* 158(4): 570–574.

Chapter 14

Aseptic Packaging Council. 2003. The award-winning, Earth smart packaging for a healthy lifestyle. www.aseptic.org/main.shtml. Accessed April 2004.

Bauman, R. W. 2004. *Microbiology.* San Francisco: Pearson Benjamin Cummings.

Bischoff, H. A., H. B. Stähelin, W. Dick, R. Akos, M. Knecht, C. Salis, M. Nebiker, R. Theiler, M. Pfeifer, B. Begerow, R. A. Lew, and M. Conzelmann. 2003. Effects of vitamin D and calcium supplementation on falls: a randomized control trial. *J Bone Min Res* 18:343–351.

Blaylock, R. L. 1996. *Excitoxins: The Taste That Kills.* Sante Fe, NM: Health Press.

Bren, L. 2004. Got milk? Make sure it's pasteurized. *FDA Consumer* 38:29–31.

Campaign for Real Milk. (n.d.). www.realmilk.com. Accessed April 2008.

Canadian Food Inspection Agency. 2002. Durable Life Information on Food Products. www.inspection.gc.ca/english/fssa/concen/ tipcon/lifee.shtml. Accessed August 2008.

Canadian Food Inspection Agency. 2003. Consolidated Health Hazard Alert: Some Products May contain Sudan I Dye. www .inspection.gc.ca/english/corpaffr/recarapp/ 2003/20031107e.shtml. Accessed April 2008.

Canadian Food Inspection Agency. 2007a. Food safety facts on campylobacter. www.inspection.gc.ca/ english/fssa/concen/cause/campye.shtml. Accessed April 2008.

Canadian Food Inspection Agency. 2007b. Food safety facts on microwave ovens. www .inspection.gc.ca/english/fssa/concen/tipcon/ microe.shtml. Accessed Aug. 2008.

Canadian Food Inspection Agency. 2008a. Avian influenza. www.inspection.gc.ca/english/ anima/heasan/disemala/avflu/avflue.shtml. Accessed April 2008.

Canadian Food Inspection Agency. 2008b. Salmonella food safety facts: Preventing foodborne illness. www.inspection.gc.ca/english/fssa/concen/ cause/salmonellae.shtml. Accessed April 2008.

Canadian General Standards Board. 2006. Organic Production Systems General Principles and Management Standards. CAN/GSB-32.310–2006. www.organicagcentre.ca/Docs/Cdn_Stds_Principles2006_e.pdf. Accessed April 2008.

Canadian Institutes of Health Research. 2003. Canadian researchers develop *E. coli* vaccine for cattle. www.cihr-irsc.gc.ca/e/19939.html. Accessed May 2005.

Center for Science in the Public Interest (CSPI). 2004a (accessed). Food safety. Chemical cuisine. CSPI's guide to food additives. www.cspinet.org/reports/chemcuisine.htm. Accessed April 2004.

Center for Science in the Public Interest (CSPI). 2004b (accessed). Tips to prevent food poisoning: CSPI's "eggspert" egg advice. www.cspinet.org/foodsafety/eggspert_advice.html. Accessed April 2004.

Centers for Disease Control and Prevention (CDC). 2003a. Division of Bacterial and Mycotic Diseases. Disease information. *Foodborne illness.* www.cdc.gov/ncidod/dbmd/diseaseinfo/foodborneinfections_g.htm. Accessed April 2004.

Currier, R. W. 1981. Raw milk and human gastrointestinal disease: Problems resulting from legalized sale of certified raw milk. *J. Pub. Health Policy* 2:226–234.

Dietitians of Canada. 2007. Current Issues: the inside story. Microbial food safety and reported consumer practices. www.dietitians.ca. Accessed April 2008.

Doering, R. 2005. Regulating organics. www.foodincanada.com. Accessed June 2005.

Eldieb, D. August 7, 2007. Neighbors have a cow over raw milk. *Daily Southtown.* www.dailysouthtown.com/news/499882,071NWS1.article. Accessed April 2008.

Food Marketing Institute. 2003. A Consumer Guide to Food Quality and Safe Handling: Meat, Poultry, Seafood, Eggs. [pamphlet]

Food Safety Network. 2008. Why are nitrates used in cured meats and are there any food safety concerns related to their use? www.foodsafetynetwork.ca/en/faq-details.php?a=1&fc=4&id=8008. Accessed April 2008.

Gillespie, I. A., G. K. Adak, S. J. O'Brien, and F. J. Bolton. 2003. Milkborne general outbreaks of infectious intestinal disease, England and Wales, 1992–2000. *Epidem. Infect.* 130:461–468.

Health Canada. 2006a. Health Canada reminds Canadians about the risks of drinking raw milk. www.hc-sc.gc.ca/ahc-asc/media/advisories-avis/_2006/2006_65_e.html. Accessed April 2008.

Health Canada. 2006b. It's your health: Infant botulism. www.hc-sc.gc.ca/iyh-vsv/diseases-maladies/botu_e.html. Accessed March 2008.

Health Canada. 2006c. It's your health: Salmonella prevention. www.hc-sc.gc.ca/iyh-vsv/food-aliment/salmonella_e.html. Accessed April 2008.

Jayarao, B. M., S. C. Donaldson, B. A. Straley, A. A. Sawant, N. V. Hegde, and J. L. Brown. 2006. A survey of foodborne pathogens in bulk tank milk and raw milk consumption among farm families in Pennsylvania. *J. Dairy Science* 89:2451–2458.

Kidney Foundation of Canada. 2002. Hemolytic uremic syndrome. www.kidney.ca/english/publications/factsheets/hemolytic.htm. Accessed February 2005.

Lacroix, B. M., K. W. M. Li, and D. A. Powell. 2003. Consumer food handling recommendations: Is thawing of turkey a food safety issue? *Can. J. Diet. Prac, Res.* 64:59–61.

Larenbeke, N. A. Van, P. Covaci, P. Schepens, and L. Hens. 2002. Food contamination with polychlorinated biphenyls and dioxins in Belgium, Effects of the body burden. *Epidemiol. Community Health* 56(11):828–830.

National Environmental Health Association. 2008. Sale and distribution of raw milk. www.neha.org/position_papers/position_raw_milk.htm. Accessed April 2008.

Oliver, S. P., B. M. Jayarao, and R. A. Almeida. 2005. Foodborne pathogens in milk and dairy farm environment: Food safety and public health implications. *Foodborne Pathogens and Disease* 2:115–129.

Perkin, M. R. 2007. Unpasteurized milk: Health or hazard. *Clin. Experim. Allergy* 37:627–630.

Public Health Agency of Canada. 2005b. Noroviruses: Fact sheet. www.phac-aspc.gc.ca/id-mi/norovirus-eng.php. Accessed April 2008.

Schafer, K. S., and S. E. Kegley. 2002. Persistent toxic chemicals in the US food supply. *J. Epidemiol. Community Health* 56:813–817.

Shephard, S. 2000. *Pickled, Potted and Canned: The Story of Food Preserving.* London: Headline Publishing.

Tauxe, R. V. 2001. Food safety and irradiation: Protecting the public from foodborne infections. *Emerging Infectious Diseases* 7:516–521.

Tortora, G. J., B. R. Funke, and C. L. Case. 2003. *Microbiology: An Introduction*, 8th ed. San Francisco: Pearson Benjamin Cummings.

U.S. Department of Agriculture (USDA). 2003, July 2. News Release: For an enjoyable Fourth, consumers should practice food safety. www.usda.gov/news/releases/2003/07/0239.htm. Accessed July 2003.

U.S. Food and Drug Administration (FDA). 2003. Draft advice for women who are pregnant, or who might become pregnant, and nursing mothers, about avoiding harm to your baby or young child from mercury in fish and shellfish. www.fda.gov/oc/opacom/mehgadvisory 1208.html. Accessed February 2004.

U.S. Food and Drug Administration (FDA). 2007. FDA finalizes report on 2006 spinach outbreak. FDA News. www.fda.gov/bbs/topics/NEWS/2007/NEW01593.html. Accessed April 2008.

University of Florida. 2002. *E.coli* 0157:H7: A Potential Health Concern. http://edis.ifas.ufl.edu/BODY_SS197. Accessed May 2005.

Wier, E., J. Mitchell, S. Reballato, and D. Fortuna. 2007. Raw milk and the protection of the public health. *Can. Med.l Assoc. J.* 177:721–722.

Winter, R. 1994. *A Consumer's Dictionary of Food Additives.* New York: Three Rivers Press.

World Health Organization. 2005a. Avian influenza fact sheet. www.who.int/csr/disease/avian_influenza/avian_faqs/en/index.html#poultry. Accessed April 2008.

World Health Organization. 2005b. Cumulative number of confirmed human cases of avian influenza A since 28 January 2004. www.who.int/csr/disease/avian_influenza/country/cases_table_2005_01_21/en/. Accessed May 2005.

Chapter 15

American Academy of Pediatrics, Policy Statement, Committee on Nutrition. 2000. Hypoallergenic Infant Formulas (RE0005). www.aap.org/policy/re0005.html

Arenz, S., R. Ruckerl, B. Koletzko, and R. von Kries. 2004. Breast-feeding and childhood obesity—a systematic review. *Int. J. Obes.* 28:1247–1256.

Barnet, B., A. K. Duggan, and M. Devoe. 2003. Reduced low birth weight for teenagers receiving prenatal care at a school-based health center: effect of access and comprehensive care. *J. Adolesc. Health* 33(5):349–358.

Benyshek, D. C., J. F. Martin, and C. S. Johnston. 2001. A reconsideration of the origins of type 2 diabetes epidemic among Native Americans and the implications for intervention policy. *Med. Anthropol.* 20(1):25–64.

Berlanga, M. R., G. Salazar, C. Garcia, and J. Hernandez. 2002. Maternal smoking effects on infant growth. *Food & Nutrition Bulletin* 23 (3 Suppl):142–145.

Centers for Disease Control and Prevention (CDC). 2003. Folic Acid: Topic Home. www.cdc.gov.node.do/id/0900f3ec80010af9. Accessed April 2004.

Cross, N. A., L. S. Hillman, S. H. Allen, G. F. Krause, and N. E. Vieira. 1995. Calcium homeostasis and bone metabolism during pregnancy, lactation, and postweaning: A longitudinal study. *Am. J. Clin. Nutr.* 61:514–523.

Dabelea, D., R. L. Hanson, P. H. Bennett, J. Roumain, W. C. Knowler, and D. J. Pettitt. 1998. Increasing prevalence of type 2 diabetes in American Indian children. *Diabetologia* 41:904–910.

Davidsson, L., A. Almgren, B. Sandstrom, and R. F. Hurrell. 1995. Zinc absorption in adult humans. The effect of iron fortification. *Br. J. Nutr.* 74:417–425.

Elliot, J. 2003. Breastfeeding could save lives. BBC News, http://news.bbc.co.uk/1/hi/health/2973845.stm.

Ernst, E. 2002. Herbal medicinal products during pregnancy: Are they safe? *Br. J. Obstet. Gynaecol.* 109:227–235.

Harder, T., R. Bergmann, G. Kallischnigg, and A. Plagemann. 2005. Duration of breastfeeding and risk of overweight: a meta-analysis. *Am. J. Epidemiol.* 162:397–403.

Harding, J. E. 2001. The nutritional basis of the fetal origins of adult disease. *Int. J. Epidemiol.* 30:15–23.

Health Canada. 2004. Exclusive Breastfeeding Duration - 2004 Health Canada Recommendation. http://www.hc-sc.gc.ca/fn-an/nutrition/child-enfant/infant-nourisson/excl_bf_dur-dur_am_excl-eng.php. Accessed September 2008.

Health Canada. 2005. *Nutrition for a Healthy Pregnancy - National Guidelines for the Childbearing Years.* www.hc-sc.gc.ca/fn-an/nutrition/prenatal/national_guidelines-lignes_directrices_nationales-06g_e.html. Accessed May 2008.

Health Canada. 2006. *It's Your Health: Fetal Alcohol Spectrum Disorder.* www.hc-sc.gc.ca/iyh-vsv/diseases-maladies/fasd-etcaf_e.html. Accessed May 2008.

Health Canada. 2007. *Nutrition for Healthy Term Infants - Statement of the Joint Working Group: Canadian Paediatric Society, Dietitians of Canada and Health Canada*. www.hc-sc.gc.ca/fn-an/pubs/infant. Accessed May 2008.

Health Canada. 2008. *Nutrients of Special Concern for a Healthy Pregnancy*. www.hc-sc.gc.ca/fn-an/consultation/init/prenatal/folate-cons_e.html. Accessed April 2008.

Institute of Medicine, Food and Nutrition Board. 1997. *Dietary Reference Intakes for Calcium, Phosphorus, Magnesium, Vitamin D, and Fluoride*. Washington, DC: National Academies Press.

Institute of Medicine, Food and Nutrition Board. 1998. *Dietary Reference Intakes for Thiamin, Riboflavin, Niacin, Vitamin B₆, Folate, Vitamin B₁₂, Pantothenic Acid, Biotin, and Choline*. Washington, DC: National Academies Press.

Institute of Medicine, Food and Nutrition Board. 2004. *Dietary Reference for Water, Potassium, Sodium, Chloride, and Sulfate*. Washington, DC: National Academies Press.

Jackson, D. J., M. Chopra, C. Witten, and M. J. Sengwana. 2003. HIV and infant feeding: Issues in developed and developing countries. *Journal of Obstetric, Gynecologic, and Neonatal Nursing* 32(1):117–127.

Mitra, K., and M. K. Chowdhury. 2002. Maternal malnutrition, perinatal mortality and fetal pathology: A clinicopathological study. *Journal of the Indian Medical Association*, February, 2002. www.jimaonline.org/Feb2002/report04.html. Accessed January 2004.

Mostello, D., T. K. Catlin, L. Roman, W. L. Holcomb Jr., and T. Leet. 2002. Preeclampsia in the parous woman: Who is at risk? *Am. J. Obstet. Gynecol.* 187(2):425–429.

Olds, S. B., M. L. London, P. W. Ladewig, and M. R. Davidson. 2003. *Maternal-Newborn Nursing and Women's Health Care*, 7th ed. Upper Saddle River, NJ: Prentice Hall Health.

Porter, D. V. 2003. Breastfeeding: Impact on health, employment, and society. CRS Report for Congress. Congressional Research Service. The Library of Congress. www.breastfeeding.org/law/CRS1.pdf. Accessed April 2004.

Ray, J. G., J. Goodman, P. R. A. O'Mahoney, M. M. Mamdani, and D. Jiang. 2008. High rate of maternal vitamin B12 deficiency nearly a decade after Canadian folic acid flour fortification. *QJMed.* doi:10.1093/qjmed/hcn031. Accessed May 2008.

Ray, J. G., P. R. Wyatt, M. D. Thompson, M. J. Vermeulen, C. Meier, P.-Y. Wong, S. A. Farrell, and D. E. C. Cole. 2007. Vitamin B12 and the risk of neural tube defects in a folic-acid-fortified population. *Epidem.* 18:362–366.

Reuters. 2000. Peers encourage third world women to breastfeed. www.durhamobgyn.com/viewArticle?ID522184.

U.S. Food and Drug Administration (FDA). 1997. Preventing Iron Poisoning in Children. FDA Backgrounder. www.fda.gov/opacom/backgrounders/ironbg.html. Accessed January 2004.

Uauy, R., and P. Mena. 1999. Requirements for long-chain polyunsaturated fatty acids in the preterm infant. *Curr. Opin. Pediatr.* 11(2):115–120.

UNICEF (United Nations Childrens' Fund). 2004. Maternal nutrition and low birth weight. www.unicef.org/nutrition/index_lowbirthweight.html. Accessed January 2004.

UNICEF. 2003. Protecting, promoting and supporting breastfeeding. www.unicef.org/nutrition/index_breastfeeding.html. Accessed January 2004.

von Dadelszen, P. 2000. The Etiology of Nausea and Vomiting in Pregnancy. In First International Congress on NVP. www.nvp-volumes.org/index.htm. Accessed April 2004.

Weimer, D. R. 2003. Summary of state breastfeeding laws. CRS Report for Congress. Congressional Research Service. The Library of Congress. www.breastfeeding.org/law/CRS2.pdf

Whittaker, P. 1998. Iron and zinc interactions in humans. *Am. J. Clin. Nutr.* 68:442S–446S.

Yeo, S., and S. T. Davidge. 2001. Possible beneficial effect of exercise, by reducing oxidative stress, on the incidence of preeclampsia. *J. Women's Health Gender-Based Med.* 10(10):983–989.

Chapter 16

American Dietetic Association. January 27, 2005. Balance food marketing to children with nutrition education messages, American Dietetic Association advises Institute of Medicine. www.eatright.org/Public/Media/PublicMedia_21509.cfm. Accessed June 2005.

Bailey, I. 2001. *National Post*. Daughters, 9 and 5, Starving on a Vegan Diet, Father Claims. http://fact.on.ca/news/news0103/np010305.htm. Accessed April 2004.

Barberger-Gateau P., L. Letenneur, V. Deschamps, K. Peres, J.-F. Dartigues, and S. Renaud. 2002. Fish, meat, and risk of dementia: Cohort study. *Br. Med. J.* 325:932–934.

Beresford, S. A., and C. J. Boushey. 1997. Homocysteine, folic acid, and cardiovascular disease risk. In *Preventive Nutrition: The Comprehensive Guide for Health Professionals,* edited by A. Bendich and R. J. Deckelbaum. Totowa, NJ: Humana Press.

Centers for Disease Control and Prevention. 2000. National Center for Chronic Disease Prevention and Health Promotion. Tobacco Information and Prevention Source (TIPS). Facts on Youth Smoking, Health, and Performance. www .cdc.gov/tobacco/research_data/youth/ ythsprt.htm. Accessed April 2004.

Centers for Disease Control and Prevention. 2001. Neurologic impairment in children associated with maternal dietary deficiency of cobalamin. *Morbid. Mortal. Wkly. Rep.* 52(04):61–64.

Eakin, J. M., and V. S. Tarasuk. 2003. Charitable food assistance as symbolic gesture: An ethnographic study of food banks in Ontario. *Social Sc. and Med.* 22:1505–1515.

Heaney, R. P., and K. Rafferty. 2001. Carbonated beverages and urinary calcium excretion. *Am. J. Clin. Nutr.* 74:343–347.

Institute of Medicine, Food and Nutrition Board. 1997. *Dietary Reference Intakes for Calcium, Phosphorus, Magnesium, Vitamin D, and Fluoride.* Washington, DC: National Academies Press.

Institute of Medicine, Food and Nutrition Board. 1998. *Dietary Reference Intakes for Thiamin, Riboflavin, Niacin, Vitamin B_6, Folate, Vitamin B_{12}, Pantothenic Acid, Biotin, and Choline.* Washington, DC: National Academies Press.

Institute of Medicine, Food and Nutrition Board. 2000. *Dietary Reference Intakes for Vitamin C, Vitamin E, Selenium, and Carotenoids.* Washington, DC: National Academies Press.

Institute of Medicine, Food and Nutrition Board. 2001. *Dietary Reference Intakes for Vitamin A, Vitamin K, Arsenic, Boron, Chromium, Copper, Iodine, Iron, Manganese, Molybdenum, Nickel, Silicon, Vanadium, and Zinc.* Washington, DC: National Academies Press.

Institute of Medicine, Food and Nutrition Board. 2002. *Dietary Reference Intakes for Energy, Carbohydrates, Fiber, Fat, Protein and Amino Acids (Macronutrients).* Washington, DC: The National Academy of Sciences.

Institute of Medicine, Food and Nutrition Board. 2004a. *Dietary Reference Intakes for Water, Potassium, Sodium, Chloride, and Sulfate.* Washington, DC: National Academies Press.

Kaplan, R. J., C. E. Greenwood, G. Winocur, and T. M. S. Wolever. 2001. Dietary protein, carbohydrate, and fat enhance memory performance in the healthy elderly. *Am. J. Clin. Nutr.* 74:687–693.

Kim, W. Y., M. Hur, M. S. Cho, and H. S. Lee. 2003. Effect of olfactory function on nutritional status of Korean elderly women. *Nutr. Res.* 23:723–734.

Kuchler, F., E. Golan, N. V. Jayachandran, and S. R. Crutchfield. June 2005. Obesity policy and the law of unintended consequences. *Amber Waves.* www.ers.usda.gov/AmberWaves/June05/Features/ ObesityPolicy.htm. Accessed June 2005.

Mangels, R. 2001. The Vegetarian Resource Group. Vegetarianism in a Nutshell. Feeding Vegan Kids. www.vrg.org/nutshell/kids.htm. Accessed April 2004.

McIntyre, J., *Food and Drink Weekly.* March 21, 2005. Legislation could limit "junk food" advertising aimed at children. www.findarticles.com/p/ articles/mi_m0EUY/is_11_11/ai_n13482067# continue. Accessed June 2005.

Morris, M. C., D. A. Evans, J. L. Bienias, C. C. Tangney, D. A. Bennett, R. S. Wilson, N. Aggarwal, and J. Schneider. 2003. Consumption of fish and n-3 fatty acids and risk of incident Alzheimer disease. *Arch. Neurol.* 60:940–946.

Polan, E. U., and D. R. Taylor. 2003. *Journey Across the Lifespan,* 2nd ed. Philadelphia: F. A. Davis.

Roberts, S. B. and G. E. Dallal. 2001. The new childhood growth charts. *Nutr. Rev.* 59:31–36.

Second Opinions. 2002. Vegan Child Abuse. www.second-opinions.co.uk/child_abuse.html. Accessed April 2004.

Shields, M. 2005. *Nutrition: Findings from the Canadian Community Health Survey. Measured Obesity: Overweight Canadian children and adolescents,* issue no. 1. Cat. No. 82–620-MWE, Statistics Canada. www.statcan.ca/english/ research/82–620-MIE/82–620-MIE2005001 .htm. Accessed July 2005.

Statistics Canada. 2005. Canadian Community Health Survey. Food Security. www.statcan.ca/english/ research/82–620-MIE/2005001/tables/ t006_en.pdf. Accessed July 2005.

Tarasuk, V. S. 2001. A critical examination of community-based responses to household food insecurity in Canada. *Health Ed. Behav.* 28:487–499.

Tarasuk, V. S., and G. H. Beaton. 1999. Women's dietary intakes in the context of household food insecurity. *J. Nutr.* 12:672–679.

Tarasuk, V. S., and N. T. Vozoris. 2003. Household food insufficiency is associated with poorer health. *J. Nutr.* 133:120–126.

Tarasuk, V. S., N. Dachner, and J. Li. 2005. Homeless youth in Toronto are nutritionally vulnerable. *J. Nutr.* 135:1926–1933.

Torgan, C. 2002. Childhood Obesity on the Rise. The NIH Word on Health. www.nih.gov/news/.

USDA Food and Nutrition Service. 2003. School Breakfast Program. Healthy Eating Helps You Make the Grade. www.fns.usda.gov/cnd/Breakfast/SchoolBfastCampaign/theresearch.html. Accessed April 2004.

USDA/ARS Children's Nutrition Research Center at Baylor College of Medicine. 1999. Consumer News—Facts and Answers. Hunger Hinders School Performance. www.kidsnutrition.org/consumer/archives/breakfast-fuel.htm. Accessed April 2004.

Appendices

The following table of nutrient values is taken from the EvaluEat diet analysis software that is included with every new copy of this text. The foods in the table are just a fraction of the foods provided in the software. When using the software you can quickly find foods shown here by entering the EvaluEat code in the search field. Values are obtained from the USDA Nutrient Database for Standard Reference, Release 16. A "0" indicates that nutrient value is determined to be zero; a blank space indicates that nutrient information is not available.

Amt = serving amount; **Wt** = weight; **Ener** = energy; **Prot** = protein; **Carb** = carbohydrate; **Fiber** = dietary fiber; **Fat** = total fat; **Mono** = mono-unsaturated fat; **Poly** = poly-unsaturated fat; **Sat** = saturated fat; **Chol** = cholesterol; **Calc** = calcium; **Iron** = iron; **Mag** = magnesium; **Phos** = phosphate; **Sodi** = sodium; **Zinc** = zinc; **Vit A** = vitamin A; **Vit C** = vitamin C; **Thia** = thiamin; **Ribo** = riboflavin; **Niac** = niacin; **Vit B$_6$** = vitamin B$_6$; **Vit B$_{12}$**-vitamin B$_{12}$; **Vit E** = vitamin E; **Fol** = folate; **Alc** = alcohol.

EvaluEat Code	Food Name	Amt	Wt (g)	Energy (kcal)	Prot (g)	Carb (g)	Fiber (g)	Fat (g)	Mono (g)	Poly (g)	Sat (g)
2047	Salt, table (sodium chloride)	1 tsp	6	0	0	0	0	0	0	0	0
4609	Animal fat, bacon grease	1 tbsp	12.8	114.8	0	0	0	12.736	5.744	1.426	4.993
4542	Animal fat, chicken	1 cup	205	1845	0	0	0	204.59	91.635	42.845	61.09
43388	Apple cider-flavored drink, powder, low calorie, with vitamin C, prepared	1 fl. oz.	29.8	0.298	0	0.089	0	0	0	0	0
9357	Apricots, canned, heavy syrup, drained	1 fruit	122	101.26	0.781	25.998	3.294	0.134	0.055	0.026	0.009
7921	Bacon and beef sticks	1 oz	28	145.6	8.148	0.224	0	12.376	6.132	1.204	4.48
43212	Bacon bits, meatless	1 cup	186	885.36	59.52	53.196	18.972	48.174	11.578	25.199	7.542
16104	Bacon, vegetarian, meatless	1 strip	5	15.5	0.534	0.316	0.13	1.476	0.355	0.772	0.231
18005	Bagel, cinnamon-raisin	1 bagel (4" dia)	89	243.86	8.722	49.128	2.047	1.513	0.156	0.597	0.244
18003	Bagel, egg	1 large bagel (4-1/2" dia)	131	364.18	13.886	69.43	3.013	2.751	0.55	0.841	0.552
18504	Bagel, Lender's Bagel Shop Blueberry	1 bagel (4" dia)	102	264.18	10.71	53.377	1.734	1.53	0.408	0.51	0.306
18007	Bagel, oatbran	1 bagel (4" dia)	89	226.95	9.523	47.437	3.204	1.068	0.222	0.433	0.17
18001	Bagel, plain/onion/poppy/sesame, enriched	1 bagel (4" dia)	89	244.75	9.345	47.526	2.047	1.424	0.117	0.619	0.196
43449	Baked beans, canned, no salt added	1 fl. oz.	29.8	31.29	1.43	6.142	1.639	0.119	0.01	0.051	0.031
42182	Bean beverage	1 oz	28.34	9.636	0.794	1.644	0	0	0	0	0
16115	Bean flour, soy, fullfat, raw	1 cup, stirred	84	366.24	29.014	29.56	8.064	17.346	3.831	9.792	2.509
16119	Bean meal, soy, defatted, raw	1 cup	122	413.58	54.839	48.971		2.916	0.499	1.275	0.327
16112	Bean sauce, fermented soy product, Miso	1 cup	275	566.5	32.478	76.89	14.85	16.693	3.688	9.427	2.414
16113	Bean sauce, fermented soy product, Natto	1 cup	175	371	31.01	25.13	9.45	19.25	4.253	10.868	2.784
16114	Bean sauce, fermented soy product, Tempeh	1 cup	166	320.38	30.776	15.587		17.928	4.98	6.353	3.685
16424	Bean sauce, soy & wheat (Shoyu) low sodium	1 tbsp	18	9.54	0.931	1.532	0.144	0.014	0.002	0.006	0.002
16124	Bean sauce, soy (Tamari)	1 tsp	6	3.6	0.631	0.334	0.048	0.006	0.001	0.003	0.001
16375	Beans, baby lima, mature seed, boiled w/salt	1 cup	182	229.32	14.633	42.424	14.014	0.692	0.062	0.308	0.16
16008	Beans, baked w/franks, canned	1 cup	259	367.78	17.483	39.86	17.871	17.016	7.33	2.165	6.092
16006	Beans, baked, plain or vegetarian, canned	1 cup	254	236.22	12.167	52.121	12.7	1.143	0.099	0.493	0.295
16015	Beans, black, mature seeds, boiled w/o salt	1 cup	172	227.04	15.239	40.781	14.964	0.929	0.081	0.397	0.239
16353	Beans, broadbeans (Fava) mature seed, boiled w/salt	1 cup	170	187	12.92	33.405	9.18	0.68	0.134	0.279	0.112
43112	Beans, chili, barbeque, ranch style, cooked	1 cup	186	180.42	9.3	31.527	7.812	1.86	0.143	1.032	0.27

Chol (g)	Calc (mg)	Iron (mg)	Mag (mg)	Phos (mg)	Pota (mg)	Sodi (mg)	Zinc (mg)	Vit A (RAE)	Vit C (mg)	Thia (mg)	Ribo (mg)	Niac (mg)	Vit B_6 (mg)	Vit B_{12} (µg)	Vit E (mg)	Fol (µg)	Alc (g)
0	1.44	0.02	0.06	0	0.48	2325.48	0.006	0	0	0	0	0	0	0	0	0	0
12.16	0	0	0	0	0	19.2	0.014	0	0	0	0	0	0	0	0.077	0	0
174.25	0	0	0	0	0	0	0	0	0	0	0	0	0	0	5.535	0	0
0	3.278	0.009	0.298	3.576	0		0.009	0		0	0	0	0	0	0	0	0
0	12.2	0.366	8.54	15.86	174.46	4.88	0.134	178.1	3.782	0.026	0.029	0.459	0.067	0	1.086	2.44	0
28.56	3.92	0.521	4.76	39.76	107.8	397.6	0.904	0	0	0.168	0.08	1.363	0.14	0.532	0.078	0.56	0
0	187.86	1.339	176.7	403.62	269.7	3292.2	3.478	0	3.534	1.116	0.13	2.976	0.149	2.232	12.834	236.2	0
0	1.15	0.121	0.95	3.5	8.5	73.25	0.021	0.2	0	0.22	0.024	0.378	0.024	0	0.345	2.1	0
0	16.91	3.382	24.92	89	131.72	286.58	1.006	18.69	0.623	0.342	0.247	2.741	0.055	0	0.276	98.79	0
31.44	17.03	5.214	32.75	110.04	89.08	661.55	1.009	43.23	0.786	0.702	0.308	4.51	0.114	0.21		115.3	0
0	57.12	1.836			158.1	427.38			0	0.265	0.204	4.08	0.061	0		75.48	
0	10.68	2.741	27.59	97.9	102.35	451.23	0.801	0.89	0.178	0.295	0.301	2.634	0.038	0	0.294	87.22	0
0	65.86	3.168	25.81	85.44	89.89	475.26	0.783	0	0	0.479	0.28	4.06	0.045	0	0.258	94.34	0
0	14.9	0.086	9.536	30.992	88.208	0.298	0.417	1.49	0.924	0.045	0.018	0.128	0.039	0	0.158	7.152	0
0	4.818	0.354	13.603	26.073	95.506	0.567	0.105	0	0	0.043	0.028	0.176	0.028	0	0.068	17	0
0	173.04	5.351	360.36	414.96	2112.6	10.92	3.293	5.04	0	0.488	0.974	3.629	0.387	0	1.638	289.8	0
0	297.68	16.714	373.32	855.22	3037.8	3.66	6.173	2.44	0	0.843	0.306	3.156	0.694	0		369.67	0
0	181.5	7.535	115.5	420.75	451	10029.23	9.13	11	0	0.267	0.688	2.365	0.591	0	0.027	90.75	0
0	379.75	15.05	201.25	304.5	1275.75	12.25	5.302	0	22.75	0.28	0.332	0	0.227	0	0.018	14	0
0	184.26	4.482	134.46	441.56	683.92	14.94	1.892	0	0	0.129	0.594	4.382	0.357	0.133		39.84	0
0	3.06	0.364	6.12	19.8	32.4	599.94	0.067	0	0	0.009	0.023	0.605	0.031	0	0	2.88	0
0	1.2	0.143	2.4	7.8	12.72	335.16	0.026	0	0	0.004	0.009	0.237	0.012	0	0	1.08	0
0	52.78	4.368	96.46	231.14	729.82	434.98	1.875	0	0	0.293	0.1	1.201	0.142	0		273	0
15.54	124.32	4.481	72.52	269.36	608.65	1113.7	4.843	10.36	5.957	0.15	0.145	2.334	0.119	0	1.191	77.7	0
0	127	0.737	81.28	264.16	751.84	1008.38	3.556	12.7	7.874	0.389	0.152	1.087	0.34	0	1.346	60.96	0
0	46.44	3.612	120.4	240.8	610.6	1.72	1.926	0	0	0.42	0.101	0.869	0.119	0		256.3	0
0	61.2	2.55	73.1	212.5	455.6	409.7	1.717	1.7	0.51	0.165	0.151	1.209	0.122	0	0.034	176.8	0
0	57.66	3.46	83.7	286.44	837	1348.5	3.72	1.86	3.162	0.074	0.279	0.67	0.502	0.019	0.391	48.36	0

EvaluEat Code	Food Name	Amt	Wt (g)	Energy (kcal)	Prot (g)	Carb (g)	Fiber (g)	Fat (g)	Mono (g)	Poly (g)	Sat (g)
16137	Beans, hummus, garbanzo or chickpea spread, homemade	1 tbsp	15	26.55	0.729	3.018	0.6	1.289	0.737	0.312	0.168
16029	Beans, kidney, mature seeds, canned	1 cup	256	207.36	13.312	38.093	8.96	0.794	0.061	0.44	0.115
16033	Beans, kidney, red, mature seeds, boiled w/o salt	1 cup	177	224.79	15.346	40.356	13.098	0.885	0.069	0.487	0.127
16072	Beans, large lima, mature seeds, boiled w/o salt	1 cup	188	216.2	14.664	39.254	13.16	0.714	0.064	0.321	0.167
16073	Beans, large lima, mature seeds, canned	1 cup	241	190.39	11.881	35.933	11.568	0.41	0.036	0.178	0.094
16070	Beans, lentils, mature seeds, boiled w/o salt	1 cup	198	229.68	17.86	39.857	15.642	0.752	0.127	0.347	0.105
16081	Beans, mung, mature seeds, boiled w/o salt	1 cup	202	212.1	14.18	38.683	15.352	0.768	0.109	0.259	0.234
16080	Beans, mung, mature seeds, raw	1 tbsp	13	45.11	3.102	8.141	2.119	0.149	0.021	0.05	0.045
16038	Beans, navy, mature seeds, boiled w/o salt	1 cup	182	258.44	15.834	47.884	11.648	1.037	0.091	0.448	0.269
16039	Beans, navy, mature seeds, canned	1 cup	262	296.06	19.729	53.579	13.362	1.127	0.1	0.487	0.293
16044	Beans, pinto, mature seeds, canned	1 cup	240	206.4	11.664	36.6	11.04	1.944	0.389	0.694	0.401
16109	Beans, soy, mature seeds, boiled w/o salt	1 cup	172	297.56	28.621	17.08	10.32	15.428	3.407	8.71	2.231
16108	Beans, soy, mature seeds, raw	1 cup	186	773.76	67.871	56.098	17.298	37.088	8.191	20.934	5.364
16110	Beans, soy, mature seeds, roasted w/salt	1 cup	172	810.12	60.578	57.706	30.444	43.688	9.649	24.663	6.319
16162	Beans, soy, tofu, Mori-Nu, silken, firm	1 slice	84	52.08	5.796	2.016	0.084	2.268	0.453	1.247	0.341
16164	Beans, soy, tofu, Mori-Nu, silken, lite firm	1 slice	84	31.08	5.292	0.924	0	0.672	0.114	0.377	0.112
16161	Beans, soy, tofu, Mori-Nu, silken, soft	1 slice	84	46.2	4.032	2.436	0.084	2.268	0.438	1.302	0.3
16129	Beans, soy, tofu, nigari, fried	1 oz	28.35	76.829	4.873	2.974	1.106	5.721	1.263	3.229	0.827
16050	Beans, white, mature seeds, boiled w/o salt	1 cup	179	248.81	17.417	44.911	11.277	0.626	0.055	0.272	0.163
16051	Beans, white, mature seeds, canned	1 cup	262	306.54	19.021	57.483	12.576	0.76	0.065	0.322	0.194
16048	Beans, yellow, mature seeds, boiled w/o salt	1 cup	177	254.88	16.213	44.728	18.408	1.912	0.166	0.825	0.494
51696	Beef & onion patty, flame broiled, Lean Magic product #9676	1 piece	74	138.38	17.094	1.939	1.036	6.727	2.857	0.276	2.633
51738	Beef & turkey, flame broiled patty w/teriyaki sauce, Lean Magic 30 product #9128	1 piece	20	28.2	3.892	1.672	0.26	0.72	0.306	0.099	0.248
51737	Beef & turkey, flame broiled rib-B-Q w/BBQ sauce, Rib-B-Q lean magic 30	1 piece	85	115.6	14.348	8.024	1.36	3.094	1.301	0.42	1.008
13168	Beef bottom round, all grades, lean (1/4"trim) braised	3 oz	85	177.65	26.852	0	0	6.97	3.052	0.264	2.355
13160	Beef bottom round, all grades, lean & fat (1/4"trim) braised	3 oz	85	233.75	24.361	0	0	14.365	6.247	0.544	5.415
13319	Beef brain, pan fried	3 oz	85	166.6	10.684	0	0	13.456	3.383	1.964	3.179
13022	Beef brisket, whole, all grades, lean & fat (1/4"trim) braised	3 oz	85	327.25	19.975	0	0	26.826	11.815	0.961	10.523
13345	Beef cured breakfast strip, cooked	3 slices	34	152.66	10.642	0.476	0	11.696	5.729	0.537	4.879
13322	Beef heart, simmered	3 oz	85	133.45	24.208	0.128	0	4.021	0.859	0.837	1.193
13324	Beef kidney, simmered	3 oz	85	128.35	23.18	0	0	3.953	0.604	0.703	0.906
13327	Beef liver, pan fried	1 slice (yield from 112 g raw liver)	81	141.75	21.481	4.18	0	3.791	0.529	0.471	1.209
22529	Beef pot pie, frozen	1 package	198	449.46	13.266	44.154	2.178	24.354	9.682	2.673	8.514
7956	Beef sausage, fresh, cooked	1 hot dog	52	172.64	9.469	0.182	0	14.55	6.572	0.345	5.671
7954	Beef sausage, pre-cooked	1 hot dog	52	210.6	8.06	0.016	0	19.536	8.521	0.457	7.851
13458	Beef short loin, porterhouse steak, all grades, lean & fat (1/4"trim) broiled	3 oz	85	279.65	19.134	0	0	21.964	9.822	0.849	8.642
13472	Beef short loin, T-bone steak, all grades, lean & fat (1/4"trim) broiled	3 oz	85	260.1	19.949	0	0	19.363	8.63	0.701	7.582
13270	Beef short loin, top loin, all grades, lean (1/4" trim) broiled	3 oz	85	175.95	24.327	0	0	7.99	3.213	0.264	3.052

Chol (g)	Calc (mg)	Iron (mg)	Mag (mg)	Phos (mg)	Pota (mg)	Sodi (mg)	Zinc (mg)	Vit A (RAE)	Vit C (mg)	Thia (mg)	Ribo (mg)	Niac (mg)	Vit B6 (mg)	Vit B12 (µg)	Vit E (mg)	Fol (µg)	Alc (g)
0	7.35	0.236	4.35	16.5	25.95	36.3	0.164	0	1.185	0.013	0.008	0.06	0.06	0	0.113	8.85	0
0	69.12	3.149	79.36	268.8	657.92	888.32	1.408	0	3.072	0.279	0.184	1.285	0.177	0		125.4	0
0	49.56	5.204	79.65	251.34	713.31	3.54	1.894	0	2.124	0.283	0.103	1.023	0.212	0	1.54	230.1	0
0	31.96	4.493	80.84	208.68	955.04	3.76	1.786	0	0	0.303	0.103	0.791	0.303	0	0.338	156	0
0	50.61	4.362	93.99	178.34	530.2	809.76	1.566	0	0	0.133	0.082	0.629	0.219	0		120.5	0
0	37.62	6.593	71.28	356.4	730.62	3.96	2.515	0	2.97	0.335	0.145	2.099	0.352	0	0.218	358.4	0
0	54.54	2.828	96.96	199.98	537.32	4.04	1.697	2.02	2.02	0.331	0.123	1.166	0.135	0	0.303	321.2	0
0	17.16	0.876	24.57	47.71	161.98	1.95	0.348	0.78	0.624	0.081	0.03	0.293	0.05	0	0.066	81.25	0
0	127.4	4.514	107.38	285.74	669.76	1.82	1.929	0	1.638	0.368	0.111	0.966	0.298	0		254.8	0
0	123.14	4.847	123.14	351.08	754.56	1173.76	2.017	0	1.834	0.369	0.144	1.276	0.27	0	2.044	162.4	0
0	103.2	3.504	64.8	220.8	583.2	705.6	1.656	0	2.16	0.242	0.151	0.701	0.178	0	1.416	144	0
0	175.44	8.841	147.92	421.4	885.8	1.72	1.978	0	2.924	0.267	0.49	0.686	0.402	0	0.602	92.88	0
0	515.22	29.202	520.8	1309.44	3342.42	3.72	9.095	0	11.16	1.626	1.618	3.019	0.701	0	1.581	697.5	0
0	237.36	6.708	249.4	624.36	2528.4	280.36	5.401	17.2	3.784	0.172	0.249	2.425	0.358	0	1.565	362.9	0
0	26.88	0.865	22.68	75.6	162.96	30.24	0.512	0	0	0.085	0.034	0.207	0.009	0	0.16		0
0	30.24	0.63	8.4	68.04	52.92	71.4	0.277	0	0	0.034	0.017	0.092	0	0	0.05		0
0	26.04	0.689	24.36	52.08	151.2	4.2	0.437	0	0	0.084	0.034	0.252	0.009	0	0.168		0
0	105.462	1.381	17.01	81.365	41.391	4.536	0.564	0.284	0	0.048	0.014	0.028	0.028	0	0.011	7.655	0
0	161.1	6.623	112.77	202.27	1004.19	10.74	2.47	0	0	0.211	0.082	0.251	0.166	0	1.736	145	0
0	191.26	7.834	133.62	238.42	1189.48	13.1	2.934	0	0	0.252	0.097	0.296	0.197	0		170.3	0
0	109.74	4.39	130.98	323.91	575.25	8.85	1.876	0	3.186	0.331	0.182	1.253	0.228	0		143.4	0
42.18	23.68	2.153	28.86	240.5	283.42	313.02	5.025		0.518	0.139	0.152	2.917	0.278	1.643	0.068	5.18	0
8.2	6.2	0.43	6.6	45.8	59.2	127.4	0.878		0	0.034	0.023	0.561	0.058	0.264	0.005	0.4	0
28.9	33.15	1.87	26.35	202.3	244.8	560.15	3.179		1.275	0.144	0.086	2.356	0.264	1.403	0.046	1.7	0
81.6	4.25	2.941	21.25	231.2	261.8	43.35	4.658	0	0	0.06	0.221	3.468	0.306	2.1	0.119	9.35	0
81.6	5.1	2.652	18.7	208.25	239.7	42.5	4.174	0	0	0.06	0.204	3.171	0.281	1.997	0.162	8.5	0
1695.75	7.65	1.887	12.75	328.1	300.9	134.3	1.148	0	2.805	0.111	0.221	3.213	0.331	12.92		5.1	0
79.9	6.8	1.904	15.3	158.95	196.35	51.85	4.335	0	0	0.051	0.153	2.55	0.204	1.938	0.204	5.1	0
40.46	3.06	1.068	9.18	80.24	140.08	766.02	2.166	0	0	0.031	0.088	2.2	0.105	1.173	0.099	2.72	0
180.2	4.25	5.423	17.85	215.9	186.15	50.15	2.439	0	0	0.086	1.029	5.678	0.208	9.18	0.247	4.25	0
608.6	16.15	4.93	10.2	258.4	114.75	79.9	2.414	0	0	0.136	2.525	3.332	0.332	21.165	0.068	70.55	0
308.61	4.86	4.998	17.82	392.85	284.31	62.37	4.236	6273	0.567	0.143	2.774	14.155	0.832	67.335	0.373	210.6	0
37.62						736.56											
42.64	5.72	0.816	7.28	73.32	134.16	339.04	2.278	6.76	0	0.025	0.078	1.872	0.163	1.045	0.125	1.56	0
43.16	7.8	0.796	6.76	96.2	121.68	473.2	1.518	13	0.364	0.015	0.061	1.669	0.1	1.056	0.255	2.6	0
61.2	6.8	2.278	17	150.45	216.75	52.7	3.511	0	0	0.077	0.178	3.272	0.284	1.793	0.187	5.95	0
55.25	5.95	2.626	18.7	157.25	239.7	56.95	3.655	0	0	0.079	0.183	3.367	0.286	1.811	0.178	5.95	0
64.6	6.8	2.1	22.95	185.3	336.6	57.8	4.437	0	0	0.077	0.17	4.539	0.357	1.7	0.119	6.8	0

EvaluEat Code	Food Name	Amt	Wt (g)	Energy (kcal)	Prot (g)	Carb (g)	Fiber (g)	Fat (g)	Mono (g)	Poly (g)	Sat (g)
13262	Beef short loin, top loin, all grades, lean & fat (1/4" trim) broiled	3 oz	85	243.95	21.726	0	0	16.796	7.064	0.604	6.647
13340	Beef tongue, simmered	3 oz	85	236.3	16.397	0	0	18.955	8.587	0.557	6.906
13341	Beef tripe, raw	1 oz	28.35	23.247	3.422	0	0	1.046	0.435	0.051	0.366
13012	Beef, all cuts, all grades, lean (1/4"trim) cooked	3 oz	85	183.6	25.143	0	0	8.424	3.545	0.289	3.222
13004	Beef, all cuts, all grades, lean & fat (1/4"trim) cooked	3 oz	85	259.25	22.049	0	0	18.309	7.837	0.663	7.259
43384	Beef, bologna, reduced sodium	1 fl. oz.	29.8	93.274	3.487	0.596	0	8.463	3.963	0.313	3.479
13870	Beef, bottom round, all grades, lean & fat (1/8" trim) roasted	1 piece, cooked, (yield from 1 lb raw meat)	338	736.84	89.266	0	0	39.343	16.778	1.518	14.933
13953	Beef, bottom sirloin, tri-tip roast, separable lean and fat, 0"trim, all grades, cooked, roasted	3 oz (1 serving)	85	176.8	22.142	0	0	9.41	4.659	0.309	3.46
13055	Beef, brisket, flat half, separable lean and fat, 1/8"trim, select, cooked, braised	3 oz	85	238	24.625	0	0	14.765	6.359	0.546	5.855
13034	Beef, chuck, arm pot roast, all grades, lean & fat (1/4"trim) braised	3 oz	85	282.2	23.316	0	0	20.239	8.679	0.774	7.973
13050	Beef, chuck, blade roast, all grades, lean & fat (1/4"trim) braised	3 oz	85	293.25	22.585	0	0	21.837	9.435	0.782	8.695
23553	Beef, chuck, clod roast, separable lean and fat, trimmed to 1/4"fat, all grades, cooked, roasted	3 oz (1 serving)	85	205.7	20.587	0	0	13.107	5.952	0.521	4.877
23555	Beef, chuck, clod steak, separable lean and fat, trimmed to 1/4"fat, all grades, cooked, braised	3 oz (1 serving)	85	231.2	22.262	0	0	15.071	6.809	0.599	5.694
23547	Beef, chuck, tender steak, separable lean and fat, trimmed to 0"fat, all grades, cooked, broiled	3 oz (1 serving)	85	136	21.99	0	0	4.692	2.256	0.329	1.59
23523	Beef, chuck, top blade, separable lean and fat, trimmed to 0"fat, USDA Choice, cooked, broiled	3 oz (1 serving)	85	192.95	21.905	0	0	10.991	5.329	0.39	3.538
22698	Beef, corned beef hash, canned entree/Hormel	1 cup	236	387.04	20.603	21.877	2.596	24.166	12.414	0.708	10.195
22908	Beef, corned beef hash, canned, with potato	100 grams	100	164	8.73	9.27	1.1	10.24	5.26	0.3	4.32
51658	Beef, country fried finger/Pierre product #3813	1 piece	26	82.16	4.334	4.009	0.364	5.486	1.704	1.897	1.372
51613	Beef, country fried nugget/Pierre product #1935	1 piece	14.2	48.706	2.424	2.256	0.185	3.385	1.113	1.078	0.9
51605	Beef, country fried patty/Pierre product #1840	1 piece	108	356.4	17.55	16.459	1.512	24.786	7.951	7.957	6.515
51602	Beef, country fried steak/Pierre product #1610	1 piece	108	356.4	16.859	14.083	0.432	25.607	9.168	6.324	7.897
13358	Beef, cured, smoked, chopped	1 slice (1 oz)	28	37.24	5.653	0.521	0	1.238	0.512	0.064	0.507
13360	Beef, cured, thin sliced	10 slices	28	42.84	8.708	0.773	0	0.543	0.235	0.02	0.266
13350	Beef, dried, cured	10 slices	28	42.84	8.708	0.773	0	0.543	0.235	0.02	0.267
13176	Beef, eye of round, all grades, lean & fat (1/4"trim) roasted	3 oz	85	194.65	22.772	0	0	10.838	4.658	0.391	4.233
13682	Beef, eye of round, Prime, lean & fat (1/2"trim) roasted	3 oz	85	212.5	22.958	0	0	12.708	5.67	0.459	5.117
13096	Beef, eye/small end ribs (10−12 ribs), Choice, lean & fat (1/4"trim) broiled	1 steak	236	625.4	62.729	0	0	39.554	16.197	1.468	15.354
51718	Beef, flame broiled fajita/Lean Magic Wonderbites Dipper product #9974	1 piece	18	32.58	3.897	1.089	0.27	1.483	0.626	0.062	0.576
51663	Beef, flame broiled meatloaf/Lean Magic product #3825	1 piece	74	148	16.643	4.151	0.814	7.2	3.092	0.362	2.793
51677	Beef, flame broiled patty/Pierre product #3871	1 piece	69	158.01	16.187	1.546	1.035	9.536	4.082	0.386	3.782

Chol (g)	Calc (mg)	Iron (mg)	Mag (mg)	Phos (mg)	Pota (mg)	Sodi (mg)	Zinc (mg)	Vit A (RAE)	Vit C (mg)	Thia (mg)	Ribo (mg)	Niac (mg)	Vit B$_6$ (mg)	Vit B$_{12}$ (µg)	Vit E (mg)	Fol (µg)	Alc (g)
67.15	7.65	1.896	19.55	164.9	296.65	53.55	3.885	0	0	0.068	0.153	3.995	0.315	1.649	0.017	5.95	0
112.2	4.25	2.218	12.75	123.25	156.4	55.25	34.77	0	1.105	0.019	0.25	2.967	0.132	2.661	0.255	5.95	0
34.587	19.562	0.167	3.686	18.144	18.995	27.5	0.403	0	0	0	0.018	0.25	0.004	0.394	0.026	1.418	0
73.1	7.65	2.542	22.1	198.05	306	56.95	5.891	0	0	0.085	0.204	3.511	0.315	2.244	0.119	6.8	0
74.8	8.5	2.227	18.7	172.55	266.05	52.7	4.972	0	0	0.068	0.178	3.094	0.281	2.074	0.17	5.95	0
16.688	3.576	0.417	2.98	24.436	46.19	203.236	0.596	0	0	0.018	0.039	0.784	0.054	0.42	0.057	1.49	0
253.5	20.28	7.301	57.46	554.32	723.32	118.3	14.97	0	0	0.206	0.477	15.602	1.173	4.969	1.386	27.04	0
71.4	16.15	1.411	18.7	170.85	274.55	45.05	3.97	0	0	0.06	0.107	5.893	0.463	1.301	0.34	6.8	0
60.35	14.45	2.04	16.15	153	201.45	41.65	5.882	0	0	0.054	0.134	3.549	0.242	1.632	0.425	7.65	0
84.15	8.5	2.644	16.15	187	209.1	51	5.814	0	0	0.06	0.204	2.703	0.238	2.508	0.187	7.65	0
88.4	11.05	2.635	16.15	170	196.35	54.4	7.072	0	0	0.06	0.204	2.057	0.221	1.938	0.17	4.25	0
63.75	6.8	2.388	17	166.6	286.45	56.95	4.854	0	0	0.069	0.192	2.726	0.217	2.405	0.119	7.65	0
79.9	7.65	2.831	16.15	175.95	220.15	48.45	5.772	0	0	0.057	0.192	2.428	0.205	2.329	0.094	6.8	0
53.55	6.8	2.491	19.55	192.95	249.05	60.35	6.647	0	0	0.094	0.196	3.087	0.273	2.882	0.136	6.8	0
49.3	5.95	2.355	20.4	182.75	255	57.8	7.446	0	0	0.094	0.195	3.076	0.272	2.873	0.153	6.8	0
75.52	44.84	2.36	30.68		405.92	1003	3.304	2.124									0
32	19	1	13	56	172	425	1.4	0	0.9	0.069	0.05	1.572	0.231	0.41	0.04	7	0
9.88	8.32	0.783	7.02	60.06	71.76	125.58	1.191		0	0.08	0.064	1.083	0.066	0.387	0.548	9.36	0
5.254	5.538	0.454	3.834	34.932	39.192	71.284	0.626		0	0.044	0.039	0.563	0.036	0.25	0.298	6.106	0
42.12	34.56	3.208	29.16	246.24	293.76	519.48	4.828		0	0.329	0.261	4.441	0.27	1.588	2.272	38.88	0
51.84	15.12	2.657	12.96	177.12	217.08	376.92	3.402		0	0.211	0.233	3.776	0.159	1.512	1.859	37.8	0
12.88	2.24	0.798	5.88	50.68	105.56	352.24	1.1	0	0	0.023	0.049	1.282	0.098	0.484		2.24	0
22.12	1.68	0.781	5.6	61.04	69.16	781.2	1.229	0	0	0.016	0.059	0.914	0.081	0.554	0.031	2.52	0
22.12	1.4	0.812	6.16	54.88	81.48	781.2	1.112	0	0	0.017	0.062	0.927	0.069	0.661	0	2.24	0
61.2	5.1	1.564	20.4	176.8	307.7	50.15	3.689	0	0	0.068	0.136	2.967	0.298	1.785	0.153	5.95	0
61.2	5.1	1.573	21.25	178.5	311.1	50.15	3.723	0	0	0.068	0.138	2.986	0.298	1.793		5.95	0
297.36	42.48	4.248	51.92	474.36	769.36	125.08	11.3	0	0	0.156	0.276	17.013	1.251	4.13	1.109	18.88	0
9.36	6.3	0.531	7.2	57.24	67.68	85.86	1.195	0.054		0.035	0.036	0.689	0.065	0.38	0.012	0.9	0
41.44	25.9	2.079	23.68	142.08	244.94	399.6	4.359	2.072		0.109	0.155	2.53	0.242	1.643	0.073	7.4	0
41.4	24.15	2.105	29.67	228.39	276	291.18	4.975	0		0.149	0.146	2.904	0.275	1.615	0.042	3.45	0

EvaluEat Code	Food Name	Amt	Wt (g)	Energy (kcal)	Prot (g)	Carb (g)	Fiber (g)	Fat (g)	Mono (g)	Poly (g)	Sat (g)
51683	Beef, flame broiled steak/Pierre product #9010	1 piece	74	248.64	17.856	0.326	0	18.944	8.161	0.712	7.586
13067	Beef, flank, choice, lean & fat (0″ trim) broiled	1 steak	387	781.74	106.62	0	0	36.03	14.516	1.409	14.861
23580	Beef, ground, 75% lean meat/25% fat, crumbles, cooked, pan-browned	3 oz	85	235.45	22.338	0	0	15.478	7.131	0.386	6.027
23575	Beef, ground, 80% lean meat/20% fat, crumbles, cooked, pan-browned	3 oz	85	231.2	22.95	0	0	14.756	6.542	0.428	5.586
23570	Beef, ground, 85% lean meat/15% fat, crumbles, cooked, pan-browned	3 oz	85	217.6	23.57	0	0	13.005	5.605	0.406	4.925
23565	Beef, ground, 90% lean meat/10% fat, crumbles, cooked, pan-browned	3 oz	85	195.5	24.183	0	0	10.234	4.316	0.315	4.053
23560	Beef, ground, 95% lean meat/5% fat, crumbles, cooked, pan-browned	3 oz	85	164.05	24.795	0	0	6.443	2.825	0.328	3.022
13299	Beef, ground, extra lean, broiled, well done	3 oz	85	225.25	24.293	0	0	13.43	5.882	0.502	5.279
13306	Beef, ground, lean, broiled, well done	3 oz	85	238	23.97	0	0	14.994	6.562	0.561	5.891
13313	Beef, ground, regular, broiled, well done	3 oz	85	248.2	23.12	0	0	16.541	7.242	0.621	6.503
13113	Beef, large end ribs (6–9 ribs) all grades, lean (1/4″ trim) roasted	yield from 1 lb raw meat	210	497.7	57.813	0	0	27.72	11.592	0.798	11.067
13101	Beef, large end ribs (6–9 ribs) all grades, lean & fat (1/4″ trim) roasted	yield from 1 lb raw meat	293	1069.5	66.335	0	0	87.226	37.358	3.047	35.189
23545	Beef, loin, bottom sirloin butt, tri-tip steak, separable lean and fat (0″ trim) all grades	3 oz	85	225.25	25.475	0	0	12.903	6.599	0.457	4.851
23540	Beef, plate, inside skirt steak, separable lean and fat, trimmed to 0″ fat, all grades, broiled	3 oz	85	187	22.211	0	0	10.243	5.147	0.371	3.966
13979	Beef, plate, outside skirt steak, separable lean only, trimmed to 0″ fat, all grades, broiled	3 oz	85	198.05	20.553	0	0	12.215	6.273	0.51	5.075
13952	Beef, rib eye, small end (ribs 10–12), separable lean and fat, 0″ trim, all grades, cooked, broiled	3 oz	85	209.95	23.18	0	0	12.529	5.129	0.465	4.862
23626	Beef, rib, small end ribs (ribs 10–12), separable lean only, 1/8″ trim, Choice, cooked, broiled	3 oz	85	171.7	24.047	0	0	7.693	3.07	0.275	2.928
22721	Beef, roast beef hash, canned entree/Hormel	3 oz	236	384.68	21.311	22.916	3.54	23.647	11.281	0.637	9.912
23592	Beef, round, top round, separable lean only, 1/8″ trim, select, cooked, broiled	3 oz	85	150.45	26.869	0	0	3.953	1.652	0.16	1.362
23002	Beef, short loin, porterhouse steak, all grades, lean & fat (1/8″ trim) broiled	3 oz	85	252.45	19.984	0	0	18.556	8.152	0.697	7.157
23006	Beef, short loin, T-bone steak, all grades, lean & fat (1/8″ trim) broiled	3 oz	85	238	20.681	0	0	16.549	7.259	0.595	6.426
23630	Beef, short loin, top loin, separable lean only, 1/8″ trim, Choice, cooked, broiled	3 oz	85	170.85	24.786	0	0	7.182	2.867	0.257	2.734
13148	Beef, short ribs, Choice, lean & fat, braised	3 oz	85	400.35	18.334	0	0	35.683	16.048	1.301	15.13
13124	Beef, small end ribs (10–12 ribs) all grades, lean & fat (1/4″ trim) broiled	3 oz	85	285.6	20.137	0	0	22.083	9.486	0.765	8.942
13238	Beef, tenderloin, all grades, lean & fat (1/4″ trim) broiled	3 oz	85	247.35	21.471	0	0	17.221	7.064	0.655	6.758
13192	Beef, tip round, all grades, lean & fat (1/4″ trim) roasted	3 oz	85	198.9	22.874	0	0	11.254	4.684	0.433	4.267
13427	Beef, top round, all grades, lean & fat (1/4″ trim) braised	3 oz	85	210.8	28.756	0	0	9.716	4.012	0.4	3.672
13278	Beef, top sirloin, all grades, lean & fat (1/4″ trim) broiled	3 oz	85	219.3	23.639	0	0	13.099	5.636	0.502	5.219

Chol (g)	Calc (mg)	Iron (mg)	Mag (mg)	Phos (mg)	Pota (mg)	Sodi (mg)	Zinc (mg)	Vit A (RAE)	Vit C (mg)	Thia (mg)	Ribo (mg)	Niac (mg)	Vit B$_6$ (mg)	Vit B$_{12}$ (µg)	Vit E (mg)	Fol (µg)	Alc (g)
64.38	7.4	1.791	14.8	229.4	208.68	284.9	3.826		0	0.053	0.144	2.398	0.211	1.717	0.057	4.44	0
197.37	69.66	6.966	85.14	777.87	1261.62	205.11	18.54	0	0	0.267	0.468	28.913	2.125	7.043	1.509	34.83	0
75.65	28.9	2.236	18.7	181.9	300.9	79.05	5.245	0	0	0.039	0.159	4.543	0.365	2.499	0.408	10.2	0
75.65	23.8	2.363	19.55	192.1	323	77.35	5.44	0	0	0.038	0.161	4.956	0.364	2.431	0.408	9.35	0
76.5	18.7	2.491	21.25	202.3	345.95	75.65	5.627	0	0	0.037	0.162	5.37	0.364	2.372	0.4	8.5	0
75.65	13.6	2.618	22.95	212.5	368.05	73.95	5.814	0	0	0.037	0.164	5.783	0.364	2.304	0.374	6.8	0
75.65	7.65	2.746	23.8	223.55	390.15	72.25	6.001	0	0	0.036	0.166	6.197	0.364	2.244	0.34	5.95	0
84.15	7.65	2.355	21.25	161.5	313.65	69.7	5.465		0	0.06	0.272	4.972	0.272	2.176	0.153	9.35	0
85.85	10.2	2.082	20.4	154.7	296.65	75.65	5.27		0	0.051	0.204	5.075	0.255	2.312	0.173	9.35	0
85.85	10.2	2.329	18.7	162.35	277.95	79.05	4.938		0	0.034	0.178	5.499	0.255	2.788	0.196	8.5	0
170.1	16.8	5.922	52.5	438.9	749.7	153.3	15.67	0	0	0.189	0.462	9.345	0.546	5.481	0.294	18.9	0
249.05	29.3	6.768	55.67	498.1	843.84	187.52	16.7	0	0	0.205	0.527	10.577	0.674	6.798	0.674	20.51	0
57.8	10.2	3.094	22.1	225.25	371.45	61.2	5.993	0	0	0.109	0.243	3.591	0.377	2.405	0.145	8.5	0
51	9.35	2.355	20.4	195.5	245.65	63.75	6.146	0	0	0.077	0.162	3.183	0.273	3.162	0.085	5.95	0
49.3	8.5	2.261	21.25	187.85	334.05	79.9	4.862	0	0	0.101	0.166	3.681	0.421	3.655	0.094	6.8	0
94.35	17	1.488	19.55	180.2	289	47.6	4.19	0	0	0.063	0.111	6.168	0.485	1.36	0.382	6.8	0
72.25	13.6	1.632	20.4	186.15	299.2	49.3	4.514	0	0	0.064	0.123	7.095	0.501	1.505	0.357	7.65	0
73.16	42.48	2.36	33.04		431.88	792.96	3.304		1.888								0
51.85	5.95	2.261	18.7	175.95	229.5	36.55	4.735	0	0	0.065	0.145	4.621	0.354	1.377	0.289	9.35	0
60.35	6.8	2.329	19.55	158.95	272.85	54.4	3.893	0	0	0.085	0.187	3.46	0.298	1.828	0.17	5.95	0
52.7	6.8	2.405	20.4	164.05	285.6	56.1	3.978	0	0	0.085	0.187	3.519	0.298	1.845	0.162	5.95	0
67.15	13.6	1.675	21.25	192.1	307.7	51	4.649	0	0	0.065	0.127	7.313	0.516	1.547	0.349	8.5	0
79.9	10.2	1.964	12.75	137.7	190.4	42.5	4.148	0	0	0.043	0.128	2.084	0.187	2.227	0.247	4.25	0
71.4	11.05	1.862	18.7	148.75	276.25	52.7	4.752	0	0	0.077	0.153	3.391	0.281	2.457	0.187	5.95	0
73.1	6.8	2.678	22.1	178.5	312.8	50.15	4.148	0	0	0.094	0.221	2.992	0.331	2.049	0.162	5.1	0
69.7	5.1	2.338	21.25	191.25	305.15	53.55	5.525	0	0	0.077	0.213	2.992	0.315	2.346	0.145	5.95	0
76.5	4.25	2.652	20.4	180.2	267.75	38.25	3.638	0	0	0.06	0.204	3.069	0.23	2.21	0.145	7.65	0
76.5	9.35	2.601	24.65	188.7	311.1	53.55	4.972	0	0	0.094	0.23	3.341	0.349	2.287	0.153	7.65	0

EvaluEat Code	Food Name	Amt	Wt (g)	Energy (kcal)	Prot (g)	Carb (g)	Fiber (g)	Fat (g)	Mono (g)	Poly (g)	Sat (g)
13073	Beef, whole ribs (6–12 ribs) all grades, lean & fat (1/4" trim) roasted	3 oz	85	304.3	19.125	0	0	24.659	10.6	0.876	9.945
14169	Beverage mix, carob flavor, dry, prep w/milk	1 cup (8 fl. oz.)	256	192	8.09	22.221	1.024	7.962	1.989	0.484	4.554
14177	Beverage mix, chocolate flavor, dry mix, prep w/milk	1 cup (8 fl. oz.)	266	226.1	8.592	31.681	1.064	8.618	2.205	0.495	4.948
14318	Beverage mix, chocolate malted milk powder, no added nutrients, prep w/milk	1 cup (8 fl. oz.)	265	225.25	8.931	29.68	1.325	8.719	2.192	0.551	4.99
14312	Beverage mix, natural malt powder, no added nutrients, prep w/milk	1 cup (8 fl. oz.)	265	233.2	10.229	27.109	0.265	9.593	2.393	0.731	5.403
14351	Beverage mix, strawberry flavor, dry, prep w/milk	1 cup (8 fl. oz.)	266	234.08	7.98	32.718	0	8.246	2.357	0.303	5.081
14006	Beverage, alcoholic, beer, light	1 can or bottle (12 fl. oz.)	354	99.12	0.708	4.602	0	0	0	0	0
14003	Beverage, alcoholic, beer, regular	1 can	356	117.48	1.068	5.732	0.356	0.214	0	0	0
14534	Beverage, alcoholic, coffee liqueur 63 proof	1 jigger (1.5 fl. oz.)	52	160.16	0.052	16.744	0	0.156	0.011	0.055	0.055
14415	Beverage, alcoholic, coffee w/cream liqueur, 34 proof	1 jigger (1.5 fl. oz.)	47	153.69	1.316	9.823	0	7.379	2.095	0.314	4.542
14034	Beverage, alcoholic, creme de menthe, 72 proof	1 jigger (1.5 fl. oz.)	50	185.5	0	20.8	0	0.15	0.007	0.083	0.007
14010	Beverage, alcoholic, daiquiri, prep from recipe	1 cocktail (2 fl. oz.)	60	111.6	0.036	4.164	0.06	0.036	0.004	0.01	0.004
14049	Beverage, alcoholic, distilled spirits, gin 90 proof	1 jigger (1.5 fl. oz.)	42	110.46	0	0	0	0	0	0	0
14050	Beverage, alcoholic, distilled spirits, rum 80 proof	1 jigger (1.5 fl. oz.)	42	97.02	0	0	0	0	0	0	0
14051	Beverage, alcoholic, distilled spirits, vodka 80 proof	1 jigger (1.5 fl. oz.)	42	97.02	0	0	0	0	0	0	0
14052	Beverage, alcoholic, distilled spirits, whiskey 86 proof	1 jigger	42	105	0	0.042	0	0	0	0	0
14014	Beverage, alcoholic, martini, prepared from recipe	1 cocktail (2 fl. oz.)	60	145.8	0.024	1.224	0	0	0	0	0
14017	Beverage, alcoholic, pina colada, prep from recipe	1 cocktail (4.5 fl. oz.)	141	245.34	0.592	31.951	0.423	2.651	0.116	0.047	2.307
43479	Beverage, alcoholic, rice (sake)	1 oz	28.34	37.976	0.142	1.417	0	0	0	0	0
14084	Beverage, alcoholic, wine (all table)	1 glass (3.5 fl. oz.)	103	79.31	0.206	3.296	0	0	0	0	0
43154	Beverage, alcoholic, wine, cooking	1 cup	186	93	0.93	11.718	0	0	0	0	0
14536	Beverage, alcoholic, wine, dry dessert	1 glass (3.5 fl. oz.)	103	156.56	0.206	12.02	0	0	0	0	0
14096	Beverage, alcoholic, wine, red	1 glass (3.5 fl. oz.)	103	74.16	0.206	1.751	0	0	0	0	0
14104	Beverage, alcoholic, wine, rose	1 glass (3.5 fl. oz.)	103	73.13	0.206	1.442	0	0	0	0	0
14057	Beverage, alcoholic, wine, sweet dessert	1 glass (3.5 fl. oz.)	103	164.8	0.206	14.101	0	0	0	0	0
14106	Beverage, alcoholic, wine, white	1 glass (3.5 fl. oz.)	103	70.04	0.103	0.824	0	0	0	0	0
14182	Beverage, chocolate syrup w/o added nutrients, prep w/milk	1 cup (8 fl. oz.)	282	253.8	8.657	36.04	0.846	8.347	2.087	0.485	4.74
14390	Beverage, cocoa mix w/aspartame, dry, low kcal, prep w/H$_2$O	1 packet dry mix with 6 fl. oz. water	192	55.68	2.419	10.445	0.96	0.442	0.146	0.013	0
14194	Beverage, cocoa mix, dry, w/o added nutrients, prep w/H$_2$O	1 oz packet with 6 fl. oz. water	206	113.3	1.669	23.978	1.03	1.133	0.375	0.035	0.672
14195	Beverage, cocoa, hot cocoa mix w/marshmallows/Carnation	1 envelope	28	111.72	1.347	24.254	0.504	1.025	0.307	0.376	0.412
14418	Beverage, coffee mix w/sugar (cappuccino) dry, prep w/H$_2$O	6 fl. oz. H$_2$O & 2 rounded tsp mix	192	61.44	0.384	10.752	0	2.112	0.123	0.038	1.83
14419	Beverage, coffee mix w/sugar (French) dry, prep w/H$_2$O	6 fl. oz. H$_2$O & 2 rounded tsp mix	189	56.7	0.567	6.615	0	3.402	0.198	0.062	2.947
14420	Beverage, coffee mix w/sugar (mocha) dry, prep w/H$_2$O	6 fl. oz. & 2 round tsp mix	188	50.76	0.564	8.46	0.188	1.88	0.109	0.034	1.609
14232	Beverage, coffee mix, Kraft Intl Sugar-Free Fat-Free Low-Calorie French Vanilla	1 NLEA serving	7	25.41	0.217	5.32	0.343	0.343			0.056
14209	Beverage, coffee, brewed	1 cup (8 fl. oz.)	237	9.48	0.332	0	0	1.801	0	0	0

Chol (g)	Calc (mg)	Iron (mg)	Mag (mg)	Phos (mg)	Pota (mg)	Sodi (mg)	Zinc (mg)	Vit A (RAE)	Vit C (mg)	Thia (mg)	Ribo (mg)	Niac (mg)	Vit B$_6$ (mg)	Vit B$_{12}$ (µg)	Vit E (mg)	Fol (µg)	Alc (g)
71.4	9.35	1.989	17	148.75	255.85	53.55	4.548	0	0	0.06	0.145	2.899	0.196	2.159		5.95	0
25.6	250.88	0.64	25.6	204.8	335.36	117.76	0.947	69.12	0	0.108	0.445	0.353	0.102	1.075		12.8	0
23.94	252.7	0.798	47.88	234.08	457.52	154.28	1.277	69.16	0.266	0.114	0.479	0.378	0.09	1.064	0.16	13.3	0
26.5	259.7	0.557	39.75	241.15	455.8	159	1.087	68.9	0.265	0.143	0.488	0.686	0.122	1.113	0.159	23.85	0
31.8	310.05	0.239	45.05	280.9	484.95	209.35	1.14	87.45	0.53	0.215	0.641	1.375	0.175	1.219	0.329	21.2	0
31.92	292.6	0.213	31.92	228.76	369.74	127.68	0.931	69.16	2.394	0.093	0.42	0.221	0.104	0.878		13.3	0
0	17.7	0.142	17.7	42.48	63.72	10.62	0.106	0	0	0.032	0.106	1.388	0.12	0.035	0	14.16	11.328
0	17.8	0.071	21.36	46.28	89	14.24	0.036	0	0	0.021	0.093	1.613	0.178	0.071	0	21.36	12.816
0	0.52	0.031	1.56	3.12	15.6	4.16	0.016	0	0	0.002	0.006	0.075	0	0		0	13.52
27.26	7.52	0.061	0.94	23.5	15.04	43.24	0.075	81.31	0.094	0.005	0.027	0.037	0.005	0.038	0.211	0.94	6.486
0	0	0.035	0	0	0	2.5	0.02	0	0	0	0	0.002	0	0	0	0	14.9
0	1.8	0.054	1.2	3	12.6	3	0.024	0	0.96	0.008	0.003	0.031	0.005	0	0.018	1.2	13.86
0	0	0	0	0	0	0.84	0	0	0	0	0	0	0	0	0	0	15.918
0	0	0.05	0	2.1	0.84	0.42	0.029	0	0	0.003	0	0	0	0	0	0	14.028
0	0	0.004	0	2.1	0.42	0.42	0	0	0	0.002	0.003	0	0	0		0	14.028
0	0	0.008	0	1.26	0.42	0	0.008	0	0	0.003	0	0.021	0	0		0	15.12
0	0.6	0.024	1.2	1.2	9.6	1.8	0.006	0	0	0.002	0.002	0.022	0	0	0	0	20.34
0	11.28	0.296	11.28	9.87	100.11	8.46	0.183	0	6.909	0.041	0.024	0.166	0.063	0	0.028	16.92	13.959
0	1.417	0.028	1.7	1.7	7.085	0.567	0.006	0	0	0	0	0	0	0	0	0	4.563
0	8.24	0.36	9.27	13.39	86.52	6.18	0.062	0	0	0.004	0.016	0.076	0.025	0.01	0	1.03	9.579
0	16.74	0.744	18.6	27.9	163.68	1164.36	0.149	0	0	0	0.019	0.186	0.037	0	0	1.86	6.138
0	8.24	0.247	9.27	9.27	94.76	9.27	0.072	0	0	0.019	0.019	0.219	0	0	0	0	15.759
0	8.24	0.443	13.39	14.42	115.36	5.15	0.093	0	0	0.005	0.029	0.083	0.035	0.01		2.06	9.579
0	8.24	0.391	10.3	15.45	101.97	5.15	0.062	0	0	0.004	0.016	0.076	0.025	0.01		1.03	9.579
0	8.24	0.247	9.27	9.27	94.76	9.27	0.072	0	0	0.019	0.019	0.219	0	0	0	0	15.759
0	9.27	0.33	10.3	14.42	82.4	5.15	0.072	0	0	0.004	0.005	0.069	0.014	0		0	9.579
25.38	250.98	0.902	50.76	253.8	408.9	132.54	1.213	70.5	0	0.11	0.465	0.386	0.09	1.072	0.141	14.1	0
0	90.24	0.749	32.64	134.4	405.12	170.88	0.518	26.88	0.192	0.04	0.209	0.163	0.048	0.25	0.058	1.92	0
2.06	45.32	0.35	24.72	88.58	201.88	146.26	0.433	0	0.412	0.027	0.161	0.167	0.033	0.371	0.144	0	0
1.68	41.16	0.238	16.24	57.96	141.96	96.04	0.204	0	0	0.028	0.118	0.104	0.031	0.118	0.043	1.12	0
0	7.68	0.154	9.6	26.88	119.04	103.68	0.077		0	0.015	0.006	0.323	0	0		0	0
0	7.56	0.019	1.89	41.58	136.08	30.24	0.038		0	0	0.002	0.675	0	0		0	0
0	7.52	0.244	9.4	28.2	118.44	35.72	0.15		0	0.004	0.004	0.259	0	0		0	0
0	4.34	0.057		16.1	71.75	65.03			0								
0	2.37	0.024	4.74	7.11	113.76	2.37	0.024	0	0	0	0.118	0	0.002	0	0.047	4.74	0

EvaluEat Code	Food Name	Amt	Wt (g)	Energy (kcal)	Prot (g)	Carb (g)	Fiber (g)	Fat (g)	Mono (g)	Poly (g)	Sat (g)
14201	Beverage, coffee, brewed, prepared with tap water, decaffeinated	1 cup (8 fl. oz.)	237	9.48	0.332	0	0	1.801	0	0	0
14219	Beverage, coffee, instant powder, decaffeinated, prep	6 fl. oz.	179	3.58	0.215	0.77	0	0	0	0.002	0.002
14215	Beverage, coffee, instant	6 fl. oz.	179	3.58	0.179	0.609	0	0	0	0.004	0.004
14400	Beverage, cola w/caffeine	1 can (12 fl. oz.)	370	155.4	0.185	39.775	0	0	0	0	0
1057	Beverage, eggnog	1 cup	254	342.9	9.677	34.392	0	18.999	5.672	0.861	11.285
14119	Beverage, mixed vegetable and fruit juice drink	1 oz	28.34	32.024	0.071	7.935	0.17	0.014	0.001	0.006	0.002
14137	Beverage, Nestea Ice Tea, lemon flavor	1 cup (8 fl. oz.)	240	88.8	0	20.4	0	0.72			0.058
14121	Beverage, soft drink, club soda	1 can or bottle (16 fl. oz.)	474	0	0	0	0	0	0	0	0
14146	Beverage, soft drink, cola, low calorie, with aspartame, caffeine free	1 can or bottle (16 fl. oz.)	474	4.74	0.474	0.474	0	0	0	0	0
14416	Beverage, soft drink, cola, w/aspartame, low calorie	1 bottle 16 fl. oz.	474	4.74	0.474	0.474	0	0	0	0	0
14148	Beverage, soft drink, cola, with higher caffeine	1 can or bottle (16 fl. oz.)	492	206.64	0.246	52.89	0	0	0	0	0
14130	Beverage, soft drink, cream soda	1 can or bottle (16 fl. oz.)	494	251.94	0	65.702	0	0	0	0	0
14136	Beverage, soft drink, ginger ale	1 can or bottle (16 fl. oz.)	488	165.92	0	42.798	0	0	0	0	0
14142	Beverage, soft drink, grape	1 can or bottle (12 fl. oz.)	372	159.96	0	41.664	0	0	0	0	0
14145	Beverage, soft drink, lemon-lime	1 can or bottle (16 fl. oz.)	491	196.4	0	51.064	0	0	0	0	0
14150	Beverage, soft drink, orange	1 can or bottle (16 fl. oz.)	496	238.08	0	61.008	0	0	0	0	0
14153	Beverage, soft drink, pepper type	1 can or bottle (16 fl. oz.)	491	201.31	0	51.064	0	0.491	0	0	0.344
14157	Beverage, soft drink, root beer	1 can or bottle (16 fl. oz.)	493	202.13	0	52.258	0	0	0	0	0
14376	Beverage, tea mix, instant w/lemon flavor, w/saccharin, dry	1 cup (8 fl. oz.)	237	4.74	0.047	1.043	0	0	0	0.002	0
14369	Beverage, tea mix, Instant w/lemon, unsweetened, dry	1 cup (8 fl. oz.)	238	4.76	0	0.952	0	0	0	0.002	0
14355	Beverage, tea, brewed	1 cup (8 fl. oz.)	237	2.37	0	0.711	0	0	0.002	0.009	0.005
14352	Beverage, tea, brewed, prepared with tap water, decaffeinated	1 cup (8 fl. oz.)	237	2.37	0	0.711	0	0	0.002	0.009	0.005
14545	Beverage, tea, chamomile, brewed	1 cup (8 fl. oz.)	237	2.37	0	0.474	0	0	0.002	0.012	0.005
14381	Beverage, tea, herbal (not chamomile) brewed	1 cup (8 fl. oz.)	237	2.37	0	0.474	0	0	0.002	0.012	0.005
14429	Beverage, water	1 cup (8 fl. oz.)	237	0	0	0	0	0	0	0	0
14155	Beverage, water, carbonated, tonic (quinine)	1 fl. oz.	30.5	10.37	0	2.684	0	0	0	0	0
14553	Beverage, wine, non-alcoholic	1 fl. oz.	29	1.74	0.145	0.319	0	0	0	0	0
18629	Biscuit, buttermilk, refrigerated dough/Pillsbury	1 serving	64	154.24	4.992	30.4		1.408	0.605	0.312	0.285
18017	Biscuit, mixed grain, refrigerated dough	1 biscuit (2-1/2"dia)	44	115.72	2.684	20.856		2.464	1.29	0.387	0.601
18013	Biscuit, plain or buttermilk, refrigerated dough, baked, reduced fat	1 biscuit (2–1/4"dia)	21	62.79	1.638	11.634	0.399	1.092	0.587	0.164	0.272

Chol (g)	Calc (mg)	Iron (mg)	Mag (mg)	Phos (mg)	Pota (mg)	Sodi (mg)	Zinc (mg)	Vit A (RAE)	Vit C (mg)	Thia (mg)	Ribo (mg)	Niac (mg)	Vit B6 (mg)	Vit B12 (µg)	Vit E (mg)	Fol (µg)	Alc (g)
0	2.37	0.024	4.74	7.11	113.76	2.37	0.024	0	0	0	0.118	0	0.002	0	0.047	4.74	0
0	5.37	0.107	8.95	7.16	82.34	3.58	0	0	0	0	0.025	0.505	0	0	0	0	0
0	7.16	0.072	5.37	5.37	53.7	3.58	0.018	0	0	0	0.002	0.422	0	0	0	0	0
0	11.1	0.074	3.7	48.1	3.7	14.8	0.037	0	0	0	0	0	0	0	0	0	0
149.86	330.2	0.508	48.26	276.86	419.1	137.16	1.168	114.3	3.81	0.086	0.483	0.267	0.127	1.143	0.508	2.54	0
0	2.834	0.065	1.417	1.984	51.012	5.668	0.026	29.47	7.085	0.003	0.004	0.044	0.01	0	0.045	1.134	0
						0											0
0	23.7	0.047	4.74	0	9.48	99.54	0.474	0	0	0	0	0	0	0	0	0	0
0	18.96	0.142	4.74	42.66	0	28.44	0.379	0	0	0.024	0.109	0	0	0	0	0	0
0	14.22	0.142	4.74	52.14	28.44	23.7	0	0	0	0.024	0.109	0	0	0	0	0	0
0	14.76	0.098	4.92	63.96	4.92	19.68	0.049	0	0	0	0	0	0	0	0	0	0
0	24.7	0.247	4.94	0	4.94	59.28	0.346	0	0	0	0	0	0	0	0	0	0
0	14.64	0.878	4.88	0	4.88	34.16	0.244	0	0	0	0	0	0	0	0	0	0
0	11.16	0.298	3.72	0	3.72	55.8	0.26	0	0	0	0	0	0	0	0	0	0
0	9.82	0.344	4.91	0	4.91	54.01	0.245	0	0	0	0	0.074	0	0	0	0	0
0	24.8	0.298	4.96	4.96	9.92	59.52	0.496	0	0	0	0	0	0	0	0	0	0
0	14.73	0.196	0	54.01	4.91	49.1	0.196	0	0	0	0	0	0	0	0	0	0
0	24.65	0.247	4.93	0	4.93	64.09	0.345	0	0	0	0	0	0	0	0	0	0
0	7.11	0.118	2.37	2.37	30.81	23.7	0.024	0	0	0	0.002	0.047	0.002	0	0	0	0
0	4.76	0.024	4.76	2.38	49.98	14.28	0.071	0	0	0	0.019	0.09	0.005	0	0	0	0
0	0	0.047	7.11	2.37	87.69	7.11	0.047	0	0	0	0.033	0	0	0	0	11.85	0
0	0	0.047	7.11	2.37	87.69	7.11	0.047	0	0	0	0.033	0	0	0	0	11.85	0
0	4.74	0.19	2.37	0	21.33	2.37	0.095	2.37	0	0.024	0.009	0	0	0	0	2.37	0
0	4.74	0.19	2.37	0	21.33	2.37	0.095	0	0	0.024	0.009	0	0	0	0	2.37	0
0	4.74	0	2.37	0	0	4.74	0	0	0	0	0	0	0	0	0	0	0
0	0.305	0.003	0	0	0	1.22	0.031	0	0	0	0	0	0	0	0	0	0
0	2.61	0.116	2.9	4.35	25.52	2.03	0.023	0	0	0	0.003	0.029	0.006	0	0	0.29	0
		1.549				547.2											0
0	7.48	1.21	13.2	103.84	200.64	294.8	0.264	0	0	0.172	0.092	1.496	0.029	0		36.52	0
0	3.99	0.649	3.57	97.65	38.85	304.71	0.097	0	0	0.088	0.049	0.724	0.006	0	0.015	17.43	0

EvaluEat Code	Food Name	Amt	Wt (g)	Energy (kcal)	Prot (g)	Carb (g)	Fiber (g)	Fat (g)	Mono (g)	Poly (g)	Sat (g)
9043	Blackberry juice, canned	1 cup	144	54.72	0.432	11.232	0.144	0.864	0.084	0.495	0.026
42129	Bologna, beef and pork, low-fat	1 oz	28.34	65.182	3.259	0.737	0	5.47	2.592	0.464	2.071
42161	Bologna, beef, low-fat	1 oz	28.34	65.182	3.599	0.879	0	5.356	2.594	0.205	2.269
20034	Bran, oat, cooked	1 cup	219	87.6	7.03	25.054	5.694	1.883	0.637	0.742	0.357
7924	Bratwurst, pork, beef and turkey, lite, smoked	1 serving (2.33 oz)	66	122.76	9.537	1.069	0	8.93	4.729	0.558	3.16
18376	Bread crumbs, dry, grated, seasoned	1 oz	28.35	104.05	4.026	19.958	1.191	0.737	0.274	0.187	0.206
18079	Bread crumbs, plain, grated, dry	1 oz	28.35	111.98	3.785	20.406	1.276	1.503	0.29	0.584	0.341
18080	Bread sticks, plain	1 stick, small (approx 4-1/4" long)	5	20.6	0.6	3.42	0.15	0.475	0.178	0.181	0.071
18085	Bread stuffing, corn, dry mix, prep	.5 cup	100	179	2.9	21.9	2.9	8.8	3.856	2.706	1.755
18082	Bread stuffing, plain, dry mix, prep	.5 cup	100	178	3.2	21.7	2.9	8.6	3.808	2.604	1.734
18019	Bread, banana, Elfin Loaves/Keebler	1 slice	60	195.6	2.58	32.76	0.66	6.3	2.688	1.878	1.342
18023	Bread, corn, dry mix, prepared	1 piece	60	188.4	4.32	28.86	1.44	6	3.084	0.734	1.643
18270	Bread, corn, hushpuppies, homemade	1 cup	152	512.24	11.704	69.92	4.256	20.52	4.96	10.973	3.204
18627	Bread, crusty Italian Bread w/garlic/PepFarm	1 serving	50	186	4.15	20.8		9.6	3.918	1.832	2.411
18027	Bread, egg	1 slice (5" x 3" x 1/2")	40	114.8	3.8	19.12	0.92	2.4	0.921	0.442	0.637
18029	Bread, french/vienna/sourdough	1 slice, medium (4" x 2-1/2" x 1-3/4")	64	175.36	5.632	33.216	1.92	1.92	0.778	0.444	0.41
18604	Bread, garlic, frozen/Campione	1 serving	28	101.36	2.38	12.404	1.316	4.704			0.756
18641	Bread, hamburger rolls/Wonder	1 serving	43	117.39	3.47	21.861	1.118	1.785	0.365	0.936	0.436
18031	Bread, indian (Navajo) Fry	1 piece (10-1/2" dia)	160	526.4	11.36	85.28	2.88	15.2	6.381	4.141	3.701
18032	Bread, Irish soda, homemade, prepared from recipe	1 oz	28.35	82.215	1.871	15.876	0.737	1.418	0.567	0.419	0.315
18033	Bread, Italian	1 slice, medium	20	54.2	1.76	10	0.54	0.7	0.162	0.278	0.171
18035	Bread, mixed grain/7-grain/whole grain	1 slice, large	32	80	3.2	14.848	2.048	1.216	0.488	0.295	0.258
18037	Bread, oatbran	1 slice	30	70.8	3.12	11.94	1.35	1.32	0.477	0.508	0.209
18049	Bread, oatbran, reduced kcal	1 slice	23	46.23	1.84	9.499	2.76	0.736	0.157	0.384	0.102
18039	Bread, oatmeal	1 slice	27	72.63	2.268	13.095	1.08	1.188	0.426	0.46	0.19
18041	Bread, pita, white, enriched	1 pita, large (6-1/2" dia)	60	165	5.46	33.42	1.32	0.72	0.063	0.321	0.1
18042	Bread, pita, whole wheat	1 pita, large (6-1/2" dia)	64	170.24	6.272	35.2	4.736	1.664	0.223	0.675	0.262
18044	Bread, pumpernickel	1 slice, regular	26	65	2.262	12.35	1.69	0.806	0.242	0.322	0.114
18047	Bread, raisin, enriched	1 slice	26	71.24	2.054	13.598	1.118	1.144	0.596	0.177	0.281
18060	Bread, rye	1 slice	32	82.88	2.72	15.456	1.856	1.056	0.42	0.256	0.2
18064	Bread, wheat (includes wheat berry)	1 slice	25	65	2.275	11.8	1.075	1.025	0.43	0.227	0.223
18066	Bread, wheat bran	1 slice	36	89.28	3.168	17.208	1.44	1.224	0.582	0.234	0.28
18068	Bread, wheat germ	1 slice	28	73.08	2.688	13.524	0.588	0.812	0.357	0.187	0.184
18055	Bread, wheat, reduced kcal	1 slice	23	45.54	2.093	10.028	2.76	0.529	0.058	0.223	0.079
18069	Bread, white, commercially prep, crumbs/cubes/slices	1 slice	25	66.5	1.91	12.653	0.6	0.822	0.17	0.339	0.179
18057	Bread, white, reduced kcal	1 slice	23	47.61	2.001	10.189	2.231	0.575	0.248	0.129	0.126
18075	Bread, whole wheat, commercially prep	1 slice	28	68.88	2.716	12.908	1.932	1.176	0.47	0.281	0.257
43100	Breakfast bars, oats, sugar, raisins, coconut (include granola bar)	1 cup	186	863.04	18.228	124.062	5.766	32.736	3.595	3.039	23.603

Chol (g)	Calc (mg)	Iron (mg)	Mag (mg)	Phos (mg)	Pota (mg)	Sodi (mg)	Zinc (mg)	Vit A (RAE)	Vit C (mg)	Thia (mg)	Ribo (mg)	Niac (mg)	Vit B_6 (mg)	Vit B_{12} (µg)	Vit E (mg)	Fol (µg)	Alc (g)
0	17.28	0.691	30.24	17.28	194.4	1.44	0.59	11.52	16.27	0.017	0.026	0.642	0.03	0	1.296	14.4	0
11.053	3.117	0.187	3.401	51.295	44.21	314.007	0.425	0	0	0.048	0.037	0.72	0.051	0.371	0.062	1.417	0
10.486	2.551	0.283	3.401	50.445	41.66	319.675	0.519	0	0.283	0.014	0.028	0.709	0.043	0.397	0.054	1.417	0
0	21.9	1.927	87.6	260.61	201.48	2.19	1.161	0	0	0.35	0.074	0.315	0.055	0		13.14	0
36.96	9.24	0.62	9.24	87.12	162.36	648.12	1.769	0	0	0.059	0.11	1.219	0.141	1.056	0.03	3.3	0
0.284	28.067	0.902	10.773	37.706	76.545	751.275	0.258	1.134	0.113	0.045	0.048	0.774	0.042	0.011		30.9	0
0	51.881	1.369	12.191	46.778	55.566	207.522	0.411	0	0	0.274	0.114	1.881	0.034	0.099	0.023	30.34	0
0	1.1	0.214	1.6	6.05	6.2	32.85	0.044	0	0	0.029	0.028	0.264	0.004	0	0.051	8.1	0
0	26	0.94	13	34	62	455	0.23	78	0.8	0.117	0.092	1.247	0.038	0.01	0.85	97	0
0	32	1.09	12	42	74	543	0.28	118	0	0.136	0.107	1.475	0.04	0.01	1.4	39	0
25.8	12.6	0.84	8.4	34.8	80.4	181.2	0.21	63.6	1.02	0.103	0.12	0.868	0.09	0.06	1.071	19.8	0
36.6	43.8	1.14	12	225.6	76.8	466.8	0.378	26.4	0.06	0.146	0.162	1.234	0.062	0.096		33	0
68.4	422.56	4.621	36.48	287.28	218.88	1015.36	1.003	62.32	0.304	0.535	0.505	4.229	0.155	0.289	1.915	135.3	0
5.5		1.185				200											
20.4	37.2	1.216	7.6	42.4	46	196.8	0.316	25.2	0	0.175	0.174	1.939	0.026	0.04	0.104	42	0
0	48	1.619	17.28	67.2	72.32	389.76	0.557	0	0	0.333	0.211	3.039	0.028	0	0.192	94.72	0
		0.302				154											
	37.41	0.955				256.28											
0	372.8	5.76	25.6	251.2	118.4	1112	0.8	0	0	0.688	0.486	5.818	0.043	0	1.235	118.4	0
5.103	22.964	0.763	6.521	32.319	75.411	112.833	0.162	13.61	0.227	0.084	0.076	0.682	0.024	0.014	0.3	13.33	0
0	15.6	0.588	5.4	20.6	22	116.8	0.172	0	0	0.095	0.058	0.876	0.01	0	0.058	38.2	0
0	29.12	1.11	16.96	56.32	65.28	155.84	0.406	0	0.096	0.13	0.109	1.397	0.107	0.022	0.109	37.76	0
0	19.5	0.936	10.5	42.3	44.1	122.1	0.267	0.6	0	0.151	0.104	1.449	0.022	0	0.132	24.3	0
0	13.11	0.725	12.65	31.97	23.46	80.73	0.241	0	0	0.081	0.047	0.865	0.024	0	0.064	18.63	0
0	17.82	0.729	9.99	34.02	38.34	161.73	0.275	1.35	0	0.108	0.065	0.847	0.018	0.008	0.13	16.74	0
0	51.6	1.572	15.6	58.2	72	321.6	0.504	0	0	0.359	0.196	2.779	0.02	0	0.18	64.2	0
0	9.6	1.958	44.16	115.2	108.8	340.48	0.973	0	0	0.217	0.051	1.818	0.17	0	0.39	22.4	0
0	17.68	0.746	14.04	46.28	54.08	174.46	0.385	0	0	0.085	0.079	0.804	0.033	0	0.109	24.18	0
0	17.16	0.754	6.76	28.34	59.02	101.4	0.187	0	0.026	0.088	0.103	0.901	0.018	0	0.073	27.56	0
0	23.36	0.906	12.8	40	53.12	211.2	0.365	0	0.128	0.139	0.107	1.218	0.024	0	0.106	35.2	0
0	26.25	0.827	11.5	37.5	50.25	132.5	0.26	0	0	0.105	0.07	1.031	0.024	0	0.072	22.75	0
0	26.64	1.105	29.16	66.6	81.72	174.96	0.486	0	0	0.143	0.103	1.585	0.063	0	0.115	37.8	0
0	24.92	0.966	7.84	33.88	71.12	154.84	0.274	0	0.056	0.103	0.105	1.259	0.022	0.02	0.143	33.04	0
0	18.4	0.681	8.97	23.46	28.06	117.53	0.258	0	0.023	0.097	0.068	0.894	0.029	0	0.055	20.93	0
0	37.75	0.935	5.75	24.75	25	170.25	0.185	0	0	0.114	0.083	1.096	0.021	0	0.055	27.75	0
0	21.62	0.734	5.29	27.83	17.48	104.19	0.308	0	0.115	0.094	0.066	0.837	0.01	0.064	0.044	21.85	0
0	20.16	0.924	24.08	64.12	70.56	147.56	0.543	0	0	0.098	0.057	1.074	0.05	0.003	0.087	14	0
0	111.6	5.915	187.86	515.22	606.36	517.08	2.976	14.88	1.86	0.521	0.205	3.255	0.651	0	4.352	150.7	0

EvaluEat Code	Food Name	Amt	Wt (g)	Energy (kcal)	Prot (g)	Carb (g)	Fiber (g)	Fat (g)	Mono (g)	Poly (g)	Sat (g)
11097	Broccoli raab, cooked	.5 cup	92	30.36	3.524	2.87	2.576	0.478			
11096	Broccoli raab, raw	.5 cup	92	20.24	2.916	2.622	2.484	0.451	0.024	0.12	0.046
4601	Butter, light, stick, with salt	1 tbsp	12.8	63.872	0.422	0	0	7.053	2.039	0.262	4.393
4602	Butter, light, stick, without salt	1 tbsp	12.8	63.872	0.422	0	0	7.053	2.039	0.262	4.393
1001	Butter, regular (with salt)	1 tbsp	14.2	101.81	0.121	0.009	0	11.518	4.735	0.407	5.799
1145	Butter, unsalted	1 tbsp	14.2	101.81	0.121	0.009	0	11.518	2.985	0.432	7.294
1002	Butter, whipped (with salt)	1 tbsp	9.4	67.398	0.08	0.006	0	7.624	2.202	0.283	4.746
43143	Cabbage, japanese style, fresh, pickled	1 cup	186	55.8	2.976	10.546	5.766	0.186	0.015	0.089	0.024
43144	Cabbage, mustard, salted	1 cup	186	52.08	2.046	10.472	5.766	0.186	0.013	0.089	0.024
18086	Cake, angelfood, commercially prep	1 piece (1/12 of 12 oz cake)	28	72.24	1.652	16.184	0.42	0.224	0.02	0.103	0.034
18090	Cake, boston cream pie, commercially prep	1 piece (1/6 of pie)	92	231.84	2.208	39.468	1.288	7.82	4.18	0.928	2.249
18096	Cake, chocolate w/chocolate icing, commercially prep	1 piece (1/8 of 18 oz cake)	64	234.88	2.624	34.944	1.792	10.496	5.606	1.181	3.053
18101	Cake, chocolate, homemade, w/o icing	1 piece (1/12 of 9" dia)	95	340.1	5.035	50.73	1.52	14.345	5.737	2.623	5.158
18116	Cake, gingerbread, homemade	1 piece (1/9 of 8" square)	74	263.44	2.886	36.408		12.136	5.272	3.12	3.05
18120	Cake, pound, commercially prep w/butter	1 piece (1/12 of 12 oz cake)	28	108.64	1.54	13.664	0.14	5.572	1.652	0.299	3.237
18452	Cake, snack/cupcakes, chocolate w/frosting, low-fat	1 cupcake	43	131.15	1.849	28.896	1.849	1.591	0.795	0.209	0.466
18127	Cake, snack-type cream filled, chocolate w/icing	1 cupcake	50	188	1.7	30.15	0.4	7.25	2.845	2.618	1.429
18133	Cake, sponge, commercially prep	1 piece (1/12 of 16 oz cake)	38	109.82	2.052	23.218	0.19	1.026	0.361	0.17	0.305
18102	Cake, white w/coconut icing, homemade	1 piece (1/12 of 9" dia)	112	398.72	4.928	70.784	1.12	11.536	4.135	2.421	4.365
18139	Cake, white, homemade, w/o icing	1 piece (1/12 of 9" dia)	74	264.18	3.996	42.328	0.592	9.176	3.929	2.33	2.419
18140	Cake, yellow w/chocolate icing, commercially prep	1 piece (1/8 of 18 oz cake)	64	242.56	2.432	35.456	1.152	11.136	6.14	1.352	2.98
18146	Cake, yellow, homemade, w/o icing	1 piece (1/12 of 8" dia)	68	245.48	3.604	36.04	0.476	9.928	4.236	2.428	2.668
9426	Candied fruit	1 oz	28.34	90.971	0.099	23.449	0.453	0.02	0.002	0.006	0.003
43031	Candies, chocolate covered, caramel with nuts	1 cup	186	874.2	17.67	112.8	7.998	39.06	17.566	10.851	8.662
43058	Candies, hard, dietetic or low calorie (sorbitol)	1 cup	186	697.5	0	173.72	0	0	0	0	0
19236	Candies, Hershey's milk chocolate with almond bites	17 pieces	39	214.5	3.806	19.89	1.404	13.935	5.608	0.944	6.782
19279	Candies, milk chocolate coated coffee beans	1 NLEA serving	6	30.78	0.445	3.745	0.342	1.565	0.35	0.051	0.749
19068	Candies, Nestle, Bit-O'-Honey candy chews	18 pieces	40	160	0.84	32.4	0	3	0.781	0.25	2
43046	Candies, nougat	1 cup	186	740.28	6.194	171.85	6.138	3.106	0	0	3.101
19159	Candy bar, 3 Musketeers/M&M Mars	1 bar (.8 oz)	23	95.68	0.736	17.664	0.414	2.967	0.987	0.104	1.495
19065	Candy bar, Almond Joy/Hershey	1 package (1.76 oz)	49	234.71	2.024	29.16	2.45	13.196	2.577	0.578	8.619
19111	Candy bar, Baby Ruth/Nestle	1 bar (0.75 oz)	21	97.44	1.491	12.978	0.504	5.25	1.356	0.694	2.583
19069	Candy bar, Butterfinger Bar and Dessert Topping	1 bar fun size	21	99.96	1.218	15.223	0.357	3.99	1.025	0.517	2.151
19075	Candy bar, Caramello/Hershey	1 bar (1.25 oz)	35	161.7	2.167	22.333	0.42	7.417	1.851	0.22	4.452
19109	Candy bar, Kit Kat Wafer/Hershey	1 bar (1.5 oz)	42	217.14	2.692	26.951	0.798	11.386	2.012	0.214	7.346

Chol (g)	Calc (mg)	Iron (mg)	Mag (mg)	Phos (mg)	Pota (mg)	Sodi (mg)	Zinc (mg)	Vit A (RAE)	Vit C (mg)	Thia (mg)	Ribo (mg)	Niac (mg)	Vit B$_6$ (mg)	Vit B$_{12}$ (µg)	Vit E (mg)	Fol (µg)	Alc (g)
	108.56	1.168	24.84	75.44	315.56	51.52	0.497	208.8	34.04	0.155	0.129	1.854	0.202		2.328	65.32	
	99.36	1.969	20.24	67.16	180.32	30.36	0.708	120.5	18.58	0.149	0.119	1.123	0.157		1.49	76.36	
13.568	6.144	0.14	0.64	4.352	9.088	57.6	0.033	59.52	0	0.001	0.009	0.003	0.001	0.017	0.202	0.128	0
13.568	6.144	0.14	0.64	4.352	9.088	4.608	0.033	59.52	0	0.001	0.009	0.003	0.001	0.017	0.202	0.128	0
30.53	3.408	0.003	0.284	3.408	3.408	81.792	0.013	97.13	0	0.001	0.005	0.006	0	0.024	0.329	0.426	0
30.53	3.408	0.003	0.284	3.408	3.408	1.562	0.013	97.13	0	0.001	0.005	0.006	0	0.024	0.329	0.426	0
20.586	2.256	0.015	0.188	2.162	2.444	77.738	0.005	64.3	0	0	0.003	0.004	0	0.012	0.218	0.282	0
0	89.28	0.911	22.32	79.98	1586.58	515.22	0.372	16.74	1.302	0	0.074	0.335	0.186	0	0.223	78.12	0
0	124.62	1.302	27.9	50.22	457.56	1333.62	0.558	91.14	0	0.074	0.167	1.339	0.558	0	0.037	133.9	0
0	39.2	0.146	3.36	8.96	26.04	209.72	0.02	0	0	0.029	0.137	0.247	0.009	0.017		9.8	0
34.04	21.16	0.35	5.52	45.08	35.88	132.48	0.147	22.08	0.184	0.375	0.248	0.176	0.024	0.147	0.138	12.88	0
26.88	27.52	1.408	21.76	78.08	128	213.76	0.442	16.64	0.064	0.017	0.085	0.369	0.026	0.09		10.88	0
55.1	57	1.53	30.4	100.7	133	299.25	0.655	38	0.19	0.134	0.202	1.08	0.039	0.152	1.512	25.65	0
23.68	52.54	2.131	51.8	39.96	324.86	241.98	0.289	10.36	0.074	0.141	0.12	1.286	0.141	0.044		24.42	0
61.88	9.8	0.386	3.08	38.36	33.32	111.44	0.129	41.72	0	0.038	0.064	0.367	0.012	0.07		11.48	0
0	15.48	0.662	10.75	78.69	96.32	177.59	0.237	0	0	0.015	0.057	0.307	0.003	0		6.45	0
8.5	36.5	1.68	20.5	46.5	61	212.5	0.255	2.5	0	0.111	0.147	1.214	0.012	0.03	1.09	20	0
38.76	26.6	1.034	4.18	52.06	37.62	92.72	0.194	16.72	0	0.092	0.102	0.734	0.02	0.091	0.091	17.86	0
1.12	100.8	1.299	13.44	78.4	110.88	318.08	0.37	13.44	0.112	0.143	0.212	1.191	0.032	0.067	0.134	34.72	0
1.48	96.2	1.125	8.88	68.82	70.3	241.98	0.237	11.1	0.148	0.138	0.179	1.134	0.016	0.059	0.089	28.12	0
35.2	23.68	1.331	19.2	103.04	113.92	215.68	0.397	21.12	0	0.077	0.1	0.798	0.021	0.109	1.455	14.08	0
36.72	99.28	1.115	8.16	79.56	61.88	233.24	0.306	27.2	0.136	0.124	0.158	0.99	0.024	0.109	0.819	23.12	0
0	5.101	0.048	1.134	1.417	16.154	27.773	0.014	0.283	0	0	0	0	0	0	0.011	0	0
0	145.08	3.162	150.66	308.76	827.7	44.64	3.478	78.12	2.604	0.074	0.298	8.854	0.298	0	2.046	171.1	0
0	0	0	0	0	0	0	0	0	0	0	0	0	0	0	0	0	0
7.41	85.8	0.585	23.01	88.53	183.69	28.86	0.523		0.702	0.027	0.148	0.242	0.027		0.152	6.24	0
1.2	10.14	0.137	3.84	11.28	24.78	4.26	0.106	2.52	0	0.006	0.019	0.02	0.002	0.032	0.104	0.6	0
0	20	0.116	2.8	18	50.4	120	0.084	0	0	0	0.1	0.024	0.007	0.068	0.396	1.6	0
0	59.52	1.097	59.52	102.3	195.3	61.38	0.781	0	0.558	0.024	0.275	0.889	0.037	0.019	5.152	9.3	0
2.53	19.32	0.168	6.67	20.93	30.59	44.62	0.127	3.45	0.092	0.008	0.032	0.053	0.003	0.044	0.214	0	0
1.96	31.36	0.622		54.88	124.46	69.58			0.343						0.01		0
0.42	9.45	0.147	15.33	28.98	74.76	44.94	0.25	0	0.021	0.02	0.016	0.583	0.013	0.008	0.393	6.51	0
0	7.35	0.16	17.43	28.35	82.95	44.94	0.25	0	0	0.023	0.016	0.647	0.021	0.004	0.363	6.93	0
9.45	74.55	0.382		52.5	119.35	42.7			0.595						0.077		0
3.78	56.7	0.357	1.26	47.46	121.8	27.3	0.038	10.5	0.546	0.021	0.071	0.088	0.004	0.088	0.147	1.26	0

EvaluEat Code	Food Name	Amt	Wt (g)	Energy (kcal)	Prot (g)	Carb (g)	Fiber (g)	Fat (g)	Mono (g)	Poly (g)	Sat (g)
19110	Candy bar, Krackel/Hershey	1 bar (1.45 oz)	41	209.92	2.714	26.224	0.902	10.898	2.563	0.234	6.527
19115	Candy bar, Mars Almond/M&M Mars	1 bar (1.76 oz)	50	233.5	4.05	31.35	1	11.5	5.346	1.99	3.634
19135	Candy bar, Mars Milky Way/M&M Mars	1 bar (.8 oz)	23	97.29	1.035	16.491	0.391	3.703	1.385	0.138	1.792
19143	Candy bar, Mr. Goodbar/Hershey	1 bar (1.75 oz)	49	263.62	5.008	26.627	1.862	16.273	4.019	2.139	6.924
19118	Candy bar, Oh Henry!/Nestle	1 bar	26	120.12	2.002	17.004	0.546	6.006	1.734	0.707	1.747
19136	Candy bar, Skor Toffee Candy/Hershey	1 bar (1.4 oz)	39	208.65	1.221	24.071	0.507	12.55	3.623	0.499	7.324
19155	Candy bar, Snickers/M&M Mars	1 bar (2 oz)	57	273.03	4.56	33.75	1.425	14.011	5.958	2.803	5.127
19164	Candy bar, Special Dark Sweet Chocolate/Hershey	1 bar (1.45 oz)	41	217.71	2.271	24.358	2.665	13.284	2.107	0.18	7.868
19160	Candy bar, Twix Caramel Cookie/M&M Mars	1 package (2 oz)	57	284.43	2.622	37.381	0.627	13.902	7.638	0.485	5.072
19070	Candy, butterscotch	3 pieces	16	62.56	0.005	14.464	0	0.528	0.136	0.02	0.332
19074	Candy, caramel	1 piece	10.1	38.582	0.465	7.777	0.121	0.818	0.085	0.018	0.665
19071	Candy, carob	1 bar (3 oz)	87	469.8	7.09	48.972	3.306	27.283	0.42	0.257	25.246
19080	Candy, chocolate chips, semisweet	1 cup chips (6 oz package)	168	804.72	7.056	106.01	9.912	50.4	16.75	1.63	29.82
19078	Candy, chocolate, baking, unsweetened, square	1 square	29	145.29	3.741	8.654	4.814	15.17	4.671	0.451	9.382
19081	Candy, chocolate, sweet	1 bar (1.45 oz)	41	207.05	1.599	24.436	2.255	14.022	4.6	0.406	8.233
19011	Candy, fruit leather bar	1 bar	23	80.73	0.414	18.055	0.805	1.219	0.145	0.041	0.925
19013	Candy, fruit leather, pieces	1 package	27	94.77	0.27	22.815	0	0.27	0.141	0.052	0.062
19014	Candy, fruit leather, roll	1 large	21	77.91	0.021	17.997	0.693	0.63	0.311	0.113	0.136
19301	Candy, fudge, chocolate marshmallow nut, homemade	1 oz	28.34	133.77	0.915	19.022	0.595	5.966	1.585	1.152	2.829
19101	Candy, fudge, chocolate w/nuts, homemade	1 oz	28.34	130.65	1.241	19.26	0.709	5.365	1.052	2.099	1.71
19100	Candy, fudge, chocolate, homemade	1 piece	17	69.87	0.406	13.002	0.289	1.77	0.463	0.039	1.006
19106	Candy, gumdrops/gummy bears/fish/worm/dinosaur	10 gumdrops	36	142.56	0	35.604	0.036	0	0	0	0
19107	Candy, hard candy	1 piece	6	23.64	0	5.88	0	0.012	0	0	0
19108	Candy, jellybeans	10 large (1 oz)	28	105	0	26.194	0.056	0.014	0	0	0
19140	Candy, M&M's Peanut chocolate	1 package (1.67 oz)	47	242.52	4.451	28.416	1.598	12.333	5.17	1.974	4.856
19141	Candy, M&M's Plain chocolate	1 box (1.48 oz)	42	206.64	1.819	29.908	1.05	8.875	1.485	0.162	5.494
19116	Candy, marshmallow	1 regular	7.2	22.896	0.13	5.854	0.007	0.014	0.006	0.003	0.004
19120	Candy, milk chocolate	1 bar (1.55 oz)	44	235.4	3.366	26.136	1.496	13.05	5.819	0.358	6.271
19132	Candy, milk chocolate w/almonds	1 bar (1.45 oz)	41	215.66	3.69	21.812	2.542	14.104	5.531	0.935	6.962
19134	Candy, milk chocolate w/rice cereal	1 bar (1.4 oz)	40	198.4	2.52	25.36	1.32	10.6	3.456	0.312	6.356
19148	Candy, peanut brittle, homemade	1 oz	28.34	137.17	2.145	20.025	0.709	5.379	2.285	1.292	1.174
19151	Candy, peanut butter candy/Reese's Pieces/Hershey	10 pieces	8	39.76	0.997	4.789	0.24	1.982	0.357	0.15	1.314
19150	Candy, peanut butter cups, Reese's/Hershey	1 package (0.6 oz, 1 cup)	17	87.55	1.741	9.411	0.612	5.19	2.227	0.952	1.824
19126	Candy, peanuts, milk chocolate coated	10 pieces	40	207.6	5.24	19.76	1.88	13.4	5.168	1.732	5.84
19127	Candy, raisins, milk chocolate coated	10 pieces	10	39	0.41	6.83	0.42	1.48	0.474	0.051	0.88
19152	Candy, Rolo Caramel, milk chocolate/Hershey	1 package (1.91 oz)	54	255.96	2.743	36.693	0.486	11.302	2.03	0.211	7.787
19154	Candy, sesame crunch	1 piece	1.8	9.306	0.209	0.905	0.142	0.599	0.226	0.262	0.08
19370	Candy, Skittles, original bite size candy/M&M Mars	1 package	9979	40415	18.96	9045	0	436.08	295.38	11.975	86.618
19156	Candy, Starburst Fruit Chews/M&M Mars	1 package (2.07 oz)	59	233.64	0.236	49.855	0	4.897	2.106	1.841	0.73
19112	Candy, Twizzlers Strawberry/Hershey	4 pieces from 5 oz package	38	133	0.973	30.301	0	0.882			0
19091	Candy, York Peppermint Patty	1 patty (1.5 oz)	43	165.12	0.942	34.826	0.86	3.083	0.176	0.047	1.866
11683	Carrot, dehydrated	1 tbsp chopped	10	34.1	0.81	7.957	2.36	0.149	0.008	0.073	0.026

Chol (g)	Calc (mg)	Iron (mg)	Mag (mg)	Phos (mg)	Pota (mg)	Sodi (mg)	Zinc (mg)	Vit A (RAE)	Vit C (mg)	Thia (mg)	Ribo (mg)	Niac (mg)	Vit B$_6$ (mg)	Vit B$_{12}$ (µg)	Vit E (mg)	Fol (µg)	Alc (g)
4.51	64.78	0.435	5.33	50.43	133.25	80.36	0.201		0.328	0.021	0.078	0.107	0.016		0.033	2.46	0
8.5	84	0.55	36	117	162.5	85	0.555	7.5	0.35	0.021	0.156	0.472	0.03	0.18	3.875	4.5	0
3.22	29.9	0.175	7.82	33.12	55.43	55.2	0.163	4.14	0.23	0.008	0.051	0.08	0.012	0.074	0.287	1.38	0
4.9	53.9	0.681	23.03	79.87	193.06	20.09	0.456	17.15	0.441	0.069	0.069	1.686	0.034	0.162	1.553	18.62	0
2.34	21.06	0.161	13.26	36.4	84.24	60.06	0.299	2.6	0.052	0.006	0.042	0.728	0.022	0.052	0.536	11.44	0
20.67	50.7	0.222	3.9	23.79	59.67	123.63	0.066		0.195	0.008	0.039	0.051			0.016	1.17	0
7.41	53.58	0.433	32.49	97.47	169.86	151.62	0.889	23.94	0.342	0.072	0.111	0.901	0.034	0.188	0.627	17.1	0
2.05	12.3	0.873	12.71	20.91	205.82	2.46	0.004		0	0	0.004	0	0	0	0.078	0	0
2.85	51.3	0.462	18.24	62.13	107.73	110.01	0.57	12.54	0.228	0.068	0.109	0.429	0.013	0.165	1.106	10.83	0
1.44	0.32	0.003	0.16	0.16	0.64	62.56	0.002	4.48	0	0	0.003	0.001	0	0	0.014	0	0
0.707	13.938	0.014	1.717	11.514	21.614	24.745	0.044	0.101	0.051	0.001	0.034	0.025	0.004	0	0.28	0.505	0
2.61	263.61	1.122	31.32	109.62	550.71	93.09	3.071	0	0.435	0.087	0.155	0.905	0.113	0.87	1.027	18.27	0
0	53.76	5.258	193.2	221.76	613.2	18.48	2.722	0	0	0.092	0.151	0.717	0.059	0	0.386	5.04	0
0	29.29	5.046	94.83	116	240.7	6.96	2.793	0	0	0.043	0.029	0.393	0.008	0	0.116	8.12	0
0	9.84	1.132	46.33	60.27	118.9	6.56	0.615	0	0	0.008	0.098	0.275	0.018	0	0.107	1.23	0
0	6.67	0.184	5.06	12.65	31.74	17.71	0.044	1.38	16.1	0.01	0.007	0.023	0.069	0		0.92	0
0	4.86	0.203	3.78	6.48	44.28	108.81	0.051	1.62	15.12	0.012	0.027	0.081	0		0.151	1.08	0
0	6.72	0.212	4.2	6.51	61.74	66.57	0.04	1.26	25.2	0.015	0.004	0.021	0.063	0	0.118	0.84	0.021
6.518	13.887	0.323	13.036	24.939	47.895	27.49	0.218	21.82	0.085	0.012	0.023	0.083	0.015	0.009	0.197	2.267	0
3.401	15.304	0.558	15.587	31.741	51.012	11.619	0.402	10.77	0.057	0.019	0.027	0.09	0.025	0.02	0.185	4.534	0
2.38	7.65	0.301	6.12	11.73	22.27	7.99	0.187	7.48	0	0.004	0.014	0.03	0.002	0.015	0.031	0.68	0
0	1.08	0.144	0.36	0.36	1.8	15.84	0	0	0	0.002	0.005	0.004	0.002	0	0	0	0
0	0.18	0.018	0.18	0.18	0.3	2.28	0.001	0	0	0	0	0	0	0	0	0	0
0	0.84	0.036	0.56	1.12	10.36	14	0.014	0	0	0.001	0.003	0.002	0.001	0	0	0	0
4.23	47.47	0.54	35.72	109.51	163.09	22.56	1.133	12.22	0.235	0.048	0.074	1.922	0.041	0.075	1.203	17.86	0
5.88	44.1	0.466	14.28	47.88	85.26	25.62	0.462	11.34	0.21	0.026	0.071	0.088	0.008	0.143	0.462	2.52	0
0	0.216	0.017	0.144	0.576	0.36	5.76	0.003	0	0	0	0	0.006	0	0	0	0.072	0
10.12	83.16	1.034	27.72	91.52	163.68	34.76	0.884	21.56	0	0.049	0.131	0.17	0.016	0.273	0.889	5.28	0
7.79	91.84	0.668	36.9	108.24	182.04	30.34	0.549	18.04	0.082	0.025	0.178	0.304	0.021	0.135	1.841	5.74	0
7.6	68.4	0.3	19.6	77.2	137.2	58	0.448	24.8	0.12	0.023	0.116	0.185	0.023	0.248	0.8	6	0
3.401	7.652	0.346	11.903	30.04	47.611	126.113	0.247	11.05	0	0.038	0.012	0.75	0.022	0.003	0.726	13.04	0
0	5.52	0.039	7.04	16.56	28.72	15.52	0.092	0	0	0.014	0.018	0.485	0.009	0.01	0.087	4.4	0
1.02	13.26	0.206	10.54	27.37	58.31	53.38	0.218	2.89	0.051	0.027	0.019	0.763	0.017	0.095	0.026	8.5	0
3.6	41.6	0.524	38.4	84.8	200.8	16.4	0.956	13.6	0	0.046	0.07	1.7	0.084	0.176	1.384	3.2	0
0.3	8.6	0.171	4.5	14.3	51.4	3.6	0.081	2.4	0.02	0.008	0.016	0.04	0.008	0.018	0.102	0.7	0
6.48	78.3	0.227	0	38.34	101.52	101.52	0	18.36	0.486	0.011	0.065	0.022	0	0.146	0.481	0	0
0	11.79	0.077	4.518	7.614	5.796	3.006	0.068	0	0.002	0.01	0.003	0.067	0.01	0	0.003	0.936	0
0	0	0.998	99.79	199.58	898.11	1596.64	0.998	0	6676	0.2	2.295	1.497	0.299	0	43.908	0	0
0	2.36	0.077	0.59	4.13	1.18	33.04	0	0	31.21	0.001	0.001	0.003	0	0	0.413	0	0
0	0	0.194				109.06			0								0
0.43	4.73	0.396		0	47.73	12.04			0						0.004		0
0	21.2	0.393	11.8	34.6	254	27.5	0.157	541.6	1.46	0.053	0.042	0.657	0.104	0	0.697	5.5	0

EvaluEat Code	Food Name	Amt	Wt (g)	Energy (kcal)	Prot (g)	Carb (g)	Fiber (g)	Fat (g)	Mono (g)	Poly (g)	Sat (g)
44055	Celery flakes, dried	1 cubic inch	10.2	32.538	1.153	6.497	2.836	0.214	0.041	0.106	0.057
8053	Cereal, 100% bran (wheat bran & barley)	.333 cup									
		(1 NLEA serving)	29	83.23	3.683	22.678	8.294	0.609	0.092	0.319	0.087
8153	Cereal, 40% bran flakes/Ralston Purina	1 cup	49	158.76	5.635	39.102	6.909	0.686			
8001	Cereal, All-Bran/Kellogg	.5 cup									
		(1 NLEA serving)	30	78	3.75	22.2	9.6	0.996	0.222	0.612	0.162
8263	Cereal, Apple Cinnamon Cheerios/General Mills	.75 cup									
		(1 NLEA serving)	30	117.6	1.8	25.2	1.29	1.53	0.713	0.384	0.297
8254	Cereal, Apple Cinnamon Squares Mini-Wheats/Kellogg	.75 cup									
		(1 NLEA serving)	55	182.05	3.96	44.055	4.73	0.99	0.275	0.495	0.22
8003	Cereal, Apple Jacks/Kellogg	1 cup									
		(1 NLEA serving)	30	117	0.9	27.3	0.96	0.6	0.18	0.3	0.12
8262	Cereal, Basic 4/General Mills	1 cup									
		(1 NLEA serving)	55	201.85	4.4	42.35	3.19	2.805	0.99	1.1	0.44
8006	Cereal, Bran Chex (wheat & corn)	1 cup	49	156.31	5.047	39.053	7.938	1.372	0.254	0.671	0.198
8322	Cereal, Bran Flakes/Kraft, Post	.75 cup									
		(1 NLEA serving)	30	96	2.82	24.12	5.28	0.66			0.12
8010	Cereal, Cap'n Crunch/Quaker	.75 cup	27	108.27	1.174	22.901	0.675	1.569	0.289	0.2	0.405
8013	Cereal, Cheerios/General Mills	1 cup									
		(1 NLEA serving)	30	110.7	3.3	22.2	2.7	1.8	0.642	0.216	0.36
8139	Cereal, Cinnamon Grahams/General Mills	.75 cup	30	113.4	1.5	25.8	0.96	0.84	0.304	0.312	0.15
8215	Cereal, Cinnamon Oatmeal Squares/Quaker	1 cup									
		(1 NLEA serving)	60	226.8	6.066	47.898	4.56	2.568	0.864	1.044	0.504
8272	Cereal, Cinnamon Toast Crunch/General Mills	.75 cup									
		(1 NLEA serving)	30	126.6	1.5	23.7	1.2	3.3	1.539	1.015	0.54
8014	Cereal, Cocoa Krispies/Kellogg	.75 cup									
		(1 NLEA serving)	31	118.11	1.054	27.001	0.992	0.992	0.124	0.071	0.617
8271	Cereal, Cocoa Puffs/General Mills	1 cup									
		(1 NLEA serving)	30	117	1.2	26.4	0.69	0.96	0.501	0.184	0.21
8028	Cereal, Complete Wheat Bran Flakes/Kellogg	.75 cup									
		(1 NLEA serving)	29	92.22	2.9	22.91	5.075	0.58	0.145	0.319	0.116
8295	Cereal, Corn Blasts/Quaker	1 cup	33	132.66	1.416	28.034	0.726	1.904	1.033	0.343	0.508
8019	Cereal, Corn Chex	1 cup									
		(1 NLEA serving)	30	111.9	2.1	25.8	0.6	0.27	0.059	0.101	0.06
8020	Cereal, Corn Flakes/Kellogg	1 cup									
		(1 NLEA serving)	28	101.08	1.96	24.08	0.98	0.224	0.031	0.09	0.053
8093	Cereal, corn grits, instant, plain, prep/Quaker	1 cup	245	166.6	3.945	36.897	2.205	0.465	0.066	0.14	0.047
8161	Cereal, corn grits, white, regular/quick, enriched, prep w/salt	1 cup	242	142.78	3.436	31.145	0.726	0.46	0.116	0.201	0.061
8068	Cereal, Corn Pops/Kellogg	1 cup									
		(1 NLEA serving)	31	117.8	1.147	27.9	0.248	0.226	0.084	0.071	0.071
8023	Cereal, Cracklin' Oat Bran/Kellogg	.75 cup									
		(1 NLEA serving)	55	224.95	4.565	39.27	6.435	8.03	4.565	1.155	2.31
8168	Cereal, Cream of Rice, prep w/salt	1 cup	244	126.88	2.196	28.06	0.244	0.244	0.076	0.066	0.049
8171	Cereal, Cream of Wheat, instant, prep w/salt	1 cup	241	149.42	4.434	31.523	1.446	0.578	0.08	0.323	0.092
8169	Cereal, Cream of Wheat, regular, prep w/salt	1 cup	251	125.5	3.665	26.932	1.004	0.477	0.063	0.259	0.075

Chol (g)	Calc (mg)	Iron (mg)	Mag (mg)	Phos (mg)	Pota (mg)	Sodi (mg)	Zinc (mg)	Vit A (RAE)	Vit C (mg)	Thia (mg)	Ribo (mg)	Niac (mg)	Vit B₆ (mg)	Vit B₁₂ (µg)	Vit E (mg)	Fol (µg)	Alc (g)
0	59.874	0.799	19.992	41.004	447.576	146.37	0.283	9.996	8.823	0.045	0.051	0.473	0.047	0	0.566	10.91	0
0	22.04	8.1	80.62	235.77	274.63	120.93	3.75	225	0	0.374	0.426	5	0.502	0	0.673	100.1	0
0	22.54	7.791	117.6	272.93	286.16	456.19	2.038		25.97	0.637	0.735	8.624	0.882	2.597		173	0
0	99	4.8	114	339	339	77.4	1.8	157.5	6	0.36	0.42	4.8	1.8	6	0.369	393	0
0	99.9	4.5	20.1	65.1	57.6	120.3	3.75	150.3	6	0.375	0.426	5.01	0.501	1.5	0.15	200.1	0
0	20.9	16.225	48.4	154	166.1	19.8	1.485	0	0	0.385	0.44	5.005	0.495	1.485	0.303	110	0
0	7.5	4.17	16.5	37.5	36	142.5	1.5	46.8	13.8	0.51	0.39	4.62	0.45	1.38	0.048	93	0
0	196.35	3.52	40.15	231.55	154.55	315.7	2.97	117.7	0	0.297	0.336	3.905	0.391	1.155	0.594	78.65	0
0	29.4	13.994	69.09	172.97	216.09	345.45	6.483		25.97	0.637	0.265	8.624	0.882	2.597	0.563	173	0
0	16.8	8.1	64.2	152.4	184.8	219.6	1.5		0	0.375	0.426	5.001	0.501	1.5		99.9	
0	4.05	5.16	15.12	45.09	54	202.23	4.285	1.89	0	0.427	0.481	5.711	0.57	0	0.248	420.1	0
0	99.9	8.1	39.9	99.9	96.3	273	3.75	150.3	6	0.375	0.426	5.01	0.501	1.5	0.105	200.1	0
0	99.9	4.5	8.1	20.1	44.1	236.7	3.75	150.3	6	0.375	0.426	5.01	0.501	1.5	0.093	99.9	0
0	116.4	16.86	64.8	201.6	250.2	263.4	4.128	165	6.6	0.408	0.462	5.502	0.546	0	2.214	420	0
0	99.9	4.5	8.1	80.1	42.6	206.1	3.75	150.3	6	0.375	0.426	5.01	0.501	1.5	0.342	99.9	0
0	39.99	4.65	11.78	30.38	49.91	190.03	1.488	152.5	15	0.372	0.434	4.96	0.496	1.519	0.192	102	0
0	99.9	4.5	8.1	20.1	50.4	171.3	3.75	0	6	0.375	0.426	5.01	0.501	1.5	0.063	99.9	0
0	15.37	17.98	40.6	156.6	171.1	207.35	15.23	228.5	60.03	1.566	1.711	20.01	2.03	6.003	26.874	403.1	0
0	10.89	4.95	17.49	60.06	63.69	239.91	4.125		13.2	0.413	0.465	5.498	0.548	0	0.304	109.9	0
0	99.9	9	8.4	21.6	24.9	287.7	3.75	150.6	6	0.375	0.426	5.01	0.501	1.5	0.054	200.1	0
0	1.96	8.4	3.08	14	25.2	203	0.076	150.4	6.16	0.364	0.428	5.012	0.504	1.512	0.039	102.2	0
0	14.7	14.234	17.15	51.45	68.6	514.5	0.318	0	0	0.279	0.333	3.959	0.098	0	0.049	83.3	0
0	7.26	1.452	12.1	26.62	50.82	539.66	0.169	0	0	0.201	0.133	1.747	0.051	0	0.048	79.86	0
0	5.27	1.922	2.17	9.61	26.35	119.66	1.519	151	6.014	0.372	0.434	4.991	0.496	1.519	0.034	102	0
0	22.55	2.035	67.65	178.75	247.5	157.3	1.705	252.5	17.6	0.424	0.479	5.665	0.561	1.705	0.77	112.8	0
0	7.32	0.488	7.32	41.48	48.8	422.12	0.39	0	0	0	0	0.976	0.066	0	0.049	7.32	0
0	154.24	11.954	14.46	43.38	48.2	363.91	0.41	559.1	0	0.559	0.506	7.454	0.745	0	0.048	149.4	0
0	112.95	9.764	12.55	95.38	45.18	336.34	0.351	0	0	0.143	0.065	1.358	0.03	0	0.05	30.12	0

EvaluEat Code	Food Name	Amt	Wt (g)	Energy (kcal)	Prot (g)	Carb (g)	Fiber (g)	Fat (g)	Mono (g)	Poly (g)	Sat (g)
8259	Cereal, Crispix/Kellogg	1 cup (1 NLEA serving)	29	109.33	1.972	24.94	0.145	0.232	0.058	0.116	0.058
8173	Cereal, Farina, enriched, prep w/salt	1 cup	233	111.84	3.309	24.395	0.699	0.163	0.023	0.07	0.023
8244	Cereal, Fiber One/General Mills	.5 cup (1 NLEA serving)	30	59.1	2.4	24.3	14.4	0.81	0.132	0.41	0.12
8030	Cereal, Froot Loops/Kellogg	1 cup (1 NLEA serving)	30	117.9	1.02	26.25	0.93	1.23	0.129	0.204	0.456
8069	Cereal, Frosted Flakes/Kellogg	.75 cup (1 NLEA serving)	31	113.77	1.023	27.993	0.992	0.161	0.028	0.081	0.053
8319	Cereal, Frosted Mini-Wheats, bite size/Kellogg	1 cup, bite size	55	189.2	5.555	44.55	5.5	0.88	0.132	0.55	0.198
8327	Cereal, Fruit & Fiber Dates, Raisins & Walnuts/Kraft, Post	1 cup (1 NLEA serving)	55	211.75	3.905	41.91	5.335	3.08			0.44
8037	Cereal, granola (oats & wheat germ) homemade	1 cup	122	597.8	18.141	64.599	10.492	29.719	9.324	13.066	5.535
8329	Cereal, Grape-Nuts/Kraft, Post	.5 cup (1 NLEA serving)	58	208.22	6.264	47.154	5.046	1.102			0.232
8333	Cereal, Honey Bunches of Oats Honey Roasted/Kraft, Post	.75 cup (1 NLEA serving)	30	118.2	2.13	24.57	1.47	1.65			0.24
8242	Cereal, Just Right w/crunchy nuggets/Kellogg	1 cup (1 NLEA serving)	55	204.05	4.235	46.035	2.805	1.485	0.275	1.045	0.11
8048	Cereal, Kix/General Mills	1.333 cup (1 NLEA serving)	30	113.1	1.8	25.8	0.9	0.6	0.159	0.2	0.15
8049	Cereal, Life, plain/Quaker	.75 cup (1 NLEA serving)	32	120	3.174	24.992	2.112	1.402	0.477	0.451	0.259
8284	Cereal, Low-Fat Granola with Raisins/Kellogg	.667 cup (1 NLEA serving)	55	201.3	4.4	44	2.75	2.75	1.375	0.55	0.825
8050	Cereal, Lucky Charms/General Mills	1 cup (1 NLEA serving)	30	114	2.1	24.9	1.5	1.14	0.252	0.288	0.24
8176	Cereal, Maltex, prep w/salt	1 cup	249	189.24	5.702	39.367	2.241	1.071	0.115	0.386	0.152
8178	Cereal, Malt-O-Meal, plain & chocolate, prep w/salt	1 cup	240	122.4	3.6	25.92	0.96	0.24			0.048
8285	Cereal, Mueslix Apple & Almond Crunch/Kellogg	3/4 cup	55	210.65	5.39	40.865	4.675	4.95	2.585	1.045	1.045
8345	Cereal, Multi-Bran Chex/General Mills	1 cup	49	165.62	3.43	41.16	6.37	1.225	0.299	0.537	0.245
8265	Cereal, Multigrain Cheerios/General Mills	1 cup	30	111.9	2.556	24.45	1.92	1.089	0.297	0.15	0.249
8207	Cereal, Multi-Grain Flakes/Healthy Choice, Kellogg	1 cup	30	103.8	2.55	25.23	2.82	0.36	0.15	0.18	0.03
8291	Cereal, Nutri-Grain Almond and Raisin/Kellogg	1 oz	28.35	104.045	2.268	22	2.268	1.616	0.737	0.822	0.057
8152	Cereal, Nutri-Grain, Wheat	1 oz	28.34	102.02	2.466	23.976	1.785	0.283	0.032	0.119	0.052
8216	Cereal, Oat Bran Cereal/Quaker	1.25 cup	57	212.04	7.057	42.687	5.643	2.913	0.895	1.163	0.519
8214	Cereal, Oatmeal Squares/Quaker	1 cup (1 NLEA serving)	56	211.68	6.182	43.87	3.976	2.419	0.812	0.986	0.504
8125	Cereal, oatmeal, instant, w/apple & cinnamon, prep/Quaker	1 packet, prepared	149	129.63	2.712	26.477	2.682	1.49	0.513	0.428	0.249
8123	Cereal, oats, instant, plain, fortified, prep	1 cup, cooked	234	128.7	5.429	22.441	3.744	2.129	0.672	0.782	0.349
8180	Cereal, oats, regular/quick/instant, cooked w/salt	1 cup	234	145.08	6.084	25.272	3.978	2.34	0.749	0.866	0.421
8196	Cereal, Pop-Tarts Crunch, frosted strawberry/Kellogg	3/4 cup	30	117.9	1.35	26.76	0	0.81	0.24	0.27	0.33
8066	Cereal, Puffed Rice/Quaker	1 cup (1 NLEA serving)	14	53.62	0.98	12.288	0.196	0.126	0.025	0.048	0.045

Chol (g)	Calc (mg)	Iron (mg)	Mag (mg)	Phos (mg)	Pota (mg)	Sodi (mg)	Zinc (mg)	Vit A (RAE)	Vit C (mg)	Thia (mg)	Ribo (mg)	Niac (mg)	Vit B$_6$ (mg)	Vit B$_{12}$ (µg)	Vit E (mg)	Fol (µg)	Alc (g)
0	6.09	8.12	7.25	26.39	37.7	209.96	1.45	150.2	5.8	0.551	0.609	6.989	0.696	2.088	0.058	279.9	0
0	9.32	1.165	4.66	27.96	30.29	766.57	0.186	0	0	0.142	0.1	1.139	0.016	0	0.023	79.22	0
0	99.9	4.5	60	150	232.2	128.7	3.75	0	6	0.375	0.426	5.01	0.501	1.5	0.213	99.9	0
0	23.4	4.23	8.7	19.2	32.7	141.3	1.41	144.9	14.1	0.36	0.39	4.68	0.48	1.41	0.144	93.9	0
0	1.55	4.495	2.48	10.54	22.63	148.49	0.056	160.3	6.2	0.372	0.465	5.022	0.496	1.55	0.016	101.4	0
0	17.6	15.4	64.9	161.7	189.75	4.4	1.76	0	0	0.407	0.456	5.39	0.539	1.617	0	107.8	0
0	23.65	5.401	66	161.7	243.65	279.95	1.502		0	0.374	0.424	5	0.501	1.502		100.1	
0	95.16	5.185	213.5	557.54	655.14	26.84	5.014	1.22	1.464	0.898	0.356	2.58	0.379	0	7.174	101.3	0
0	19.72	16.199	58	138.62	178.06	353.8	1.201		0	0.377	0.423	5	0.499	1.502		99.76	
0	6.3	8.1	16.5	48.3	51.6	192.6	0.3		0	0.375	0.426	5.001	0.501	1.5		99.9	
0	14.3	16.225	34.1	106.15	121	337.7	0.88	375.7	0	0.385	0.44	5.005	0.495	1.485	2.2	102.3	0
0	150	8.1	8.1	39.9	35.1	267.3	3.75	159.6	6.3	0.375	0.426	5.01	0.501	1.5	0.066	200.1	0
0	112	8.954	30.72	132.8	91.2	164.16	4.128	0.64	0	0.403	0.467	5.504	0.55	0	0.176	416	0
0	23.1	1.65	41.25	128.7	165	135.3	3.465	206.3	3.3	0.347	0.385	4.565	1.815	5.5	4.615	369.6	0
0	99.9	4.5	15.9	60	57.3	203.4	3.75	150.3	6	0.375	0.426	5.01	0.501	1.5	0.093	200.1	0
0	22.41	1.793	57.27	176.79	266.43	189.24	1.868	0	0	0.264	0.102	2.373	0.077	0	1.12	29.88	0
0	4.8	9.6	4.8	24	31.2	324	0.168	0	0	0.48	0.24	5.76	0.019	0		4.8	0
0	33.55	4.675	62.7	175.45	209	270.05	3.135		0	0.385	0.44	5.17	0.495	1.265	5.775	110	0
0	89.18	14.455	53.41	178.36	189.63	321.93	3.332	133.8	5.39	0.333	0.377	4.459	0.446	1.323	0.152	356.2	0
0	57	8.1	29.7	114.3	97.2	254.1	3.75		15	0.375	0.426	5.001	0.501	0	0.191	99.9	0
0	8.7	6.3	29.1	86.4	100.2	174	1.5		0	0.54	0.6	6.99	0.69	2.1	3	90	0
0	86.468	0.709	6.521	96.674	101.21	100.643	1.928		0	0.198	0.227	2.58	0.255	0.765	2.835	56.7	0
0	7.935	0.799	22.105	105.992	77.085	192.712	3.741		15.02	0.368	0.425	4.988	0.51	1.502	7.482	100	0
0	108.87	17.072	95.76	295.26	249.66	207.48	3.961	165.3	6.612	0.41	0.467	5.495	0.547	0	2.103	420.1	0
0	112.56	17.069	65.52	205.52	204.96	268.8	4.239	166.9	6.384	0.386	0.476	5.628	0.549	0	1.49	439.6	0
0	110.26	3.844	28.31	93.87	108.77	165.39	0.641	321.8	0.298	0.288	0.346	4.066	0.428	0	0.134	84.93	0
0	131.04	10.156	53.82	126.36	124.02	105.3	1.076	376.7	0	0.339	0.405	4.76	0.501	0	0.234	100.6	0
0	18.72	1.591	56.16	177.84	131.04	374.4	1.147	0	0	0.257	0.047	0.304	0.047	0		9.36	0
0	2.4	4.08	9.6	17.4	27.3	113.7	3.42		13.8	0.33	0.39	4.56	0.45	0	0.083	90	0
0	1.26	0.4	4.2	16.52	16.24	0.7	0.154	0	0	0.062	0.036	0.493	0	0	0.017	21.56	0

EvaluEat Code	Food Name	Amt	Wt (g)	Energy (kcal)	Prot (g)	Carb (g)	Fiber (g)	Fat (g)	Mono (g)	Poly (g)	Sat (g)
8060	Cereal, Raisin Bran/Kellogg	1 cup (1 NLEA serving)	61	194.59	5.185	46.543	7.259	1.525	0.305	0.885	0.336
8287	Cereal, Raisin Squares Mini-Wheats/Kellogg	.75 cup (1 NLEA serving)	55	184.8	5.17	43.56	5.17	0.88	0.192	0.495	0.192
8194	Cereal, Reese's Peanut Butter Puffs/General Mills	.75 cup (1 NLEA serving)	30	127.5	1.8	23.4	0	2.91	1.243	0.903	0.57
8064	Cereal, Rice Chex	1.25 cup (1 NLEA serving)	31	116.87	1.86	26.66	0.31	0.31	0.067	0.069	0.124
8065	Cereal, Rice Krispies/Kellogg	1.25 cup (1 NLEA serving)	33	118.8	2.046	29.04	0.132	0.429	0.132	0.175	0.122
8318	Cereal, Smart Start/Kellogg	1 cup	50	182	3.1	43	2.3	0.6	0.15	0.25	0.2
8264	Cereal, S'mores Grahams/General Mills	3/4 cup	30	117	1.677	25.59	0.84	1.2	0.393	0.15	0.177
8067	Cereal, Special K/Kellogg	1 cup (1 NLEA serving)	31	117.49	6.975	22.01	0.744	0.48	0.124	0.248	0.108
8203	Cereal, Sun Crunchers/General Mills	1 cup	55	215.6	4.857	43.742	2.2	3.157	2.046	0.33	0.341
8059	Cereal, Sweet Crunch/Quisp	1 cup	27	109.35	1.199	22.95	0.702	1.644	0.302	0.205	0.427
8088	Cereal, Team Cheerios/General Mills	1 cup (1 NLEA serving)	30	113.1	2.151	25.068	1.65	1.131	0.329	0.462	0.182
8341	Cereal, The Original Shredded Wheat'n Bran/Kraft, Post	1.25 cup (1 NLEA serving)	59	197.06	7.375	47.141	7.906	0.826			0.118
8219	Cereal, Toasted Oatmeal Cereal, Honey Nut/Quaker	1 cup (1 NLEA serving)	49	192.08	4.484	37.926	3.479	3.655	1.71	1.005	0.534
8350	Cereal, Toasty O's/Malt-o-Meal	1 cup (1 NLEA serving)	30	111.6	3.321	22.401	2.7	1.809	0.669	0.609	0.369
8247	Cereal, Total Raisin Bran/General Mills	1 cup (1 NLEA serving)	55	171.05	3.85	41.25	4.95	1.1	0.149	0.524	0.22
8077	Cereal, Total/General Mills	.75 cup (1 NLEA serving)	30	97.2	2.4	22.5	2.4	0.75	0.123	0.273	0.159
8078	Cereal, Trix/General Mills	1 cup (1 NLEA serving)	30	117.3	0.9	26.7	0.9	1.14	0.596	0.274	0.18
8305	Cereal, Waffle Crisp/Post	1 cup (1 NLEA serving)	30	129	1.8	23.97	0.54	2.94	1.291	1.225	0.42
8082	Cereal, Wheat Chex	1 cup (1 NLEA serving)	30	103.5	3	24.3	3.3	0.6	0.079	0.242	0.12
8157	Cereal, wheat, puffed, fortified	1 cup	12	43.68	1.764	9.552	0.528	0.144			0.024
8147	Cereal, wheat, shredded, large biscuit	2 biscuits (1 NLEA serving)	46	156.4	5.235	36.138	5.336	1.104	0.161	0.58	0.207
8089	Cereal, Wheaties/General Mills	1 cup (1 NLEA serving)	30	106.5	3	24.3	3	0.96	0.286	0.35	0.18
1163	Cheese fondue	1 cup	215	492.35	30.594	8.106	0	28.961	7.66	1.041	18.75
44048	Cheese food, imitation	1 cubic inch	10.2	14.382	2.285	0.898	0	0.133	0.039	0.005	0.083
19434	Cheese puffs and twists, corn based, low-fat	1 oz	28.35	122.47	2.41	20.511	3.033	3.43	0.992	1.627	0.595
43276	Cheese spread, cream cheese base	1 cup	186	548.7	13.206	6.51	0	53.196	15.012	1.921	33.517
1004	Cheese, blue	1 oz	28.35	100.08	6.067	0.663	0	8.148	2.205	0.227	5.293
1006	Cheese, brie	1 cubic inch	17	56.78	3.528	0.076	0	4.706	1.362	0.14	2.96

Chol (g)	Calc (mg)	Iron (mg)	Mag (mg)	Phos (mg)	Pota (mg)	Sodi (mg)	Zinc (mg)	Vit A (RAE)	Vit C (mg)	Thia (mg)	Ribo (mg)	Niac (mg)	Vit B_6 (mg)	Vit B_{12} (µg)	Vit E (mg)	Fol (µg)	Alc (g)
0	29.28	4.636	82.96	258.64	372.1	361.73	1.549	154.9	0.427	0.39	0.439	5.185	0.519	1.549	0.476	103.7	0
0	21.45	15.4	43.45	155.65	264.55	3.3	1.54	0	0	0.391	0.44	5.17	0.517	1.595	0.286	104	0
0	99.9	4.5	15.9	20.1	41.7	166.5	3.75	150.3	6	0.375	0.426	5.01	0.501	1.5	0.36	99.9	0
0	103.23	9.3	9.3	35.34	30.38	291.71	3.875	155.3	6.2	0.387	0.44	5.177	0.518	1.55	0.016	206.8	0
0	5.28	1.815	13.2	45.87	43.89	318.78	0.462	153.1	6.369	0.376	0.462	5.049	0.495	1.485	0.036	104	0
0	17	18	32	101	102	280.5	15.1	231	15.5	1.55	1.7	20	2	6	20.135	402.5	0
0	14.4	4.5	10.8	40.5	48	212.4	3.75		15	0.375	0.426	5.001	0.501	0	0.218	99.9	0
0	9.3	8.37	19.22	67.89	60.76	223.51	0.899	230.3	20.99	0.527	0.589	7.13	1.984	6.045	7.074	399.9	0
0	85.25	4.499	43.45	171.6	129.8	380.05	0.798		15.02	0.374	0.424	5	0.501	0	0.056	99.55	0
0	2.97	4.96	14.85	45.36	51.03	200.07	4.134	10.8	2.916	0.413	0.467	5.511	0.551	0	0.184	420.1	0
	105.9	4.5	21.6	78.3	69.6	223.5	3.75		6	0.375	0.426	5.001	0.501	1.5	0.159	202.5	
0	26.55	2.466	80.83	234.82	247.8	2.95	1.929		0	0.153	0.071	3.723	0.195	0		27.14	
0	133.28	6.806	60.27	166.11	180.81	215.6	5.39	215.6	1.47	0.588	0.666	7.183	0.715	0	2.68	436.6	0
0	39.9	8.1	32.1	99.9	93.9	284.1	3.75	375.3	15	0.375	0.426	5.001	0.501	0	0.189	99.9	0
0	999.9	17.985	40.15	100.1	354.2	239.25	15.02	150.2	0	1.502	1.699	20.02	2.002	5.995	20.301	399.9	0
0	999.9	18	24	80.1	89.4	191.7	15	150.3	60	1.5	1.701	20.01	2.001	6	20.133	399.9	0
0	99.9	4.5	3.6	20.1	17.4	194.1	3.75	150.3	6	0.375	0.426	5.01	0.501	1.5	0.597	99.9	0
0	6	1.8	11.7	33.9	33.6	129.6	0.408	221.1	0	0.375	0.426	5.001	0.501	0	0.225	99.9	0
0	60	8.7	24	90	112.5	267.3	2.4	90	3.6	0.225	0.255	3	0.3	0.9	0.216	240	0
0	3.36	3.804	17.4	42.6	41.76	0.48	0.283	0	0	0.312	0.216	4.236	0.02	0		3.84	0
0	20.24	1.509	62.56	164.68	170.66	5.52	1.426	0	9.246	0.142	0.115	2.636	1.467	0	0.304	27.14	0
0	0	8.1	32.1	99.9	111	217.5	7.5	150.3	6	0.75	0.849	9.99	0.999	3	0.186	200.1	0
96.75	1023.4	0.839	49.45	657.9	225.75	283.8	4.214	234.4	0	0.058	0.421	0.409	0.118	1.785		17.2	0.645
0.612	56.304	0.093	3.57	50.898	34.272	126.378	0.336	1.02	0	0.003	0.049	0.015	0.013	0.125	0.001	0.816	0
0.284	101.21	0.363	11.624	101.21	81.081	364.298	0.607	12.47	6.067	0.153	0.173	2.024	0.201	0.607	1.205	27.5	0
167.4	132.06	2.102	11.16	169.26	208.32	1251.78	0.949	634.3	0	0.037	0.353	1.767	0.074	0.744	1.432	22.32	0
21.263	149.688	0.088	6.521	109.715	72.576	395.483	0.754	56.13	0	0.008	0.108	0.288	0.047	0.346	0.071	10.21	0
17	31.28	0.085	3.4	31.96	25.84	106.93	0.405	29.58	0	0.012	0.088	0.065	0.04	0.28	0.041	11.05	0

EvaluEat Code	Food Name	Amt	Wt (g)	Energy (kcal)	Prot (g)	Carb (g)	Fiber (g)	Fat (g)	Mono (g)	Poly (g)	Sat (g)
1007	Cheese, camembert	1 oz	28.35	85.05	5.613	0.13	0	6.878	1.991	0.205	4.326
1009	Cheese, cheddar	1 cup, shredded	113	455.39	28.137	1.446	0	37.448	10.612	1.064	23.834
1168	Cheese, cheddar or colby, low-fat	1 cup, shredded	113	195.49	27.516	2.158	0	7.91	2.353	0.251	4.906
1012	Cheese, cottage, creamed, large or small curd	4 oz	113	116.39	14.114	3.028	0	5.096	1.452	0.157	3.224
1015	Cheese, cottage, lowfat, 2% fat	4 oz	113	101.7	15.526	4.102	0	2.181	0.622	0.067	1.38
1014	Cheese, cottage, nonfat, uncreamed, dry, large or small curd	4 oz	113	96.05	19.515	2.091	0	0.475	0.124	0.017	0.308
1017	Cheese, cream	1 tbsp	14.5	50.605	1.095	0.386	0	5.056	1.427	0.183	3.185
1186	Cheese, cream, fat-free	1 oz	28.34	27.206	4.084	1.644	0	0.385	0.094	0.017	0.255
1018	Cheese, edam	1 oz	28.35	101.21	7.085	0.405	0	7.881	2.303	0.189	4.982
1019	Cheese, feta	1 oz	28.35	74.844	4.029	1.16	0	6.033	1.311	0.168	4.237
1020	Cheese, fontina	1 cup, shredded	108	420.12	27.648	1.674	0	33.631	9.382	1.786	20.732
1022	Cheese, gouda	1 oz	28.35	100.93	7.07	0.629	0	7.779	2.196	0.186	4.994
1188	Cheese, Kraft Cheez Whiz pasteurized process cheese sauce	2 tbsp	33	91.08	3.96	3.036	0.099	6.93			4.323
1190	Cheese, Kraft Free Singles American nonfat pasteurized process cheese product	1 slice	21	31.08	4.767	2.457	0.042	0.21			0.147
1165	Cheese, Mexican, queso anejo	1 oz	28.35	105.75	6.078	1.313	0	8.499	2.418	0.255	5.396
1025	Cheese, monterey	1 cup, shredded	113	421.49	27.662	0.768	0	34.216	9.889	1.016	21.545
1028	Cheese, mozzarella, part skim milk	1 oz	28.35	72.009	6.878	0.785	0	4.513	1.279	0.134	2.867
1026	Cheese, mozzarella, whole milk	1 oz	28.35	85.05	6.285	0.621	0	6.336	1.863	0.217	3.729
1030	Cheese, muenster	1 cup, shredded	113	415.84	26.453	1.266	0	33.945	9.843	0.747	21.598
1032	Cheese, parmesan, grated	1 tbsp	5	21.55	1.923	0.203	0	1.431	0.419	0.059	0.865
42205	Cheese, pasteurized process, cheddar or American, fat-free	1 cup	186	275.28	41.85	24.924	0	1.488	0.426	0.047	0.937
1035	Cheese, provolone	1 oz	28.35	99.509	7.252	0.607	0	7.547	2.096	0.218	4.842
1037	Cheese, ricotta, part skim milk	1 cup	246	339.48	28.019	12.644	0	19.459	5.692	0.64	12.12
1036	Cheese, ricotta, whole milk	1 cup	246	428.04	27.7	7.478	0	31.931	8.922	0.947	20.406
1038	Cheese, romano	1 oz	28.35	109.72	9.015	1.029	0	7.637	2.222	0.168	4.852
1039	Cheese, roquefort	1 oz	28.35	104.61	6.107	0.567	0	8.686	2.402	0.374	5.461
1040	Cheese, Swiss	1 oz	28.35	107.73	7.635	1.525	0	7.881	2.062	0.276	5.04
18147	Cheesecake, commercially prep	1 piece (1/6 of 17 oz cake)	80	256.8	4.4	20.4	0.32	18	6.907	1.282	7.937
18148	Cheesecake, no bake mix, prep	1 piece (1/12 of 9" dia)	99	271.26	5.445	35.145	1.881	12.573	4.474	0.8	6.624
9367	Cherries, sweet, canned, heavy syrup, drained	1 fruit (2-1/4" high x 2-1/2" dia)	122	101.26	0.891	25.705	3.05	0.256	0.06	0.067	0.049
5028	Chicken liver, simmered	1 container, cooked, yield from 400 g raw liver	256	427.52	62.618	2.227	0	16.666	3.625	3.249	5.274
22703	Chicken & dumplings, canned/Sweet Sue	1 serving	240	218.4	15.12	22.8	2.64	7.44	2.952	1.625	1.795
7932	Chicken breast, fat-free, mesquite flavor, sliced	1 serving 2 slices	42	33.6	7.056	0.945	0	0.164	0.067	0.025	0.055
7933	Chicken breast, oven-roasted, fat-free, sliced	1 serving 2 slices	42	33.18	7.052	0.911	0	0.164	0.051	0.031	0.055
5026	Chicken heart, simmered	1 cup, chopped or diced	145	268.25	38.295	0.145	0	11.484	2.914	3.335	3.277
22527	Chicken pie, frozen/Stouffers	1 package yields	283	571.66	23.206	36.507	3.113	37.073	12.367	10.443	10.726
5058	Chicken, broiler or fryer, breast w/skin, batter fried	1/2 breast, bone removed	140	364	34.776	12.586	0.42	18.48	7.644	4.312	4.928

Chol (g)	Calc (mg)	Iron (mg)	Mag (mg)	Phos (mg)	Pota (mg)	Sodi (mg)	Zinc (mg)	Vit A (RAE)	Vit C (mg)	Thia (mg)	Ribo (mg)	Niac (mg)	Vit B_6 (mg)	Vit B_{12} (µg)	Vit E (mg)	Fol (µg)	Alc (g)
20.412	109.998	0.094	5.67	98.375	53.015	238.707	0.675	68.32	0	0.008	0.138	0.179	0.064	0.369	0.06	17.58	0
118.65	814.73	0.768	31.64	578.56	110.74	701.73	3.514	299.5	0	0.031	0.424	0.09	0.084	0.938	0.328	20.34	0
23.73	468.95	0.475	18.08	546.92	74.58	691.56	2.057	67.8	0	0.014	0.25	0.058	0.051	0.554	0.068	12.43	0
16.95	67.8	0.158	5.65	149.16	94.92	457.65	0.418	49.72	0	0.024	0.184	0.142	0.076	0.701	0.045	13.56	0
9.04	77.97	0.181	6.78	170.63	108.48	458.78	0.475	23.73	0	0.027	0.209	0.163	0.086	0.802	0.023	14.69	0
7.91	36.16	0.26	4.52	117.52	36.16	14.69	0.531	10.17	0	0.028	0.16	0.175	0.093	0.938	0	16.95	0
15.95	11.6	0.174	0.87	15.08	17.255	42.92	0.078	53.07	0	0.002	0.029	0.015	0.007	0.061	0.043	1.885	0
2.267	52.429	0.051	3.968	122.996	46.194	154.453	0.249	79.07	0	0.014	0.049	0.045	0.014	0.156	0.003	10.49	0
25.232	207.239	0.125	8.505	151.956	53.298	273.578	1.063	68.89	0	0.01	0.11	0.023	0.022	0.437	0.068	4.536	0
25.232	139.766	0.184	5.387	95.54	17.577	316.386	0.816	35.44	0	0.044	0.239	0.281	0.12	0.479	0.051	9.072	0
125.28	594	0.248	15.12	373.68	69.12	864	3.78	281.9	0	0.023	0.22	0.162	0.09	1.814	0.292	6.48	0
32.319	198.45	0.068	8.222	154.791	34.304	232.187	1.106	46.78	0	0.009	0.095	0.018	0.023	0.437	0.068	5.954	0
24.75	118.47	0.063		265.98	79.2	540.54	0.541		0.132		0.079						
3.36	149.52	0.01		193.83	49.56	272.58	0.525		0.042		0.059						
29.768	192.78	0.133	7.938	125.874	24.665	320.639	0.833	15.31	0	0.006	0.059	0.009	0.013	0.391	0.074	0.284	0
100.57	842.98	0.814	30.51	501.72	91.53	605.68	3.39	223.74	0	0.017	0.441	0.105	0.089	0.938	0.294	20.34	0
18.144	221.697	0.062	6.521	131.261	23.814	175.487	0.782	36.01	0	0.005	0.086	0.03	0.02	0.232	0.04	2.552	0
22.397	143.168	0.125	5.67	100.359	21.546	177.755	0.828	50.75	0	0.009	0.08	0.029	0.01	0.646	0.054	1.985	0
108.48	810.21	0.463	30.51	528.84	151.42	709.64	3.175	336.7	0	0.015	0.362	0.116	0.063	1.661	0.294	13.56	0
4.4	55.45	0.045	1.9	36.45	6.25	76.45	0.193	6	0	0.001	0.024	0.006	0.002	0.113	0.013	0.5	0
20.46	1281.54	0.521	66.96	1740.96	535.68	2842.08	6.361	818.4	0	0.112	0.893	0.391	0.167	2.083	0.502	50.22	0
19.562	214.326	0.147	7.938	140.616	39.123	248.346	0.916	66.91	0	0.005	0.091	0.044	0.021	0.414	0.065	2.835	0
76.26	669.12	1.082	36.9	450.18	307.5	307.5	3.296	263.22	0	0.052	0.455	0.192	0.049	0.713	0.172	31.98	0
125.46	509.22	0.935	27.06	388.68	258.3	206.64	2.854	295.2	0	0.032	0.48	0.256	0.106	0.836	0.271	29.52	0
29.484	301.644	0.218	11.624	215.46	24.381	340.2	0.731	27.22	0	0.01	0.105	0.022	0.024	0.318	0.065	1.985	0
25.515	187.677	0.159	8.505	111.132	25.799	512.852	0.59	83.35	0	0.011	0.166	0.208	0.035	0.181		13.892	0
26.082	224.249	0.057	10.773	160.745	21.83	54.432	1.236	62.37	0	0.018	0.084	0.026	0.024	0.947	0.108	1.701	0
44	40.8	0.504	8.8	74.4	72	165.6	0.408	113.6	0.32	0.022	0.154	0.156	0.042	0.136	1.265	14.4	0
28.71	170.28	0.465	18.81	231.66	208.89	376.2	0.455	95.04	0.495	0.12	0.26	0.488	0.051	0.307		29.7	0
0	12.2	0.427	10.98	24.4	180.56	3.66	0.122	14.64	4.392	0.027	0.052	0.483	0.038	0	0.281	6.1	0
1441.28	28.16	29.773	64	1036.8	673.28	194.56	10.19	10191	71.424	0.745	5.102	28.275	1.933	43.136	2.099	1480	0
36		2.568				945.6											0
15.12	1.68	0.126	15.12	107.52	132.72	436.8	0.252	0	0	0.006	0.01	1.152	0.05	0.029	0.022	0.42	0
15.12	2.52	0.134	3.78	25.2	28.14	456.54	0.126	0	0	0.008	0.012	1.44	0.063	0.038	0.028	0.42	0
350.9	27.55	13.094	29	288.55	191.4	69.6	10.59	11.6	2.61	0.102	1.074	4.064	0.464	10.571		116	0
76.41	101.88	3				942.39											0
119	28	1.75	33.6	259	281.4	385	1.33	28	0	0.161	0.204	14.732	0.602	0.42	1.484	21	0

EvaluEat Code	Food Name	Amt	Wt (g)	Energy (kcal)	Prot (g)	Carb (g)	Fiber (g)	Fat (g)	Mono (g)	Poly (g)	Sat (g)
5060	Chicken, broiler or fryer, breast w/skin, roasted	1 cup, chopped or diced	140	275.8	41.72	0	0	10.892	4.242	2.324	3.066
5063	Chicken, broiler or fryer, breast, no skin, fried	1/2 breast, bone and skin removed	86	160.82	28.758	0.439	0	4.051	1.479	0.92	1.109
5064	Chicken, broiler or fryer, breast, no skin, roasted	1 cup, chopped or diced	140	231	43.428	0	0	4.998	1.736	1.078	1.414
5035	Chicken, broiler or fryer, dark meat w/skin, batter fried	yield from 1 lb ready-to-cook chicken	167	497.66	36.489	15.665		31.129	12.659	7.398	8.266
5037	Chicken, broiler or fryer, dark meat w/skin, roasted	yield from 1 lb ready-to-cook chicken	101	255.53	26.23	0	0	15.938	6.252	3.525	4.414
5044	Chicken, broiler or fryer, dark meat, no skin, fried	1 cup	140	334.6	40.586	3.626	0	16.268	6.048	3.878	4.368
5045	Chicken, broiler or fryer, dark meat, no skin, roasted	1 cup, chopped or diced	140	287	38.318	0	0	13.622	4.984	3.164	3.724
5067	Chicken, broiler or fryer, drumstick w/skin, batter fried	1 drumstick, bone removed	72	192.96	15.804	5.962	0.216	11.34	4.63	2.729	2.981
5069	Chicken, broiler or fryer, drumstick w/skin, roasted	1 drumstick, bone removed	52	112.32	14.056	0	0	5.798	2.21	1.3	1.586
5072	Chicken, broiler or fryer, drumstick, no skin, fried	yield from 1 lb ready-to-cook chicken	25	48.75	7.155	0	0	2.02	0.735	0.493	0.533
5073	Chicken, broiler or fryer, drumstick, no skin, roasted	1 drumstick, bone and skin removed	44	75.68	12.448	0	0	2.49	0.823	0.603	0.651
5021	Chicken, broiler or fryer, giblets, floured, fried	1 cup, chopped or diced	145	401.65	47.183	6.307	0	19.517	6.409	4.901	5.51
5022	Chicken, broiler or fryer, giblets, simmered	1 cup, chopped or diced	145	229.1	39.368	0.624	0	6.525	1.395	1.177	1.917
5024	Chicken, broiler or fryer, gizzard, simmered	1 cup, chopped or diced	145	211.7	44.066	0	0	3.886	0.766	0.512	0.972
5076	Chicken, broiler or fryer, leg w/skin, batter fried	1 leg, bone removed	158	431.34	34.397	13.778	0.474	25.549	10.396	6.083	6.762
5078	Chicken, broiler or fryer, leg w/skin, roasted	1 leg, bone removed	114	264.48	29.594	0	0	15.344	5.974	3.42	4.241
5081	Chicken, broiler or fryer, leg, no skin, fried	1 leg, bone and skin removed	94	195.52	26.677	0.611	0	8.761	3.224	2.087	2.341
5082	Chicken, broiler or fryer, leg, no skin, roasted	1 leg, bone and skin removed	95	181.45	25.679	0	0	8.009	2.897	1.872	2.175
5030	Chicken, broiler or fryer, light meat w/skin, batter fried	1/2 chicken, bone removed	188	520.76	44.274	17.86		29.027	11.976	6.768	7.746
5032	Chicken, broiler or fryer, light meat w/skin, roasted	1/2 chicken, bone removed	132	293.04	38.306	0	0	14.322	5.623	3.049	4.026
5040	Chicken, broiler or fryer, light meat, no skin, fried	1 cup	140	268.8	45.948	0.588	0	7.756	2.758	1.764	2.128
5041	Chicken, broiler or fryer, light meat, no skin, roasted	1 cup, chopped or diced	140	242.2	43.274	0	0	6.314	2.156	1.372	1.778

Chol (g)	Calc (mg)	Iron (mg)	Mag (mg)	Phos (mg)	Pota (mg)	Sodi (mg)	Zinc (mg)	Vit A (RAE)	Vit C (mg)	Thia (mg)	Ribo (mg)	Niac (mg)	Vit B$_6$ (mg)	Vit B$_{12}$ (µg)	Vit E (mg)	Fol (µg)	Alc (g)
117.6	19.6	1.498	37.8	299.6	343	99.4	1.428	37.8	0	0.092	0.167	17.794	0.784	0.448	0.378	5.6	0
78.26	13.76	0.98	26.66	211.56	237.36	67.94	0.929	6.02	0	0.068	0.108	12.713	0.55	0.318	0.361	3.44	0
119	21	1.456	40.6	319.2	358.4	103.6	1.4	8.4	0	0.098	0.16	19.197	0.84	0.476	0.378	5.6	0
148.63	35.07	2.405	33.4	242.15	308.95	492.65	3.474	51.77	0	0.195	0.364	9.364	0.417	0.451		30.06	0
91.91	15.15	1.374	22.22	169.68	222.2	87.87	2.515	60.6	0	0.067	0.209	6.423	0.313	0.293		7.07	0
134.4	25.2	2.086	35	261.8	354.2	135.8	4.074	33.6	0	0.13	0.349	9.898	0.518	0.462		12.6	0
130.2	21	1.862	32.2	250.6	336	130.2	3.92	30.8	0	0.102	0.318	9.167	0.504	0.448	0.378	11.2	0
61.92	12.24	0.972	14.4	105.84	133.92	193.68	1.678	18.72	0	0.081	0.155	3.669	0.194	0.202		12.96	0
47.32	6.24	0.692	11.96	91	119.08	46.8	1.492	15.6	0	0.036	0.112	3.117	0.177	0.166	0.14	4.16	0
23.5	3	0.33	6	46.5	62.25	24	0.805	4.5	0	0.019	0.059	1.536	0.097	0.087	0.123	2.25	0
40.92	5.28	0.572	10.56	80.96	108.24	41.8	1.399	7.92	0	0.033	0.103	2.673	0.172	0.15	0.119	3.96	0
646.7	26.1	14.964	36.25	414.7	478.5	163.85	9.092	5194	12.62	0.141	2.21	15.931	0.885	19.3		549.6	0
640.9	20.3	10.208	20.3	419.05	324.8	97.15	6.134	2542	18.13	0.207	1.525	9.606	0.576	13.688	0.667	372.7	0
536.5	24.65	4.626	4.35	274.05	259.55	81.2	6.409	0	0	0.038	0.305	4.524	0.103	1.508	0.29	7.25	0
142.2	28.44	2.212	31.6	240.16	298.62	440.82	3.429	42.66	0	0.183	0.349	8.584	0.427	0.442		28.44	0
104.88	13.68	1.516	26.22	198.36	256.5	99.18	2.964	44.46	0	0.078	0.243	7.063	0.376	0.342	0.308	7.98	0
93.06	12.22	1.316	23.5	181.42	238.76	90.24	2.801	18.8	0	0.078	0.232	6.287	0.367	0.32		8.46	0
89.3	11.4	1.244	22.8	173.85	229.9	86.45	2.717	18.05	0	0.071	0.22	6.003	0.352	0.304	0.257	7.6	0
157.92	37.6	2.369	41.36	315.84	347.8	539.56	1.993	45.12	0	0.212	0.276	17.213	0.733	0.526		30.08	0
110.88	19.8	1.505	33	264	299.64	99	1.624	43.56	0	0.079	0.156	14.697	0.686	0.422		3.96	0
126	22.4	1.596	40.6	323.4	368.2	113.4	1.778	12.6	0	0.102	0.176	18.711	0.882	0.504		5.6	0
119	21	1.484	37.8	302.4	345.8	107.8	1.722	12.6	0	0.091	0.162	17.389	0.84	0.476	0.378	5.6	0

EvaluEat Code	Food Name	Amt	Wt (g)	Energy (kcal)	Prot (g)	Carb (g)	Fiber (g)	Fat (g)	Mono (g)	Poly (g)	Sat (g)
5007	Chicken, broiler or fryer, meat & skin, batter fried	yield from 1 lb ready-to-cook chicken	280	809.2	63.112	26.376	0.84	48.58	19.852	11.48	12.908
5009	Chicken, broiler or fryer, meat & skin, roasted	1 cup, chopped or diced	140	334.6	38.22	0	0	19.04	7.476	4.158	5.306
5012	Chicken, broiler or fryer, meat only, no skin, fried	1 cup, chopped or diced	140	306.6	42.798	2.366	0.14	12.768	4.69	3.01	3.444
5013	Chicken, broiler or fryer, meat only, no skin, roasted	1 cup, chopped or diced	140	266	40.502	0	0	10.374	3.724	2.366	2.856
5092	Chicken, broiler or fryer, thigh w/skin, batter fried	1 thigh, bone removed	86	238.22	18.585	7.809	0.258	14.216	5.762	3.354	3.793
5094	Chicken, broiler or fryer, thigh w/skin, roasted	1 thigh, bone removed	62	153.14	15.537	0	0	9.604	3.813	2.12	2.685
5097	Chicken, broiler or fryer, thigh, no skin, fried	1 thigh, bone and skin removed	52	113.36	14.654	0.614	0	5.356	1.986	1.264	1.446
5098	Chicken, broiler or fryer, thigh, no skin, roasted	1 thigh, bone and skin removed	52	108.68	13.489	0	0	5.658	2.158	1.29	1.576
5002	Chicken, broiler or fryer, whole, batter fried	1 chicken	1028	2991.5	234.8	92.828		180.21	73.296	42.662	48.008
5001	Chicken, broiler or fryer, whole, raw	1 chicken	1046	2228	191.73	1.36	0	155.12	63.597	33.367	44.35
5004	Chicken, broiler or fryer, whole, roasted	1 chicken	682	1595.9	182.64	0.409	0	90.501	35.259	19.778	25.234
5101	Chicken, broiler or fryer, wing w/skin, batter fried	1 wing, bone removed	49	158.76	9.736	5.361	0.147	10.687	4.39	2.484	2.857
5103	Chicken, broiler or fryer, wing w/skin, roasted	1 wing, bone removed	34	98.6	9.132	0	0	6.616	2.598	1.408	1.853
5106	Chicken, broiler or fryer, wing, no skin, fried	1 wing, bone and skin removed	20	42.2	6.03	0	0	1.83	0.616	0.414	0.5
5107	Chicken, broiler or fryer, wing, no skin, roasted	1 wing, bone and skin removed	21	42.63	6.397	0	0	1.707	0.548	0.374	0.475
22697	Chicken, chicken salad ready to serve sandwich salad/Libby Spreadable	1 serving	118	171.1	5.782	11.918		11.092	3.457	4.224	2.301
5335	Chicken, feet, boiled	1 cup chopped or diced, cooked	174	374.1	33.756	0.348	0	25.404	9.57	5.185	6.821
5277	Chicken, meat only w/broth, canned	1 can (5 oz)	142	234.3	30.913	0	0	11.289	4.473	2.485	3.124
43128	Chicken, meatless	1 cup	186	416.64	43.97	6.77	6.696	23.678	5.072	13.528	3.385
51608	Chicken, nugget, breaded/Pierre product #1879	1 piece	14.2	46.718	2.378	1.889	0.156	3.321	0.977	1.478	0.653
22904	Chili con carne w/beans, canned entree	1 serving	222	255.3	20.18	24.487	8.214	8.147	2.153	1.443	2.109
16059	Chili w/beans, canned	1 cup	256	286.72	14.618	30.49	11.264	14.054	5.97	0.927	6.021
22705	Chili w/o beans, canned entree/Hormel	1 cup	236	193.52	16.992	17.912	3.068	6.561	2.242	0.85	2.195
22720	Chili, vegetarian chili w/beans, canned entree/Hormel	1 cup	247	205.01	11.93	38.013	9.88	0.692	0.074	0.395	0.124
18606	Chocolate cake, snack cake, chocolate creme filling, Ding Dongs/Hostess	1 serving	80	368	3.12	45.36	1.84	19.36	3.992	1.198	11.036
19124	Chocolate, baking, Mexican, squares	1 tablet	20	85.2	0.728	15.482	0.8	3.118	1.009	0.232	1.721
14198	Cocoa mix, No Sugar Added Hot Cocoa Mix/Carnation	1 serving	15	54.75	4.304	8.433	0.75	0.426	0.136	0.014	0.203
14197	Cocoa mix, Rich Chocolate Hot Cocoa Mix/Carnation	1 serving	28	112	1.296	24.237	0.672	1.109	0.348	0.265	0.291
1105	Cocoa, hot, homemade w/whole milk	1 cup	250	192.5	8.8	26.575	2.5	5.825	1.692	0.085	3.577
18103	Coffee cake, cheese	1 piece (1/6 of 16 oz cake)	76	257.64	5.32	33.668	0.76	11.552	5.418	1.25	4.097

Chol (g)	Calc (mg)	Iron (mg)	Mag (mg)	Phos (mg)	Pota (mg)	Sodi (mg)	Zinc (mg)	Vit A (RAE)	Vit C (mg)	Thia (mg)	Ribo (mg)	Niac (mg)	Vit B6 (mg)	Vit B12 (µg)	Vit E (mg)	Fol (µg)	Alc (g)
243.6	58.8	3.836	58.8	434	518	817.6	4.676	78.4	0	0.322	0.529	19.72	0.868	0.784	3.472	50.4	0
123.2	21	1.764	32.2	254.8	312.2	114.8	2.716	65.8	0	0.088	0.235	11.882	0.56	0.42	0.378	7	0
131.6	23.8	1.89	37.8	287	359.8	127.4	3.136	25.2	0	0.119	0.277	13.528	0.672	0.476	0.644	9.8	0
124.6	21	1.694	35	273	340.2	120.4	2.94	22.4	0	0.097	0.249	12.842	0.658	0.462	0.378	8.4	0
79.98	15.48	1.247	18.06	133.3	165.12	247.68	1.754	24.94	0	0.102	0.195	4.915	0.224	0.241		16.34	0
57.66	7.44	0.831	13.64	107.88	137.64	52.08	1.463	29.76	0	0.042	0.131	3.946	0.192	0.18	0.167	4.34	0
53.04	6.76	0.759	13.52	103.48	134.68	49.4	1.451	10.92	0	0.046	0.133	3.702	0.198	0.172		4.68	0
49.4	6.24	0.681	12.48	95.16	123.76	45.76	1.336	10.4	0	0.038	0.12	3.393	0.182	0.161	0.14	4.16	0
1058.84	215.88	18.401	215.88	1624.24	1953.2	2919.52	19.64	1861	4.112	1.162	2.549	72.813	3.29	8.532		329	0
941.4	115.06	13.703	209.2	1558.54	1976.94	732.2	15.48	2427	27.2	0.638	1.946	69.444	3.556	11.611	3.849	313.8	0
729.74	102.3	11.321	156.86	1241.24	1445.84	538.78	14.73	1303	3.41	0.43	1.528	53.933	2.592	6.411	2.251	197.8	0
38.71	9.8	0.632	7.84	59.29	67.62	156.8	0.676	16.66	0	0.052	0.074	2.58	0.147	0.123		8.82	0
28.56	5.1	0.432	6.46	51.34	62.56	27.88	0.619	15.98	0	0.014	0.044	2.26	0.143	0.099	0.092	1.02	0
16.8	3	0.228	4.2	32.8	41.6	18.2	0.424	3.6	0	0.009	0.026	1.448	0.118	0.068		0.8	0
17.85	3.36	0.244	4.41	34.86	44.1	19.32	0.449	3.78	0	0.01	0.027	1.536	0.124	0.071	0.057	0.84	0
30.68						552.24											0
146.16	153.12	1.583	8.7	144.42	53.94	116.58	1.201	52.2	0	0.104	0.348	0.696	0.017	0.818	0.47	149.6	0
88.04	19.88	2.244	17.04	157.62	195.96	714.26	2.002	48.28	2.84	0.021	0.183	8.987	0.497	0.412	0.369	5.68	0
0	65.1	6.082	31.62	623.1	100.44	1318.74	1.302	0	0	1.269	0.459	2.704	1.302	4.055	4.985	141.4	0
5.538	5.112	0.315	3.408	31.95	29.962	98.974	0.349		0	0.043	0.035	0.888	0.038	0.099	0.386	4.118	0
24.42	66.6	3.308	55.5	193.14	608.28	1032.3	2.42	44.4	0.888	0.153	0.149	2.073	0.186	0.577	0.284	57.72	0
43.52	120.32	8.781	115.2	394.24	934.4	1336.32	5.12	43.52	4.352	0.123	0.269	0.916	0.338	0	1.459	58.88	0
35.4	49.56	2.596	37.76		349.28	969.96	2.596		0								0
0	96.33	3.458	81.51		802.75	778.05	1.729		1.235								0
13.6	3.2	1.84				240.8											0
0	6.8	0.436	19	28.4	79.4	0.6	0.252	0	0.02	0.011	0.021	0.366	0.007	0	0.072	1	0
2.85	123.45	0.39	27	135	288.15	142.05	0.599	0	0.405	0.056	0.218	0.183	0.053	0.447	0.013	5.85	0
1.68	40.04	0.28	27.44	70.84	194.32	101.64	0.358	0	0	0.027	0.116	0.155	0.03	0.104	0.042	1.96	0
20	262.5	1.2	57.5	262.5	492.5	110	1.575	127.5	0.5	0.098	0.455	0.333	0.1	1.05	0.075	12.5	0
64.6	44.84	0.486	11.4	76.76	219.64	257.64	0.448	65.36	0.076	0.08	0.095	0.518	0.044	0.258	1.186	29.64	0

EvaluEat Code	Food Name	Amt	Wt (g)	Energy (kcal)	Prot (g)	Carb (g)	Fiber (g)	Fat (g)	Mono (g)	Poly (g)	Sat (g)
18105	Coffee cake, creme w/chocolate icing	1 piece (1/6 of 19 oz cake)	90	297.9	4.5	48.42	1.8	9.72	5.098	1.319	2.55
14210	Coffee, brewed, espresso, restaurant-prep	1 oz	28.34	2.551	0.003	0.434	0	0.051	0	0.026	0.026
14202	Coffee, brewed, espresso, restaurant-prepared, decaffeinated	1 cup (8 fl. oz.)	237	21.33	0.024	3.626	0	0.427	0	0.218	0.218
2055	Condiment, horseradish, prep	1 tbsp	15	7.2	0.177	1.694	0.495	0.104	0.02	0.051	0.014
2046	Condiment, mustard, prepared, yellow	1 tsp or 1 packet	5	3.3	0.198	0.389	0.16	0.155	0.107	0.029	0.008
11945	Condiment, pickle relish, sweet	1 tbsp	15	19.5	0.056	5.258	0.165	0.071	0.031	0.018	0.008
11935	Condiment, tomato catsup	1 tbsp	15	14.25	0.271	3.582	0.195	0.089	0.014	0.036	0.012
18150	Cookie, animal crackers/Arrowroot/Tea Biscuits	1 oz	28.35	126.44	1.956	21.007	0.312	3.912	2.173	0.531	0.982
18151	Cookie, brownies, commercially prep/Little Debbie	1 square, large (2-3/4" sq x 7/8")	56	226.8	2.688	35.784	1.176	9.128	5.02	1.265	2.372
18154	Cookie, brownies, homemade	1 brownie (2" square)	24	111.84	1.488	12.048		6.984	2.601	2.259	1.757
18159	Cookie, chocolate chip, enriched, commercially prep	1 cookie	12	57.72	0.648	8.016	0.3	2.712	1.401	0.284	0.897
18378	Cookie, chocolate chip, homemade w/butter	1 cookie, medium (2-1/4" dia)	16	78.08	0.912	9.312		4.544	1.319	0.727	2.251
18158	Cookie, chocolate chip, lower fat, commercially prep	1 cookie	10	45.3	0.58	7.33	0.36	1.54	0.609	0.465	0.381
18160	Cookie, chocolate chip, soft, commercially prep	1 cookie	15	68.7	0.525	8.865	0.48	3.645	1.955	0.525	1.112
18608	Cookie, Chocolate Graham Selects/Keebler	1 serving	31	144.15	2.201	22.258		5.146			0.958
18169	Cookie, coconut macaroons, homemade	1 cookie, medium (2" dia)	24	96.96	0.864	17.328	0.432	3.048	0.132	0.034	2.697
18170	Cookie, fig bar	1 individual package (2 oz package containing 2 3" bars)	57	198.36	2.109	40.413	2.622	4.161	1.712	1.58	0.64
18171	Cookie, fortune	1 cookie	8	30.24	0.336	6.72	0.128	0.216	0.108	0.037	0.054
18172	Cookie, ginger snaps	1 cookie	7	29.12	0.392	5.383	0.154	0.686	0.376	0.096	0.172
18609	Cookie, Golden Vanilla Wafers/Keebler	1 serving	31	147.25	1.612	21.607		6.045			1.11
18174	Cookie, graham crackers, chocolate coated	1 cracker (2-1/2" square)	14	67.76	0.812	9.31	0.434	3.248	1.076	0.145	1.873
18173	Cookie, graham crackers, plain/honey/cinnamon	1 large rectangular piece or 2 squares or 4 small rectangular pieces	14	59.22	0.966	10.752	0.392	1.414	0.572	0.536	0.213
18175	Cookie, Ladyfingers/Egg Jumbo w/lemon juice & rind	1 cookie	11	40.15	1.166	6.567	0.11	1.001	0.468	0.177	0.382
18612	Cookie, Little Debbie Nutty Bars, Chocolate Covered Wafers w/Peanut Butter	1 serving	57	312.36	4.56	31.464		18.696			3.585
18177	Cookie, molasses	1 large (3-1/2" to 4" dia)	32	137.6	1.792	23.616	0.32	4.096	2.282	0.553	1.028
18178	Cookie, oatmeal, commercially prep	1 cookie, big (3-1/2" to 4" dia)	25	112.5	1.55	17.175	0.7	4.525	2.506	0.636	1.13
18184	Cookie, oatmeal, homemade w/raisins	1 cookie (2-5/8" dia)	15	65.25	0.975	10.26		2.43	1.033	0.755	0.485
18185	Cookie, peanut butter, commercially prep	1 cookie	15	71.55	1.44	8.835	0.27	3.54	1.855	0.828	0.673
18189	Cookie, peanut butter, homemade	1 cookie (3" dia)	20	95	1.8	11.78		4.76	2.166	1.445	0.888
18186	Cookie, peanut butter, soft, commercially prep	1 cookie	15	68.55	0.795	8.655	0.255	3.66	2.077	0.477	0.922

Chol (g)	Calc (mg)	Iron (mg)	Mag (mg)	Phos (mg)	Pota (mg)	Sodi (mg)	Zinc (mg)	Vit A (RAE)	Vit C (mg)	Thia (mg)	Ribo (mg)	Niac (mg)	Vit B$_6$ (mg)	Vit B$_{12}$ (µg)	Vit E (mg)	Fol (µg)	Alc (g)
62.1	34.2	0.459	13.5	67.5	70.2	290.7	0.396	33.3	0.09	0.072	0.067	0.756	0.037	0.18		36.9	0
0	0.567	0.037	22.672	1.984	32.591	3.968	0.014	0	0.057	0	0.05	1.476	0.001	0	0.006	0.283	0
0	4.74	0.308	189.6	16.59	272.55	33.18	0.118	0	0.474	0.002	0.419	12.341	0.005	0	0.047	2.37	0
0	8.4	0.063	4.05	4.65	36.9	47.1	0.124	0	3.735	0.001	0.004	0.058	0.011	0	0.002	8.55	0
0	4	0.093	1.9	4.4	7.55	56	0.03	0.35	0.145	0.003	0.001	0.023	0.004	0	0.015	0.4	0
0	0.45	0.131	0.75	2.1	3.75	121.65	0.021	1.35	0.15	0	0.005	0.035	0.002	0	0.014	0.15	0
0	2.7	0.076	2.85	4.95	57.3	166.95	0.039	7.05	2.265	0.002	0.07	0.225	0.022	0	0.219	2.25	0
0	12.191	0.78	5.103	32.319	28.35	111.416	0.181	0	0	0.099	0.092	0.984	0.006	0.014	0.034	29.2	0
9.52	16.24	1.26	17.36	56.56	83.44	174.72	0.403	11.2	0	0.143	0.118	0.964	0.02	0.039	0.084	26.32	0
17.52	13.68	0.442	12.72	31.68	42.24	82.32	0.233	42.24	0.072	0.034	0.046	0.236	0.023	0.038		6.96	0
0	3	0.337	3.72	12.96	16.2	37.8	0.077	0	0	0.027	0.034	0.326	0.007	0.001	0.017	6.96	0
11.2	6.08	0.397	8.8	16	35.36	54.56	0.15	22.24	0.032	0.029	0.028	0.218	0.013	0.013		5.28	0
0	1.9	0.307	2.8	8.4	12.3	37.7	0.07	0	0	0.029	0.027	0.277	0.026	0		7	0
0	2.25	0.362	5.25	7.5	13.95	48.9	0.069	0	0	0.016	0.03	0.243	0.024	0		5.85	0
						110.67											0
0	1.68	0.18	5.04	10.32	37.44	59.28	0.17	0	0	0.003	0.026	0.031	0.024	0.007	0.036	0.96	0
0	36.48	1.653	15.39	35.34	117.99	199.5	0.222	5.13	0.171	0.09	0.124	1.068	0.043	0.051	0.37	19.95	0
0.16	0.96	0.115	0.56	2.8	3.28	21.92	0.014	0.08	0	0.015	0.01	0.147	0.001	0.001	0.002	5.28	0
0	5.39	0.448	3.43	5.81	24.22	45.78	0.038	0	0	0.014	0.021	0.226	0.007	0	0.068	6.09	0
						119.66											0
0	8.12	0.501	8.12	18.76	29.26	40.74	0.136	0.7	0	0.02	0.03	0.305	0.01	0	0.038	2.8	0
0	3.36	0.522	4.2	14.56	18.9	84.7	0.113	0	0	0.031	0.044	0.577	0.009	0	0.046	6.44	0
40.15	5.17	0.394	1.32	19.03	12.43	16.17	0.125	0.33	0.407	0.031	0.047	0.231	0.013	0.082	0.069	6.6	0
						127.11								1.14			0
0	23.68	2.058	16.64	30.4	110.72	146.88	0.144	0	0	0.114	0.084	0.97	0.033	0	0.035	28.48	0
0	9.25	0.645	8.25	34.5	35.5	95.75	0.198	1.25	0.125	0.067	0.058	0.557	0.016	0	0.065	14.75	0
4.95	15	0.398	6.3	24.15	35.85	80.7	0.129	21.45	0.075	0.037	0.025	0.189	0.011	0.012		4.5	0
0.15	5.25	0.377	6.75	12.9	25.05	62.25	0.079	0.45	0	0.026	0.027	0.641	0.013	0.006	0.33	10.8	0
6.2	7.8	0.446	7.8	23.2	46.2	103.6	0.164	27.4	0.02	0.044	0.042	0.703	0.017	0.018		11	0
0	1.8	0.134	4.8	13.05	16.05	50.4	0.083	0	0	0.037	0.025	0.324	0.004	0		10.05	0

EvaluEat Code	Food Name	Amt	Wt (g)	Energy (kcal)	Prot (g)	Carb (g)	Fiber (g)	Fat (g)	Mono (g)	Poly (g)	Sat (g)
18166	Cookie, sandwich, chocolate, cream filled	1 cookie	10	47.2	0.47	7.03	0.32	2.06	0.856	0.725	0.366
18190	Cookie, sandwich, peanut butter, regular	1 cookie	14	66.92	1.232	9.184	0.266	2.954	1.567	0.531	0.699
18210	Cookie, sandwich, vanilla, cream filled	1 cookie, oval (3-1/8" x 1-1/4" x 3/8")	15	72.45	0.675	10.815	0.225	3	1.266	1.133	0.447
18193	Cookie, shortbread, pecan, commercially prep	1 cookie (2" dia)	14	75.88	0.686	8.162	0.252	4.55	2.608	0.577	1.149
18192	Cookie, shortbread, plain, commercially prep	1 cookie (1-5/8" square)	8	40.16	0.488	5.16	0.144	1.928	1.074	0.259	0.488
18209	Cookie, sugar wafer, cream filled	1 wafer, large (3-1/2" x 1" x 1/2")	9	45.99	0.369	6.309	0.054	2.187	0.93	0.824	0.326
18206	Cookie, sugar, refrig dough, baked	1 cookie 1 pre-sliced cookie dough	23	111.32	1.081	15.088	0.184	5.313	2.992	0.665	1.358
18213	Cookie, vanilla wafer	1 wafer	6	28.38	0.258	4.266	0.12	1.164	0.665	0.146	0.296
18524	Cookies, Archway Home Style, Coconut Macaroon	1 serving	22	106.04	0.854	12.353	0.506	6.142	0.418	0.077	5.436
18555	Cookies, Archway Home Style, fat-free Oatmeal Raisin	1 serving	31	106.33	1.435	24.363	0.93	0.493	0.174	0.211	0.105
18557	Cookies, Archway Home Style, fat-free Sugar Cookies	1 serving	20	70.8	0.88	16.58	0.24	0.158	0.042	0.066	0.052
18535	Cookies, Archway Home Style, Molasses	1 serving	26	103.48	1.178	18.184	0.312	2.98	1.118	0.208	0.733
18541	Cookies, Archway Home Style, Peanut Butter	1 serving	21	100.8	1.89	12.281	0.588	5.099	2.144	0.888	1.132
18548	Cookies, Archway Home Style, Sugar	1 serving	24	98.4	1.231	16.555	0.264	3.084	1.145	0.202	0.761
13348	Corned beef brisket, canned	1 oz	28.35	70.875	7.683	0	0	4.233	1.69	0.179	1.752
20027	Cornstarch	1 cup	128	487.68	0.333	116.83	1.152	0.064	0.02	0.032	0.012
18214	Cracker, cheese	1 cup, bite size	62	311.86	6.262	36.084	1.488	15.686	7.505	1.533	5.81
18216	Cracker, crispbread, rye	1 cracker	10	36.6	0.79	8.22	1.65	0.13	0.017	0.056	0.014
18217	Cracker, Matzo, plain	1 matzo	28	110.6	2.8	23.436	0.84	0.392	0.036	0.169	0.063
18219	Cracker, Matzo, whole wheat	1 matzo	28	98.28	3.668	22.092	3.304	0.42	0.054	0.183	0.068
18220	Cracker, melba toast rounds, plain	1 cracker	3	11.7	0.363	2.298	0.189	0.096	0.023	0.038	0.013
18221	Cracker, melba toast, rye or pumpernickel	1 toast	5	19.45	0.58	3.865	0.4	0.17	0.045	0.067	0.023
18620	Cracker, Original Premium Saltine Crackers/Nabisco	1 serving	14	58.8	1.526	9.954	0.364	1.428	0.819	0.241	0.259
18228	Cracker, oyster/soda/soup	1 cup	45	195.3	4.14	32.175	1.35	5.31	2.89	0.756	1.319
18621	Cracker, Ritz/Nabisco	1 serving	16	78.72	1.152	10.272	0.304	3.664	2.872	0.283	0.627
18224	Cracker, rusk toast	1 rusk	10	40.7	1.35	7.23		0.72	0.276	0.231	0.138
18425	Cracker, saltine/oyster/soda/soup, low salt	1 cup	45	195.3	4.14	32.175	1.35	5.31	2.89	0.756	1.319
18230	Cracker, sandwich, cheese filled	1 cracker	7	33.39	0.651	4.319	0.133	1.477	0.788	0.18	0.429
18215	Cracker, sandwich, cheese w/peanut butter filling	1 sandwich	6.5	32.24	0.807	3.688	0.221	1.633	0.845	0.331	0.286
18231	Cracker, sandwich, peanut butter filled	1 sandwich	6.5	32.11	0.746	3.795	0.149	1.595	0.895	0.303	0.319
18652	Cracker, Snackwell Wheat Cracker/Nabisco	1 serving	15	62.25	1.191	11.55	0.585	1.5			
18624	Cracker, Wheat Thins, baked/Nabisco	1 serving	29	136.3	2.407	20.039	0.87	5.8	2.03	0.36	0.925
18235	Cracker, whole wheat	10 Triscuit Bits	10	44.3	0.88	6.86	1.05	1.72	0.588	0.66	0.339
18429	Cracker, whole wheat, low sodium	10 Triscuit Bits	10	44.3	0.88	6.86	1.05	1.72	0.588	0.66	0.339
18434	Crackers, cheese, Cheez-its/Goldfish, low sodium	1 gold fish	0.6	3.018	0.061	0.349	0.014	0.152	0.071	0.015	0.058
18457	Crackers, saltines, fat-free, low-sodium	6 saltines	30	117.9	3.15	24.69	0.81	0.48	0.043	0.206	0.073
9079	Cranberries, dried, sweetened	1 cup, whole	95	292.6	0.067	78.242	5.415	1.301	0.188	0.625	0.098
42136	Cream substitute, powdered, light	1 oz	28.34	122.15	0.538	20.802	0	4.449	3.259	0.056	1.077
1058	Cream, filled cream, nonbutterfat sour dressing, cultured	1 tbsp	12	21.36	0.39	0.562	0	1.988	0.235	0.056	1.593
1049	Cream, half and half	1 tbsp	15	19.5	0.444	0.645	0	1.725	0.498	0.064	1.074

Chol (g)	Calc (mg)	Iron (mg)	Mag (mg)	Phos (mg)	Pota (mg)	Sodi (mg)	Zinc (mg)	Vit A (RAE)	Vit C (mg)	Thia (mg)	Ribo (mg)	Niac (mg)	Vit B$_6$ (mg)	Vit B$_{12}$ (µg)	Vit E (mg)	Fol (µg)	Alc (g)
0	2.6	0.388	4.5	9.8	17.5	60.4	0.081	0	0	0.008	0.018	0.207	0.002	0.003	0.158	5.1	0
0	7.42	0.364	6.86	26.32	26.88	51.52	0.148	0.14	0.014	0.045	0.037	0.523	0.019	0.032	0.262	8.54	0
0	4.05	0.332	2.1	11.25	13.65	52.35	0.06	0	0	0.039	0.036	0.404	0.003	0	0.24	7.5	0
4.62	4.2	0.34	2.52	11.9	10.22	39.34	0.081	0.14	0	0.041	0.031	0.347	0.003	0.001		8.82	0
1.6	2.8	0.219	1.36	8.64	8	36.4	0.042	1.44	0	0.026	0.026	0.267	0.006	0.007	0.026	5.6	0
0	1.62	0.176	0.99	5.04	5.31	13.23	0.032	0	0	0.009	0.018	0.219	0.001	0	0.176	4.68	0
7.36	20.7	0.423	1.84	43.01	37.49	107.64	0.062	2.76	0	0.042	0.028	0.555	0.005	0.016	0.048	16.1	0
0	1.5	0.133	0.72	3.84	6.42	18.36	0.02	0	0	0.022	0.013	0.179	0.001	0.002		2.58	0
0	3.3	0.354			57.42	38.28			0	0.007	0.013	0.067				1.1	
0	11.47	0.983			86.8	164.92			0	0.081	0.043	0.505				14.57	
0	2.6	0.436			11.6	80.4			0	0.062	0.04	0.504				15.2	
8.06	8.58	1.136			29.12	143.78			0	0.073	0.06	0.658					
7.77	7.35	0.571			43.89	84.84			0	0.05	0.042	0.918					
5.04	7.2	0.528			19.92	162.24			0	0.074	0.055	0.588					
24.381	3.402	0.59	3.969	31.469	38.556	285.201	1.012	0	0	0.006	0.042	0.689	0.037	0.459	0.043	2.552	0
0	2.56	0.602	3.84	16.64	3.84	11.52	0.077	0	0	0	0	0	0	0	0	0	0
8.06	93.62	2.957	22.32	135.16	89.9	616.9	0.701	17.98	0	0.353	0.265	2.896	0.343	0.285	0.037	94.24	0
0	3.1	0.243	7.8	26.9	31.9	26.4	0.239	0	0	0.024	0.014	0.104	0.021	0	0.081	4.7	0
0	3.64	0.885	7	24.92	31.36	0.56	0.19	0	0	0.108	0.081	1.09	0.032	0	0.017	4.76	0
0	6.44	1.302	37.52	85.4	88.48	0.56	0.731	0	0	0.102	0.076	1.515	0.045	0	0.374	9.8	0
0	2.79	0.111	1.77	5.88	6.06	24.87	0.06	0	0	0.012	0.008	0.123	0.003	0	0.013	3.72	0
0	3.9	0.184	1.95	9.15	9.65	44.95	0.068	0	0	0.024	0.014	0.236	0.004	0	0.032	4.25	0
0	27.02	0.727	2.94	13.86	13.86	177.8			0	0.046	0.062	0.612	0.007			11.76	0
0	53.55	2.43	12.15	47.25	57.6	585.9	0.346	0	0	0.254	0.208	2.362	0.017	0	0.054	55.8	0
0	23.52	0.648	3.2	48	14.88	124.16	0.232		0	0.04	0.049	0.61	0.006	0		9.6	0
7.8	2.7	0.272	3.6	15.3	24.5	25.3	0.11	1.2	0	0.04	0.04	0.463	0.005	0.018		8.7	0
0	53.55	2.43	12.15	47.25	325.8	286.2	0.346	0	0	0.254	0.208	2.362	0.017	0	0.054	55.8	0
0.14	17.99	0.167	2.52	28.42	30.03	98.07	0.043	1.19	0.007	0.031	0.048	0.264	0.003	0.007	0.015	7	0
0	3.25	0.177	3.64	17.42	14.17	46.15	0.068	0	0	0.036	0.019	0.379	0.01	0.018	0.154	6.11	0
0	5.265	0.18	3.575	17.81	13.975	46.67	0.073	0	0	0.032	0.018	0.397	0.01	0.001	0.134	5.59	0
	22.35	0.585	6.9	49.5	28.5	150	0.323		0	0.042	0.055				0		
0	23.2	1.073	15.08	60.32	56.26	167.62			0	0.087	0.087	1.16	0.025			12.18	0
0	5	0.308	9.9	29.5	29.7	65.9	0.215	0	0	0.02	0.01	0.452	0.018	0	0.086	2.8	0
0	5	0.308	9.9	29.5	29.7	24.7	0.215	0	0	0.02	0.01	0.452	0.018	0	0.086	2.8	0
0.078	0.906	0.029	0.216	1.308	0.636	2.748	0.007	0.102	0	0.003	0.003	0.028	0.003	0.003	0.002	0.534	0
0	6.6	2.316	7.8	33.9	34.5	190.8	0.282	0	0	0.155	0.177	1.714	0.026	0	0.036	37.2	0
0	9.5	0.503	4.75	7.6	38	2.85	0.104	0	0.19	0.007	0.015	0.941	0.036	0	1.016	0	0
0	0.283	0.009	0	38.542	255.627	64.899	0.006	0.283	0	0	0	0	0	0	0.074	0.283	0
0.6	13.56	0.004	1.2	10.44	19.44	5.76	0.044	0.36	0.108	0.005	0.02	0.009	0.002	0.04	0.161	1.44	0
5.55	15.75	0.011	1.5	14.25	19.5	6.15	0.076	14.55	0.135	0.005	0.022	0.012	0.006	0.05	0.05	0.45	0

EvaluEat Code	Food Name	Amt	Wt (g)	Energy (kcal)	Prot (g)	Carb (g)	Fiber (g)	Fat (g)	Mono (g)	Poly (g)	Sat (g)
1053	Cream, heavy whipping	1 cup, whipped	120	414	2.46	3.348	0	44.4	12.823	1.649	27.638
1052	Cream, light whipping	1 cup, whipped	120	350.4	2.604	3.552	0	37.092	10.912	1.061	23.204
1056	Cream, sour, cultured	1 tbsp	12	25.68	0.379	0.512	0	2.515	0.726	0.093	1.566
1074	Cream, sour, imitation, cultured	1 oz	28.35	58.968	0.68	1.88	0	5.534	0.167	0.016	5.044
1055	Cream, sour, reduced fat (half and half) cultured	1 tbsp	15	20.25	0.441	0.639	0	1.8	0.52	0.067	1.12
1054	Cream, whipped cream topping, pressurized	1 tbsp	3	7.71	0.096	0.375	0	0.667	0.193	0.025	0.415
18242	Croutons, plain	.5 oz	14.2	57.794	1.69	10.437	0.724	0.937	0.434	0.181	0.214
18243	Croutons, seasoned	1 package, fast food	10	46.5	1.08	6.35	0.5	1.83	0.95	0.237	0.525
19205	Custard, egg, dry mix prep w/reduced fat (2%) milk	100 grams	100	111	4.08	17.42	0	2.74	0.852	0.197	1.357
19170	Custard, egg, dry mix prep w/whole milk	100 grams	100	121	4.04	17.29	0	4.01	1.201	0.244	2.122
9421	Dates, medjool	1 cup, drained	178	493.06	3.222	133.45	11.926	0.267			
18251	Donut, cake, chocolate w/sugar or glaze	1 doughnut (3-3/4" dia)	60	250.2	2.7	34.44	1.32	11.94	6.767	1.486	3.079
18249	Donut, cake, plain w/chocolate icing	1 doughnut, large (approx 3-1/2" dia)	57	270.18	2.85	27.36	1.14	17.67	9.976	2.158	4.621
18250	Donut, cake, plain w/sugar or glaze	1 doughnut, medium (approx 3" dia)	45	191.7	2.34	22.86	0.675	10.305	5.714	1.309	2.667
18248	Donut, cake, plain/old-fashioned	1 doughnut, medium (3-1/4" dia)	47	197.87	2.35	23.359	0.705	10.763	4.37	3.704	1.704
18253	Donut, French cruller, glazed	1 cruller (3" dia)	41	168.92	1.271	24.395	0.492	7.503	4.283	0.937	1.913
18254	Donut, yeast leavened, cream filled	1 doughnut oval (3-1/2" x 2-1/2")	85	306.85	5.44	25.5	0.68	20.825	10.268	2.62	4.615
18255	Donut/Honey Bun, yeast leavened, glazed	1 doughnut, large (approx 4-1/4" dia)	75	302.25	4.8	33.225	0.9	17.1	9.649	2.176	4.36
43287	Dove, cooked (includes squab)	1 cup	186	407.34	44.454	0	0	24.18	10.159	5.083	6.955
5143	Duck liver, domestic, raw	1 liver	44	59.84	8.246	1.553	0	2.042	0.312	0.277	0.634
5140	Duck, domestic, meat & skin, roasted	1 cup, chopped or diced	140	471.8	26.586	0	0	39.69	18.06	5.11	13.538
5142	Duck, domestic, meat, no skin, roasted	1 cup, chopped or diced	140	281.4	32.872	0	0	15.68	5.18	2.002	5.838
1142	Egg substitute, frozen	.25 cup	60	96	6.774	1.92	0	6.666	1.461	3.745	1.158
1143	Egg substitute, liquid	1 cup	251	210.84	30.12	1.606	0	8.308	2.249	4.024	1.654
1144	Egg substitute, powdered	.7 oz	20	88.8	11.1	4.36	0	2.6	1.068	0.337	0.753
1124	Egg, white, raw	1 large	33	17.16	3.597	0.241	0	0.056	0	0	0
1128	Egg, whole, fried	1 large	46	92.5	6.27	0.405	0		2.919	1.224	1.975
1129	Egg, whole, hard-cooked	1 large	50	77.5	6.29	0.56	0	5.305	2.039	0.707	1.633
1131	Egg, whole, poached	1 large	50	73.5	6.265	0.38	0	4.95	1.898	0.679	1.543
1132	Egg, whole, scrambled	1 large	61	101.26	6.765	1.342	0	7.448	2.908	1.31	2.244
1125	Egg, yolk, raw, fresh	1 large	17	54.74	2.696	0.61	0	4.512	1.995	0.715	1.624
43146	Eggplant, pickled	1 cup	186	91.14	1.674	18.172	4.65	1.302	0.117	0.547	0.26
18260	English muffin, mixed grain/granola	1 muffin	66	155.1	6.006	30.558	1.848	1.188	0.546	0.369	0.152
18258	English muffin, plain/sourdough, enriched	1 muffin	57	133.95	4.389	26.22	1.539	1.026	0.172	0.506	0.148
18264	English muffin, wheat	1 muffin	57	127.11	4.959	25.536	2.622	1.14	0.16	0.475	0.164

Chol (g)	Calc (mg)	Iron (mg)	Mag (mg)	Phos (mg)	Pota (mg)	Sodi (mg)	Zinc (mg)	Vit A (RAE)	Vit C (mg)	Thia (mg)	Ribo (mg)	Niac (mg)	Vit B$_6$ (mg)	Vit B$_{12}$ (µg)	Vit E (mg)	Fol (µg)	Alc (g)
164.4	78	0.036	8.4	74.4	90	45.6	0.276	493.2	0.72	0.026	0.132	0.047	0.031	0.216	1.272	4.8	0
133.2	82.8	0.036	8.4	73.2	116.4	40.8	0.3	334.8	0.72	0.029	0.15	0.05	0.034	0.24	1.056	4.8	0
5.28	13.92	0.007	1.32	10.2	17.28	6.36	0.032	21.24	0.108	0.004	0.018	0.008	0.002	0.036	0.072	1.32	0
0	0.851	0.111	1.701	12.758	45.644	28.917	0.335	0	0	0	0	0	0	0	0.21	0	0
5.85	15.6	0.011	1.5	14.25	19.35	6.15	0.075	15.3	0.135	0.005	0.022	0.01	0.002	0.045	0.051	1.65	0
2.28	3.03	0.002	0.33	2.67	4.41	3.9	0.011	5.64	0	0.001	0.002	0.002	0.001	0.009	0.019	0.09	0
0	10.792	0.579	4.402	16.33	17.608	99.116	0.126	0	0	0.088	0.039	0.772	0.004	0		18.74	0
0.7	9.6	0.282	4.2	14	18.1	123.8	0.094	0.7	0	0.051	0.042	0.465	0.008	0.014	0.04	10.5	0
48	145	0.35	19	138	224	89	0.52	61	0.8	0.054	0.213	0.128	0.069	0.45		9	0
53	143	0.35	19	136	221	88	0.51	37	0.8	0.054	0.211	0.126	0.068	0.44		9	0
	113.92	1.602	96.12	110.36	1238.88	1.78	0.783	12.46	0	0.089	0.107	2.866	0.443			26.7	
34.2	127.8	1.362	20.4	97.2	63.6	204	0.342	7.2	0.06	0.027	0.042	0.282	0.016	0.06	0.126	27	0
34.77	19.95	1.402	22.8	115.14	111.72	244.53	0.348	3.99	0.114	0.072	0.06	0.741	0.029	0.137	0.211	26.79	0
14.4	27	0.477	7.65	52.65	45.9	180.9	0.198	1.35	0.045	0.105	0.089	0.68	0.012	0.108		20.7	0
17.39	20.68	0.917	9.4	126.43	59.69	256.62	0.259	17.86	0.094	0.104	0.113	0.871	0.026	0.127	0.907	24.44	0
4.51	10.66	0.992	4.92	50.43	31.98	141.45	0.107	0.82	0	0.074	0.094	0.873	0.008	0.021	0.066	17.22	0
20.4	21.25	1.556	17	64.6	68	262.65	0.68	9.35	0	0.287	0.126	1.906	0.058	0.119	0.247	59.5	0
4.5	32.25	1.53	16.5	69.75	81	256.5	0.577	3	0.075	0.273	0.161	2.139	0.043	0.068	0.262	36.75	0
215.76	31.62	10.993	48.36	617.52	476.16	106.02	7.124	52.08	5.394	0.521	0.651	14.136	1.06	0.763	0.112	11.16	0
226.6	4.84	13.433	10.56	118.36	101.2	61.6	1.351	5273	1.98	0.247	0.392	2.86	0.334	23.76		324.7	0
117.6	15.4	3.78	22.4	218.4	285.6	82.6	2.604	88.2	0	0.244	0.377	6.755	0.252	0.42	0.98	8.4	0
124.6	16.8	3.78	28	284.2	352.8	91	3.64	32.2	0	0.364	0.658	7.14	0.35	0.56	0.98	14	0
1.2	43.8	1.188	9	43.2	127.8	119.4	0.588	6.6	0.3	0.072	0.232	0.084	0.08	0.204	0.954	9.6	0
2.51	133.03	5.271	22.59	303.71	828.3	444.27	3.263	45.18	0	0.276	0.753	0.276	0.008	0.753	0.678	37.65	0
114.4	65.2	0.632	13	95.6	148.8	160	0.364	73.8	0.16	0.045	0.352	0.115	0.029	0.704	0.252	25	0
0	2.31	0.026	3.63	4.95	53.79	54.78	0.01	0	0	0.001	0.145	0.035	0.002	0.03	0	1.32	0
210.2	27.1	0.911	5.98	95.7	67.6	93.8	0.552	91.1	0	0.035	0.238	0.035	0.071	0.639	0.561	23.5	0
212	25	0.595	5	86	63	62	0.525	84.5	0	0.033	0.257	0.032	0.06	0.555	0.515	22	0
211	26.5	0.915	6	95	66.5	147	0.55	69.5	0	0.034	0.238	0.035	0.071	0.64	0.48	23.5	0
214.72	43.31	0.732	7.32	103.7	84.18	170.8	0.61	87.23	0.122	0.032	0.267	0.048	0.072	0.47	0.519	18.3	0
209.78	21.93	0.464	0.85	66.3	18.53	8.16	0.391	64.77	0	0.03	0.09	0.004	0.06	0.332	0.439	24.82	0
0	46.5	1.432	11.16	16.74	22.32	3113.64	0.428	5.58	0	0.093	0.13	1.228	0.26	0	0.056	37.2	0
0	129.36	1.993	27.06	53.46	102.96	274.56	0.917	0	0	0.284	0.207	2.365	0.025	0	0	52.8	0
0	99.18	1.425	11.97	75.81	74.67	264.48	0.399	0	0	0.252	0.16	2.214	0.025	0.023	0.177	54.15	0
0	101.46	1.636	21.09	60.99	106.02	217.74	0.61	0	0	0.246	0.166	1.913	0.05	0	0.256	36.48	0

EvaluEat Code	Food Name	Amt	Wt (g)	Energy (kcal)	Prot (g)	Carb (g)	Fiber (g)	Fat (g)	Mono (g)	Poly (g)	Sat (g)
21069	Fast food, burrito w/apples or cherries	1 burrito, small	74	230.88	2.501	34.98		9.524	3.42	1.055	4.569
21060	Fast food, burrito w/beans	2 pieces	217	447.02	14.062	71.436		13.497	4.739	1.196	6.888
21061	Fast food, burrito w/beans & cheese	2 pieces	186	377.58	15.066	54.963		11.699	2.483	1.784	6.849
21064	Fast food, burrito w/beans, cheese & beef	2 pieces	203	330.89	14.575	39.686		13.297	4.458	1.019	7.15
21066	Fast food, burrito w/beef	2 pieces	220	523.6	26.598	58.52		20.812	7.41	0.854	10.459
21035	Fast food, chicken, breaded, fried, dark meat (drumstick or thigh)	2 pieces	148	430.68	30.074	15.703		26.699	10.93	6.323	7.049
21036	Fast food, chicken, breaded, fried, light meat (breast or wing)	2 pieces	163	493.89	35.713	19.576		29.519	12.228	6.786	7.844
21037	Fast food, chicken, breaded, fried, no bone, plain	1 piece	18	54.18	3.06	2.594	0	3.499	1.78	0.78	0.79
21038	Fast food, chicken, breaded, fried, no bone, w/BBQ sauce	6 pieces	130	330.2	17.147	25.025		17.966	8.765	2.389	5.57
21042	Fast food, chili con carne	1 cup (8 fl. oz.)	253	255.53	24.617	21.935		8.273	3.408	0.529	3.431
21071	Fast food, chimichanga w/beef & cheese	1 chimichanga	183	442.86	20.057	39.327		23.442	9.434	0.728	11.178
21043	Fast food, clams (shellfish) breaded, fried	.75 cup	115	450.8	12.822	38.813		26.404	11.44	6.773	6.603
21128	Fast food, corn on the cob w/butter	1 ear	146	154.76	4.468	31.945		3.431	1.004	0.612	1.643
21046	Fast food, crab cake (shellfish)	1 cake	60	159.6	11.25	5.112	0.24	10.35	4.308	3.078	2.244
21015	Fast food, Danish pastry, cheese	1 pastry	91	353.08	5.833	28.692		24.625	15.601	2.423	5.123
21016	Fast food, Danish pastry, cinnamon	1 pastry	88	349.36	4.805	46.851		16.72	10.593	1.646	3.479
21017	Fast food, Danish pastry, fruit	1 pastry	94	334.64	4.756	45.064		15.933	10.096	1.568	3.315
21074	Fast food, enchilada w/cheese	1 enchilada	163	319.48	9.633	28.541		18.843	6.311	0.817	10.588
21075	Fast food, enchilada w/cheese & beef	1 enchilada	192	322.56	11.923	30.47		17.645	6.146	1.388	9.047
21076	Fast food, enchirito w/cheese, beef & beans	1 enchirito	193	343.54	17.891	33.794		16.077	6.518	0.328	7.948
21019	Fast food, English muffin w/butter	1 muffin	63	189	4.87	30.36		5.758	1.532	1.348	2.43
21024	Fast food, French toast sticks	5 pieces	141	513.24	8.277	57.852	2.679	29.046	12.648	9.941	4.709
21023	Fast food, French toast w/butter	2 slices	135	356.4	10.341	36.045		18.765	7.074	2.444	7.749
21077	Fast food, frijoles (beans) w/cheese	1 cup	167	225.45	11.373	28.707		7.782	2.617	0.696	4.075
21116	Fast food, ham & cheese sandwich	1 sandwich	146	351.86	20.688	33.346		15.476	6.738	1.375	6.437
21117	Fast food, ham, egg & cheese sandwich	1 sandwich	143	347.49	19.248	30.945		16.302	5.744	1.69	7.4
21202	Fast food, hamburger, large, one meat patty w/condiments	1 sandwich	172	426.56	23.1	36.825	2.064	21.001	9.307	1.594	7.926
21119	Fast food, hot dog w/chili, plain	1 sandwich	114	296.4	13.509	31.293		13.441	6.595	1.188	4.854
21120	Fast food, hot dog w/corn flour coating, corn dog	1 sandwich	175	460.25	16.8	55.79		18.9	9.109	3.497	5.161
21118	Fast food, hot dog, plain	1 sandwich	98	242.06	10.388	18.032		14.543	6.853	1.706	5.109
21129	Fast food, hush puppies	5 pieces	78	256.62	4.875	34.897		11.591	7.819	0.388	2.686
21033	Fast food, ice cream sundae, hot fudge	1 sundae	158	284.4	5.641	47.669	0	8.627	2.331	0.807	5.023
14346	Fast food, milk beverage, chocolate shake/McDonald's	1 medium shake (16 fl. oz.)	333	422.91	11.322	68.265	6.327	12.321	3.58	0.466	7.702
21078	Fast food, nachos w/cheese	1 portion (6–8 nachos)	113	345.78	9.097	36.33		18.95	7.994	2.233	7.78
21080	Fast food, nachos w/cheese, beans, ground beef & peppers	1 portion (6–8 nachos)	255	568.65	19.788	55.819		30.702	10.98	5.689	12.487
21130	Fast food, onion rings, breaded, fried	1 portion (8–9 onion rings)	83	275.56	3.702	31.324		15.513	6.651	0.665	6.953
21048	Fast food, oysters (shellfish) battered/breaded, fried	6 pieces	139	368.35	12.538	39.879		17.931	6.921	4.638	4.579
21025	Fast food, pancakes w/butter & syrup	2 cakes	232	519.68	8.259	90.898		13.99	5.269	1.958	5.851
21049	Fast food, pizza w/cheese	1 slice	63	140.49	7.68	20.5		3.213	0.99	0.491	1.54
21050	Fast food, pizza w/cheese, meat & vegetables	1 slice	79	184.07	13.011	21.291		5.364	2.543	0.915	1.535

Chol (g)	Calc (mg)	Iron (mg)	Mag (mg)	Phos (mg)	Pota (mg)	Sodi (mg)	Zinc (mg)	Vit A (RAE)	Vit C (mg)	Thia (mg)	Ribo (mg)	Niac (mg)	Vit B$_6$ (mg)	Vit B$_{12}$ (µg)	Vit E (mg)	Fol (µg)	Alc (g)
3.7	15.54	1.073	7.4	14.8	104.34	211.64	0.4	20.72	0.74	0.17	0.178	1.857	0.074	0.511		24.42	0
4.34	112.84	4.514	86.8	97.65	653.17	985.18	1.519	17.36	1.953	0.629	0.608	4.058	0.304	1.085		86.8	0
27.9	213.9	2.269	79.98	180.42	496.62	1166.22	1.637	98.58	1.674	0.223	0.707	3.571	0.242	0.893		74.4	0
123.83	129.92	3.735	50.75	140.07	410.06	990.64	2.355	150.2	5.075	0.305	0.711	3.857	0.223	1.096		75.11	0
63.8	83.6	6.094	81.4	173.8	739.2	1491.6	4.73	13.2	1.1	0.242	0.924	6.446	0.308	1.958		129.8	0
165.76	35.52	1.598	37	239.76	445.48	754.8	3.241	66.6	0	0.133	0.429	7.208	0.326	0.829		25.16	0
148.33	60.31	1.483	37.49	306.44	565.61	974.74	1.548	57.05	0	0.147	0.293	11.981	0.571	0.668		29.34	0
10.44	2.34	0.16	4.14	49.14	51.84	87.12	0.169	0.9	0	0.02	0.027	1.269	0.052	0.052	0.221	5.22	0
61.1	20.8	1.456	24.7	214.5	318.5	829.4	1.118	16.9	0.78	0.104	0.156	7.02	0.338	0.299		29.9	0
134.09	68.31	5.186	45.54	197.34	690.69	1006.94	3.567	83.49	1.518	0.126	1.138	2.479	0.329	1.138		45.54	0
51.24	237.9	3.843	60.39	186.66	203.13	957.09	3.367	131.8	2.745	0.384	0.86	4.667	0.22	1.299		91.5	0
87.4	20.7	3.048	31.05	238.05	265.65	833.75	1.633	36.8	0	0.207	0.264	2.863	0.034	1.104		42.55	0
5.84	4.38	0.876	40.88	108.04	359.16	29.2	0.905	33.58	6.862	0.248	0.102	2.175	0.321	0		43.8	0
82.2	202.2	1.116	25.2	226.8	162	491.4	2.124	93	0.18	0.055	0.075	1.166	0.149	4.398		24.6	0
20.02	70.07	1.847	15.47	80.08	116.48	319.41	0.628	44.59	2.639	0.264	0.209	2.548	0.055	0.228		54.6	0
27.28	36.96	1.795	14.08	73.92	95.92	326.48	0.484	5.28	2.552	0.255	0.194	2.2	0.053	0.22		54.56	0
18.8	21.62	1.401	14.1	68.62	109.98	332.76	0.479	25.38	1.598	0.291	0.207	1.795	0.056	0.235		31.02	0
44.01	324.37	1.32	50.53	133.66	239.61	784.03	2.51	99.43	0.978	0.082	0.424	1.907	0.391	0.75		65.2	0
40.32	228.48	3.072	82.56	167.04	574.08	1319.04	2.688	97.92	1.344	0.096	0.403	2.515	0.269	1.018		67.2	0
50.18	218.09	2.393	71.41	223.88	559.7	1250.64	2.76	88.78	4.632	0.174	0.695	2.991	0.212	1.621		94.57	0
12.6	102.69	1.588	13.23	85.05	69.3	386.19	0.422	31.5	0.756	0.252	0.315	2.615	0.038	0.019	0.126	56.7	0
74.73	77.55	2.961	26.79	122.67	126.9	499.14	0.931	0	0	0.226	0.254	2.961	0.254	0.071	2.326	255.2	0
116.1	72.9	1.89	16.2	145.8	176.85	513	0.594	136.4	0.135	0.581	0.5	3.915	0.054	0.365		72.9	0
36.74	188.71	2.238	85.17	175.35	604.54	881.76	1.737	35.07	1.503	0.134	0.334	1.486	0.2	0.685		111.9	0
58.4	129.94	3.241	16.06	151.84	290.54	770.88	1.372	96.36	2.774	0.307	0.482	2.686	0.204	0.54	0.292	75.92	0
245.96	211.64	3.103	25.74	346.06	210.21	1005.29	1.988	165.9	2.717	0.429	0.558	4.204	0.157	1.23	0.586	75.79	0
70.52	134.16	4.145	34.4	213.28	395.6	731	4.764	5.16	2.58	0.342	0.284	6.562	0.246	2.58	0.034	61.92	0
51.3	19.38	3.283	10.26	191.52	166.44	479.94	0.775	3.42	2.736	0.217	0.399	3.739	0.046	0.296		72.96	0
78.75	101.5	6.177	17.5	166.25	262.5	973	1.313	59.5	0	0.28	0.7	4.165	0.087	0.438		103.25	0
44.1	23.52	2.313	12.74	97.02	143.08	670.32	1.98	0	0.098	0.235	0.274	3.646	0.049	0.51		48.02	0
134.94	68.64	1.427	16.38	190.32	187.98	964.86	0.429	8.58	0	0	0.023	2.028	0.101	0.172		57.72	0
20.54	206.98	0.585	33.18	227.52	395	181.7	0.948	58.46	2.37	0.063	0.3	1.074	0.126	0.648	0.664	9.48	0
43.29	376.29	1.032	56.61	339.66	666	323.01	1.365	86.58	1.332	0.193	0.816	0.536	0.167	1.132	0.366	16.65	0
18.08	272.33	1.277	55.37	275.72	171.76	815.86	1.785	149.2	1.243	0.192	0.373	1.537	0.203	0.825		10.17	0
20.4	385.05	2.78	96.9	387.6	451.35	1800.3	3.646	436.1	4.845	0.23	0.688	3.34	0.408	1.02		38.25	0
14.11	73.04	0.847	15.77	86.32	129.48	429.94	0.349	0.83	0.581	0.083	0.1	0.921	0.058	0.124	0.332	54.78	0
108.42	27.8	4.462	23.63	195.99	182.09	676.93	15.64	108.4	4.17	0.306	0.347	4.42	0.028	1.015		30.58	0
58	127.6	2.622	48.72	475.6	250.56	1104.32	1.021	81.2	3.48	0.394	0.557	3.387	0.116	0.232	1.392	51.04	0
9.45	116.55	0.58	15.75	112.77	109.62	335.79	0.813	73.71	1.26	0.183	0.164	2.482	0.044	0.334		34.65	0
20.54	101.12	1.533	18.17	131.14	178.54	382.36	1.114	58.46	1.58	0.213	0.174	1.959	0.095	0.363		32.39	0

EvaluEat Code	Food Name	Amt	Wt (g)	Energy (kcal)	Prot (g)	Carb (g)	Fiber (g)	Fat (g)	Mono (g)	Poly (g)	Sat (g)
21051	Fast food, pizza w/pepperoni	1 slice	71	181.05	10.125	19.866		6.958	3.14	1.165	2.236
21132	Fast food, potato, baked, topped w/cheese & bacon	1 piece	299	451.49	18.418	44.431		25.893	9.715	4.751	10.133
21131	Fast food, potato, baked, topped w/cheese sauce	1 piece	296	473.6	14.622	46.502		28.742	10.7	6.044	10.558
21135	Fast food, potato, baked, topped w/sour cream & chives	1 piece	302	392.6	6.674	50.011		22.318	7.873	3.316	10.011
21138	Fast food, potato, French fried w/vegetable oil	1 large	169	577.98	7.267	67.279	5.915	31.147	17.99	5.288	6.507
21139	Fast food, potato, mashed	.333 cup	80	66.4	1.848	12.896		0.968	0.281	0.234	0.383
21026	Fast food, potatoes, hash brown	.5 cup	72	151.2	1.944	16.15		9.216	3.858	0.47	4.324
21122	Fast food, roast beef sandwich w/cheese	1 sandwich	176	473.44	32.226	45.373		18.005	3.661	3.502	9.029
21121	Fast food, roast beef sandwich, plain	1 sandwich	139	346.11	21.503	33.443		13.761	6.804	1.706	3.606
4021	Fast food, salad dressing, Italian, w/salt, diet (2 kcal/tsp)	1 tbsp	15	11.25	0.071	0.686	0	0.957	0.329	0.256	0.068
4025	Fast food, salad dressing, mayonnaise, soybean oil, w/salt	1 tbsp	13.8	98.946	0.152	0.538	0	10.792	2.705	5.889	1.64
21127	Fast food, salad, cole slaw	.75 cup	99	146.52	1.455	12.751		10.969	2.42	6.394	1.606
21140	Fast food, salad, potato	.333 cup	95	108.3	1.453	12.853		5.728	1.605	2.869	0.978
21083	Fast food, salad, taco	1.5 cup	198	279.18	13.226	23.582		14.771	5.16	1.748	6.823
21084	Fast food, salad, taco w/chili con carne	1.5 cup	261	289.71	17.409	26.57		13.128	4.539	1.537	6
21002	Fast food, sandwich, biscuit w/egg	1 biscuit	136	372.64	11.601	31.906	0.816	22.073	9.073	6.4	4.729
21003	Fast food, sandwich, biscuit w/egg & bacon	1 biscuit	150	457.5	16.995	28.59	0.75	31.095	13.44	7.47	7.95
21004	Fast food, sandwich, biscuit w/egg & ham	1 biscuit	192	441.6	20.429	30.317	0.768	27.034	10.963	7.699	5.914
21005	Fast food, sandwich, biscuit w/egg & sausage	1 biscuit	180	581.4	19.152	41.148	0.9	38.7	16.398	4.446	14.976
21007	Fast food, sandwich, biscuit w/egg, cheese & bacon	1 biscuit	144	476.64	16.258	33.422		31.392	14.226	3.495	11.398
21008	Fast food, sandwich, biscuit w/ham	1 biscuit	113	386.46	13.391	43.787	0.791	18.419	4.833	1.037	11.408
21009	Fast food, sandwich, biscuit w/sausage	1 biscuit	124	484.84	12.115	40.04	1.364	31.781	12.82	3.026	14.22
21093	Fast food, sandwich, cheeseburger (2 patty) condiments & vegetables	1 sandwich	166	416.66	21.248	35.192		21.082	7.809	2.658	8.717
21092	Fast food, sandwich, cheeseburger (2 patty) plain	1 sandwich	155	457.25	27.667	22.056		28.474	11.008	1.914	12.997
21097	Fast food, sandwich, cheeseburger, large, one meat patty w/bacon & condiments	1 sandwich	195	608.4	32	37.128		36.758	14.488	2.711	16.243
21098	Fast food, sandwich, cheeseburger, large, one meat patty w/condiments & vegetables	1 sandwich	219	562.83	28.185	38.391		32.938	12.61	2.026	15.039
21103	Fast food, sandwich, chicken filet w/cheese	1 sandwich	228	631.56	29.412	41.587		38.76	13.65	9.948	12.449
21102	Fast food, sandwich, chicken filet, plain	1 sandwich	182	515.06	24.115	38.693		29.448	10.41	8.383	8.527
21011	Fast food, sandwich, croissant w/egg & cheese	1 croissant	127	368.3	12.789	24.308		24.701	7.541	1.367	14.065
21012	Fast food, sandwich, croissant w/egg, cheese & bacon	1 croissant	129	412.8	16.228	23.646		28.354	9.176	1.758	15.432
21013	Fast food, sandwich, croissant w/egg, cheese & ham	1 croissant	152	474.24	18.924	24.198		33.577	11.392	2.359	17.475
21020	Fast food, sandwich, English muffin w/cheese & sausage	1 muffin	115	393.3	15.341	29.164	1.495	24.265	10.081	2.694	9.851
21021	Fast food, sandwich, English muffin w/egg, cheese & Canadian bacon	1 sandwich	137	289.07	16.687	26.742	1.507	12.59	4.67	1.558	4.665
21105	Fast food, sandwich, fish w/tartar sauce	1 sandwich	158	431.34	16.938	41.017		22.768	7.693	8.248	5.235
21106	Fast food, sandwich, fish w/tartar sauce & cheese	1 sandwich	183	523.38	20.606	47.635		28.603	8.919	9.432	8.14
21114	Fast food, sandwich, hamburger, large (2 patty) w/condiments & vegetables	1 sandwich	226	540.14	34.284	40.273		26.555	10.328	2.796	10.518
21113	Fast food, sandwich, hamburger, large, one meat patty w/condiments & vegetables	1 sandwich	218	512.3	25.833	40.003		27.359	11.423	2.202	10.42
21109	Fast food, sandwich, hamburger, one patty w/condiments & vegetables	1 sandwich	110	279.4	12.914	27.291		13.475	5.29	2.577	4.131

Chol (g)	Calc (mg)	Iron (mg)	Mag (mg)	Phos (mg)	Pota (mg)	Sodi (mg)	Zinc (mg)	Vit A (RAE)	Vit C (mg)	Thia (mg)	Ribo (mg)	Niac (mg)	Vit B_6 (mg)	Vit B_{12} (μg)	Vit E (mg)	Fol (μg)	Alc (g)
14.2	64.61	0.937	8.52	75.26	152.65	266.96	0.518	52.54	1.633	0.135	0.234	3.046	0.057	0.185		36.92	0
29.9	307.97	3.139	68.77	346.84	1178.06	971.75	2.153	188.4	28.7	0.269	0.239	3.977	0.748	0.329		29.9	0
17.76	310.8	3.019	65.12	319.68	1166.24	381.84	1.894	251.6	26.05	0.237	0.207	3.345	0.71	0.178		26.64	0
24.16	105.7	3.111	69.46	184.22	1383.16	181.2	0.906	265.8	33.82	0.272	0.181	3.715	0.785	0.211		33.22	0
0	23.66	1.318	65.91	218.01	1164.41	334.62	0.794	0	19.6	0.135	0.068	4.817	0.605	0	2.569	11.83	0
1.6	16.8	0.376	14.4	44	235.2	181.6	0.256	8.8	0.32	0.072	0.04	0.96	0.184	0.04		6.4	0
9.36	7.2	0.482	15.84	69.12	267.12	290.16	0.216	1.44	5.472	0.079	0.014	1.073	0.166	0.014	0.122	7.92	0
77.44	183.04	5.051	40.48	401.28	344.96	1633.28	5.368	58.08	0	0.387	0.458	5.896	0.334	2.059		63.36	0
51.43	54.21	4.226	30.58	239.08	315.53	792.3	3.392	11.12	2.085	0.375	0.306	5.866	0.264	1.223		56.99	0
0.9	1.35	0.098	0.6	1.65	12.75	204.9	0.029	0.15	0	0	0.002	0	0.011	0	0.03	0	0
5.244	2.484	0.069	0.138	3.864	4.692	78.384	0.022	11.59	0	0	0	0.001	0.08	0.036	0.72	1.104	0
4.95	33.66	0.723	8.91	35.64	177.21	267.3	0.198	35.64	8.316	0.04	0.03	0.079	0.109	0.178		38.61	0
57	13.3	0.693	7.6	53.2	256.5	311.6	0.19	28.5	1.045	0.067	0.104	0.257	0.142	0.114		23.75	0
43.56	192.06	2.277	51.48	142.56	415.8	762.3	2.693	71.28	3.564	0.099	0.356	2.455	0.218	0.634		83.16	0
5.22	245.34	2.662	52.2	153.99	391.5	884.79	3.289	258.4	3.393	0.157	0.496	2.532	0.522	0.731		91.35	0
244.8	81.6	2.897	19.04	387.6	238	890.8	0.993	179.5	0.136	0.303	0.487	2.153	0.112	0.626	3.264	57.12	0
352.5	189	3.735	24	238.5	250.5	999	1.635	106.5	2.7	0.135	0.225	2.4	0.135	1.035	1.965	60	0
299.52	220.8	4.55	30.72	316.8	318.72	1382.4	2.227	236.2	0	0.672	0.595	1.997	0.269	1.19	2.285	65.28	0
302.4	154.8	3.96	25.2	489.6	320.4	1141.2	2.16	160.2	0	0.504	0.45	3.6	0.198	1.368	2.844	64.8	0
260.64	164.16	2.549	20.16	459.36	230.4	1260	1.541	190.1	1.584	0.302	0.432	2.304	0.101	1.051		53.28	0
24.86	160.46	2.723	22.6	553.7	196.62	1432.84	1.65	30.51	0.113	0.508	0.316	3.48	0.136	0.034	1.661	38.42	0
34.72	127.72	2.579	19.84	446.4	198.4	1071.36	1.55	12.4	0.124	0.397	0.285	3.274	0.112	0.508	1.364	45.88	0
59.76	170.98	3.42	29.88	242.36	335.32	1050.78	3.486	71.38	1.66	0.349	0.282	8.051	0.183	1.926		61.42	0
110.05	232.5	3.41	32.55	373.55	308.45	635.5	4.96	99.2	0	0.248	0.372	6.014	0.248	2.309	1.193	68.2	0
111.15	161.85	4.739	44.85	399.75	331.5	1043.25	6.825	81.9	2.145	0.312	0.41	6.63	0.312	2.34		85.8	0
87.6	205.86	4.665	43.8	310.98	444.57	1108.14	4.599	140.2	7.884	0.394	0.46	7.38	0.285	2.562	1.183	81.03	0
77.52	257.64	3.625	43.32	405.84	332.88	1238.04	2.896	164.2	2.964	0.41	0.456	9.074	0.41	0.456		109.4	0
60.06	60.06	4.677	34.58	232.96	353.08	957.32	1.875	30.94	8.918	0.328	0.237	6.807	0.2	0.382		100.1	0
215.9	243.84	2.197	21.59	347.98	173.99	551.18	1.753	276.9	0.127	0.191	0.381	1.511	0.102	0.775		46.99	0
215.43	150.93	2.193	23.22	276.06	201.24	888.81	1.896	141.9	2.193	0.348	0.335	2.193	0.116	0.864		45.15	0
212.8	144.4	2.128	25.84	335.92	272.08	1080.72	2.174	130.7	11.4	0.517	0.304	3.192	0.228	1.003		45.6	0
58.65	167.9	2.254	24.15	186.3	215.05	1036.15	1.679	101.2	1.265	0.701	0.253	4.14	0.149	0.678	1.265	66.7	0
234.27	150.7	2.439	23.29	269.89	198.65	728.84	1.562	176.7	1.781	0.495	0.448	3.335	0.147	0.671	0.562	68.5	0
55.3	83.74	2.607	33.18	211.72	339.7	614.62	0.995	33.18	2.844	0.332	0.221	3.397	0.111	1.074	0.869	85.32	0
67.71	184.83	3.495	36.6	311.1	353.19	938.79	1.171	129.93	2.745	0.458	0.421	4.227	0.11	1.08	1.83	91.5	0
122.04	101.7	5.853	49.72	314.14	569.52	791	5.673	4.52	1.13	0.362	0.384	7.571	0.542	4.068		76.84	0
87.2	95.92	4.927	43.6	233.26	479.6	824.04	4.883	23.98	2.616	0.414	0.371	7.281	0.327	2.376		82.84	0
26.4	62.7	2.629	22	124.3	226.6	503.8	2.057	4.4	1.65	0.231	0.198	3.685	0.121	0.88		51.7	0

EvaluEat Code	Food Name	Amt	Wt (g)	Energy (kcal)	Prot (g)	Carb (g)	Fiber (g)	Fat (g)	Mono (g)	Poly (g)	Sat (g)
21107	Fast food, sandwich, hamburger, plain	1 sandwich	90	274.5	12.321	30.51		11.817	5.456	0.918	4.141
14347	Fast food, shake, vanilla/McDonald's	1 medium shake (16 fl. oz.)	333	369.63	11.655	59.607	0.333	9.99	2.87	0.37	6.187
21059	Fast food, shrimp (shellfish) breaded, fried	6–8 shrimp	164	454.28	18.876	40		24.895	17.379	0.645	5.379
21123	Fast food, steak sandwich	1 sandwich	204	459	30.335	51.959		14.076	5.345	3.346	3.815
21124	Fast food, submarine sandwich, cold cuts	1 sandwich	228	456	21.842	51.049		18.628	8.226	2.282	6.808
21126	Fast food, submarine sandwich, tuna salad	1 sandwich	256	583.68	29.696	55.373		27.981	13.402	7.296	5.33
21082	Fast food, taco	1 large	263	568.08	31.77	41.107		31.613	10.115	1.475	17.484
21085	Fast food, tostada w/beans & cheese	1 piece	144	223.2	9.605	26.525		9.864	3.054	0.749	5.367
21087	Fast food, tostada w/beef & cheese	1 piece	163	314.59	18.99	22.771		16.349	3.345	0.975	10.395
4002	Fat, animal, lard, pork	1 tbsp	12.8	115.46	0	0	0	12.8	5.773	1.434	5.018
6963	Fish broth	.5 cup	125	20	2.5	0.5	0	0.75	0.151	0.203	0.178
43129	Fish sticks, meatless	1 cup	186	539.4	42.78	16.74	11.346	33.48	8.139	17.358	5.299
15187	Fish, bass, freshwater, cooked w/dry heat	3 oz	85	124.1	20.553	0	0	4.021	1.56	1.156	0.851
15188	Fish, bass, striped, cooked w/dry heat	3 oz	85	105.4	19.32	0	0	2.542	0.719	0.854	0.553
15008	Fish, carp, raw	3 oz	85	107.95	15.156	0	0	4.76	1.979	1.216	0.921
15011	Fish, catfish, channel, breaded & fried	3 oz	85	194.65	15.377	6.834	0.595	11.331	4.769	2.826	2.795
15235	Fish, catfish, channel, farmed, cooked w/dry heat	3 oz	85	129.2	15.912	0	0	6.817	3.532	1.183	1.521
15012	Fish, caviar, black/red, granular	1 tbsp	16	40.32	3.936	0.64	0	2.864	0.741	1.185	0.65
15016	Fish, cod, Atlantic, baked/broiled (dry heat)	3 oz	85	89.25	19.406	0	0	0.731	0.105	0.248	0.143
15192	Fish, cod, Pacific, cooked w/dry heat	3 oz	85	89.25	19.508	0	0	0.689	0.089	0.266	0.088
15026	Fish, eel, baked or broiled (dry heat)	3 oz	85	200.6	20.103	0	0	12.708	7.835	1.032	2.57
15034	Fish, haddock, baked or broiled (dry heat)	3 oz	85	95.2	20.604	0	0	0.791	0.128	0.263	0.142
15035	Fish, haddock, smoked	3 oz	85	98.6	21.445	0	0	0.816	0.133	0.273	0.147
15037	Fish, halibut, Atlantic & Pacific, baked or broiled (dry heat)	3 oz	85	119	22.687	0	0	2.499	0.822	0.799	0.354
15196	Fish, halibut, Greenland, cooked w/dry heat	3 oz	85	203.15	15.657	0	0	15.079	9.131	1.49	2.637
15040	Fish, herring, Atlantic, baked or broiled (dry heat)	3 oz	85	172.55	19.576	0	0	9.852	4.072	2.325	2.223
15197	Fish, herring, Pacific, cooked w/dry heat	3 oz	85	212.5	17.859	0	0	15.122	7.486	2.64	3.548
15121	Fish, light tuna, canned in H$_2$O, drained	3 oz	85	98.6	21.684	0	0	0.697	0.135	0.286	0.199
15119	Fish, light tuna, canned in oil, drained	3 oz	85	168.3	24.76	0	0	6.979	2.507	2.452	1.304
15047	Fish, mackerel, Atlantic, baked or broiled (dry heat)	3 oz	85	222.7	20.273	0	0	15.139	5.955	3.655	3.55
15200	Fish, mackerel, king, cooked w/dry heat	3 oz	85	113.9	22.1	0	0	2.176	0.832	0.501	0.395
15058	Fish, ocean perch, Atlantic, baked or broiled (dry heat)	3 oz	85	102.85	20.298	0	0	1.776	0.681	0.465	0.266
15230	Fish, octopus, common, cooked w/moist heat	3 oz	85	139.4	25.347	3.74	0	1.768	0.275	0.405	0.385
15061	Fish, perch, baked or broiled (dry heat)	3 oz	85	99.45	21.131	0	0	1.003	0.166	0.401	0.201
15063	Fish, pike, northern, baked or broiled (dry heat)	3 oz	85	96.05	20.987	0	0	0.748	0.171	0.22	0.128
15204	Fish, pike, walleye, cooked w/dry heat	3 oz	85	101.15	20.859	0	0	1.326	0.32	0.487	0.271
15205	Fish, pollock, Atlantic, cooked w/dry heat	3 oz	85	100.3	21.182	0	0	1.071	0.122	0.529	0.145
15067	Fish, pollock, walleye, baked or broiled	3 oz	85	96.05	19.984	0	0	0.952	0.148	0.445	0.196
15069	Fish, pompano, Florida, baked or broiled (dry heat)	3 oz	85	179.35	20.137	0	0	10.319	2.818	1.239	3.824
15071	Fish, rockfish, Pacific, baked or broiled (dry heat)	3 oz	85	102.85	20.434	0	0	1.709	0.38	0.505	0.403
15207	Fish, roe, cooked w/dry heat	3 oz	85	173.4	24.327	1.632	0	6.995	1.81	2.893	1.586
15232	Fish, roughy, orange, cooked w/dry heat	3 oz	85	75.65	16.023	0	0	0.765	0.523	0.014	0.02

Chol (g)	Calc (mg)	Iron (mg)	Mag (mg)	Phos (mg)	Pota (mg)	Sodi (mg)	Zinc (mg)	Vit A (RAE)	Vit C (mg)	Thia (mg)	Ribo (mg)	Niac (mg)	Vit B6 (mg)	Vit B12 (µg)	Vit E (mg)	Fol (µg)	Alc (g)
35.1	63	2.403	18.9	102.6	144.9	387	1.998	0	0	0.333	0.27	3.717	0.063	0.891	0.495	53.1	0
36.63	406.26	0.3	39.96	339.66	579.42	273.06	1.199	123.2	2.664	0.15	0.606	0.616	0.173	1.199	0.2	16.65	0
200.08	83.64	2.952	39.36	344.4	183.68	1446.48	1.214	36.08	0	0.213	0.902	0	0.066	0.148		100	0
73.44	91.8	5.161	48.96	297.84	524.28	797.64	4.529	20.4	5.508	0.408	0.367	7.303	0.367	1.571		89.76	0
36.48	189.24	2.508	68.4	287.28	394.44	1650.72	2.576	70.68	12.31	1.003	0.798	5.495	0.137	1.094		86.64	0
48.64	74.24	2.637	79.36	220.16	335.36	1292.8	1.869	46.08	3.584	0.461	0.333	11.341	0.23	1.613		102.4	0
86.79	339.27	3.708	107.83	312.97	728.51	1233.47	6.049	165.7	3.419	0.237	0.684	4.944	0.368	1.604		105.2	0
30.24	210.24	1.886	59.04	116.64	403.2	542.88	1.901	44.64	1.296	0.101	0.331	1.325	0.158	0.691		43.2	0
40.75	216.79	2.869	63.57	179.3	572.13	896.5	3.684	50.53	2.608	0.098	0.554	3.146	0.228	1.174		74.98	0
12.16	0	0	0	0	0	0	0.014	0	0	0	0	0	0	0	0.077	0	0
0	37.5	0.262	1.25	37.5	107.5	397.5	0.125	1.25	0	0	0.037	1.712	0.012	0.125	0.188	5	0
0	176.7	3.72	42.78	837	1116	911.4	2.604	0	0	2.046	1.674	22.32	2.79	7.812	7.347	189.7	0
73.95	87.55	1.623	32.3	217.6	387.6	76.5	0.706	29.75	1.785	0.074	0.077	1.294	0.117	1.964		14.45	0
87.55	16.15	0.918	43.35	215.9	278.8	74.8	0.433	26.35	0	0.098	0.031	2.174	0.294	3.748		8.5	0
56.1	34.85	1.054	24.65	352.75	283.05	41.65	1.258	7.65	1.36	0.098	0.047	1.394	0.162	1.301	0.535	12.75	0
68.85	37.4	1.215	22.95	183.6	289	238	0.731	6.8	0	0.062	0.113	1.94	0.162	1.615		25.5	0
54.4	7.65	0.697	22.1	208.25	272.85	68	0.892	12.75	0.68	0.357	0.062	2.136	0.139	2.38		5.95	0
94.08	44	1.901	48	56.96	28.96	240	0.152	89.76	0	0.03	0.099	0.019	0.051	3.2	1.12	8	0
46.75	11.9	0.417	35.7	117.3	207.4	66.3	0.493	11.9	0.85	0.075	0.067	2.136	0.241	0.892	0.689	6.8	0
39.95	7.65	0.281	26.35	189.55	439.45	77.35	0.433	8.5	2.55	0.021	0.043	2.112	0.393	0.884		6.8	0
136.85	22.1	0.544	22.1	235.45	296.65	55.25	1.768	966.5	1.53	0.156	0.043	3.814	0.065	2.457	4.335	14.45	0
62.9	35.7	1.148	42.5	204.85	339.15	73.95	0.408	16.15	0	0.034	0.038	3.937	0.294	1.182		11.05	0
65.45	41.65	1.19	45.9	213.35	352.75	648.55	0.425	18.7	0	0.04	0.042	4.312	0.34	1.36	0.468	12.75	0
34.85	51	0.91	90.95	242.25	489.6	58.65	0.45	45.9	0	0.059	0.077	6.055	0.337	1.164	0.927	11.9	0
50.15	3.4	0.723	28.05	178.5	292.4	87.55	0.433	15.3	0	0.062	0.088	1.635	0.412	0.816		0.85	0
65.45	62.9	1.199	34.85	257.55	356.15	97.75	1.079	30.6	0.595	0.095	0.254	3.505	0.296	11.169	1.164	10.2	0
84.15	90.1	1.224	34.85	248.2	460.7	80.75	0.578	29.75	0	0.062	0.218	2.398	0.441	8.177		5.1	0
25.5	9.35	1.301	22.95	138.55	201.45	287.3	0.655	14.45	0	0.027	0.063	11.288	0.298	2.542	0.281	3.4	0
15.3	11.05	1.182	26.35	264.35	175.95	300.9	0.765	19.55	0	0.032	0.102	10.54	0.094	1.87	0.74	4.25	0
63.75	12.75	1.335	82.45	236.3	340.85	70.55	0.799	45.9	0.34	0.135	0.35	5.823	0.391	16.15		1.7	0
57.8	34	1.938	34.85	270.3	474.3	172.55	0.612	214.2	1.36	0.098	0.493	8.893	0.433	15.3		7.65	0
45.9	116.45	1.003	33.15	235.45	297.5	81.6	0.519	11.9	0.68	0.111	0.114	2.071	0.23	0.978		8.5	0
81.6	90.1	8.109	51	237.15	535.5	391	2.856	76.5	6.8	0.048	0.065	3.213	0.551	30.6	1.02	20.4	0
97.75	86.7	0.986	32.3	218.45	292.4	67.15	1.215	8.5	1.445	0.068	0.102	1.615	0.119	1.87		5.1	0
42.5	62.05	0.604	34	239.7	281.35	41.65	0.731	20.4	3.23	0.057	0.065	2.38	0.115	1.955		14.45	0
93.5	119.85	1.419	32.3	228.65	424.15	55.25	0.672	20.4	0	0.265	0.166	2.381	0.117	1.964		14.45	0
77.35	65.45	0.502	73.1	240.55	387.6	93.5	0.51	10.2	0	0.046	0.191	3.386	0.281	3.128		2.55	0
81.6	5.1	0.238	62.05	409.7	328.95	98.6	0.51	21.25	0	0.063	0.065	1.403	0.059	3.57	0.672	3.4	0
54.4	36.55	0.57	26.35	289.85	540.6	64.6	0.586	30.6	0	0.578	0.128	3.23	0.196	1.02		14.45	0
37.4	10.2	0.45	28.9	193.8	442	65.45	0.45	60.35	0	0.037	0.071	3.331	0.23	1.02	1.326	8.5	0
407.15	23.8	0.655	22.1	437.75	240.55	99.45	1.088	77.35	13.94	0.235	0.807	1.863	0.157	9.809		78.2	0
22.1	32.3	0.196	32.3	217.6	327.25	68.85	0.816	20.4	0	0.098	0.156	3.106	0.294	1.964		6.8	0

EvaluEat Code	Food Name	Amt	Wt (g)	Energy (kcal)	Prot (g)	Carb (g)	Fiber (g)	Fat (g)	Mono (g)	Poly (g)	Sat (g)
15237	Fish, salmon, Atlantic, farmed, cooked w/dry heat	3 oz	85	175.1	18.785	0	0	10.498	3.767	3.762	2.128
15209	Fish, salmon, Atlantic, wild, cooked w/dry heat	3 oz	85	154.7	21.624	0	0	6.911	2.292	2.768	1.068
15087	Fish, salmon, sockeye w/bone, canned, drained	3 oz	85	130.05	17.399	0	0	6.214	2.688	1.605	1.397
15086	Fish, salmon, sockeye, baked or broiled (dry heat)	3 oz	85	183.6	23.214	0	0	9.325	4.497	2.048	1.629
15092	Fish, sea bass, baked or broiled (dry heat)	3 oz	85	105.4	20.086	0	0	2.176	0.462	0.81	0.557
15214	Fish, sea trout, cooked w/dry heat	3 oz	85	113.05	18.241	0	0	3.936	0.963	0.79	1.099
15096	Fish, shark, battered, fried	3 oz	85	193.8	15.8	5.431	0	11.7	5.045	3.146	2.724
15100	Fish, smelt, rainbow, baked or broiled (dry heat)	3 oz	85	105.4	19.21	0	0	2.635	0.699	0.965	0.492
15102	Fish, snapper, baked or broiled (dry heat)	3 oz	85	108.8	22.355	0	0	1.462	0.274	0.5	0.31
15176	Fish, squid, fried	3 oz	85	148.75	15.249	6.622	0	6.358	2.337	1.816	1.596
15105	Fish, sturgeon, baked or broiled	3 oz	85	114.75	17.595	0	0	4.403	2.113	0.752	0.997
15106	Fish, sturgeon, smoked	3 oz	85	147.05	26.52	0	0	3.74	2.003	0.371	0.881
15111	Fish, swordfish, baked or broiled (dry heat)	3 oz	85	131.75	21.582	0	0	4.369	1.684	1.005	1.195
15241	Fish, trout, rainbow, farmed, cooked w/dry heat	3 oz	85	143.65	20.63	0	0	6.12	1.782	1.98	1.789
15116	Fish, trout, rainbow, wild, cooked w/dry heat	3 oz	85	127.5	19.482	0	0	4.947	1.484	1.556	1.376
15128	Fish, tuna salad	1 cup	205	383.35	32.882	19.29	0	18.983	5.918	8.45	3.165
15118	Fish, tuna, bluefin, baked or broiled (dry heat)	3 oz	85	156.4	25.424	0	0	5.338	1.745	1.567	1.37
15221	Fish, tuna, yellowfin, fresh, cooked w/dry heat	3 oz	85	118.2	25.5	0	0	1.037	0.167	0.309	0.256
15222	Fish, turbot, European, cooked w/dry heat	3 oz	85	103.7	17.493	0	0	3.213			
15126	Fish, white tuna, canned in H$_2$0, drained	3 oz	85	108.8	20.077	0	0	2.525	0.666	0.943	0.673
15124	Fish, white tuna, canned in oil, drained	3 oz	85	158.1	22.551	0	0	6.868	2.773	2.526	1.088
15223	Fish, whitefish, cooked w/dry heat	3 oz	85	146.2	20.799	0	0	6.384	2.175	2.342	0.988
15133	Fish, whiting, baked or broiled (dry heat)	3 oz	85	98.6	19.958	0	0	1.437	0.378	0.499	0.34
15225	Fish, yellowtail, cooked w/dry heat	3 oz	85	158.95	25.22	0	0	5.712			
2050	Flavoring, vanilla extract	1 tsp	4.2	12.096	0.003	0.531	0	0.003	0	0	0
20003	Flour, arrowroot	1 cup	128	456.96	0.384	112.83	4.352	0.128	0.003	0.058	0.024
20130	Flour, barley flour or meal	1 cup	148	510.6	15.54	110.29	14.948	2.368	0.303	1.141	0.496
20011	Flour, buckwheat, whole groat	1 cup	120	402	15.144	84.708	12	3.72	1.139	1.139	0.812
20017	Flour, corn, masa, enriched	1 cup	114	416.1	10.648	86.948	10.944	4.309	1.137	1.965	0.606
20070	Flour, triticale, whole grain	1 cup	130	439.4	17.134	95.082	18.98	2.353	0.238	1.032	0.413
20081	Flour, wheat, white, all purpose, bleached, enriched	1 cup	125	455	12.913	95.387	3.375	1.225	0.109	0.516	0.194
20082	Flour, wheat, white, all purpose, self-rise, enriched	1 cup	125	442.5	12.363	92.775	3.375	1.213	0.108	0.512	0.192
20083	Flour, wheat, white, bread, enriched	1 cup	137	494.57	16.413	99.366	3.288	2.274	0.192	0.996	0.334
20084	Flour, wheat, white, cake, enriched	1 cup unsifted, dipped	137	495.94	11.234	106.9	2.329	1.178	0.1	0.519	0.174
20080	Flour, whole wheat, whole grain	1 cup	120	406.8	16.44	87.084	14.64	2.244	0.278	0.935	0.386
7945	Frankfurter, beef, heated	1 serving	52	169.52	6.001	1.96	0	15.319	7.447	0.553	5.947
18268	French toast, frozen	1 piece	59	125.67	4.366	18.939	0.649	3.599	1.204	0.724	0.904
18269	French toast, homemade w/reduced fat (2%) milk	1 slice	65	148.85	5.005	16.25		7.02	2.941	1.686	1.77
22606	Frozen dinner, cacciatore chicken, pasta w/chicken breast pieces & vegetables in cacci	1 serving	354	265.5	21.983	35.86	4.956	3.965	2.372	0.637	0.991
22602	Frozen dinner, creamed spinach/Stouffer	1 cup	250	337.5	7	18	4.5	26.25	5.67	8.98	7.4
22603	Frozen dinner, spinach au gratin/The Budget Gourmet	1 serving	155	221.65	6.665	11.47	2.325	16.585			7.595
22601	Frozen dinner, Stir Fry 2, white rice & vegetables w/Oriental soy sauce/Hanover	1 serving	137	130.15	4.521	26.989	2.466	0.411			

Chol (g)	Calc (mg)	Iron (mg)	Mag (mg)	Phos (mg)	Pota (mg)	Sodi (mg)	Zinc (mg)	Vit A (RAE)	Vit C (mg)	Thia (mg)	Ribo (mg)	Niac (mg)	Vit B6 (mg)	Vit B12 (µg)	Vit E (mg)	Fol (µg)	Alc (g)
53.55	12.75	0.289	25.5	214.2	326.4	51.85	0.366	12.75	3.145	0.289	0.115	6.838	0.55	2.38		28.9	0
60.35	12.75	0.876	31.45	217.6	533.8	47.6	0.697	11.05	0	0.234	0.414	8.565	0.802	2.592		24.65	0
37.4	203.15	0.901	24.65	277.1	320.45	457.3	0.867	45.05	0	0.014	0.164	4.658	0.255	0.255	1.36	8.5	0
73.95	5.95	0.468	26.35	234.6	318.75	56.1	0.433	53.55	0	0.183	0.145	5.67	0.186	4.93		4.25	0
45.05	11.05	0.315	45.05	210.8	278.8	73.95	0.442	54.4	0	0.111	0.128	1.615	0.391	0.255		5.1	0
90.1	18.7	0.298	34	272.85	371.45	62.9	0.493	29.75	0	0.059	0.176	2.485	0.393	2.941		5.1	0
50.2	42.5	0.944	36.5	164.9	131.8	103.7	0.408	45.9	0	0.061	0.082	2.366	0.255	1.029	0	12.8	0
76.5	65.45	0.978	32.3	250.75	316.2	65.45	1.802	14.45	0	0.009	0.124	1.501	0.145	3.375		4.25	0
39.95	34	0.204	31.45	170.85	443.7	48.45	0.374	29.75	1.36	0.045	0.003	0.294	0.391	2.975		5.1	0
221	33.15	0.859	32.3	213.35	237.15	260.1	1.479	9.35	3.57	0.048	0.389	2.212	0.049	1.046		11.9	0
65.45	14.45	0.765	38.25	230.35	309.4	58.65	0.459	223.55	0	0.068	0.077	8.585	0.196	2.125	0.535	14.45	0
68	14.45	0.791	39.95	238.85	322.15	628.15	0.476	238	0	0.077	0.077	9.435	0.23	2.465	0.425	17	0
42.5	5.1	0.884	28.9	286.45	313.65	97.75	1.25	34.85	0.935	0.037	0.099	10.022	0.324	1.717		1.7	0
57.8	73.1	0.281	27.2	226.1	374.85	35.7	0.417	73.1	2.805	0.201	0.068	7.472	0.337	4.224		20.4	0
58.65	73.1	0.323	26.35	228.65	380.8	47.6	0.433	12.75	1.7	0.129	0.082	4.905	0.294	5.355		16.15	0
26.65	34.85	2.05	38.95	364.9	364.9	824.1	1.148	49.2	4.51	0.064	0.144	13.735	0.166	2.46		16.4	0
41.65	8.5	1.113	54.4	277.1	274.55	42.5	0.655	643.5	0	0.236	0.26	8.959	0.446	9.248		1.7	0
49.3	17.9	0.799	54.4	208.2	483.7	40	0.57	17	0.85	0.426	0.048	10.1	0.882	0.51	0	1.7	0
52.7	19.55	0.391	55.25	140.25	259.25	163.2	0.238	10.2	1.445	0.065	0.082	2.277	0.206	2.159		7.65	0
35.7	11.9	0.825	28.05	184.45	201.45	320.45	0.408	5.1	0	0.007	0.037	4.929	0.184	0.994	0.723	1.7	0
26.35	3.4	0.553	28.9	226.95	283.05	336.6	0.4	4.25	0	0.014	0.067	9.943	0.366	1.87	1.955	4.25	0
65.45	28.05	0.4	35.7	294.1	345.1	55.25	1.079	33.15	0	0.145	0.131	3.269	0.294	0.816		14.45	0
71.4	52.7	0.357	22.95	242.25	368.9	112.2	0.45	28.9	0	0.058	0.051	1.419	0.153	2.21	0.255	12.75	0
60.35	24.65	0.535	32.3	170.85	457.3	42.5	0.57	26.35	2.465	0.149	0.043	7.41	0.157	1.063		3.4	0
0	0.462	0.005	0.504	0.252	6.216	0.378	0.005	0	0	0	0.004	0.018	0.001	0	0	0	1.445
0	51.2	0.422	3.84	6.4	14.08	2.56	0.09	0	0	0.001	0	0	0.006	0		8.96	0
0	47.36	3.966	142.08	438.08	457.32	5.92	2.96	0	0	0.548	0.169	9.278	0.586	0	0.844	11.84	0
0	49.2	4.872	301.2	404.4	692.4	13.2	3.744	0	0	0.5	0.228	7.38	0.698	0	0.384	64.8	0
0	160.74	8.219	125.4	254.22	339.72	5.7	2.029	0	0	1.629	0.858	11.221	0.422	0	0.171	265.6	0
0	45.5	3.367	198.9	417.3	605.8	2.6	3.458	0	0	0.491	0.172	3.718	0.524	0	1.17	96.2	0
0	18.75	5.8	27.5	135	133.75	2.5	0.875	0	0	0.981	0.618	7.38	0.055	0	0.075	228.8	0
0	422.5	5.838	23.75	743.75	155	1587.5	0.775	0	0	0.843	0.517	7.29	0.063	0	0.063	245	0
0	20.55	6.042	34.25	132.89	137	2.74	1.164	0	0	1.112	0.701	10.349	0.051	0	0.548	250.71	0
0	19.18	10.028	21.92	116.45	143.85	2.74	0.849	0	0	1.222	0.589	9.302	0.045	0	0.027	254.8	0
0	40.8	4.656	165.6	415.2	486	6	3.516	0	0	0.536	0.258	7.638	0.409	0	0.984	52.8	0
29.12	6.24	0.811	7.28	88.92	76.44	600.08	1.222	0		0.02	0.075	1.224	0.048	0.858	0.104	3.64	0
48.38	63.13	1.304	10.03	82.01	79.06	292.05	0.454	31.86	0.177	0.163	0.225	1.606	0.293	0.991	0.395	30.68	0
75.4	65	1.085	11.05	76.05	87.1	311.35	0.435	80.6	0.195	0.133	0.209	1.058	0.048	0.201		27.95	0
31.86	53.1	2.23		254.88	750.48	552.24											0
32.5	282.5					670											0
41.85	243.35	1.953				654.1			27.13								0
						635.68			16.3								0

EvaluEat Code	Food Name	Amt	Wt (g)	Energy (kcal)	Prot (g)	Carb (g)	Fiber (g)	Fat (g)	Mono (g)	Poly (g)	Sat (g)
22618	Frozen meal, barbecue glazed chicken & sauce w/mixed vegetables/WW Ultimate 200	1 package	209	217.36	18.81	25.916		4.389	1.559	1.099	0.995
22613	Frozen meal, beef & bean burrito/Las Campanas	1 serving	114	296.4	8.664	38.19	0.798	12.084	5.518	0.787	4.184
22682	Frozen meal, beef & bean chimichanga/Fiesta Cafe	1 package	227	422.22	24.062	55.615	6.129	11.577	3.882	3.473	2.156
22402	Frozen meal, beef macaroni/Healthy Choice	1 serving	240	211.2	14.136	33.456	4.56	2.232	1.2	0.336	0.672
22578	Frozen meal, beef pot roast w/whipped potatoes/Stouffer Lean Cuisine Homestyle	1 package	255	206.55	17.34	22.44	3.57	5.355	2.285	0.808	1.306
22616	Frozen meal, beef sirloin salisbury steak w/red skinned potatoes & vegetables/Budget Gourmet	1 package	311	261.24	18.349	33.899	7.153	5.909	1.754	0.936	2.018
22686	Frozen meal, beef stir fry kit: white rice, oriental vegetables, beef strips, Oriental	1 package	810	866.7	51.597	141.59		9.963			
22677	Frozen meal, beef stroganoff and noodles w/carrots & peas/Marie Callender	1 package	368	599.84	30.397	58.696	4.416	27.011	11.96	3.974	11.077
22577	Frozen meal, chicken & vegetables w/vermicelli/Stouffer's Lean Cuisine	1 package	297	252.45	18.711	32.076	5.049	5.643	2.132	1.384	1.028
22581	Frozen meal, chicken a l'orange in sauce w/broccoli & rice/Stouffer's Lean Cuisine	1 package	255	267.75	24.48	38.505		1.785	0.502	0.413	0.418
22610	Frozen meal, chicken alfredo w/fettucini & vegetables/Stouffer's Lunch Express	1 package	272	372.64	19.04	32.64	3.808	18.496	6.256	2.394	6.99
22575	Frozen meal, chicken cordon bleu, filled w/cheese & ham/Barber Food	1 package	340	697	51.68	29.58		41.48	16.694	6.562	11.526
22615	Frozen meal, chicken enchilada & mexican rice w/monterey jack cheese sauce/Stouffer's	1 package	283	376.39	12.452	48.393	4.528	14.716	4.415	3.707	3.368
22687	Frozen meal, chicken fajita kit/Tyson	1 package	756	914.76	56.624	122.77		23.209	9.148	4.158	5.897
22688	Frozen meal, chicken mesquite w/BBQ sauce, corn medley & potatoes au gratin/Tyson	1 package	255	321.3	17.773	44.956	4.335	7.752	2.729	0.484	2.601
22906	Frozen meal, chicken pot pie, frozen entree	1 serving	217	483.91	13.042	42.706	1.736	29.1	12.478	4.488	9.667
22587	Frozen meal, chicken teriyaki w/rice, mixed vegetables w/butter sauce & apple cherry compote	1 package	312	268.32	17.066	37.097	2.808	5.616	2.153	0.468	2.995
22690	Frozen meal, cosmic chicken nuggets w/macaroni & cheese, corn, chocolate pudding	1 package	257	524.28	17.733	52.942	3.084	26.728	10.717	5.962	6.605
22619	Frozen meal, country roast turkey w/mushrooms in brown gravy & rice pilaf/Healthy Choice	1 package	240	223.2	18.984	27.84	3.12	3.936	1.8	0.888	1.248
22579	Frozen meal, creamed chipped beef/Stouffer's	1 package	311	435.4	24.569	17.727		29.545	8.739	2.923	12.533
22614	Frozen meal, escalloped chicken & noodles/Stouffer's	1 package	283	418.84	16.98	31.413		25.187	7.669	13.556	6.566
22617	Frozen meal, French recipe chicken breast, vegetables & potatoes in red wine sauce/Budget Gourmet	1 package	255	178.5	22.95	9.18	6.12	5.61	2.703	0.482	1.446
22710	Frozen meal, gravy & sliced beef, mashed potatoes & carrots/Freezer Queen	1 package	255	206.55	15.3	25.5	3.57	4.845	1.25	1.709	1.3
22585	Frozen meal, homestyle stuffed cabbage w/meat in tomato sauce & whipped pots/Stouffer's	1 package	269	199.06	11.567	25.824	6.456	5.649	2.375	0.748	1.681
22673	Frozen meal, Italian sausage lasagna/Budget Gourmet	1 package	298	455.94	20.562	39.932	2.98	23.84	9.774	1.997	8.165
22570	Frozen meal, lasagna w/meat & sauce/Stouffer's	1 package	595	767.55	51.765	73.185	8.925	29.75	9.639	1.547	13.03
22576	Frozen meal, macaroni & beef in tomato sauce/Stouffer's Lean Cuisine	1 package	283	249.04	13.867	36.507	3.396	5.377	2.057	0.702	1.636

Chol (g)	Calc (mg)	Iron (mg)	Mag (mg)	Phos (mg)	Pota (mg)	Sodi (mg)	Zinc (mg)	Vit A (RAE)	Vit C (mg)	Thia (mg)	Ribo (mg)	Niac (mg)	Vit B$_6$ (mg)	Vit B$_{12}$ (µg)	Vit E (mg)	Fol (µg)	Alc (g)
48.07		1.087				405.46			21.53								0
12.54		3.112				579.12											0
36.32		6.81				803.58			5.902								0
14.4	45.6	2.712	36	134.4	364.8	444	1.224	55.2	58.08	0.276	0.156	3.108	0.194	0.12	1.68	105.6	0
38.25						494.7											0
43.54		3.048				494.49			51								0
						3167.1			50.22								0
69.92	69.92	1.803				1140.8			0								0
23.76	103.95	1.336				582.12			14.55								0
45.9						359.55			18.11								0
57.12	146.88					587.52			24.21								0
163.2	292.4					1526.6											0
25.47	254.7					1001.82			15.28								0
90.72						2472.12			73.33								0
25.5						793.05			0								0
41.23	32.55	2.062	23.87	119.35	256.06	857.15	1.02	256.7	1.519	0.254	0.356	4.13	0.202	0.152	3.847	41.23	0
43.68	37.44	1.092		224.64	424.32	602.16			12.17								0
48.83	205.6	2.853				974.03											0
26.4	21.6	1.032				436.8											0
108.85	472.72	2.27				1545.67											0
76.41	116.03	1.132				1211.24											0
25.5						864.45											
30.6						647.7		530.4									0
24.21	104.91					411.57			52.99								0
47.68	315.88	2.682				902.94											0
113.05	636.65					2034.9											0
22.64		2.179				563.17			157.3								0

EvaluEat Code	Food Name	Amt	Wt (g)	Energy (kcal)	Prot (g)	Carb (g)	Fiber (g)	Fat (g)	Mono (g)	Poly (g)	Sat (g)
22675	Frozen meal, meat loaf w/tomato sauce, mashed potatoes & carrots in seasoned sauce/Budget Gourmet	1 package	453	611.55	29.083	33.567	6.342	40.045	17.305	7.248	15.493
22586	Frozen meal, Mexican w/tamales, beef enchiladas & chili sauce, beans & rice	1 package	376	507.6	13.912	68.432	8.272	19.928	7.708	2.707	6.768
22571	Frozen meal, original fried chicken meal w/mashed potatoes & corn in seasoned sauce	1 package	228	469.68	21.455	35.089	2.052	27.041	15.367	2.44	9.257
22569	Frozen meal, pepper, stuffed w/beef in tomato sauce/Stouffer's	1 package	439	377.54	15.804	41.705	10.536	16.243	7.507	1.058	5.444
22672	Frozen meal, roast turkey medallions & mushrooms in sauce w/rice & vegetables/WW Smart	1 package	240	213.6	15.12	34.56	3.12	1.68	0.43	0.451	0.446
22712	Frozen meal, roasted chicken w/garlic sauce, pasta & vegetable medley/Tyson	1 package	255	214.2	16.932	21.522	3.57	6.707	2.346	2.142	1.3
22595	Frozen meal, scrambled eggs & sausage w/hashed brown potatoes	1 package	177	361.08	12.567	17.169	1.416	26.904	12.673	3.628	7.345
22580	Frozen meal, spaghetti w/meat sauce/Stouffer's Lean Cuisine	1 package	326	312.96	14.344	50.53	5.542	5.868	2.282	1.324	1.353
22608	Frozen meal, spaghetti w/meatballs & pomodoro sauce, low-fat/Michelina's	1 package	284	312.4	13.632	48.564	6.248	7.1	2.627	1.051	2.212
22573	Frozen meal, Swedish meatballs w/pasta/Stouffer's Lean Cuisine	1 package	258	276.06	21.672	31.218	2.58	7.224	2.34	1.04	2.423
22599	Frozen meal, turkey w/gravy & dressing w/broccoli/Marie Callender	1 package	397	504.19	31.045	51.848		19.016	8.178	1.747	9.091
42185	Frozen yogurts, chocolate, nonfat milk, with low calorie sweetener	1 cup	186	199.02	8.184	36.642	3.72	1.488	0.398	0.056	0.939
42187	Frozen yogurts, flavors other than chocolate	1 cup	186	236.22	5.58	40.176	0	6.696	1.834	0.186	4.326
14127	Fruit beverage mix, Kool-Aid, sugar free w/aspartame & vit C, dry mix, cherry flavor	.125 envelope	1.2	3.48	0.073	1.019		0.004			
14275	Fruit beverage mix, Kraft Kool-Aid Sugar Sweetened Tropical Punch, powder	1 NLEA serving	17	63.75	0	16.252	0	0			0
14297	Fruit beverage mix, Lemonade Flavor Drink, dry, prep w/H$_2$O	8 fl. oz.	266	111.72	0	28.728	0	0	0.005	0.011	0.045
14290	Fruit beverage mix, Lemonade w/aspartame, low kcal, dry, prep	8 fl. oz.	237	4.74	0.047	1.232	0	0	0	0.002	0
14408	Fruit beverage mix, orange flavor drink, dry, prep w/H$_2$O	8 fl. oz.	271	132.79	0	34.281	0.271	0	0	0	0
14403	Fruit beverage mix, orange flavor, Tang, dry mix	8 fl. oz.	25	91.5	0	24.6	0.075	0	0	0	0
14263	Fruit beverage, citrus drink, frozen concentrate, prep w/H$_2$O	8 fl. oz.	248	124	0.446	30.231	0.248	0.124	0	0	0
14242	Fruit beverage, cranberry cocktail, bottled	8 fl. oz.	253	144.21	0	36.432	0.253	0.253	0.035	0.111	0.023
14431	Fruit beverage, cranberry juice cocktail, frozen concentrate, prep w/H$_2$O	8 fl. oz.	250	137.5	0	35	0.25	0	0	0	0
14241	Fruit beverage, cranberry-grape drink, bottled	8 fl. oz.	245	137.2	0.49	34.3	0.245	0.245	0.01	0.056	0.081
14267	Fruit beverage, fruit punch, canned	8 fl. oz.	248	116.56	0	29.686	0.496	0	0.005	0.007	0
14269	Fruit beverage, fruit punch, frozen concentrate, prep w/H$_2$O	8 fl. oz.	247	113.62	0.148	28.8	0.247	0	0.002	0.005	0.002
14277	Fruit beverage, grape drink, canned	8 fl. oz.	250	112.5	0.025	28.875	0	0	0	0.003	0.003
14406	Fruit beverage, juice drink, frozen concentrate, prep	8 fl. oz.	248	124	0.248	30.256	0.248	0.496	0.06	0.122	0.062
14543	Fruit beverage, lemonade, pink, frozen conc, prep w/H$_2$O	8 fl. oz.	247	98.8	0.247	25.935	0	0	0.005	0.032	0.015
14293	Fruit beverage, lemonade, white, frozen, prep w/H$_2$O	8 fl. oz.	248	131.44	0.223	34.05	0.248	0.149	0.005	0.042	0.02
14303	Fruit beverage, limeade, frozen concentrate, prep w/H$_2$O	8 fl. oz.	247	103.74	0.099	26.108	0	0.025	0	0	0

Chol (g)	Calc (mg)	Iron (mg)	Mag (mg)	Phos (mg)	Pota (mg)	Sodi (mg)	Zinc (mg)	Vit A (RAE)	Vit C (mg)	Thia (mg)	Ribo (mg)	Niac (mg)	Vit B$_6$ (mg)	Vit B$_{12}$ (µg)	Vit E (mg)	Fol (µg)	Alc (g)
113.25	77.01	3.941				1943.37			7.701								0
26.32	240.64	2.858				1812.32			4.888								0
88.92	38.76	1.368				1500.24			1.368								0
43.9						1154.57			173								0
24		1.416				504											0
28.05		1.556				466.65											0
283.2		1.664				771.72											0
13.04		2.119				609.62			34.88								0
14.2		2.925				1011.04			8.804								0
46.44		2.064				562.44											0
79.4	131.01	4.367				2036.61			23.82								0
7.44	295.74	0.074	74.4	239.94	630.54	150.66	0.911	3.72	1.302	0.074	0.335	0.372	0.074	0.911	0.149	22.32	0
24.18	186	0.856	18.6	165.54	290.16	117.18	0.521	91.14	1.302	0.074	0.335	0.13	0.074	0.13	0.167	7.44	0
						5.064			6.72								0
0	27.88	0.012		12.75	0.34	1.53			6.001								
0	29.26	0.053	2.66	2.66	2.66	18.62	0.08	0	34.05	0	0.003	0	0	0		0	0
0	52.14	0.095	2.37	23.7	0	4.74	0.024	0	5.925	0	0	0	0	0	0	0	0
0	138.21	0.027	2.71	51.49	65.04	10.84	0.027	208.7	79.95	0	0.236	2.772	0.276	0	0	0	0
0	92.25	0.018	0	42.25	47.5	2	0.01		60	0	0.17	2	0.2	0	2.013	0	0
0	12.4	0.124	9.92	9.92	121.52	4.96	0.05	2.48	36.21	0.04	0.02	0.151	0.04	0	0.05	7.44	0
0	7.59	0.38	5.06	5.06	45.54	5.06	0.177	0	89.56	0.023	0.023	0.089	0.048	0	0	0	0
0	12.5	0.225	5	2.5	35	7.5	0.1	2.5	24.75	0.018	0.022	0.03	0.035	0		0	0
0	19.6	0.024	7.35	9.8	58.8	7.35	0.098	0	78.4	0.024	0.044	0.294	0.069	0		2.45	0
0	19.84	0.223	7.44	7.44	62	94.24	0.025	4.96	73.41	0.055	0.057	0.052	0.027	0	0.05	9.92	0
0	9.88	0.222	4.94	2.47	32.11	9.88	0.049	0	108.2	0.025	0.032	0.052	0.015	0		2.47	0
0	5	0.45	2.5	0	30	15	0.3	0	85.25	0.003	0.01	0.025	0.005	0	0	0	0
0	17.36	0.57	9.92	0	190.96	12.4	0.546	0	13.89	0.002	0.161	0.146	0.032	0		0	0
0	7.41	0.395	4.94	4.94	37.05	7.41	0.099	0	9.633	0.015	0.052	0.04	0.015	0		4.94	0
0	9.92	0.521	4.96	7.44	49.6	7.44	0.074	0	12.9	0.02	0.069	0.055	0.017	0	0.025	2.48	0
0	7.41	0.025	2.47	2.47	22.23	4.94	0.025	0	5.928	0.005	0.007	0.02	0.01	0	0	2.47	0

EvaluEat Code	Food Name	Amt	Wt (g)	Energy (kcal)	Prot (g)	Carb (g)	Fiber (g)	Fat (g)	Mono (g)	Poly (g)	Sat (g)
14323	Fruit beverage, orange drink, canned	8 fl. oz.	248	126.48	0	31.992	0	0	0.005	0.007	0.005
14334	Fruit beverage, pineapple & grapefruit juice drink, canned	8 fl. oz.	250	117.5	0.5	29	0.25	0.25	0.025	0.07	0.015
14341	Fruit beverage, pineapple & orange juice drink, canned	8 fl. oz.	250	125	3.25	29.5	0.25	0	0	0	0
9100	Fruit cocktail (peach, pineapple, pear, grape & cherry)canned in heavy syrup	1 cup	248	181.04	0.967	46.897	2.48	0.174	0.032	0.077	0.025
9097	Fruit cocktail (peach, pineapple, pear, grape & cherry)canned in juice	1 cup	237	109.02	1.09	28.108	2.37	0.024	0.005	0.009	0.002
9016	Fruit juice, apple, canned or bottled, unsweetened w/o added vit C	1 cup	248	116.56	0.149	28.966	0.248	0.273	0.012	0.082	0.047
9018	Fruit juice, apple, frozen concentrate, unsweetened w/o added vit C, prep	1 cup	239	112.33	0.335	27.581	0.239	0.239	0.005	0.074	0.043
9036	Fruit juice, apricot nectar, canned w/o added vit C	1 cup	251	140.56	0.929	36.119	1.506	0.226	0.095	0.043	0.015
9124	Fruit juice, grapefruit, canned, sweetened	1 cup	250	115	1.45	27.825	0.25	0.225	0.03	0.052	0.03
9123	Fruit juice, grapefruit, canned, unsweetened	1 cup	247	93.86	1.284	22.131	0.247	0.247	0.032	0.057	0.032
9126	Fruit juice, grapefruit, frozen concentrate, unsweetened, prep	1 cup	247	101.27	1.359	24.033	0.247	0.321	0.044	0.079	0.047
9152	Fruit juice, lemon, fresh	1 fl. oz.	30.5	7.625	0.116	2.632	0.122	0	0	0	0
9160	Fruit juice, lime, fresh	1 fl. oz.	30.8	8.316	0.136	2.775	0.123	0.031	0.003	0.008	0.003
9207	Fruit juice, orange, canned, unsweetened	1 cup	249	104.58	1.469	24.527	0.498	0.349	0.062	0.085	0.045
9206	Fruit juice, orange, fresh	1 cup	248	111.6	1.736	25.792	0.496	0.496	0.089	0.099	0.06
9215	Fruit juice, orange, frozen concentrate, unsweetened, prep	1 cup	249	112.05	1.693	26.842	0.498	0.149	0.025	0.03	0.017
9217	Fruit juice, orange-grapefruit, canned, unsweetened	1 cup	247	106.21	1.482	25.392	0.247	0.247	0.042	0.047	0.027
9229	Fruit juice, papaya nectar, canned	1 cup	250	142.5	0.425	36.275	1.5	0.375	0.103	0.087	0.117
9232	Fruit juice, passion fruit, purple, fresh	1 cup	247	125.97	0.963	33.592	0.494	0.124	0.015	0.072	0.01
9251	Fruit juice, peach nectar, canned w/o added vit C	1 cup	249	134.46	0.672	34.661	1.494	0.05	0.02	0.027	0.005
9273	Fruit juice, pineapple, canned, unsweetened w/o added vit C	1 cup	250	140	0.8	34.45	0.5	0.2	0.022	0.07	0.012
9294	Fruit juice, prune, canned	1 cup	256	181.76	1.562	44.672	2.56	0.077	0.054	0.018	0.008
9223	Fruit juice, tangerine, canned, sweetened	1 cup	249	124.5	1.245	29.88	0.498	0.498	0.045	0.062	0.032
9105	Fruit salad (peach, pineapple, pear, apricot & cherry)canned in heavy syrup	1 cup	255	186.15	0.867	48.73	2.55	0.178	0.036	0.079	0.025
9103	Fruit salad (peach, pineapple, pear, apricot & cherry)canned in juice	1 cup	249	124.5	1.27	32.494	2.49	0.075	0.012	0.027	0.01
9003	Fruit, apple w/skin, raw	1 large (3-1/4" dia) (approx 2 per lb)	212	110.24	0.551	29.277	5.088	0.36	0.015	0.108	0.059
9004	Fruit, apple, peeled, raw, medium	1 medium (2-3/4" dia) (approx 3 per lb)	128	61.44	0.346	16.333	1.664	0.166	0.006	0.047	0.027
9007	Fruit, apple, slices, sweetened, canned, drained	1 cup slices	204	136.68	0.367	34.068	3.468	1	0.041	0.294	0.163
9402	Fruit, applesauce, canned, sweetened w/added vit C	1 cup	255	193.8	0.459	50.771	3.06	0.459	0.018	0.138	0.076
9401	Fruit, applesauce, canned, unsweetened w/added vit C	1 cup	244	104.92	0.415	27.548	2.928	0.122	0.005	0.034	0.02
9027	Fruit, apricot w/skin, canned in heavy syrup	1 cup, halves	258	214.14	1.367	55.393	4.128	0.206	0.085	0.039	0.013
9024	Fruit, apricot w/skin, canned in juice	1 cup, halves	244	117.12	1.537	30.11	3.904	0.098	0.041	0.017	0.007
9035	Fruit, apricot, frozen, sweetened	1 cup	242	237.16	1.694	60.742	5.324	0.242	0.106	0.048	0.017
9023	Fruit, apricot, peeled, canned in H_2O	1 cup, whole, without pits	227	49.94	1.566	12.44	2.497	0.068	0.03	0.014	0.005

Chol (g)	Calc (mg)	Iron (mg)	Mag (mg)	Phos (mg)	Pota (mg)	Sodi (mg)	Zinc (mg)	Vit A (RAE)	Vit C (mg)	Thia (mg)	Ribo (mg)	Niac (mg)	Vit B$_6$ (mg)	Vit B$_{12}$ (µg)	Vit E (mg)	Fol (µg)	Alc (g)
0	14.88	0.694	4.96	2.48	44.64	39.68	0.223	2.48	84.57	0.015	0.007	0.077	0.022	0	0.05	9.92	0
0	17.5	0.775	15	15	152.5	35	0.15	0	115	0.075	0.04	0.667	0.105	0	0.025	22.5	0
0	12.5	0.675	15	10	115	7.5	0.15	2.5	56.25	0.075	0.047	0.517	0.117	0	0.075	22.5	0
0	14.88	0.719	12.4	27.28	218.24	14.88	0.198	24.8	4.712	0.045	0.047	0.928	0.124	0	0.992	7.44	0
0	18.96	0.498	16.59	33.18	225.15	9.48	0.213	35.55	6.399	0.028	0.038	0.955	0.121	0	0.948	7.11	0
0	17.36	0.918	7.44	17.36	295.12	7.44	0.074	0	2.232	0.052	0.042	0.248	0.074	0	0.025	0	0
0	14.34	0.621	11.95	16.73	301.14	16.73	0.096	0	1.434	0.007	0.036	0.091	0.079	0	0.024	0	0
0	17.57	0.954	12.55	22.59	286.14	7.53	0.226	165.7	1.506	0.023	0.035	0.653	0.055	0	0.778	2.51	0
0	20	0.9	25	27.5	405	5	0.15	0	67.25	0.1	0.058	0.798	0.05	0	0.1	25	0
0	17.29	0.494	24.7	27.17	377.91	2.47	0.222	0	72.12	0.104	0.049	0.571	0.049	0	0.099	24.7	0
0	19.76	0.346	27.17	34.58	335.92	2.47	0.124	0	83.24	0.101	0.054	0.536	0.109	0	0.099	9.88	0
0	2.135	0.009	1.83	1.83	37.82	0.305	0.015	0.305	14.03	0.009	0.003	0.031	0.016	0	0.046	3.965	0
0	2.772	0.009	1.848	2.156	33.572	0.308	0.018	0.616	9.024	0.006	0.003	0.031	0.013	0	0.046	2.464	0
0	19.92	1.096	27.39	34.86	435.75	4.98	0.174	22.41	85.66	0.149	0.07	0.782	0.219	0	0.498	44.82	0
0	27.28	0.496	27.28	42.16	496	2.48	0.124	24.8	124	0.223	0.074	0.992	0.099	0	0.099	74.4	0
0	22.41	0.249	24.9	39.84	473.1	2.49	0.124	12.45	96.86	0.197	0.045	0.503	0.11	0	0.498	109.6	0
0	19.76	1.136	24.7	34.58	390.26	7.41	0.173	14.82	71.88	0.138	0.074	0.83	0.057	0	0.346	34.58	0
0	25	0.85	7.5	0	77.5	12.5	0.375	45	7.5	0.015	0.01	0.375	0.022	0	0.6	5	0
0	9.88	0.593	41.99	32.11	686.66	14.82	0.124	88.92	73.61	0	0.324	3.606	0.124	0	0.025	17.29	0
0	12.45	0.473	9.96	14.94	99.6	17.43	0.199	32.37	13.2	0.007	0.035	0.717	0.017	0	0.722	2.49	0
0	42.5	0.65	32.5	20	335	2.5	0.275	0	26.75	0.138	0.055	0.642	0.24	0	0.05	57.5	0
0	30.72	3.021	35.84	64	706.56	10.24	0.538	0	10.5	0.041	0.179	2.01	0.558	0	0.307	0	0
0	44.82	0.498	19.92	34.86	443.22	2.49	0.075	32.37	54.78	0.149	0.05	0.249	0.08	0	0.374	12.45	0
0	15.3	0.714	12.75	22.95	204	15.3	0.178	63.75	6.12	0.038	0.054	0.885	0.082	0	1.02	7.65	0
0	27.39	0.623	19.92	34.86	288.84	12.45	0.349	74.7	8.217	0.027	0.035	0.886	0.067	0		7.47	0
0	12.72	0.254	10.6	23.32	226.84	2.12	0.085	6.36	9.752	0.036	0.055	0.193	0.087	0	0.382	6.36	0
0	6.4	0.09	5.12	14.08	115.2	0	0.064	2.56	5.12	0.024	0.036	0.116	0.047	0	0.064	0	0
0	8.16	0.469	4.08	10.2	138.72	6.12	0.061	6.12	0.816	0.018	0.02	0.149	0.09	0	0.428	0	0
0	10.2	0.892	7.65	17.85	155.55	71.4	0.102	2.55	4.335	0.033	0.071	0.479	0.066	0		2.55	0
0	7.32	0.293	7.32	17.08	183	4.88	0.073	2.44	51.73	0.032	0.061	0.459	0.063	0		2.44	0
0	23.22	0.774	18.06	30.96	361.2	10.32	0.284	160	7.998	0.052	0.057	0.97	0.139	0	1.548	5.16	0
0	29.28	0.732	24.4	48.8	402.6	9.76	0.268	207.4	11.96	0.044	0.046	0.839	0.132	0	1.464	4.88	0
0	24.2	2.178	21.78	45.98	554.18	9.68	0.242	203.3	21.78	0.048	0.097	1.936	0.145	0	2.154	4.84	0
0	18.16	1.226	20.43	36.32	349.58	24.97	0.25	206.6	4.086	0.045	0.054	0.992	0.123	0		4.54	0

EvaluEat Code	Food Name	Amt	Wt (g)	Energy (kcal)	Prot (g)	Carb (g)	Fiber (g)	Fat (g)	Mono (g)	Poly (g)	Sat (g)
9028	Fruit, apricot, peeled, canned in heavy syrup	1 cup, whole, without pits	258	214.14	1.316	55.341	4.128	0.232	0.095	0.044	0.015
9021	Fruit, apricot, raw	1 apricot	35	16.8	0.49	3.892	0.7	0.136	0.06	0.027	0.009
9038	Fruit, avocado, California, peeled, raw	1 fruit without skin and seed	173	288.91	3.391	14.947	11.764	26.659	16.952	3.484	3.678
9040	Fruit, banana, peeled, raw, mashed/sliced	1 medium (7" to 7-7/8" long)	118	105.02	1.286	26.951	3.068	0.389	0.038	0.086	0.132
9048	Fruit, blackberries, frozen, unsweetened	1 cup, unthawed	151	96.64	1.782	23.662	7.55	0.649	0.062	0.37	0.023
9042	Fruit, blackberries, raw	1 cup	144	61.92	2.002	13.838	7.632	0.706	0.068	0.403	0.02
9054	Fruit, blueberries, frozen, unsweetened	1 cup, unthawed	155	79.05	0.651	18.863	4.185	0.992	0.141	0.432	0.082
9050	Fruit, blueberries, raw	1 cup	145	82.65	1.073	21.01	3.48	0.479	0.068	0.212	0.041
9056	Fruit, boysenberries, canned in heavy syrup	1 cup	256	225.28	2.534	57.114	6.656	0.307	0.031	0.174	0.01
9057	Fruit, boysenberries, frozen, unsweetened	1 cup, unthawed	132	66	1.452	16.091	6.996	0.343	0.033	0.195	0.012
9059	Fruit, breadfruit, peeled, raw	1 cup	220	226.6	2.354	59.664	10.78	0.506	0.075	0.145	0.106
9060	Fruit, carambola (starfruit) raw	1 cup, cubes	137	45.21	0.74	10.727	3.699	0.479	0.042	0.262	0.032
9066	Fruit, cherries, sour, red, canned in heavy syrup	1 cup	256	232.96	1.869	59.571	2.816	0.256	0.067	0.074	0.054
9068	Fruit, cherries, sour, red, frozen, unsweetened	1 cup, unthawed	155	71.3	1.426	17.081	2.48	0.682	0.186	0.205	0.155
9064	Fruit, cherries, sour/tart, red, canned in H$_2$O	1 cup	244	87.84	1.879	21.814	2.684	0.244	0.066	0.073	0.056
9074	Fruit, cherries, sweet, canned in heavy syrup	1 cup, pitted	253	209.99	1.518	53.813	3.795	0.38	0.104	0.114	0.086
9072	Fruit, cherries, sweet, canned in juice	1 cup, pitted	250	135	2.275	34.525	3.75	0.05	0.012	0.015	0.01
9070	Fruit, cherries, sweet, raw	1 cup, with pits	117	73.71	1.24	18.732	2.457	0.234	0.055	0.061	0.044
9078	Fruit, cranberries, raw	1 cup, chopped	110	50.6	0.429	13.42	5.06	0.143	0.02	0.06	0.012
9081	Fruit, cranberry sauce, canned, sweetened	1 slice (1/2" thick, approx 8 slices per can)	57	86.07	0.114	22.173	0.57	0.086	0.012	0.038	0.007
9082	Fruit, cranberry-orange relish, canned	1 cup	275	489.5	0.825	127.05	0	0.275			0.033
9084	Fruit, currant, red or white, raw	1 cup	112	62.72	1.568	15.456	4.816	0.224	0.031	0.099	0.019
9085	Fruit, currants, zante, dried	1 cup	144	407.52	5.875	106.68	9.792	0.389	0.068	0.259	0.04
9087	Fruit, dates, domestic, natural, dried	1 cup, pitted, chopped	178	501.96	4.361	133.55	14.24	0.694	0.064	0.034	0.057
9092	Fruit, figs, canned in heavy syrup	1 cup	259	227.92	0.984	59.311	5.698	0.259	0.057	0.124	0.052
9094	Fruit, figs, dried, raw	1 cup	149	371.01	4.917	95.166	14.602	1.386	0.237	0.514	0.215
9089	Fruit, figs, raw	1 large (2-1/2" dia)	64	47.36	0.48	12.275	1.856	0.192	0.042	0.092	0.038
9107	Fruit, gooseberries, raw	1 cup	150	66	1.32	15.27	6.45	0.87	0.076	0.475	0.057
9120	Fruit, grapefruit, canned in juice	1 cup	249	92.13	1.743	22.933	0.996	0.224	0.03	0.052	0.03
9111	Fruit, grapefruit, red, white or pink, peeled, raw	1/2 medium (approx 4" dia)	128	40.96	0.806	10.342	1.408	0.128	0.017	0.031	0.018
9131	Fruit, grapes, American type (slip skin) raw	1 cup	92	61.64	0.58	15.778	0.828	0.322	0.013	0.094	0.105
9139	Fruit, guava, common, raw	1 fruit	90	45.9	0.738	10.692	4.86	0.54	0.049	0.228	0.155
9148	Fruit, kiwifruit (Chinese gooseberry) peeled, raw	1 fruit without skin, medium	76	46.36	0.866	11.142	2.28	0.395	0.036	0.218	0.022
9149	Fruit, kumquat, raw	1 fruit without refuse	19	13.49	0.357	3.021	1.235	0.163	0.029	0.032	0.02
9165	Fruit, lychee (litchi) shelled, dried	1 fruit	2.5	6.925	0.095	1.767	0.115	0.03	0.008	0.009	0.007

Chol (g)	Calc (mg)	Iron (mg)	Mag (mg)	Phos (mg)	Pota (mg)	Sodi (mg)	Zinc (mg)	Vit A (RAE)	Vit C (mg)	Thia (mg)	Ribo (mg)	Niac (mg)	Vit B$_6$ (mg)	Vit B$_{12}$ (µg)	Vit E (mg)	Fol (µg)	Alc (g)
0	23.22	1.109	20.64	33.54	345.72	28.38	0.258	160	7.224	0.049	0.059	1.073	0.139	0		5.16	0
0	4.55	0.136	3.5	8.05	90.65	0.35	0.07	33.6	3.5	0.01	0.014	0.21	0.019	0	0.311	3.15	0
0	22.49	1.055	50.17	93.42	877.11	13.84	1.176	12.11	15.22	0.13	0.247	3.308	0.497	0	3.408	107.3	0
0	5.9	0.307	31.86	25.96	422.44	1.18	0.177	3.54	10.27	0.037	0.086	0.785	0.433	0	0.118	23.6	0
0	43.79	1.208	33.22	45.3	211.4	1.51	0.377	9.06	4.681	0.044	0.069	1.823	0.092	0	1.767	51.34	0
0	41.76	0.893	28.8	31.68	233.28	1.44	0.763	15.84	30.24	0.029	0.037	0.93	0.043	0	1.685	36	0
0	12.4	0.279	7.75	17.05	83.7	1.55	0.108	3.1	3.875	0.05	0.057	0.806	0.091	0	0.744	10.85	0
0	8.7	0.406	8.7	17.4	111.65	1.45	0.232	4.35	14.07	0.054	0.059	0.606	0.075	0	0.826	8.7	0
0	46.08	1.101	28.16	25.6	230.4	7.68	0.486	5.12	15.87	0.067	0.074	0.589	0.097	0	1.818	87.04	0
0	35.64	1.122	21.12	35.64	183.48	1.32	0.29	3.96	4.092	0.07	0.049	1.012	0.074	0	1.148	83.16	0
0	37.4	1.188	55	66	1078	4.4	0.264	0	63.8	0.242	0.066	1.98	0.22	0	0.22	30.8	0
0	5.48	0.356	12.33	21.92	223.31	2.74	0.151	4.11	29.04	0.038	0.037	0.563	0.137	0	0.206	19.18	0
0	25.6	3.328	15.36	25.6	238.08	17.92	0.154	92.16	5.12	0.041	0.1	0.43	0.113	0	0.589	20.48	0
0	20.15	0.821	13.95	24.8	192.2	1.55	0.155	68.2	2.635	0.068	0.053	0.212	0.104	0	0.078	7.75	0
0	26.84	3.343	14.64	24.4	239.12	17.08	0.171	92.72	5.124	0.041	0.1	0.432	0.107	0	0.561	19.52	0
0	22.77	0.885	22.77	45.54	366.85	7.59	0.253	20.24	9.108	0.053	0.101	1.002	0.076	0	0.582	10.12	0
0	35	1.45	30	55	327.5	7.5	0.25	15	6.25	0.045	0.06	1.015	0.075	0	0.575	10	0
0	15.21	0.421	12.87	24.57	259.74	0	0.082	3.51	8.19	0.032	0.039	0.18	0.057	0	0.082	4.68	0
0	8.8	0.275	6.6	14.3	93.5	2.2	0.11	3.3	14.63	0.013	0.022	0.111	0.063	0	1.32	1.1	0
0	2.28	0.125	1.71	3.42	14.82	16.53	0.029	1.14	1.14	0.009	0.012	0.057	0.008	0	0.473	0.57	0
0	30.25	0.55	11	22	104.5	88		11	49.5	0.082	0.055	0.275		0			0
0	36.96	1.12	14.56	49.28	308	1.12	0.258	2.24	45.92	0.045	0.056	0.112	0.078	0	0.112	8.96	0
0	123.84	4.694	59.04	180	1284.48	11.52	0.95	5.76	6.768	0.23	0.204	2.326	0.426	0	0.158	14.4	0
0	69.42	1.816	76.54	110.36	1167.68	3.56	0.516	0	0.712	0.093	0.117	2.268	0.294	0	0.089	33.82	0
0	69.93	0.725	25.9	25.9	256.41	2.59	0.285	5.18	2.59	0.057	0.096	1.109	0.181	0	0.311	5.18	0
0	241.38	3.025	101.32	99.83	1013.2	14.9	0.82	0	1.788	0.127	0.122	0.922	0.158	0	0.521	13.41	0
0	22.4	0.237	10.88	8.96	148.48	0.64	0.096	4.48	1.28	0.038	0.032	0.256	0.072	0	0.07	3.84	0
0	37.5	0.465	15	40.5	297	1.5	0.18	22.5	41.55	0.06	0.045	0.45	0.12	0	0.555	9	0
0	37.35	0.523	27.39	29.88	420.81	17.43	0.199	0	84.41	0.072	0.045	0.62	0.05	0	0.224	22.41	0
0	15.36	0.115	10.24	10.24	177.92	0	0.09	58.88	44.03	0.046	0.026	0.32	0.054	0	0.166	12.8	0
0	12.88	0.267	4.6	9.2	175.72	1.84	0.037	4.6	3.68	0.085	0.052	0.276	0.101	0	0.175	3.68	0
0	18	0.279	9	22.5	255.6	2.7	0.207	27.9	165	0.045	0.045	1.08	0.129	0	0.657	12.6	0
0	25.84	0.236	12.92	25.84	237.12	2.28	0.106	3.04	70.45	0.021	0.019	0.259	0.048	0	1.11	19	0
0	11.78	0.163	3.8	3.61	35.34	1.9	0.032	2.85	8.341	0.007	0.017	0.082	0.007	0	0.029	3.23	0
0	0.825	0.043	1.05	4.525	27.75	0.075	0.007	0	4.575	0	0.014	0.078	0.002	0	0.008	0.3	0

EvaluEat Code	Food Name	Amt	Wt (g)	Energy (kcal)	Prot (g)	Carb (g)	Fiber (g)	Fat (g)	Mono (g)	Poly (g)	Sat (g)
9164	Fruit, lychee (litchi) shelled, raw	1 fruit	9.6	6.336	0.08	1.587	0.125	0.042	0.012	0.013	0.01
9176	Fruit, mango, peeled, raw	1 cup, sliced	165	107.25	0.841	28.05	2.97	0.446	0.167	0.084	0.109
9185	Fruit, melon balls (cantaloupe & honeydew) frozen	1 cup, unthawed	173	57.09	1.453	13.736	1.211	0.433	0.01	0.17	0.111
9181	Fruit, melon, cantaloupe (musk) peeled, pieces/balls, raw	1 wedge, large (1/8 of large melon)	102	34.68	0.857	8.323	0.918	0.194	0.003	0.083	0.052
9183	Fruit, melon, casaba, peeled, raw	1 cup, cubes	170	47.6	1.887	11.186	1.53	0.17	0.003	0.066	0.043
9184	Fruit, melon, honeydew, peeled, wedges, raw	1 wedge (1/8 of 6" to 7" dia melon)	160	57.6	0.864	14.544	1.28	0.224	0.005	0.094	0.061
9188	Fruit, mixed (prune, apricot & pear) dried	1 package (11 oz)	293	711.99	7.208	187.7	22.854	1.436	0.68	0.322	0.117
9191	Fruit, nectarine, raw	1 fruit (2-1/2" dia)	136	59.84	1.442	14.348	2.312	0.435	0.12	0.154	0.034
9193	Fruit, olives, ripe, pitted, canned	1 tbsp	8.4	9.66	0.071	0.526	0.269	0.897	0.663	0.077	0.119
9200	Fruit, orange, all varieties, peeled, raw	1 fruit (2-5/8" dia)	131	61.57	1.231	15.392	3.144	0.157	0.03	0.033	0.02
9226	Fruit, papayas, peeled, cubed/mashed, raw	1 medium (5-1/8" long x 3" dia)	304	118.56	1.854	29.822	5.472	0.426	0.116	0.094	0.131
9231	Fruit, passion fruit/granadilla, purple, peeled, raw	1 fruit	18	17.46	0.396	4.208	1.872	0.126	0.015	0.074	0.011
9241	Fruit, peach, canned in heavy syrup	1 cup	262	193.88	1.179	52.243	3.406	0.262	0.092	0.123	0.026
9238	Fruit, peach, canned in juice	1 cup	250	110	1.575	28.925	3.25	0.075	0.03	0.04	0.01
9250	Fruit, peach, frozen, sweetened	1 cup, thawed	250	235	1.575	59.95	4.5	0.325	0.12	0.16	0.035
9236	Fruit, peach, peeled, raw	1 medium (2-1/2" dia) (approx 4 per lb)	98	38.22	0.892	9.349	1.47	0.245	0.066	0.084	0.019
9257	Fruit, pear, canned in heavy syrup	1 cup	266	196.84	0.532	50.992	4.256	0.346	0.072	0.08	0.019
9254	Fruit, pear, canned in juice	1 cup, halves	248	124	0.843	32.091	3.968	0.174	0.035	0.037	0.01
9252	Fruit, pear, raw	1 pear, medium (approx 2-1/2 per lb)	166	96.28	0.631	25.664	5.146	0.199	0.043	0.048	0.01
9265	Fruit, persimmon, native, raw	1 fruit	25	31.75	0.2	8.375		0.1			
9270	Fruit, pineapple, canned in heavy syrup	1 cup, crushed, sliced, or chunks	254	198.12	0.889	51.308	2.032	0.279	0.033	0.102	0.023
9268	Fruit, pineapple, canned in juice	1 cup, crushed, sliced, or chunks	249	149.4	1.046	39.093	1.992	0.199	0.025	0.072	0.015
9278	Fruit, plantain, peeled, cooked	1 cup, mashed	200	232	1.58	62.3	4.6	0.36	0.03	0.066	0.138
9284	Fruit, plum, purple, canned in heavy syrup	1 cup, pitted	258	229.62	0.929	59.959	2.322	0.258	0.17	0.057	0.021
9282	Fruit, plum, purple, canned in juice	1 cup, pitted	252	146.16	1.285	38.178	2.268	0.05	0.035	0.013	0.005
9279	Fruit, plum, raw	1 fruit (2-1/8" dia)	66	30.36	0.462	7.537	0.924	0.185	0.088	0.029	0.011
9286	Fruit, pomegranates, peeled, raw	1 fruit (3-3/8" dia)	154	104.72	1.463	26.442	0.924	0.462	0.071	0.097	0.059
9287	Fruit, prickly pear, peeled, raw	1 cup	149	61.09	1.088	14.259	5.364	0.76	0.112	0.317	0.1
9288	Fruit, prunes, canned in heavy syrup	5 fruits with liquid	86	90.3	0.748	23.908	3.268	0.172	0.112	0.037	0.014
9291	Fruit, prunes, dried	1 prune	8.4	20.16	0.183	5.366	0.596	0.032	0.004	0.005	0.007
9295	Fruit, pummelo, peeled, raw	1 fruit	609	231.42	4.628	58.586	6.09	0.244			
9296	Fruit, quinces, peeled, raw	1 fruit	92	52.44	0.368	14.076	1.748	0.092	0.033	0.046	0.009
9298	Fruit, raisins, seedless	1 cup (not packed)	145	433.55	4.451	114.81	5.365	0.667	0.074	0.054	0.084
9302	Fruit, raspberries, raw	1 cup	123	63.96	1.476	14.686	7.995	0.799	0.079	0.461	0.023
9306	Fruit, raspberries, red, frozen, sweetened	1 cup, unthawed	250	257.5	1.75	65.4	11	0.4	0.037	0.222	0.012

Chol (g)	Calc (mg)	Iron (mg)	Mag (mg)	Phos (mg)	Pota (mg)	Sodi (mg)	Zinc (mg)	Vit A (RAE)	Vit C (mg)	Thia (mg)	Ribo (mg)	Niac (mg)	Vit B$_6$ (mg)	Vit B$_{12}$ (µg)	Vit E (mg)	Fol (µg)	Alc (g)
0	0.48	0.03	0.96	2.976	16.416	0.096	0.007	0	6.864	0.001	0.006	0.058	0.01	0	0.007	1.344	0
0	16.5	0.214	14.85	18.15	257.4	3.3	0.066	62.7	45.71	0.096	0.094	0.964	0.221	0	1.848	23.1	0
0	17.3	0.502	24.22	20.76	484.4	53.63	0.294	154	10.73	0.287	0.038	1.107	0.183	0	0.26	44.98	0
0	9.18	0.214	12.24	15.3	272.34	16.32	0.184	172.4	37.43	0.042	0.019	0.749	0.073	0	0.051	21.42	0
0	18.7	0.578	18.7	8.5	309.4	15.3	0.119	0	37.06	0.025	0.053	0.394	0.277	0	0.085	13.6	0
0	9.6	0.272	16	17.6	364.8	28.8	0.144	4.8	28.8	0.061	0.019	0.669	0.141	0	0.032	30.4	0
0	111.34	7.94	114.27	225.61	2332.28	52.74	1.465	357.5	11.13	0.129	0.46	5.646	0.466	0		11.72	0
0	8.16	0.381	12.24	35.36	273.36	0	0.231	23.12	7.344	0.046	0.037	1.53	0.034	0	1.047	6.8	0
0	7.392	0.277	0.336	0.252	0.672	73.248	0.018	1.68	0.076	0	0	0.003	0.001	0	0.139	0	0
0	52.4	0.131	13.1	18.34	237.11	0	0.092	14.41	69.69	0.114	0.052	0.369	0.079	0	0.236	39.3	0
0	72.96	0.304	30.4	15.2	781.28	9.12	0.213	167.2	187.9	0.082	0.097	1.028	0.058	0	2.219	115.5	0
0	2.16	0.288	5.22	12.24	62.64	5.04	0.018	11.52	5.4	0	0.023	0.27	0.018	0	0.004	2.52	0
0	7.86	0.707	13.1	28.82	241.04	15.72	0.236	44.54	7.336	0.029	0.063	1.609	0.05	0	1.284	7.86	0
0	15	0.675	17.5	42.5	320	10	0.275	47.5	9	0.02	0.043	1.455	0.047	0	1.225	7.5	0
0	7.5	0.925	12.5	27.5	325	15	0.125	35	235.5	0.032	0.087	1.632	0.045	0	1.55	7.5	0
0	5.88	0.245	8.82	19.6	186.2	0	0.167	15.68	6.468	0.024	0.03	0.79	0.025	0	0.715	3.92	0
0	13.3	0.585	10.64	18.62	172.9	13.3	0.213	0	2.926	0.027	0.059	0.644	0.037	0	0.213	2.66	0
0	22.32	0.719	17.36	29.76	238.08	9.92	0.223	0	3.968	0.027	0.027	0.496	0.035	0	0.198	2.48	0
0	14.94	0.282	11.62	18.26	197.54	1.66	0.166	1.66	6.972	0.02	0.041	0.261	0.046	0	0.199	11.62	0
0	6.75	0.625		6.5	77.5	0.25			16.5					0			0
0	35.56	0.965	40.64	17.78	264.16	2.54	0.305	2.54	18.8	0.229	0.064	0.729	0.188	0	0.025	12.7	0
0	34.86	0.697	34.86	14.94	303.78	2.49	0.249	4.98	23.66	0.237	0.047	0.707	0.184	0	0.025	12.45	0
0	4	1.16	64	56	930	10	0.26	90	21.8	0.092	0.104	1.512	0.48	0	0.26	52	0
0	23.22	2.167	12.9	33.54	234.78	49.02	0.181	33.54	1.032	0.041	0.098	0.751	0.07	0	0.464	7.74	0
0	25.2	0.857	20.16	37.8	388.08	2.52	0.277	126	7.056	0.058	0.149	1.192	0.068	0	0.454	7.56	0
0	3.96	0.112	4.62	10.56	103.62	0	0.066	11.22	6.27	0.018	0.017	0.275	0.019	0	0.172	3.3	0
0	4.62	0.462	4.62	12.32	398.86	4.62	0.185	7.7	9.394	0.046	0.046	0.462	0.162	0	0.924	9.24	0
0	83.44	0.447	126.65	35.76	327.8	7.45	0.179	2.98	20.86	0.021	0.089	0.685	0.089	0	0.015	8.94	0
0	14.62	0.353	12.9	22.36	194.36	2.58	0.163	34.4	2.408	0.029	0.105	0.745	0.175	0		0	0
0	3.612	0.078	3.444	5.796	61.488	0.168	0.037	3.276	0.05	0.004	0.016	0.158	0.017	0	0.036	0.336	0
0	24.36	0.67	36.54	103.53	1315.44	6.09	0.487	0	371.5	0.207	0.164	1.34	0.219	0			0
0	10.12	0.644	7.36	15.64	181.24	3.68	0.037	1.84	13.8	0.018	0.028	0.184	0.037	0	0.506	2.76	0
0	72.5	2.726	46.4	146.45	1086.05	15.95	0.319	0	3.335	0.154	0.181	1.111	0.252	0	0.174	7.25	0
0	30.75	0.849	27.06	35.67	185.73	1.23	0.517	2.46	32.23	0.039	0.047	0.736	0.068	0	1.07	25.83	0
0	37.5	1.625	32.5	42.5	285	2.5	0.45	7.5	41.25	0.047	0.113	0.575	0.085	0	1.8	65	0

EvaluEat Code	Food Name	Amt	Wt (g)	Energy (kcal)	Prot (g)	Carb (g)	Fiber (g)	Fat (g)	Mono (g)	Poly (g)	Sat (g)
9310	Fruit, rhubarb, frozen, cooked w/sugar	1 cup	240	278.4	0.936	74.88	4.8	0.12	0.024	0.06	0.034
9307	Fruit, rhubarb, raw	1 cup, diced	122	25.62	1.098	5.539	2.196	0.244	0.048	0.121	0.065
9319	Fruit, strawberries, frozen, whole, sweetened	1 cup, thawed	255	198.9	1.326	53.55	4.845	0.357	0.048	0.173	0.018
9316	Fruit, strawberries, halves/slices, raw	1 cup, halves	152	48.64	1.018	11.674	3.04	0.456	0.065	0.236	0.023
9322	Fruit, tamarind, raw	1 fruit (3"x 1")	2	4.78	0.056	1.25	0.102	0.012	0.004	0.001	0.005
9326	Fruit, watermelon, balls, raw	1 cup, balls	154	46.2	0.939	11.627	0.616	0.231	0.057	0.077	0.025
17345	Game meat, deer, loin, separable lean only, 1"steak, cooked, broiled	1 serving (3 oz)	85	127.5	25.67	0	0	2.023	0.298	0.088	0.746
17157	Game, bison, roasted	3 oz	85	121.55	24.174	0	0	2.057	0.808	0.204	0.774
5308	Game, cornish game hen w/skin, roasted	1/2 bird	129	335.4	28.728	0	0	23.491	10.32	4.644	6.515
5310	Game, cornish game hens, no skin, roasted	1/2 bird	110	147.4	25.63	0	0	4.257	1.364	1.034	1.089
5145	Game, duck, wild, breast, no skin, raw	1/2 breast, bone and skin removed	83	102.09	16.476	0	0	3.527	1.004	0.481	1.096
5144	Game, duck, wild, meat & skin, raw	1/2 duck	270	569.7	47.034	0	0	41.04	18.36	5.454	13.608
5157	Game, quail, meat & skin, raw	1 quail	109	209.28	21.397	0	0	13.135	4.556	3.248	3.684
17178	Game, rabbit, domestic, composite, roasted	3 oz	85	167.45	24.701	0	0	6.843	1.845	1.326	2.04
5160	Game, squab/pigeon, meat & skin, raw	1 squab	199	585.06	36.755	0	0	47.362	19.343	6.109	16.776
5282	Goose liver pate/pate de fois gras, smoked, canned	1 oz	28.35	130.98	3.232	1.324	0	12.429	7.26	0.238	4.097
5147	Goose, domestic, meat & skin, roasted	1 cup, chopped or diced	140	427	35.224	0	0	30.688	14.35	3.528	9.618
5149	Goose, domestic, meat only, no skin, roasted	yield from 1 lb ready-to-cook goose	143	340.34	41.427	0	0	18.118	6.206	2.202	6.521
20006	Grain, barley, pearled, cooked	1 cup	157	193.11	3.548	44.305	5.966	0.691	0.089	0.336	0.146
20013	Grain, bulgar, cooked	1 cup	182	151.06	5.606	33.816	8.19	0.437	0.056	0.178	0.076
20314	Grain, corn, white	1 cup	166	605.9	15.637	123.27		7.868	2.077	3.591	1.107
20014	Grain, corn, yellow	1 cup	166	605.9	15.637	123.27	12.118	7.868	2.077	3.591	1.107
20038	Grain, oats	1 cup	156	606.84	26.348	103.38	16.536	10.764	3.398	3.955	1.899
20037	Grain, rice, brown, long grain, cooked	1 cup	195	216.45	5.031	44.772	3.51	1.755	0.638	0.63	0.351
20041	Grain, rice, brown, medium grain, cooked	1 cup	195	218.4	4.524	45.845	3.51	1.618	0.585	0.577	0.322
20055	Grain, rice, white, glutinous, cooked	1 cup	174	168.78	3.515	36.697	1.74	0.331	0.122	0.12	0.068
20345	Grain, rice, white, long grain, enriched, cooked w/salt	1 cup	158	205.4	4.25	44.509	0.632	0.442	0.139	0.12	0.122
20049	Grain, rice, white, long grain, precooked/instant, enriched, cooked	1 cup	165	161.7	3.399	35.096	0.99	0.264	0.084	0.073	0.073
20051	Grain, rice, white, medium grain, cooked	1 cup	186	241.8	4.427	53.177	0.558	0.391	0.121	0.104	0.106
20066	Grain, semolina, enriched	1 cup	167	601.2	21.176	121.63	6.513	1.753	0.207	0.718	0.25
20067	Grain, sorghum	1 cup	192	650.88	21.696	143.29		6.336	1.907	2.63	0.877
20068	Grain, tapioca, pearl, dry	1 cup	152	544.16	0.289	134.81	1.368	0.03	0.008	0.005	0.008
20078	Grain, wheat germ, crude	1 cup	115	414	26.622	59.57	15.18	11.178	1.57	6.911	1.915
20087	Grain, wheat, sprouted	1 cup	108	213.84	8.089	45.932	1.188	1.372	0.163	0.602	0.222
6114	Gravy, au jus, canned	1 cup	238	38.08	2.856	5.95	0	0.476	0.19	0.024	0.238
6116	Gravy, beef, canned	1 cup	233	123.49	8.737	11.207	0.932	5.499	2.241	0.186	2.686
6119	Gravy, chicken, canned	1 cup	238	188.02	4.593	12.9	0.952	13.59	6.069	3.57	3.356
6579	Gravy, Home Style Savory Brown Gravy, canned/Heinz	.25 cup	60	24.6	0.9	3.414		0.78	0.276	0.037	0.324
6121	Gravy, mushroom, canned	1 cup	238	119	2.999	13.019	0.952	6.45	2.785	2.428	0.952
6125	Gravy, turkey, canned	1 cup	238	121.38	6.188	12.138	0.952	4.998	2.142	1.166	1.476

Chol (g)	Calc (mg)	Iron (mg)	Mag (mg)	Phos (mg)	Pota (mg)	Sodi (mg)	Zinc (mg)	Vit A (RAE)	Vit C (mg)	Thia (mg)	Ribo (mg)	Niac (mg)	Vit B$_6$ (mg)	Vit B$_{12}$ (µg)	Vit E (mg)	Fol (µg)	Alc (g)
0	348	0.504	28.8	19.2	230.4	2.4	0.192	9.6	7.92	0.043	0.055	0.48	0.048	0	0.648	12	0
0	104.92	0.268	14.64	17.08	351.36	4.88	0.122	6.1	9.76	0.024	0.037	0.366	0.029	0	0.464	8.54	0
0	28.05	1.198	15.3	30.6	249.9	2.55	0.127	2.55	100.7	0.038	0.196	0.747	0.071	0	0.612	10.2	0
0	24.32	0.638	19.76	36.48	232.56	1.52	0.213	1.52	89.38	0.036	0.033	0.587	0.071	0	0.441	36.48	0
0	1.48	0.056	1.84	2.26	12.56	0.56	0.002	0.04	0.07	0.009	0.003	0.039	0.001	0	0.002	0.28	0
0	10.78	0.37	15.4	16.94	172.48	1.54	0.154	43.12	12.47	0.051	0.032	0.274	0.069	0	0.077	4.62	0
67.15	5.1	3.477	25.5	235.45	338.3	48.45	3.086	0	0	0.238	0.436	9.143	0.643	1.556	0.527	7.65	0
69.7	6.8	2.907	22.1	177.65	306.85	48.45	3.128	0	0	0.085	0.23	3.154	0.34	2.431	0.306	6.8	0
168.99	16.77	1.174	23.22	188.34	316.05	82.56	1.922	41.28	0.645	0.086	0.257	7.607	0.396	0.361	0.464	2.58	0
116.6	14.3	0.847	20.9	163.9	275	69.3	1.683	22	0.66	0.083	0.25	6.9	0.394	0.33	0.264	2.2	0
63.91	2.49	3.743	18.26	154.38	222.44	47.31	0.614	13.28	5.146	0.345	0.257	2.859	0.523	0.631		20.75	0
216	13.5	11.232	54	453.6	672.3	151.2	2.079	70.2	14.04	0.948	0.726	8.956	1.431	1.755	1.893	56.7	0
82.84	14.17	4.327	25.07	299.75	235.44	57.77	2.638	79.57	6.649	0.266	0.283	8.216	0.654	0.469	0.764	8.72	0
69.7	16.15	1.929	17.85	223.55	325.55	39.95	1.929	0	0	0.077	0.178	7.166	0.4	7.055		9.35	0
189.05	23.88	7.045	43.78	493.52	396.01	107.46	4.378	145.3	10.35	0.422	0.446	12.032	0.816	0.796		11.94	0
42.525	19.845	1.559	3.686	56.7	39.123	197.6	0.261	283.8	0.567	0.025	0.085	0.712	0.017	2.665		17.01	0
127.4	18.2	3.962	30.8	378	460.6	98	3.668	29.4	0	0.108	0.452	5.835	0.518	0.574	2.436	2.8	0
137.28	20.02	4.104	35.75	441.87	554.84	108.68	4.533	17.16	0	0.132	0.558	5.836	0.672	0.701		17.16	0
0	17.27	2.088	34.54	84.78	146.01	4.71	1.287	0	0	0.13	0.097	3.239	0.181	0	0.016	25.12	0
0	18.2	1.747	58.24	72.8	123.76	9.1	1.037	0	0	0.104	0.051	1.82	0.151	0	0.018	32.76	0
0	11.62	4.499	210.82	348.6	476.42	58.1	3.669	0	0	0.639	0.334	6.021	1.033	0			0
0	11.62	4.499	210.82	348.6	476.42	58.1	3.669	18.26	0	0.639	0.334	6.021	1.033	0	0.813	31.54	0
0	84.24	7.363	276.12	815.88	669.24	3.12	6.193	0	0	1.19	0.217	1.499	0.186	0	1.092	87.36	0
0	19.5	0.819	83.85	161.85	83.85	9.75	1.229	0	0	0.187	0.049	2.98	0.283	0	0.058	7.8	0
0	19.5	1.033	85.8	150.15	154.05	1.95	1.209	0	0	0.199	0.023	2.594	0.291	0		7.8	0
0	3.48	0.244	8.7	13.92	17.4	8.7	0.713	0	0	0.035	0.023	0.505	0.045	0	0.07	1.74	0
0	15.8	1.896	18.96	67.94	55.3	603.56	0.774	0	0	0.258	0.021	2.332	0.147	0	0.063	91.64	0
0	13.2	1.039	8.25	23.1	6.6	4.95	0.396	0	0	0.124	0.076	1.452	0.016	0	0.016	115.5	0
0	5.58	2.771	24.18	68.82	53.94	0	0.781	0	0	0.311	0.03	3.413	0.093	0		107.9	0
0	28.39	7.281	78.49	227.12	310.62	1.67	1.753	0	0	1.354	0.954	10.003	0.172	0	0.434	305.6	0
0	53.76	8.448		551.04	672	11.52		0	0	0.455	0.273	5.62		0			0
0	30.4	2.402	1.52	10.64	16.72	1.52	0.182	0	0	0.006	0	0	0.012	0	0	6.08	0
0	44.85	7.199	274.85	968.3	1025.8	13.8	14.13	0	0	2.164	0.574	7.835	1.495	0		323.2	0
0	30.24	2.311	88.56	216	182.52	17.28	1.782	0	2.808	0.243	0.167	3.334	0.286	0	0.054	41.04	0
0	9.52	1.428	4.76	71.4	192.78	119	2.38	0	2.38	0.048	0.143	2.142	0.024	0.238		4.76	0
6.99	13.98	1.631	4.66	69.9	188.73	1304.8	2.33	2.33	0	0.075	0.084	1.538	0.023	0.233	0.047	4.66	0
4.76	47.6	1.119	4.76	69.02	259.42	1373.26	1.904	2.38	0	0.04	0.102	1.054	0.024	0.238	0.309	4.76	0
2.4						351.6											0
0	16.66	1.571	4.76	35.7	252.28	1356.6	1.666	0	0	0.079	0.15	1.597	0.048	0		28.56	0
4.76	9.52	1.666	4.76	69.02	259.42	1373.26	1.904	0	0	0.048	0.19	3.094	0.024	0.238	0.119	4.76	0

EvaluEat Code	Food Name	Amt	Wt (g)	Energy (kcal)	Prot (g)	Carb (g)	Fiber (g)	Fat (g)	Mono (g)	Poly (g)	Sat (g)
22700	Hamburger Helper, cheeseburger macaroni, dry mix/Betty Crocker	1 serving	45	177.75	4.95	28.935		4.68			1.269
2003	Herb, basil, ground	1 tsp, leaves	0.7	1.757	0.101	0.427	0.283	0.028	0.003	0.015	0.002
2004	Herb, bay leaf, crumbled	1 tsp, crumbled	0.6	1.878	0.046	0.45	0.158	0.05	0.01	0.014	0.014
11215	Herb, garlic, raw	1 tsp	2.8	4.172	0.178	0.926	0.059	0.014	0	0.007	0.002
11216	Herb, ginger root, peeled, sliced, raw	5 slices (1" dia)	11	8.8	0.2	1.955	0.22	0.082	0.017	0.017	0.022
2029	Herb, parsley, dried	1 tsp	0.3	0.828	0.067	0.155	0.091	0.013	0.01	0.001	0
2036	Herb, rosemary, dried	1 tsp	1.2	3.972	0.059	0.769	0.511	0.183	0.036	0.028	0.088
2042	Herb, thyme, ground	1 tbsp, leaves	2.7	7.452	0.246	1.726	0.999	0.201	0.013	0.032	0.074
18271	Ice cream cone, cake or wafer	1 cone	4	16.68	0.324	3.16	0.12	0.276	0.074	0.131	0.049
18272	Ice cream cone, sugar, rolled	1 cone	10	40.2	0.79	8.41	0.17	0.38	0.147	0.145	0.057
19270	Ice cream, chocolate	.5 cup (4 fl. oz.)	66	142.56	2.508	18.612	0.792	7.26	2.119	0.271	4.488
19264	Ice cream, Eskimo Pie Vanilla Ice Cream Bar w/dark chocolate coating	1 bar	50	165.5	2.05	12.25		12.05			7.25
19262	Ice cream, Klondike Vanilla Ice Cream Bar w/chocolate coating	1 bar (5 fl. oz.)	148	488.4	6.216	35.668		35.668			19.388
19096	Ice cream, light, vanilla, soft serve	.5 cup (4 fl. oz.)	88	110.88	4.312	19.184	0	2.288	0.669	0.088	1.434
19271	Ice cream, strawberry	.5 cup (4 fl. oz.)	66	126.72	2.112	18.216	0.594	5.544			3.425
19095	Ice cream, vanilla	.5 cup	72	144.7	2.52	17	0.504	7.92	2.138	0.325	4.889
7934	Kielbasa, polish, turkey and beef, smoked	2 oz	56	126.56	7.336	2.184	0	9.856	4.631	1.305	3.489
17004	Lamb, domestic, choice, composite, lean (1/4" trim) cooked	3 oz	85	175.1	23.987	0	0	8.092	3.545	0.527	2.89
17002	Lamb, domestic, choice, composite, lean & fat (1/4" trim) cooked	3 oz	85	249.9	20.842	0	0	17.799	7.497	1.284	7.506
18369	Leavening agent, baking powder, double acting, Na Al sulfate	1 tsp	4.6	2.438	0	1.274	0.009	0	0	0	0
18372	Leavening agent, baking soda	1 tsp	4.6	0	0	0	0	0	0	0	0
18373	Leavening agent, cream of tartar	1 tsp	3	7.74	0	1.845	0.006	0	0	0	0
18375	Leavening agent, yeast, Baker's, active	1 tsp	4	11.8	1.532	1.528	0.84	0.184	0.102	0	0.024
11257	Lettuce, red leaf, raw	.5 cup	60	9.6	0.798	1.356	0.54	0.132			
7274	Lunch meat, beef pastrami, cooked, smoked, chopped, pressed/Carl Budding	2 oz	57	80.37	11.172	0.57	0	3.705		0.171	1.71
7272	Lunch meat, beef, smoked, sliced/Carl Budding	2 oz	57	79.23	11.001	0.342	0	3.705		0.171	1.482
7043	Lunch meat, beef, thin slices	1 oz	28.35	50.18	7.969	1.619	0	1.089	0.476	0.057	0.468
7202	Lunch meat, bologna (beef light)/Oscar Mayer	1 slice	28	56	3.29	1.568	0	4.06	2.005	0.132	1.63
7007	Lunch meat, bologna (beef)	1 slice	28	87.08	2.876	1.114	0	7.893	3.421	0.217	3.118
7207	Lunch meat, braunschweiger liver sausage, sliced/Oscar Mayer	1 slice	28	92.68	3.99	0.728	0.056	8.218	4.334	1.044	3.063
7250	Lunch meat, chicken breast, oven roasted deluxe/Louis Rich	1 serving	28	28.28	5.124	0.7	0	0.56	0.23	0.089	0.151
7270	Lunch meat, corned beef, cooked, chopped, pressed/Carl Budding	2 oz	57	80.94	11.001	0.57	0	3.876		0.171	1.596
7253	Lunch meat, franks (turkey & chicken)/Louis Rich	1 serving	45	84.6	5.04	2.385	0	6.075	2.499	1.423	1.728
7029	Lunch meat, ham, slices, regular (11% fat)	1 serving	56	91.28	9.296	2.145	0.728	4.816	2.438	0.442	1.644
7041	Lunch meat, liver sausage (liverwurst)	1 slice (2-1/2" dia x 1/4" thick)	18	58.68	2.538	0.396	0	5.13	2.401	0.468	1.908
7222	Lunch meat, old fashioned loaf/Oscar Mayer	1 serving	28	64.68	3.668	2.24	0	4.564	2.201	0.739	1.568
7051	Lunch meat, olive loaf (pork)	2 slices	57	133.95	6.726	5.244	0	9.405	4.486	1.1	3.334

Chol (g)	Calc (mg)	Iron (mg)	Mag (mg)	Phos (mg)	Pota (mg)	Sodi (mg)	Zinc (mg)	Vit A (RAE)	Vit C (mg)	Thia (mg)	Ribo (mg)	Niac (mg)	Vit B₆ (mg)	Vit B₁₂ (µg)	Vit E (mg)	Fol (µg)	Alc (g)
4.05						913.5											0
0	14.791	0.294	2.954	3.43	24.031	0.238	0.041	3.283	0.428	0.001	0.002	0.049	0.016	0	0.052	1.918	0
0	5.004	0.258	0.72	0.678	3.174	0.138	0.022	1.854	0.279	0	0.003	0.012	0.01	0	0.011	1.08	0
0	5.068	0.048	0.7	4.284	11.228	0.476	0.032	0	0.874	0.006	0.003	0.02	0.035	0	0	0.084	0
0	1.76	0.066	4.73	3.74	45.65	1.43	0.037	0	0.55	0.003	0.004	0.082	0.018	0	0.029	1.21	0
0	4.404	0.294	0.747	1.053	11.415	1.356	0.014	1.527	0.366	0.001	0.004	0.024	0.003	0	0.021	0.54	0
0	15.36	0.351	2.64	0.84	11.46	0.6	0.039	1.872	0.734	0.006	0.005	0.012	0.021	0	0.024	3.684	0
0	51.03	3.337	5.94	5.427	21.978	1.485	0.167	5.13	1.35	0.014	0.011	0.133	0.015	0	0.202	7.398	0
0	1	0.144	1.04	3.88	4.48	5.72	0.027	0	0	0.01	0.014	0.177	0.001	0	0.031	6.92	0
0	4.4	0.443	3.1	10.3	14.5	32	0.075	0	0	0.051	0.041	0.507	0.005	0	0.007	14	0
22.44	71.94	0.614	19.14	70.62	164.34	50.16	0.383	77.88	0.462	0.028	0.128	0.149	0.036	0.191	0.198	10.56	0
14	59.5					34											0
39.96	211.64					108.04											0
10.56	138.16	0.053	12.32	106.48	194.48	61.6	0.466	25.52	0.792	0.046	0.174	0.104	0.04	0.44	0.053	5.28	0
19.14	79.2	0.139	9.24	66	124.08	39.6	0.224	63.36	5.082	0.03	0.168	0.112	0.033	0.198		7.92	0
31.7	92.2	0.065	10.1	75.6	143.3	57.6	0.497	85	0.432	0.03	0.173	0.084	0.035	0.281	0.216	3.6	0.144
39.2		0.694				672		0	8.288								0
78.2	12.75	1.743	22.1	178.5	292.4	64.6	4.48	0	0	0.085	0.238	5.372	0.136	2.218	0.162	19.55	0
82.45	14.45	1.598	19.55	159.8	263.5	61.2	3.791	0	0	0.085	0.213	5.661	0.111	2.168	0.119	15.3	0
0	270.296	0.507	1.242	100.786	0.92	487.6	0	0	0	0	0	0	0	0	0	0	0
0	0	0	0	0	0	1258.56	0	0	0	0	0	0	0	0	0	0	0
0	0.24	0.112	0.06	0.15	495	1.56	0.013	0	0	0	0	0	0	0	0	0	0
0	2.56	0.664	3.92	51.6	80	2	0.256	0	0.012	0.094	0.219	1.59	0.062	0.001	0	93.6	0
	19.8	0.72	7.2	16.8	112.2	15	0.12	225	2.22	0.038	0.046	0.193	0.06		0.09	21.6	
37.05	9.69	1.396			208.05	601.92				0.051	0.131	2.337					0
38.19	7.98	1.288			191.52	815.67				0.051	0.137	2.2					0
11.624	3.119	0.765	5.387	47.628	121.622	407.957	1.128	0	0	0.023	0.054	1.494	0.096	0.729	0.054	3.119	0
12.32	3.64	0.342	3.92	49.84	43.68	322.28	0.535	0	0							3.64	0
15.68	8.68	0.308	3.92	48.16	48.16	302.4	2.548	3.64	4.256	0.007	0.028	0.704	0.048	0.356	0.098	2.52	0
49.84	2.52	2.943	3.92	55.72	56.56	324.52	0.952	1322	2.52	0.064	0.448	2.573	0.092	5.258		13.16	0
13.72	1.96	0.322	6.72	74.48	74.2	332.64	0.204		0								0
37.05	9.69	1.368			200.64	764.94				0.051	0.137	2.394					0
41.4	58.95	0.981	10.35	66.15	72	511.2	0.837		0								0
31.92	13.44	0.571	12.32	85.68	160.72	730.24	0.756	0	2.24	0.351	0.1	1.626	0.184	0.235	0.045	3.92	0
28.44	4.68	1.152	2.16	41.4	30.6	154.8	0.414	1495	0	0.049	0.185	0.774	0.034	2.423		5.4	0
17.08	31.64	0.37	6.44	58.24	82.32	331.52	0.524		0								0
21.66	62.13	0.308	10.83	72.39	169.29	845.88	0.787	34.2	0	0.168	0.148	1.046	0.131	0.718	0.142	1.14	0

EvaluEat Code	Food Name	Amt	Wt (g)	Energy (kcal)	Prot (g)	Carb (g)	Fiber (g)	Fat (g)	Mono (g)	Poly (g)	Sat (g)
13355	Lunch meat, pastrami (beef)	1 slice (1 oz)	28	97.72	4.827	0.854	0	8.17	4.052	0.277	2.918
7052	Lunch meat, pastrami (turkey)	2 slices	57	80.37	10.465	0.946	0	3.54	1.168	0.906	1.032
7225	Lunch meat, pork sausage links, cooked/Oscar Mayer	1 serving, 2 links	48	164.64	7.824	0.48	0	14.64	7.104	1.766	5.131
7226	Lunch meat, salami beef cotto/Oscar Mayer	1 serving, 2 slices	46	94.76	6.532	0.874	0	7.222	3.179	0.359	3.1
7232	Lunch meat, smokie links sausage/Oscar Mayer	1 serving	43	129.86	5.332	0.731	0	11.739	5.663	1.195	4.033
7276	Lunch meat, Spam, pork with ham, minced, canned/Hormel	1 serving, 2 oz	56	173.6	7.414	1.697	0	15.254	7.717	1.652	5.533
7238	Lunch meat, summer sausage thuringer cervalat/Oscar Mayer	1 serving, 2 slices	46	139.84	6.854	0.414	0	12.282	5.585	1.025	4.934
7254	Lunch meat, turkey bacon/Louis Rich	1 serving	14	35	2.114	0.231	0	2.842	1.051	0.658	0.738
7255	Lunch meat, turkey bologna/Louis Rich	1 serving	28	51.52	3.164	1.358	0	3.696	1.487	1.005	1.061
7079	Lunch meat, turkey breast meat	1 slice	28	26.88	2.044	3.822	0.56	0.378	0.151	0.092	0.118
7080	Lunch meat, turkey ham, cured	1 serving , .99 oz	28	35.28	4.9	0.571	0.056	1.355	0.533	0.369	0.427
7266	Lunch meat, turkey salami/Louis Rich	1 serving	28	41.16	4.284	0.112	0	2.632	0.881	0.656	0.779
7242	Lunch meat, wieners (beef franks) bun length/Oscar Mayer	1 serving, 1 link	57	184.68	6.327	1.511	0	17.157	8.333	0.547	7.142
7243	Lunch meat, wieners (beef franks) fat-free/Oscar Mayer	1 serving	50	39	6.6	2.55	0	0.25	0.095	0.024	0.112
7241	Lunch meat, wieners (beef franks)/Oscar Mayer	1 serving	45	147.15	5.108	1.057	0	13.617	6.633	0.612	5.607
22005	Macaroni and Cheese Dinner, Kraft Original Flavor, unprepared	1 NLEA serving (makes about 1 cup prepared)	70	259	11.34	47.53	1.47	2.59			1.26
20100	Macaroni, enriched, cooked	1 cup elbow shaped	140	197.4	6.678	39.676	1.82	0.938	0.111	0.382	0.133
9328	Maraschino cherries, canned, drained	1 cup, balls	154	254.1	0.339	64.634	4.928	0.323	0.075	0.085	0.06
4067	Margarine, hard, corn, soybean-hydrogenated & cottonseed-hydrogenated w/salt	1 tsp	4.7	33.793	0.042	0.042	0	3.783	1.73	1.18	0.705
4611	Margarine, regular, tub, composite, 80% fat, with salt	1 tbsp	12.8	91.648	0.102	0.077	0	10.291	4.616	3.565	1.66
20322	Meal, corn, white, degermed, enriched	1 cup	138	505.08	11.702	107.2	10.212	2.277	0.569	0.98	0.31
20022	Meal, corn, yellow, degermed, enriched	1 cup	138	505.08	11.702	107.2	10.212	2.277	0.569	0.98	0.31
1110	Milk shake, thick, chocolate	1 container (10.6 oz)	300	357	9.15	63.45	0.9	8.1	2.34	0.3	5.043
1111	Milk shake, thick, vanilla	1 container (11 oz)	313	350.56	12.082	55.558	0	9.484	2.739	0.354	5.903
1088	Milk, buttermilk, lowfat, cultured	1 cup	245	98	8.109	11.736	0	2.156	0.622	0.081	1.343
1107	Milk, human, mature breast	1 cup	246	172.2	2.534	16.949	0	10.775	4.079	1.223	4.942
1082	Milk, lowfat, 1% fat w/added vitamin A	1 cup	244	102.48	8.223	12.176	0	2.367	0.676	0.085	1.545
1104	Milk, lowfat, 1% fat, chocolate	1 cup	250	157.5	8.1	26.1	1.25	2.5	0.75	0.087	1.54
1154	Milk, nonfat, dry w/added vit A	.25 cup	30	108.6	10.848	15.594	0	0.231	0.06	0.009	0.15
1097	Milk, nonfat, skim, evaporated, canned	1 cup	256	199.68	19.328	29.056	0	0.512	0.159	0.015	0.31
1085	Milk, nonfat/fat-free, skim w/added vit A	1 cup	245	83.3	8.257	12.152	0	0.196	0.115	0.017	0.287
1079	Milk, reduced fat, 2% fat w/added vitamin A	1 cup	244	122	8.052	11.419	0	4.807	2.042	0.166	2.35
16120	Milk, soy, fluid	1 cup	245	120.05	9.188	11.368	3.185	5.096	0.799	2.041	0.524
1095	Milk, sweetened condensed, canned	1 cup	306	982.26	24.205	166.46	0	26.622	7.427	1.031	16.787
1077	Milk, whole, 3.25% fat	1 cup	244	146.4	7.857	11.029	0	7.93	1.981	0.476	4.551
1102	Milk, whole, chocolate	1 cup	250	207.5	7.925	25.85	2	8.475	2.475	0.31	5.26
1153	Milk, whole, evaporated, canned, w/added vit A	.5 cup	126	168.84	8.581	12.65	0	9.526	2.942	0.309	5.785
1106	Milk, whole, goat	1 cup	244	168.36	8.686	10.858	0	10.102	2.706	0.364	6.507
15250	Mollusks, conch, baked or broiled	3 oz	85	110.5	22.355	1.445	0	1.02	0.284	0.233	0.315
18274	Muffin, blueberry, commercially prep	1 medium	113	313.01	6.215	54.24	2.938	7.345	2.228	2.819	1.579

Chol (g)	Calc (mg)	Iron (mg)	Mag (mg)	Phos (mg)	Pota (mg)	Sodi (mg)	Zinc (mg)	Vit A (RAE)	Vit C (mg)	Thia (mg)	Ribo (mg)	Niac (mg)	Vit B$_6$ (mg)	Vit B$_{12}$ (µg)	Vit E (mg)	Fol (µg)	Alc (g)
26.04	2.52	0.529	5.04	42	63.84	343.56	1.193	0	0	0.027	0.048	1.418	0.05	0.493	0.07	1.96	0
30.78	5.13	0.946	7.98	114	148.2	595.65	1.231	0	0	0.031	0.142	2.01	0.154	0.137	0.125	2.85	0
36.96	7.68	0.826	8.64	75.84	114.24	401.28	1.248	0									0
38.18	3.22	1.247	7.82	103.04	95.22	602.14	0.961	0									0
27.09	4.3	0.503	7.31	103.2	77.4	433.01	0.899	0									0
39.2	7.84	0.504	7.84		128.24	766.64	1.008	0	0.504							1.68	0
38.64	4.14	1.03	6.9	59.8	104.88	657.8	0.98		0	0.106	0.133	2.019	0.138	1.73		2.3	0
12.6	5.6	0.203	2.66	27.86	29.12	169.82	0.353	0	0							1.12	0
18.76	34.72	0.459	6.16	54.88	42.56	301.56	0.518	0	0							1.68	0
3.36	3.08	0.33	5.88	45.36	58.52	47.04	0.372	0	0	0.003	0.01	0.489	0.036	0.025	0.025	1.12	0
20.16	2.24	0.655	6.16	82.32	80.36	311.92	0.725	1.96	0	0.008	0.042	0.593	0.059	0.064	0.179	1.96	0
21.28	11.2	0.35	6.16	74.48	60.48	281.12	0.65		0								0
33.63	7.41	0.889	8.55	59.85	90.06	584.25	1.283	0	0							6.27	0
15	10	0.975	9.5	64.5	233.5	463.5	1.205		0								0
25.2	4.5	0.603	5.85	63	58.5	461.25	0.985	0	0	0.015	0.045	1.031	0.032	0.734		2.7	0
9.8	92.4	2.562		264.6	296.1	561.4			0.35	0.672	0.413	4.536				65.1	
0	9.8	1.96	25.2	75.6	43.4	1.4	0.742	0	0	0.286	0.137	2.341	0.049	0	0.084	107.8	0
0	83.16	0.662	6.16	4.62	32.34	6.16	0.4	3.08	0	0	0	0.006	0.008	0	0.077	0	0
0	1.41	0	0.141	1.081	1.974	44.321	0	38.49	0.009	0	0.002	0.001	0	0.005	0.517	0.047	0
0	3.328	0	0.256	2.56	4.864	138.112	0	104.8	0.013	0.001	0.004	0.003	0.001	0.01	0.64	0.128	0
0	6.9	5.699	55.2	115.92	223.56	4.14	0.994	0	0	0.987	0.562	6.947	0.355	0	0.207	321.5	0
0	6.9	5.699	55.2	115.92	223.56	4.14	0.994	15.18	0	0.987	0.562	6.947	0.355	0	0.207	321.5	0
33	396	0.93	48	378	672	333	1.44	54	0	0.141	0.666	0.372	0.075	0.96	0.15	15	0
37.56	456.98	0.313	37.56	359.95	572.79	297.35	1.221	78.25	0	0.094	0.61	0.457	0.131	1.628	0.157	21.91	0
9.8	284.2	0.123	26.95	218.05	369.95	257.25	1.029	17.15	2.45	0.083	0.377	0.142	0.083	0.539	0.123	12.25	0
34.44	78.72	0.074	7.38	34.44	125.46	41.82	0.418	150.1	12.3	0.034	0.089	0.435	0.027	0.123	0.197	12.3	0
12.2	263.52	0.854	26.84	217.16	290.36	122	2.123	141.5	0	0.049	0.451	0.227	0.09	1.074	0.024	12.2	0
7.5	287.5	0.6	32.5	257.5	425	152.5	1.025	145	2.25	0.095	0.415	0.317	0.103	0.85	0.05	12.5	0
6	377.1	0.096	33	290.4	538.2	160.5	1.224	195.9	2.04	0.124	0.465	0.285	0.108	1.209	0	15	0
10.24	742.4	0.742	69.12	499.2	849.92	294.4	2.304	302.1	3.072	0.115	0.791	0.445	0.141	0.614	0	23.04	0
4.9	222.95	1.225	22.05	181.3	237.65	107.8	2.082	149.5	0	0.11	0.446	0.23	0.091	1.298	0.024	12.25	0
19.52	270.84	0.244	26.84	224.48	341.6	114.68	1.171	134.2	0.488	0.095	0.451	0.224	0.093	1.122	0.073	12.2	0
0	9.8	1.421	46.55	120.05	345.45	29.4	0.564	4.9	0	0.394	0.171	0.36	0.1	0	0.024	4.9	0
104.04	869.04	0.581	79.56	774.18	1135.26	388.62	2.876	226.4	7.956	0.275	1.273	0.643	0.156	1.346	0.49	33.66	0
24.4	246.44	0.073	24.4	204.96	324.52	104.92	0.927	68.32	0	0.107	0.447	0.261	0.088	1.074	0.146	12.2	0
30	280	0.6	32.5	252.5	417.5	150	1.025	65	2.25	0.093	0.405	0.313	0.1	0.825	0.15	12.5	0
36.54	328.86	0.239	30.24	255.78	381.78	133.56	0.97	141.1	2.394	0.059	0.398	0.244	0.063	0.202		10.08	0
26.84	326.96	0.122	34.16	270.84	497.76	122	0.732	139.1	3.172	0.117	0.337	0.676	0.112	0.171	0.171	2.44	0
55.25	83.3	1.199	202.3	184.45	138.55	130.05	1.454	5.95	0	0.051	0.068	0.884	0.051	4.463	5.381	152.2	0
33.9	64.41	1.819	18.08	222.61	138.99	505.11	0.554	25.99	1.243	0.158	0.136	1.243	0.025	0.655	0.938	83.62	0

EvaluEat Code	Food Name	Amt	Wt (g)	Energy (kcal)	Prot (g)	Carb (g)	Fiber (g)	Fat (g)	Mono (g)	Poly (g)	Sat (g)
18279	Muffin, corn, commercially prep	1 medium	113	344.65	6.667	57.517	3.842	9.492	2.378	3.633	1.53
18283	Muffin, oatbran	1 medium	113	305.1	7.91	54.579	5.198	8.362	1.915	4.666	1.228
18639	Muffin, Thomas' English Muffins, plain/Best Foods	1 serving	57	131.67	4.959	25.992		0.855	1.052	1.86	0.697
20134	Noodles, rice, cooked	1 cup	176	191.84	1.602	43.824	1.76	0.352	0.046	0.04	0.04
22702	Noodles, alfredo egg noodles in a creamy sauce, dry mix/Lipton	1 cup	93	388.74	14.415	58.032		10.974	3.586	1.157	4.25
20113	Noodles, Chinese, chow mein	1 cup	45	237.15	3.771	25.893	1.755	13.842	3.46	7.799	1.973
20110	Noodles, egg, enriched, cooked w/salt	1 cup	160	212.8	7.6	39.744	1.76	2.352	0.688	0.653	0.496
20115	Noodles, Japanese, soba, cooked	1 cup	114	112.86	5.768	24.442		0.114	0.03	0.035	0.022
12062	Nuts, almonds, dried, blanched	1 tbsp	9.1	52.871	1.997	1.815	0.946	4.606	2.938	1.097	0.354
12566	Nuts, almonds, oil roast, blanched w/salt	1 oz (24 whole kernels)	28.35	173.79	5.398	5.109	3.175	16.026	10.406	3.363	1.519
12077	Nuts, beechnuts, dried	1 oz	28.35	163.3	1.758	9.497		14.175	6.206	5.695	1.621
12078	Nuts, brazilnuts, dried, unblanched	1 oz (6–8 kernels)	28.35	185.98	4.06	3.479	2.126	18.833	6.959	5.834	4.291
12084	Nuts, butternuts, dried	1 oz	28.35	173.5	7.059	3.416	1.332	16.154	2.955	12.117	0.37
12087	Nuts, cashew nuts, raw	1 oz	28.35	160.46	5.165	7.691	0.936	13.302	7.218	2.379	2.361
12585	Nuts, cashews, dry roasted w/salt	1 oz	28.35	162.73	4.34	9.268	0.851	13.14	7.744	2.222	2.596
12094	Nuts, chestnuts, Chinese, dried	1 oz	28.35	102.91	1.933	22.612		0.513	0.268	0.133	0.075
12116	Nuts, coconut cream, canned (liquid expressed from grated meat)	1 cup	296	568.32	7.962	24.716	6.512	52.451	2.232	0.574	46.51
12119	Nuts, coconut water (liquid from coconuts)	1 cup	240	45.6	1.728	8.904	2.64	0.48	0.019	0.005	0.422
12109	Nuts, coconut, sweetened, flakes, dried	1 cup	74	350.76	2.427	35.217	3.182	23.791	1.012	0.26	21.097
12108	Nuts, coconut, unsweetened, dried	1 oz	28.35	187.11	1.95	6.705	4.621	18.294	0.778	0.2	16.221
12122	Nuts, filberts/hazelnuts, dry roasted, unblanched, w/o salt	1 oz	28.35	183.14	4.261	4.99	2.665	17.69	13.213	2.399	1.279
12132	Nuts, macadamia nuts, dry roasted, without salt added	1 oz (10–12 kernels)	28.35	203.55	2.208	3.793	2.268	21.569	16.804	0.425	3.387
12635	Nuts, mixed w/peanuts, dry roasted w/salt	1 oz	28.35	168.4	4.905	7.187	2.552	14.586	8.9	3.053	1.956
12142	Nuts, pecans, dried	1 oz (20 halves)	28.35	195.9	2.6	3.929	2.722	20.403	11.567	6.128	1.752
12147	Nuts, pine nut, pignolias, dried	1 oz (167 kernels)	28.35	190.8	3.881	3.708	1.049	19.383	5.32	9.674	1.389
12652	Nuts, pistachios, dry roasted w/salt	1 oz (49 kernels)	28.35	161.03	6.053	7.592	2.92	13.032	6.865	3.94	1.575
12154	Nuts, walnut, black, dried	1 oz	28.35	175.2	6.821	2.809	1.928	16.727	4.254	9.944	0.955
4589	Oil, fish, cod liver	1 tbsp	13.6	122.67	0	0	0	13.6	6.353	3.066	3.075
4582	Oil, vegetable, canola	1 tbsp	14	123.76	0	0	0	14	8.246	4.144	0.994
4047	Oil, vegetable, coconut	1 tbsp	13.6	117.23	0	0	0	13.6	0.789	0.245	11.764
4518	Oil, vegetable/salad/cooking, corn	1 tbsp	13.6	120.22	0	0	0	13.6	3.291	7.983	1.727
4053	Oil, vegetable/salad/cooking, olive	1 tbsp	13.5	119.34	0	0	0	13.5	9.977	1.35	1.816
4042	Oil, vegetable/salad/cooking, peanut	1 tbsp	13.5	119.34	0	0	0	13.5	6.237	4.32	2.282
4510	Oil, vegetable/salad/cooking, safflower, linoleic >70%	1 tbsp	13.6	120.22	0	0	0	13.6	1.952	10.149	0.844
4511	Oil, vegetable/salad/cooking, safflower, oleic >70%	1 tbsp	13.6	120.22	0	0	0	13.6	10.152	1.952	0.844
4058	Oil, vegetable/salad/cooking, sesame	1 tbsp	13.6	120.22	0	0	0	13.6	5.399	5.671	1.931
4044	Oil, vegetable/salad/cooking, soybean	1 tbsp	13.6	120.22	0	0	0	13.6	3.169	7.874	1.958
11294	Onions, sweet, raw	1 oz	28.34	9.636	0.227	2.14	0.255	0.023			
11292	Onions, young green, tops only	1 tbsp chopped	6	1.86	0.108	0.339	0.21	0.006	0.001	0.002	0.001
18499	Pancake/waffle, buttermilk, Eggo/Kellogg	1 oz	28.34	66.032	1.7	10.798	0.312	1.896	0.833	0.604	0.408

Chol (g)	Calc (mg)	Iron (mg)	Mag (mg)	Phos (mg)	Pota (mg)	Sodi (mg)	Zinc (mg)	Vit A (RAE)	Vit C (mg)	Thia (mg)	Ribo (mg)	Niac (mg)	Vit B_6 (mg)	Vit B_{12} (μg)	Vit E (mg)	Fol (μg)	Alc (g)
29.38	83.62	3.175	36.16	320.92	77.97	588.73	0.61	58.76	0	0.308	0.368	2.302	0.095	0.102	0.904	90.4	0
0	71.19	4.746	177.41	424.88	572.91	444.09	2.079	0	0	0.296	0.107	0.475	0.182	0.011	0.746	100.6	0
	76.38	1.704				210.33		0	0.057					0.205	0.994	82.65	0
0	7.04	0.246	5.28	35.2	7.04	33.44	0.44	0	0	0.032	0.007	0.127	0.011	0		5.28	0
104.16	118.11	2.809				1646.1											0
0	9	2.128	23.4	72.45	54	197.55	0.63	0	0	0.26	0.189	2.677	0.049	0	1.566	40.5	0
52.8	19.2	2.544	30.4	110.4	44.8	11.2	0.992	9.6	0	0.298	0.133	2.379	0.058	0.144	0.256	102.4	0
0	4.56	0.547	10.26	28.5	39.9	68.4	0.137	0	0	0.107	0.03	0.581	0.046	0		7.98	0
0	19.656	0.339	25.025	43.68	62.517	2.548	0.284	0	0	0.018	0.051	0.333	0.011	0	2.249	2.73	0
0	54.999	1.503	82.215	163.58	196.466	219.996	0.403		0.284	0.022	0.079	1.106	0.026	0	1.573	18	0
0	0.284	0.697	0	0	288.32	10.773	0.102	0	4.394	0.086	0.105	0.249	0.194	0		32.04	0
0	45.36	0.689	106.596	205.538	186.827	0.851	1.151	0	0.198	0.175	0.01	0.084	0.029	0	1.624	6.237	0
0	15.026	1.14	67.19	126.441	119.354	0.284	0.887	1.701	0.907	0.109	0.042	0.296	0.159	0	0.992	18.71	0
0	10.49	1.894	82.782	168.116	187.11	3.402	1.639	0	0.142	0.12	0.016	0.301	0.118	0	0.255	7.088	
0	12.758	1.701	73.71	138.915	160.178	181.44	1.588	0	0	0.057	0.057	0.397	0.073	0	0.261	19.56	0
0	8.222	0.649	38.84	43.943	205.821	1.418	0.4	4.536	16.59	0.074	0.083	0.369	0.189	0		31.19	0
0	2.96	1.51	50.32	65.12	298.96	148	1.776	0	5.328	0.065	0.118	0.112	0.086	0	0.385	41.44	0
0	57.6	0.696	60	48	600	252	0.24	0	5.76	0.072	0.137	0.192	0.077	0	0	7.2	0
0	10.36	1.332	35.52	74	233.84	189.44	1.295	0	0	0.022	0.015	0.222	0.193	0	0.281	5.92	0
0	7.371	0.941	25.515	58.401	153.941	10.49	0.57	0	0.425	0.017	0.028	0.171	0.085	0	0.125	2.552	0
0	34.871	1.242	49.046	87.885	214.043	0	0.709	0.851	1.077	0.096	0.035	0.581	0.176	0	4.332	24.95	0
0	19.845	0.751	33.453	56.133	102.911	1.134	0.366	0	0.198	0.201	0.025	0.645	0.102	0	0.162	2.835	0
0	19.845	1.049	63.788	123.323	169.25	189.662	1.077	0	0.113	0.057	0.057	1.332	0.084	0	3.101	14.18	0
0	19.845	0.717	34.304	78.53	116.235	0	1.284	0.851	0.312	0.187	0.037	0.331	0.06	0	0.397	6.237	0
0	4.536	1.568	71.159	163.013	169.25	0.567	1.829	0.284	0.227	0.103	0.064	1.244	0.027	0	2.645	19	0
0	31.185	1.191	34.02	137.498	295.407	114.818	0.652	3.686	0.652	0.238	0.045	0.404	0.361	0	0.547	14.18	0
0	17.294	0.885	56.984	145.436	148.271	0.567	0.955	0.567	0.482	0.016	0.037	0.133	0.165	0	0.51	8.789	0
77.52	0	0	0	0	0	0	0	4080	0			0	0	0	0	0	0
0	0	0	0	0	0	0	0	0	0	0	0	0	0	0	2.394	0	0
0	0	0.005	0	0	0	0	0	0	0	0	0	0	0	0	0.012	0	0
0	0	0	0	0	0	0	0	0	0	0	0	0	0	0	1.945	0	0
0	0.135	0.089	0	0	0.135	0.405	0	0	0	0	0	0	0	0	1.937	0	0
0	0	0.004	0	0	0	0	0.001	0	0	0	0	0	0	0	2.118	0	0
0	0	0	0	0	0	0	0	0	0	0	0	0	0	0	4.638	0	0
0	0	0	0	0	0	0	0	0	0	0	0	0	0	0	4.638	0	0
0	0	0	0	0	0	0	0	0	0	0	0	0	0	0	0.19	0	0
0	0	0.003	0	0	0	0	0	0	0	0	0	0	0	0	1.253	0	0
	5.668	0.074	2.551	7.652	33.725	2.267	0.037	0	1.36	0.012	0.006	0.038	0.037			6.518	0
0	3.66	0.115	1.2	1.98	15.6	0.24	0.027	12	2.736	0.004	0.008	0.012	0.004	0	0.013	0.84	0
3.117	9.919	0.879	5.101	96.639	29.19	150.202	0.17		0.397	0.074	0.082	0.978	0.099	0.292	0	14.74	0

EvaluEat Code	Food Name	Amt	Wt (g)	Energy (kcal)	Prot (g)	Carb (g)	Fiber (g)	Fat (g)	Mono (g)	Poly (g)	Sat (g)
18294	Pancakes, blueberry, homemade	1 pancake (4" dia)	38	84.36	2.318	11.02		3.496	0.88	1.582	0.755
18390	Pancakes, buttermilk, homemade	1 pancake (4" dia)	38	86.26	2.584	10.906		3.534	0.897	1.705	0.696
18293	Pancakes, plain, homemade	1 pancake (4" dia)	38	86.26	2.432	10.754		3.686	0.94	1.69	0.806
18288	Pancakes, plain/buttermilk, frozen	1 pancake (6" dia)	73	167.17	3.796	31.828	1.314	2.409	0.881	0.703	0.56
22515	Pasta, beef ravioli in tomato & meat sauce, canned entree/Chef Boyardee	1 serving	244	229.36	8.369	36.893	3.66	5.392	2.001	0.22	2.489
22516	Pasta, beefaroni, macaroni w/beef in tomato sauce, canned entree/Chef Boyardee	1 serving	212	184.44	8.247	31.143	2.968	2.947	1.272	0.254	1.187
22517	Pasta, mini beef ravioli in tomato & meat sauce, canned entree/Chef Boyardee	1 package	425	403.75	14.833	68.51	5.525	7.99	3.4	0.298	2.975
22518	Pasta, spaghetti & meatballs in tomato sauce, canned entree/Chef Boyardee	1 package	425	442	16.065	60.307	3.825	15.3	6.503	0.68	6.843
20121	Pasta, spaghetti, enriched, cooked w/o salt	1 cup	140	197.4	6.678	39.676	2.38	0.938	0.111	0.382	0.133
20125	Pasta, spaghetti, whole wheat, cooked	1 cup	140	173.6	7.462	37.156	6.3	0.756	0.105	0.298	0.139
22701	Pasta, whole wheat macaroni and cheese dinner, dry mix/Hodgson Mill	1 package	206	774.56	29.046	142.55	15.656	9.682			2.822
18635	Pastry, cinnamon rolls w/icing, refrigerated dough/Pillsbury	1 serving	44	150.04	2.376	23.892		5.016			1.25
18237	Pastry, cream puff/eclair shell, homemade	1 eclair (5" x 2" x 1-3/4")	48	173.76	4.32	10.944	0.384	12.432	5.341	3.542	2.688
18239	Pastry, croissant, butter	1 croissant, mini	28	113.68	2.296	12.824	0.728	5.88	1.547	0.306	3.265
18241	Pastry, croissant, cheese	1 croissant, small	42	173.88	3.864	19.74	1.092	8.778	2.734	1.001	4.464
18245	Pastry, Danish, cheese	1 pastry	71	265.54	5.68	26.412	0.71	15.549	8.032	1.828	4.824
18246	Pastry, Danish, fruit (apple/cinnamon/raisin/lemon/ raspberry/strawberry) enriched	1 toaster strudel	53	196.63	2.862	25.334	1.007	9.805	5.314	1.253	2.576
18247	Pastry, Danish, nut (almond/raisin nut/cinnamon nut)	1 pastry (4-1/4" dia)	65	279.5	4.615	29.705	1.3	16.38	8.895	2.783	3.784
18257	Pastry, eclair/cream puff, homemade, custard filled w/chocolate icing	1 cream puff (3-1/2" x 2")	112	293.44	7.168	27.104	0.672	17.584	7.262	4.422	4.613
18338	Pastry, phyllo dough	1 sheet dough	19	56.81	1.349	9.994	0.361	1.14	0.598	0.175	0.279
18354	Pastry, strudel, apple	1 piece	71	194.54	2.343	29.181	1.562	7.952	2.32	3.774	1.451
16097	Peanut butter, chunky w/salt	2 tbsp	32	188.48	8.022	6.749	2.112	15.904	7.539	4.532	3.066
16098	Peanut butter, smooth w/salt	2 tbsp	32	191.68	7.99	5.894	1.888	16.73	7.919	4.764	3.209
16390	Peanuts, all types, dry roasted w/o salt	1 oz	28.35	165.85	6.713	6.098	2.268	14.079	6.985	4.449	1.954
16090	Peanuts, all types, dry roasted w/salt	1 oz	28.35	165.85	6.713	6.098	2.268	14.079	6.985	4.449	1.954
16087	Peanuts, all types, raw	1 oz	28.35	160.75	7.314	4.573	2.41	13.96	6.926	4.411	1.937
16138	Peas, chickpea/garbanzo, falafel, homemade	1 patty (approx 2-1/4" dia)	17	56.61	2.263	5.413		3.026	1.729	0.707	0.405
16158	Peas, chickpea/garbanzo, hummus, commercial	1 tbsp	14	23.24	1.106	2.001	0.84	1.344	0.565	0.506	0.201
16363	Peas, cowpea, common (blackeyed, crowder, southern) mature seed, boiled w/salt	1 cup	171	198.36	13.218	35.5	11.115	0.906	0.075	0.385	0.236
16065	Peas, cowpeas, common (blackeyed, crowder, southern) mature seed, canned w/pork	1 cup	240	199.2	6.576	39.672	7.92	3.84	1.574	0.55	1.452

Chol (g)	Calc (mg)	Iron (mg)	Mag (mg)	Phos (mg)	Pota (mg)	Sodi (mg)	Zinc (mg)	Vit A (RAE)	Vit C (mg)	Thia (mg)	Ribo (mg)	Niac (mg)	Vit B_6 (mg)	Vit B_{12} (μg)	Vit E (mg)	Fol (μg)	Alc (g)
21.28	78.28	0.654	6.08	57.38	52.44	156.56	0.205	19	0.836	0.074	0.103	0.579	0.019	0.076		13.68	0
22.04	59.66	0.646	5.7	52.82	55.1	198.36	0.236	11.4	0.152	0.078	0.111	0.599	0.017	0.068		14.44	0
22.42	83.22	0.684	6.08	60.42	50.16	166.82	0.213	20.52	0.114	0.076	0.107	0.595	0.017	0.084		14.44	0
6.57	45.26	2.54	10.22	271.56	53.29	371.57	0.482	21.17	0.219	0.277	0.342	2.927	0.058	0.131	0.204	32.85	0
14.64	19.52	2.416			353.8	1173.64			0.244								0
16.96	16.96	1.505				799.24			0.424								0
29.75	38.25	4.08				2018.75			0.425								0
38.25	29.75	3.145				1666			1.7								0
0	9.8	1.96	25.2	75.6	43.4	1.4	0.742	0	0	0.286	0.137	2.341	0.049	0	0.084	107.8	0
0	21	1.484	42	124.6	61.6	4.2	1.134	0	0	0.151	0.063	0.99	0.111	0	0.42	7	0
16.48	234.84	5.397				1258.66											0
						334.4											0
94.08	17.28	0.97	5.76	57.12	46.56	267.36	0.35	133.4	0	0.099	0.173	0.752	0.036	0.187	1.349	25.44	0
18.76	10.36	0.568	4.48	29.4	33.04	208.32	0.21	57.68	0.056	0.109	0.067	0.613	0.016	0.045	0.235	24.64	0
23.94	22.26	0.903	10.08	54.6	55.44	233.1	0.395	85.68	0.084	0.22	0.136	0.907	0.031	0.134	0.605	31.08	0
11.36	24.85	1.136	10.65	76.68	69.58	319.5	0.497	24.85	0.071	0.135	0.185	1.42	0.028	0.121	0.241	42.6	0
60.42	24.38	0.938	7.95	47.17	43.99	187.62	0.286	7.95	2.067	0.139	0.117	1.056	0.023	0.048	0.18	24.91	0
29.9	61.1	1.17	20.8	71.5	61.75	235.95	0.565	5.85	1.105	0.143	0.156	1.495	0.068	0.136	0.533	53.95	0
142.24	70.56	1.322	16.8	119.84	131.04	377.44	0.683	222.9	0.336	0.129	0.298	0.895	0.066	0.381	2.251	48.16	0
0	2.09	0.61	2.85	14.25	14.06	91.77	0.093	0	0	0.103	0.065	0.774	0.006	0	0.015	16.72	0
4.26	10.65	0.298	6.39	23.43	105.79	190.99	0.135	4.26	1.207	0.028	0.018	0.234	0.033	0.156	1.008	19.88	0
0	16.96	0.653	62.08	125.44	201.92	150.4	1.04	0	0	0.04	0.036	4.38	0.144	0	2.454	29.44	0
0	15.04	0.602	56	105.92	176.64	160	0.938	0	0	0.027	0.034	4.289	0.145	0	2.454	23.68	0
0	15.309	0.641	49.896	101.493	186.543	1.701	0.938	0	0	0.124	0.028	3.834	0.073	0	1.965	41.11	0
0	15.309	0.641	49.896	101.493	186.543	230.486	0.938	0	0	0.124	0.028	3.834	0.073	0	2.211	41.11	0
0	26.082	1.298	47.628	106.596	199.868	5.103	0.927	0	0	0.181	0.038	3.421	0.099	0	2.362	68.04	0
0	9.18	0.581	13.94	32.64	99.45	49.98	0.255	0.17	0.272	0.025	0.028	0.177	0.021	0		15.81	0
0	5.32	0.342	9.94	24.64	31.92	53.06	0.256	0.28	0	0.025	0.009	0.081	0.028	0		11.62	0
0	41.04	4.292	90.63	266.76	475.38	410.4	2.206	1.71	0.684	0.345	0.094	0.846	0.171	0	0.479	355.7	0
16.8	40.8	3.408	103.2	230.4	427.2	840	2.496	0	0.48	0.151	0.12	1.034	0.108	0		122.4	0

EvaluEat Code	Food Name	Amt	Wt (g)	Energy (kcal)	Prot (g)	Carb (g)	Fiber (g)	Fat (g)	Mono (g)	Poly (g)	Sat (g)
16386	Peas, split, mature seed, boiled w/salt	1 cup	196	231.28	16.346	41.356	16.268	0.764	0.159	0.323	0.106
6962	Peppers, hot, chili, immature green, canned, chili sauce	.5 cup	125	25	0.875	6.25	2.375	0.125	0.085	0.015	0.016
6961	Peppers, hot, chili, mature red, canned, chili sauce	.5 cup	125	26.25	1.125	4.875	0.875	0.75	0.514	0.093	0.1
11339	Peppers, sweet, green, sauteed	1 oz	28.34	35.992	0.221	1.196	0.51	3.358	0.662	1.672	0.451
11921	Peppers, sweet, red, sauteed	1 oz	28.34	41.093	0.295	1.862	0.51	3.613	0.735	1.839	0.501
11942	Pickles, cucumber, fresh, (bread and butter pickles)	1 slice	7	5.39	0.063	1.253	0.105	0.014	0	0.006	0.004
18398	Pie crust, chocolate wafer cookie type, chilled	1 piece (1/8 of 9" crust)	28	141.68	1.428	15.232	0.42	8.708	4.124	2.16	1.885
18618	Pie crust, cookie type Nilla Wafer, ready to use/Nabisco	1 serving	28	143.64	0.98	17.668	0.252	7.588	5.236	0.378	1.442
18335	Pie crust, frozen, baked	1 piece (1/8 of 9" crust)	16	82.24	0.704	7.936	0.16	5.248	2.514	0.645	1.693
18399	Pie crust, graham cracker cookie type, chilled	1 piece (1/8 of 9" crust)	30	145.2	1.23	19.17	0.45	7.32	3.343	2.031	1.528
18336	Pie crust, homemade, baked	1 piece (1/8 of 9" crust)	23	121.21	1.472	10.925	0.391	7.958	3.489	2.098	1.983
18628	Pie, apple turnover, frozen, ready to bake/Pepperidge Farm	1 serving	89	283.91	3.738	31.239	1.602	16.02			4.032
18301	Pie, apple, enriched, commercially prep	1 piece (1/8 of 9" dia)	125	296.25	2.375	42.5	2	13.75	5.485	2.747	4.746
18304	Pie, banana cream, homemade	1 piece (1/8 of 9" dia)	144	387.36	6.336	47.376	1.008	19.584	8.235	4.74	5.412
18305	Pie, blueberry, commercially prep	1 piece (1/8 of 9" dia)	125	290	2.25	43.625	1.25	12.5	5.305	4.405	2.099
18308	Pie, cherry, commercially prep	1 piece (1/8 of 9" dia)	125	325	2.5	49.75	1	13.75	7.296	2.569	3.203
18310	Pie, chocolate creme, commercially prep	1 piece (1/4 of 6" pie)	99	300.96	2.574	33.264	1.98	19.206	11.006	2.374	4.918
18312	Pie, chocolate mousse, no bake mix	1 piece (1/8 of 9" dia)	95	247	3.325	28.12		14.63	4.83	0.773	7.785
18313	Pie, coconut creme, commercially prep	1 piece (1/6 of 7" pie)	64	190.72	1.344	23.808	0.832	10.624	4.646	0.988	4.465
18317	Pie, egg custard, commercially prep	1 piece (1/6 of 8" pie)	105	220.5	5.775	21.84	1.68	12.18	5.037	3.909	2.466
18320	Pie, lemon meringue, commercially prep	1 piece (1/6 of 8" pie)	113	302.84	1.695	53.336	1.356	9.831	3.034	4.122	1.996
18322	Pie, mince, homemade	1 piece (1/8 of 9" dia)	165	476.85	4.29	79.2	4.29	17.82	7.679	4.689	4.425
18323	Pie, peach	1 piece (1/6 of 8" pie)	117	260.91	2.223	38.493	0.936	11.7	4.962	4.386	1.764
18324	Pie, pecan, commercially prep	1 piece (1/6 of 8" pie)	113	452	4.52	64.636	3.955	20.905	12.137	3.596	4.006
18326	Pie, pumpkin, commercially prep	1 piece (1/6 of 8" pie)	109	228.9	4.251	29.757	2.943	10.355	4.395	3.434	1.946
18328	Pie, vanilla creme, homemade	1 piece (1/8 of 9" dia)	126	350.28	6.048	41.076	0.756	18.144	7.614	4.332	5.078
22531	Pizza Rolls Pizza Snacks, hamburger, frozen/Totinos	1 serving	85	231.2	9.35	26.435		9.775			

Chol (g)	Calc (mg)	Iron (mg)	Mag (mg)	Phos (mg)	Pota (mg)	Sodi (mg)	Zinc (mg)	Vit A (RAE)	Vit C (mg)	Thia (mg)	Ribo (mg)	Niac (mg)	Vit B$_6$ (mg)	Vit B$_{12}$ (µg)	Vit E (mg)	Fol (µg)	Alc (g)
0	27.44	2.528	70.56	194.04	709.52	466.48	1.96	0	0.784	0.372	0.11	1.744	0.094	0	0.059	127.4	0
0	6.25	0.5	15	17.5	705	31.25	0.188	36.25	85	0.037	0.037	0.875	0.175	0	0.425	15	0
0	11.25	0.625	15	20	705	31.25	0.188	28.75	37.5	0.012	0.113	0.75	0.175	0	0.45	13.75	0
0	2.267	0.085	2.267	4.251	37.976	4.818	0.017	3.968	50.16	0.012	0.014	0.165	0.056	0	0.397	0.567	
	1.984	0.133	3.401	6.518	54.696	5.951	0.043	39.11	46.14	0.016	0.031	0.27	0.103	0	0.876	0.567	0
0	2.24	0.028	0.14	1.89	14	47.11	0.003	0.49	0.63	0	0.002	0	0.001	0	0.011	0.28	0
0.28	8.4	0.84	11.2	29.4	47.04	188.16	0.23	59.08	0	0.043	0.058	0.599	0.001	0.006	0.792	14.84	0
2.8	11.48	0.496	2.24	23.24	19.32	62.72	0.078			0.046	0.054	0.696	0.006	0.031		8.4	0
0	3.36	0.362	2.88	9.44	17.6	103.52	0.054	0	0	0.045	0.061	0.39	0.011	0.003	0.421	8.8	0
0	6	0.636	5.4	19.2	25.8	168	0.138	57.3	0	0.031	0.052	0.627	0.011	0.006	0.684	10.2	0
0	2.3	0.665	3.22	15.41	15.41	124.66	0.101	0	0	0.09	0.064	0.761	0.006	0	0.071	15.41	0
		1.219				176.22											0
0	13.75	0.563	8.75	30	81.25	332.5	0.2	40	4	0.035	0.034	0.329	0.047	0.012	1.9	33.75	0
73.44	108	1.498	23.04	132.48	237.6	345.6	0.691	87.84	2.304	0.2	0.298	1.518	0.192	0.36	0.576	38.88	0
0	10	0.375	6.25	28.75	62.5	406.25	0.2	55	3.375	0.012	0.037	0.375	0.046	0.012	1.3	33.75	0
0	15	0.6	10	36.25	101.25	307.5	0.225	65	1.125	0.029	0.036	0.25	0.051	0.012	0.95	33.75	0
4.95	35.64	1.059	20.79	67.32	125.73	134.64	0.228	0	0	0.036	0.106	0.671	0.02	0.01	2.707	12.87	0
33.25	73.15	1.026	30.4	219.45	270.75	437	0.57	117.8	0.475	0.048	0.14	0.565	0.028	0.199		24.7	0
0	18.56	0.512	12.8	54.4	41.6	163.2	0.301	17.28	0	0.032	0.051	0.128	0.044	0.077	0.096	4.48	0
34.65	84	0.609	11.55	117.6	111.3	252	0.546	59.85	0.63	0.041	0.218	0.307	0.05	0.451	0.987	21	0
50.85	63.28	0.689	16.95	118.65	100.57	164.98	0.554	57.63	3.616	0.07	0.236	0.733	0.034	0.192	1.198	27.12	0
0	36.3	2.458	23.1	69.3	334.95	419.1	0.363	1.65	9.735	0.248	0.173	1.962	0.107	0	0.248	37.95	0
0	9.36	0.585	7.02	25.74	146.25	315.9	0.105	11.7	1.053	0.071	0.039	0.234	0.027	0	1.1	33.93	0
36.16	19.21	1.175	20.34	87.01	83.62	479.12	0.644	57.63	1.243	0.103	0.138	0.281	0.024	0.113	0.362	38.42	0
21.8	65.4	0.861	16.35	77.39	167.86	307.38	0.491	488.3	1.09	0.06	0.167	0.204	0.062	0.283	1.123	26.16	0
78.12	113.4	1.285	16.38	131.04	158.76	327.6	0.668	104.6	0.63	0.175	0.272	1.24	0.062	0.378	0.567	32.76	0
						417.35											0

EvaluEat Code	Food Name	Amt	Wt (g)	Energy (kcal)	Prot (g)	Carb (g)	Fiber (g)	Fat (g)	Mono (g)	Poly (g)	Sat (g)
22533	Pizza Rolls Pizza Snacks, pepperoni, frozen/Totinos	1 serving	141	384.93	14.382	39.48	2.256	18.894	9.236	2.214	4.991
22554	Pizza, deluxe French bread w/sausage, pepperoni & mushroom, frozen/Stouffer's	1 serving	175	428.75	16.1	44.45	3.5	20.65	8.715	2.52	6.37
22542	Pizza, deluxe w/sausage, green & red pepper & mushrooms, frozen/Celeste	1 serving	167	385.77	16.7	33.233		20.708	7.615	2.421	8.116
22556	Pizza, original pepperoni, frozen, 12"/Tombstone	1 serving	113	311.88	14.464	28.25		15.707	5.311	2.045	6
22557	Pizza, original sausage & mushroom, frozen/Tombstone	1 serving	132	306.24	14.388	31.152		13.728	4.435	2.086	5.069
22903	Pizza, pepperoni, frozen	1 serving	146	400.04	16.191	36.208	2.336	21.112	8.439	2.438	7.066
22902	Pizza, sausage & pepperoni, frozen	1 serving	146	385.44	15.768	36.179	2.336	19.695	7.796	2.599	6.336
22598	Pizza, supreme, sausage, mushrooms, pepperoni, frozen/Red Baron	1 serving	136	344.08	13.6	31.824		18.088	7.167	2.475	6.093
43572	Popcorn, microwave, low-fat and sodium	1 cup	148	634.92	18.648	108.62	21.016	14.06	6.046	5.287	2.094
19436	Popcorn, sugar syrup/caramel, fat-free	1 bag (6 oz)	170	647.7	3.4	153.1	4.25	2.38	0.442	1.078	0.34
10193	Pork back rib, fresh, lean & fat, roasted	1 piece, cooked (yield from 1 lb raw meat)	219	810.3	53.129	0	0	64.78	29.477	5.081	24.068
10857	Pork bacon, Canadian style / Hormel	1 serving	56	68.32	9.453	1.047		2.766	1.394	0.347	1.025
10124	Pork bacon, cured, broiled, pan-fried, or roasted	1 slice, cooked	8	43.28	2.963	0.114	0	3.342	1.482	0.364	1.099
10188	Pork composite (leg/loin/shoulder/sparerib) fresh, lean & fat, cooked	3 oz	85	232.05	23.434	0	0	14.603	6.494	1.233	5.287
10227	Pork composite (loin & shoulder blade) fresh, lean & fat, cooked	3 oz	85	214.2	23.613	0	0	12.546	5.568	1.003	4.505
10134	Pork ham, cured, boneless, extra lean (5% fat) roasted	3 oz	85	123.25	17.791	1.275	0	4.701	2.227	0.459	1.538
10136	Pork ham, cured, boneless, regular fat (11% fat) roasted	3 oz	85	151.3	19.227	0	0	7.667	3.774	1.199	2.652
7953	Pork sausage, pre-cooked	1 serving (1 hot dog)	52	196.56	7.535	0	0	18.221	7.888	2.532	6.064
10863	Pork, fresh, variety meats and by-products, stomach, cooked, simmered	1 serving	56	84.56	11.984	0.05	0	4.066	1.191	0.413	1.674
10220	Pork, ground, fresh, cooked	3 oz	85	252.45	21.837	0	0	17.655	7.863	1.59	6.562
10173	Pork, pig's feet, fresh, simmered	3 oz	85	197.2	18.649	0	0	13.642	6.804	1.309	3.692
19823	Potato chips, without salt, reduced fat	1 cup	146	711.02	10.366	98.988	8.906	30.368	7.008	15.972	6.074
11358	Potatoes, red, flesh and skin, baked	1 potato, large (3" to 4-1/4"dia)	299	266.11	6.877	58.574	5.382	0.449	0.006	0.129	0.078
11356	Potatoes, russet, flesh and skin, baked	1 potato, large	299	290.03	7.864	64.106	6.877	0.389	0.006	0.129	
43109	Pretzels, soft	1 cup	186	628.68	15.252	129.07	3.162	5.766	1.992	1.763	1.293
19311	Pudding, banana, ready-to-eat	1 can (5 oz)	142	180.34	3.408	30.104	0.142	5.112	2.173	1.889	0.795
19183	Pudding, chocolate, ready-to-eat	1 can (5 oz)	142	197.38	3.834	32.66	1.42	5.68	2.414	2.031	1.008
19187	Pudding, flan (caramel custard) dry mix	1 portion, amount to make 1/2 cup	21	73.08	0	19.236	0	0	0	0	0
19289	Pudding, Kraft, JELL-O fat-free Pudding Snacks, vanilla, ready-to-eat	1 NLEA serving	113	103.96	2.373	23.165	0.113	0.226			0.226
19276	Pudding, Kraft, JELL-O fat-free Sugar Free Instant, vanilla, asp & ace, powder	1 NLEA serving	8	26.48	0.064	6.232	0.104	0.072			0.008
19277	Pudding, Kraft, JELL-O Sugar Free Cook & Serve, chocolate, asp & ace, powder	1 NLEA serving	10	31	0.61	7.45	0.93	0.3			0.16
19193	Pudding, rice, ready-to-eat	1 can (5 oz)	142	231.46	2.84	31.24	0.142	10.65	4.558	3.962	1.661

Chol (g)	Calc (mg)	Iron (mg)	Mag (mg)	Phos (mg)	Pota (mg)	Sodi (mg)	Zinc (mg)	Vit A (RAE)	Vit C (mg)	Thia (mg)	Ribo (mg)	Niac (mg)	Vit B$_6$ (mg)	Vit B$_{12}$ (µg)	Vit E (mg)	Fol (µg)	Alc (g)
31.02	102.93					865.74											0
33.25	231	2.712				840			29.93								0
36.74	280.56					764.86											0
31.64	202.27					551.44											0
26.4	200.64					718.08											0
33.58	0	2.613	24.82	221.92	221.92	878.92	1.781	45.26	1.752	0.371	0.352	3.616	0.105	0.058	1.644	54.02	0
30.66	191.26	2.774	26.28	207.32	255.5	854.1	1.606	64.24	3.212	0.372	0.329	3.631	0.098	0.35	1.407	51.1	0
23.12	223.04	2.285				738.48											0
0	16.28	3.374	223.48	390.72	356.68	725.2	5.668	10.36	0	0.518	0.163	3.064	0.252	0	7.415	25.16	0
0	30.6	1.36	45.9	93.5	187	486.2	1.054	3.4	0	0.065	0.099	0.581	0.08	0	0.221	6.8	0
258.42	98.55	3.022	45.99	427.05	689.85	221.19	7.38	6.57	0.657	0.935	0.438	7.774	0.672	1.402		6.57	0
27.44	3.36	0.504	10.64		156.24	568.96	1.008		0.784								0
8.8	0.88	0.115	2.64	42.64	45.2	184.8	0.28	0.88	0	0.032	0.021	0.888	0.028	0.098	0.025	0.16	0
77.35	21.25	0.935	20.4	197.2	300.9	52.7	2.465	1.7	0.255	0.655	0.279	4.187	0.335	0.655	0.17	5.1	0
73.1	20.4	0.842	20.4	192.95	307.7	48.45	2.227	1.7	0.255	0.722	0.275	4.216	0.343	0.629	0.204	5.1	0
45.05	6.8	1.258	11.9	166.6	243.95	1022.55	2.448	0	0	0.641	0.172	3.42	0.34	0.553	0.213	2.55	0
50.15	6.8	1.139	18.7	238.85	347.65	1275	2.1	0	0	0.621	0.281	5.228	0.264	0.595	0.264	2.55	0
38.48	71.24	0.478	6.76	143	159.64	391.04	0.78	9.88	0.364	0.108	0.081	2.106	0.077	0.369	0.276	0.52	0
176.96	8.4	0.689	8.4	72.24	47.6	22.4	1.635	0	0	0.022	0.105	0.773	0.012	0.269	0.05	1.68	0
79.9	18.7	1.097	20.4	192.1	307.7	62.05	2.729	1.7	0.595	0.6	0.187	3.575	0.332	0.459	0.178	5.1	0
90.95	0	0.833	4.25	69.7	28.05	62.05	0.892	0	0	0.014	0.048	0.497	0.032	0.349	0.077	1.7	0
0	30.66	1.971	129.94	281.78	2546.24	11.68	1.475	0	37.52	0.307	0.394	10.22	0.978	0	7.986	14.6	0
0	26.91	2.093	83.72	215.28	1629.55	23.92	1.196	2.99	37.67	0.215	0.149	4.769	0.634	0	0.12	80.73	0
0	53.82	3.199	89.7	212.29	1644.5	23.92	1.046	2.99	38.57	0.2	0.144	4.031	1.058	0	0.12	32.89	0
5.58	42.78	7.291	39.06	146.94	163.68	2611.44	1.748	0	0	0.763	0.539	7.942	0.037	0	1.004	44.64	0
0	120.7	0.185	11.36	97.98	156.2	278.32	0.398	8.52	0.71	0.028	0.209	0.231	0.03	0.256		2.84	0
4.26	127.8	0.724	29.82	113.6	255.6	183.18	0.596	14.2	2.556	0.037	0.22	0.493	0.04	0	0.412	4.26	0
0	5.04	0.017	0	0.21	32.13	90.72	0.008	0	0	0	0	0	0	0		0	0
2.26	85.88	0.045		115.26	123.17	240.69			0.339								
0	11.76	0.006		189.44	2.48	332.32			0								
0	6.9	1.183		21.2	139	108.5			0								
1.42	73.84	0.426	11.36	96.56	85.2	120.7	0.696	35.5	0.71	0.026	0.102	0.229	0.041	0.298	1.954	4.26	0

EvaluEat Code	Food Name	Amt	Wt (g)	Energy (kcal)	Prot (g)	Carb (g)	Fiber (g)	Fat (g)	Mono (g)	Poly (g)	Sat (g)
19218	Pudding, tapioca, ready-to-eat	1 can (5 oz)	142	168.98	2.84	27.548	0.142	5.254	2.244	1.931	0.852
19201	Pudding, vanilla, ready-to-eat	4 oz	113	145.77	2.599	24.747	0	4.068	1.74	1.514	0.644
43282	Quail, cooked, total edible	1 cup	186	435.24	46.686	0	0	26.226	9.097	6.486	7.356
14342	Rice beverage, Rice Dream, canned/Imagine Foods	1 cup	245	120.05	0.417	24.843	0	1.985	1.345	0.309	0.167
18344	Roll, dinner, egg	1 roll (2-1/2" dia)	35	107.45	3.325	18.2	1.295	2.24	1.026	0.395	0.552
18396	Roll, dinner, plain, homemade w/reduced fat (2%) milk	1 roll (2-1/2" dia)	35	110.6	2.975	18.69	0.665	2.555	1.008	0.702	0.628
18347	Roll, dinner, wheat	1 roll (1 oz)	28	76.44	2.408	12.88	1.064	1.764	0.871	0.31	0.419
18349	Roll, french	1 roll	38	105.26	3.268	19.076	1.216	1.634	0.745	0.317	0.366
18350	Roll, hamburger/hot dog, plain	1 roll	43	119.97	4.085	21.264	0.903	1.862	0.478	0.846	0.47
18348	Roll, hamburger/hot dog, whole wheat	1 medium (2-1/2" dia)	36	95.76	3.132	18.396	2.7	1.692	0.432	0.778	0.301
18353	Roll, hard/kaiser	1 roll (3-1/2" dia)	57	167.01	5.643	30.039	1.311	2.451	0.646	0.98	0.345
4017	Salad dressing, 1000 Island, regular, w/salt	1 tbsp	16	59.2	0.174	2.342	0.128	5.61	1.261	2.915	0.815
4635	Salad dressing, 1000 Island dressing, fat-free	1 tbsp	14.6	19.272	0.08	4.273	0.482	0.212	0.05	0.092	0.029
4539	Salad dressing, blue/roquefort cheese, regular w/salt	1 tbsp	15	75.6	0.72	1.11	0	7.845	1.845	4.17	1.485
4367	Salad dressing, French dressing, fat-free	1 tbsp	14	18.48	0.028	4.5	0.308	0.038	0.02	0.009	0.005
4142	Salad dressing, French, low-fat, no salt, diet (5 kcal/tsp)	1 tbsp	16	37.28	0.093	4.685	0.176	2.154	0.944	0.805	0.176
4120	Salad dressing, French, regular w/salt	1 tbsp	16	73.12	0.123	2.493	0	7.17	1.349	3.365	0.904
4636	Salad dressing, Italian dressing, fat-free	1 tbsp	14.6	6.862	0.142	1.278	0.088	0.127	0.034	0.028	0.043
4114	Salad dressing, Italian, regular w/salt	1 tbsp	14.7	42.777	0.056	1.533	0	4.17	0.928	1.902	0.658
4641	Salad dressing, mayonnaise, light	1 tbsp	14.6	47.304	0.128	1.197	0	4.831	1.178	2.621	0.761
4026	Salad dressing, mayonnaise, regular, safflower/soybean oil, w/salt	1 tbsp	13.8	98.946	0.152	0.373	0	10.957	1.794	7.59	1.187
4012	Salad dressing, Miracle Whip Light Dressing / Kraft	1 tbsp	16	36.96	0.096	2.304	0.016	2.976			0.464
4638	Salad dressing, ranch dressing, fat-free	1 tbsp	14.6	17.374	0.036	3.87	0.015	0.28	0.065	0.117	0.075
4640	Salad dressing, ranch dressing, reduced fat	1 tbsp	14.6	32.85	0.15	2.365	0.131	2.526	0.792	0.633	0.194
4015	Salad dressing, Russian w/salt	1 tbsp	15	74.1	0.24	1.56	0	7.62	1.77	4.41	1.095
4016	Salad dressing, sesame seed	1 tbsp	15	66.45	0.465	1.29	0.15	6.78	1.785	3.765	0.93
4135	Salad dressing, vinegar & oil, homemade	1 tbsp	16	71.84	0	0.4	0	8.016	2.368	3.856	1.456
22534	Sandwich, Hot Pockets, beef & cheddar stuffed, frozen	1 serving	142	403.28	16.33	39.192		20.164	6.658	1.221	8.804
22535	Sandwich, Hot Pockets, Croissant Pocket w/chicken, broccoli, & cheddar, frozen	1 serving	128	300.8	11.392	38.912	1.408	11.008	4.378	1.664	3.354
22538	Sandwich, Lean Pockets, glazed chicken supreme stuffed, frozen	1 serving	128	232.96	9.856	34.176		6.272	2.483	0.952	1.92
22364	Sandwich, Sausage Biscuits, breakfast sandwich, frozen/Jimmy Dean	1	48	192.48	4.752	11.568	0.72	14.112			4.306
6140	Sauce, Bulls Eye Original Barbecue/Ridgs	2 tbsp	36	63	0.432	15.156		0.072			
6930	Sauce, cheese, ready-to-eat	.25 cup	63	109.62	4.227	4.303	0.315	8.373	2.408	1.637	3.786
6139	Sauce, Chunky Chili Dip, Salsa, canned/LaVictoria	2 tbsp	30	9.3	0.237	1.962	0.15	0.048			
6901	Sauce, Deluxe Marinara Sauce/Contadina	1 cup	250	145	3.05	17.375	3	7.05	3.428	2.06	1.1
6275	Sauce, Enchilada Sauce/LaVictoria	.25 cup	60	19.8	0.192	2.772	0.42	0.87			
6179	Sauce, fish, ready-to-eat	1 tbsp	18	6.3	0.911	0.655	0	0.002	0	0.001	0.001
6269	Sauce, Green Chile Salsa, mild/LaVictoria	2 tbsp	30	7.5	0.39	1.29	0.12	0.075			
6273	Sauce, Green Salsa Jalapena/LaVictoria	2 tbsp	30	9.6	0.276	1.41	0.27	0.327			
6260	Sauce, Green Taco Sauce, medium/LaVictoria	1 tbsp	15	4.5	0.119	0.873	0.09	0.054			

Chol (g)	Calc (mg)	Iron (mg)	Mag (mg)	Phos (mg)	Pota (mg)	Sodi (mg)	Zinc (mg)	Vit A (RAE)	Vit C (mg)	Thia (mg)	Ribo (mg)	Niac (mg)	Vit B_6 (mg)	Vit B_{12} (µg)	Vit E (mg)	Fol (µg)	Alc (g)
1.42	119.28	0.327	11.36	112.18	136.32	225.78	0.383	0	0.568	0.031	0.139	0.443	0.027	0.298	0.426	4.26	0
7.91	99.44	0.147	9.04	76.84	127.69	152.55	0.282	6.78	0	0.025	0.157	0.285	0.012	0.113	0	0	0
159.96	27.9	8.24	40.92	518.94	401.76	96.72	5.766	130.2	4.278	0.409	0.558	14.731	1.153	0.67	1.302	11.16	0
0	19.6	0.196	9.8	34.3	68.6	85.75	0.245	0	1.225	0.076	0.012	1.909	0.044	0	1.764	90.65	0
17.5	20.65	1.232	8.75	35.35	36.4	190.75	0.392	1.75	0	0.184	0.181	1.15	0.019	0.084	0.126	64.4	0
12.25	21	1.036	6.65	44.1	53.2	145.25	0.245	30.45	0.07	0.138	0.143	1.207	0.021	0.049	0.339	31.5	0
0	49.28	0.994	10.08	29.12	32.2	95.2	0.252	0	0	0.121	0.076	1.14	0.021	0	0.101	16.8	0
0	34.58	1.03	7.6	31.92	43.32	231.42	0.342	0	0	0.199	0.114	1.654	0.015	0	0.114	42.94	0
0	59.34	1.428	9.03	26.66	40.42	205.97	0.284	0	0	0.172	0.137	1.786	0.031	0.086	0.03	47.73	0
0	38.16	0.871	30.6	80.64	97.92	172.08	0.724	0	0	0.089	0.055	1.324	0.07	0	0.324	10.8	0
0	54.15	1.87	15.39	57	61.56	310.08	0.536	0	0	0.272	0.192	2.416	0.02	0	0.239	54.15	0
4.16	2.72	0.189	1.28	4.32	17.12	138.08	0.042	1.76	0	0.231	0.009	0.067	0	0	0.182	0	0
0.73	1.606	0.041	0.584	0.146	17.812	106.434	0.013	0.146	0	0.034	0.007	0.038	0	0	0.109	1.752	0
2.55	12.15	0.03	0	11.1	5.55	164.1	0.041	10.05	0.3	0.002	0.015	0.015	0.006	0.041	0.9	4.2	0
0	0.7	0.081	0.42	0	11.76	111.86	0.014	0.56	0	0.002	0.004	0.016	0	0	0.003	1.96	0
0	1.76	0.139	1.28	2.56	17.12	4.8	0.032	4.32	0	0.004	0.008	0.075	0.009	0	0.458	0.32	0
0	3.84	0.128	0.8	3.04	10.72	133.76	0.046	3.68	0	0.003	0.008	0.03	0	0.022	0.8	0	0
0.292	4.38	0.058	0.73	15.914	14.892	164.834	0.053	0.584	0.058	0.005	0.008	0.02	0	0.045	0.111	1.752	0
0	1.029	0.093	0.441	1.323	7.056	243.138	0.019	0.294	0	0.002	0.003	0	0.009	0	0.735	0	0
5.11	1.168	0.047	0.292	5.11	5.84	98.258	0.026	3.066	0	0.003	0	0	0	0	0.448	0.584	0
8.142	2.484	0.069	0.138	3.864	4.692	78.384	0.017	11.59	0	0	0	0.001	0.08	0.036	3.036	1.104	0
4.16	0.8	0.027		2.08	3.68	131.36			0						0.14		
1.022	7.3	0.153	1.168	16.498	16.206	110.23	0.058	0.146	0	0.004	0.004	0.001	0.004	0	0.026	0.876	0
3.066	18.25	0.127	0.876	28.178	19.272	136.072	0.091	2.628	0.102	0.003	0.004	0.001	0.004	0	0.234	0.584	0
2.7	2.85	0.09	0.3	5.55	23.55	130.2	0.065	2.25	0.9	0.008	0.008	0.09	0.005	0.045	0.603	1.5	0
0	2.85	0.09	0	5.55	23.55	150	0.015	0.3	0	0	0	0	0	0	0.75	0	0
0	0	0	0	0	1.28	0.16	0	0	0	0	0	0	0	0	0.738	0	0
52.54	336.54	2.925				905.96											0
37.12		3.802				651.52			6.272								0
23.04	121.6					561.92											0
15.84	37.92	0.792				440.64											0
						301.68											0
18.27	115.92	0.132	5.67	98.91	18.9	521.64	0.617	50.4	0.252	0.004	0.072	0.015	0.011	0.088	0.2	2.52	0
	4.2	0.012				147.9			3.15								0
0	47.5	1.5	30	65	517.5	937.5	0.325		17.5	0.108	0.08	1.43	0.21	0	0	22.5	0
0	7.2	0.072				394.8			2.64								0
0	7.74	0.14	31.5	1.26	51.84	1389.6	0.036	0.72	0.09	0.002	0.01	0.416	0.071	0.086	0	9.18	0
	4.5	0.273				172.2			4.02								0
0	4.8	0.12				180			3.6								0
0	1.2	0.008				95.1			0.72								0

EvaluEat Code	Food Name	Amt	Wt (g)	Energy (kcal)	Prot (g)	Carb (g)	Fiber (g)	Fat (g)	Mono (g)	Poly (g)	Sat (g)
6175	Sauce, hoisin	1 tbsp	16	35.2	0.53	7.053	0.448	0.542	0.154	0.272	0.091
6555	Sauce, hollandaise, with butterfat, dehydrated, prepared with water	1 cup (8 fl. oz.)	244	224.48	4.441	12.956	0.732	18.593	5.588	0.878	10.931
6308	Sauce, Kraft Barbecue Sauce Hickory Smoke	2 tbsp	34	39.44	0.17	8.908	0.306	0.102			0
6307	Sauce, Kraft Barbecue Sauce Original	2 tbsp	34	39.44	0.17	8.874	0.306	0.102			0
6136	Sauce, mole poblano, homemade	1 cup, sauce	242	396.88	8.567	31.315	10.164	26.499			
6278	Sauce, Nacho Cheese Sauce with Jalapeno Pepper, medium/LaVictoria	.25 cup	72	122.4	1.31	7.387	0.216	9.713	4.553	1.788	2.692
6933	Sauce, Old World Style Smooth Pasta Sauce, Traditional, jar/Ragu	.5 cup	125	80	1.875	12.112	2.625	2.625	0.546	1.29	0.362
6176	Sauce, oyster	1 tbsp	18	9.18	0.243	1.966	0.054	0.045	0.013	0.012	0.008
6931	Sauce, pasta, spaghetti/marinara	1 cup	250	142.5	3.55	20.55	4	5.15	2.175	1.805	0.737
6168	Sauce, pepper or hot	1 tsp	4.7	0.517	0.024	0.082	0.014	0.017	0.001	0.009	0.002
6151	Sauce, plum	1 tbsp	19	34.96	0.169	8.134	0.133	0.198	0.046	0.112	0.029
6274	Sauce, Red Salsa Jalapena/LaVictoria	2 tbsp	30	12	0.435	2.172	0.39	0.177			
6257	Sauce, Red Taco Sauce, mild/LaVictoria	1 tbsp	16	6.72	0.214	1.314	0.08	0.067			
6265	Sauce, Salsa Picante, mild/LaVictoria	2 tbsp	30	8.1	0.357	1.446	0.09	0.087			
6164	Sauce, salsa	1 cup	259	72.52	3.289	16.162	4.144	0.622	0.065	0.298	0.078
6132	Sauce, Sweet N' Sour, ready-to-eat/Nestle Chef-Mate	1 serving	33	40.26	0.158	8.181	0.264	0.785	0.229	0.377	0.122
6133	Sauce, Szechuan, ready-to-eat/Nestle Chef-Mate	1 tbsp	16	20.8	0.23	2.922	0.048	0.912	0.264	0.439	0.119
6112	Sauce, teriyaki	1 tbsp	18	15.12	1.067	2.871	0.018	0	0	0	0
6166	Sauce, white, medium, homemade	1 cup	250	367.5	9.6	22.925	0.5	26.575	11.05	7.155	7.135
6971	Sauce, worcestershire	.5 cup	125	83.75	0	24.325	0	0	0	0	0
7002	Sausage, beerwurst, beer salami (beef)	2 oz (1 slice)	56	154.56	7.84	2.106	0.504	12.617	5.659	1.165	4.725
7005	Sausage, blood	1 slice	25	94.5	3.65	0.322	0	8.625	3.975	0.865	3.35
7013	Sausage, bratwurst (pork) cooked	1 link cooked	85	281.35	11.662	2.074	0	24.803	12.495	2.244	8.6
7019	Sausage, chorizo (pork & beef)	1 link (4"long)	60	273	14.46	1.116	0	22.962	11.04	2.076	8.628
7023	Sausage, frankfurter (wiener) (beef & pork)	1 frankfurter (5 in long x 3/4 in dia, 10 per lb)	45	137.25	5.188	0.774	1.08	12.438	6.151	1.229	4.846
7022	Sausage, frankfurter (wiener) (beef)	1 frankfurter	45	148.5	5.058	1.827	0	13.306	6.437	0.532	5.26
7024	Sausage, frankfurter (wiener) (chicken)	1 frankfurter	45	115.65	5.819	3.055	0	8.766	3.816	1.818	2.493
7025	Sausage, frankfurter (wiener) (turkey)	1 frankfurter	45	101.7	6.426	0.67	0	7.965	2.511	2.25	2.65
7089	Sausage, Italian, (pork) cooked	1 link, 4/lb	83	268.09	16.625	1.245	0	21.331	9.918	2.731	7.528
7037	Sausage, kielbasa (kolbassy) (pork, beef & NFD Milk)	1 oz	28.35	87.885	3.759	0.607	0	7.697	3.668	0.873	2.809
7038	Sausage, knockwurst (knackwurst) (pork & beef)	1 link	72	221.04	7.992	2.304	0	19.944	9.223	2.102	7.351
7057	Sausage, pepperoni (pork & beef)	1 serving, 15 slices	29	135.14	5.901	1.172	0.435	11.681	5.523	0.764	4.667
7059	Sausage, Polish (pork)	1 sausage (10" long x 1-1/4"dia)	227	740.02	32.007	3.7	0	65.194	30.69	6.992	23.449
7919	Sausage, turkey, breakfast links, mild	1 serving	56	131.6	8.635	0.874	0	10.13	2.801	1.85	4.002
16107	Sausage, vegetarian, meatless	1 link	25	64.25	4.633	2.46	0.7	4.54	1.125	2.32	0.732
12220	Seeds, flax seed	1 tbsp	12	59.04	2.34	4.11	3.348	4.08	0.824	2.693	0.384
12016	Seeds, pumpkin/squash kernels, roasted w/o salt	1 oz	28.35	147.99	9.347	3.807	1.106	11.944	3.714	5.445	2.259
12166	Seeds, sesame, tahini made w/roasted & toasted kernels	1 tbsp	15	89.25	2.55	3.179	1.395	8.064	3.045	3.535	1.129

Chol (g)	Calc (mg)	Iron (mg)	Mag (mg)	Phos (mg)	Pota (mg)	Sodi (mg)	Zinc (mg)	Vit A (RAE)	Vit C (mg)	Thia (mg)	Ribo (mg)	Niac (mg)	Vit B_6 (mg)	Vit B_{12} (µg)	Vit E (mg)	Fol (µg)	Alc (g)
0.48	5.12	0.162	3.84	6.08	19.04	258.4	0.051	0	0.064	0.001	0.035	0.187	0.01	0	0.045	3.68	0
48.8	117.12	0.854	7.32	119.56	117.12	1473.76	0.732	144	0.244	0.049	0.171	0.054	0.488	0.732	0.683	12.2	0
0	5.1	0.211		3.06	27.54	417.52			0.068								0
0	5.1	0.211		3.06	27.54	424.32			0.068								0
	58.08	4.477	77.44	198.44	788.92	324.28	1.113	363	0	0.053	0	3.969	0.607			67.76	0
3.6	64.08	0.864				550.8			1.152								0
		1.025				756.25											0
0	5.76	0.032	0.72	3.96	9.72	491.94	0.016	0	0.018	0.002	0.022	0.265	0.003	0.074	0	2.7	0
0	55	1.8	42.5	80	737.5	1030	0.425	92.5	20	0.135	0.1	2.655	0.285	0	5.1	27.5	0
0	0.376	0.023	0.235	0.517	6.768	124.221	0.005	0.376	3.516	0.002	0.004	0.012	0.007	0	0.006	0.282	0
0	2.28	0.272	2.28	4.18	49.21	102.22	0.036	0.38	0.095	0.003	0.016	0.193	0.015	0	0.037	1.14	0
0	6.3	0.051				146.1			9.63								0
0	3.36	0.029				104.8			2.864								0
0	4.5	0.033				178.8			1.83								0
0	77.7	2.512	33.67	67.34	551.67	1124.06	0.647	88.06	36	0.104	0.083	2.15	0.311	0	3.056	41.44	0
0	5.94	0.281	2.31	2.97	21.78	116.49	0.026		0	0.009	0.005	0.066	0.015	0	0.066	0.66	0
0	1.76	0.12	1.6	5.92	12.8	218.08	0.019		0.256	0.002	0.005	0.096	0.008	0.118	0.069	0.64	0
0	4.5	0.306	10.98	27.72	40.5	689.94	0.018	0	0	0.005	0.013	0.229	0.018	0	0	3.6	0
17.5	295	0.825	35	245	390	885	1.025	225	2	0.172	0.463	1.005	0.1	0.7	0.7	20	0
0	133.75	6.625	16.25	75	1000	1225	0.237	6.25	16.25	0.087	0.162	0.875	0	0	0.1	10	0
34.72	15.12	0.969	10.64	75.6	136.64	409.92	1.238	0	0.336	0.138	0.097	1.666	0.129	0.65	0.106	2.8	0
30	1.5	1.6	2	5.5	9.5	170	0.325	0	0	0.018	0.032	0.3	0.01	0.25	0.032	1.25	0
62.9	23.8	0.45	17.85	191.25	220.15	719.1	2.117	0	0	0.531	0.221	3.94	0.348	0.68	0.017	2.55	0
52.8	4.8	0.954	10.8	90	238.8	741	2.046	0	0	0.378	0.18	3.079	0.318	1.2	0.132	1.2	0
22.5	4.95	0.517	4.5	38.7	75.15	504	0.828	8.1	0	0.09	0.054	1.185	0.058	0.585	0.112	1.8	0
23.85	6.3	0.679	6.3	72	70.2	513	1.107	0	0	0.018	0.066	1.067	0.04	0.774	0.09	2.25	0
45.45	42.75	0.9	4.5	48.15	37.8	616.5	0.468	17.55	0	0.03	0.052	1.39	0.144	0.108	0.099	1.8	0
48.15	47.7	0.828	6.3	60.3	80.55	641.7	1.399	0	0	0.018	0.081	1.859	0.104	0.126	0.279	3.6	0
64.74	19.92	1.245	14.94	141.1	252.32	765.26	1.984	0	1.66	0.517	0.193	3.457	0.274	1.079	0.207	4.15	0
18.995	12.474	0.411	4.536	41.958	76.829	305.046	0.573	0	0	0.065	0.061	0.816	0.051	0.456	0.062	1.418	0
43.2	7.92	0.475	7.92	70.56	143.28	669.6	1.195	0	0	0.246	0.101	1.968	0.122	0.85	0.41	1.44	0
34.22	6.09	0.418	5.22	51.04	91.35	518.52	0.792	0	0.203	0.154	0.067	1.571	0.113	0.455	0.084	1.74	0
158.9	27.24	3.269	31.78	308.72	537.99	1988.52	4.381	0	2.27	1.14	0.336	7.816	0.431	2.225		4.54	0
33.6	17.92	0.599	14	103.6	110.32	327.6	1.193	0	17.02	0.04	0.097	2.058	0.213	0.241	0.186	4.48	0
0	15.75	0.93	9	56.25	57.75	222	0.365	0	0	0.586	0.101	2.799	0.207	0	0.525	6.5	0
0	23.88	0.746	43.44	59.76	81.72	4.08	0.5	0	0.156	0.02	0.019	0.168	0.111	0	0.038	33.36	0
0	12.191	4.235	151.389	332.262	228.501	5.103	2.109	5.387	0.51	0.06	0.09	0.494	0.026	0	0	16.16	0
0	63.9	1.342	14.25	109.8	62.1	17.25	0.693	0.45	0	0.183	0.071	0.817	0.022	0	0.038	14.7	0

EvaluEat Code	Food Name	Amt	Wt (g)	Energy (kcal)	Prot (g)	Carb (g)	Fiber (g)	Fat (g)	Mono (g)	Poly (g)	Sat (g)
12023	Seeds, sesame, whole, dried	1 tbsp	9	51.57	1.596	2.111	1.062	4.47	1.688	1.96	0.626
12037	Seeds, sunflower kernels, dry roast w/o salt	1 oz	28.35	165	5.48	6.824	3.147	14.118	2.695	9.323	1.48
15156	Shellfish, abalone, fried	3 oz	85	160.65	16.685	9.393	0	5.763	2.33	1.425	1.399
15159	Shellfish, clams, boiled/steamed (moist heat)	20 small	190	281.2	48.545	9.747	0	3.705	0.327	1.049	0.357
15158	Shellfish, clams, breaded & fried	3 oz	85	171.7	12.104	8.781		9.477	3.863	2.439	2.281
15160	Shellfish, clams, canned, drained	3 oz	85	125.8	21.718	4.361	0	1.658	0.146	0.469	0.16
15157	Shellfish, clams, raw	1 cup (with liquid and clams)	227	167.98	28.988	5.834	0	2.202	0.182	0.64	0.213
15137	Shellfish, crab, Alaskan king, boiled/steamed	1 leg	134	129.98	25.929	0	0	2.064	0.248	0.718	0.178
15138	Shellfish, crab, Alaskan king, imitation surimi	3 oz	85	86.7	10.217	8.687	0	1.113	0.17	0.57	0.221
15243	Shellfish, crayfish, farmed, cooked w/moist heat	3 oz	85	73.95	14.892	0	0	1.105	0.213	0.351	0.184
15229	Shellfish, cuttlefish, cooked w/moist heat	3 oz	85	134.3	27.608	1.394	0	1.19	0.138	0.228	0.201
15148	Shellfish, lobster, northern, boiled/steamed (moist heat)	3 oz	85	83.3	17.425	1.088	0	0.502	0.136	0.077	0.091
15165	Shellfish, mussel, blue, boiled/steamed	3 oz	85	146.2	20.23	6.281	0	3.808	0.862	1.03	0.723
15170	Shellfish, oyster, east, canned	1 oyster	8	5.52	0.565	0.313	0	0.198	0.02	0.059	0.05
15168	Shellfish, oyster, eastern, breaded & fried	6 medium	88	173.36	7.718	10.226		11.07	4.138	2.915	2.813
15245	Shellfish, oyster, eastern, farmed, raw	6 medium	84	49.56	4.385	4.645	0	1.302	0.128	0.496	0.372
15171	Shellfish, oyster, Pacific, raw	1 medium	50	40.5	4.725	2.475	0	1.15	0.179	0.447	0.255
15173	Shellfish, scallops, breaded, fried	2 large	31	66.65	5.602	3.14		3.391	1.394	0.885	0.827
15151	Shellfish, shrimp, boiled/steamed (moist heat)	4 large	22	21.78	4.6	0	0	0.238	0.043	0.097	0.064
15150	Shellfish, shrimp, breaded & fried	4 large	30	72.6	6.417	3.441	0.12	3.684	1.144	1.526	0.626
19097	Sherbet, orange	.5 cup (4 fl. oz.)	74	106.56	0.814	22.496	2.442	1.48	0.392	0.059	0.858
4615	Shortening, household, composite	1 tbsp	12.8	113.15	0	0	0	12.8	5.711	3.952	2.568
4031	Shortening, vegetable fat, soy hydrogenated & cottonseed hydrogenated	1 tbsp	12.8	113.15	0	0	0	12.8	5.696	3.341	3.2
19400	Snack, banana chips	1 oz	28.35	147.14	0.652	16.556	2.183	9.526	0.553	0.179	8.213
19002	Snack, beef jerky	1 piece, large	20	82	6.64	2.2	0.36	5.12	2.261	0.202	2.17
18501	Snack, cereal bar, mixed berry/Kellogg	1 oz	28.34	104.86	1.219	20.632	0.538	2.154	1.417	0.312	0.425
19033	Snack, Chex Snack Mix	1 oz (approx 2/3 cup)	28.35	120.49	3.119	18.456	1.588	4.905			1.568
19004	Snack, corn chips, BBQ flavor	1 oz	28.35	148.27	1.985	15.933	1.474	9.27	2.688	4.584	1.264
19003	Snack, corn chips, plain	1 oz	28.35	152.81	1.871	16.131	1.389	9.469	2.739	4.672	1.29
19401	Snack, Corn Nuts, BBQ flavor	1 oz	28.35	123.61	2.552	20.327	2.381	4.054	2.087	0.913	0.731
19009	Snack, Corn Nuts, plain	1 oz	28.35	126.44	2.41	20.372	1.956	4.434	2.682	0.865	0.689
19008	Snack, corn puffs or twists, cheese flavor	1 oz	28.35	157.06	2.155	15.252	0.312	9.752	5.749	1.349	1.868
19420	Snack, granola bar, hard, peanut butter	1 bar	24	115.92	2.352	14.952	0.696	5.712	1.68	2.899	0.768
19015	Snack, granola bar, hard, plain	1 bar (1 oz)	28	131.88	2.828	18.032	1.484	5.544	1.226	3.374	0.664
19017	Snack, granola bar, hard, w/chocolate chips	1 bar	24	105.12	1.752	17.304	1.056	3.912	0.631	0.305	2.738
19024	Snack, granola bar, soft, chocolate chip, milk chocolate cover	1 bar (1.25 oz)	35	163.1	2.03	22.33	1.19	8.715	2.72	0.637	4.977
19406	Snack, granola bar, soft, nut & raisin	1 bar (1 oz)	28	127.12	2.24	17.808	1.568	5.712	1.182	1.546	2.671
19020	Snack, granola bar, soft, plain	1 bar (1 oz)	28	124.04	2.072	18.844	1.288	4.816	1.067	1.49	2.027
19407	Snack, meat-based sticks, smoked	1 stick	20	110	4.3	1.08		9.92	4.094	0.884	4.16
19031	Snack, Oriental mix, rice-based	1 oz	28.35	143.45	4.907	14.634	3.742	7.252	2.795	3.017	1.073

Chol (g)	Calc (mg)	Iron (mg)	Mag (mg)	Phos (mg)	Pota (mg)	Sodi (mg)	Zinc (mg)	Vit A (RAE)	Vit C (mg)	Thia (mg)	Ribo (mg)	Niac (mg)	Vit B$_6$ (mg)	Vit B$_{12}$ (µg)	Vit E (mg)	Fol (µg)	Alc (g)
0	87.75	1.31	31.59	56.61	42.12	0.99	0.698	0	0	0.071	0.022	0.406	0.071	0	0.023	8.73	0
0	19.845	1.077	36.572	327.443	240.975	0.851	1.5	0.284	0.397	0.03	0.07	1.996	0.228	0	6.03	67.19	0
79.9	31.45	3.23	47.6	184.45	241.4	502.35	0.808	1.7	1.53	0.187	0.111	1.615	0.128	0.586		11.9	0
127.3	174.8	53.124	34.2	642.2	1193.2	212.8	5.187	324.9	41.99	0.285	0.809	6.373	0.209	187.891		55.1	0
51.85	53.55	11.824	11.9	159.8	277.1	309.4	1.241	77.35	8.5	0.085	0.207	1.754	0.051	34.229		30.6	0
56.95	78.2	23.766	15.3	287.3	533.8	95.2	2.321	153.9	18.79	0.128	0.362	2.851	0.094	84.057	0.527	24.65	0
77.18	104.42	31.735	20.43	383.63	712.78	127.12	3.11	204.3	29.51	0.182	0.484	4.007	0.136	112.229	0.704	36.32	0
71.02	79.06	1.018	84.42	375.2	351.08	1436.48	10.21	12.06	10.18	0.071	0.074	1.796	0.241	15.41		68.34	0
17	11.05	0.331	36.55	239.7	76.5	714.85	0.281	17	0	0.027	0.023	0.153	0.025	1.36	0.085	1.7	0
116.45	43.35	0.944	28.05	204.85	202.3	82.45	1.258	12.75	0.425	0.04	0.068	1.417	0.114	2.635		9.35	0
190.4	153	9.214	51	493	541.45	632.4	2.941	172.6	7.225	0.014	1.47	1.861	0.23	4.59		20.4	0
61.2	51.85	0.331	29.75	157.25	299.2	323	2.482	22.1	0	0.006	0.056	0.91	0.065	2.644	0.85	9.35	0
47.6	28.05	5.712	31.45	242.25	227.8	313.65	2.27	77.35	11.56	0.255	0.357	2.55	0.085	20.4		64.6	0
4.4	3.6	0.536	4.32	11.12	18.32	8.96	7.276	7.2	0.4	0.012	0.013	0.1	0.008	1.53	0.068	0.72	0
71.28	54.56	6.116	51.04	139.92	214.72	366.96	76.67	80.08	3.344	0.132	0.178	1.452	0.056	13.754		27.28	0
21	36.96	4.855	27.72	78.12	104.16	149.52	31.85	6.72	3.948	0.088	0.055	1.064	0.05	13.608		15.12	0
25	4	2.555	11	81	84	53	8.31	40.5	4	0.034	0.116	1.005	0.025	8	0.425	5	0
18.91	13.02	0.254	18.29	73.16	103.23	143.84	0.329	7.13	0.713	0.013	0.034	0.467	0.043	0.409		11.47	0
42.9	8.58	0.68	7.48	30.14	40.04	49.28	0.343	14.96	0.484	0.007	0.007	0.57	0.028	0.328	0.304	0.88	0
53.1	20.1	0.378	12	65.4	67.5	103.2	0.414	17.1	0.45	0.039	0.041	0.921	0.029	0.561		5.4	0
0	39.96	0.104	5.92	29.6	71.04	34.04	0.355	7.4	4.292	0.023	0.066	0.056	0.02	0.089	0.022	5.18	0
0	0	0	0	0	0	0	0	0	0	0	0	0	0	0	0.102	0	0
0	0	0	0	0	0	0	0	0	0	0	0	0	0	0	0.102	0	0
0	5.103	0.354	21.546	15.876	151.956	1.701	0.213	1.134	1.786	0.024	0.005	0.201	0.074	0	0.068	3.969	0
9.6	4	1.084	10.2	81.4	119.4	442.6	1.622	0	0	0.031	0.028	0.346	0.036	0.198	0.098	26.8	0
0	11.053	1.389	7.368	27.773	53.279	84.17	1.162		0	0.283	0.312	3.826	0.397	0	0	30.61	0
0	9.923	7.002	17.861	53.015	76.262	288.32	0.593	1.985	13.47	0.441	0.141	4.774	0.441	3.515		14.18	0
0	37.139	0.437	21.83	58.685	66.906	216.311	0.301	8.789	0.482	0.021	0.06	0.466	0.065	0		11.06	0
0	36.005	0.374	21.546	52.448	40.257	178.605	0.357	1.418	0	0.008	0.041	0.335	0.069	0	0.386	5.67	0
0	4.82	0.482	30.902	80.231	81.081	276.696	0.533	4.82	0.113	0.099	0.04	0.427	0.053	0		0	0
0	2.552	0.473	32.036	77.963	78.813	155.642	0.505	0	0	0.012	0.037	0.48	0.065	0	0.561	0	0
1.134	16.443	0.666	5.103	30.618	47.061	297.675	0.108	1.701	0.057	0.075	0.1	0.916	0.038	0.04	1.205	34.02	0
0	9.84	0.576	13.2	33.36	69.84	67.92	0.3	0.24	0.048	0.05	0.022	0.473	0.023	0		4.32	0
0	17.08	0.826	27.16	77.56	94.08	82.32	0.568	2.24	0.252	0.074	0.033	0.443	0.024	0		6.44	0
0	18.48	0.732	17.28	48.96	60.24	82.56	0.463	0.48	0.024	0.043	0.024	0.133	0.014	0.002		3.12	0
1.75	36.05	0.815	23.1	69.65	109.55	70	0.455	2.45	0	0.032	0.087	0.252	0.035	0.199		9.1	0
0.28	23.52	0.61	25.48	67.48	109.76	71.12	0.448	0.56	0	0.053	0.053	0.731	0.034	0.067		8.4	0
0.28	29.4	0.717	20.72	64.4	91	77.84	0.42	0	0	0.083	0.046	0.144	0.028	0.109		6.72	0
26.6	13.6	0.68	4.2	36	51.4	296	0.484	2.6	1.36	0.028	0.087	0.908	0.041	0.2		0	0
0	15.309	0.692	33.453	74.277	92.988	117.086	0.754	0	0.085	0.088	0.04	0.873	0.02	0	1.588	10.77	0

EvaluEat Code	Food Name	Amt	Wt (g)	Energy (kcal)	Prot (g)	Carb (g)	Fiber (g)	Fat (g)	Mono (g)	Poly (g)	Sat (g)
19036	Snack, popcorn cakes	1 cake	10	38.4	0.97	8.01	0.29	0.31	0.092	0.135	0.048
19034	Snack, popcorn, air-popped	1 cup	8	30.56	0.96	6.232	1.208	0.336	0.088	0.152	0.046
19039	Snack, popcorn, caramel coated, no peanuts	1 oz	28.35	122.19	1.077	22.425	1.474	3.629	0.816	1.27	1.023
19040	Snack, popcorn, cheese flavor	1 cup	11	57.86	1.023	5.676	1.089	3.652	1.067	1.691	0.705
19035	Snack, popcorn, oil-popped, yellow corn	1 cup	11	55	0.99	6.292	1.1	3.091	0.899	1.476	0.538
19041	Snack, pork skins, plain	1 oz	28.35	154.51	17.379	0	0	8.874	4.19	1.032	3.223
19042	Snack, potato chips, BBQ flavor	1 oz	28.35	139.2	2.183	14.969	1.247	9.185	1.854	4.641	2.282
19422	Snack, potato chips, light	1 oz	28.35	133.53	2.013	18.966	1.673	5.897	1.361	3.101	1.179
19811	Snack, potato chips, plain, no salt	1 oz	28.35	151.96	1.985	14.997	1.361	9.809	2.79	3.45	3.107
19411	Snack, potato chips, plain, salted	1 oz	28.35	151.96	1.985	14.997	1.276	9.809	2.79	3.45	3.107
19043	Snack, potato chips, sour cream & onion	1 oz	28.35	150.54	2.296	14.6	1.474	9.611	1.735	4.939	2.52
19814	Snack, pretzel, hard, plain, no salt	10 twists	60	228.6	5.46	47.52	1.68	2.1	0.816	0.732	0.45
19047	Snack, pretzel, hard, plain, salted	10 twists	60	228.6	5.46	47.52	1.92	2.1	0.816	0.732	0.45
19053	Snack, rice cake, brown rice & sesame seed	2 cakes	18	70.56	1.368	14.67	0.972	0.684	0.198	0.207	0.097
19051	Snack, rice cake, brown rice, plain	2 cakes	18	69.66	1.476	14.67	0.756	0.504	0.185	0.178	0.103
19524	Snack, taco chips	1 oz	28.35	141.18	0.652	19.306	2.041	7.059	1.256	3.651	1.823
19057	Snack, tortilla chips, nacho flavor	1 oz	28.35	141.18	2.211	17.69	1.503	7.258	4.278	1.004	1.389
19056	Snack, tortilla chips, plain	1 oz	28.35	142.03	1.985	17.832	1.843	7.428	4.38	1.029	1.423
19058	Snack, tortilla chips, ranch flavor	1 oz	28.35	138.92	2.155	18.314	1.106	6.747	3.983	0.936	1.293
19059	Snack, trail mix, regular	1 cup	150	693	20.7	67.35		44.1	18.795	14.475	8.325
19062	Snack, trail mix, regular, chocolate chip, salted nuts & seeds	1 cup	146	706.64	20.732	65.554		46.574	19.768	16.483	8.906
19269	Snacks, Fruit Roll Ups, berry flavored w/vit C/ General Mills-Betty Crocker	2 rolls	28	104.44	0.028	23.856		0.98	0.483	0.026	0.277
19423	Snacks, potato chips, fat-free, made with olestra	1 oz	28.35	75.128	1.88	16.783	1.106	0.198	0.071	0.081	0.045
19438	Snacks, Rice Krispies Treat Squares/Kellogg	1 oz	28.34	117.33	0.964	22.814	0.17	2.551	0.709	1.445	0.397
6190	Soup, bean & ham, canned, reduced sodium, prepared with water or ready-to-serve	1 cup	128	94.72	5.363	17.485	5.12	1.318	0.531	0.344	0.323
6474	Soup, bean w/bacon, dry, made w/H₂O	1 cup	265	106	5.485	16.377	9.01	2.147	0.928	0.159	0.954
6978	Soup, beef and mushroom, low sodium, chunk style	.5 cup	125	86.25	5.375	11.975	0.25	2.875	0.493	0.085	2.026
6199	Soup, beef barley, canned/Progresso Healthy Classics	1 cup	241	142.19	11.327	20.003	3.133	1.928	0.689	0.251	0.747
6008	Soup, beef broth or bouillon, canned	1 cup	240	16.8	2.736	0.096	0	0.528	0.216	0.024	0.264
6547	Soup, beef mushroom, canned, made w/H₂O	1 cup	244	73.2	5.783	6.344	0.244	3.001	1.244	0.122	1.488
6070	Soup, beef, chunky, canned	1 cup	240	170.4	11.736	19.56	1.44	5.136	2.136	0.216	2.544
6478	Soup, cauliflower, dry, made w/H₂O	1 cup	256	69.12	2.893	10.726		1.715	0.742	0.64	0.256
6411	Soup, cheese, canned, made w/H₂O	1 cup	247	155.61	5.409	10.522	0.988	10.473	2.964	0.296	6.669
6413	Soup, chicken broth, canned, made w/H₂O	1 cup	240	38.4	4.848	0.912	0	1.368	0.576	0.264	0.384
6417	Soup, chicken gumbo, canned, made w/H₂O	1 cup	244	56.12	2.635	8.369	1.952	1.44	0.659	0.342	0.317
6549	Soup, chicken mushroom, canned, made w/H₂O	1 cup	244	131.76	4.392	9.272	0.244	9.15	4.026	2.318	2.391
6018	Soup, chicken noodle, chunky, canned	1 cup	240	175.2	12.72	17.04	3.84	6	2.664	1.512	1.392
6022	Soup, chicken rice, chunky, ready-to-eat, canned	1 cup	240	127.2	12.264	12.984	0.96	3.192	1.44	0.672	0.96
6024	Soup, chicken vegetable, chunky, canned	1 cup	240	165.6	12.312	18.888		4.824	2.16	1.008	1.44
6015	Soup, chicken, chunky, canned	1 cup	240	170.4	12.144	16.512	1.44	6.336	2.832	1.32	1.896
6203	Soup, cream of broccoli, canned, ready-to-eat/Progresso Healthy Classics	1 cup	244	87.84	2.367	13.322	2.44	2.806	0.92	0.573	0.659
6410	Soup, cream of celery, canned, made w/H₂O	1 cup	244	90.28	1.659	8.833	0.732	5.588	1.293	2.513	1.415

Chol (g)	Calc (mg)	Iron (mg)	Mag (mg)	Phos (mg)	Pota (mg)	Sodi (mg)	Zinc (mg)	Vit A (RAE)	Vit C (mg)	Thia (mg)	Ribo (mg)	Niac (mg)	Vit B$_6$ (mg)	Vit B$_{12}$ (µg)	Vit E (mg)	Fol (µg)	Alc (g)
0	0.9	0.187	15.9	27.7	32.7	28.8	0.399	0.4	0	0.008	0.018	0.601	0.018	0	0.029	1.8	0
0	0.8	0.213	10.48	24	24.08	0.32	0.275	0.8	0	0.016	0.023	0.156	0.02	0	0.023	1.84	0
1.418	12.191	0.493	9.923	23.531	30.902	58.401	0.164	0.567	0	0.018	0.02	0.624	0.008	0.003	0.34	1.418	0
1.21	12.43	0.246	10.01	39.71	28.71	97.79	0.221	4.18	0.055	0.014	0.027	0.16	0.026	0.058	0.013	1.21	0
0	1.1	0.306	11.88	27.5	24.75	97.24	0.29	0.88	0.033	0.015	0.015	0.17	0.023	0	0.551	1.87	0
26.933	8.505	0.249	3.119	24.098	36.005	521.073	0.159	3.402	0.142	0.028	0.08	0.439	0.007	0.181	0.15	0	0
0	14.175	0.55	21.263	52.731	357.494	212.625	0.266	3.119	9.611	0.061	0.061	1.33	0.176	0	1.418	23.53	0
0	5.954	0.383	25.232	54.716	494.424	139.482	0.02	0	7.286	0.059	0.076	1.985	0.19	0	1.551	7.655	0
0	6.804	0.462	18.995	46.778	361.463	2.268	0.309	0	8.817	0.047	0.056	1.085	0.187	0	2.583	12.76	0
0	6.804	0.462	18.995	46.778	361.463	168.399	0.309	0	8.817	0.047	0.056	1.085	0.187	0	2.583	12.76	0
1.985	20.412	0.454	20.979	49.896	377.339	177.188	0.278	3.969	10.58	0.054	0.057	1.142	0.189	0.284		17.58	0
0	21.6	2.592	21	67.8	87.6	173.4	0.51	0	0	0.277	0.374	3.151	0.07	0	0.21	102.6	0
0	21.6	2.592	21	67.8	87.6	1029	0.51	0	0	0.277	0.374	3.151	0.07	0	0.21	102.6	0
0	2.16	0.284	24.48	67.5	52.2	40.86	0.54	0	0.54	0.009	0.015	1.297	0.028	0		3.24	0
0	1.98	0.268	23.58	64.8	52.2	58.68	0.54	0	0	0.011	0.03	1.405	0.027	0	0.223	3.78	0
0	17.01	0.34	23.814	37.139	214.043	96.957	0.108	1.985	1.418	0.049	0.008	0.146	0.124	0	3.215	5.67	0
0.851	41.675	0.405	23.247	69.174	61.236	200.718	0.34	6.804	0.51	0.036	0.054	0.406	0.081	0.014		3.969	0
0	43.659	0.431	24.948	58.118	55.85	149.688	0.434	1.134	0	0.021	0.052	0.363	0.081	0	1.001	2.835	0
0.284	39.974	0.414	25.232	67.757	69.174	173.502	0.352	4.253	0.255	0.03	0.067	0.412	0.057	0		4.82	0
0	117	4.575	237	517.5	1027.5	343.5	4.83	1.5	2.1	0.693	0.297	7.068	0.447	0		106.5	0
5.84	159.14	4.949	235.06	565.02	946.08	176.66	4.584	2.92	1.898	0.603	0.327	6.431	0.378	0		94.9	0
						88.76			33.6								0
0	9.639	0.422	23.247	46.778	365.715	184.842	0.272	0	8.363	0.098	0.02	1.304	0.519	0	0	8.505	0
0	0.85	0.36	3.684	11.903	11.053	99.473	0.142	91.82	0	0.359	0.387	4.615	0.255	0	0	30.89	0
2.56	48.64	1.306	24.32	16.64	202.24	239.36	0.678	44.8	1.408	0.072	0.037	0.415	0.059	0.038	0.499	37.12	0
2.65	55.65	1.325	29.15	90.1	325.95	927.5	0.689	2.65	1.06	0.053	0.265	0.398	0.026	0.026	0.557	7.95	0
7.5	16.25	1.213	2.5	62.5	175	31.25	1.375	122.5	3.75	0.05	0.138	1.413	0.075	0.325	0.275	6.25	0
19.28	28.92	1.856	31.33	118.09	366.32	469.95	1.542		3.615	0.128	0.125	2.919	0.186	0.362	0.268	24.1	0
0	14.4	0.408	4.8	31.2	129.6	782.4	0	0	0	0.005	0.05	1.872	0.024	0.168	0	4.8	0
7.32	4.88	0.878	9.76	34.16	153.72	941.84	1.464	0	4.636	0.039	0.056	0.954	0.049	0.195		9.76	0
14.4	31.2	2.328	4.8	120	336	866.4	2.64	129.6	6.96	0.058	0.151	2.705	0.132	0.624	0.672	14.4	0
0	10.24	0.512	2.56	51.2	104.96	842.24	0.256	0	2.56	0.077	0.077	0.512	0.026	0.179		2.56	0
29.64	140.79	0.741	4.94	135.85	153.14	958.36	0.642	296.4	0	0.017	0.136	0.398	0.025	0		4.94	0
0	9.6	0.504	2.4	72	206.4	763.2	0.24	0	0	0.01	0.07	3.293	0.024	0.24	0.048	4.8	0
4.88	24.4	0.903	4.88	24.4	75.64	954.04	0.366	7.32	4.88	0.024	0.049	0.664	0.063	0.024	0.366	4.88	0
9.76	29.28	0.878	9.76	26.84	153.72	941.84	0.976	56.12	0	0.024	0.112	1.63	0.049	0.049		0	0
19.2	24	1.44	9.6	72	108	849.6	0.96	67.2	0	0.072	0.168	4.32	0.048	0.312	0.336	38.4	0
12	33.6	1.872	9.6	72	108	888	0.96	292.8	3.84	0.024	0.098	4.104	0.048	0.312	0.576	4.8	0
16.8	26.4	1.464	9.6	105.6	367.2	1068	2.16	300	5.52	0.041	0.166	3.29	0.096	0.24		12	0
28.8	24	1.656	7.2	108	168	849.6	0.96	64.8	1.2	0.082	0.166	4.224	0.048	0.24	0.312	4.8	0
4.88	41.48	1.22	14.64	39.04	161.04	578.28	0.268		5.856	0.029	0.059	0.317	0.073	0	0.383	29.28	0
14.64	39.04	0.634	7.32	36.6	122	949.16	0.146	56.12	0.244	0.029	0.049	0.332	0.012	0.244	0.903	2.44	0

EvaluEat Code	Food Name	Amt	Wt (g)	Energy (kcal)	Prot (g)	Carb (g)	Fiber (g)	Fat (g)	Mono (g)	Poly (g)	Sat (g)
6443	Soup, cream of mushroom, canned, made w/H$_2$O	1 cup	244	129.32	2.318	9.296	0.488	8.979	1.708	4.221	2.44
6453	Soup, cream of potato, canned, made w/H$_2$O	1 cup	244	73.2	1.757	11.468	0.488	2.367	0.561	0.415	1.22
6582	Soup, Cup Noodles, ramen, chicken flavor, dry/Nissin	1 container, individual	64	296.32	5.568	36.8		14.08			6.253
6036	Soup, gazpacho, canned	1 cup	244	46.36	7.076	4.392	0.488	0.244	0.024	0.073	0.024
6449	Soup, green pea, canned, made w/H$_2$O	1 cup	250	165	8.6	26.5	2.75	2.925	1	0.375	1.4
6490	Soup, leek, dry, made w/H$_2$O	1 cup	254	71.12	2.108	11.43	3.048	2.057	0.864	0.076	1.016
6428	Soup, Manhattan clam chowder, canned, made w/H$_2$O	1 cup	244	78.08	2.196	12.224	1.464	2.22	0.383	1.291	0.383
6440	Soup, minestrone, canned, made w/H$_2$O	1 cup	241	81.94	4.266	11.231	0.964	2.506	0.699	1.109	0.554
6445	Soup, onion, canned, made w/H$_2$O	1 cup	241	57.84	3.76	8.17	0.964	1.735	0.747	0.651	0.265
6583	Soup, ramen noodle, any flavor, dehydrated, dry	1 container, individual	64	289.92	5.952	41.92	1.536	10.944	4.096	1.667	4.883
6180	Soup, shark fin, restaurant-prep	1 cup	216	99.36	6.912	8.208	0	4.32	1.259	0.737	1.082
6451	Soup, split pea w/ham, canned, made w/H$_2$O	1 cup	253	189.75	10.322	27.957	2.277	4.402	1.796	0.632	1.771
6174	Soup, stock, fish, homemade	1 cup	233	39.61	5.266	0	0	1.887	0.55	0.322	0.473
6499	Soup, tomato vegetable, dry, made w/H$_2$O	1 cup	241	53.02	1.904	9.736	0.482	0.819	0.289	0.072	0.362
6559	Soup, tomato, canned, made w/H$_2$O	1 cup	244	85.4	2.05	16.592	0.488	1.928	0.439	0.952	0.366
6466	Soup, turkey vegetable, canned, made w/H$_2$O	1 cup	241	72.3	3.085	8.628	0.482	3.037	1.326	0.675	0.892
6471	Soup, vegetable beef, canned, made w/H$_2$O	1 cup	244	78.08	5.588	10.175	0.488	1.903	0.805	0.122	0.854
6974	Soup, vegetable chicken, low sodium	.5 cup	125	86.25	6.375	10.95	0.5	2.5	1.119	0.523	0.746
6468	Soup, vegetarian vegetable, canned, made w/H$_2$O	1 cup	241	72.3	2.097	11.978	0.482	1.928	0.819	0.723	0.289
1180	Sour cream, fat-free	1 oz	28.34	20.972	0.879	4.421	0	0	0	0	0
1179	Sour cream, light	1 oz	28.34	38.542	0.992	2.012	0	3.004	0.879	0.113	1.87
43133	Soyburger	1 cup	186	332.94	33.313	24.924	8.556	11.104	2.055	4.382	1.337
2001	Spice, allspice, ground	1 tsp	1.9	4.997	0.116	1.37	0.41	0.165	0.013	0.045	0.048
2002	Spice, anise seed	1 tsp	2.1	7.077	0.37	1.05	0.307	0.334	0.205	0.066	0.012
2007	Spice, celery seed	1 tsp	2	7.84	0.361	0.827	0.236	0.505	0.319	0.074	0.044
2009	Spice, chili powder	1 tsp	2.6	8.164	0.319	1.421	0.889	0.436	0.093	0.194	0.077
2010	Spice, cinnamon, ground	1 tsp	2.3	6.003	0.089	1.837	1.249	0.073	0.011	0.012	0.015
2011	Spice, cloves, ground	1 tsp	2.1	6.783	0.126	1.285	0.718	0.421	0.031	0.149	0.114
2013	Spice, coriander seed	1 tsp	1.8	5.364	0.223	0.99	0.754	0.32	0.244	0.031	0.018
2014	Spice, cumin seed	1 tsp	2.1	7.875	0.374	0.929	0.22	0.468	0.295	0.069	0.032
2015	Spice, curry powder	1 tsp	2	6.5	0.253	1.163	0.664	0.276	0.111	0.051	0.045
2016	Spice, dill seed	1 tsp	2.1	6.405	0.336	1.159	0.443	0.305	0.198	0.021	0.015
2018	Spice, fennel seed	1 tsp	2	6.9	0.316	1.046	0.796	0.297	0.198	0.034	0.01
2020	Spice, garlic powder	1 tsp	2.8	9.296	0.47	2.036	0.277	0.021	0	0.011	0.004
2021	Spice, ginger, ground	1 tsp	1.8	6.246	0.164	1.274	0.225	0.107	0.018	0.024	0.035
2024	Spice, mustard seed, yellow	1 tsp	3.3	15.477	0.823	1.153	0.485	0.949	0.654	0.178	0.048
2025	Spice, nutmeg, ground	1 tsp	2.2	11.55	0.128	1.084	0.458	0.799	0.071	0.008	0.571
2026	Spice, onion powder	1 tsp	2.4	8.328	0.243	1.936	0.137	0.025	0.004	0.011	0.004
2028	Spice, paprika	1 tsp	2.1	6.069	0.31	1.171	0.785	0.272	0.026	0.175	0.044
2030	Spice, pepper, black	1 tsp	2.1	5.355	0.23	1.361	0.557	0.068	0.021	0.024	0.021

Chol (g)	Calc (mg)	Iron (mg)	Mag (mg)	Phos (mg)	Pota (mg)	Sodi (mg)	Zinc (mg)	Vit A (RAE)	Vit C (mg)	Thia (mg)	Ribo (mg)	Niac (mg)	Vit B6 (mg)	Vit B12 (µg)	Vit E (mg)	Fol (µg)	Alc (g)
2.44	46.36	0.512	4.88	48.8	100.04	880.84	0.586	14.64	0.976	0.046	0.09	0.725	0.015	0.049	0.952	4.88	0
4.88	19.52	0.488	2.44	46.36	136.64	1000.4	0.634	70.76	0	0.034	0.037	0.539	0.037	0.049	0.024	2.44	0
		2.182				1433.6											0
0	24.4	0.976	7.32	36.6	224.48	739.32	0.244	14.64	7.076	0.049	0.024	0.927	0.146	0	0.439	19.52	0
0	27.5	1.95	40	125	190	917.5	1.7	10	1.75	0.108	0.068	1.24	0.052	0	0.375	2.5	0
2.54	30.48	0.508	10.16	30.48	88.9	965.2	0.229	2.54	2.54	0.051	0.025	0.254	0.025	0.025	0.178	7.62	0
2.44	26.84	1.635	12.2	41.48	187.88	578.28	0.976	56.12	3.904	0.029	0.039	0.817	0.1	4.05	0.342	9.76	0
2.41	33.74	0.916	7.23	55.43	313.3	910.98	0.747	118.1	1.205	0.053	0.043	0.942	0.099	0	0.072	36.15	0
0	26.51	0.675	2.41	12.05	67.48	1053.17	0.603	0	1.205	0.034	0.024	0.6	0.048	0	0.193	14.46	0
0	10.24	2.733	15.36	69.12	76.8	742.4	0.403	0.64	0	0.422	0.282	3.456	0.039	0.006	1.299	94.08	0
4.32	21.6	2.03	15.12	45.36	114.48	1082.16	1.771	0	0.216	0.058	0.084	1.065	0.056	0.41	6.86	19.44	0
7.59	22.77	2.277	48.07	212.52	399.74	1006.94	1.316	22.77	1.518	0.147	0.076	1.475	0.068	0.253		2.53	0
2.33	6.99	0.023	16.31	130.48	335.52	363.48	0.14	4.66	0.233	0.077	0.177	2.763	0.086	1.608	0.396	4.66	0
0	7.23	0.603	19.28	28.92	98.81	1091.73	0.169	9.64	5.784	0.055	0.043	0.752	0.048	0	0.337	9.64	0
0	12.2	1.757	7.32	34.16	263.52	695.4	0.244	29.28	66.37	0.088	0.051	1.418	0.112	0	2.318	14.64	0
2.41	16.87	0.771	4.82	40.97	175.93	906.16	0.603	122.9	0	0.029	0.039	1.005	0.048	0.169	0.142	4.82	0
4.88	17.08	1.122	4.88	41.48	173.24	790.56	1.537	95.16	2.44	0.037	0.049	1.032	0.076	0.317	0.366	9.76	0
8.75	13.75	0.763	5	55	191.25	43.75	1.125	172.5	2.875	0.025	0.087	1.712	0.05	0.125	0.375	22.5	0
0	21.69	1.084	7.23	33.74	209.67	821.81	0.458	115.7	1.446	0.053	0.046	0.916	0.055	0	0.41	9.64	0
2.551	35.425	0	2.834	26.923	36.559	39.959	0.142	20.69	0	0.011	0.043	0.02	0.006	0.085	0	3.117	0
9.919	39.959	0.02	2.834	20.121	60.081	20.121	0.142	25.51	0.255	0.011	0.034	0.02	0.006	0.119	0.085	3.117	0
0	53.94	3.906	33.48	639.84	334.8	1023	3.348	0	0	1.674	1.116	18.6	2.232	4.464	3.218	145.1	0
0	12.559	0.134	2.565	2.147	19.836	1.463	0.019	0.513	0.745	0.002	0.001	0.054	0.004	0	0.02	0.684	0
0	13.566	0.776	3.57	9.24	30.261	0.336	0.111	0.336	0.441	0.007	0.006	0.064	0.014	0	0.022	0.21	0
0	35.34	0.898	8.8	10.94	28	3.2	0.139	0.06	0.342	0.007	0.006	0.061	0.018	0	0.021	0.2	0
0	7.228	0.37	4.42	7.878	49.816	26.26	0.07	38.56	1.667	0.009	0.021	0.205	0.095	0	0.755	2.6	0
0	28.244	0.876	1.288	1.403	11.5	0.598	0.045	0.322	0.655	0.002	0.003	0.03	0.007	0	0.022	0.667	0
0	13.566	0.182	5.544	2.205	23.142	5.103	0.023	0.567	1.697	0.002	0.006	0.031	0.012	0	0.179	1.953	0
0	12.762	0.294	5.94	7.362	22.806	0.63	0.085	0	0.378	0.004	0.005	0.038		0		0	0
0	19.551	1.394	7.686	10.479	37.548	3.528	0.101	1.344	0.162	0.013	0.007	0.096	0.009	0	0.07	0.21	0
0	9.56	0.592	5.08	6.98	30.86	1.04	0.081	0.98	0.228	0.005	0.006	0.069	0.023	0	0.44	3.08	0
0	31.836	0.343	5.376	5.817	24.906	0.42	0.109	0.063	0.441	0.009	0.006	0.059	0.005	0	0.022	0.21	0
0	23.92	0.371	7.7	9.74	33.88	1.76	0.074	0.14	0.42	0.008	0.007	0.121	0.009	0			0
0	2.24	0.077	1.624	11.676	30.828	0.728	0.074	0	0.504	0.013	0.004	0.019	0.082	0	0.018	0.056	0
0	2.088	0.207	3.312	2.664	24.174	0.576	0.085	0.126	0.126	0.001	0.003	0.093	0.015	0	0.324	0.702	0
0	17.193	0.329	9.834	27.753	22.506	0.165	0.188	0.099	0.099	0.018	0.013	0.26	0.014	0	0.095	2.508	0
0	4.048	0.067	4.026	4.686	7.7	0.352	0.047	0.11	0.066	0.008	0.001	0.029	0.004	0	0	1.672	0
0	8.712	0.061	2.928	8.16	22.632	1.296	0.056	0	0.353	0.01	0.001	0.016	0.029	0	0.006	3.984	0
0	3.717	0.495	3.885	7.245	49.224	0.714	0.085	55.38	1.493	0.014	0.037	0.322	0.084	0	0.626	2.226	0
0	9.177	0.606	4.074	3.633	26.439	0.924	0.03	0.315	0.441	0.002	0.005	0.024	0.007	0	0.015	0.21	0

EvaluEat Code	Food Name	Amt	Wt (g)	Energy (kcal)	Prot (g)	Carb (g)	Fiber (g)	Fat (g)	Mono (g)	Poly (g)	Sat (g)
2033	Spice, poppy seed	1 tsp	2.8	14.924	0.505	0.663	0.28	1.252	0.178	0.863	0.136
2037	Spice, saffron	1 tsp	0.7	2.17	0.08	0.458	0.027	0.041	0.003	0.014	0.011
2043	Spice, turmeric, ground	1 tsp	2.2	7.788	0.172	1.428	0.464	0.217	0.037	0.048	0.069
22905	Stew, beef stew, canned entree	1 serving	232	218.08	11.461	15.706	3.48	12.482	5.522	0.51	5.15
18355	Sweet roll, cheese	1 roll	66	237.6	4.686	28.842	0.792	12.078	5.978	1.341	3.999
18358	Sweet roll, cinnamon w/icing, refrigerated dough, baked	1 roll	30	108.6	1.62	16.83		3.96	2.226	0.518	1.004
18356	Sweet roll, cinnamon-raisin, commercially prep	1 large	83	308.76	5.146	42.247	1.992	13.612	3.982	6.203	2.556
19163	Sweet, chewing gum	1 stick	3	7.41	0	1.982	0.072	0.009	0.002	0.004	0.001
19711	Sweet, frosting, chocolate creamy	1/12 package	38	150.86	0.418	24.016	0.228	6.688	3.428	0.809	2.101
19228	Sweet, frosting, cream cheese flavor	2 tbsp	33	136.95	0.033	22.216	0	5.709	1.239	2.03	1.5
19715	Sweet, frosting, vanilla, creamy	1/12 package	38	159.22	0.038	26.372	0.038	6.384	3.333	0.866	1.858
19294	Sweet, fruit butter, apple	1 tbsp	17	29.41	0.066	7.271	0.255	0	0	0	0
19173	Sweet, gelatin, dry, prep w/H$_2$O	.5 cup	135	83.7	1.647	19.156	0	0	0	0	0
19290	Sweet, gelatin, Kraft, JELL-O Sugar Free Dessert, strawberry, powder	1 NLEA serving	2.5	8.325	1.42	0.123	0	0.003			0
19296	Sweet, honey, strained/extracted	1 tbsp	21	63.84	0.063	17.304	0.042	0	0	0	0
19283	Sweet, ice popsicle	1 bar (1.75 fl. oz.)	52	37.44	0	9.828	0	0	0	0	0
19297	Sweet, jams & preserves	1 tbsp	20	55.6	0.074	13.772	0.22	0.014	0.008	0	0.002
19300	Sweet, jellies	1 packet (0.5 oz)	14	37.24	0.021	9.793	0.14	0.003	0	0.001	0.001
19303	Sweet, marmalade, orange	1 tbsp	20	49.2	0.06	13.26	0.14	0	0	0	0
19304	Sweet, molasses	1 tbsp	20	58	0	14.946	0	0.02	0.006	0.01	0.004
19334	Sweet, sugar, brown	1 tsp packed	4.6	17.342	0	4.477	0	0	0	0	0
19335	Sweet, sugar, granulated, white	1 tsp	4.2	16.254	0	4.199	0	0	0	0	0
19340	Sweet, sugar, maple	1 tsp	3	10.62	0.003	2.727	0	0.006	0.002	0.003	0.001
19336	Sweet, sugar, powdered/confectioner's, white	1 tsp	2.5	9.725	0	2.49	0	0.003	0.001	0.001	0
19113	Sweet, syrup w/butter, pancake	1 tbsp	20	59.2	0	14.82	0	0.32	0.094	0.012	0.202
19348	Sweet, syrup, chocolate, fudge-type	2 tbsp	38	133	1.748	23.902	1.064	3.382	1.466	0.106	1.512
19351	Sweet, syrup, corn, hi-fructose	1 tbsp	19	53.39	0	14.44	0	0	0	0	0
19350	Sweet, syrup, corn, light	1 tbsp	20	58.6	0	15.926	0	0.02	0	0	0
19353	Sweet, syrup, maple	1 tbsp	20	52.2	0	13.418	0	0.04	0.013	0.02	0.007
19129	Sweet, syrup, pancake	1 tbsp	20	46.8	0	12.294	0.14	0	0	0	0
19128	Sweet, syrup, pancake, reduced-kcal	1 tbsp	15	24.6	0	6.645	0	0	0	0	0
19355	Sweet, syrup, sorghum	1 tbsp	21	60.9	0	15.729	0	0	0	0	0
19364	Sweet, topping, butterscotch or caramel	2 tbsp	41	103.32	0.615	27.019	0.369	0.041	0.008	0	0.045
19137	Sweet, topping, strawberry	2 tbsp	42	106.68	0.084	27.846	0.294	0.042	0.006	0.021	0.002
43026	Syrups, dietetic	1 cup	186	74.4	1.488	91.512	5.58	0	0	0	0
18277	Toaster muffin, blueberry	1 muffin	33	103.29	1.518	17.589	0.594	3.135	0.713	1.766	0.461
18281	Toaster muffin, corn	1 muffin	33	114.18	1.749	19.107	0.528	3.729	0.866	2.087	0.555
18361	Toaster pastry, brown sugar—cinnamon	1 pastry	50	206	2.55	34.05	0.5	7.1	4.016	0.901	1.819
18475	Toaster pastry, Pop Tart, Apple Cinnamon/Kellogg	1 pastry	52	205.4	2.288	37.45	0.572	5.304	3.052	1.352	0.879
18491	Toaster pastry, Pop Tart, Frosted Apple Cinnamon, low-fat/Kellogg	1 pastry	52	191.36	2.184	39.988	0.572	2.86	1.456	0.832	0.572

Chol (g)	Calc (mg)	Iron (mg)	Mag (mg)	Phos (mg)	Pota (mg)	Sodi (mg)	Zinc (mg)	Vit A (RAE)	Vit C (mg)	Thia (mg)	Ribo (mg)	Niac (mg)	Vit B₆ (mg)	Vit B₁₂ (µg)	Vit E (mg)	Fol (µg)	Alc (g)
0	40.544	0.263	9.268	23.772	19.6	0.588	0.286	0	0.084	0.024	0.005	0.027	0.012	0	0.031	1.624	0
0	0.777	0.078	1.848	1.764	12.068	1.036	0.008	0.189	0.566	0.001	0.002	0.01	0.007	0	0.012	0.651	0
0	4.026	0.911	4.246	5.896	55.55	0.836	0.096	0	0.57	0.003	0.005	0.113	0.04	0	0.068	0.858	0
37.12	27.84	1.647	32.48	127.6	403.68	946.56	1.902	192.6	10.21	0.167	0.142	2.856	0.299	0.858	0.172	25.52	0
50.16	77.88	0.502	12.54	64.68	90.42	235.62	0.416		0.132	0.099	0.086	0.548	0.046	0.198		28.38	
0	10.2	0.795	3.6	104.4	18.9	249.6	0.102	0	0.06	0.123	0.073	1.087	0.01	0.015		16.5	
54.78	59.76	1.328	14.11	63.08	92.13	317.89	0.49	51.46	1.66	0.269	0.22	1.979	0.089	0.116	1.652	59.76	0
0	0	0	0	0	0.06	0.03	0	0	0	0	0	0	0	0	0	0	0
0	3.04	0.54	7.98	22.42	74.48	69.54	0.11		0	0.005	0.006	0.045	0.002	0		0	0
0	0.99	0.053	0.66	0.99	11.55	63.03	0.007	0	0	0	0.002	0.004	0	0	1.401	0	0
0	1.14	0.042	0.38	1.14	14.06	34.2	0		0	0	0.002	0.004	0	0		0	0
0	2.38	0.053	0.85	1.19	15.47	2.55	0.01	0.17	0.17	0.001	0.004	0.011	0.006	0	0.003	0.17	0
0	4.05	0.027	1.35	29.7	1.35	101.25	0.014	0	0	0	0.008	0.001	0	0		1.35	0
0.025	0.525	0.029		34.025	0.45	57.05		0									
0	1.26	0.088	0.42	0.84	10.92	0.84	0.046	0	0.105	0	0.008	0.025	0.005	0	0	0.42	0
0	0	0	0.52	0	2.08	6.24	0.01	0	0	0	0	0	0	0	0	0	0
0	4	0.098	0.8	3.8	15.4	6.4	0.012	0.2	1.76	0.003	0.015	0.007	0.004	0	0.024	2.2	0
0	0.98	0.027	0.84	0.84	7.56	4.2	0.004	0	0.126	0	0.004	0.005	0.003	0	0	0.28	0
0	7.6	0.03	0.4	0.8	7.4	11.2	0.008	0.6	0.96	0.001	0.005	0.01	0.004	0	0.012	1.8	0
0	41	0.944	48.4	6.2	292.8	7.4	0.058	0	0	0.008	0	0.186	0.134	0	0	0	0
0	3.91	0.088	1.334	1.012	15.916	1.794	0.008	0	0	0	0	0.004	0.001	0	0	0.046	0
0	0.042	0	0	0	0.084	0	0	0	0	0	0.001	0	0	0	0	0	0
0	2.7	0.048	0.57	0.09	8.22	0.33	0.182	0	0	0	0	0.001	0	0	0	0	0
0	0.025	0.001	0	0	0.05	0.025	0	0	0	0	0	0	0	0	0	0	0
0.8	0.4	0.018	0.4	2	0.6	19.6	0.008	2.8	0	0.002	0.002	0.004	0	0	0.006	0	0
0.76	38	0.597	24.32	63.84	171.38	131.48	0.319	1.9	0.038	0.027	0.107	0.139	0.029	0.106	0.946	1.9	0
0	0	0.006	0	0	0	0.38	0.004	0	0	0	0.004	0	0	0	0	0	0
0	0.6	0.01	0.4	0.4	0.8	24.2	0.004	0	0	0.002	0.002	0.004	0.002	0	0	0	0
0	13.4	0.24	2.8	0.4	40.8	1.8	0.832	0	0	0.001	0.002	0.006	0	0	0	0	0
0	0.6	0.006	0.4	1.8	3	16.4	0.016	0	0	0.001	0.002	0.002	0.001	0	0	0	0
0	0.15	0.003	0	6.45	0.45	30	0.003	0	0	0.002	0.001	0.003	0	0	0	0	0
0	31.5	0.798	21	11.76	210	1.68	0.086	0	0	0.021	0.033	0.021	0.141	0	0	0	0
0.41	21.73	0.082	2.87	19.27	34.44	143.09	0.078	11.07	0.123	0.005	0.039	0.016	0.006	0.037		0.82	0
0	2.52	0.118	1.68	2.1	21.42	8.82	0.025	0.42	5.754	0.005	0.01	0.068	0.005	0	0.042	2.52	0
0	0	0	0	0	0	39.06	0	0	0	0	0	0	0	0	0	0	0
1.98	4.29	0.168	3.96	19.47	27.39	157.74	0.129	31.02	0	0.079	0.096	0.667	0.009	0.007	0.3	21.45	0
4.29	6.27	0.485	4.62	49.83	30.36	141.9	0.129	5.94	0	0.102	0.122	0.762	0.016	0.01		18.81	0
0	17	2.015	12	66.5	57	212	0.315	148	0.05	0.186	0.288	2.287	0.213	0.11		14.5	0
0	11.96	1.82	5.72	27.56	47.32	173.68	0.338		0	0.151	0.172	1.976	0.198	0	0	41.6	0
0	5.72	1.82	4.68	21.32	28.08	205.92	0.156		0	0.156	0.156	1.976	0.208	0	0	52	0

EvaluEat Code	Food Name	Amt	Wt (g)	Energy (kcal)	Prot (g)	Carb (g)	Fiber (g)	Fat (g)	Mono (g)	Poly (g)	Sat (g)
18495	Toaster pastry, Pop Tart, Frosted Chocolate Fudge, low fat/Kellogg	1 pastry	52	190.32	2.652	39.52	0.572	3.016	1.248	0.884	0.52
18482	Toaster pastry, Pop Tart, Frosted Chocolate Fudge/Kellogg	1 pastry	52	201.24	2.652	37.336	0.572	4.836	2.704	1.144	0.988
3930	Toddler formula, Mead Johnson Next Step Soy, prepared from powder	1 fl. oz.	30.5	20.13	0.641	2.159	0	0.885	0.339	0.169	0.381
43476	Tofu yogurt	1 oz	28.34	26.64	0.992	4.523	0.057	0.51	0.113	0.288	0.073
19125	Topping, chocolate-flavored hazelnut spread	1 oz	28.34	153.32	1.533	17.616	1.53	8.425	4.614	1.919	1.528
22901	Tortellini, pasta with cheese filling	1 cup	236	724.52	31.86	110.92	4.484	17.063	4.876	1.088	8.496
18449	Tortilla, corn, w/o salt, ready to cook	1 tortilla, medium (approx 6" dia)	26	57.72	1.482	12.116	1.352	0.65	0.169	0.292	0.087
18364	Tortilla, flour, ready-to-cook	1 tortilla, medium (approx 6" dia)	46	149.5	4.002	25.576	1.518	3.266	1.733	0.489	0.803
18360	Tortilla, taco shell, baked	1 large (6-1/2" dia)	21	98.28	1.512	13.104	1.575	4.746	1.876	1.784	0.681
42130	Turkey bacon, cooked	1 oz	28.34	108.26	8.389	0.879	0	7.907	3.089	1.929	2.351
22706	Turkey chili w/beans, canned entree/Hormel	1 cup	247	202.54	18.723	25.565	6.422	2.766	0.42	1.21	0.667
5172	Turkey giblets, simmered	1 cup, chopped or diced	145	288.55	30.291	1.16	0	17.197	7.183	1.827	5.688
5174	Turkey gizzard, simmered	1	84	103.32	18.245	0.319	0	3.251	1.016	0.423	0.977
42128	Turkey ham, sliced, extra lean, prepackaged or deli-sliced	1 oz	28.34	33.441	5.555	0.425	0	1.077	0.245	0.322	0.361
5176	Turkey heart, simmered	1 heart	21	27.3	4.509	0.143	0	0.974	0.239	0.25	0.271
5178	Turkey liver, simmered	1 liver	83	226.59	16.617	1.004	0	17.048	7.56	1.678	5.766
5292	Turkey patty, breaded, fried	1 medium slice (approx 3" x 2" x 1/4")	28	79.24	3.92	4.396	0.14	5.04	2.092	1.319	1.313
22528	Turkey pot pie, frozen	1 serving	397	698.72	25.805	70.269	4.367	34.936	13.736	5.479	11.434
5296	Turkey roast, light & dark meat, no bone, frozen, seasoned, cooked	1 cup, chopped or diced	135	209.25	28.782	4.144	0	7.803	1.62	2.241	2.565
5286	Turkey w/gravy, frozen	1 cup	240	160.8	14.112	11.064	0	6.312	2.328	1.128	2.04
5218	Turkey, fryer/roaster, breast w/skin, roasted	1 unit (yield from 1 lb ready-to-cook turkey)	98	149.94	28.489	0	0	3.136	1.176	0.745	0.853
5220	Turkey, fryer/roaster, breast, no skin, roasted	1 unit (yield from 1 lb ready-to-cook turkey)	87	117.45	26.152	0	0	0.644	0.113	0.174	0.209
5208	Turkey, fryer/roaster, dark meat w/skin, roasted	1 unit (yield from 1 lb ready-to-cook turkey)	106	192.92	29.351	0	0	7.484	2.406	1.993	2.247
5206	Turkey, fryer/roaster, light meat w/skin, roasted	1 unit (yield from 1 lb ready-to-cook turkey)	123	201.72	35.387	0	0	5.633	2.091	1.341	1.538
5306	Turkey, ground, cooked	1 patty (4 oz, raw)	82	192.7	22.435	0	0	10.783	4.01	2.649	2.78
7900	Turkey, pork, and beef sausage, low-fat, smoked	1 frankfurter	56	56.56	4.48	6.44	0.336	1.4	0.577	0.185	0.476
17203	Veal liver, braised	1 slice (yield from 116 g raw liver)	80	153.6	22.736	3.016	0	5.008	0.917	0.831	1.589
17204	Veal liver, pan fried	1 slice (yield from 99 g raw liver)	67	129.31	18.338	2.995	0	4.362	0.8	0.745	1.413

Chol (g)	Calc (mg)	Iron (mg)	Mag (mg)	Phos (mg)	Pota (mg)	Sodi (mg)	Zinc (mg)	Vit A (RAE)	Vit C (mg)	Thia (mg)	Ribo (mg)	Niac (mg)	Vit B_6 (mg)	Vit B_{12} (µg)	Vit E (mg)	Fol (µg)	Alc (g)
0	13.52	1.82	14.56	39.52	61.88	248.56	0.26		0	0.156	0.156	1.976	0.208	0	0	52	0
0	19.76	1.82	15.08	43.68	82.16	202.8	0.26		0	0.156	0.156	1.976	0.208	0	0	52	0
0	23.18	0.36	1.525	17.995	29.89	8.845	0.241	17.69	2.41	0.016	0.018	0.201	0.018	0.058	0.4	3.05	0
0	33.441	0.3	11.336	10.769	13.32	9.919	0.088	0.567	0.709	0.017	0.006	0.068	0.006	0	0.088	1.7	0
0	30.607	1.241	18.138	43.077	115.344	11.619	0.3	0.283	0	0.034	0.048	0.121	0.024	0.079	1.406	3.968	0
99.12	358.72	3.54	49.56	500.32	210.04	811.84	2.407	89.68	0	0.739	0.732	6.363	0.101	0.378	0.378	174.6	0
0	45.5	0.364	16.9	81.64	40.04	2.86	0.244	0	0	0.029	0.019	0.389	0.057	0	0.04	29.64	0
0	57.5	1.518	11.96	57.04	60.26	219.88	0.327	0	0	0.244	0.135	1.643	0.023	0	0.258	47.84	0
0	33.6	0.525	22.05	52.08	37.59	77.07	0.294	0	0	0.048	0.011	0.283	0.062	0	0.349	27.51	0
27.773	2.551	0.598	8.219	130.364	111.943	647.569	0.859	0	0	0.017	0.068	1	0.091	0.102	0.292	2.551	0
34.58	116.09	3.458	69.16		681.72	1197.95	2.717		1.482								0
419.05	8.7	11.18	26.1	334.95	391.5	92.8	4.524	15569	19.87	0.039	2.179	10.147	0.842	48.213	0.116	485.8	0
170.52	5.88	4.158	14.28	129.36	278.88	56.28	2.831	0	5.292	0.011	0.174	3.587	0.089	6.787	0.042	10.92	0
18.988	1.417	0.383	5.668	86.154	84.737	294.169	0.669	0	0	0.014	0.071	1	0.065	0.074	0.111	1.7	0
38.64	1.47	1.092	5.46	54.39	61.11	18.9	0.934	3.99	0.588	0.007	0.218	0.71	0.089	4.557	0.01	1.68	0
322.04	4.15	8.881	14.11	244.02	175.13	46.48	2.175	18758	18.76	0.032	2.291	8.466	0.863	48.306	0.091	573.5	0
17.36	3.92	0.616	4.2	75.6	77	224	0.403	3.08	0	0.028	0.053	0.644	0.056	0.062	0.353	7.84	0
63.52		3.97				1389.5											0
71.55	6.75	2.201	29.7	329.4	402.3	918	3.429	0	0	0.063	0.22	8.466	0.365	2.052	0.513	6.75	0
43.2	33.6	2.232	19.2	194.4	146.4	1329.6	1.68	31.2	0	0.058	0.305	4.318	0.24	0.576		9.6	0
88.2	14.7	1.539	27.44	211.68	273.42	51.94	1.735	0	0	0.04	0.132	6.823	0.5	0.363		5.88	0
72.21	10.44	1.331	25.23	194.88	254.04	45.24	1.514	0	0	0.037	0.114	6.519	0.487	0.339	0.078	5.22	0
124.02	28.62	2.47	24.38	201.4	251.22	80.56	4.06	0	0	0.051	0.249	3.551	0.35	0.392		9.54	0
116.85	22.14	1.98	31.98	252.15	322.26	70.11	2.558	0	0	0.047	0.171	7.718	0.603	0.443		7.38	0
83.64	20.5	1.583	19.68	160.72	221.4	87.74	2.345	0	0	0.044	0.138	3.952	0.32	0.271	0.279	5.74	0
11.76	5.6	1.232	8.96	41.44	136.08	445.76	0.672	0	1.064	0.073	0.045	0.868	0.056	0.157	0.05	3.36	0
408.8	4.8	4.088	16	368	263.2	62.4	8.984	16916	0.88	0.146	2.288	10.52	0.734	67.68	0.544	264.8	0
324.95	4.69	4.007	15.41	323.61	236.51	56.95	7.973	13450	0.469	0.119	2.05	9.615	0.597	48.575	0.402	234.5	0

EvaluEat Code	Food Name	Amt	Wt (g)	Energy (kcal)	Prot (g)	Carb (g)	Fiber (g)	Fat (g)	Mono (g)	Poly (g)	Sat (g)
17223	Veal tongue, braised	3 oz	85	171.7	21.973	0	0	8.585	3.919	0.323	3.697
17089	Veal, composite, lean & fat, cooked	3 oz	85	196.35	25.585	0	0	9.682	3.74	0.68	3.638
17143	Veal, ground, broiled	3 oz	85	146.2	20.723	0	0	6.426	2.414	0.468	2.584
11655	Vegetable juice, carrot, canned	1 cup	236	94.4	2.242	21.924	1.888	0.354	0.017	0.168	0.064
11886	Vegetable juice, tomato, canned w/o salt	1 cup	243	41.31	1.847	10.303	0.972	0.122	0.022	0.058	0.019
11001	Vege, alfalfa seeds, sprouted, raw	1 tbsp	3	0.87	0.12	0.113	0.075	0.021	0.002	0.012	0.002
11697	Vege, arrowroot, raw	1 cup, sliced	120	78	5.088	16.068	1.56	0.24	0.005	0.11	0.047
11702	Vege, artichokes (globe or French) boiled w/salt, drained	1 artichoke, medium	120	60	4.176	13.416	6.48	0.192	0.006	0.082	0.044
11009	Vege, artichokes (globe or French) frozen	1 package (9 oz)	255	96.9	6.707	19.788	9.945	1.097	0.031	0.456	0.252
11959	Vege, arugula/roquette, raw	1 leaf	2	0.5	0.052	0.073	0.032	0.013	0.001	0.006	0.002
11705	Vege, asparagus, boiled w/salt, drained	4 spears (1/2" base)	60	13.2	1.44	2.466	1.2	0.132	0.006	0.082	0.043
11015	Vege, asparagus, canned, drained	1 spear (about 5" long)	18	3.42	0.385	0.443	0.288	0.117	0.004	0.051	0.026
11011	Vege, asparagus, raw	1 spear, large (7-1/4" to 8-1/2")	20	4	0.44	0.776	0.42	0.024	0.001	0.018	0.009
11712	Vege, bamboo shoots, boiled w/salt, drained	1 cup (1/2" slices)	120	14.4	1.836	2.304	1.2	0.264	0.006	0.118	0.061
11028	Vege, bamboo shoots, canned, drained	1 cup (1/8" slices)	131	24.89	2.253	4.218	1.834	0.524	0.012	0.233	0.121
11026	Vege, bamboo shoots, raw	1 cup (1/2" slices)	151	40.77	3.926	7.852	3.322	0.453	0.011	0.202	0.104
11626	Vege, bean sprouts, mung, mature seeds, sprouted, canned, drained	1 cup	125	15	1.75	2.675	1	0.075	0.01	0.025	0.02
11973	Vege, beans, fava, in pod, raw	1 cup	126	110.88	9.979	22.214		0.92	0.131	0.431	0.149
11716	Vege, beans, lima, baby, immature seeds, frozen, boiled w/salt, drained	.5 cup	90	94.5	5.985	17.505	5.4	0.27	0.015	0.13	0.061
11033	Vege, beans, lima, immature seeds, canned, solids & liquid	.5 cup	124	88.04	5.047	16.529	4.464	0.36	0.02	0.172	0.082
11720	Vege, beans, pinto, immature seeds, boiled w/salt, drained	1 package (10 oz)	284	460.08	26.44	87.699	24.424	1.363	0.099	0.784	0.165
11723	Vege, beans, snap, green, boiled w/salt, drained	1 cup	125	43.75	2.362	9.863	4	0.35	0.014	0.181	0.08
11056	Vege, beans, snap, green, canned, drained	1 cup	135	27	1.553	6.075	2.565	0.135	0.005	0.069	0.03
11052	Vege, beans, snap, green, raw	1 cup	110	34.1	2.002	7.854	3.74	0.132	0.005	0.065	0.029
11725	Vege, beans, snap, yellow, boiled w/salt, drained	1 cup	125	43.75	2.362	9.85	4.125	0.35	0.014	0.181	0.08
11932	Vege, beans, snap, yellow, canned, regular pack, drained	1 cup	135	27	1.553	6.075	1.755	0.135	0.005	0.069	0.03
11722	Vege, beans, snap, yellow, raw	1 cup	110	34.1	2.002	7.854	3.74	0.132	0.005	0.065	0.029
11736	Vege, beet greens, boiled w/salt, drained	1 cup (1" pieces)	144	38.88	3.701	7.862	4.176	0.288	0.055	0.101	0.045
11086	Vege, beet greens, raw	1 cup	38	8.36	0.836	1.645	1.406	0.049	0.01	0.017	0.008
11734	Vege, beets, boiled w/salt, drained	.5 cup slices	85	37.4	1.428	8.466	1.7	0.153	0.03	0.054	0.024
11084	Vege, beets, canned, drained	1 cup, diced	157	48.67	1.429	11.32	2.669	0.22	0.044	0.08	0.036
11080	Vege, beets, peeled, raw	1 cup	136	58.48	2.19	13.002	3.808	0.231	0.045	0.083	0.037
11609	Vege, beets, pickled, canned, solids & liquid	1 cup slices	227	147.55	1.816	36.956	5.902	0.182	0.036	0.066	0.03
11088	Vege, broadbeans, immature seeds, raw	1 cup	109	78.48	6.104	12.753	4.578	0.654	0.019	0.338	0.15
22600	Vege, broccoli in cheese flavored sauce, frozen/Green Giant	1 cup	168	112.56	3.864	14.952		4.2	1.695	0.425	0.806
11741	Vege, broccoli stalks, raw	1 stalk	114	31.92	3.397	5.974		0.399	0.027	0.19	0.062
11742	Vege, broccoli, boiled w/salt, chopped, drained	.5 cup, chopped	78	21.84	2.324	3.947	2.574	0.273	0.019	0.13	0.042
11969	Vege, broccoli, Chinese, cooked	1 cup	88	19.36	1.003	3.353	2.2	0.634	0.044	0.29	0.097
11745	Vege, Brussels sprouts, boiled w/salt, drained	.5 cup	78	31.98	1.989	6.763	2.028	0.398	0.03	0.203	0.082
11098	Vege, Brussels sprouts, raw	1 cup	88	37.84	2.974	7.876	3.344	0.264	0.02	0.135	0.055

Chol (g)	Calc (mg)	Iron (mg)	Mag (mg)	Phos (mg)	Pota (mg)	Sodi (mg)	Zinc (mg)	Vit A (RAE)	Vit C (mg)	Thia (mg)	Ribo (mg)	Niac (mg)	Vit B_6 (mg)	Vit B_{12} (µg)	Vit E (mg)	Fol (µg)	Alc (g)
202.3	7.65	1.776	15.3	141.1	137.7	54.4	3.834	0	5.1	0.06	0.298	1.25	0.128	4.505		7.65	0
96.9	18.7	0.978	22.1	203.15	276.25	73.95	4.046	0	0	0.051	0.272	6.774	0.264	1.335	0.34	12.75	0
87.55	14.45	0.842	20.4	184.45	286.45	70.55	3.289	0	0	0.06	0.23	6.826	0.331	1.079	0.128	9.35	0
0	56.64	1.086	33.04	99.12	689.12	68.44	0.425	2256	20.06	0.217	0.13	0.911	0.512	0	2.738	9.44	0
0	24.3	1.045	26.73	43.74	556.47	24.3	0.365	55.89	44.47	0.114	0.075	1.635	0.27	0	0.778	48.6	0
0	0.96	0.029	0.81	2.1	2.37	0.18	0.028	0.24	0.246	0.002	0.004	0.014	0.001	0	0.001	1.08	0
0	7.2	2.664	30	117.6	544.8	31.2	0.756	1.2	2.28	0.172	0.071	2.032	0.319	0		405.6	0
0	54	1.548	72	103.2	424.8	397.2	0.588	10.8	12	0.078	0.079	1.201	0.133	0	0.228	61.2	0
0	48.45	1.275	68.85	147.9	632.4	119.85	0.816	20.4	13.52	0.148	0.357	2.193	0.209	0		321.3	0
0	3.2	0.029	0.94	1.04	7.38	0.54	0.009	2.38	0.3	0.001	0.002	0.006	0.001	0	0.009	1.94	0
0	13.8	0.546	8.4	32.4	134.4	144	0.36	30	4.62	0.097	0.083	0.65	0.047	0		89.4	0
0	2.88	0.329	1.8	7.74	30.96	51.66	0.072	7.38	3.312	0.011	0.018	0.172	0.02	0	0.056	17.28	0
0	4.8	0.428	2.8	10.4	40.4	0.4	0.108	7.6	1.12	0.029	0.028	0.196	0.018	0	0.226	10.4	0
0	14.4	0.288	3.6	24	639.6	288	0.564	0	0	0.024	0.06	0.36	0.118	0		2.4	0
0	10.48	0.419	5.24	32.75	104.8	9.17	0.851	1.31	1.441	0.034	0.034	0.183	0.178	0	0.825	3.93	0
0	19.63	0.755	4.53	89.09	804.83	6.04	1.661	1.51	6.04	0.227	0.106	0.906	0.362	0	1.51	10.57	0
0	17.5	0.538	11.25	40	33.75	175	0.35	0	0.375	0.037	0.087	0.275	0.04	0	0.05	12.5	0
0	46.62	1.953	41.58	162.54	418.32	31.5	1.26	21.42	4.662	0.168	0.365	2.834	0.131	0		186.5	0
0	25.2	1.764	50.4	100.8	369.9	238.5	0.495	7.2	5.22	0.063	0.049	0.693	0.104	0	0.576	14.4	0
0	34.72	1.996	42.16	88.04	353.4	312.48	0.794	9.92	9.052	0.036	0.053	0.66	0.077	0	0.36	19.84	0
0	147.68	7.696	153.36	284	1834.64	905.96	1.96	0	1.988	0.778	0.307	1.795	0.551	0		96.56	0
0	57.5	1.6	31.25	48.75	373.75	298.75	0.45	43.75	12.13	0.093	0.121	0.768	0.07	0	0.563	41.25	0
0	35.1	1.215	17.55	25.65	147.15	353.7	0.391	29.7	6.48	0.02	0.076	0.271	0.05	0	0.378	43.2	0
0	40.7	1.144	27.5	41.8	229.9	6.6	0.264	38.5	17.93	0.092	0.115	0.827	0.081	0	0.451	40.7	0
0	57.5	1.6	31.25	48.75	373.75	298.75	0.45	5	12.13	0.093	0.121	0.768	0.07	0	0.563	41.25	0
0	35.1	1.215	17.55	25.65	147.15	338.85	0.391	6.75	6.48	0.02	0.076	0.271	0.05	0	0.391	43.2	0
0	40.7	1.144	27.5	41.8	229.9	6.6	0.264	5.5	17.93	0.092	0.115	0.827	0.081	0		40.7	0
0	164.16	2.736	97.92	59.04	1308.96	686.88	0.72	367.2	35.86	0.168	0.416	0.719	0.19	0		20.16	0
0	44.46	0.977	26.6	15.58	289.56	85.88	0.144	120.1	11.4	0.038	0.084	0.152	0.04	0	0.57	5.7	0
0	13.6	0.672	19.55	32.3	259.25	242.25	0.298	387.6	3.06	0.023	0.034	0.281	0.057	0	1.836	68	0
0	23.55	2.857	26.69	26.69	232.36	304.58	0.33	1.57	6.437	0.016	0.063	0.246	0.089	0	0.047	47.1	0
0	21.76	1.088	31.28	54.4	442	106.08	0.476	2.72	6.664	0.042	0.054	0.454	0.091	0	0.054	148.2	0
0	24.97	0.931	34.05	38.59	335.96	599.28	0.59	2.27	5.221	0.023	0.109	0.57	0.113	0		61.29	0
0	23.98	2.071	41.42	103.55	272.5	54.5	0.632	19.62	35.97	0.185	0.12	1.635	0.041	0		104.6	0
						806.4			59.47								0
0	54.72	1.003	28.5	75.24	370.5	30.78	0.456	22.8	106.2	0.074	0.136	0.727	0.181	0	1.892	80.94	0
0	31.2	0.523	16.38	52.26	228.54	204.36	0.351	76.44	32.76	0.049	0.096	0.431	0.156	0	1.131	84.24	0
0	88	0.493	15.84	36.08	229.68	6.16	0.343	72.16	24.82	0.084	0.128	0.385	0.062	0	0.422	87.12	0
0	28.08	0.936	15.6	43.68	247.26	200.46	0.257	28.08	48.36	0.083	0.062	0.473	0.139	0		46.8	0
0	36.96	1.232	20.24	60.72	342.32	22	0.37	33.44	74.8	0.122	0.079	0.656	0.193	0	0.774	53.68	0

EvaluEat Code	Food Name	Amt	Wt (g)	Energy (kcal)	Prot (g)	Carb (g)	Fiber (g)	Fat (g)	Mono (g)	Poly (g)	Sat (g)
11109	Vege, cabbage heads, raw	1 cup, chopped	89	21.36	1.282	4.966	2.047	0.107	0.008	0.053	0.014
11112	Vege, cabbage heads, red, raw	1 cup, chopped	89	27.59	1.273	6.559	1.869	0.142	0.017	0.111	0.03
11752	Vege, cabbage, red, boiled w/salt, drained	.5 cup, shredded	75	15.75	0.787	3.48	1.5	0.15	0.011	0.071	0.02
11751	Vege, cabbage, boiled w/salt, drained	.5 cup, shredded	75	16.5	0.765	3.345	1.425	0.322	0.022	0.147	0.04
11754	Vege, cabbage, pak-choi (Chinese) boiled w/salt, drained	1 cup, shredded	170	20.4	2.652	3.026	1.7	0.272	0.02	0.131	0.036
11119	Vege, cabbage, pe-tsai (Chinese) raw	1 cup, shredded	76	12.16	0.912	2.455	0.912	0.152	0.017	0.055	0.033
11960	Vege, carrots, baby, raw	1 medium	10	3.5	0.064	0.824	0.18	0.013	0.001	0.006	0.002
11757	Vege, carrots, boiled w/salt, drained	.5 cup slices	78	27.3	0.593	6.412	2.34	0.14	0.005	0.069	0.023
11128	Vege, carrots, canned, drained	1 cup, sliced	146	36.5	0.934	8.088	2.19	0.277	0.013	0.134	0.053
11124	Vege, carrots, chopped/grated, raw	1 cup, chopped	128	52.48	1.19	12.262	3.84	0.307	0.015	0.131	0.041
11134	Vege, cassava (manioc) raw	1 cup	206	329.6	2.802	78.404	3.708	0.577	0.155	0.099	0.152
11135	Vege, cauliflower head, raw	1 cup	100	25	1.98	5.3	2.5	0.1	0.014	0.099	0.032
11761	Vege, cauliflower, boiled w/salt, drained	.5 cup (1" pieces)	62	14.26	1.141	2.548	1.674	0.279	0.02	0.135	0.043
11764	Vege, celery, boiled w/salt, drained	1 cup, diced	150	27	1.245	6.015	2.4	0.24	0.045	0.113	0.06
11143	Vege, celery, raw	1 cup, diced	120	16.8	0.828	3.564	1.92	0.204	0.038	0.097	0.052
11765	Vege, chard, Swiss, boiled w/salt, drained	1 cup, chopped	175	35	3.29	7.227	3.675	0.14			
11151	Vege, chicory, witloof (Belgian endive) raw	1 head	53	9.01	0.477	2.12	1.643	0.053	0.001	0.023	0.013
11768	Vege, collards, boiled w/salt, drained	1 cup, chopped	190	49.4	4.009	9.329	5.32	0.684	0.049	0.329	0.089
11161	Vege, collards, raw	1 cup, chopped	36	10.8	0.882	2.048	1.296	0.151	0.011	0.072	0.02
11167	Vege, corn ears, yellow, sweet, raw	1 ear, medium	90	77.4	2.898	17.118	2.43	1.062	0.312	0.503	0.164
11908	Vege, corn, white, sweet, canned, vacuum/regular pack	.5 cup	105	82.95	2.53	20.412	2.1	0.525	0.154	0.249	0.081
11900	Vege, corn, white, sweet, ears, raw	1 ear, large	143	122.98	4.605	27.199	3.861	1.687	0.496	0.799	0.26
11770	Vege, corn, yellow, sweet, boiled w/salt, drained	1 cup	164	177.12	5.445	41.18	4.592	2.099	0.613	0.989	0.323
11176	Vege, corn, yellow, sweet, canned, vacuum/regular pack	.5 cup	105	82.95	2.53	20.412	2.1	0.525	0.154	0.249	0.081
11174	Vege, corn, yellow, sweet, cream style, regular pack, canned	1 cup	256	184.32	4.454	46.413	3.072	1.075	0.315	0.507	0.166
11777	Vege, cowpeas (blackeyes), immature seeds, boiled w/salt, drained	1 cup	165	160.05	5.231	33.528	8.25	0.627	0.056	0.266	0.158
11203	Vege, cress, garden, raw	1 cup	50	16	1.3	2.75	0.55	0.35	0.119	0.114	0.012
11205	Vege, cucumber, raw	.5 cup slices	52	7.8	0.338	1.888	0.26	0.057	0.002	0.028	0.018
11207	Vege, dandelion greens, raw	1 cup, chopped	55	24.75	1.485	5.06	1.925	0.385	0.008	0.168	0.094
11783	Vege, eggplant (brinjal) boiled w/salt, drained	1 cup (1" cubes)	99	34.65	0.822	8.643	2.475	0.228	0.02	0.092	0.044
11213	Vege, endive (escarole) raw	.5 cup, chopped	25	4.25	0.313	0.837	0.775	0.05	0.001	0.022	0.012
11957	Vege, fennel bulb, raw	1 cup, sliced	87	26.97	1.079	6.342	2.697	0.174			
11987	Vege, fungi, mushroom, oyster, raw	1 large	148	54.76	6.127	9.206	3.552	0.755			
11798	Vege, fungi, mushroom, shiitake, boiled w/salt, drained	4 mushrooms	72	39.6	1.123	10.282	1.512	0.158	0.049	0.022	0.04
11266	Vege, fungi, mushrooms, brown, Italian, or crimini, raw	1 piece	14	3.08	0.35	0.577	0.084	0.014	0	0.006	0.002
11264	Vege, fungi, mushrooms, canned, caps/slices, drained	1 can	132	33	2.468	6.719	3.168	0.383	0.007	0.149	0.05
11265	Vege, fungi, mushrooms, portabella, raw	1 oz	28.34	7.368	0.709	1.437	0.425	0.057	0.001	0.022	0.007
11260	Vege, fungi, mushrooms, slices, raw	1 medium	18	3.96	0.56	0.583	0.216	0.061	0.001	0.025	0.008
11961	Vege, hearts of palm, canned	1 cup	146	40.88	3.679	6.745	3.504	0.905	0.15	0.295	0.19
11790	Vege, kale, boiled w/salt, drained	1 cup, chopped	130	36.4	2.47	7.319	2.6	0.52	0.039	0.251	0.068
11233	Vege, kale, raw	1 cup, chopped	67	33.5	2.211	6.707	1.34	0.469	0.035	0.226	0.061
11793	Vege, kohlrabi, boiled w/salt, drained	1 cup slices	165	47.85	2.97	11.038	1.815	0.182	0.013	0.087	0.023
11241	Vege, kohlrabi, peeled, raw	1 cup	135	36.45	2.295	8.37	4.86	0.135	0.009	0.065	0.018

Chol (g)	Calc (mg)	Iron (mg)	Mag (mg)	Phos (mg)	Pota (mg)	Sodi (mg)	Zinc (mg)	Vit A (RAE)	Vit C (mg)	Thia (mg)	Ribo (mg)	Niac (mg)	Vit B6 (mg)	Vit B12 (µg)	Vit E (mg)	Fol (µg)	Alc (g)
0	41.83	0.525	13.35	20.47	218.94	16.02	0.16	8.01	28.66	0.045	0.036	0.267	0.085	0	0.134	38.27	0
0	40.05	0.712	14.24	26.7	216.27	24.03	0.196	49.84	50.73	0.057	0.061	0.372	0.186	0	0.098	16.02	0
0	27.75	0.262	8.25	21.75	105	183	0.113	0.75	25.8	0.026	0.015	0.15	0.105	0		9.75	0
0	23.25	0.127	6	11.25	72.75	191.25	0.068	5.25	15.08	0.043	0.041	0.212	0.085	0	0.09	15	0
0	158.1	1.768	18.7	49.3	630.7	459	0.289	360.4	44.2	0.054	0.107	0.728	0.282	0	0.153	69.7	0
0	58.52	0.236	9.88	22.04	180.88	6.84	0.175	12.16	20.52	0.03	0.038	0.304	0.176	0	0.091	60.04	0
0	3.2	0.089	1	2.8	23.7	7.8	0.017	69	0.84	0.003	0.004	0.056	0.01	0		3.3	0
0	23.4	0.265	7.8	23.4	183.3	235.56	0.156	659.1	2.808	0.051	0.034	0.503	0.119	0	0.803	1.56	0
0	36.5	0.934	11.68	35.04	261.34	353.32	0.38	814.7	3.942	0.026	0.044	0.806	0.164	0	1.08	13.14	0
0	42.24	0.384	15.36	44.8	409.6	88.32	0.307	770.6	7.552	0.084	0.074	1.258	0.177	0	0.845	24.32	0
0	32.96	0.556	43.26	55.62	558.26	28.84	0.7	2.06	42.44	0.179	0.099	1.759	0.181	0	0.391	55.62	0
0	22	0.44	15	44	303	30	0.28	1	46.4	0.057	0.063	0.526	0.222	0	0.08	57	0
0	9.92	0.205	5.58	19.84	88.04	150.04	0.112	0.62	27.47	0.026	0.032	0.254	0.107	0	0.043	27.28	0
0	63	0.63	18	37.5	426	490.5	0.21	43.5	9.15	0.065	0.071	0.479	0.129	0	0.525	33	0
0	48	0.24	13.2	28.8	312	96	0.156	26.4	3.72	0.025	0.068	0.384	0.089	0	0.324	43.2	0
0	101.5	3.955	150.5	57.75	960.75	726.25	0.578	535.5	31.5	0.06	0.15	0.63	0.149	0	3.307	15.75	0
0	10.07	0.127	5.3	13.78	111.83	1.06	0.085	0.53	1.484	0.033	0.014	0.085	0.022	0		19.61	0
0	266	2.204	38	57	220.4	478.8	0.437	771.4	34.58	0.076	0.201	1.092	0.243	0	1.672	176.7	0
0	52.2	0.068	3.24	3.6	60.84	7.2	0.047	119.9	12.71	0.019	0.047	0.267	0.059	0	0.814	59.76	0
0	1.8	0.468	33.3	80.1	243	13.5	0.405	9	6.12	0.18	0.054	1.53	0.049	0	0.063	41.4	0
0	5.25	0.441	24.15	67.2	195.3	285.6	0.483	0	8.505	0.043	0.077	1.225	0.058	0		51.45	0
0	2.86	0.744	52.91	127.27	386.1	21.45	0.643	0	9.724	0.286	0.086	2.431	0.079	0	0.1	65.78	0
0	3.28	1	52.48	168.92	408.36	414.92	0.787	21.32	10.17	0.353	0.118	2.647	0.098	0	0.148	75.44	0
0	5.25	0.441	24.15	67.2	195.3	285.6	0.483	4.2	8.505	0.043	0.077	1.225	0.058	0	0.042	51.45	0
0	7.68	0.973	43.52	130.56	343.04	729.6	1.357	10.24	11.78	0.064	0.136	2.458	0.161	0	0.179	115.2	0
0	211.2	1.848	85.8	84.15	689.7	396	1.699	66	3.63	0.167	0.244	2.315	0.107	0	0.363	209.6	0
0	40.5	0.65	19	38	303	7	0.115	173	34.5	0.04	0.13	0.5	0.123	0	0.35	40	0
0	8.32	0.146	6.76	12.48	76.44	1.04	0.104	2.6	1.456	0.014	0.017	0.051	0.021	0	0.016	3.64	0
0	102.85	1.705	19.8	36.3	218.35	41.8	0.226	135.9	19.25	0.105	0.143	0.443	0.138	0	2.635	14.85	0
0	5.94	0.248	10.89	14.85	121.77	236.61	0.119	1.98	1.287	0.075	0.02	0.594	0.085	0	0.406	13.86	0
0	13	0.207	3.75	7	78.5	5.5	0.198	27	1.625	0.02	0.019	0.1	0.005	0	0.11	35.5	0
0	42.63	0.635	14.79	43.5	360.18	45.24	0.174	6.09	10.44	0.009	0.028	0.557	0.041	0		23.49	0
0	8.88	2.575	29.6	208.68	763.68	45.88	1.154	2.96	0	0.081	0.533	5.297	0.181	0		69.56	0
0	2.16	0.317	10.08	20.88	84.24	172.8	0.958	0	0.216	0.027	0.122	1.08	0.114	0		15.12	0
0	2.52	0.056	1.26	16.8	62.72	0.84	0.154	0	0	0.013	0.069	0.532	0.015	0.014	0.016	1.96	
0	14.52	1.043	19.8	87.12	170.28	561	0.95	0	0	0.112	0.028	2.103	0.081	0	0.013	15.84	0
0	2.267	0.17	3.117	36.842	137.166	1.7	0.17	0	0	0.022	0.136	1.275	0.028	0.014	0.037	6.235	
0	0.54	0.094	1.62	15.3	56.52	0.72	0.094	0	0.432	0.016	0.075	0.694	0.021	0.007	0.002	2.88	0
0	84.68	4.57	55.48	94.9	258.42	621.96	1.679	0	11.53	0.016	0.083	0.638	0.032	0		56.94	0
0	93.6	1.17	23.4	36.4	296.4	336.7	0.312	885.3	53.3	0.069	0.091	0.65	0.179	0	1.105	16.9	0
0	90.45	1.139	22.78	37.52	299.49	28.81	0.295	515.2	80.4	0.074	0.087	0.67	0.182	0	0.536	19.43	0
0	41.25	0.66	31.35	74.25	561	424.05	0.512	3.3	89.1	0.066	0.033	0.643	0.254	0	0.858	19.8	0
0	32.4	0.54	25.65	62.1	472.5	27	0.041	2.7	83.7	0.068	0.027	0.54	0.203	0	0.648	21.6	0

EvaluEat Code	Food Name	Amt	Wt (g)	Energy (kcal)	Prot (g)	Carb (g)	Fiber (g)	Fat (g)	Mono (g)	Poly (g)	Sat (g)
11246	Vege, leeks (bulb & lower leaf-portion) raw	1 leek	89	54.29	1.335	12.593	1.602	0.267	0.004	0.148	0.036
11795	Vege, leeks (bulbs & lower leaves) boiled w/salt, drained	1 leek	124	38.44	1.004	9.449	1.24	0.248	0.004	0.138	0.033
11250	Vege, lettuce, butterhead (Boston/bibb) leaves, raw	1 leaf, medium	7.5	0.975	0.101	0.167	0.083	0.016	0.001	0.009	0.002
11251	Vege, lettuce, cos/romaine, raw	1 inner leaf	10	1.7	0.123	0.329	0.21	0.03	0.001	0.016	0.004
11252	Vege, lettuce, iceberg, head, raw	1 head, medium	539	53.9	4.366	11.265	5.39	0.593	0.022	0.296	0.075
11253	Vege, lettuce, looseleaf, raw	1 leaf	10	1.5	0.136	0.279	0.13	0.015	0.001	0.008	0.002
11799	Vege, mustard greens, boiled w/salt, drained	1 cup, chopped	140	21	3.164	2.94	2.8	0.336	0.154	0.064	0.017
11270	Vege, mustard greens, raw	1 cup, chopped	56	14.56	1.512	2.744	1.848	0.112	0.052	0.021	0.006
11803	Vege, okra, boiled w/salt, drained	.5 cup slices	80	17.6	1.496	3.608	2	0.168	0.022	0.037	0.036
11278	Vege, okra, raw	1 cup	100	31	2	7.03	3.2	0.1	0.017	0.027	0.026
11296	Vege, onion rings, breaded, par fried, frozen, oven heated	10 rings, large	71	288.97	3.791	27.094	0.923	18.957	7.715	3.63	6.095
11805	Vege, onions, boiled w/salt, chopped, drained	1 cup	210	92.4	2.856	21.315	2.94	0.399	0.057	0.153	0.065
11282	Vege, onions, chopped, raw	1 cup, chopped	160	67.2	1.472	16.176	2.24	0.128	0.037	0.099	0.042
11291	Vege, onions, spring (tops & bulb) chopped, raw	1 cup, chopped	100	32	1.83	7.34	2.6	0.19	0.027	0.074	0.032
11808	Vege, parsnip, boiled w/salt, drained	.5 cup, sliced	78	63.18	1.03	15.233	3.12	0.234	0.087	0.037	0.039
11298	Vege, parsnip, peeled, raw	1 cup, sliced	133	99.75	1.596	23.927	6.517	0.399	0.149	0.063	0.067
11318	Vege, peas & carrots, canned, regular pack, solids & liquid	1 cup	255	96.9	5.534	21.624	5.1	0.688	0.059	0.329	0.125
11809	Vege, peas w/edible pod-snow/sugar, boiled w/salt, drained	1 cup	160	67.2	5.232	11.28	4.48	0.368	0.037	0.16	0.07
11300	Vege, peas w/edible pod-snow/sugar, raw	1 cup, chopped	98	41.16	2.744	7.399	2.548	0.196	0.021	0.087	0.038
11811	Vege, peas, green, boiled w/salt, drained	1 cup	160	134.4	8.576	25.024	8.8	0.352	0.03	0.163	0.062
11308	Vege, peas, green, canned, regular pack, drained	1 cup	170	117.3	7.514	21.386	6.97	0.595	0.053	0.277	0.105
11304	Vege, peas, green, raw	1 cup	145	117.45	7.859	20.967	7.395	0.58	0.051	0.271	0.103
11980	Vege, pepper, chili, green, canned	1 cup	139	29.19	1.001	6.394	2.363	0.375	0.024	0.213	0.039
11979	Vege, pepper, jalapeno, raw	1 cup, sliced	90	27	1.215	5.319	2.52	0.558	0.03	0.287	0.056
11977	Vege, pepper, serrano, raw	1 pepper	6.1	1.952	0.106	0.409	0.226	0.027	0.001	0.014	0.004
11333	Vege, pepper, sweet, green, chopped/sliced, raw	1 medium	119	23.8	1.023	5.522	2.023	0.202	0.01	0.074	0.069
11821	Vege, pepper, sweet, red, raw	1 medium	119	30.94	1.178	7.176	2.38	0.357	0.008	0.186	0.07
11951	Vege, pepper, sweet, yellow, raw	1 medium	186	50.22	1.86	11.755	1.674	0.391			0.058
11937	Vege, pickles, cucumber, dill	1 medium	65	11.7	0.403	2.678	0.78	0.123	0.002	0.05	0.031
11940	Vege, pickles, cucumber, sweet, gherkins	1 gherkin (2-3/4" long)	25	29.25	0.093	7.952	0.275	0.065	0.001	0.026	0.017
11943	Vege, pimiento, canned	1 tbsp	12	2.76	0.132	0.612	0.228	0.036	0.002	0.019	0.005
11383	Vege, potato mashed, granules w/milk, prep w/water & margarine	1 cup	210	243.6	4.599	33.768	2.73	10.059	4.105	2.824	2.541
11672	Vege, potato pancakes, homemade	1 pancake	76	206.72	4.682	21.766	1.52	11.582	3.526	4.971	2.313
11414	Vege, potato salad, homemade	1 cup	250	357.5	6.7	27.925	3.25	20.5	6.2	9.342	3.572
11373	Vege, potato, au gratin, homemade w/butter	1 cup	245	323.4	12.397	27.612	4.41	18.596	5.265	0.676	11.596
11833	Vege, potato, boiled w/o skin & w/salt	1 medium	167	143.62	2.856	33.417	3.34	0.167	0.003	0.072	0.043
11376	Vege, potato, canned, drained	1 cup	180	108	2.538	24.498	4.14	0.378	0.009	0.16	0.097
11838	Vege, potato, french fries, frozen, oven heated, w/salt	10 strips	50	100	1.585	15.595	1.6	3.78	2.381	0.389	0.631
11391	Vege, potato, hashed brown, plain, frozen, cooked	1 patty, (approx 3" x 1-1/2" x 1/2")	29	63.22	0.916	8.149	0.58	3.335	1.49	0.384	1.303
11387	Vege, potato, scalloped, mix, prep w/H$_2$O, whole milk & butter	1 cup (unprepared)	245	227.85	5.194	31.287	2.695	10.535	2.972	0.475	6.451

Chol (g)	Calc (mg)	Iron (mg)	Mag (mg)	Phos (mg)	Pota (mg)	Sodi (mg)	Zinc (mg)	Vit A (RAE)	Vit C (mg)	Thia (mg)	Ribo (mg)	Niac (mg)	Vit B$_6$ (mg)	Vit B$_{12}$ (µg)	Vit E (mg)	Fol (µg)	Alc (g)
0	52.51	1.869	24.92	31.15	160.2	17.8	0.107	73.87	10.68	0.053	0.027	0.356	0.207	0	0.819	56.96	0
0	37.2	1.364	17.36	21.08	107.88	305.04	0.074	2.48	5.208	0.032	0.025	0.248	0.14	0		29.76	0
0	2.625	0.093	0.975	2.475	17.85	0.375	0.015	12.45	0.278	0.004	0.005	0.027	0.006	0	0.014	5.475	0
0	3.3	0.097	1.4	3	24.7	0.8	0.023	29	2.4	0.007	0.007	0.031	0.007	0	0.013	13.6	0
0	107.8	1.886	43.12	118.58	819.28	48.51	0.862	86.24	21.02	0.199	0.113	0.668	0.248	0	0.162	301.8	0
0	3.6	0.086	1.3	2.9	19.4	2.8	0.018	37	1.8	0.007	0.008	0.038	0.009	0	0.029	3.8	0
0	103.6	0.98	21	57.4	282.8	352.8	0.154	442.4	35.42	0.057	0.088	0.606	0.137	0	1.694	102.2	0
0	57.68	0.818	17.92	24.08	198.24	14	0.112	294	39.2	0.045	0.062	0.448	0.101	0	1.126	104.7	0
0	61.6	0.224	28.8	25.6	108	4.8	0.344	11.2	13.04	0.106	0.044	0.697	0.15	0	0.216	36.8	0
0	81	0.8	57	63	303	8	0.6	19	21.1	0.2	0.06	1	0.215	0	0.36	88	0
0	22.01	1.2	13.49	57.51	91.59	266.25	0.298	7.81	0.994	0.199	0.099	2.563	0.055	0		46.86	0
0	46.2	0.504	23.1	73.5	348.6	501.9	0.441	0	10.92	0.088	0.048	0.347	0.271	0	0.042	31.5	0
0	35.2	0.304	16	43.2	230.4	4.8	0.256	0	10.24	0.077	0.04	0.133	0.235	0	0.032	30.4	0
0	72	1.48	20	37	276	16	0.39	50	18.8	0.055	0.08	0.525	0.061	0	0.55	64	0
0	28.86	0.452	22.62	53.82	286.26	191.88	0.203	0	10.14	0.065	0.04	0.565	0.073	0		45.24	0
0	47.88	0.785	38.57	94.43	498.75	13.3	0.785	0	22.61	0.12	0.067	0.931	0.12	0	1.982	89.11	0
0	58.65	1.912	35.7	117.3	255	663	1.479	737	16.83	0.189	0.135	1.482	0.224	0		45.9	0
0	67.2	3.152	41.6	88	384	384	0.592	86.4	76.64	0.205	0.122	0.862	0.23	0	0.624	46.4	0
0	42.14	2.038	23.52	51.94	196	3.92	0.265	52.92	58.8	0.147	0.078	0.588	0.157	0	0.382	41.16	0
0	43.2	2.464	62.4	187.2	433.6	382.4	1.904	64	22.72	0.414	0.238	3.234	0.346	0	0.224	100.8	0
0	34	1.615	28.9	113.9	294.1	428.4	1.207	45.9	16.32	0.206	0.133	1.244	0.109	0	0.051	74.8	0
0	36.25	2.132	47.85	156.6	353.8	7.25	1.798	55.1	58	0.386	0.191	3.03	0.245	0	0.189	94.25	0
0	50.04	1.849	5.56	15.29	157.07	551.83	0.125	8.34	47.54	0.014	0.042	0.872	0.167	0		75.06	0
0	9	0.63	17.1	27.9	193.5	0.9	0.207	36	39.87	0.13	0.051	1.005	0.457	0	0.423	42.3	0
0	0.671	0.052	1.342	2.44	18.605	0.61	0.016	2.867	2.739	0.003	0.005	0.094	0.031	0	0.042	1.403	0
0	11.9	0.405	11.9	23.8	208.25	3.57	0.155	21.42	95.68	0.068	0.033	0.571	0.267	0	0.44	13.09	0
0	8.33	0.512	14.28	30.94	251.09	2.38	0.298	186.8	226.1	0.064	0.101	1.165	0.346	0	1.88	21.42	0
0	20.46	0.856	22.32	44.64	394.32	3.72	0.316	18.6	341.3	0.052	0.047	1.655	0.312	0		48.36	0
0	5.85	0.344	7.15	13.65	75.4	833.3	0.091	5.85	1.235	0.009	0.019	0.039	0.008	0	0.058	0.65	0
0	1	0.147	1	3	8	234.75	0.02	2.25	0.3	0.002	0.008	0.043	0.004	0	0.023	0.25	0
0	0.72	0.202	0.72	2.04	18.96	1.68	0.023	15.96	10.19	0.002	0.007	0.074	0.026	0	0.083	0.72	0
4.2	67.2	0.441	42	130.2	325.5	361.2	0.504	98.7	13.65	0.189	0.181	1.814	0.336	0.21	1.071	16.8	0
72.96	18.24	1.186	25.08	84.36	597.36	386.08	0.631	5.32	16.72	0.103	0.131	1.629	0.288	0.144		17.48	0
170	47.5	1.625	37.5	130	635	1322.5	0.775	80	25	0.192	0.15	2.225	0.353	0		17.5	0
56.35	291.55	1.568	49	276.85	970.2	1060.85	1.691	156.8	24.26	0.157	0.284	2.433	0.426	0		26.95	0
0	13.36	0.518	33.4	66.8	547.76	402.47	0.451	0	12.36	0.164	0.032	2.191	0.449	0	0.017	15.03	0
0	9	2.268	25.2	50.4	412.2	394.2	0.504	0	9.18	0.122	0.023	1.647	0.338	0	0.09	10.8	0
0	4	0.62	11	41	209	133	0.2	0	5.05	0.056	0.014	1.044	0.154	0		6	0
0	4.35	0.438	4.93	20.88	126.44	9.86	0.093	0	1.827	0.032	0.006	0.702	0.037	0	0.055	2.03	0
26.95	88.2	0.931	34.3	137.2	497.35	835.45	0.613	85.75	8.085	0.047	0.137	2.521	0.103	0	0.368	24.5	0

EvaluEat Code	Food Name	Amt	Wt (g)	Energy (kcal)	Prot (g)	Carb (g)	Fiber (g)	Fat (g)	Mono (g)	Poly (g)	Sat (g)
11830	Vege, potato, skin only, baked w/salt	1 skin	58	114.84	2.488	26.715	4.582	0.058	0.001	0.025	0.015
11426	Vege, pumpkin pie mix, canned	1 cup	270	280.8	2.943	71.253	22.41	0.351	0.043	0.019	0.175
11846	Vege, pumpkin, canned w/salt	1 cup	245	83.3	2.695	19.796	7.105	0.686	0.091	0.037	0.358
11952	Vege, radicchio, raw	1 cup, shredded	40	9.2	0.572	1.792	0.36	0.1	0.004	0.044	0.024
11430	Vege, radish, oriental (daikon) raw	1 radish (7" long)	338	60.84	2.028	13.858	5.408	0.338	0.057	0.152	0.101
11429	Vege, radish, slices, raw	1 large (1" to 1-1/4" dia)	9	1.44	0.061	0.306	0.144	0.009	0.002	0.004	0.003
11851	Vege, rutabaga, boiled w/salt, drained	.5 cup, mashed	120	46.8	1.548	10.488		0.264	0.032	0.114	0.035
11439	Vege, sauerkraut, canned, solids & liquid	1 cup	142	26.98	1.292	6.078	3.55	0.199	0.018	0.087	0.05
11445	Vege, seaweed, kelp, raw	2 tbsp (1/8 cup)	10	4.3	0.168	0.957	0.13	0.056	0.01	0.005	0.025
11667	Vege, seaweed, spirulina, dried	1 cup	15	43.5	8.621	3.585	0.54	1.158	0.101	0.312	0.398
11677	Vege, shallots, peeled, raw	1 tbsp, chopped	10	7.2	0.25	1.68		0.01	0.001	0.004	0.002
11658	Vege, spinach egg souffle, homemade	1 cup	136	218.96	10.989	2.829		18.36	6.835	3.082	7.148
11854	Vege, spinach, boiled w/salt, drained	1 cup	180	41.4	5.346	6.75	4.32	0.468	0.013	0.194	0.076
11461	Vege, spinach, canned, drained	1 cup	214	49.22	6.013	7.276	5.136	1.07	0.03	0.447	0.173
11457	Vege, spinach, raw	1 cup	30	6.9	0.858	1.089	0.66	0.117	0.003	0.05	0.019
11864	Vege, squash, acorn, peeled, baked w/salt	1 cup, cubes	205	114.8	2.296	29.889	9.02	0.287	0.02	0.121	0.059
11866	Vege, squash, butternut, baked w/salt	1 cup, cubes	205	82	1.845	21.504		0.185	0.014	0.078	0.039
11870	Vege, squash, spaghetti, baked or boiled w/salt, drained	1 cup	155	41.85	1.023	10.013	2.17	0.403	0.034	0.195	0.096
11857	Vege, squash, summer, all varieties, boiled w/salt, drained	1 cup, sliced	180	36	1.638	7.758	2.52	0.558	0.041	0.236	0.115
11863	Vege, squash, winter, all varieties, baked w/salt	1 cup, cubes	205	79.95	1.824	17.938	5.74	1.291	0.096	0.543	0.266
11477	Vege, squash, zucchini w/skin, slices, raw	1 cup, chopped	124	19.84	1.5	4.154	1.364	0.223	0.017	0.094	0.046
11861	Vege, squash, zucchini w/skin, boiled w/salt, drained	.5 cup, sliced	90	14.4	0.576	3.537	1.26	0.045	0.004	0.019	0.009
11871	Vege, succotash (corn & lima beans) boiled w/salt, drained	1 cup	192	220.8	9.734	46.81		1.536	0.298	0.732	0.284
11875	Vege, sweet potato, baked in skin w/salt	1 medium (2" dia, 5" long, raw)	114	102.6	2.291	23.609	3.762	0.171	0.001	0.073	0.039
11647	Vege, sweet potato, canned w/syrup, drained	1 cup	196	211.68	2.509	49.706	5.88	0.627	0.024	0.276	0.135
11878	Vege, taro, cooked w/salt	1 cup, sliced	132	187.44	0.686	45.672	6.732	0.145	0.012	0.061	0.03
11954	Vege, tomatillos, raw	1 medium	34	10.88	0.326	1.986	0.646	0.347	0.053	0.142	0.047
11887	Vege, tomato paste, canned w/salt	1 can (6 oz)	170	139.4	7.344	32.147	7.65	0.799	0.141	0.381	0.182
11888	Vege, tomato puree, canned w/salt	1 cup	250	95	4.125	22.45	4.75	0.525	0.078	0.215	0.072
11549	Vege, tomato sauce, canned	1 cup	245	78.4	3.234	18.056	3.675	0.588	0.091	0.24	0.083
11533	Vege, tomato, red, canned, stewed	1 cup	255	66.3	2.321	15.785	2.55	0.484	0.074	0.196	0.066
11531	Vege, tomato, red, canned, whole	1 cup	240	40.8	1.92	9.384	2.16	0.312	0.05	0.13	0.043
11883	Vege, tomato, red, cherry, ripe, raw, June–October	1 cup	149	31.29	1.266	6.914	1.639	0.492	0.075	0.201	0.067
11529	Vege, tomato, red, ripe, whole, raw	1 cup, chopped or sliced	180	32.4	1.584	7.056	2.16	0.36	0.09	0.243	0.081
11955	Vege, tomato, sun-dried	1 cup	54	139.32	7.619	30.11	6.642	1.604	0.263	0.602	0.23
11696	Vege, tomato, yellow, raw	1 tomato	212	31.8	2.078	6.318	1.484	0.551	0.085	0.229	0.076
11891	Vege, turnip greens, boiled w/salt, drained	1 cup, chopped	144	28.8	1.642	6.278	5.04	0.331	0.022	0.131	0.076
11889	Vege, turnip, boiled w/salt, drained	1 cup, cubes	156	32.76	1.108	7.644	3.12	0.125	0.008	0.066	0.012
11990	Vege, wasabi, root, raw	1 cup, sliced	130	141.7	6.24	30.602	10.14	0.819			
11590	Vege, waterchestnut, Chinese, canned, solids & liquid	.5 cup, sliced	70	35	0.616	8.61	1.75	0.042	0.001	0.018	0.011
11591	Vege, watercress, raw	1 cup, chopped	34	3.74	0.782	0.439	0.17	0.034	0.003	0.012	0.009
11897	Vege, yam, boiled or baked w/salt	1 cup, cubes	136	157.76	2.026	37.509	5.304	0.19	0.007	0.082	0.039

Chol (g)	Calc (mg)	Iron (mg)	Mag (mg)	Phos (mg)	Pota (mg)	Sodi (mg)	Zinc (mg)	Vit A (RAE)	Vit C (mg)	Thia (mg)	Ribo (mg)	Niac (mg)	Vit B_6 (mg)	Vit B_{12} (µg)	Vit E (mg)	Fol (µg)	Alc (g)
0	19.72	4.083	24.94	58.58	332.34	149.06	0.284	0.58	7.83	0.071	0.061	1.778	0.356	0	0.023	12.76	0
0	99.9	2.862	43.2	121.5	372.6	561.6	0.729	1121	9.45	0.043	0.319	1.01	0.429	0		94.5	0
0	63.7	3.405	56.35	85.75	504.7	590.45	0.417	2702	10.29	0.059	0.132	0.899	0.137	0		29.4	0
0	7.6	0.228	5.2	16	120.8	8.8	0.248	0.4	3.2	0.006	0.011	0.102	0.023	0	0.904	24	0
0	91.26	1.352	54.08	77.74	767.26	70.98	0.507	0	74.36	0.068	0.068	0.676	0.155	0	0	94.64	0
0	2.25	0.031	0.9	1.8	20.97	3.51	0.025	0	1.332	0.001	0.004	0.023	0.006	0	0	2.25	0
0	57.6	0.636	27.6	67.2	391.2	304.8	0.42	0	22.56	0.098	0.049	0.858	0.122	0	0.384	18	0
0	42.6	2.087	18.46	28.4	241.4	938.62	0.27	1.42	20.87	0.03	0.031	0.203	0.185	0	0.142	34.08	0
0	16.8	0.285	12.1	4.2	8.9	23.3	0.123	0.6	0.3	0.005	0.015	0.047	0	0	0.087	18	0
0	18	4.275	29.25	17.7	204.45	157.2	0.3	4.35	1.515	0.357	0.551	1.923	0.055	0	0.75	14.1	0
0	3.7	0.12	2.1	6	33.4	1.2	0.04	6	0.8	0.006	0.002	0.02	0.034	0		3.4	0
183.6	229.84	1.346	38.08	231.2	201.28	762.96	1.292	266.6	2.992	0.091	0.305	0.477	0.12	1.36		80.24	0
0	244.8	6.426	156.6	100.8	838.8	550.8	1.368	943.2	17.64	0.171	0.425	0.882	0.436	0	3.744	262.8	0
0	271.78	4.922	162.64	94.16	740.44	57.78	0.984	1049	30.6	0.034	0.295	0.83	0.214	0	4.152	209.7	0
0	29.7	0.813	23.7	14.7	167.4	23.7	0.159	140.7	8.43	0.023	0.057	0.217	0.058	0	0.609	58.2	0
0	90.2	1.906	88.15	92.25	895.85	492	0.348	43.05	22.14	0.342	0.027	1.806	0.398	0		38.95	0
0	84.05	1.23	59.45	55.35	582.2	492	0.266	717.5	30.96	0.148	0.035	1.986	0.254	0		38.95	0
0	32.55	0.527	17.05		181.35	393.7	0.31	9.3	5.425	0.059	0.034	1.255	0.153	0		12.4	0
0	48.6	0.648	43.2	70.2	345.6	426.6	0.702	246.6	9.9	0.079	0.074	0.923	0.117	0	0.126	36	0
0	28.7	0.677	16.4	41	895.85	485.85	0.533	364.9	19.68	0.174	0.049	1.437	0.148	0		57.4	0
0	18.6	0.434	21.08	47.12	324.88	12.4	0.36	12.4	21.08	0.06	0.176	0.604	0.27	0	0.149	35.96	0
0	11.7	0.315	19.8	36	227.7	215.1	0.162	50.4	4.14	0.037	0.037	0.385	0.07	0	0.108	15.3	0
0	32.64	2.918	101.76	224.64	787.2	485.76	1.21	28.8	15.74	0.323	0.184	2.548	0.223	0		63.36	0
0	43.32	0.787	30.78	61.56	541.5	280.44	0.365	1096	22.34	1.65	0.121	1.695	0.326	0	0.809	6.84	0
0	33.32	1.862	23.52	49	378.28	76.44	0.314	701.7	21.17	0.049	0.074	0.666	0.122	0	0.549	15.68	0
0	23.76	0.95	39.6	100.32	638.88	331.32	0.356	0	6.6	0.141	0.037	0.673	0.437	0		25.08	0
0	2.38	0.211	6.8	13.26	91.12	0.34	0.075	2.04	3.978	0.015	0.012	0.629	0.019	0	0.129	2.38	0
0	61.2	5.066	71.4	141.1	1723.8	1343	1.071	129.2	37.23	0.102	0.26	5.229	0.367	0	7.31	20.4	0
0	45	4.45	57.5	100	1097.5	997.5	0.9	65	26.5	0.063	0.2	3.665	0.315	0	4.925	27.5	0
0	31.85	2.499	39.2	63.7	810.95	1283.8	0.49	41.65	17.15	0.059	0.162	2.389	0.238	0	5.096	22.05	0
0	86.7	3.391	30.6	51	527.85	563.55	0.433	22.95	20.15	0.117	0.089	1.821	0.043	0	2.116	12.75	0
0	74.4	2.328	26.4	45.6	451.2	307.2	0.336	14.4	21.6	0.108	0.113	1.764	0.216	0	1.704	19.2	0
0	7.45	0.67	16.39	35.76	330.78	13.41	0.134	46.19	38.74	0.088	0.072	0.936	0.119	0	0.507	22.35	0
0	18	0.486	19.8	43.2	426.6	9	0.306	75.6	22.86	0.067	0.034	1.069	0.144	0	0.972	27	0
0	59.4	4.909	104.76	192.24	1850.58	1131.3	1.075	23.76	21.17	0.285	0.264	4.887	0.179	0	0.005	36.72	0
0	23.32	1.039	25.44	76.32	546.96	48.76	0.594	0	19.08	0.087	0.1	2.499	0.119	0		63.6	0
0	197.28	1.152	31.68	41.76	292.32	381.6	0.202	548.6	39.46	0.065	0.104	0.592	0.259	0	2.707	169.9	0
0	34.32	0.343	12.48	29.64	210.6	446.16	0.312	0	18.1	0.042	0.036	0.466	0.105	0		14.04	0
0	166.4	1.339	89.7	104	738.4	22.1	2.106	2.6	54.47	0.17	0.148	0.966	0.356	0		23.4	0
0	2.8	0.609	3.5	13.3	82.6	5.6	0.266	0	0.91	0.008	0.017	0.252	0.111	0	0.35	4.2	0
0	40.8	0.068	7.14	20.4	112.2	13.94	0.037	79.9	14.62	0.031	0.041	0.068	0.044	0	0.34	3.06	0
0	19.04	0.707	24.48	66.64	911.2	331.84	0.272	8.16	16.46	0.129	0.038	0.751	0.31	0	0.517	21.76	0

EvaluEat Code	Food Name	Amt	Wt (g)	Energy (kcal)	Prot (g)	Carb (g)	Fiber (g)	Fat (g)	Mono (g)	Poly (g)	Sat (g)
11601	Vege, yam, peeled, raw	1 cup, cubes	150	177	2.295	41.82	6.15	0.255	0.009	0.114	0.056
11603	Vege, yambean (jicama) peeled, slices, raw	1 cup, sliced	120	45.6	0.864	10.584	5.88	0.108	0.006	0.052	0.025
14187	Vegetable beverage, clam & tomato juice, canned	1 can (5.5 oz)	166	79.68	0.996	18.177	0.332	0.332	0.013	0.033	0.08
11578	Vegetable juice cocktail, canned	1 cup	242	45.98	1.525	11.011	1.936	0.218	0.034	0.092	0.031
11159	Vegetable salad, coleslaw, homemade	.5 cup	60	41.4	0.774	7.446	0.9	1.566	0.425	0.811	0.231
11894	Vegetables, mixed, frozen, boiled w/salt, drained	.5 cup	91	53.69	2.603	11.912	4.004	0.137	0.009	0.066	0.028
43134	Vegetarian fillets	1 cup	186	539.4	42.78	16.74	11.346	33.48	8.139	17.358	5.299
43137	Vegetarian meatloaf or patties	1 cup	186	366.42	39.06	14.88	8.556	16.74	4.07	8.679	2.65
43136	Vegetarian stew	1 cup	186	228.78	31.62	13.02	2.046	5.58	1.356	2.892	0.883
22121	Vegetarian, Better'n Burgers/vegan burgers, frozen/Worthington, Morningstar	1 patty	85	90.95	13.906	7.531	4.25	0.535	0.318	0.173	0.107
22122	Vegetarian, breakfast patties/Worthington, Morningstar	1 patty	38	79.42	9.918	3.716	1.976	2.77	0.688	1.319	0.509
22120	Vegetarian, burger crumbles/Worthington, Morningstar	1 cup	110	231	22.154	6.622	5.06	12.925	4.628	4.925	3.257
22215	Vegetarian, chili w/beans, canned entree/Nestle Chef-Mate	1 cup	253	412.39	17.735	29.044	11.132	25.022	10.747	1.397	10.93
22119	Vegetarian, deli franks/Worthington, Morningstar	1 serving	45	111.6	10.386	3.699	2.745	6.16	1.953	3.314	0.893
22118	Vegetarian, garden patties, frozen/Worthington, Morningstar	1 patty	67	119.26	11.209	10.204	4.02	3.765	1.065	2.161	0.539
22125	Vegetarian, Harvest Burger, original flavor, vegetable protein patty	1 patty	90	137.7	18	7.02	5.67	4.14	2.135	0.265	1.017
22223	Vegetarian, macaroni and cheese, canned entree/Nestle Chef-Mate	1 cup	253	283.36	10.803	35.42	3.289	11.005	3.026	0.524	6.199
22128	Vegetarian, Natural Touch Vegan Burgers, frozen/Worthington	1 patty	85	90.95	13.906	7.531	4.25	0.535	0.318	0.173	0.107
22123	Vegetarian, Spicy Black Bean Burger/Worthington, Morningstar	1 patty	78	114.66	11.786	15.202	4.758	0.78	0.25	0.351	0.179
2048	Vinegar, cider	1 tbsp	15	2.1	0	0.885	0	0	0	0	0
2053	Vinegar, distilled	1 tbsp	13	1.56	0	0.65	0	0	0	0	0
48052	Vital wheat gluten	1 cup	148	547.6	111.24	20.409	0.888	2.738	0.231	1.199	0.403
18505	Waffle, Eggo Lowfat Homestyle/Kellogg	1 waffle, round (4"dia)	35	82.6	2.471	15.453	0.35	1.246	0.35	0.375	0.315
18367	Waffle, plain, homemade	1 waffle, round (7"dia)	75	218.25	5.925	24.675		10.575	2.641	5.089	2.149
18365	Waffle, plain/buttermilk, frozen, ready-to-heat	1 waffle square	39	97.89	2.301	15.054	0.858	3.042	1.23	1.081	0.505
1072	Whipped dessert topping, nondairy, pressurized can	1 tbsp	4	10.56	0.039	0.643	0	0.892	0.077	0.01	0.756
1073	Whipped dessert topping, nondairy, semi-solid, frozen	1 tbsp	4	12.72	0.05	0.922	0	1.012	0.065	0.021	0.871
42135	Whipped topping, frozen, low-fat	1 oz	28.34	62.348	0.85	6.688	0	3.713	0.237	0.076	3.195
43406	Yeast extract spread	1 fl. oz.	29.8	47.084	8.284	3.516	0.894	0	0	0	0
19393	Yogurt, frozen, chocolate, soft serve	.5 cup (4 fl. oz.)	72	115.2	2.88	17.928	1.584	4.32	1.26	0.158	2.614
43261	Yogurt, fruit variety, nonfat	1 cup	186	174.84	8.184	35.34	0	0.372	0.093	0.03	0.221
1121	Yogurt, lowfat w/fruit, 10 g protein/8 oz	1 cup (8 fl. oz.)	245	249.9	10.707	46.673	0	2.646	0.728	0.076	1.708
1117	Yogurt, lowfat, plain, 12 g protein/8 oz	1 cup (8 fl. oz.)	245	154.35	12.863	17.248	0	3.797	1.044	0.108	2.45
1116	Yogurt, whole milk, plain, 8 g protein/8 oz	1 cup (8 fl. oz.)	245	149.45	8.502	11.417	0	7.963	2.188	0.225	5.135

Chol (g)	Calc (mg)	Iron (mg)	Mag (mg)	Phos (mg)	Pota (mg)	Sodi (mg)	Zinc (mg)	Vit A (RAE)	Vit C (mg)	Thia (mg)	Ribo (mg)	Niac (mg)	Vit B₆ (mg)	Vit B₁₂ (µg)	Vit E (mg)	Fol (µg)	Alc (g)
0	25.5	0.81	31.5	82.5	1224	13.5	0.36	10.5	25.65	0.168	0.048	0.828	0.44	0	0.585	34.5	0
0	14.4	0.72	14.4	21.6	180	4.8	0.192	1.2	24.24	0.024	0.035	0.24	0.05	0	0.552	14.4	0
0	19.92	0.996	36.52	129.48	149.4	600.92	1.793	18.26	6.806	0.066	0.05	0.315	0.139	50.796		26.56	0
0	26.62	1.016	26.62	41.14	467.06	653.4	0.484	188.8	67.03	0.104	0.068	1.757	0.339	0	12.1	50.82	0
4.8	27	0.354	6	19.2	108.6	13.8	0.12	31.8	19.62	0.04	0.037	0.163	0.076	0		16.2	0
0	22.75	0.746	20.02	46.41	153.79	246.61	0.446	194.7	2.912	0.065	0.109	0.774	0.067	0		17.29	0
0	176.7	3.72	42.78	837	1116	911.4	2.604	0	0	2.046	1.674	22.32	2.79	7.812	6.417	189.7	0
0	53.94	3.906	33.48	639.84	334.8	1023	3.348	0	0	1.674	1.116	18.6	2.232	4.464	3.218	145.1	0
0	57.66	2.418	236.22	409.2	223.2	744	2.046	87.42	0	1.302	1.116	22.32	2.046	4.092	0.911	191.6	0
0	86.7	2.899	16.15	181.05	433.5	382.5	0.748		0	0.256	0.553	4.113	0.198	0	0.009	245.7	0
0.76	18.24	1.919	1.14	106.4	101.84	259.16	0.369		0	5.385	0.133	1.835	0.19	1.497	0.298		0
0	79.2	6.402	2.2	173.8	178.2	476.3	1.639		0	9.922	0.352	2.981	0.539	4.367	0.689		0
55.66	88.55	4.832	45.54	166.98	511.06	1171.39	3.871		0.759	0.106	0.202	3.476	0.228	1.442	1.209		0
0.45	17.1	0.608	3.6	42.3	49.95	430.65	0.378		0	0.144	0.022	0	0.012	0.009	1.256		0
0.67	48.24	1.213	29.48	123.95	179.56	381.9	0.576	134	0	6.465	0.101	0	0	0	0.549	58.96	0
0	101.7	3.852	70.2	225	432	411.3	8.073		0	0.315	0.198	6.3	0.387	0	1.557	21.6	0
27.83	202.4	1.923	32.89	250.47	151.8	1343.43	1.569		0	0.319	0.331	2.505	0.071	0.202	0.159		0
0	86.7	2.899	16.15	181.05	433.5	382.5	0.748		0	0.256	0.553	4.113	0.198	0	0.009	245.7	0
0.78	56.16	1.841	43.68	149.76	269.1	499.2	0.928		0	8.057	0.14	0	0.211	0.07	0.359		0
0	0.9	0.09	3.3	1.35	15	0.15	0	0	0	0	0	0	0	0	0	0	0
0	0	0	2.86	0	1.95	0.13	0	0	0	0	0	0	0	0	0	0	0
0	210.16	7.696	37	384.8	148	42.92	1.258	0	0	0	0	0	0	0	0	0	0
8.75	20.3	1.946	23.8	28.35	50.05	154.7			0	0.308	0.259	2.593	0.164	0.549		26.95	
51.75	191.25	1.732	14.25	142.5	119.25	383.25	0.51	48.75	0.3	0.197	0.26	1.555	0.042	0.188		34.5	0
12.48	86.19	1.657	8.19	155.61	47.58	291.72	0.214	149	0	0.178	0.196	1.826	0.369	0.928	0.246	23.79	0
0	0.2	0.001	0.04	0.72	0.76	2.48	0	0.16	0	0	0	0	0	0	0.034	0	0
0	0.24	0.005	0.08	0.32	0.72	1	0.001	0.28	0	0	0	0	0	0	0.038	0	0
0.567	20.121	0.028	1.984	20.972	28.623	20.405	0.028	1.134	0	0.006	0.026	0.028	0.006	0.057	0.142	0.85	0
0	25.628	1.103	53.64	30.992	774.8	1072.8	0.626	0	0	2.891	4.261	28.906	0.387	0.149		301	0
3.6	105.84	0.9	19.44	100.08	187.92	70.56	0.353	31.68	0.216	0.026	0.152	0.22	0.053	0.209	0.097	7.92	0
3.72	282.72	0.13	27.9	221.34	360.84	107.88	1.376	3.72	1.302	0.074	0.335	0.186	0.074	0.874	0.112	16.74	0
9.8	372.4	0.171	36.75	291.55	477.75	142.1	1.813	24.5	1.715	0.091	0.436	0.233	0.098	1.151	0.049	22.05	0
14.7	448.35	0.196	41.65	352.8	573.3	171.5	2.181	34.3	1.96	0.108	0.524	0.279	0.12	1.372	0.073	26.95	0
31.85	296.45	0.123	29.4	232.75	379.75	112.7	1.446	66.15	1.225	0.071	0.348	0.184	0.078	0.907	0.147	17.15	0

Appendix B *Calculations and Conversions*

Calculation and Conversion Aids

Commonly Used Metric Units

millimetre (mm): one-thousandth of a metre (0.001)
centimetre (cm): one-hundredth of a metre (0.01)
kilometre (km): one-thousand times a metre (1000)
kilogram (kg): one-thousand times a gram (1000)
milligram (mg): one-thousandth of a gram (0.001)
microgram (μg): one-millionth of a gram (0.000001)
millilitre (mL): one-thousandth of a litre (0.001)

International Units

Some vitamin supplements may report vitamin content as International Units (IU).

To convert IU to:

- Micrograms of vitamin D (cholecalciferol), divide the IU value by 40 or multiply by 0.025.
- Milligrams of vitamin E (alpha-tocopherol), divide the IU value by 1.5 if vitamin E is from natural sources. Divide the IU value by 2.22 if vitamin E is from synthetic sources.
- Vitamin A: 1 IU = 0.3 μg retinol or 3.6 μg beta-carotene

Retinol Activity Equivalents

Retinol activity equivalents (RAE) are a standardized unit of measure for vitamin A. RAE account for the various differences in bioavailability from sources of vitamin A. Many supplements will report vitamin A content in IU, as shown above, or retinol equivalents (RE).

1 RAE = 1 μg retinol
          12 μg beta-carotene
          24 μg other vitamin A carotenoids

To calculate RAE from the RE value of vitamin carotenoids in foods, divide RE by 2.
For vitamin A supplements and foods fortified with vitamin A, 1 RE = 1 RAE.

Folate

Folate is measured as dietary folate equivalents (DFE). DFE account for the different factors affecting bioavailability of folate sources.

1 DFE = 1 μg food folate
          0.6 μg folate from fortified foods
          0.5 μg folate supplement taken on an empty stomach
          0.6 μg folate as a supplement consumed with a meal

To convert micrograms of synthetic folate, such as that found in supplements or fortified foods, to DFE:

μg synthetic folate × 1.7 = μg DFE

For naturally occurring food folate, such as spinach, each microgram of folate equals 1 microgram DFE:

μg folate = μg DFE

Conversion Factors

Original Unit	Multiply by	To Get
grams	28.3495	ounces avdp
pounds	0.0625	ounces
kilograms	0.4536	pounds
ounces	16	pounds
ounces	0.0353	grams
pounds	0.002205	grams
pounds	2.2046	kilograms
pints (dry)	1.8162	litres
pints (liquid)	2.1134	litres
quarts (dry)	0.9081	litres
quarts (liquid)	1.0567	litres
gallons (imperial)	0.2642	litres
litres	0.5506	pints (dry)
litres	0.4732	pints (liquid)
litres	1.1012	quarts (dry)
litres	0.9463	quarts (liquid)
litres	3.7853	gallons (Imperial)
inches	0.0394	millimetres
inches	0.3937	centimetres
feet	0.03281	centimetres
millimetres	25.4000	inches
centimetres	2.5400	inches
metres	0.0254	inches
metres	0.3048	feet
feet	3.2808	metres
yards	1.0936	metres
cubic metres	0.0283	cubic feet
cubic feet	35.03145	cubic metres
cubic yards	1.3079	cubic metres
cubic metres	0.7646	cubic yards

Length: Imperial and Metric Equivalents

¼ inch = 0.6 centimetres
1 inch = 2.5 centimetres
1 foot = 0.3048 metre
       = 30.48 centimetres
1 yard = 0.91144 metre
1 millimetre = 0.03937 inch
1 centimetre = 0.3937 inch
1 decimetre = 3.937 inches
1 metre = 39.37 inches
       = 1.094 yards
1 micron = 0.00003937 inch

Weights and Measures

Food Measurement Equivalencies from U.S. to Metric

Capacity

¼ teaspoon = 1.25 millilitres
½ teaspoon = 2.5 millilitres
1 teaspoon = 5 millilitres
1 tablespoon = 15 millilitres
1 fluid ounce = 28.4 millilitres
¼ cup = 65 millilitres
⅓ cup = 80 millilitres
½ cup = 125 millilitres
1 cup = 250 millilitres
1 U.S. pint (2 cups) = 473 millilitres
1 quart (4 cups) = 0.95 litre
1 litre (1.06 quarts) = 1000 millilitres
1 gallon (4 quarts) = 3.84 litres

Weight

0.035 ounce = 1 gram
1 ounce = 28 grams
¼ pound (4 ounces) = 114 grams
1 pound (16 ounces) = 454 grams
2.2 pounds (35 ounces) = 1 kilogram

Food Measurement Equivalents

3 teaspoons = 1 tablespoon
½ tablespoon = 1½ teaspoons
2 tablespoons = ⅛ cup
4 tablespoons = ¼ cup
5 tablespoons + 1 teaspoon = ⅓ cup
8 tablespoons = ½ cup
10 tablespoons + 2 teaspoons = ⅔ cup
12 tablespoons = ¾ cup
16 tablespoons = 1 cup
2 cups = 1 pint
4 cups = 1 quart
2 pints = 1 quart
4 quarts = 1 gallon

Volumes and Capacities

1 cup = 8 fluid ounces
½ liquid pint
1 millilitre = 0.061 cubic inches
1 litre = 1.057 liquid quarts
0.908 dry quart
61.024 cubic inches
1 U.S. gallon = 231 cubic inches
3.785 litres
0.833 British gallon
128 U.S fluid ounces
1 British Imperial gallon = 277.42 cubic inches
1.201 U.S gallons
4.546 litres
160 British fluid ounces
1 U.S. ounce, liquid or fluid = 1.805 cubic inches
29.574 millilitres
1.041 British fluid ounces
1 pint, dry = 33.600 cubic inches
0.551 litre
1 pint, liquid = 28.875 cubic inches
0.473 litre
1 U.S. quart, dry = 67.201 cubic inches
1.101 litres
1 U.S. quart, liquid = 57.75 cubic inches
0.946 litre
1 British quart = 69.354 cubic inches
1.032 U.S. quarts, dry
1.201 U.S. quarts, liquid

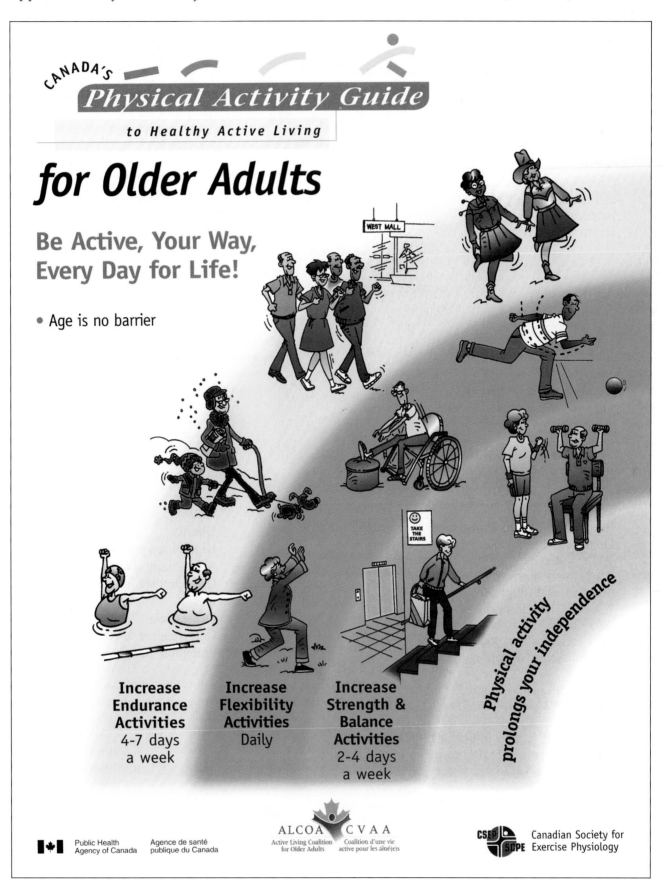

CANADA'S
Physical Activity Guide
to Healthy Active Living

for Older Adults

Be Active, Your Way, Every Day for Life!

- Age is no barrier

WEST MALL

TAKE THE STAIRS

Physical activity prolongs your independence

Increase Endurance Activities
4-7 days a week

Increase Flexibility Activities
Daily

Increase Strength & Balance Activities
2-4 days a week

Public Health Agency of Canada   Agence de santé publique du Canada

ALCOA   CVAA
Active Living Coalition for Older Adults   Coalition d'une vie active pour les aîné(e)s

CSEP SCPE   Canadian Society for Exercise Physiology

Being active is very safe for most people

Start slowly and build up – listen to your body. Accumulate 30 to 60 minutes of moderate physical activity most days. Minutes count – add it up 10 minutes at a time. Not sure? Consult with a health-care professional.

Choose a variety of activities from each of these three groups:

Endurance
- Continuous activities that make you feel warm and breathe deeply
- Increase your energy
- Improve your heart, lungs, and circulatory system

Flexibility
- Gentle reaching, bending, and stretching
- Keep your muscles relaxed and joints mobile
- Move more easily and be more agile

Strength & Balance
- Lift weights, do resistance activities
- Improve balance and posture
- Keep muscles and bones strong
- Prevent bone loss

Getting started is easier than you think

- Build physical activity into your daily routine.
- Do the activities you are doing now, more often.
- Walk wherever and whenever you can.
- Start slowly with easy stretching.
- Move around frequently.
- Take the stairs instead of the elevator.
- Carry home the groceries.
- Find activities that you enjoy.
- Try out a class in your community.

For a free copy of the companion *Handbook* and more information: **1-888-334-9769**, or *Web site:* **www.healthcanada.ca/paguide**

> **Eating well is also important. Follow *Canada's Food Guide to Healthy Eating* to make wise food choices.**

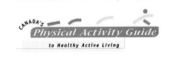

No changes permitted. Permission to photocopy this document in its entirety not required.
Cat. No. H39-429/1999-1E ISBN 0-662-27781-3

Benefits increase as physical activity increases

Benefits when starting out:
- Meet new people
- Feel more relaxed
- Sleep better
- Have more fun

Benefits from regular physical activity:
- Continued independent living
- Better physical and mental health
- Improved quality of life
- More energy
- Move with fewer aches and pains
- Better posture and balance
- Improved self-esteem
- Weight maintenance
- Stronger muscles and bones
- Relaxation and reduced stress

Scientists have proved that

Being active reduces the risk of:
- Heart disease
- Falls and injuries
- Obesity
- High blood pressure
- Adult-onset diabetes
- Osteoporosis
- Stroke
- Depression
- Colon cancer
- Premature death

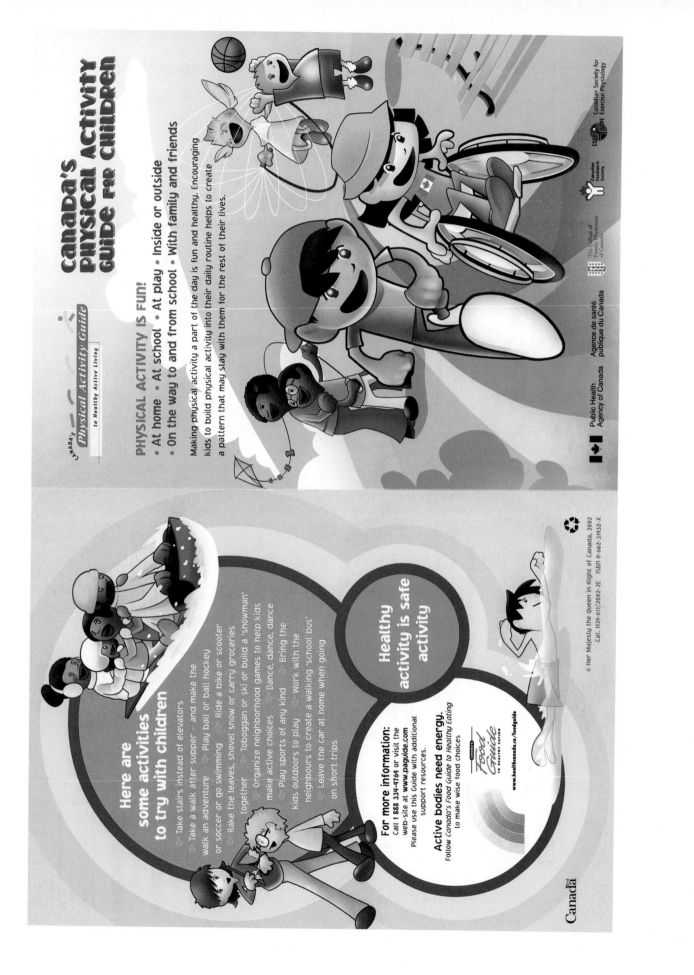

Canada's Physical Activity Guide for Children

CANADA'S *Physical Activity Guide*
to Healthy Active Living

PHYSICAL ACTIVITY IS FUN!

- At home • At school • At play • Inside or outside
- On the way to and from school • With family and friends

Making physical activity a part of the day is fun and healthy. Encouraging kids to build physical activity into their daily routine helps to create a pattern that may stay with them for the rest of their lives.

Here are some activities to try with children

- Take stairs instead of elevators
- Take a walk after supper — and make the walk an adventure
- Play ball or ball hockey
- Ride a bike or scooter or soccer or go swimming
- Rake the leaves, shovel snow or carry groceries together
- Toboggan or ski or build a 'snowman'
- Organize neighborhood games to help kids make active choices
- Dance, dance, dance
- Play sports of any kind
- Bring the kids outdoors to play
- Work with the neighbours to create a walking 'school bus' on short trips
- Leave the car at home when going

Healthy activity is safe activity

For more information:
Call 1 888 334-9769 or visit the web-site at **www.paguide.com**
Please use this Guide with additional support resources.

Active bodies need energy.
Follow *Canada's Food Guide to Healthy Eating* to make wise food choices

Food Guide TO HEALTHY EATING

www.healthcanada.ca/foodguide

Public Health Agency of Canada — Agence de santé publique du Canada

The College of Family Physicians of Canada

Canadian Paediatric Society

CSEP SCPE Canadian Society for Exercise Physiology

© Her Majesty the Queen in Right of Canada, 2002
Cat. H39-611/2002-2E   ISBN 0-662-31932-X

Canada

The Benefits of Regular Activity

- Builds strong bones and strengthens muscles
- Maintains flexibility
- Achieves a healthy weight
- Promotes good posture and balance
- Improves fitness
- Meet new friends
- Strengthens the heart
- Improves physical self-esteem
- Increases relaxation
- Enhances healthy growth and development

Endurance
Flexibility
Strength

All contribute to a healthy body

Combine 3 types of physical activity for best results:

1. **Endurance** activities that strengthen the heart and lungs such as running, jumping and swimming.
2. **Flexibility** activities that encourage children to bend, stretch and reach such as gymnastics and dancing.
3. **Strength** building activities that build strong muscles and bones such as climbing or swinging across the playground ladder.

CALL TO ACTION

for parents, educators, physicians and community leaders

Canada's Guidelines for INCREASING Physical Activity in Children

This Guide will help children:

- **INCREASE** time **CURRENTLY** spent on physical activity, starting with 30 minutes **MORE** per day (See CHART BELOW)
- **REDUCE** "non active" time spent on TV, video, computer games and surfing the Internet, starting with 30 minutes **LESS** per day (See CHART BELOW)

Build up physical activity throughout the day in periods of at least 5 to 10 minutes

	Daily INCREASE in moderate* physical activity (Minutes)		Daily INCREASE in vigorous** physical activity (Minutes)		Total Daily INCREASE in physical activity (Minutes)	Daily DECREASE in non-active time (Minutes)
Month 1	at least 20	+	10	=	30	30
Month 2	at least 30	+	15	=	45	45
Month 3	at least 40	+	20	=	60	60
Month 4	at least 50	+	25	=	75	75
Month 5	at least 60	+	30	=	90	90

Congratulations! Daily active time is part of a healthy lifestyle.

* Moderate physical activity examples
- brisk walking • swimming
- skating • playing outdoors
- bike riding

** Vigorous physical activity examples
- running • soccer

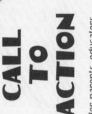

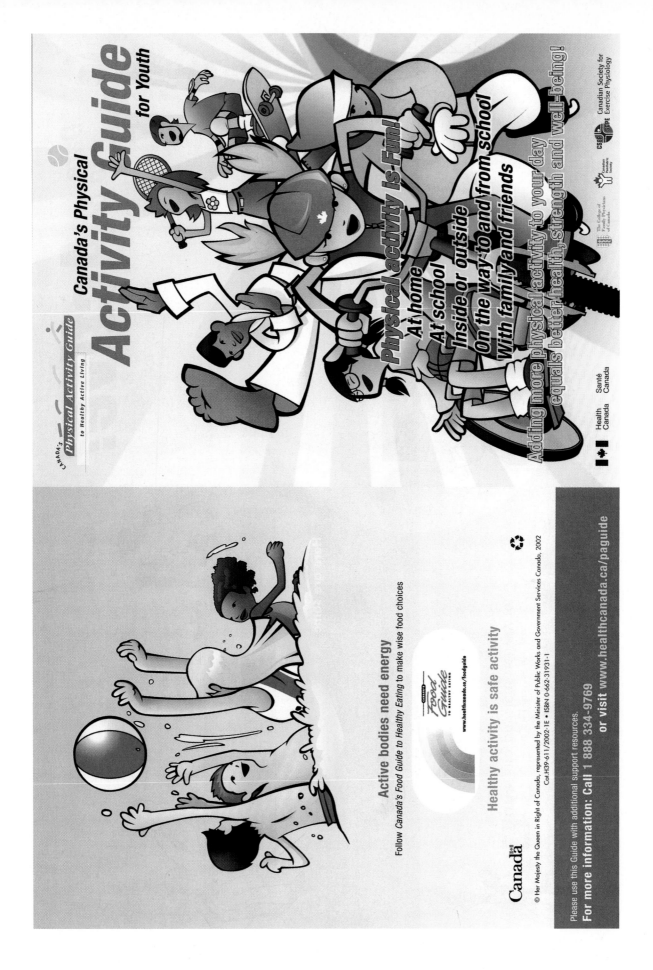

Dare to be Active!

Tune into physical activity to:

- Meet new friends
- Improve physical self-esteem
- Achieve a healthy weight
- Build strong bones and strengthen muscles
- Maintain flexibility

- Promote good posture and balance
- Improve fitness
- Strengthen the heart
- Increase relaxation
- Promote healthy growth and development

Here's the SCOOP!

– Combine three types of physical activity for best results:

1. **Endurance** activities that make you breathe deeper, your heart beat faster, and make you feel warm.
2. **Flexibility** activities like bending, stretching and reaching that keep your joints moving.
3. **Strength** activities that build your muscles and bones.

Let's Get ACTIVE!

Canada's Guidelines for **INCREASING** Physical Activity in Youth

This Guide will help you:

1. **INCREASE** time **CURRENTLY** spent on physical activity, starting with 30 minutes **MORE** per day (See CHART BELOW)
2. **REDUCE** "non active" time spent on TV, video, computer games and surfing the Internet, starting with 30 minutes **LESS** per day (See CHART BELOW)

Build up physical activity throughout the day in periods of at least 5 to 10 minutes

MONTH	Daily INCREASE in moderate* activity (Minutes)	Daily INCREASE in vigorous** activity (Minutes)	Total Daily INCREASE in physical activity (Minutes)	Daily DECREASE in non-active time (Minutes)
Month 1	at least 20	+ 10	= 30	30
Month 2	at least 30	+ 15	= 45	45
Month 3	at least 40	+ 20	= 60	60
Month 4	at least 50	+ 25	= 75	75
Month 5	at least 60	+ 30	= 90	90

Congratulations!

Daily active time is part of a healthy lifestyle.

*Moderate physical activity examples
- Brisk walking, skating, bike riding

**Vigorous physical activity examples
- Running, supervised weight training, basketball, soccer

Here are some ideas to get you started

Decide to take the first step – It's all up to you – And YOU can DO it!

- Walk more – to school, to the mall, to the park, to your friend's house
- Walk, run or bike instead of getting a drive with mom or dad
- Take the dog for a walk
- Run, jump, skateboard, snow-board, ski, skate or toboggan
- Play sports
- Go skating, swimming, bike riding or bowling
- Rake the leaves, shovel snow or carry the groceries
- Take a class like yoga, hip hop, aerobics or gymnastics
- Check out some activities at the community centre
- Be active with your friends
- Put on some music and move
- Stretch your muscles every day
- Try something new like wall climbing or dance classes

Choose activities you like or think you might like.

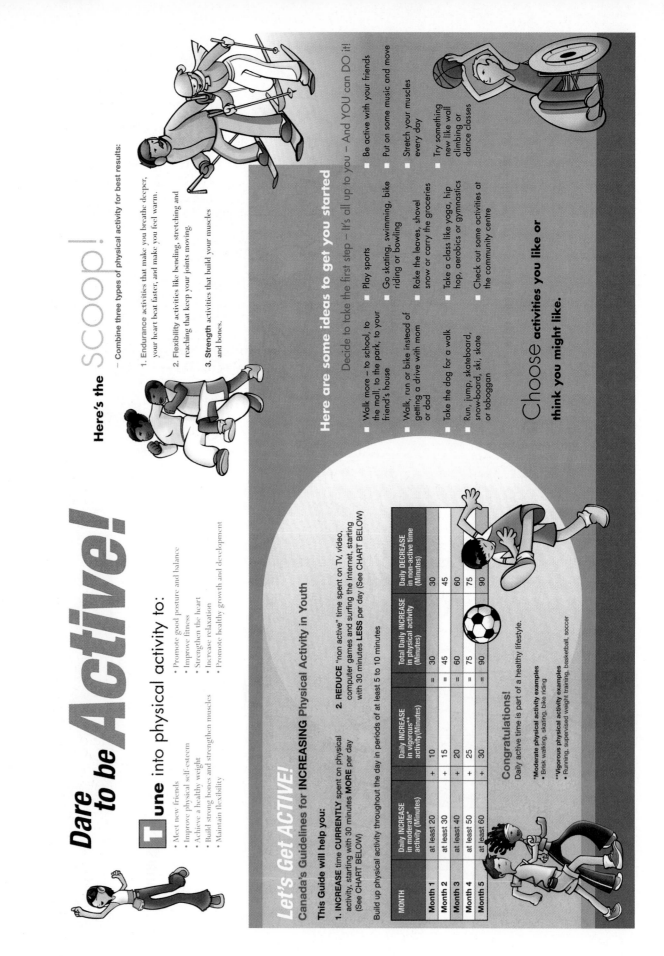

Nutrient Classification	Nutrient	Primary Functions	Recommended Intake	Toxicity Symptoms/ Side Effects	Deficiency Symptoms/ Side Effects	Chapter Reference
Water-soluble vitamin	Thiamin vitamin B_1	Part of the coenzyme thiamin pyrophosphate (TPP) involved in carbohydrate metabolism Coenzyme involved in branched-chain amino acid metabolism	RDA: Men = 1.2 mg/day Women = 1.1 mg/day	None known at this time	Beriberi Anorexia and weight loss Apathy Decreased short-term memory Confusion and irritability Muscle weakness Enlarged heart	10
Water-soluble vitamin	Riboflavin vitamin B_2	Coenzymes involved in oxidation-reduction reactions, including flavin mononucleotide (FMN) and flavin adenine dinucleotide (FAD).	RDA: Men = 1.3 mg/day Women = 1.1 mg/day	None known at this time	Ariboflavinosis Sore throat Swelling of mouth and throat Cheilosis Angular stomatitis Glossitis (magenta tongue) Seborrheic dermatitis Anemia	10
Water-soluble vitamin	Niacin (nicotinamide and nicotinic acid)	Coenzymes in carbohydrate and fatty acid metabolism, including nicotinamide adenine dinucleotide (NAD^+ and NADH) and nicotinamide adenine dinucleotide phosphate ($NADP^+$) Plays role in DNA replication and repair and cell differentiation	RDA: Men = 16 mg/day Women = 14 mg/day	Flushing Liver dysfunction and damage Glucose intolerance Blurred vision and edema of eyes	Pellagra Pigmented rash Vomiting Constipation or diarrhea Bright red tongue Depression Apathy Headache Fatigue Loss of memory	10
Water-soluble vitamin	Vitamin B_6 (pyridoxine)	Part of coenzyme (pyridoxal phosphate, or PLP) involved in amino acid metabolism, synthesis of blood cells, and carbohydrate metabolism	RDA: Men aged 19 to 50 = 1.3 mg/day Men aged > 50 = 1.7 mg/day Women aged 19 to 50 = 1.3 mg/day Women aged > 50 = 1.5 mg/day	Sensory neuropathy Lesions of the skin	Seborrheic dermatitis Microcytic anemia Convulsions Depression and confusion	10
Water-soluble vitamin	Folate (folic acid)	Coenzyme tetrahydrofolate (THF) (or tetrahydrofolic acid, THFA) involved in DNA synthesis and amino acid metabolism Involved in the metabolism of homocysteine	RDA: Men = 400 µg/day Women = 400 µg/day	Masks symptoms of vitamin B_{12} deficiency Neurological damage	Macrocytic anemia Weakness and fatigue Difficulty concentrating Irritability Headache Palpitations Shortness of breath Elevated levels of homocysteine in the blood Neural tube defects in the developing fetus	10

continued

Nutrient Classification	Nutrient	Primary Functions	Recommended Intake	Toxicity Symptoms/Side Effects	Deficiency Symptoms/Side Effects	Chapter Reference
Water-soluble vitamin	Vitamin B_{12} (cobalamin)	Part of coenzymes that assist with formation of blood, nervous system function, and homocysteine metabolism	RDA: Men = 2.4 µg/day Women = 2.4 µg/day	None known at this time	Pernicious anemia; Pale skin; Diminished energy and low exercise tolerance; Fatigue; Shortness of breath; Palpitations; Tingling and numbness in extremities; Abnormal gait; Memory loss; Poor concentration; Disorientation; Dementia	10
Water-soluble vitamin	Pantothenic Acid	Component of coenzymes (coenzyme A) that assist with fatty acid metabolism	AI: Men = 5 mg/day Women = 5 mg/day	None known at this time	Rare; only seen in people fed diets with virtually no pantothenic acid	10
Water-soluble vitamin	Biotin	Component of coenzymes involved in carbohydrate, fat, and protein metabolism	AI: Men = 30 µg/day Women = 30 µg/day	None known at this time	Red, scaly skin rash; Depression; Lethargy; Hallucinations; Paresthesia of the extremities	10
Water-soluble vitamin	Vitamin C	Antioxidant in extracellular fluid and lungs; Regenerates oxidized vitamin E; Reduces formation of nitrosamines in stomach; Assists with collagen synthesis; Enhances immune function; Assists in the synthesis of hormones, neurotransmitters, and DNA; Enhances absorption of iron	RDA: Men = 90 mg Women = 75 mg Smokers = 35 mg more per day than RDA	Nausea and diarrhea; Nosebleeds; Abdominal cramps; Increased oxidative damage; Increased formation of kidney stones in those with kidney disease	Scurvy; Bleeding gums and joints; Loose teeth; Weakness; Hemorrhaging of hair follicles; Poor wound healing; Swollen ankles and wrists; Diarrhea; Bone pain and fractures; Depression; Anemia	8
Fat-soluble vitamin	Vitamin A	Necessary for our ability to adjust to changes in light; Protects colour vision; Cell differentiation; Necessary for sperm production in men and fertilization in women; Contributes to healthy bone growth	RDA: Men = 900 µg Women = 700 µg	Spontaneous abortions and birth defects of fetus in pregnant women; Loss of appetite; Blurred vision; Hair loss; Abdominal pain, nausea, diarrhea; Liver and nervous system damage	Night blindness; Xerophthalmia, which leads to permanent blindness; Impaired immunity and increased risk of illness and infection; Inability to reproduce; Failure of normal growth	8
Fat-soluble vitamin	Vitamin D	Regulates blood calcium levels; Maintains bone health; Cell differentiation	AI (based on the assumption that a person does not get adequate sun exposure): Men aged 19 to 50 = 5 µg/day	Hypercalcemia, including weakness, loss of appetite, diarrhea, mental confusion, vomiting, excessive urine output, extreme thirst, and formation of calcium deposits in kidney, heart, and liver	Rickets (in children), leading to bone weakness and deformities; Osteomalcia (in adults), leading to bone weakness and increased rate of fractures	9

continued

Nutrient Classification	Nutrient	Primary Functions	Recommended Intake	Toxicity Symptoms/ Side Effects	Deficiency Symptoms/ Side Effects	Chapter Reference
			Men aged 50 to 70 = 10 µg/day Men aged > 70 = 15 µg/day Women aged 19 to 50 = 5 µg/day Women aged 50 to 70 = 10 µg/day Women aged > 70 = 15 µg/day	Increased bone loss	Osteoporosis, leading to increased rate of fractures	
Fat-soluble vitamin	Vitamin E	Protects cell membranes from oxidation Protects polyunsaturated fatty acids (PUFAs) from oxidation Protects vitamin A from oxidation Protects white blood cells and enhances immune function Improves absorption of vitamin A	RDA: Men = 15 mg alpha-tocopherol Women = 15 mg alpha-tocopherol	Inhibition of blood clotting Increased risk of hemorrhagic stroke Intestinal discomfort	Red blood cell hemolysis Anemia Impairment of nerve transmission Muscle weakness and degeneration Leg cramps Difficulty walking Fibrocystic breast disease	8
Fat-soluble vitamin	Vitamin K	Serves as a coenzyme during production of specific proteins that assist in blood coagulation and bone metabolism	AI: Men = 120 µg/day Women = 90 µg/day	No known side effects or toxicity symptoms from consuming excess vitamin K	Reduced ability to form blood clots, leading to excessive bleeding and easy bruising Effect on bone health is controversial	9 and 10
Major mineral	Sodium	Major positively charged electrolyte in extracellular fluid Maintains proper acid–base balance Assists with transmission of nerve signals Aids muscle contraction Assists in the absorption of glucose and other nutrients	AI: Men = 1.5 g/day (1500 mg/day) Women = 1.5 g/day (1500 mg/day)	Water retention High blood pressure May increase loss of calcium in urine	Muscle cramps Loss of appetite Dizziness Fatigue Nausea Vomiting Mental confusion	7
Major mineral	Potassium	Major positively charged electrolyte in intracellular fluid Regulates contraction of muscles Regulates transmission of nerve impulses Assists in maintaining healthy blood pressure levels	AI: Men = 4.7 g/day (4700 mg/day) Women = 4.7 g/day (4700 mg/day)	Muscle weakness Vomiting Irregular heartbeat	Muscle weakness Muscle paralysis Mental confusion	7
Major mineral	Phosphorus	Major negatively charged electrolyte in intracellular fluid Maintains proper fluid balance Plays critical role in bone formation as a major component of hydroxyapatite crystals Component of ATP, which provides energy for our bodies Helps regulate biochemical reactions by activating and inactivating enzymes	RDA: Men = 700 mg/day Women = 700 mg/day	High blood phosphorus levels Muscle spasms Convulsions Low blood calcium levels	Low blood phosphorus levels Muscle weakness Muscle damage Bone pain Dizziness	7 and 9

continued

Nutrient Classification	Nutrient	Primary Functions	Recommended Intake	Toxicity Symptoms/Side Effects	Deficiency Symptoms/Side Effects	Chapter Reference
		Major part of genetic materials (DNA, RNA) A component in cell membranes, LDL, and HDL				
Major mineral	Calcium	Primary component of bone and teeth structure Helps maintain optimal acid–base balance Maintains normal nerve transmission Supports muscle contraction and relaxation Regulates blood pressure, blood clotting, and various hormones and enzymes	AI: Men aged 19 to 50 = 1000 mg/day Men aged > 50 = 1200 mg/day Women aged 19 to 50 = 1000 mg/day Women aged > 50 = 1200 mg/day	Potential mineral imbalances; calcium can interfere with absorption of iron, zinc, and magnesium Shock Kidney failure Fatigue Mental confusion	Osteoporosis Bone fractures Convulsions and muscle spasms Heart failure Bleeder's disease	9
Major mineral	Magnesium	An essential component of bone tissue Influences formation of hydroxyapatite crystals and bone growth Cofactor for more than 300 enzyme systems, including ATP, DNA and protein synthesis and vitamin D metabolism and action Supports muscle contraction and blood clotting	RDA: Men aged 19 to 30 = 400 mg/day Men aged > 30 = 420 mg/day Women aged 19 to 30 = 310 mg/day Women aged > 30 = 320 mg/day	No known toxicity symptoms of consuming excess in diet Toxicity from pharmacological use includes diarrhea, nausea, abdominal cramps; in severe cases, massive dehydration, cardiac arrest, and death can result	Hypomagnesemia, resulting in low blood calcium levels, muscle cramps, spasms or seizures, nausea, weakness, irritability, and confusion Chronic diseases such as heart disease, high blood pressure, osteoporosis, and type 2 diabetes	9
Major mineral	Sulphur	Component of B vitamins thiamin and biotin As part of the amino acids methionine and cysteine, helps stabilize the three-dimensional shapes of proteins in our bodies Assists liver in the detoxification of alcohol and various drugs Assists in maintaining acid–base balance	No DRI	No known symptoms	No known symptoms	10
Trace mineral	Chloride	Assists with maintaining fluid balance Aids in preparing food for digestion (as HCl) Helps kill bacteria Assists in the transmission of nerve impulses	AI: Men = 2.3 g/day (2300 mg/day) Women = 2.3 g/day (2300 mg/day)	Vomiting	Dangerous changes in pH Irregular heartbeat	7
Trace mineral	Selenium	Part of glutathione peroxidase, an antioxidant enzyme Indirectly spares vitamin E from oxidation Assists in production of thyroid hormone Assists in maintaining immune function	RDA: Men = 55 µg/day Women = 55 µg/day	Brittle hair and nails Skin rashes Vomiting, nausea Weakness Cirrhosis of liver	Keshan disease: a specific form of heart disease Kashin-Beck disease: deforming arthritis Impaired immune function Increased risk of viral infections Infertility Depression, hostility Muscle pain and wasting	8

continued

Nutrient Classification	Nutrient	Primary Functions	Recommended Intake	Toxicity Symptoms/ Side Effects	Deficiency Symptoms/ Side Effects	Chapter Reference
Trace mineral	Fluoride	Maintains health of teeth and bones Protects teeth against dental caries Stimulates new bone growth	AI: Men = 4 mg/day Women = 3 mg/day	Teeth fluorosis, which causes staining and pitting of teeth Skeletal fluorosis, which ranges from mild to severe; causes joint pain and stiffness, and in extreme cases can cause crippling, wasting of muscles, and osteoporosis of the extremities	High occurrence of dental caries and tooth decay Low fluoride intakes may also be associated with lower bone density	9
Trace mineral	Iodine	Critical for synthesis of thyroid hormones Assists in temperature regulation, maintenance of resting metabolic rate, and supports reproduction and growth	RDA: Men = 150 µg/day Women = 150 µg/day	Goitre, or enlargement of thyroid gland	Goitre, or enlargement of thyroid gland Hypothyroidism, which includes decreased body temperature, inability to tolerate cold temperatures, weight gain, fatigue, and sluggishness Iodine deficiency during pregnancy causes a form of mental retardation in the infant called cretinism	10
Trace mineral	Chromium	Enhances the ability of insulin to transport glucose from the bloodstream into the cells Plays an important role in the metabolism of RNA and DNA Important for healthy immune function and growth	AI: Men aged 19 to 50 = 35 µg/day Men aged > 50 = 30 µg/day Women aged 19 to 50 = 25 µg/day Women aged > 50 = 20 µg/day	No known symptoms	Inhibition of uptake of glucose by the cells, leading to rise in blood glucose and insulin Elevated blood lipid levels Damage to brain and nervous system	10
Trace minerals	Manganese	Coenzyme involved in energy metabolism and in the formation of urea Assists in the synthesis of the protein matrix found in bone tissue and in building cartilage An integral component of superoxide dismutase, an antioxidant enzyme	AI: Men = 2.3 mg/day Women = 1.8 mg/day	Impairment of the neuromuscular system, causing muscle spasms and tremors	Impaired growth and reproductive function Reduced bone density and impaired skeletal growth Impaired glucose and lipid metabolism Skin rash	10
Trace mineral	Iron	As a component of hemoglobin, assists with oxygen transport in our blood As a component of myoglobin, assists in the transport of oxygen into muscle cells Coenzyme for enzymes involved in energy metabolism Part of the antioxidant enzyme system that combats free radicals	RDA: Men aged 19 to 50 years = 8 mg/day Men aged > 50 = 8 mg/day Women aged 19 to 50 = 18 mg/day Women aged > 50 = 8 mg/day	Nausea Vomiting Diarrhea Dizziness, confusion Rapid heartbeat Damage to heart, central nervous system, liver, kidneys Death	First stage of iron deficiency: decrease in iron stores with no physical symptoms Second stage of iron deficiency: decrease in iron transport, causing reduced work capacity Third stage of iron deficiency: anemia, causing impaired work performance, general fatigue, pale skin, depressed immune function, impaired cognitive and nerve function, and impaired memory	10

continued

Nutrient Classification	Nutrient	Primary Functions	Recommended Intake	Toxicity Symptoms/Side Effects	Deficiency Symptoms/Side Effects	Chapter Reference
Trace mineral	Zinc	Coenzyme that assists with hemoglobin production Part of superoxide dismutase antioxidant enzyme system that combats free radicals Facilitates folding of proteins, which assists in gene regulation Plays role in cell replication and normal growth and sexual maturation Plays a role in proper development and function of immune system	RDA: Men = 11 mg/day Women = 8 mg/day	Intestinal pain and cramps Nausea Vomiting Loss of appetite Diarrhea Headaches Depressed immune function Reduced absorption of copper	Growth retardation Diarrhea Delayed sexual maturation and impotence Eye and skin lesions Hair loss Impaired appetite Increased incidence of illness and infections	10
Trace mineral	Copper	Coenzyme in metabolic pathways that produce energy Coenzyme that assists in production of collagen and elastin Part of superoxide dismutase antioxidant enzyme system that combats free radicals Component of ceruloplasmin, which allows for the proper transport of iron	RDA: Men = 900 µg/day Women = 900 µg/day	Abdominal pain and cramps Nausea Diarrhea Vomiting Liver damage occurs in extreme cases that result from Wilson's disease and other rare disorders	Anemia Reduced levels of white blood cells Osteoporosis in infants and growing children	10

Appendix E *Foods Containing Caffeine*

Source: Values are obtained from the USDA Nutrient Database for Standard Reference, Release 16.

Beverages

Food Name	Serving	Caffeine/serving (mg)
Beverage Mix, chocolate flavour, dry mix, prep w/milk	1 cup (8 fl. oz.)	7.98
Beverage Mix, chocolate malt powder, fortified, prepared w/milk	1 cup (8 fl. oz.)	5.3
Beverage Mix, chocolate malted milk powder, no added nutrients, prepared w/milk	1 cup (8 fl. oz.)	7.95
Beverage, chocolate syrup w/o added nutrients, prepared w/milk	1 cup (8 fl. oz.)	5.64
Beverage, chocolate syrup, fortified, mixed w/milk	1 cup milk and 1 Tbsp syrup	2.63
Cocoa Mix w/aspartame and calcium and phosphorus, no sodium or vitamin A, low Cal, dry, prepared	6 fl. oz. water and 0.53 oz packet	15.36
Cocoa Mix w/aspartame, dry, low Cal, prepared w/water	1 packet dry mix with 6 fl. oz. water	1.92
Cocoa Mix, dry mix	1 serving (3 heaping tsp or 1 envelope)	5.04
Cocoa Mix, dry, w/o added nutrients, prepared w/water	1 oz packet with 6 fl. oz. water	4.12
Cocoa Mix, fortified, dry, prepared w/water	6 fl. oz. H_2O and 1 packet	6.27
Cocoa, dry powder, high-fat or breakfast, plain	1 piece	6.895
Cocoa, hot, homemade w/whole milk	1 cup	5
Coffee Liqueur 53 proof	1 fl. oz.	9.048
Coffee Liqueur 63 proof	1 fl. oz.	9.048
Coffee w/Cream Liqueur, 34 proof	1 fl. oz.	2.488
Coffee Mix w/sugar (cappuccino) dry, prepared w/water	6 fl. oz. H_2O and 2 rounded tsp mix	74.88
Coffee Mix w/sugar (French) dry, prepared w/water	6 fl. oz. H_2O and 2 rounded tsp mix	51.03
Coffee Mix w/sugar (mocha) dry, prepared w/water	6 fl. oz. and 2 round tsp mix	33.84
Coffee, brewed	1 cup (8 fl. oz.)	85.32
Coffee, brewed, prepared with tap water, decaffeinated	1 cup (8 fl. oz.)	2.37
Coffee, instant, prepared	1 fl. oz.	7.748
Coffee, instant, regular, powder, half the caffeine	1 cup (8 fl. oz.)	3723.27
Coffee, instant powder, decaffeinated, prepared	6 fl. oz.	1.79
Coffee and cocoa (mocha) powder, with whitener and low calorie sweetener	1 cup	405.48
Coffee, brewed, espresso, restaurant-prepared	1 ounce	60.081
Coffee, brewed, espresso, restaurant-prepared, decaffeinated	1 cup (8 fl. oz.)	2.37
Energy drink, with caffeine, niacin, pantothenic acid, vitamin B_6	1 fl. oz.	9.517
Milk Beverage Mix, dairy drink w/aspartame, low Cal, dry, prep	6 fl. oz.	4.08
Milk, low-fat, 1% fat, chocolate	1 cup	5
Milk, whole, chocolate	1 cup	5
Soft Drink, cola w/caffeine	1 fl. oz.	3.1
Soft Drink, cola, w/higher caffeine	1 fl. oz.	8.37
Soft Drink, cola or Pepper type, low Cal w/saccharin and caffeine	1 fl. oz.	3.256
Soft Drink, cola, low Cal w/saccharin and aspartame, w/caffeine	1 fl. oz.	4.144
Soft Drink, lemon-lime soda, w/caffeine	1 fl. oz.	4.605
Soft Drink, low Cal, not cola or Pepper, with aspartame and caffeine	1 fl. oz.	4.44
Soft Drink, Pepper type	1 fl. oz.	3.07
Tea Mix, instant w/lemon flavour, w/saccharin, dry, prepared	1 cup (8 fl. oz.)	16.59
Tea Mix, instant w/lemon, unsweetened, dry, prepared	1 cup (8 fl. oz.)	26.18
Tea Mix, instant w/sugar and lemon, dry, no added vitamin C, prepared	1 cup (8 fl. oz.)	28.49
Tea Mix, instant, unsweetened, dry, prepared	1 cup (8 fl. oz.)	30.81
Tea, brewed	1 cup (8 fl. oz.)	47.4
Tea, brewed, prepared with tap water, decaffeinated	1 cup (8 fl. oz.)	2.37
Tea, instant, unsweetened, powder, decaffeinated	1 tsp	1.183
Tea, instant, w/sugar, lemon-flavoured, w/added vitamin C, dry prepared	1 cup (8 fl. oz.)	28.49
Tea, instant, with sugar, lemon-flavoured, decaf, no added vitamin	1 cup	9.1

Cake, Cookies, and Desserts

Food Name	Serving	Caffeine/serving (mg)
Brownies, commercially prepared, Little Debbie	1 oz	0.567
Cake, chocolate pudding, dry mix	1 oz	1.701
Cake, chocolate, dry mix, regular	1 oz	3.118
Cake, German chocolate pudding, dry mix	1 oz	1.985
Cake, marble pudding, dry mix	1 oz	1.985
Candies, chocolate covered, caramel with nuts	1 cup	35.34
Candies, chocolate covered, dietetic or low Calorie	1 cup	16.74
Candy, milk chocolate w/almonds	1 bar (1.45 oz)	9.02
Candy, milk chocolate w/rice cereal	1 bar (1.4 oz)	9.2
Candy, raisins, milk chocolate coated	1 cup	45
Chocolate Chips, semisweet	1 cup chips (6 oz package)	104.16
Chocolate, baking, unsweetened, square	1 cup, grated	105.6
Chocolate, baking, Mexican, squares	1 tablet	2.8
Chocolate, sweet	1 oz	18.711
Cookie Cake, Snackwell Fat Free Devil's Food, Nabisco	1 serving	1.28
Cookie, Snackwell Caramel Delights, Nabisco	1 serving	1.44
Cookie, chocolate chip, enriched, commercially prepared	1 oz	3.118
Cookie, chocolate chip, homemade w/margarine	1 oz	4.536
Cookie, chocolate chip, lower fat, commercially prepared	1 oz	1.985
Cookie, chocolate chip, refrigerated dough	1 portion, dough spoon from roll	2.61
Cookie, chocolate chip, soft, commercially prepared	1 oz	1.985
Cookie, chocolate wafers	1 cup, crumbs	7.84
Cookie, graham crackers, chocolate coated	1 oz	13.041
Cookie, sandwich, chocolate, cream filled	1 oz	3.686
Cookie, sandwich, chocolate, cream filled, special dietary	1 oz	0.85
Cupcakes, chocolate w/frosting, low-fat	1 oz	0.567
Donut, cake, chocolate w/sugar or glaze	1 oz	0.284
Donut, cake, plain w/chocolate icing	1 oz	0.567
Fast Food, ice cream sundae, hot fudge	1 sundae	1.58
Fast Food, milk beverage, chocolate shake	1 cup (8 fl. oz.)	1.66
Frosting, chocolate, creamy, ready to eat	2 Tbsp creamy	0.82
Frozen Yogurts, chocolate	1 cup	5.58
Fudge, chocolate w/nuts, homemade	1 ounce	1.984
Granola Bar, soft, milk chocolate coated, peanut butter	1 ounce	0.85
Granola Bar, with coconut, chocolate coated	1 cup	5.58
Ice Cream, chocolate	1 individual (3.5 fl. oz.)	1.74
Ice Cream, chocolate, light	1 ounce	0.85
Ice Cream, chocolate, rich	1 cup	5.92
M&M's Peanut Chocolate	1 cup	18.7
M&M's Plain Chocolate	1 cup	22.88
Milk chocolate	1 cup chips	33.6
Milk chocolate coated coffee beans	1 NLEA serving	48
Milk Dessert, frozen, fat-free milk, chocolate	1 ounce	0.85
Milk Shake, thick, chocolate	1 fl. oz.	0.568
Pastry, eclair/cream puff, homemade, custard filled w/chocolate	1 oz	0.567
Pie Crust, chocolate wafer cookie type, chilled	1 crust, single 9″	11.15
Pie, chocolate mousse, no bake mix	1 oz	0.284
Pudding, chocolate, instant dry mix prep w/reduced fat (2%) milk	1 ounce	0.283
Pudding, chocolate, regular dry mix prep w/reduced fat (2%) milk	1 ounce	0.567
Pudding, chocolate, ready-to-eat, fat free	1 ounce	0.567
Syrups, chocolate, genuine chocolate flavour, light, Hershey	2 tbsp	1.05
Topping, chocolate-flavoured hazelnut spread	1 ounce	1.984
Yogurt, chocolate, non-fat milk	1 ounce	0.567
Yogurt, frozen, chocolate, soft serve	.5 cup (4 fl. oz.)	2.16

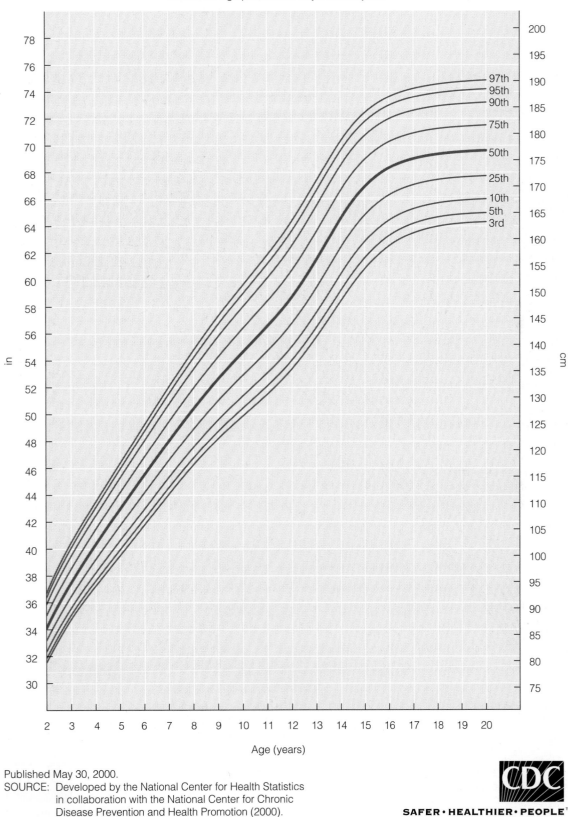

CDC Growth Charts: United States

Stature-for-age percentiles: Boys, 2 to 20 years

Published May 30, 2000.
SOURCE: Developed by the National Center for Health Statistics
in collaboration with the National Center for Chronic
Disease Prevention and Health Promotion (2000).

http://www.cdc.gov/nchs/data/nhanes/growthcharts/set1/chart07.pdf

CDC
SAFER · HEALTHIER · PEOPLE™

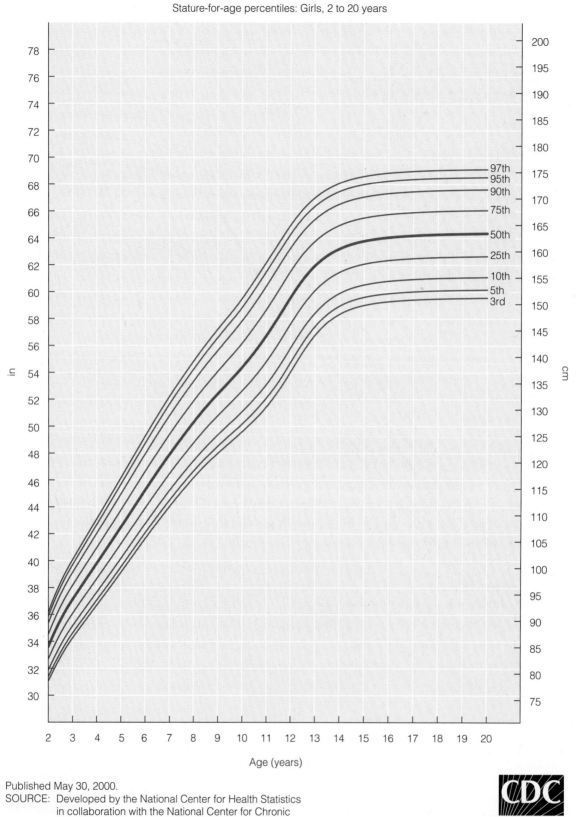

CDC Growth Charts: United States
Stature-for-age percentiles: Girls, 2 to 20 years

Published May 30, 2000.
SOURCE: Developed by the National Center for Health Statistics
in collaboration with the National Center for Chronic
Disease Prevention and Health Promotion (2000).

http://www.cdc.gov/nchs/data/nhanes/growthcharts/set1/char14.pdf

CDC

SAFER · HEALTHIER · PEOPLE™

.

Appendix G *Organizations and Resources*

Academic Journals

Canadian Journal of Dietetic Practice and Research
Dietitians of Canada
480 University Avenue, Suite 604
Toronto, ON M5G 1V2
(416) 596-0857
www.dietitians.ca/public/content/research/journal.asp

Journal of the American Dietetic Association
Elsevier, Health Services Division
Subscription Customer Service
6277 Sea Harbor Drive
Orlando, FL 32887
(800) 654-2452
www.adajournal.org/

American Journal of Clinical Nutrition
9650 Rockville Pike
Bethesda, MD 20814-3998
(301) 634-7038
www.ajcn.org/

International Journal of Sport Nutrition and Exercise Metabolism
Human Kinetics
P.O. Box 5076
Champaign, IL 61825-5076
(800) 747-4457
www.humankinetics.com/IJSNEM

International Journal for Behavioral Nutrition and Physical Activity (ISBNPA)
www.ijbnpa.org/

Journal of Nutrition
A. Catharine Ross, Editor
Pennsylvania State University
Department of Nutritional Sciences
126-S Henderson Building
University Park, PA 16802-6504
(814) 865-4721
www.nutrition.org/

Journal of Nutrition Education and Behavior
Stephanie Wallner, Managing Editor
Colorado State University
502 W. Lake Street, Campus Delivery 1571
Fort Collins, CO 80523-1571
(970) 491-3060
www.jneb.org

Nutrition Research
Elsevier: Journals Customer Service
6277 Sea Harbor Drive
Orlando, FL 32887
(877) 839-7126
www.journals.elsevierhealth.com/periodicals/NTR

Nutrition
Elsevier: Journals Customer Service
6277 Sea Harbor Drive
Orlando, FL 32887
(877) 839-7126
www.journals.elsevierhealth.com/periodicals/NUT

Nutrition Reviews
International Life Sciences Institute
Subscription Office
P.O. Box 830430
Birmingham, AL 35283
(800) 633-4931
www.ilsi.org/Press/NutritionReviews/default.htm

Obesity Research
North American Association for the Study of Obesity (NAASO)
8630 Fenton Street, Suite 918
Silver Spring, MD 20910
(301) 563-6526
www.obesityresearch.org/

International Journal of Obesity
Journal of the International Association for the Study of Obesity
Nature Publishing Group
The Macmillan Building
4 Crinan Street
London NI 9XW
United Kingdom
www.nature.com/ijo/

Journal of the American Medical Association
American Medical Association
P.O. Box 10946
Chicago, IL 60610-0946
(800) 262-2350
jama.ama-assn.org/

New England Journal of Medicine
10 Shattuck Street
Boston, MA 02115-6094
(617) 734-9800
content.nejm.org/

Canadian Government

Health Canada (General Inquiries)
Address Locator 0900C2
Ottawa, ON K1A 0K9
(613) 957-2991
Toll-free: 1-866-225-0709
www.hc-sc.gc.ca/english/

It's Your Health
Health Canada (General Inquiries)
Address Locator 0900C2
Ottawa, ON K1A 0K9
(613) 957-2991
Toll-free: 1-866-225-0709
www.hc-sc.gc.ca/iyh-vsv/index_e.html

Public Health Agency of Canada
130 Colonnade Road
Address Locator 6501H
Ottawa, ON K1A 0K9
www.phac-aspc.gc.ca/new_e.html

Centre for Chronic Disease Prevention and Control, Public Health Agency of Canada
130 Colonnade Road
Address Locator 6501H
Ottawa, ON K1A 0K9
www.phac-aspc.gc.ca/ccdpc-cpcmc/index_e.html

Integrated Pan-Canadian Healthy Living Strategy, Public Health Agency of Canada
130 Colonnade Road
Address Locator 6501H
Ottawa, ON K1A 0K9
www.healthyliving-viesaine.ca

Natural Health Products Directorate, Health Products and Food Branch, Health Canada (General Inquiries)
Address Locator 0900C2
Ottawa, ON K1A 0K9
(613) 957-2991
Toll free: 1-866-225-0709
www.hc-sc.gc.ca/hpfb-dgpsa/nhpd-dpsn

Health Products and Food Branch – Food and Nutrition
Sir Frederick G. Banting Research Centre
Tunney's Pasture (2203A)
Ottawa, ON K1A 0L2
(613) 957-0352
www.hc-sc.gc.ca/fn-an/index_e.html

Agriculture and Agri-Food Canada (AAFC)
Public Information Request Service
Sir John Carling Building
930 Carling Avenue
Ottawa, ON K1A 0L2
(613) 759-1000
Email: info@agr.gc.ca
www.agr.gc.ca/

Canadian Food Inspection Agency
59 Camelot Drive
Ottawa, ON K1A 0Y9
(613) 225-2342
www.inspection.gc.ca/english/toce.shtml

Health Canada and the Canadian Food Inspection Agency's Canadian Nutrient File
Food Directorate
Health Products and Food Branch
Health Canada (General Inquiries)
Address Locator 0900C2
Ottawa, ON K1A 0K9
(613) 957-2991
Toll-free: 1-866-225-0709
www.hc-sc.gc.ca/fn-an/nutrition/fiche-nutri-data/index_e.html

Health Canada's Food Allergen Program
Bureau of Chemical Safety
Food Directorate
Health Products and Food Branch
Health Canada
Banting Building, AL: 2203D
Ottawa, ON K1A 0L2
Phone: (613) 957-0944
www.hc-sc.gc.ca/fn-an/securit/allerg/index_e.html

Environment Canada: Mercury and the Environment
70 Crémazie St.
Gatineau, QC K1A 0H3
(819) 997-2800 or 1 800 668-6767
Email: mercury@ec.gc.ca
www.ec.gc.ca/MERCURY/EN/fc.cfm

Nutrition Policies and Dietary Guidance in Canada
Food Directorate
Health Products and Food Branch
Health Canada (General Inquiries)
Address Locator 0900C2
Ottawa, ON K1A 0K9
(613) 957-2991
Toll-free: 1-866-225-0709
www.hc-sc.gc.ca/fn-an/nutrition/diet-guide-nutri/nut_pol_diet_guid-pol_nut_lig_direc_e.html

Dietary Reference Intakes Tables
Food Directorate
Health Products and Food Branch
Health Canada (General Inquiries)
Address Locator 0900C2
Ottawa, ON K1A 0K9
(613) 957-2991
Toll-free: 1-866-225-0709
www.hc-sc.gc.ca/fn-an/nutrition/reference/table/index_e.html

Canadian Community Health Survey Update
Food Directorate
Health Products and Food Branch
Health Canada (General Inquiries)
Address Locator 0900C2
Ottawa, ON K1A 0K9
(613) 957-2991
Toll-free: 1-866-225-0709
www.hc-sc.gc.ca/fn-an/surveill/nutrition/commun/index_e.html

Canadian Nutrition and Health Professional Organizations

Canadian Cancer Society
Suite 200, 10 Alcorn Avenue
Toronto, ON M4V 3B1
(416) 961-7223
Email: ccs@cancer.ca
www.cancer.ca

Canadian Institute for Health Information
CIHI Ottawa
495 Richmond Road, Suite 600
Ottawa, ON K2A 4H6
(613) 241-7860
www.cihi.ca/

Canadian Council of Food and Nutrition
3800 Steeles Avenue West, Suite 301A
Woodbridge, ON L4L 4G9
(905) 265-9124
www.ccfn.ca/index.asp

Canadian Public Health Association
1565 Carling Avenue, Suite 400
Ottawa, ON K1Z 8R1
(613) 725-3769
www.cpha.ca/

Canadian Fitness and Lifestyle Research Institute
201-185 Somerset Street West
Ottawa, ON K2P 0J2
(613) 233-5528
www.cflri.ca/cflri/cflri.html

Chronic Disease Prevention Alliance of Canada (CDPAC)
1010-116 Albert Street
Ottawa, ON K1P 5G3
(613) 565-2522 x307
info@CDPAC.ca
www.cdpac.ca

Canadian Diabetes Association
National Life Building
1400-522 University Avenue
Toronto, ON M5G 2R5
(800) 226-8464
www.diabetes.ca/

National Eating Disorder Information Centre
ES 7-421, 200 Elizabeth Street
Toronto, ON M5G 2C4
(866) NEDIC-20
Email: nedic@uhn.on.ca
www.nedic.ca/

Canadian Pediatric Society
2305 St. Laurent Boulevard
Ottawa, ON K1G 4J8
(613) 526-9397
www.cps.ca/

Canadian Society of Nutritional Sciences
www.nutritionalsciences.ca/

Canadian Society of Nutritional Management
650 King Street East, Suite 207
Oshawa, ON L1H 1G5
(905) 728-0429
http://csnm.org/

Dietitians of Canada
480 University Avenue, Suite 604
Toronto, ON M5G 1V2
(416) 596-0857
www.dietitians.ca/

Irritable Bowel Syndrome Association of Canada
P.O. Box 94074
Toronto, ON M4N 3R1
Email: ibsa@ibsassociation.ca
www.ibsassociation.ca

Canadian Digestive Health Foundation
2902 South Sheridan Way
Oakville, ON L6J 7L6
(866) 819-2333
www.cdhf.ca

Canadian Society of Intestinal Research
855 West 12th Avenue
Vancouver, BC V5Z 1M9
(866) 600-4875
www.badgut.com

Crohn's and Colitis Foundation of Canada
60 St. Clair Avenue East, Suite 600
Toronto, ON M4T 1N5
(800) 387-1479
www.ccfc.ca

The Kidney Foundation of Canada
5165 Sherbrooke Street West, Suite 300
Montreal, QC H4A 1T6
(800) 361-7494
www.kidney.ca

Canadian Celiac Association
5170 Dixie Road, Suite 204
Mississauga, ON L4W 1E3
(800) 363-7296
www.celiac.ca

**Canadian Society of Allergy and
Clinical Immunology**
774 Echo Drive
Ottawa ON K1S 5N8
(613) 730-6272
www.csaci.medical.org

Allergy/Asthma Information Association
P.O. Box 100
Toronto, ON M9W 5K9
(800) 611-7011
www.aaia.ca

Anaphylaxis Canada
416 Moore Avenue, Suite 306
Toronto, ON M4G 1C9
(416) 785-5666
www.anaphylaxis.ca

Heart and Stroke Foundation of Canada
222 Queen Street, Suite 1402
Ottawa, ON K1P 5V9
(613) 569-4361
www.heartandstroke.ca

Canadian Dental Association
1815 Alta Vista Drive
Ottawa, ON K1G 3Y6
(613) 523-1770
www.cda-adc.ca

The Foundation Fighting Blindness
60 St.Clair Avenue East, Suite 703
Toronto, ON M4T 1N5
(800) 461-3331
www.ffb.ca

Osteoporosis Society of Canada
33 Laird Drive
Toronto, ON M4G 3S8
(800) 463-6842
www.osteoporosis.ca

The Canadian National Institute for the Blind
1929 Bayview Avenue
Toronto, ON M4G 3E8
(416) 486-2500
www.cnib.ca

Other Canadian Resources

Motherisk
Hospital for Sick Children
555 University Ave.
Toronto, ON M5G 1X8
Alcohol and Substance Use Helpline
(877) 327-4636

Nausea and Vomiting of Pregnancy Helpline
(800) 436-8477
HIV and HIV Treatment in Pregnancy
(888) 246-5840
Motherisk's Home Line
(416) 813-6780
www.motherisk.org/

Healthy Eating Is in Store for You
Developed by the Canadian Diabetes Association and
Dietitians of Canada.
www.healthyeatingisinstore.ca

McDonald's Canada
McDonald's Restaurants of Canada Limited
McDonald's Place
Toronto, ON M3C 3L4
(416) 443-1000
www.mcdonalds.ca/en/food/calculator.aspx

Burger King Restaurants of Canada
401 The West Mall, 7th Floor
Etobicoke, ON M9C-5J4
(877) 271-0493
www.burgerking.ca/en/1133/index.php

**Health Check™
The Heart and Stroke Foundation of Canada**
222 Queen Street, Suite 1402
Ottawa, ON K1P 5V9
(613) 569-4361 ext. 324
www.healthcheck.org

5-to-10-a-Day for Better Health
Kerstin Ring, Senior Manager, Communications
Canadian Cancer Society
(416) 934-5664
www.5to10aday.com/eng/

Aging—International

Osteoporosis Society of Canada
33 Laird Drive
Toronto, ON M4G 3S8
(416) 696-2663
www.osteoporosis.ca

Administration on Aging
U.S. Health & Human Services
200 Independence Avenue, SW
Washington, DC 20201
(877) 696-6775
www.aoa.gov

American Association of Retired Persons (AARP)
601 E Street, NW
Washington, DC 20049
(888) 687-2277
www.aarp.org

Health and Age
Sponsored by the Novartis Foundation for Gerontology
and the Web-based Health Education Foundation.
Robert Griffith, MD, Executive Director
573 Vista de la Ciudad
Santa Fe, NM 87501
www.healthandage.com

National Council on the Aging
300 D Street, SW, Suite 801
Washington, DC 20024
(202) 479-1200
www.ncoa.org

International Osteoporosis Foundation
5 Rue Perdtemps
1260 Nyon
Switzerland
41 22 994 01 00
www.osteofound.org

Osteogenesis Imperfecta Foundation
804 W. Diamond Avenue, Suite 210
Gaithersburg, MD 20878
(800) 981-2663
www.oif.org

National Institute on Aging
Building 31, Room 5C27
31 Center Drive, MSC 2292
Bethesda, MD 20892
(301) 496-1752
www.nia.nih.gov

**Osteoporosis and Related Bone Diseases
National Resource Center**
2 AMS Circle
Bethesda, MD 20892-3676
(800) 624-BONE
www.osteo.org

American Geriatrics Society
The Empire State Building
350 Fifth Avenue, Suite 801
New York, NY 10118
(212) 308-1414
www.americangeriatrics.org/

National Osteoporosis Foundation
1232 22nd Street, NW
Washington, DC 20037-1292
(202) 223-2226
www.nof.org/

Alcohol and Drug Abuse—U.S.

National Institute on Drug Abuse
6001 Executive Boulevard, Room 5213
Bethesda, MD 20892-9561
(301) 443-1124
www.nida.nih.gov

National Institute on Alcohol Abuse and Alcoholism
5635 Fishers Lane, MSC 9304
Bethesda, MD 20892-9304
www.niaaa.nih.gov

Alcoholics Anonymous
Grand Central Station
P.O. Box 459
New York, NY 10163
www.alcoholics-anonymous.org

Narcotics Anonymous
P.O. Box 9999
Van Nuys, California 91409
(818) 773-9999
www.na.org/

National Council on Alcoholism and Drug Dependence
22 Cortlandt Street, Suite 801
New York, NY 10007-3128
(212) 269-7797
www.ncadd.org/

National Clearinghouse for Alcohol and Drug Information
11420 Rockville Pike
Rockville, MD 20852
(800) 729-6686
www.health.org/

Disordered Eating/Eating Disorders—U.S.

American Psychiatric Association
1000 Wilson Boulevard, Suite 1825
Arlington, VA 22209-3901
(703) 907-7300
www.psych.org/

Harvard Eating Disorders Center
WACC 725
15 Parkman Street
Boston, MA 02114
(617) 236-7766
www.hedc.org/

National Institute of Mental Health
Public Information and Communications Branch
6001 Executive Boulevard, Room 8184, MSC 9663
Bethesda, MD 20892-9663
(866) 615-6464
www.nimh.nih.gov

National Association of Anorexia Nervosa and Associated Disorders (ANAD)
P.O. Box 7
Highland Park, IL 60035
(847) 831-3438
www.anad.org

National Eating Disorders Association
603 Stewart Street, Suite 803
Seattle, WA 98101
(206) 382-3587
www.nationaleatingdisorders.org/p.asp?WebPage_ID=337

International Eating Disorder Referral Organization
2923 Sandy Pointe, Suite 6
Del Mar, CA 92014-2052
(858) 792-7463
www.edreferral.com/

Anorexia Nervosa and Related Eating Disorders, Inc. (ANRED)
Affiliated with the National Eating Disorders Association.
Email: jarinor@rio.com
www.anred.com/

Overeaters Anonymous
P.O. Box 44020
Rio Rancho, NM 87174-4020
(505) 891-2664
www.oa.org/

Exercise, Physical Activity, and Sports—U.S.

American College of Sports Medicine (ACSM)
P.O. Box 1440
Indianapolis, IN 46206-1440
(317) 637-9200
www.acsm.org/

American Physical Therapy Association (APTA)
1111 North Fairfax Street
Alexandria, VA 22314-1488
(800) 999-APTA (2782)
www.apta.org

Gatorade Sports Science Institute (GSSI)
617 West Main Street
Barrington, IL 60010
(800) 616-GSSI
www.gssiweb.com/

National Coalition for Promoting Physical Activity (NCPPA)
1100 H Street, NW, Suite 510
Washington, DC 20005
(202) 454-7522
www.ncppa.org/

Sports, Cardiovascular and Wellness Nutritionists (SCAN)
Chris Rosenbloom, PhD, RD (SCAN Chair)
Office of the Dean
Georgia State University
P.O. Box 3995
Atlanta, GA 30302-3995
(404) 651-1102
www.scandpg.org/

President's Council on Physical Fitness and Sports
Department of Health and Human Services
Department W
200 Independence Avenue, SW, Room 738-H
Washington, DC 20201-0004
(202) 690-9000
www.fitness.gov/

American Council on Exercise
4851 Paramount Drive
San Diego, CA 92123
(800) 825-3636
www.acefitness.org/

IDEA Health & Fitness Association
10455 Pacific Center Court
San Diego, CA 92121-4339
(800) 999-4332, ext. 7
www.ideafit.com

International Society of Sports Nutrition
Maelu Fleck, Executive Director
600 Pembrook Drive
Woodland Park, CO 80863
(866) 472-4650
www.sportsnutritionsociety.org/

International Society for Behavioral Nutrition and Physical Activity (ISBNPA)
www.isbnpa.org/

Food Safety—U.S.

International Food Information Council
1100 Connecticut Avenue, NW, Suite 430
Washington, DC 20036
(202) 296-6540
www.ific.org/about/contact.cfm

Food Marketing Institute
655 15th Street, NW
Washington, DC 20005
(202) 452-8444
www.fmi.org/

Agency for Toxic Substances and Disease Registry (ATSDR)
ATSDR Information Center
Mailstop E-29
1600 Clifton Road
Atlanta, GA 30333
(888) 422-8737
www.atsdr.cdc.gov/

Food Allergy and Anaphylaxis Network
11781 Lee Jackson Highway, Suite 160
Fairfax, VA 22033-3309
(800) 929-4040
http://foodallergy.org/

Foodsafety.gov
www.foodsafety.gov

The USDA Food Safety and Inspection Service
Food Safety and Inspection Service
United States Department of Agriculture
Washington, DC 20250
www.fsis.usda.gov

Center for Science in the Public Interest: Food Safety
1875 Connecticut Avenue, NW
Washington, DC 20009
(202) 332-9110
www.cspinet.org/foodsafety/index.html

Center for Food Safety and Applied Nutrition
5100 Paint Branch Parkway
College Park, MD 20740-3835
(888) SAFEFOOD
www.cfsan.fda.gov

Food Safety Project
Sam Beattie, PhD, Food Safety Extension Specialist
Department of Food Science and Human Nutrition
Iowa State University Extension
122A MacKay Hall
Ames, IA, 50011-1120
(515) 294-3357
www.extension.iastate.edu/foodsafety/

Organic Consumers Association
6101 Cliff Estate Road
Little Marais, MN 55614
(218) 226-4164
www.organicconsumers.org

Infancy and Childhood—U.S.

Administration for Children and Families
370 L'Enfant Promenade, SW
Washington, DC 20201
www.acf.dhhs.gov/

The American Academy of Pediatrics
141 Northwest Point Boulevard
Elk Grove Village, IL 60007
(847) 434-4000
www.aap.org/

Kidnetic.com
International Food Information Council
1100 Connecticut Avenue, NW, Suite 430
Washington, DC 20036
Email: contactus@kidnetic.com
www.kidnectic.com

Kidshealth: The Nemours Foundation
12735 West Gran Bay Parkway
Jacksonville, FL 32258
(866) 390-3610
www.kidshealth.org

National Center for Education in Maternal Health and Child Health
Georgetown University
Box 571272
Washington, DC 20057
(202) 784-9770
www.ncemch.org

Birth Defects Research for Children, Inc.
930 Woodcock Road, Suite 225
Orlando, FL 32803
(407) 895-0802
www.birthdefects.org

USDA/ARS Children's Nutrition Research Center at Baylor College of Medicine
1100 Bates Street
Houston, TX 77030
(713) 798-7098
www.kidsnutrition.org

Keep Kids Healthy.com
www.keepkidshealthy.com

International Agencies

UNICEF
Canada Square
2200 Yonge Street, Suite 1100
Toronto, ON M4S 2C6
(416) 482-4444
www.unicef.ca/

World Health Organization
Avenue Appia 20
1211 Geneva 27
Switzerland
41 22 791 21 11
www.who.int/en/

The Stockholm Convention on Persistent Organic Pollutants
11-13 Chemin des Anémones
1219 Châtelaine
Geneva, Switzerland
41 22 917 8191
www.pops.int/

Food and Agricultural Organization of the United Nations
Viale delle Terme di Caracalla
00100 Rome, Italy
39 06 57051
www.fao.org/

International Food Information Council Foundation
1100 Connecticut Avenue, NW, Suite 430
Washington, DC 20036
(202) 296-6540
www.ific.org/

Pregnancy and Lactation—U.S.

San Diego County Breastfeeding Coalition
c/o Children's Hospital and Health Center
3020 Children's Way, MC 5073
San Diego, CA 92123-4282
(800) 371-MILK
www.breastfeeding.org

National Alliance for Breastfeeding Advocacy
Barbara Heiser, Executive Director
9684 Oak Hill Drive
Ellicott City, MD 21042-6321
OR
Marsha Walker, Executive Director
254 Conant Road
Weston, MA 02493-1756
www.naba-breastfeeding.org/

American College of Obstetricians and Gynecologists
409 12th Street, SW,
P.O. Box 96920
Washington, DC 20090-6920
(202) 638-5577
www.acog.org/

La Leche League
1400 N. Meacham Road
Schaumburg, IL 60173-4808
(847) 519-7730
www.lalecheleague.org

National Organization on Fetal Alcohol Syndrome
900 17th Street, NW, Suite 910
Washington, DC 20006
(800) 66 NOFAS
www.nofas.org

March of Dimes Birth Defects Foundation
1275 Mamaroneck Avenue
White Plains, NY 10605
(888) 663-4637
http://modimes.com

Professional Organizations—U.S.

Association of Departments and Programs of Nutrition (ADPN)
Dr. Jeanne H. Freeland-Graves
A2700
Division of Nutritional Sciences
University of Texas at Austin
Austin, TX 78712-1097
http://andpnet.org/

North American Association for the Study of Obesity (NAASO)
8630 Fenton Street, Suite 918
Silver Spring, MD 20910
(301) 563-6526
www.naaso.org/

American Dental Association
211 East Chicago Avenue
Chicago, IL 60611-2678
(312) 440-2500
www.ada.org/

American Heart Association
National Center
7272 Greenville Avenue
Dallas, TX 75231
(800) 242-8721
www.americanheart.org/

American Dietetic Association (ADA)
120 South Riverside Plaza, Suite 2000
Chicago, IL 60606-6995
(800) 877-1600
www.eatright.org

The American Society for Clinical Nutrition (ASCN)
9650 Rockville Pike
Bethesda, MD 20814-3998
(301) 634-7110
www.ascn.org/

The Society for Nutrition Education
7150 Winton Drive, Suite 300
Indianapolis, IN 46268
(800) 235-6690
www.sne.org/

American College of Nutrition
300 South Duncan Avenue, Suite 225
Clearwater, FL 33755
(727) 446-6086
www.amcollnutr.org/

American Obesity Association
1250 24th Street, NW, Suite 300
Washington, DC 20037
(800) 98-OBESE
www.obesity.org/

American Council on Health and Science
1995 Broadway
Second Floor
New York, NY 10023-5860
(212) 362-7044
www.acsh.org/

The American Society for Nutrition (ASN)
9650 Rockville Pike, Suite 4500
Bethesda, MD 20814
(301) 634-7050
www.asnutrition.org/

American Diabetes Association
ATTN: National Call Center
1701 North Beauregard Street
Alexandria, VA 22311
(800) 342-2383
www.diabetes.org/

Institute of Food Technologists
525 West Van Buren, Suite 1000
Chicago, IL 60607
(312) 782-8424
www.ift.org

ILSI Human Nutrition Institute
One Thomas Circle, Ninth Floor
Washington, DC 20005
(202) 659-0524
http://hni.ilsi.org

Trade Organizations

American Meat Institute
1150 Connecticut Avenue, NW, 12th floor
Washington, DC 20036
(202) 587-4200
www.meatami.com/

National Dairy Council
10255 W. Higgins Road, Suite 900
Rosemont, IL 60018
(312) 240-2880
www.nationaldairycouncil.org/

United Fresh Fruit and Vegetable Association
1901 Pennsylvania Ave. NW, Suite 1100
Washington, DC 20006
(202) 303-3400
www.uffva.org/

USA Rice Federation
Washington, DC
4301 North Fairfax Drive, Suite 425
Arlington, VA 22203
(703) 236-2300
www.usarice.com

U.S. Government

The USDA National Organic Program
Agricultural Marketing Service
USDA-AMS-TMP-NOP
Room 4008-South Building
1400 Independence Avenue, SW
Washington, DC 20250-0020
(202) 720-3252
www.ams.usda.gov

U.S. Department of Health and Human Services
200 Independence Avenue, SW
Washington, DC 20201
(202) 619-0257
www.os.dhhs.gov/

Food and Drug Administration
5600 Fishers Lane
Rockville, MD 20857
(888) 463-6332
www.fda.gov/

Environmental Protection Agency
Ariel Rios Building
1200 Pennsylvania Avenue, NW
Washington, DC 20460
(202) 272-0167
www.epa.gov/

Federal Trade Commission
600 Pennsylvania Avenue, NW
Washington, DC 20580
(202) 326-2222
www.ftc.gov

Partnership for Healthy Weight Management
www.consumer.gov/weightloss

Office of Dietary Supplements
National Institutes of Health
6100 Executive Boulevard, Room 3B01, MSC 7517
Bethesda, MD 20892
(301) 435-2920
http://dietary-supplements.info.nih.gov

Nutrient Data Laboratory Homepage
Beltsville Human Nutrition Center
10300 Baltimore Avenue
Building 307-C Room 117
BARC-East
Beltsville, MD 20705
(301) 504-8157
www.ars.usda.gov/ba/bhnrc/ndl

National Digestive Diseases Information Clearinghouse
2 Information Way
Bethesda, MD 20892-3570
(800) 891-5389
http://digestive.niddk.nih.gov

The National Cancer Institute
NCI Public Inquiries Office
Suite 3036A
6116 Executive Boulevard, MSC 8322
Bethesda, MD 20892-8322
(800) 4-CANCER
www.cancer.gov/

The National Eye Institute
Information Office
31 Center Drive MSC 2510
Bethesda, MD 20892-2510
www.nei.nih.gov/

The National Heart, Lung, and Blood Institute
Building 31, Room 5A52
31 Center Drive MSC 2486
Bethesda, MD 20892
(301) 592-8573
www.nhlbi.nih.gov/index.htm

Institute of Diabetes and Digestive and Kidney Diseases
Office of Communications and Public Liaison
NIDDK, NIH, Building 31, Room 9A04
Center Drive, MSC 2560
Bethesda, MD 20892
(301) 496-4000
www.niddk.nih.gov/

National Center for Complementary and Alternative Medicine
NCCAM Clearinghouse
P.O. Box 7923
Gaithersburg, MD 20898
(888) 644-6226
http://nccam.nih.gov/

U.S. Department of Agriculture (USDA)
14th Street, SW
Washington, DC 20250
(202) 720-2791
www.usda.gov/

Centers for Disease Control and Prevention (CDC)
Department of Health and Human Services
1600 Clifton Rd
Atlanta, GA 30333
(404) 639-3311 / Public Inquiries: (800) 311-3435
www.cdc.gov/

National Institutes of Health (NIH)
9000 Rockville Pike
Bethesda, MD 20892
(301) 496-4000
www.nih.gov/

Food and Nutrition Information Center
Agriculture Research Service, USDA
National Agricultural Library, Room 105
10301 Baltimore Avenue
Beltsville, MD 20705-2351
(301) 504-5719
www.nal.usda.gov/fnic/

Nutrition.gov (A Service of the National Agricultural Library, U.S. Department of Agriculture)
National Agricultural Library
Food and Nutrition Information Center
Nutrition.gov Staff
10301 Baltimore Avenue
Beltsville, MD 20705-2351
www.nutrition.gov/

National Institute of Allergy and Infectious Diseases
NIAID Office of Communications and Public Liaison
6610 Rockledge Drive, MSC 6612
Bethesda, MD 20892-6612
(301) 496-5717
www.niaid.nih.gov

Weight and Health Management—U.S.

The Vegetarian Resource Group
P.O. Box 1463
Baltimore, MD 21203
(410) 366-8343
www.vrg.org

American Obesity Association
1250 24th Street, NW, Suite 300
Washington, DC 20037
(202) 776-7711
www.obesity.org/

Anemia Lifeline
(888) 722-4407
www.anemia.com

The Arc
1010 Wayne Avenue, Suite 650
Silver Spring, MD 20910
(301) 565-3842
Email: info@thearc.org
www.thearc.org

Bottled Water Web
Best Cellars, LLC
P.O. Box 5658
Santa Barbara, CA 93150
(805) 879-1564
www.bottledwaterweb.com/

The Food and Nutrition Board
Institute of Medicine
500 Fifth Street, NW
Washington, DC 20001
(202) 334-2352
www.iom.edu/topic.asp?id=3708

The Calorie Control Council
www.caloriecontrol.org/

TOPS (Take Pounds Off Sensibly)
4575 South Fifth Street
P.O. Box 07360
Milwaukee, WI 53207
(800) 932-8677
www.tops.org

Shape Up America!
15009 Native Dancer Road
North Potomac, MD 20878
(240) 631-6533
www.shapeup.org

World Hunger

Center on Hunger, Poverty, and Nutrition Policy
Friedman School of Nutrition Science and Policy
Tufts University
Medford, MA 02155
(617) 627-3020
www.tufts.edu/nutrition/

Freedom from Hunger
1644 DaVinci Court
Davis, Ca 95616
(800) 708-2555
http://freefromhunger.org/

Oxfam Canada
250 City Centre Avenue, Suite 400
Ottawa, ON K1R 6K7
(613) 237-5236
www.oxfam.ca/index.htm

Oxfam International Secretariat
David Byer, Chair, Jeremy Hobbs, Executive Director
Suite 20, 266 Banbury Road,
Oxford 0X2 7DL UK
44 1865 339 100
www.oxfam.org

WorldWatch Institute
1776 Massachusetts Avenue, NW
Washington, DC 20036
(202) 452-1999
www.worldwatch.org

Food First
Institute for Food and Development Policy
398 60th Street
Oakland, CA 94618
(510) 654-4400
www.foodfirst.org

The Hunger Project
Malgorzata Smelkowska, Country Director
11 O'Connor Drive
Toronto, ON M4K 2K3
(416) 429-0023
www.thp.org/index.html

U.S. Agency for International Development
Information Center
Ronald Reagan Building
Washington, DC 20523
(202) 712-0000
www.usaid.gov/

Appendix H *Dietary Reference Intake Tables*

Tolerable Upper Intake Levels (UL[a])

Vitamins

Life Stage Group	Vitamin A (µg/d)[b]	Vitamin C (mg/d)	Vitamin D (µg/d)	Vitamin E (mg/d)[c,d]	Niacin (mg/d)[d]	Vitamin B6 (mg/d)	Folate (µg/d)[d]	Choline (g/d)
Infants								
0–6 mo	600	ND[e]	25	ND	ND	ND	ND	ND
7–12 mo	600	ND	25	ND	ND	ND	ND	ND
Children								
1–3 y	600	400	50	200	10	30	300	1.0
4–8 y	900	650	50	300	15	40	400	1.0
Males, Females								
9–13 y	1700	1200	50	600	20	60	600	2.0
14–18 y	2800	1800	50	800	30	80	800	3.0
19–70 y	3000	2000	50	1000	35	100	1000	3.5
>70 y	3000	2000	50	1000	35	100	1000	3.5
Pregnancy								
≤18 y	2800	1800	50	800	30	80	800	3.0
19–50 y	3000	2000	50	1000	35	100	1000	3.5
Lactation								
≤18 y	2800	1800	50	800	30	80	800	3.0
19–50 y	3000	2000	50	1000	35	100	1000	3.5

Elements

Life Stage Group	Boron (mg/d)	Calcium (g/d)	Copper (µg/d)	Fluoride (mg/d)	Iodine (µg/d)	Iron (mg/d)	Magnesium (mg/d)[f]	Manganese (mg/d)	Molybdenum (µg/d)	Nickel (mg/d)	Phosphorus (g/d)	Selenium (µg/d)	Vanadium (mg/d)[g]	Zinc (mg/d)
Infants														
0–6 mo	ND	ND	ND	0.7	ND	40	ND	ND	ND	ND	ND	45	ND	4
7–12 mo	ND	ND	ND	0.9	ND	40	ND	ND	ND	ND	ND	60	ND	5
Children														
1–3 y	3	2.5	1000	1.3	200	40	65	2	300	0.2	3	90	ND	7
4–8 y	6	2.5	3000	2.2	300	40	110	3	600	0.3	3	150	ND	12
Males, Females														
9–13 y	11	2.5	5000	10	600	40	350	6	1100	0.6	4	280	ND	23
14–18 y	17	2.5	8000	10	900	45	350	9	1700	1.0	4	400	ND	34
19–70 y	20	2.5	10 000	10	1,100	45	350	11	2000	1.0	4	400	1.8	40
>70 y	20	2.5	10 000	10	1,100	45	350	11	2000	1.0	3	400	1.8	40
Pregnancy														
≤18 y	17	2.5	8000	10	900	45	350	9	1700	1.0	3.5	400	ND	34
19–50 y	20	2.5	10 000	10	1,100	45	350	11	2000	1.0	3.5	400	ND	40
Lactation														
≤18 y	17	2.5	8000	10	900	45	350	9	1700	1.0	4	400	ND	34
19–50 y	20	2.5	10 000	10	1,100	45	350	11	2000	1.0	4	400	ND	40

Source: Adapted from the Dietary Reference Intakes series, National Academies Press. Copyright 1997, 1998, 2000, 2001, by the National Academy of Sciences. These reports may be accessed via www.nap.edu. Courtesy of the National Academies Press, Washington D.C.

[a] UL = The maximum level of daily nutrient intake that is likely to pose no risk of adverse effects. Unless otherwise specified, the UL represents total intake from food, water, and supplements. Due to lack of suitable data, ULs could not be established for vitamin K, thiamin, riboflavin, vitamin B12, pantothenic acid, biotin, or carotenoids. In the absence of ULs, extra caution may be warranted in consuming levels above recommended intakes.

[b] As preformed vitamin A only.

[c] As α-tocopherol; applies to any form of supplemental α-tocopherol.

[d] The ULs for vitamin E, niacin, and folate apply to synthetic forms obtained from supplements, fortified foods, or a combination of the two.

[e] ND = Not determinable due to lack of data of adverse effects in this age group and concern with regard to lack of ability to handle excess amounts. Source of intake should be from food only to prevent high levels of intake.

[f] The ULs for magnesium represent intake from a pharmacological agent only and do not include intake from food and water.

[g] Although vanadium in food has not been shown to cause adverse effects in humans, there is no justification for adding vanadium to food, and vanadium supplements should be used with caution. The UL is based on adverse effects in laboratory animals, and this data could be used to set a UL for adults but not children and adolescents.

Life Stage Group	Carbohydrate— Total Digestible (g/d)	Total Fibre (g/d)	Total Fat (g/d)	n-6 polyunsaturated fatty acids (linoleic acid) (g/d)	n-3 polyunsaturated fatty acids (α-linolenic acid) (g/d)	Protein and Amino Acids (g/d) [a]
Macronutrients						
Infants						
0–6 mo	60* (ND[b])[c]	ND	31*	4.4* (ND)	0.5* (ND)	9.1* (ND)
7–12 mo	95* (ND)	ND	30*	4.6* (ND)	0.5* (ND)	13.5 (ND)
Children						
1–3 y	130 (45–65)	19*	(30–40)	7* (5–10)	0.7* (0.6–1.2)	13 (5–20)
4–8 y	130 (45–65)	25*	(25–35)	10* (5–10)	0.9* (0.6–1.2)	19 (10–30)
Males						
9–13 y	130 (45–65)	31*	(25–35)	12* (5–10)	1.2* (0.6–1.2)	34 (10–30)
14–18 y	130 (45–65)	38*	(25–35)	16* (5–10)	1.6* (0.6–1.2)	52 (10–30)
19–30 y	130 (45–65)	38*	(20–35)	17* (5–10)	1.6* (0.6–1.2)	56 (10–35)
31–50 y	130 (45–65)	38*	(20–35)	17* (5–10)	1.6* (0.6–1.2)	56 (10–35)
51–70 y	130 (45–65)	30*	(20–35)	14* (5–10)	1.6* (0.6–1.2)	56 (10–35)
> 70 y	130 (45–65)	30*	(20–35)	14* (5–10)	1.6* (0.6–1.2)	56 (10–35)
Females						
9–13 y	130 (45–65)	26*	(25–35)	10* (5–10)	1.0* (0.6–1.2)	34 (10–30)
14–18 y	130 (45–65)	26*	(25–35)	11* (5–10)	1.1* (0.6–1.2)	46 (10–30)
19–30 y	130 (45–65)	25*	(20–35)	12* (5–10)	1.1* (0.6–1.2)	46 (10–35)
31–50 y	130 (45–65)	25*	(20–35)	12* (5–10)	1.1* (0.6–1.2)	46 (10–35)
51–70 y	130 (45–65)	21*	(20–35)	11* (5–10)	1.1* (0.6–1.2)	46 (10–35)
> 70 y	130 (45–65)	21*	(20–35)	11* (5–10)	1.1* (0.6–1.2)	46 (10–35)
Pregnancy						
≤ 18 y	175 (45–65)	28*	(20–35)	13* (5–10)	1.4* (0.6–1.2)	71 (10–35)
19–30 y	175 (45–65)	28*	(20–35)	13* (5–10)	1.4* (0.6–1.2)	71 (10–35)
31–50 y	(45–65)	28*	(20–35)	13* (5–10)	1.4* (0.6–1.2)	71 (10–35)
Lactation						
≤ 18 y	210 (45–65)	29*	(20–35)	13* (5–10)	1.3* (0.6–1.2)	71 (10–35)
19–30 y	210 (45–65)	29*	(20–35)	13* (5–10)	1.3* (0.6–1.2)	71 (10–35)
31–50 y	210 (45–65)	29*	(20–35)	13* (5–10)	1.3* (0.6–1.2)	71 (10–35)

Sources: Adapted from the Dietary Reference Intakes series, National Academies Press. Copyright 1997, 1998, 2000, 2001, by the National Academy of Sciences. These reports may be accessed via www.nap.edu. Courtesy of the National Academies Press, Washington D.C.

Note: This table is adapted from the DRI reports, see www.nap.edu. It lists Recommended Dietary Allowances (RDAs), with Adequate Intakes (AIs) indicated by an asterisk (*), and Acceptable Macronutrient Distribution Range (AMDR) data provided in parentheses. RDAs and AIs may both be used as goals for individual intake. RDAs are set to meet the needs of almost all (97 to 98 percent) individuals in a group. For healthy breastfed infants, the AI is the mean intake. The AI for other life stage and gender groups is believed to cover the needs of all individuals in the group, but lack of data prevent being able to specify with confidence the percentage of individuals covered by this intake.

[a] Based on 1.5 g/kg/day for infants, 1.1 g/kg/day for 1–3 y, 0.95 g/kg/day for 4–13 y, 0.85 g/kg/day for 14–18 y, 0.8 g/kg/day for adults, and 1.1 g/kg/day for pregnant (using pre-pregnancy weight) and lactating women.

[b] ND = Not determinable due to lack of data of adverse effects in this age group and concern with regard to lack of ability to handle excess amounts. Source of intake should be from food only to prevent high levels of intake.

[c] Data in parentheses are Acceptable Macronutrient Distribution Range (AMDR). This is the range of intake for a particular energy source that is associated with reduced risk of chronic disease while providing intakes of essential nutrients. If an individual consumes in excess of the AMDR, there is a potential of increasing the risk of chronic diseases and/or insufficient intakes of essential nutrients.

Dietary Reference Intakes: RDA, AI*

Life Stage Group	Vitamin A (μg/d)[a]	Vitamin D (μg/d)[b]	Vitamin E (mg/d)[c]	Vitamin K (μg/d)	Thiamin (mg/d)	Riboflavin (mg/d)	Niacin (mg/d)[d]	Pantothenic Acid (mg/d)	Biotin (μg/d)	Vitamin B$_6$ (mg/d)	Folate (μg/d)[e]	Vitamin B$_{12}$ (μg/d)	Vitamin C (mg/d)	Choline (mg/d)
Infants														
0–6 mo	400*	5*	4*	2.0*	0.2*	0.3*	2*	1.7*	5*	0.1*	65*	0.4*	40*	125*
7–12 mo	500*	5*	5*	2.5*	0.3*	0.4*	4*	1.8*	6*	0.3*	80*	0.5*	50*	150*
Children														
1–3 y	300	5*	6	30*	0.5	0.5	6	2*	8*	0.5	150	0.9	15	200*
4–8 y	400	5*	7	55*	0.6	0.6	8	3*	12*	0.6	200	1.2	25	250*
Males														
9–13 y	600	5*	11	60*	0.9	0.9	12	4*	20*	1.0	300	1.8	45	375*
14–18 y	900	5*	15	75*	1.2	1.3	16	5*	25*	1.3	400	2.4	75	550*
19–30 y	900	5*	15	120*	1.2	1.3	16	5*	30*	1.3	400	2.4	90	550*
31–50 y	900	5*	15	120*	1.2	1.3	16	5*	30*	1.3	400	2.4	90	550*
51–70 y	900	10*	15	120*	1.2	1.3	16	5*	30*	1.7	400	2.4	90	550*
> 70 y	900	15*	15	120*	1.2	1.3	16	5*	30*	1.7	400	2.4	90	550*
Females														
9–13 y	600	5*	11	60*	0.9	0.9	12	4*	20*	1.0	300	1.8	45	375*
14–18 y	700	5*	15	75*	1.0	1.0	14	5*	25*	1.2	400	2.4	65	400*
19–30 y	700	5*	15	90*	1.1	1.1	14	5*	30*	1.3	400	2.4	75	425*
31–50 y	700	5*	15	90*	1.1	1.1	14	5*	30*	1.3	400	2.4	75	425*
51–70 y	700	10*	15	90*	1.1	1.1	14	5*	30*	1.5	400	2.4	75	425*
> 70 y	700	15*	15	90*	1.1	1.1	14	5*	30*	1.5	400	2.4	75	425*
Pregnancy														
≤ 18 y	750	5*	15	75*	1.4	1.4	18	6*	30*	1.9	600	2.6	80	450*
19–30 y	770	5*	15	90*	1.4	1.4	18	6*	30*	1.9	600	2.6	85	450*
31–50 y	770	5*	15	90*	1.4	1.4	18	6*	30*	1.9	600	2.6	85	450*
Lactation														
≤ 18 y	1200	5*	19	75*	1.4	1.4	17	7*	35*	2.0	500	2.8	115	550*
19–30 y	1300	5*	19	90*	1.4	1.4	17	7*	35*	2.0	500	2.8	120	550*
31–50 y	1300	5*	19	90*	1.4	1.4	17	7*	35*	2.0	500	2.8	120	550*

Sources: Adapted from the Dietary Reference Intakes series, National Academies Press. Copyright 1997, 1998, 2000, 2001, by the National Academy of Sciences. These reports may be accessed via www.nap.edu. Courtesy of the National Academies Press, Washington D.C.

Note: This table is adapted from the DRI reports; see www.nap.edu. It lists Recommended Dietary Allowances (RDAs), with Adequate Intakes (AIs) indicated by an asterisk (*). RDAs and AIs may both be used as goals for individual intake. RDAs are set to meet the needs of almost all (97 to 98 percent) individuals in a group. For healthy breastfed infants, the AI is the mean intake. The AI for other life stage and gender groups is believed to cover the needs of all individuals in the group, but lack of data prevent being able to specify with confidence the percentage of individuals covered by this intake.

[a] Given as retinal activity equivalents (RAEs).
[b] Also known as calciferol. The DRI values are based on the absence of adequate exposure to sunlight.
[c] Also known as α-tocopherol.
[d] Given as niacin equivalents (NE), except for infants 0–6 months, which are expressed as preformed niacin.
[e] Given as dietary folate equivalents (DFE).

Dietary Reference Intakes: RDA, AI*

Life Stage Group	Calcium (mg/d)	Phosphorus (mg/d)	Magnesium (mg/d)	Iron (mg/d)	Zinc (mg/d)	Selenium (µg/d)	Iodine (µg/d)	Copper (µg/d)	Manganese (mg/d)	Fluoride (mg/d)	Chromium (µg/d)	Molybdenum (µg/d)
Infants												
0–6 mo	210*	100*	30*	0.27*	2*	15*	110*	200*	0.003*	0.01*	0.2*	2*
7–12 mo	270*	275*	75*	11	3	20*	130*	220*	0.6*	0.5*	5.5*	3*
Children												
1–3 y	500*	460	80	7	3	20	90	340	1.2*	0.7*	11*	17
4–8 y	800*	500	130	10	5	30	90	440	1.5*	1*	15*	22
Males												
9–13 y	1300*	1250	240	8	8	40	120	700	1.9*	2*	25*	34
14–18 y	1300*	1250	410	11	11	55	150	890	2.2*	3*	35*	43
19–30 y	1000*	700	400	8	11	55	150	900	2.3*	4*	35*	45
31–50 y	1000*	700	420	8	11	55	150	900	2.3*	4*	35*	45
51–70 y	1200*	700	420	8	11	55	150	900	2.3*	4*	30*	45
> 70 y	1200*	700	420	8	11	55	150	900	2.3*	4*	30*	45
Females												
9–13 y	1300*	1250	240	8	8	40	120	700	1.6*	2*	21*	34
14–18 y	1300*	1250	360	15	9	55	150	890	1.6*	3*	24*	43
19–30 y	1000*	700	310	18	8	55	150	900	1.8*	3*	25*	45
31–50 y	1000*	700	320	18	8	55	150	900	1.8*	3*	25*	45
51–70 y	1200*	700	320	8	8	55	150	900	1.8*	3*	20*	45
> 70 y	1200*	700	320	8	8	55	150	900	1.8*	3*	20*	45
Pregnancy												
≤ 18 y	1300*	1250	400	27	12	60	220	1000	2.0*	3*	29*	50
19–30 y	1000*	700	350	27	11	60	220	1000	2.0*	3*	30*	50
31–50 y	1000*	700	360	27	11	60	220	1000	2.0*	3*	30*	50
Lactation												
≤ 18 y	1300*	1250	360	10	13	70	290	1300	2.6*	3*	44*	50
19–30 y	1000*	700	310	9	12	70	290	1300	2.6*	3*	45*	50
31–50 y	1000*	700	320	9	12	70	290	1300	2.6*	3*	45*	50

Sources: Adapted from the Dietary Reference Intakes series, National Academies Press. Copyright 1997, 1998, 2000, 2001, by the National Academy of Sciences. These reports may be accessed via www.nap.edu. Courtesy of the National Academies Press, Washington D.C.

Note: This table is adapted from the DRI reports; see www.nap.edu. It lists Recommended Dietary Allowances (RDAs), with Adequate Intakes (AIs) indicated by an asterisk (*). RDAs and AIs may both be used as goals for individual intake. RDAs are set to meet the needs of almost all (97 to 98 percent) individuals in a group. For healthy breastfed infants, the AI is the mean intake. The AI for other life stage and gender groups is believed to cover the needs of all individuals in the group, but lack of data prevents being able to specify with confidence the percentage of individuals covered by this intake.

ADEQUATE NUTRIENTS WITHIN CALORIE NEEDS

- Consume a variety of nutrient-dense foods and beverages within and among the basic food groups while choosing foods that limit the intake of saturated and trans fats, cholesterol, added sugars, salt, and alcohol.

- Meet recommended intakes within energy needs by adopting a balanced eating pattern, such as the U.S. Department of Agriculture (USDA) Food Guide or the Dietary Approaches to Stop Hypertension (DASH) Eating Plan.

WEIGHT MANAGEMENT

- To maintain body weight in a healthy range, balance Calories from foods and beverages with Calories expended.

- To prevent gradual weight gain over time, make small decreases in food and beverage Calories and increase physical activity.

PHYSICAL ACTIVITY

- Engage in regular physical activity and reduce sedentary activities to promote health, psychological well-being, and a healthy body weight.

- To reduce the risk of chronic disease in adulthood: Engage in at least 30 minutes of moderate-intensity physical activity, above usual activity, at work or home on most days of the week.

- For most people, greater health benefits can be obtained by engaging in physical activity of more vigorous intensity or longer duration.

- To help manage body weight and prevent gradual, unhealthy body weight gain in adulthood: Engage in approximately 60 minutes of moderate- to vigorous-intensity activity on most days of the week while not exceeding caloric intake requirements.

- To sustain weight loss in adulthood: Participate in at least 60 to 90 minutes of daily moderate-intensity physical activity while not exceeding caloric intake requirements. Some people may need to consult with a health care provider before participating in this level of activity.

- Achieve physical fitness by including cardiovascular conditioning, stretching exercises for flexibility, and resistance exercises or calisthenics for muscle strength and endurance.

FOOD GROUPS TO ENCOURAGE

- Consume a sufficient amount of fruits and vegetables while staying within energy needs. Two cups (500 mL) of fruit and 2$\frac{1}{2}$ (625 mL) cups of vegetables per day are recommended for a reference 2000-Calorie (8400 kJ) intake, with higher or lower amounts depending on the Calorie level.

- Choose a variety of fruits and vegetables each day. In particular, select from all five vegetable subgroups (dark green, orange, legumes, starchy vegetables, and other vegetables) several times a week.

- Consume 3 or more ounce-equivalents of whole-grain products per day, with the rest of the recommended grains coming from enriched or whole-grain products. In general, at least half the grains should come from whole grains.

- Consume 750 mL (3 cups) per day of fat-free or low-fat milk or equivalent milk products.

FATS

- Consume fewer than 10% of Calories from saturated fatty acids and less than 300 mg/day of cholesterol, and keep trans fatty acid consumption as low as possible.

- Keep total fat intake between 20% to 35% of Calories, with most fats coming from sources of polyunsaturated and monounsaturated fatty acids, such as fish, nuts, and vegetable oils.

- When selecting and preparing meat, poultry, dry beans, and milk or milk products, make choices that are lean, low-fat, or fat-free.

- Limit intake of fats and oils high in saturated and/or trans fatty acids, and choose products low in such fats and oils.

CARBOHYDRATES

- Choose fibre-rich fruits, vegetables, and whole grains often.

- Choose and prepare foods and beverages with few added sugars or caloric sweeteners, such as amounts suggested by the USDA Food Guide and the DASH Eating Plan.

- Reduce the incidence of dental caries by practising good oral hygiene and consuming sugar- and starch-containing foods and beverages less frequently.

SODIUM AND POTASSIUM

- Consume less than 2300 mg (approximately 5 mL or 1 tsp of salt) of sodium per day.

- Choose and prepare foods with little salt. At the same time, consume potassium-rich foods, such as fruits and vegetables.

continued

ALCOHOLIC BEVERAGES

- Those who choose to drink alcoholic beverages should do so sensibly and in moderation—defined as the consumption of up to one drink per day for women and up to two drinks per day for men.

- Alcoholic beverages should not be consumed by some individuals, including those who cannot restrict their alcohol intake, women of childbearing age who may become pregnant, pregnant and lactating women, children and adolescents, individuals taking medications that can interact with alcohol, and those with specific medical conditions.

- Alcoholic beverages should be avoided by individuals engaging in activities that require attention, skill, or coordination, such as driving or operating machinery.

FOOD SAFETY

- To avoid microbial food-borne illness:

  - Clean hands, food contact surfaces, and fruits and vegetables. Meat and poultry should not be washed or rinsed.

  - Separate raw, cooked, and ready-to-eat foods while shopping, preparing, or storing foods.

  - Cook foods to a safe temperature to kill microorganisms.

  - Chill (refrigerate) perishable food promptly and defrost foods properly.

  - Avoid raw (unpasteurized) milk or any products made from unpasteurized milk, raw or partially cooked eggs or foods containing raw eggs, raw or undercooked meat and poultry, unpasteurized juices, and raw sprouts.

Note: The Dietary Guidelines for Americans 2005 contains additional recommendations for specific populations. The full document is available at www.healthierus.gov/dietaryguidelines.
Source: U.S. Department of Health and Human Services and Department of Agriculture, 2005, www.health.gov/dietaryguidelines/dga2005/document/pdf/brochure.pdf (accessed January 2005).

Answers to Review Questions

Please find answers to Review Questions 11–15 of each chapter on MyNutritionLab, www.pearsoned.ca/mynutritionlab.

Chapter 1

1. **d.** micronutrients.
2. **d.** All of the above.
3. **c.** contain 90 Calories (370 kJ) of energy.
4. **d.** "A high-protein diet increases the risk for porous bones," is an example of a hypothesis.
5. **d.** all of the above
6. False. Vitamins do not provide any energy, although many vitamins are critical to the metabolic processes that assist us in generating energy from carbohydrates, fats, and proteins.
7. True.
8. True.
9. True.
10. True.

Chapter 2

1. **d.** The % daily values of select nutrients in a serving of the packaged food.
2. **b.** provides enough of the energy, nutrients, and fibre to maintain a person's health.
3. **d.** protein and iron.
4. **a.** is a "heart-healthy" choice.
5. **b.** Foods with a lot of nutrients relative to their energy content, such as fish, are more nutritious choices than foods with fewer nutrients such as candy.
6. False. All foods are required to carry Nutrition Facts tables, but nutrient content claims and health claims are optional.
7. True. Although the traditional Mediterranean diet is relatively high in fat, it is mostly "heart-healthy" types of fats (monounsaturated and polyunsaturated). Research suggests that the type of fat is as important as the amount of fat in a diet.
8. False. Manufacturers can choose from a range of serving sizes for their products, but these are not necessarily the same as the serving sizes on *Canada's Food Guide to Healthy Eating.*
9. False. The Other Foods category on *Canada's Food Guide to Healthy Eating* contains foods that are high in fat and/or sugar, and should be eaten only occasionally.
10. False. The %DV on a Nutrition Facts table tells you what proportion of the recommended amount of a nutrient is supplied by one serving of the food, for an adult consuming a 2000-Calorie (8400 kJ) diet.

Chapter 3

1. **c.** atoms, molecules, cells, tissues, organs, systems
2. **d.** emulsifies fats.
3. **c.** hypothalamus.
4. **a.** seepage of gastric acid into the esophagus.
5. **a.** a bean and cheese burrito
6. True.
7. True.
8. False. Vitamins and minerals are not really "digested" the same way that macronutrients are. These compounds do not have to be broken down because they are small enough to be readily absorbed by the small intestine. For example, fat-soluble vitamins, such as vitamins A, D, E, and K, are soluble in lipids and are absorbed into the intestinal cells along with the fats in our foods. Water-soluble vitamins, such as the B vitamins and vitamin C, typically undergo some type of active transport process that helps ensure the vitamin is absorbed by the small intestine. Minerals are absorbed all along the small intestine, and in some cases in the large intestine as well, by a wide variety of mechanisms.
9. False. A person with celiac disease cannot tolerate products with gluten, a protein found in wheat, rye, and barley.
10. False. Cells are the smallest units of life. Atoms are the smallest units of matter in nature.

Chapter 4

1. **b.** the potential of foods to raise blood glucose and insulin levels.
2. **d.** carbon, hydrogen, and oxygen.
3. **b.** how much glucose has been in the bloodstream over the past three months.
4. **a.** monosaccharides.
5. **a.** phenylketonuria.
6. False. Sugar alcohols are considered nutritive sweeteners because they contain 2 to 4 kcal of energy per gram.
7. True.
8. False. A person with lactose intolerance has a difficult time tolerating milk and other dairy products. This person does not have an allergy to milk, as he or she does not exhibit an immune response indicative of an allergy. Instead, this person does not digest lactose completely, which causes intestinal distress and symptoms such as gas, bloating, diarrhea, and nausea.
9. False. Plants store glucose as starch.
10. False. Salivary amylase breaks starches into maltose and shorter polysaccharides.

Chapter 5

1. **d.** found in flaxseeds, soy milk, and fish.
2. **b.** exercise regularly.
3. **a.** lipoprotein lipase.
4. **d.** high-density lipoproteins.
5. **a.** monounsaturated fats.
6. True.
7. False. Fat is an important source of energy during rest and during exercise, and adipose tissue is our primary storage site for fat. We rely significantly on the fat stored in our adipose tissue to provide energy during rest and exercise.
8. False. A triglyceride is a lipid comprised of a glycerol molecule and three fatty acids. Thus, fatty acids are a component of triglycerides.
9. False. While most trans fatty acids result from the hydrogenation of vegetable oils by food manufacturers, a small amount of trans fatty acids are found in cow's milk.
10. False. A serving of food labeled *reduced fat* has at least 25% less fat than a standard serving, but may not have fewer calories than a full-fat version of the same food.

Chapter 6

1. **d.** mutual supplementation.
2. **a.** Rice, pinto beans, acorn squash, soy butter, and almond milk.
3. **c.** protease.
4. **b.** amine group.
5. **c.** carbon, oxygen, hydrogen, and nitrogen.
6. True.
7. False. Both shape and function are lost when a protein is denatured.
8. False. Some hormones are made from lipids.
9. False. Buffers help the body maintain acid–base balance.
10. False. Depending upon the type of sport, athletes may require the same or up to two times as much protein as nonactive people.

Chapter 7

1. **b.** It can be found in fresh fruits and vegetables.
2. **d.** A healthy infant of average weight.
3. **a.** extracellular fluid.
4. **d.** It is freely permeable to water, but impermeable to solutes.
5. **b.** Losing weight.
6. False. In addition to water, the body needs electrolytes, such as sodium and potassium, to prevent fluid imbalances during long-distance events such as a marathon. As purified water contains no electrolytes, this would not be the ideal beverage to prevent fluid imbalances during a marathon.
7. False. Our thirst mechanism is triggered by an increase in the concentration of electrolytes in our blood.
8. False. Hypernatremia is commonly caused by a rapid intake of high amounts of sodium.
9. False. Quenching our thirst does not guarantee adequate hydration. Urine that is clear or light yellow in colour is one indicator of adequate hydration.
10. False. These conditions are associated with decreased fluid loss or an increase in body fluid. Diarrhea, blood loss, and low humidity are conditions that increase fluid loss.

Chapter 8

1. **d.** It is destroyed by exposure to high heat.
2. **b.** an atom loses an electron.
3. **a.** cardiovascular disease.
4. **d.** nitrates.
5. **a.** vitamin A.
6. True.
7. True.
8. False. Vitamin C helps regenerate vitamin E.
9. True.
10. False. Pregnant women should not consume beef liver very often, as it can lead to vitamin A toxicity and potentially serious birth defects.

Chapter 9

1. **a.** calcium and phosphorus.
2. **c.** has normal bone density as compared to an average, healthy 30-year-old of the same age, sex, and race.
3. **d.** It provides the scaffolding for cortical bone.
4. **c.** a fair-skinned retired teaching living in a nursing home in Manitoba.
5. **d.** structure of bone, nerve transmission, and muscle contraction.
6. True.
7. True.
8. False. The fractures that result from osteoporosis cause an increased risk of infection and other related illnesses that can lead to premature death.
9. True.
10. False. Our body makes vitamin D by converting a cholesterol compound in our skin to the active form of vitamin D that we need to function. We do not absorb vitamin D from sunlight, but when the ultraviolet rays of the sun hit our skin, they react to eventually form calcitriol, which is considered the primary active form of vitamin D in our bodies.

Chapter 10

1. **d.** thiamin, pantothenic acid, and biotin.
2. **b.** vitamin K.
3. **b.** Iron is a component of hemoglobin, myoglobin, and certain enzymes.
4. **c.** an amino acid.
5. **d.** Choline is necessary for the synthesis of phospholipids and other components of cell membranes.
6. True.
7. True.
8. False. Iron deficiency causes iron-deficiency anemia; pernicious anemia occurs at the end stage of an autoimmune disorder that causes the loss of various cells in the stomach, which leads to a deficiency of vitamin B_{12}.
9. False. Neural tube defects occur during the first four weeks of pregnancy; this is often before a woman even knows she is pregnant. Thus, the best way for a woman to protect her fetus against neural tube defects is to make sure she is consuming adequate folate before she is pregnant.
10. False. Wilson's disease is a rare disorder that causes copper toxicity.

Chapter 11

1. **d.** body mass index.
2. **a.** basal metabolic rate, thermal effect of food, and effect of physical activity.
3. **b.** take in more energy than they expend.
4. **c.** all people have a genetic set-point for their body weight.
5. **a.** hunger.
6. False. It is the apple-shaped fat patterning, or excess fat in the trunk region, that is known to increase a person's risk for many chronic diseases.
7. True
8. False. Weight-loss medications are typically prescribed for people with a body mass index greater than or equal to 30 kg/m^2, or for people with a body mass index greater than or equal to 27 kg/m^2 who also have other significant health risk factors such as heart disease, high blood pressure, and type 2 diabetes.
9. False. Healthful weight gain includes eating more energy than you expend and also exercising to maintain both aerobic fitness and to build muscle mass.
10. True.

Chapter 12

1. **c.** 50% to 80% of your estimated maximal heart rate.
2. **a.** 1 to 3 seconds.

3. **b.** fat
4. **c.** seems to increase strength gained in resistance exercise.
5. **a.** An intensity of 12 to 15, or somewhat hard to hard, is recommended to achieve physical fitness.
6. True.
7. False. A dietary fat intake of 15% to 25% of total energy intake is generally recommended for athletes.
8. False. Carbohydrate loading involves altering duration and intensity of exercise and intake of carbohydrate such that the storage of carbohydrate is maximized.
9. False. Sports anemia is not true anemia, but a transient decrease in iron stores that occurs at the start of an exercise program. This is a result of an initial increase in plasma volume (or water in our blood) that is not matched by an increase in hemoglobin.
10. True.

Chapter 13

1. **b.** bulimia nervosa
2. **a.** increases your risk of developing a psychiatric eating disorder.
3. **d.** disordered eating, menstrual dysfunction, and osteoporosis.
4. **a.** exercise regularly.
5. **b.** I wish I could change the way I look in the mirror.
6. False. People with binge-eating disorder typically do not purge to compensate for the binge; thus, these individuals are usually overweight or obese.
7. False. Although it is suspected that media images of idealized female bodies may contribute to an increase in eating disorder in adolescent girls, there is no scientific evidence to support this suspicion.
8. True.
9. False. People with anorexia typically deny they are hungry and may lie about eating.
10. False. People who suffer from binge-eating disorder may also suffer from chronic overeating behaviours. However, chronic overeating is defined as regularly overeating without losing control, whereas binge-eating involves the loss of control during a binge episode that prevents a person from stopping him- or herself from overeating.

Chapter 14

1. **a.** oxygen, heat, and light.
2. **c.** a type of fungus used to ferment foods.
3. **b.** a flavour enhancer used in a variety of foods.
4. **c.** 48 hours.

5. **d.** cooling, canning, pasteurization, irradiation
6. False. The appropriate temperatures for cooking foods varies according to the food.
7. False. Hemolytic uremic syndrome (HUS) is caused by *E. coli* 0157:H7. Symptoms of this serious illness can include bloody diarrhea, vomiting, abdominal cramping, and fever, usually commencing between two and four days after exposure to the bacterium.
8. False. At present, Canada does not have a national mandatory regulatory system for organic production in place. About 30 different groups currently certify organic produce. In November 2004, the federal government formed the Organic Production System Task Force, and draft regulations are expected in 2006.
9. True.
10. True.

Chapter 15

1. **a.** fibre
2. **c.** oxytocin
3. **a.** fibre
4. **b.** women who begin their pregnancy underweight.
5. **d.** iron-fortified rice cereal.
6. False. These issues are most likely to occur in the first trimester of pregnancy.
7. True.
8. True.

9. True.
10. False. Exclusive breastfeeding is recommended for the first six months of age, with solid foods introduced at six months.

Chapter 16

1. **b.** vitamin D
2. **c.** 45% to 60%
3. **d.** dental caries
4. **a.** 125 mL (½ cup) of iron-fortified cooked oat cereal, 30 mL (2 Tbsp) mashed pineapple, and 250 mL (8 fl. oz.) whole milk
5. **a.** Cigarette smoking can interfere with the absorption of nutrients.
6. False. Preschool children are able to understand the basic information about which foods are more nutritious and those that should be eaten in moderation. Also, parents are important role models for preschool children.
7. True.
8. False. Although eating disorders frequently begin during adolescence, the rates of obesity are significantly higher than those for eating disorders in this age group.
9. False. There is no DRI for fat for toddlers; however, it is recommended that toddlers consume 30% to 40% of their total daily energy intake as fat.
10. True.

Glossary

A

absorption The physiologic process by which molecules of food are taken from the gastrointestinal tract into the bloodstream to be carried to different parts of the body.

acceptable daily intake (ADI) An estimate made by Health Canada of the amount of non-nutritive sweetener that someone can consume each day over a lifetime without adverse effects.

Acceptable Macronutrient Distribution Ranges (AMDR) Ranges of intakes for energy sources associated with reduced risk of chronic disease while providing adequate intakes of essential nutrients.

acetylcholine A neurotransmitter that is involved in many functions, including muscle movement and memory storage.

acidosis A disorder in which the blood becomes acidic; that is, the level of hydrogen in the blood is excessive. It can be caused by respiratory or metabolic problems.

added sugars Sugars and syrups that are added to food during processing or preparation.

adenosine triphosphate (ATP) The common currency of energy for virtually all cells of the body.

adequate diet A diet that provides enough of the energy, nutrients, and fibre to maintain a person's health.

Adequate Intake (AI) A recommended average daily nutrient intake level based on observed or experimentally determined estimates of nutrient intake by a group of healthy people.

alkalosis A disorder in which the blood becomes basic; that is, the level of hydrogen in the blood is deficient. It can be caused by respiratory or metabolic problems.

alpha-linolenic acid An essential fatty acid found in leafy green vegetables, flaxseed oil, soy oil, fish oil, fish products, and "omega-3 eggs"; an omega-3 fatty acid.

amenorrhea Lack of menstruation for at least three consecutive months in the absence of pregnancy. Primary amenorrhea is the absence of menstruation by the age of 16 years in a girl who has secondary sex characteristics, while secondary amenorrhea is the absence of the menstrual period for three or more months after menarche. The presence of amenorrhea is a criterion for the diagnosis of anorexia nervosa in females.

amino acids Nitrogen-containing molecules that combine to form proteins.

amniotic fluid The watery fluid contained within the innermost membrane of the sac containing the fetus. It cushions and protects the growing fetus.

anabolic Refers to a substance that builds muscle and increases strength.

anaerobic Means "without oxygen." Term used to refer to metabolic reactions that occur in the absence of oxygen.

anencephaly A fatal neural tube defect in which there is partial absence of brain tissue most likely caused by failure of the neural tube to close.

anorexia nervosa A serious, potentially life-threatening eating disorder that is characterized by self-starvation, which eventually leads to a deficiency in energy and essential nutrients that are required by the body to function normally. For an individual to be considered to have anorexia nervosa, he or she must be medically diagnosed by a physician and meet specific diagnostic criteria.

antibodies Defensive proteins of the immune system. Their production is prompted by the presence of bacteria, viruses, toxins, and allergens.

antioxidant A compound that has the ability to prevent the damage caused by oxidation.

anti-resorptive Characterized by an ability to slow or stop bone resorption without affecting bone formation. Anti-resorptive medications are used to reduce the rate of bone loss in people with osteoporosis.

appetite A psychological desire to consume specific foods.

ariboflavinosis A condition caused by riboflavin deficiency.

aseptic packaging Sterile packaging that does not require refrigeration or preservatives while the seal is maintained.

atom A discrete, irreducible unit of matter. It is the smallest unit of an element and is identical to all other atoms of that element.

atrophic gastritis A condition that results in low stomach-acid secretion; is estimated to occur in about 10% to 30% of adults older than 50 years of age.

B

bacteria Microorganisms that lack a true nucleus and have a chemical called peptidoglycan in their cell walls.

balanced diet A diet that contains the combinations of foods that provide the proper balance of nutrients.

basal metabolic rate (BMR) The energy the body expends to maintain its fundamental physiologic functions.

beriberi A disease caused by thiamin deficiency.

BHA (butylated hydroxyanisole) An antioxidant used primarily to stop rancidity in fats and oils.

BHT (butylated hydroxytoluene) An antioxidant used primarily to stop rancidity in fats and oils.

bile Fluid produced by the liver and stored in the gallbladder; it emulsifies fats in the small intestine.

binge eating Consumption of a large amount of food in a short time, usually accompanied by a feeling of loss of self-control.

binge-eating disorder A disorder characterized by binge eating an average of twice a week or more without compensatory behaviours, such as vomiting or excessive exercise.

bioavailability The degree to which our bodies can absorb and use any given nutrient.

biopesticides Include naturally occurring substances that control pests (biochemical pesticides), microorganisms that control pests (microbial pesticides), and pesticidal substances produced by plants containing added genetic material (plant-incorporated protectants) or PIPs.

bleaching agents Chemicals used to speed the natural process of ground flour changing from pale yellow to white.

blood volume The amount of fluid in blood.

body composition The amount of bone, muscle, and fat tissue in the body. Also, the ratio of a person's body fat to lean body mass.

body image A person's perception of his or her body's appearance and functioning.

body mass index (BMI) A measurement representing the ratio of a person's body weight to his or her height.

bolus A mouthful of chewed and moistened food that has been swallowed.

bone density The degree of compactness of bone tissue, reflecting the strength of the bones. Peak bone density is the point at which a bone is strongest.

brush border Term that describes the microvilli of the small intestine's lining. These microvilli tremendously increase the small intestine's absorptive capacity.

buffers Proteins that help maintain proper acid–base balance by attaching to, or releasing, hydrogen ions as conditions change in the body.

bulimia nervosa A serious eating disorder characterized by recurrent episodes of binge eating and recurrent inappropriate compensatory behaviours (such as self-induced vomiting; misuse of laxatives, diuretics, enemas, or other medications; fasting or excessive exercise) to prevent weight gain.

C

calcitriol (1,25-dihydroxyvitamin D) The primary active form of vitamin D in the body.

Calorie 1 Calorie = 1 kcal = 4.184 kilojoules

cancer A group of diseases characterized by cells that reproduce spontaneously and independently and may invade other tissues and organs.

carbohydrate One of the three macronutrients; a compound made up of carbon, hydrogen, and oxygen that is derived from plants and provides energy. Also, the primary fuel source for our bodies, particularly for our brain and for physical exercise.

carbohydrate loading Also known as glycogen loading. A process that involves altering training and carbohydrate intake so that muscle glycogen storage is maximized.

carcinogens Cancer-causing agents, such as certain pesticides, industrial chemicals, and pollutants. Also, any substances capable of causing the cellular mutations that lead to cancer.

cardiorespiratory fitness Fitness of the heart, lungs, and circulatory system; achieved through regular participation in aerobic-type activities.

cardiovascular disease A general term that refers to abnormal conditions involving the heart and blood vessels; cardiovascular disease can result in heart attack or stroke.

carotenoids Fat-soluble plant pigments that the body stores in the liver and adipose tissue. The body is able to convert certain carotenoids to vitamin A.

cataract A damaged portion of the eye's lens, which causes cloudiness that impairs vision.

celiac disease A genetic disorder characterized by a total intolerance for gluten that causes an immune reaction that damages the lining of the small intestine.

cell The smallest unit of matter that exhibits the properties of living things, such as growth, reproduction, and metabolism.

cell differentiation The process by which immature, undifferentiated stem cells develop into highly specialized functional cells of discrete organs and tissues.

cell membrane The boundary of an animal cell, composed of a phospholipid bilayer that separates its internal cytoplasm and organelles from the external environment.

Centers for Disease Control and Prevention (CDC) The leading federal agency in the United States that protects the health and safety of people. Its mission is to promote health and quality of life by preventing and controlling disease, injury, and disability.

cephalic phase Earliest phase of digestion in which the brain thinks about and prepares the digestive organs for the consumption of food.

childhood overweight Having a body mass index (BMI) at or above the 95th percentile.

cholecalciferol Vitamin D_3, a form of vitamin D found in animal foods and the form we synthesize from the sun.

chronic dieting Consistently and successfully restricting energy intake to maintain an average or a below average body weight.

chylomicron A lipoprotein produced in the mucosal cell of the intestine; transports dietary fat from a meal out of the intestinal tract into the lymphatic system.

chyme Semifluid mass consisting of partially digested food, water, and gastric juices.

coal tar A food additive made from thick or semisolid tar derived from bituminous coal, the byproducts of which have been found to cause cancer in animals.

coenzyme An organic compound that combines with an inactive enzyme to form an active enzyme.

cofactor A compound that is needed to allow enzymes to function properly.

colic Inconsolable infant crying that lasts for hours at a time.

collagen A protein found in all connective tissues in our body.

colostrum The first fluid made and secreted by the breasts from late in pregnancy to about a week after birth. It is rich in immune factors and protein.

complementary proteins Two or more foods that together contain all nine essential amino acids necessary for a complete protein. It is not necessary to eat complementary foods at the same meal.

complete proteins Proteins that contain all nine essential amino acids; proteins from animal sources are complete proteins. Soybeans are the only complete source of plant protein.

complex carbohydrate A nutrient compound, such as starch, glycogen, or fibre, consisting of long chains of glucose molecules.

conception (also called fertilization) The uniting of an ovum (egg) and sperm to create a fertilized egg, or zygote.

constipation A condition characterized by the absence of bowel movements for a time that is significantly longer than normal for the individual. When a bowel movement does occur, stools are usually small, hard, and difficult to pass.

cool-down Activities done after an exercise session is completed. Should be gradual and allow your body to slowly recover from exercise.

cortical bone (compact bone) A dense bone tissue that makes up the outer surface of all bones, as well as the entirety of most small bones of the body.

creatine phosphate (CP) A high-energy compound that can be broken down for energy and used to regenerate ATP.

cretinism A special form of mental retardation that occurs in infants when the mother experiences iodine deficiency during pregnancy.

cross contamination Contamination of one food by another via the unintended transfer of microbes through physical contact.

cystic fibrosis A genetic disorder that causes an alteration in chloride transport, leading to the production of thick, sticky mucus that causes life-threatening respiratory and digestive problems.

cytoplasm The liquid within an animal cell.

D

DASH diet   The diet developed in response to research into hypertension funded by the U.S. National Institutes of Health (NIH); stands for Dietary Approaches to Stop Hypertension.

deamination   The process by which an amine group is removed from an amino acid. The nitrogen is then transported in a special form to the kidneys for excretion in the urine, while the carbon skeleton is metabolized for energy or used to make other compounds.

dehydration   Depletion of body fluid that results when fluid excretion exceeds fluid intake.

denaturation   A change in the shape of a protein caused by heat, acids, bases, heavy metals, alcohol, or other substances; results in protein losing its ability to function.

denature   A term used to describe the action of unfolding proteins. Proteins must be denatured before they can be digested.

dental caries   Dental erosion and decay caused by acid-secreting bacteria in the mouth and on the teeth. The acid produced is a byproduct of bacterial metabolism of carbohydrates deposited on the teeth.

desiccant   Chemicals that prevent foods from absorbing moisture from the air.

diabetes mellitus   A chronic disease in which the body can no longer regulate glucose levels in the blood.

diarrhea   A condition characterized by the frequent passage of loose, watery stools.

dietary fibre   The indigestible carbohydrate parts of plants that form the support structure of leaves, stems, and seeds.

Dietary Reference Intakes (DRIs)   A set of nutritional reference values for Canada and the United States that apply to healthy people.

digestion   The process by which foods are broken down into their component molecules, either mechanically or chemically.

dioxins   An industrial pollutant most commonly attributed to waste incineration.

disaccharide   A carbohydrate compound consisting of two sugar molecules joined together.

disordered eating   A general term used to describe a variety of abnormal or atypical eating behaviours that are used to keep or maintain a lower body weight. Individuals with disordered eating behaviours do not have severe enough eating disturbances to be medically diagnosed with an eating disorder, such as anorexia nervosa or bulimia nervosa. The designation of "eating disorders not otherwise specified" is the medical term used to describe these individuals.

diuretic   A substance that increases fluid loss via the urine. Common diuretics include coffee, tea, cola, and other caffeine-containing beverages, as well as prescription medications for high blood pressure and other disorders.

docosahexaenoic acid (DHA)   A very long chain PUFA (22:6); critical for proper development of the central nervous system and the retina of the eyes. Found pre-formed in fish and fish oils.

dual energy x-ray absorptiometry (DXA or DEXA)   Currently the most accurate tool for measuring bone density.

E

eating disorder   A psychiatric disorder that must be clinically diagnosed by a physician and is characterized by severe disturbances in body image and eating behaviours. Anorexia nervosa and bulimia nervosa are two examples of eating disorders for which specific diagnostic criteria must be present for diagnosis.

edema   A disorder in which fluids build up in the tissue spaces of the body, causing fluid imbalances and a swollen appearance.

eicosapentaenoic acid (EPA)   A very long chain PUFA (20:5) found pre-formed in fish and fish oils. EPA and DHA appear to reduce our risk of death from a heart attack.

electrolyte   A substance that disassociates in solution into positively and negatively charged ions and is thus capable of carrying an electrical current.

electron   A negatively charged particle attracted to the nucleus of an atom.

elimination   The process by which the undigested and unabsorbed portions of food and waste products are removed from the body.

embryo   Human growth and developmental stage lasting from the third week to the end of the eighth week after fertilization.

emulsifiers   Chemicals that improve texture and smoothness in foods; stabilize oil-water mixtures.

energy cost of physical activity   The energy that is expended on body movement and muscular work above basal levels.

energy expenditure   The energy the body expends to maintain its basic functions and to perform all levels of movement and activity.

energy intake   The amount of food a person eats; in other words, it is the number of kilocalories consumed.

enteric nervous system   The nerves of the gastrointestinal (GI) tract.

enterotoxins   A type of toxin that targets the gastrointestinal tract cells.

enzymes   Small proteins that act on other chemicals to speed up body processes but are not apparently changed during those processes.

epiphyseal plates   Plates of cartilage located toward the end of long bones that provide for growth in the length of long bones.

ergocalciferol   Vitamin D_2, a form of vitamin D found exclusively in plant foods.

ergogenic aids   Substances used to improve exercise and athletic performance.

erythrocytes   The red blood cells, which are the cells that transport oxygen in our blood.

esophagus   Muscular tube of the GI tract connecting the back of the mouth to the stomach.

essential amino acids   Amino acids not produced by the body that must be obtained from food.

essential fatty acids (EFA)   Fatty acids that must be consumed in the diet because they cannot be made by our bodies. The two essential fatty acids are linoleic acid and alpha-linolenic acid.

essential nutrients   Nutrients that must come from food or nutrient supplements because they are not manufactured by the body at all or not in amounts sufficient to meet the body's needs.

Estimated Average Requirements (EAR)   The average daily nutrient intake level estimated to meet the requirement of half of the healthy individuals in a particular life stage and gender group.

Estimated Energy Requirement (EER)   The average dietary energy intake that is predicted to maintain energy balance in healthy reference adults. Also, the total amount of energy needed per day for any age group.

evaporative cooling   Another term for sweating, which is the primary way in which we dissipate heat.

exercise   A subcategory of leisure-time physical activity; any activity that is purposeful, planned, and structured.

extracellular fluid   The fluid outside the body's cells, either in the body's tissues; as the liquid portion of the blood, called plasma; or as digestive juices.

F

fat-soluble vitamins   Vitamins that are not soluble in water but are soluble in fat. These are vitamins A, D, E, and K.

fatty acids   Long chains of carbon atoms bound to each other as well as to hydrogen atoms.

female athlete triad   A condition characterized by the coexistence of three disorders in some athletic females: an eating disorder, amenorrhea, and osteoporosis.

ferritin   A storage form of iron in our bodies found primarily in the intestinal mucosa, spleen, bone marrow, and liver.

fetal alcohol spectrum disorder (FASD)   A set of serious, irreversible alcohol-related birth defects characterized by certain physical and mental abnormalities.

fetus   Human growth and developmental stage lasting from the beginning of the ninth week after conception to birth.

FIT principle   The principle used to achieve an appropriate overload for physical training. Stands for frequency, intensity, and time of activity.

5 to 10 a Day for Better Health program   A Canadian media campaign designed to make people aware of the health benefits of eating vegetables and fruits and to encourage people to eat more produce.

flavouring agents   Obtained from either natural or synthetic sources; allow manufacturers to maintain a consistent flavour from batch to batch.

flexibility   The ability to move a joint fluidly through its full range of motion.

fluid   A substance composed of molecules that move past one another freely. Fluids are characterized by their ability to conform to the shape of whatever container holds them.

fluorapatite   A mineral compound in human teeth that contains fluoride, calcium, and phosphorus and is more resistant to destruction by acids and bacteria than hydroxyapatite.

fluorosis   A condition marked by staining and pitting of the teeth; caused by an abnormally high intake of fluoride.

food additives   A substance or mixture of substances intentionally put into food to enhance its appearance, palatability, and quality.

food allergy   An allergic reaction to food, caused by an activation of the immune system.

food intolerance   Gastrointestinal discomfort caused by certain foods that is not a result of an immune system reaction.

food quality   Food characteristics, such as taste, odour, colour, and texture.

food preservatives   Chemicals that help prevent microbial growth and enzymatic deterioration.

food safety   Practices, guidelines, or legislation designed to protect our food supply from harmful substances.

food-borne illness   An illness transmitted through food or water; either by an infectious agent, by a poisonous substance, or by a protein that causes an immune reaction.

free radical   A highly unstable atom with an unpaired electron in its outermost shell.

frequency   Refers to the number of activity sessions per week you perform.

fructose   The sweetest natural sugar; a monosaccharide that occurs in fruits and vegetables. Also called levulose, or fruit sugar.

functional fibre   The indigestible forms of carbohydrate that are extracted from plants or manufactured in a laboratory and have known health benefits.

fungi   Plant-like, spore-forming organisms that can grow either as single cells or as multicellular colonies. Yeasts and moulds are two types of fungi.

G

galactose   A monosaccharide that joins with glucose to create lactose, one of the three most common disaccharides.

gallbladder   A tissue sac beneath the liver that concentrates and stores bile and secretes it into the small intestine.

gastric juice   Acidic liquid secreted within the stomach; it contains hydrochloric acid, pepsin, water, and other compounds.

gastroesophageal reflux disease (GERD)   A painful type of heartburn that occurs more than twice per week.

gastrointestinal (GI) tract   A long, muscular tube consisting of several organs: the mouth, esophagus, stomach, small intestine, and large intestine.

gene expression   The process of using a gene to make a protein.

genetic modification   Changing an organism by manipulating its genetic material.

gestation   The period of intrauterine development from conception to birth.

gestational diabetes   Insufficient insulin production or insulin resistance that results in consistently high blood glucose levels, specifically during pregnancy; condition typically resolves after birth occurs.

giardiasis   A diarrheal illness caused by the intestinal parasite *Giardia intestinalis* (or *Giardia lamblia*).

glucagon   Hormone secreted by the alpha cells of the pancreas in response to decreased blood levels of glucose. Causes breakdown of liver stores of glycogen into glucose.

gluconeogenesis   The generation of glucose from the breakdown of proteins into amino acids.

glucose   The most abundant sugar molecule; a monosaccharide generally found in combination with other sugars. The preferred source of energy for the brain and an important source of energy for all cells.

glycemic index   Rating of the potential of foods to raise blood glucose levels.

glycerol   An alcohol composed of three carbon atoms; it is the backbone of a triglyceride molecule.

glycogen   A polysaccharide stored in animals; the storage form of glucose in animals.

glycolysis   The breakdown of glucose; yields two ATP molecules and two pyruvic acid molecules for each molecule of glucose.

goiter   Enlargement of the thyroid gland; can be caused by either iodine toxicity or deficiency.

grazing   Consistently eating small meals throughout the day; done by many athletes to meet their high energy demands.

H

health   A multidimensional process that includes physical activity and occupational, social, emotional, intellectual, and spiritual health.

heartburn   The painful sensation that occurs over the sternum when hydrochloric acid backs up from the stomach into the lower esophagus.

heat cramps   Muscle spasms that occur several hours after strenuous exercise; most often occur when sweat losses and fluid intakes are high, urine volume is low, and sodium intake is inadequate.

heat exhaustion   A heat illness that is characterized by excessive sweating, weakness, nausea, dizziness, headache, and difficulty concentrating. Unchecked heat exhaustion can lead to heatstroke.

heat syncope   Dizziness that occurs when people stand for too long in the heat or when they stop suddenly after a race or stand suddenly from a lying position; results from blood pooling in the lower extremities.

heatstroke   A potentially fatal response to high temperature characterized by failure of the body's heat-regulating mechanisms. Symptoms include rapid pulse; reduced sweating; hot, dry skin; high temperature; headache; weakness; and sudden loss of consciousness. Commonly called sunstroke.

helminth   Multicellular microscopic worm.

heme   The iron-containing molecule found in hemoglobin.

heme iron   Iron that is a part of hemoglobin and myoglobin; found only in animal-based foods, such as meat, fish, and poultry.

hemoglobin   The oxygen-carrying protein found in our red blood cells; almost two thirds of all the iron in our bodies is found in hemoglobin.

hemorrhoids   Swollen varicose veins in the rectum.

hemosiderin   A storage form of iron in our bodies found primarily in the intestinal mucosa, spleen, bone marrow, and liver.

homocysteine   An amino acid that requires adequate levels of folate, vitamin B_6, and vitamin B_{12} for its metabolism. High levels of homocysteine in the blood are associated with an increased risk for vascular diseases, such as cardiovascular disease.

hormone   Chemical messenger that is secreted into the bloodstream by one of the many glands of the body and acts as a regulator of the physiologic processes at a site remote from the gland that secreted it.

humectant   Chemicals that help retain moisture in foods, keeping them soft and pliable.

hunger   A physiologic sensation that prompts us to eat.

hydrogenation   The process of adding hydrogen to unsaturated fatty acids, making them more saturated and thereby more solid at room temperature.

hydrophilic   Attracted to or soluble in water.

hydrophobic   Not attracted to or soluble in water.

hypercalcemia   A condition marked by an abnormally high concentration of calcium in the blood.

hyperkalemia   A condition in which blood potassium levels are dangerously high.

hypermagnesemia   A condition marked by an abnormally high concentration of magnesium in the blood.

hypernatremia   A condition in which blood sodium levels are dangerously high.

hypertension   A chronic condition characterized by above-average blood pressure readings; specifically, systolic blood pressure of more than 140 mm Hg or diastolic blood pressure of more than 90 mm Hg (140/90 mm Hg) when measured in a doctor's office or higher than 135/85 mm Hg when measured at home.

hypocalcemia   A condition characterized by an abnormally low concentration of calcium in the blood.

hypoglycemia   A condition marked by blood glucose levels that are below normal levels.

hypokalemia   A condition in which blood potassium levels are dangerously low.

hypomagnesemia   A condition characterized by an abnormally low concentration of magnesium in the blood.

hyponatremia   A condition in which blood sodium levels are dangerously low.

hypothalamus   A region of the forebrain below the thalamus where visceral sensations, such as hunger and thirst, are regulated.

I

incomplete proteins   Proteins that do not contain all the essential amino acids in sufficient amounts to support growth and health.

inflammatory bowel disease   A term that includes two different diseases with unknown causes that cause inflammation and swelling of the intestine: Crohn's disease and ulcerative colitis.

inorganic   A substance or nutrient that does not contain the element carbon.

insensible water loss   The loss of water from the skin in the form of sweat and from the lungs during breathing.

insoluble fibre   Components of plants that attract and cling to water. In humans, these substances speed up the movement of material through the large intestine.

insulin   Hormone secreted by the beta cells of the pancreas in response to increased blood levels of glucose. Facilitates uptake of glucose by body cells.

intensity   Refers to the amount of effort expended during the activity, or how difficult the activity is to perform.

intracellular fluid   The fluid held at any given time within the walls of the body's cells.

intrinsic factor   A protein secreted by cells of the stomach that binds to vitamin B_{12} and aids its absorption in the small intestine.

invisible fats   Fats that are hidden in foods, such as the fats found in baked goods, regular-fat dairy products, marbling in meat, and fried foods.

ion   Any electrically charged particle, either positively or negatively charged.

iron-deficiency anemia   A form of anemia that results from severe iron deficiency.

irradiation   A sterilization process utilizing gamma rays or other forms of radiation, which does not impart any radiation to the food being treated.

irritable bowel syndrome   A disorder that interferes with normal functions of the colon. Symptoms include abdominal cramps, bloating, and constipation or diarrhea.

K

Keshan disease   A heart disorder caused by selenium deficiency. It was first identified in children in the Keshan province of China.

ketoacidosis   A condition in which excessive ketones are present in the blood, causing the blood to become very acidic, which alters basic body functions and damages tissues. Untreated ketoacidosis can be fatal. This condition is found in individuals with untreated diabetes mellitus.

ketones   Substances produced during the breakdown of fat when carbohydrate intake is insufficient to meet energy needs. Provide an alternative energy source for the brain when glucose levels are low.

ketosis   The process by which the breakdown of fat during fasting results in the production of ketones.

kwashiorkor   A form of protein-energy malnutrition that is typically seen in developing countries in infants and toddlers who are weaned early because of the birth of a subsequent child. Denied breast milk, they are fed a cereal diet that provides adequate energy but inadequate protein.

L

lactase   A digestive enzyme that digests lactose into glucose and galactose.

lactation   The production of breast milk.

lacteal   A small lymph vessel located inside of the villi of the small intestine.

lactic acid   A compound that results when pyruvic acid is metabolized in the presence of insufficient oxygen.

lactose   Also called milk sugar, a disaccharide consisting of one glucose molecule and one galactose molecule. Found in milk, including human breast milk.

lactose intolerance   A disorder in which the body does not produce sufficient lactase enzyme and therefore cannot digest foods that contain lactose, such as cow's milk and fresh cheese.

large intestine   The final organ of the GI tract, consisting of cecum, colon, rectum, and anal canal, and in which most water is absorbed and feces are formed.

leisure-time physical activity   Any activity not related to a person's occupation; includes competitive sports, recreational activities, and planned exercise training.

leptin   A hormone that is produced by body fat that acts to reduce food intake and to decrease body weight and body fat.

leukocytes   The white blood cells, which protect us from infection and illness.

limiting amino acid   The essential amino acid that is missing or in the smallest supply in the amino acid pool and is thus responsible for slowing or halting protein synthesis.

linoleic acid   An essential fatty acid found in vegetable and nut oils; an omega-6 fatty acid.

lipids   An important energy source for our bodies at rest and during low-intensity exercise; a diverse group of organic substances that are insoluble in water; lipids include triglycerides, phospholipids, and sterols.

lipoprotein   A spherical compound in which fat clusters in the centre and phospholipids and proteins form the outside of the sphere.

lipoprotein lipase   An enzyme that sits on the outside of cells and breaks apart triglycerides so that their fatty acids can be removed and taken up by the cell.

liver   The largest accessory organ of the GI tract and one of the most important organs of the body. Its functions include producing bile, processing nutrient-rich blood from the small intestine, and detoxifying harmful substances.

long-chain fatty acids   Fatty acids that are 14 or more carbon atoms in length.

low birth weight   A weight of less than 2500 grams, or 2.5 kg (5.5 lb.) at birth.

low-intensity activities   Activities that cause very mild increases in breathing, sweating, and heart rate.

M

macrocytic anemia   A form of anemia manifested as the production of larger-than-normal red blood cells containing insufficient hemoglobin, which inhibits adequate transport of oxygen; also called megaloblastic anemia. Macrocytic anemia can be caused by a severe folate deficiency.

macronutrients   Nutrients that our bodies need in relatively large amounts to support normal function and health. Carbohydrates, fats, and proteins are macronutrients.

macular degeneration   A vision disorder caused by deterioration of the central portion of the retina and marked by loss or distortion of the central field of vision.

mad cow disease   A fatal brain disorder prompted by consumption of food containing prions, which are an abnormal form of protein found in the brains and other organs of infected sheep, cows, and other livestock.

major minerals   Minerals we need to consume in amounts of at least 100 milligrams per day and of which the total amount in our bodies is at least 5 grams.

malnutrition   Any condition associated with undernutrition or overnutrition.

maltase   A digestive enzyme that digests maltose into glucose.

maltose   A disaccharide consisting of two molecules of glucose. Does not generally occur independently in foods but results as a byproduct of digestion. Also called malt sugar.

marasmus   A form of protein-energy malnutrition that results from grossly inadequate intakes of protein, energy, and other nutrients.

maximal heart rate   The rate at which your heart beats during maximal intensity exercise.

medium-chain fatty acids   Fatty acids that are six to twelve carbon atoms in length.

megadose   A dose of a nutrient that is 10 or more times as large as the recommended amount.

menaquinone   The form of vitamin K produced by bacteria in the large intestine.

menarche   The beginning of menstruation, or the menstrual period.

metabolic syndrome   A syndrome characterized by high blood pressure, abnormal glucose and insulin levels, imbalance of blood fats, and large waistlines. It is strongly linked to diabetes and heart disease.

metabolic water   The water formed as a byproduct of our body's metabolic reactions.

micelle   A spherical compound made up of bile and phospholipids; traps and transports free fatty acids, monoglycerides, and free cholesterol to the mucosal cells lining the small intestine.

micronutrients   Nutrients needed in relatively small amounts to support normal health and body functions. Vitamins and some minerals are micronutrients.

minerals   Inorganic substances that are not broken down during digestion and absorption and are not destroyed by heat or light. Minerals assist in the regulation of many body processes and are classified as major minerals or trace minerals.

moderate-intensity activities   Activities that cause moderate increases in breathing, sweating, and heart rate.

moderation Eating the right amounts of foods to maintain a healthy weight and to optimize the body's metabolic processes.

monosaccharide The simplest of carbohydrates. Consists of one sugar molecule, the most common form of which is glucose.

monounsaturated fatty acids (MUFA) Fatty acids that have two carbons in the chain bound to each other with one double bond; these types of fatty acids are generally liquid at room temperature.

morning sickness Varying degrees of nausea and vomiting associated with pregnancy, most commonly in the first trimester.

MPF (meat protein factor) A special factor found in meat, fish, and poultry that enhances the absorption of non-heme iron.

multifactorial disease Any disease that may be attributable to one or more of a variety of causes.

muscle cramps Involuntary, spasmodic, and painful muscle contractions that last for many seconds or even minutes; electrolyte imbalances are often the cause of muscle cramps.

muscular endurance A subcomponent of musculoskeletal fitness defined as the ability of a muscle to maintain submaximal force levels for extended periods of time.

muscular strength A subcomponent of musculoskeletal fitness defined as the maximal force or tension level that can be produced by a muscle group.

musculoskeletal fitness Fitness of the muscles and bones.

mutual supplementation The process of combining two or more incomplete protein sources to make a complete protein.

myoglobin An iron-containing protein similar to hemoglobin except that it is found in muscle cells.

N

National Institutes of Health (NIH) The world's leading medical centre and the focal point for medical research in the United States.

neonatal A term referring to a newborn.

neural tube Embryonic tissue that forms a tube, which eventually becomes the brain and spinal cord.

neural tube defects The most common malformations of the central nervous system that occur during fetal development. A folate deficiency can cause neural tube defects.

neurotoxins A type of toxin that targets the nervous system cells.

night blindness A vitamin A deficiency disorder that results in the loss of the ability to see in dim light.

nitrates Chemicals used in meat curing to develop and stabilize the pink colour associated with cured meat; also function as antibacterial agents.

nitrites Chemicals used in meat curing to develop and stabilize the pink colour associated with cured meat; also function as antibacterial agents.

non-essential amino acids Amino acids that can be manufactured by the body in sufficient quantities and therefore do not need to be consumed regularly in our diet.

non-heme iron The form of iron that is not a part of hemoglobin or myoglobin; found in animal- and plant-based foods.

non-nutritive sweeteners Also called alternative sweeteners; manufactured sweeteners that provide little or no energy.

nucleus The positively charged central core of an atom. It is made up of two types of particles—protons and neutrons—bound tightly together. The nucleus of an atom contains essentially all of its atomic mass.

nutrient density The relative amount of nutrients per amount of energy (or number of kilocalories).

nutrients Chemicals found in foods that are critical to human growth and function.

nutrition The science that studies food and how food nourishes our bodies and influences our health.

Nutrition Facts table The table on a food package label that gives the amount of energy and a minimum of 13 key nutrients in 1 serving of the food.

nutritious diet A diet that provides the proper combination of energy and nutrients and is adequate, moderate, balanced, and varied.

nutritive sweeteners Sweeteners, such as sucrose, fructose, honey, and brown sugar, that contribute energy.

O

obesity Having excess body fat that adversely affects health, resulting in a person having a weight that is substantially greater than some accepted standard for a given height.

organ A body structure composed of two or more tissues and performing a specific function; for example, the esophagus.

organelle A tiny "organ" within a cell that performs a discrete function necessary to the cell.

organic A substance or nutrient that contains the element carbon.

osteoblasts Cells that prompt the formation of new bone matrix by laying down the collagen-containing component of bone that is then mineralized.

osteoclasts Cells that erode the surface of bones by secreting enzymes and acids that dig grooves into the bone matrix.

osteomalacia Vitamin D deficiency disease in adults, in which bones become weak and prone to fractures.

osteoporosis A disease characterized by low bone mass and deterioration of bone tissue, leading to increased bone fragility and fracture risk.

overhydration Dilution of body fluid. It results when water intake or retention is excessive.

overload principle Placing an extra physical demand on your body to improve your fitness level.

overnutrition A diet that has an imbalance of fats, carbohydrates, and proteins or simply too much energy.

overweight Having a moderate amount of excess body fat, resulting in a person having a weight that is greater than some accepted standard for a given height but is not considered obese.

ovulation The release of an ovum (egg) from a woman's ovary.

oxidation A chemical reaction in which molecules of a substance may be broken down into their component atoms. During oxidation, the atoms involved lose electrons.

P

pancreas An accessory organ located behind the stomach; it secretes digestive enzymes that break down proteins, carbohydrates, and fats.

pancreatic amylase An enzyme secreted by the pancreas into the small intestine that digests any remaining starch into maltose.

parathyroid hormone (PTH) A hormone that helps to regulate blood calcium levels.

pasteurization A form of sterilization using high temperatures for short periods.

pellagra   A disease that results from severe niacin deficiency, characterized by dermatitis, diarrhea, depression, and in later stages, dementia and sometimes death.

pepsin   An enzyme in the stomach that begins the breakdown of proteins into shorter polypeptide chains and single amino acids.

peptic ulcer   An area of the GI tract that has been eroded away by the acidic gastric juices of the stomach. The two main causes of peptic ulcers are an *H. pylori* infection or use of non-steroidal anti-inflammatory drugs.

peptidases   A set of enzymes on the surface of intestinal cells that hydrolyze peptide bonds in oligopeptides, tripeptides, and dipeptides, splitting them into single amino acids for absorption.

peptide bonds   Unique types of chemical bonds in which the amine group of one amino acid binds to the acid group of another to manufacture dipeptides and all larger peptide molecules.

percent daily values (%DV)   Information on a Nutrition Facts table that identifies how much a serving of food contributes to your overall intake of nutrients listed on the label; based on an energy intake of 2000 Calories (8400 kJ) per day.

peristalsis   Waves of squeezing and pushing contractions that move food in one direction through the length of the GI tract.

pernicious anemia   A special form of anemia that is the primary cause of a vitamin B_{12} deficiency; occurs at the end stage of an autoimmune disorder that causes the loss of various cells in the stomach.

persistent organic pollutants (POPs)   Chemicals released into the environment as a result of industry, agriculture, or improper waste disposal; automobile emissions also are considered POPs.

pesticides   Chemicals used either in the field or in storage to destroy plant, fungal, and animal pests.

pH   Stands for percentage of hydrogen. It is a measure of the acidity—or level of hydrogen—of any solution, including human blood.

phospholipids   A type of lipid with a glycerol backbone to which are attached two fatty acids and another compound that contains phosphate; unlike other lipids, phospholipids are soluble in water.

photosynthesis   The process by which plants use sunlight to fuel a chemical reaction that combines carbon dioxide and hydrogen atoms from water into glucose, which is then stored in the plants' cells.

phylloquinone   The form of vitamin K found in plants.

physical activity   Any movement produced by muscles that increases energy expenditure; includes occupational, household, leisure-time, and transportation activities.

physical fitness   The ability to carry out daily tasks with vigour and alertness, without undue fatigue, and with ample energy to enjoy leisure-time pursuits and meet unforeseen emergencies.

phytic acid   The form of phosphorus stored in plants.

phytochemicals   Chemicals found in plants (*phyto* is from the Greek word for plant), such as pigments and other substances, that have biological activity in the body.

pica   An abnormal craving to eat something not fit for food, such as clay, paint, and so on.

placenta   A pregnancy-specific organ formed from both maternal and embryonic tissues. It is responsible for oxygen, nutrient, and waste exchange between the mother and fetus.

plasma   The fluid portion of the blood; needed to maintain adequate blood volume so that blood can flow easily throughout our bodies.

platelets   Cell fragments that assist in the formation of blood clots and help stop bleeding.

polychlorinated biphenyls (PCBs)   An industrial pollutant most commonly attributed to discarded transformers.

polysaccharide   A complex carbohydrate consisting of long chains of glucose.

polyunsaturated fatty acids (PUFA)   Fatty acids that have more than one double bond in the chain; these types of fatty acids are generally liquid at room temperature.

pre-eclampsia   High blood pressure that is pregnancy specific and accompanied by protein in the urine, edema, and unexpected weight gain.

prediabetes   A condition in which fasting blood glucose levels are above normal but below the level used to diagnose type 2 diabetes; also called impaired fasting glucose.

preterm   Birth of a baby prior to 38 weeks of gestation.

prion   A protein that is closely related to a virus but is self-replicating.

pro-oxidant   A nutrient that promotes oxidation and oxidative cell and tissue damage.

proteases   A set of enzymes secreted by cells in the pancreas that hydrolyze (break apart) the peptide bonds in shorter polypeptides, splitting them into oligopeptides, tripeptides, dipeptides, and free amino acids.

protein digestibility–corrected amino acid score (PDCAAS)   A measurement of protein quality that considers the balance of essential amino acids as well as the digestibility of the protein in the food.

protein-energy malnutrition   A disorder caused by inadequate consumption of protein energy and other nutrients. It is characterized by severe wasting.

proteins   The only macronutrient that contains nitrogen; the basic building blocks of proteins are amino acids. Also, large complex molecules made up of amino acids and found as essential components of all living cells.

provitamin   An inactive form of a vitamin that the body can convert to an active form. An example is beta-carotene.

puberty   The period in life in which secondary sexual characteristics develop and people are biologically capable of reproducing.

purging   An attempt to rid the body of unwanted food by vomiting or other compensatory means, such as excessive exercise, fasting, or laxative abuse.

pyruvic acid   The primary end product of glycolysis.

R

Recommended Daily Intakes (RDI)   The amounts of vitamins and minerals used to calculate the % daily values.

Recommended Dietary Allowance (RDA)   The average daily nutrient intake level that meets the nutrient requirements of 97% to 98% of healthy individuals in a particular life stage and gender group.

reference standards   The amounts of nutrients other than vitamins and minerals; used to calculate the % daily values.

remodelling   The two-step process by which bone tissue is recycled; includes the breakdown of existing bone and the formation of new bone.

residues   Chemicals that remain in the foods we eat despite cleaning and processing.

resistance training   Exercises in which our muscles act against resistance.

resorption   The process by which the surface of bone is broken down by cells called osteoclasts.

retina   The delicate, light-sensitive membrane lining the inner eyeball and connected to the optic nerve. It contains retinal.

retinal   An active aldehyde form of vitamin A that plays an important role in healthy vision and immune function.

retinoic acid   An active acid form of vitamin A that plays an important role in cell growth and immune function.

retinol   An active alcohol form of vitamin A that plays an important role in healthy vision and immune function.

rickets   Vitamin D deficiency disease in children. Symptoms include deformities of the skeleton, such as bowed legs and knocked knees.

S

saliva   A mixture of water, mucus, enzymes, and other chemicals that moistens the mouth and food, binds food particles together, and begins the digestion of carbohydrates.

salivary amylase   An enzyme in saliva that breaks starch into smaller particles and eventually into the disaccharide maltose.

salivary glands   A group of glands found under and behind the tongue and beneath the jaw that release saliva continually, as well as in response to the thought, sight, smell, or presence of food.

salt sensitive   Those whose blood pressure increases when sodium intake is high.

saturated fatty acid (SFA)   Fatty acids that have no carbons joined together with a double bond; these types of fatty acids are generally solid at room temperature.

seizures   Uncontrollable muscle spasms caused by increased nervous system excitability that can result from electrolyte imbalances.

set-point theory   A theory that suggests that the body raises or lowers energy expenditure in response to increased and decreased food intake and physical activity. This action serves to maintain an individual's body weight within a narrow range.

short-chain fatty acids   Fatty acids fewer than six carbon atoms in length.

sickle cell anemia   A genetic disorder that causes red blood cells to be sickle, or crescent, shaped. These cells cannot travel smoothly through the blood vessels, causing cell breakage and anemia.

simple carbohydrate   Commonly called simple sugar or just sugar; a monosaccharide or disaccharide, such as glucose.

small intestine   The longest portion of the GI tract, where most digestion and absorption takes place.

soluble fibre   Natural pectins, mucilages, and gums that absorb water and form gels. In humans, these substances slow down the movement of material through the small intestine.

solvent   A substance that is capable of mixing with and breaking apart a variety of compounds. Water is an excellent solvent.

sphincter   A tight ring of muscle separating some of the organs of the GI tract and opening in response to nerve signals indicating that food is ready to pass into the next section.

spina bifida   A neural tube defect in which vertebrae of the spine are not fully developed. In the most severe form, the spinal cord nerves and their protective sheath protrude through an opening in the skin causing permanent nerve damage.

spontaneous abortion   (also called miscarriage) Natural termination of a pregnancy and expulsion of pregnancy tissues because of a genetic, developmental, or physiologic abnormality that is so severe that the pregnancy cannot be maintained.

stabilizers   Help maintain smooth texture and uniform colour and flavour in some foods.

starch   A polysaccharide stored in plants; the storage form of glucose in plants.

sterols   A type of lipid found in foods and in the body that has a ring structure; cholesterol is the most common sterol that occurs in our diets. Plant sterols block the absorption of cholesterol.

stomach   A J-shaped organ where food is partially digested, churned, and held until its release into the small intestine.

sucrase   A digestive enzyme that digests sucrose into glucose and fructose.

sucrose   A disaccharide composed of one glucose molecule and one fructose molecule. Sweeter than lactose or maltose. Also called table sugar.

sulphites   Agents that are effective as preservatives, as antioxidants, and to prevent browning. Sulphites also have antibacterial properties, are used to bleach flour, and inhibit mould growth in grapes, wine, and other foods.

system   A group of organs that work together to perform a unique function; for example, the gastrointestinal system.

T

teratogen   Any substance that can cause a birth defect.

texturizers   A chemical used to improve the texture of various foods.

thermic effect of food (TEF)   The energy expended as a result of processing food consumed.

thickening agents   Natural or chemically modified carbohydrates that absorb some of the water present in food, making the food thicker while keeping food components balanced.

thirst mechanism   A cluster of nerve cells in the hypothalamus that stimulate our conscious desire to drink fluids in response to an increase in the concentration of salt in our blood or a decrease in blood pressure and blood volume.

thrifty gene theory   A theory that suggests that some people possess a gene (or genes) that causes them to be energetically thrifty, resulting in their expending less energy at rest and during physical activity.

time of activity   How long each exercise session lasts.

tissue   A grouping of similar cells that performs a particular set of functions; for example, muscle tissue.

tocopherol   The active form of vitamin E in our bodies. Alpha-tocopherols are the forms used to establish human vitamin E requirements.

tocotrienol   A form of vitamin E that does not play an important biological role in our bodies.

Tolerable Upper Intake Level (UL)   The highest average daily nutrient intake level likely to pose no risk of adverse health effects to almost all individuals in a particular life stage and gender group.

total fibre   The sum of dietary fibre and functional fibre.

toxin   Any harmful substance; specifically, a chemical produced by a microorganism that harms tissues or causes harmful immune responses.

trabecular bone (spongy or cancellous bone)   A porous bone tissue that makes up only 20% of our skeleton and is found within the ends of the long bones, inside the spinal vertebrae, inside the flat bones (breastbone, ribs, and most bones of the skull) and inside the bones of the pelvis.

trace minerals   Minerals we need to consume in amounts less than 100 milligrams per day and of which the total amount in our bodies is less than 5 grams.

transamination   The process of transferring the amine group from one amino acid to another to manufacture a new amino acid.

transcription   The process through which messenger RNA copies genetic information from DNA in the nucleus.

transferrin   The transport protein for iron.

translation   The process that occurs when the genetic information carried by messenger RNA is translated into a chain of amino acids at the ribosome.

transport proteins   Protein molecules that help to transport substances throughout the body and across cell membranes.

triglyceride   A molecule consisting of three fatty acids attached to a three-carbon glycerol backbone.

trimester   Any one of three stages of pregnancy, each lasting 13 to 14 weeks.

T-score   A comparison of an individual's bone density to the average peak bone density of a 30-year-old healthy adult of the same sex and race. If bone density is normal, the T-score will be between +1 and –1.

tumour   Any newly formed mass of cells that are less differentiated than normal cells. Tumours can be benign (not harmful to us) or malignant (cancerous).

type 1 diabetes   A disorder in which the body cannot produce enough insulin.

type 2 diabetes   A progressive disorder in which body cells become less responsive to insulin.

U

umbilical cord   The cord containing arteries and veins that connect the baby (from the navel) to the mother via the placenta.

undernutrition   A diet that lacks energy or specific essential nutrients.

underweight   Having too little body fat to maintain health, causing a person to have a weight that is below an acceptably defined standard for a given height.

urinary tract infection   A bacterial infection of the urethra, the tube leading from the bladder to the body exterior.

V

variety   Eating many different foods each day.

vegetarianism   The practice of restricting the diet to foods of plant origin, including vegetables, fruit, grains, and nuts.

vigorous-intensity activities   Activities that produce significant increases in breathing, sweating, and heart rate; talking is difficult when exercising at a vigorous intensity.

viruses   A group of infectious agents that are much smaller than bacteria, lack independent metabolism, and need a live host to reproduce.

visible fats   Fat we can see in our foods or see added to foods, such as butter, margarine, cream, shortening, salad dressings, chicken skin, and untrimmed fat on meat.

vitamins   Organic compounds that assist us in regulating our bodies' processes.

W

warm-up   Also called preliminary exercise; includes activities that prepare you for an exercise bout, including stretching, calisthenics, and movements specific to the exercise bout.

water-soluble vitamins   Vitamins that are soluble in water. These include vitamin C and the B vitamins. Some are destroyed by heat or light.

weight cycling   The condition of successfully dieting to lose weight, regaining the weight, and repeating the cycle again.

Wernicke-Korsakoff syndrome   A form of thiamin deficiency seen in chronic alcoholics that results in mental confusion and a loss of memory.

Z

zygote   A fertilized egg (ovum) consisting of a single cell.

Index

Key terms and the pages on which they are defined appear in boldface; *t* denotes a table and *f* denotes a figure.

Credits

Photo Credits

The publisher would like to thank the following people and institutions for permission to use their © copyright materials. Every reasonable effort has been made to find copyright holders of the material in this text. The publisher would be pleased to know of any errors or omissions.

Chapter 1

p. 2 (top, bottom, and left): Dorling Kindersley; p. 2 (right): Ancil Nance/Getty Images; p. 3: Dorling Kindersley; p. 4: Lew Robertson/PictureArts/Corbis; p. 5: Lester V. Bergman/Corbis; p. 9: AP Photo/Janet Jensen; p. 10: Tom Stewart/Corbis; p. 11: Ant Strack/Corbis; p. 13: Matthew Klein/Corbis; p. 14: FoodPix/Getty Images; p. 15: Steve Terrill/Corbis; p. 16: Dorling Kindersley; p. 20: Jon Feingersh/Getty Images; p. 21: LA/Tevy Battini/Phototake; p. 22: Michael Donne/Photo Researchers; p. 25: Dorling Kindersley; p. 26: Dorling Kindersley; p. 31: © Ingram Publishing/Alamy.

Chapter 2

p. 32 (top): Health Canada, © 2003. Reproduced with the permission of the Minister of Public Works and Government Services Canada, 2005; p. 32 (centre): Michelle Garrett/Corbis; p. 32 (bottom): C Squared Studios/Getty Images; p. 33 (top): C Squared Studios/Getty Images; p. 33 (bottom): John E Kelly/Getty Images; p. 35: SW Productions/Getty Images; p. 36: Photo: Terri Rothman. Used with permission of Shoppers Drug Mart Inc. Shoppers Drug mart and Life brand are trade-marks of 911979 Alberta Ltd., used under license. p. 38: Courtesy of President's Choice®, www.presidentschoice.ca; p. 41: Health Canada. 2003. Frequently Asked Questions About Nutrition Labelling. http://hc-sc.gc.ca/fn-an/label-etiquet/nutrition/educat/te_quest-eng.php#18. Accessed September 2008; p. 47: © Reproduced with the permission of the Heart and Stroke Foundation of Canada, 2005. Health Check® is a trademark of the Heart and Stroke Foundation of Canada www.healthcheck.org; p. 51: Dorling Kindersley; p. 52: David Sacks/Getty Images; p. 53: Courtesy of Loblaw Brands Limited, www.presidentschoice.ca; p. 54: Alexander Walter/Getty Images; p. 58: Dorling Kindersley; p. 59: Dorling Kindersley; p. 61: Stock Boston; p. 63 (top): Dorling Kindersley; p. 63 (middle): Pearson Learning Photo Studio; p. 63 (bottom left and right): Pearson Learning Photo Studio; p. 65: Joe Raedle/Getty Images; p. 66 (top): Koichi Kamoshida/Getty Images; p. 66 (bottom): Sigrid Estrada/Getty Images; p. 67: C Squared Studios/Getty Images; p. 69: John E Kelly/Getty Images; p. 70: Chet Gordon/Image Works; p. 71: Reuters/Corbis.

Chapter 3

p. 76 (top): Dorling Kindersley; p. 76 (centre): Matt Bowman/Getty Images; p. 76 (bottom): Reza Estakhrian/Getty Images; p. 77: Burke/Triolo Productions/PictureArts Corporation; p. 74: Jean Luc Morales/Getty Images; p. 75: Jon Riley/Getty Images; p. 76: Howard Kingsnorth/Getty Images; p. 84: Jonelle Weaver/Getty Images; p. 87(left): Dr. David M. Phillips/Visuals Unlimited; p. 87 (right): Dr. Richard Kessel and Dr. Gene Shih/Visuals Unlimited; p. 93: Science Photo Library/Photo Researchers; p. 95: Peter Southwick/Stock Boston; p. 97: Dr. E. Walker/Photo Researchers; p. 99: Dorling Kindersley; p. 100: Dorling Kindersley/David Murray and Jules Selmes; p. 101: Peter Adams/Getty Images; p. 103: Pramod Mistry/Lonely Planet Images; p. 104: Dorling Kindersley; p. 107: Burke/Triolo Productions/PictureArts Corporation; p. 108: John E. Kelly/Getty Images; p. 109: Andrew Syred/Photo Researchers.

Chapter 4

p. 110: Dorling Kindersley; p. 111 (top and bottom): Dorling Kindersley; p. 113: Photomundo/Getty Images; p. 115: Caren Alpert/Getty Images; p. 116: Dorling Kindersley; p. 117: Robert J. Bennett/Agefotostock; p. 122: Dorling Kindersley; p. 123: Rob Lewine/Corbis; p. 124: Justin Sullivan/Getty Images; p. 125: Lars Klove Photo Service/Getty Images; p. 127: Dorling Kindersley; p. 128: Joe Raedle/Getty Images; p. 129: Philip Jones Griffiths/Magnum Photos; p. 130 (top): Jose Azel/Aurora & Quanta Productions; p. 130 (bottom): Dorling Kindersley; p. 132: Dorling Kindersley; p. 138: Kristin Piljay; p. 140: Thinkstock/Getty Images; p. 141: Kevin Winter/Getty Images; p. 143: Photo by Bayne Stanley. Reprinted with permission of Dr. Timothy Kieffer, University of British Columbia; p. 145 (top): Dorling Kindersley; p. 145 (bottom): Laura Dwight; p. 146: Dorling Kindersley; p. 149: Dorling Kindersley; p. 150: Anna Neumann/laif.

Chapter 5

p. 152 (top and centre): Dorling Kindersley; p. 152 (bottom): Corbis Digital Stock; p. 153 (top): Corbis Digital Stock; p. 153 (bottom): Dorling Kindersley; p. 154: AP Photo/Thomas Kienzle; p. 155: Dorling Kindersley; p. 156: Dorling Kindersley; p. 158: Used with permission of Parmalat Canada/Photo by Jen Handel; p. 161: Kip Peticolas/Fundamental Photographs; p. 165: Quest/Photo Researchers; p. 166 (top): Andersen Ross/Getty Images; p. 166 (bottom): Doug Pensinger/Getty Images; p. 168: Odd Andersen/Getty Images; p. 169 (top): Royalty-Free/Corbis; p. 169 (bottom): © Shutterstock; p. 170: Courtesy of Dr. Marangoni; p. 173: Spencer Platt/Getty Images; p. 174: Travis Amos/Pearson Education; p. 175: Used with permission of Parmalat Canada and courtesy of Burnbrae Farms Ltd./Photo by Jen Handel; p. 176: Dorling Kindersley; p. 180: Constantine Manos/Magnum Photos; p. 185: © Comstock/Food Icons CD; p. 186 (top): Dorling Kindersley; p. 186 (bottom): Corbis Digital Stock; p. 189: Dorling Kindersley.

Chapter 6

p. 192 (top): Corbis Digital Stock; p. 192 (centre): Royalty-Free/Corbis; p. 192 (bottom): Dorling Kindersley; p. 193 (top): Dorling Kindersley; p. 197 (bottom): Royalty-Free/Corbis; p. 194: Photo by Ryan Mah. Courtesy of Brendan Brazier. www.brendanbrazier.com; p. 199: Andrew Syed/Photo Researchers; p. 200: Dorling Kindersley; p. 201: Dorling Kindersley; p. 203: Duomo/Corbis; p. 204: Visuals Unlimited; p. 210: Dorling Kindersley; p. 213: Dorling Kindersley; p. 215: Jennifer Levy/Getty Images; p. 216: Dorling Kindersley; p. 217 (left): Alexandra Avakian/Corbis; p. 217 (right): AP WorldWide Photo; p. 219: The New York Times/The Houston Chronicle; p. 220: © Oliver Meckes/Nicole Ottawa/Photo Researchers, Inc.; p. 221: Dorling Kindersley; p. 222: Dorling Kindersley; p. 224: Royalty-Free/Corbis; p. 226: Chris Hondros/Getty Images.

Chapter 7

p. 228 (top and bottom): Dorling Kindersley; p. 228 (centre): EyeWire Collection/Getty Images; p. 229 (top and bottom): Dorling Kindersley; p. 230; Arthur Tilley/Getty Images; p. 233: Theo Allots/Corbis; p. 237: Randy Sidman-Moore/Masterfile; p. 239: James A.D. Addio/Corbis; p. 241: Layne Kennedy/Corbis; p. 242: Network Productions/The Image Works; p. 244 (top): Lars Klove/Image Bank/Getty Images; p. 244 (bottom): Marc Dietrich © iStockphotop. 247: Dorling Kindersley; p. 250: Shaun Egan/Getty Images; p. 251: Eyewire Collection; p. 253: Rick Stewart/Allsport;

p. 254: John A. Rizzo/Agefotostock; p. 257: Dorling Kindersley; p. 258: Dorling Kindersley; p. 259: Dorling Kindersley; p. 261: Photos by Martin Schwalde.

Chapter 8

p. 264 (top): Stone/Getty Images; p. 264 (centre): Michale P. Gadomski/Photo Researchers; p. 264 (bottom): Frederic Duclos/Getty Images; p. 265 (top): Stone/Getty Images; p. 265 (bottom): Dorling Kindersley; p. 267: Deborah David/Getty Images; p. 276: Dorling Kindersley; p. 278: Dorling Kindersley; p. 279 (top): © Medical-on-Line/Alamy; p. 279 (bottom): Corbis; p. 283: Dorling Kindersley; p. 285: © ISM/Phototake; p. 287: Dorling Kindersley; p. 288: Miranda Mimi Kuo; p. 291: Jeff Greenberg/PhotoEdit; p. 293: Paul Souders/Corbis; p. 294: Dorling Kindersley; p. 396: Dorling Kindersley; p. 297 (top): Ryan McVay/Getty Images; p. 297 (left): UHB Trust/Getty Images; p. 297 (right): National Eye Institute, National Institute of Health; p. 298 (left): © Sue Ford/Photo Researchers, Inc.; p. 298 (right): National Eye Institute. National Institute of Health; p. 299: Stone/Getty Images; p. 300: Stone/Getty Images; p. 301: Dorling Kindersley; p. 304: Courtesy of SISU Inc.; p. 305: Dorling Kindersley.

Chapter 9

p. 308 (top and bottom): Dorling Kindersley; p. 308 (centre): Kevin Byron/Animals Animals/Earth Scenes; p. 309 (top and bottom): Dorling Kindersley; p. 314: Pascal Alix/Photo Researchers; p. 315: Richard Ross/Getty Images; p. 318: Dorling Kindersley; p. 319: Courtesy of Vitasoy; p. 323: Peter Turnley/Corbis; p. 327: Dorling Kindersley; p. 328: Reproduced with permission by the American Journal of Clinical Nutrition. © Am J Clin Nutr. American Society for Clinical Nutrition; p. 329: Philip Maher/World Vision Canada. Reprinted with permission; p. 331: Dorling Kindersley; p. 333: Catherine Ledner/Getty Images; p. 335 (top): Spencer Jones/Getty Images; p. 335 (bottom): Larry Williams/Corbis; p. 336: National Institute of Dental Research; p. 337 (top): Yoav Levy/Phototake NYC; p. 337 (bottom): Michael Klein/Peter Arnold; p. 339: Spencer Platt/Getty Images; p. 340: Duomo/Corbis; p. 342: Dorling Kindersley; p. 344: Dorling Kindersley; p. 347: © George Doyle/MaxxImages

Chapter 10

p. 348 (top and bottom): Dorling Kindersley; p. 348 (centre): Michelle Garrett/Corbis; p. 349 (top): Dorling Kindersley; p. 349 (bottom): Dorling Kindersley; p. 355 (top): National Library of Medicine/A012411; p. 355 (bottom): Dr. Kenneth Greer/Visuals Unlimited/Getty Images. p. 356: © Dr. P. Marazzi/Science Photo Library; p. 357: Dorling Kindersley; p. 358: Robert Fiocca/PictureArts/Corbis; p. 359: Royalty-Free/Corbis; p. 359 (bottom): Dorling Kindersley; p. 360 (top): Alison Wright/Corbis; p. 360 (bottom): Lester V. Bergman/Corbis; p. 361 (top): Dorling Kindersley; p. 361 (bottom): Dorling Kindersley; p. 364 (top): Dorling Kindersley; p. 364 (bottom): Gillette; p. 366: Burke/Triolo Productions/Getty Images; p. 371: Dorling Kindersley; p. 370 (bottom): © H.H. Sandstead, The University of Texas Medical Branch, Galveston, TX; p. 371: Dorling Kindersley; p. 374 (left): © Joaquin Carrillo Farga/Photo Researchers, Inc.; p. 374 (right): © Dr. E. Walker/Photo Researchers, Inc.; p. 375: Dorling Kindersley; p. 376: Dorling Kindersley; p. 378: Dorling Kindersley; p. 379: Color Day Production/Getty Images.

Chapter 11

p. 380 (top): Lawrence Migdale; p. 380 (centre): Peter Cade/Getty Images; p. 380 (bottom): Corbis Digital Stock; p. 381 (top): Corbis Digital Stock; p. 381: Michael Newman/Photoedit; p. 383: Ryan McVay/Getty Images; p. 386: David Young-Wolff/Photoedit; p. 387: David Madison/Getty Images; p. 387: Phototake; p. 387: Life Measurement; p. 390: (both) Courtesy of Dr. Linda McCargar and the Human Nutrition Research Unit, University of Alberta; p. 391: Dorling Kindersley; p. 392: Xavier Bonghi/Getty Images; p. 398 (top): Mark Douet/Getty Images; p. 398 (bottom): Dorling Kindersley; p. 399 (top): Dorling Kindersley; p. 399 (bottom): Bruce Dale/Getty Images; p. 407 (top and second from top): Dorling Kindersley; p. 407 (second from bottom): © Igram/Ultimate Food Photography CD; p. 407 (bottom): © Comstock/Food Icons CD; p. 412: Ariel Skelley/Corbis; p. 413: AFP PHOTO/Liu Jin/Corbis; p. 414: Corbis Digital Stock; p. 416: Michael Newman/Photoedit.

Chapter 12

p. 420 (top): Mike Brinson/Getty Images; p. 420 (centre): Photolibrary.com; p. 420 (bottom): Martin King/Photolibrary.com; p. 421 (top): Mike Brinson/Getty Images; p. 421 (bottom): Emanuele Taroni/Getty Images; p. 423: Caleb Kenna/IPN/AURORA; p. 425: Photodics/Getty Images; p. 426: AP Photo/Mark Lennihan; p. 430: Will & Deni McIntyre/Photo Researchers; p. 431: Mark Romanelli/Getty Images; p. 439: Dorling Kindersley; p. 440: Jens Schlueter/Getty Images; p. 441: Photodisc/Getty Images; p. 444: Scott T. Smith/Corbis; p. 446: Dorling Kindersley; p. 452: Dorling Kindersley; p. 453: Mike Brinson/Getty Images; p. 454: Mike Brinson/Getty Images; p. 456: Emanuele Taroni/Getty Images; p. 458: Sarto/Lund/Getty Images.

Chapter 13

p. 460 (top): AP Photo/Ron Edmonds; p. 460 (centre): Donna Day/Getty Images; p. 460 (bottom): Express Newspapers/Getty Images; p. 461 (top): Express Newspapers/Getty Images; p. 461: Tony Freeman/PhotoEdit; p. 462 (bottom): Klaus Lahnstein/Getty Images; p. 468: Stockbyte/Getty Images p. 469: Laura Murray/Pearson Education; p. 472: Express Newspapers/Getty Images; p. 474: PhotoLibrary.com; p. 475: Baumgartner Olivia/Corbis Sygma; p. 480 (left): Reuters/Landov; p. 480 (right): AP Wide World Photos; p. 482: AP Photo/Thomas Kienzle; p. 487: David Young-Wolff/PhotoEdit; p. 488: Mel Yates/Getty Images; p. 489: Express Newspapers/Getty Images; p. 491: Tony Freeman/PhotoEdit; p. 493: AP Wide World Photos.

Chapter 14

p. 496 (top and centre): Dorling Kindersley; p. 496 (bottom): Michael/Prentice Hall; p. 497 (top): Dorling Kindersley; p. 497 (bottom): David Young-Wolff/PictureQuest; p. 498: © Bloomberg Photo/Gary Gardiner/Landov; p. 500: AP Photo/Gene J. Puskar; p. 501: Barry Dowsett/Photo Researchers; p. 504: Andrew Syred/Photo Researchers; p. 505: AP Images/Greg Baker; p. 506: Dorling Kindersley; p. 507 (top): Matt Meadows/Peter Arnold; p. 507 (bottom): Dorling Kindersley; p. 510: Digital Vision/Getty Images; p. 516: Owen Franken/Corbis; p. 518 (top): Hulton Archive/Getty Images; p. 518 (bottom): Digital Vision, Ltd.; p. 519: AKG/Photo Researchers; p. 522: Dorling Kindersley; p. 523: Royalty-Free/Corbis; p. 528: Dorling Kindersley; p. 530: David Young-Wolff/PictureQuest; p. 533: Getty Images

Chapter 15

p. 534 (top): Myrleen Ferguson/PhotoEdit; p. 534 (centre): Photodisc/Getty Images; p. 534 (bottom): Stockbyte; p. 535 (top): Stockbyte; p. 535 (bottom): Simon Brown/Dorling Kindersley; p. 536: Dorling Kindersley; p. 537: David Phillips/The Population

Couicl; p. 539 (top left and right): Lennart Nilsson/Albert Bonniers Forlag AB; p. 539 (bottom): Tom Galliher/Corbis; p. 541: Ron Sutherland/Photo Researchers; p. 542: Ian O'Leary/Getty Images; p. 545 (top): Medical Illustration Copyright © 2008 Nucleus Medical Art, All rights reserved. www.nucleusinc.com; p.545 (bottom): Dorling Kindersley; p. 546: Courtesy of Dr. Deborah O'Connor, Hospital for Sick Children, Toronto; p. 548: Allana Wesley White/Corbis; p. 550: Brand X Pictures/Getty Images; p. 552: Dorling Kindersley; p. 554: George Steinmetz; p. 555: Phanie/Photo Researchers; p. 560: Rick Gomez/Agefotostock; p. 561: Regine Mahaux/Image Bank/Getty Images; p. 565: © Mark Clarke/Science Photo Library; p. 566: Mel Yates/Getty Images; p. 567: Royalty-Free/Corbis; p. 569 (top): Anne Flinn Powell/Index Stock Imagery; p. 569 (bottom): Dr. Pamela Erickson; p. 570: Stockbyte; p. 572: Simon Brown/Dorling Kindersley; p. 575: Philip Gould/Corbis.

Chapter 16

p. 576 (top): Britt J. Erlanson-Messens/Getty Images; p. 576 (centre): © Michael Newman/PhotoEdit; p. 576 (bottom): Jon Riley/Getty Images; p. 577 (top): Britt J. Erlanson-Messens/Getty Images; p. 577 (bottom): Don Smetzer/Getty Images; p. 578: Michael Newman/PhotoEdit; p. 582 (top): Dorling Kindersley; p. 582 (bottom): Laura Dwight; p. 583 (top): Dorling Kindersley; p. 583 (bottom): Travis Amos/Pearson Education; p. 585: Laura Murray/Pearson Education; p. 586: Vince Streano/Corbis; p. 587: Gary Buss/Getty Images; p. 588: Jaume Gual/Age fotostock; p. 589: Holly Harris/Getty Images; p. 591 (top): Paul Barton/Corbis; p. 591 (bottom): Kidnetic.com; p. 595: Tom Stewart/Corbis; p. 596: Tom & Dee Ann McCarthy/Corbis; p. 598: Michael Krasowitz/Getty Images; p. 600: Donna Day/Getty Images; p. 603: Karen Pruess/Image Works; p. 604: Britt J. Erlanson-Messens/Getty Images; p. 606: Don Smetzer/Getty Images; p. 609: © Spencer Grant/PhotoEdit.

Additional Figure and Text Credits

p. 79: University of Guelph, Natural Hormone Has Potential to Aid Weight Loss, Researcher Finds. September 2007 News Release. www.uoguelph.ca/news/2007/09/natural_hormone.html; p. 130: Health Canada: Canadian Community Health Survey, Cycle 2.2, Nutrition (2004)—Nutrient Intakes from Food Provincial, Regional and National Summary Data Tables, Volume 1. www.hc-sc.gc.ca/fn-an/pubs/cchs-nutri-escc/index_e.html. Accessed May 2008; p. 130: Adapted from Statistics Canada publication, "Canadians' Eating Habits 2004," 2006, no. 2, Cat. No. 82-620-XIE, July 6, 2006, page 39, available at www.statcan.gc.ca/pub/82-620-m/82-620-m2006002-eng.pdf. Accessed Jan. 2008; p. 140: CFSAN/Office of Food Additive Safety. FDA Statement on European Aspartame Study. April 20, 2007. www.cfsan.fda.gov/~lrd/fpaspar2.html; p. 140: Health Canada. Comments on the Recent Study Relating to the Safety of Aspartame, May 5, 2006. http://hc-sc.gc.ca/fn-an/securit/addit/sweeten-edulcor/aspartame_statement-eng.php; p. 144: Wannamethee SG, et al. Modifiable lifestyle factors and the metabolic syndrome in older men: effects of lifestyle changes. *Journal of the American Geriatrics Society*. 2006;54(12):1909-14; Figure 5.10(a): Ed Reschke/Visuals Unlimited. Figure 5.10(b): W. Ober/Visuals Unlimited; p. 178: Health Canada. Mercury in Fish. Consumption Advice: Making Informed Choices about Fish, 2007, http://hc-sc.gc.ca/fn-an/securit/chem-chim/environ/mercur/cons-adv-etud-eng.php; p. 210: Health Canada, Canadian Community Health Survey, Cycle 2.2, Nutrition (2004) Nutrient Intakes from Food. Provincial, Regional and National Summary Data Tables, Volume 1. www.hc-sc.gc.ca/fn-an/pubs/cchs-nutri-escc/index-eng.php; p. 223: Statistics Canada. 2002. Endocrine, nutritional metabolic disease, by age, group and sex.

www.statcan.ca/english/freepub/84-208-XIE/2002/tables/table4.htm. Accessed July 2005; Figure 6.5: From Johnson, M. Human Biology, 2/e, Fig. 7.4, p. 136. Copyright © 2003 Benjamin Cummings. Used by permission of Pearson Education, Inc.; p. 249: Statistics Canada, "Canadians' Eating Habits 2004," 2006, no. 2, Cat. No. 82-620-XIE, July 6, 2006, page 39, available at www.statcan.gc.ca/pub/82-620-m/82-620-m2006002-eng.pdf. Accessed Jan. 2008; p. 253–254: Canadian Hypertension Education Program. 2008. Public Recommendations. http://hypertension.ca/bpc/wp-content/uploads/2008/02/2008publicrecommendations.pdf. Pg. 4 Accessed April 2008. Used with permission; Figure 8.1: From Campbell et al. Biology: Concepts and Connections. Copyright © 2003 Benjamin Cummings. Used by permission of Pearson Education, Inc. Figure 8.12: From Marieb, E. Human Anatomy and Physiology, 5/e. Copyright © 2003 Benjamin Cummings. Used by permission of Pearson Education, Inc. Figure 10.5: Adapted from Alerts et al., Molecular Biology of the Cell, 4/e, p. 114. Copyright © 2002. Reproduced by permission of Garland Science/Taylor & Francis Books, Inc. Also from Johnson, M. Human Biology, 2/e, Figure 7.4. Copyright © 2003 Benjamin Cummings, and from Germann, W. and Stanfield, C. Principles of Human Physiology, 2/e, Figure 16.36. Copyright © 2001 Benjamin Cummings. Both reprinted by permission of Pearson Education, Inc. Figure 12.5: From Campbell, N. Biology: Exploring Life, Figure 7.9. Copyright © 2003 Prentice Hall. Used by permission of Pearson Education, Inc. Figure 13.2: From Fig. 1, p. 36, in Stevens, J. et al. Weight-related Attitudes and Behaviors in Fourth Grade American Indian Children. Obesity Research, Vol. 7, pp. 34–42, 1999. Copyright © 1999 North American Association for the Study of Obesity. Used with permission. p. 479: Reprinted with permission from the Diagnostic and Statistical Manual of Mental Disorders, Text Revision. Copyright © 2000 American Psychiatric Association. p. 482: Reprinted with permission from the Diagnostic and Statistical Manual of Mental Disorders, Text Revision. Copyright © 2000 American Psychiatric Association. p. 482: © National Eating Disorders Association (NEDA). Used with permission. p. 485: Reprinted with permission from the Diagnostic and Statistical Manual of Mental Disorders, Text Revision. Copyright © 2000 American Psychiatric Association. p. 491–492: Otis et al., The Female Athlete Triad. Med. Science & Sports Exercise, Vol. 29, pp. I–ix, 1997. Copyright © 1997. Used with permission. pp. 495–497: From N. Piran, "Prevention of Eating Disorders" in Eating Disorders and Obesity, 2/e, pp. 367–371. Copyright © 2002 The Guilford Press. Used with permission. Figure 14.1: USDA. Figure 14.3: USDA. Figure 14.5: USDA. p. 559: Health Canada. 2004. Exclusive Breastfeeding Duration - 2004 Health Canada Recommendation. http://www.hc-sc.gc.ca/fn-an/nutrition/child-enfant/infant-nourisson/excl_bf_dur-dur_am_excl-eng.php. Accessed September 2008; Figure 15.1: Adapted from Germann, W. and Stanfield, C. Principles of Human Physiology, 2/e, Fig. 22.20a. Copyright © 2001 Benjamin Cummings. Reprinted by permission of Pearson Education, Inc. Figure 15.2: Adapted from Germann, W. and Stanfield, C. Principles of Human Physiology, 2/e, Fig. 22.21. Copyright © 2001 Benjamin Cummings. Reprinted by permission of Pearson Education, Inc. Figure 15.3: Adapted from Germann, W. and Stanfield, C. Principles of Human Physiology, 2/e, Fig. 22.22. Copyright © 2001 Benjamin Cummings. Reprinted by permission of Pearson Education, Inc. Figure 15.4: Adapted from Germann, W. and Stanfield, C. Principles of Human Physiology, 2/e, Fig. 22.25a. Copyright © 2001 Benjamin Cummings. Reprinted by permission of Pearson Education, Inc. Figure 15.6: Adapted from Germann, W. and Stanfield, C. Principles of Human Physiology, 2/e, Fig. 22.26a. Copyright © 2001 Benjamin Cummings. Reprinted by permission of Pearson Education, Inc. Figure 16.1: Adapted from Germann, W. and Stanfield, C. Principles of Human Physiology, 2/e, Fig. 20.14. Copyright © 2001 Benjamin Cummings. Reprinted by permission of

Pearson Education, Inc. p. C-1: Canada's Physical Activity Guide to Healthy Active Living for Older Adults, Public Health Agency of Canada, 1999 © Reproduced with the permission of the Minister of Public Works and Government Services Canada, 2005. p. C-2: Canada's Physical Activity Guide to Healthy Active Guide for Children, Public Health Agency of Canada, 2002 © Reproduced with the permission of the Minister of Public Works and Government Services Canada, 2005. p. C-3: Canada's Physical Activity Guide to Healthy Active Guide for Youth, Public Health Agency of Canada, 2002 © Reproduced with the permission of the Minister of Public Works and Government Services Canada, 2005. Appendix Credits: *Canada's Physical Activity Guide to Healthy Active Living for Older Adults,* Public Health Agency of Canada, 1999 © Reproduced with the permission of the Minister of Public Works and Government Services Canada, 2008; *Canada's Physical Activity Guides for Children,* Public Health Agency of Canada, 2002 © Reproduced with the permission of the Minister of Public Works and Government Services Canada, 2008; *Canada's Physical Activity Guides for Youth,* Public Health Agency of Canada, 2002 © Reproduced with the permission of the Minister of Public Works and Government Services Canada, 2008.